Davis's NCLEX-RN® Success

Third Edition

Money
<u>Back Guarantee</u>

If you are a graduate of a nursing program accredited in the United States, take the NCLEX-RN® for the first time, and do not pass after using *Davis's NCLEX-RN®* Success, return the book to **F. A. Davis Company, Customer Service, 404-420 N. 2nd Street, Philadelphia, PA 19123.** Enclose your original receipt for purchase of the book and copies of your official test results notification and your certification of graduation. We will refund the price you paid for the book. If you have any questions, please call 800-323-3555.

Davis's NCLEX-RN® Success

Third Edition

Edited by

Sally Lambert Lagerquist, RN, MS

Written by

Sally Lambert Lagerquist, RN, MS

Former Instructor of Undergraduate, Graduate, and Continuing Education in Nursing, School of Nursing, University of California, San Francisco

President, Review for Nurses, Inc., and RN Tapes Company, San Francisco, California

Janice Lloyd McMillin, RN, MSN, EdD

Former Lecturer in Perinatal Nursing, School of Nursing, California State University, Sacramento

Staff Nurse, Labor and Delivery, Methodist Hospital, Sacramento, California

Robyn Marchal Nelson, DNSc, RN

Dean, College of Nursing, West Coast University, Irvine, California

Denise Wall Parilo, RN, MSN, PhD(c)

Associate Professor, School of Nursing, California State University, Sacramento

Per Diem Staff Nurse, Pediatrics, Sutter Memorial Hospital, Sacramento, California

Kathleen E. Snider, RN, MSN, CNS

Professor of Nursing, Los Angeles Valley College, Valley Glen, California

Janis Ryan Wisherop, RN, MSN

Professor, College of San Mateo

Home Health Hospice Nurse, San Francisco, California

F.A. Davis Company • Philadelphia

F. A. Davis Company
1915 Arch Street
Philadelphia, PA 19103
www.fadavis.com

Printed in the United States of America

Last digit indicates print number: 10 9 8 7 6 5 4 3 2

Publisher, Nursing: Robert G. Martone
Director of Content Development: Darlene D. Pedersen
Sr. Project/NCLEX Editor: Padraic J. Maroney
Illustration and Design Manager: Carolyn O'Brien
Project Manager, Electronic Publishing: Tyler Baber

As new scientific information becomes available through basic and clinical research, recommended treatments and drug therapies undergo changes. The author(s) and publisher have done everything possible to make this book accurate, up to date, and in accord with accepted standards at the time of publication. The author(s), editors, and publisher are not responsible for errors or omissions or for consequences from application of the book, and make no warranty, expressed or implied, in regard to the contents of the book. Any practice described in this book should be applied by the reader in accordance with professional standards of care used in regard to the unique circumstances that may apply in each situation. The reader is advised always to check product information (package inserts) for changes and new information regarding dose and contraindications before administering any drug. Caution is especially urged when using new or infrequently ordered drugs.

Library of Congress Cataloging-in-Publication Data

Davis's NCLEX-RN® success / edited by Sally Lambert Lagerquist ; written by Sally Lambert Lagerquist . . . [et al.]. — 3rd ed.
p. ; cm.
NCLEX-RN® success
Includes bibliographical references and index.
ISBN-13: 978-0-8036-2164-0
ISBN-10: 0-8036-2164-7
I. Lagerquist, Sally L. II. Title: NCLEX-RN® success.
[DNLM: 1. Nursing Care—Examination Questions. 2. Nursing Care—Outlines. WY 18.2]

610.73076—dc23 2011038536

This book is dedicated to:

TOM – my husband,

43 years isn't enough to share all the 1001 things we want to experience. Here's to taking more time for enjoying our three granddaughters (Kaya, Kasey and Audrey), organizing our "museum" and for finally using our wedding Satsuma chinaware. Your love and devotion, your Scandinavian patience combined with your Irish good humor have been my mainstay while I cranked out 29 editions of seven different nursing books during my professional lifetime.

ELANA – our daughter,

Your creativity and talent, energy and commitment to always "giving your all" to all that you do – be it Stagewrite, parenting your two daughters, Kaya and Kasey, or fostering family unity, make you so very special.

DAN – our son-in-law,

A special thank you for putting *reviewfornurses.com* and the 6-eBookLibrary online, on smart phone or tablet device, and on DVD – making us the oldest independent, successful "all-in-one" nursing exam prep company. Your job has been never-ending and always innovative!

KALEN – our son,

Your name brings to mind some of your very special "gifts":

Kindness to and respect for generations behind you.
Ambition to seek and grow with opportunities.
Living with passion and laughter.
Embracing change, not fearing it.
Nurturing those you love (Lara and Audrey especially).

With gratitude for sharing your love, celebrations and care and concern.

*To our third generation—**the 3 granddaughters:*** **Kaya, 9, Kasey, 5, Audrey, 3** (and another grandchild on the way)—each of whom is very precious to me in her own very special way:

KAYA for your sweet, kind and thoughtful ways, and a gentle manner. You are fun and enjoyable to be with, and insightful, sensitive, sentimental and creative at the same time. (We love your notes and artwork that you leave around for us to find all over the house.)

KASEY for your enthusiasm and boundless energy as you laugh and play with us, with friends, and with your collection of dolls and stuffed animals. You delight us with your remarkable singing (on pitch! and you pick up new melodies in Swedish, Russian, Jewish, and Hawaiian really fast!). We love your affectionate and sharing ways.

AUDREY for your giant hugs and loving smiles, as well as your growth and linguistic development in the way you seek and quickly grasp and enjoy new experiences (e.g., picking the correct numerical days on your Advent calendar, learning Italian phrases, and retaining how to say "I love you" in Russian). May you continue to always enjoy both Chanukah and Christmas as part of your own cultural "diversity." May you also continue to enjoy playing with and bonding with your cousins, Kaya and Kasey.

—Sally Lambert Lagerquist

First, I thank God for His unending grace, for the many blessings in my life, and for the gift of salvation in Christ Jesus.

To my husband, Mike, who supports me in everything I do, thank you for your humor and your love. We are a great team. I look forward to a bright future with you. You are truly the best thing that ever happened to me.

To my sweet little Leilani, the light of our life, the girl who makes us smile every day, and I am truly blessed that she calls me Mommy.

To my daughter Rachel, I am proud of the nurse you have become and enjoy watching you grow in your practice.

To my son Justin, keep moving forward. I know God has a plan for your life.

To my parents, John and LaVerne Mahony, I miss you both very much and one day, I will see you again. You both always believed I was capable of achieving whatever I could dream of and for that, I am eternally grateful.

To my big brother John, thank you for being my example. You made me want to achieve even more to keep up with your great accomplishments.

To my brother Brian, who has been making God and all of heaven laugh since 1993, I miss your smile and practical jokes.

To my mentors, Dr. Mollyn Bohnen and Dr. Louise Timmer, who helped shape me as a nurse and a faculty member, I am forever grateful for your attention and encouragement.

To all the nursing students whose enthusiasm inspires me, every time I see a student cry at the birth of a child, I remember why I chose to be a perinatal nurse. It is a pleasure to mentor the next generation of nurses. I have never had a day I wanted to be anything but a nurse, and I am proud to say I am a nurse.

—Jan Lloyd McMillin

This book is dedicated—

To those who have chosen nursing as their passion, as their life work . . . one education and 1000 career choices! Thanks for choosing *NCLEX-RN® Success* to increase your knowledge for the practice of nursing. Thanks for choosing a career as a professional nurse. Nurses are the "glue" of healthcare . . . and year after year they are voted the most trusted profession by consumers. Nurses make a difference in the lives of those they care for.

This book is dedicated—

To my family which is composed of members from four generational groups—my husband Dean (the mature generation), daughters Tina (the nurse and a baby boomer) and Kelly (the musician-graphic designer and Gen Xer), and my grandsons Stirling and Sage (the millennials). Nurses are prepared to give high quality care across all generations—not just one. Our lives and our health will be better because of nurses—because of you!

Thanks to each of you for touching my life daily!

—Robyn Marchal Nelson

To my husband Chris, for always being the eager listener for a new test question and for support throughout the editing process.

To Mom, Jeri, and Joe, who took such good care of Will and Zach when I needed to write.

To Sally and Robyn, mentors and friends, who supplied humor and heart every day of this book project. You two are the best!

To nursing students, both present and past, for choosing this profession, for always doing your best, and for continuing to give me such a richly rewarding career. I hope this book helps you succeed in the next phase of your journey!

—Denise Wall Parilo

This book is gratefully dedicated:

To Terry Oleson, PhD. Thank you for your endless patience and guidance in helping me find the answers to my life's questions.

To my nursing instructors, religious and secular, who taught me that I wanted to be a pediatric nurse and had the "right stuff" with which to do it.

To my pediatric patients and their families who taught me how to be a pediatric nurse.

To my pediatric nursing students who taught me how to teach pediatric nursing.

To my friends and colleagues in the pediatric community who, with their combined experience and wisdom, gave me insight into the writing of pediatric content and taught me that there is always a "light at the end of the tunnel" and that this book was not an everlasting project.

And, finally, to Steevio Bardakjian, my resident computer genius and guru who taught me the mysteries of the computer world.

Thank you!

—Kathy Snider

I dedicate my work involved in this book first and foremost to my beautiful and loving daughters Molly and Katie. You both have always been my inspiration in everything I do and always will—I love you both more than you will ever know.

During the time in editing, authoring the chapters and developing questions for this book, my life was occupied with personal emotional distress and the most challenging experiences ever. I thank Sally Lagerquist for giving me this opportunity to have this "great distraction" and time-consuming endeavor as I coped and began a new journey in life. Sally, you are not only my partner in this book, you are a dear and loving friend. Without your ongoing support, insistence on perfection and keeping me sane through it all, I never could have been successful in achieving the final edited and authored copy.

Lastly, I dedicate this to my family, co-workers and friends, who encouraged me and cheered me on during some of the lowest points of my personal life. Without you, I could not have done this.

And, finally to my mother, Marilyn Evans, a nurse at heart and the most loving, God inspired woman on the face of the Earth. *You* are my role model in everything I do as a nurse—I have become who I am and care for my patients the way I do because of your example. Thanks for being my mom and, most of all, my very best friend.

I am forever grateful to all the wonderful people in my life.

—Janis Ryan Wisherop

ABOUT THE EDITOR/AUTHORS

Sally Lambert Lagerquist, RN, MS, is currently the author and editor of three editions of *Davis's NCLEX-RN® Success;* four editions of *Practice Questions and Answers for NCLEX-RN,* published by Review for Nurses Tapes Co.; *How to Pass Nursing Exams,* published by Review Press and later by ATI, and now available as an e-book at *www.reviewfornurses.com;* four editions of Addison Wesley's *Nursing Examination Reviews* (1977–1991); four books for the NURSENOTES, Core Content At-A-Glance series: *Psychiatric-Mental Health, Maternal-Newborn, Pediatrics,* and *Medical-Surgical,* published by Lippincott and later by ATI, and now available as e-books at *www.reviewfornurses.com;* and Little, Brown's *NCLEX-RN® Examination Review,* and Little, Brown's *Nursing Q&A: Critical-Thinking Exercises,* published by Little, Brown and Company and later by ATI, and also available as e-books at *www.reviewfornurses.com.* She is president and course coordinator of Review for Nurses, Inc. She has coordinated RN licensure exam review courses on campuses nationwide since 1976. She is presently a lecturer on test-taking techniques at workshops held for graduating senior nursing students. She has produced and developed the **NCLEX-RN® Board Game** and audio CDs, CD-ROMs, DVDs, and streaming videos on Nursing Review and Successful Test-Taking Techniques for Nurses. She originated, developed, and has presented national **satellite telecourses** for NCLEX-RN® review since June 1989. She has developed an **online** (*reviewfornurses.com*) NCLEX-RN® mobile review course (also available for smart phone or tablet device to use anywhere, anytime), and an online **P**re-NCLEX-RN® **A**ssessment **S**eries for **S**uccess (PASS™) to help candidates assess and test with the test bank to fill in gaps in knowledge as well as increase their test-taking skills. She has been a marriage, family, and child counselor and is a member of Sigma Theta Tau International. She has been a faculty member at the University of California at San Francisco School of Nursing for over 10 years, where she also received her BS and MS degrees.

Janice Lloyd McMillin, RN, MSN, EdD, is a former lecturer in perinatal nursing in the Division of Nursing at California State University, Sacramento. In addition, she currently works in Labor and Delivery at Methodist Hospital in Sacramento. She has been a lecturer for several years for Review for Nurses, Inc. She received her BA in Biology, BS in Nursing, and MS in Nursing from CSU, Sacramento. She completed her doctorate at the University of San Francisco. Her dissertation study examined the transition experiences of first-year labor and delivery nurses. She has been a perinatal nurse for over 27 years.

Robyn Marchal Nelson, DNSc, RN, is Dean of the College of Nursing at West Coast University in Irvine, California. Prior to her position at WCU, she was Chairperson and Professor in the Division of Nursing at California State University, Sacramento, and Dean, College of Health and Human Services at Touro University in Nevada. She received her BS in Nursing from Loma Linda University, her MS from Boston University, and a Doctor of Nursing Science from the University of California, San Francisco. In addition to *Davis's NCLEX-RN® Success,* she was coauthor of *NURSENOTES: Medical-Surgical Nursing,* Core Content At-A-Glance (Lippincott) and a contributor to *Nursing Q and A* (Lippincott), and has developed a number of audio and visual aids for students preparing for the licensure examination. Dr. Nelson was a lecturer for Review for Nurses, Inc., for over 20 years, both at on-site national review courses and as one of the faculty for the "first ever" nationally televised satellite review course that was offered for 7 years. She holds memberships in Sigma Theta Tau International, ANA, ANA/California, and Phi Kappa Phi. Dr. Nelson is a member of the Nurse Week (California) Advisory Board, and the academic representative to the Association of California Nurse Leaders (ACNL) Board of Directors.

Denise Wall Parilo, RN, MSN, PhD(c) is an Associate Professor in the School of Nursing at California State University, Sacramento. In addition to lecturing on pediatric nursing, she is an advisor to the Sacramento State Chapter of the California Nursing Students' Association (CNSA) and has served as coordinator of the undergraduate nursing program. Her experience ranges from pediatric intensive care to public health nursing, and she continues to work as a per diem nurse in acute care pediatrics at Sutter Memorial Hospital in Sacramento. She is a contributing author to *How to Pass Nursing Exams* by Sally Lagerquist, RN, MS, and has been a lecturer for Review for Nurses, Inc. She received both her BS in Nursing and MS in Nursing from California State University, Sacramento, and has been a Fulbright Scholar in Finland, doing community health nursing research. She is presently a doctoral student at the University of California, San Francisco School of Nursing.

Kathleen E. Snider, RN, MSN, CNS, has been a pediatric nurse for over 40 years and has a broad range of clinical and educational experience. She received her diploma in nursing from Saint Vincent's College of Nursing, Los Angeles; her baccalaureate in nursing from Mount Saint Mary's College, Los Angeles; and her master's degree in nursing from California State University, Los Angeles. She has been teaching pediatric nursing since 1976 in diploma, associate of arts, and baccalaureate nursing programs. She began teaching national licensure examination reviews in the mid-1980s and has remained active in that area ever since. She is a contributing author to two editions of *Davis's NCLEX-RN® Success* book and to ATI's *NURSENOTES: Pediatrics, Core Content At-A-Glance.* She also served as a reviewer for the 1996 Little, Brown's *Nursing Q&A Critical-Thinking Exercises* book. Kathy is currently a professor of nursing at Los Angeles Valley College, Valley Glen, California, and is the lead teacher and content expert for pediatric nursing. She is an active member in the American and California Nurses Associations, in national and local chapters of the Association of Pediatric Nurses and Practitioners, and in the Los Angeles County School Nurses Association. She has served as a District Academic Senator for the Los Angeles Community College District and as an Academic Senator at Los Angeles Valley College for over 15 years. In addition, she serves on numerous departmental and campus committees. In 1999 she received the "One of Our Own" award from the National Association of Pediatric Nurse Associates and Practitioners, Los Angeles Chapter, for service and excellence in pediatric nursing, and in 2007, she was awarded the Certificate of Distinguished Service by the Los Angeles Valley College Academic Senate.

Janis Ryan Wisherop, RN, MSN, has been a nurse for 25 years. Ms. Wisherop has been a professor with the RN program at the College of San Mateo for 18 years and has held the title of Content Expert for the Psychiatric Nursing course for that length of time. She teaches in the Medical/Surgical, Advance Medical/Surgical, Leadership/Management, and Pediatric courses as well. Ms. Wisherop has been the Faculty Advisor for the Nursing Student Association and is Assistant Director for the Nursing Program. Along with teaching, Ms. Wisherop is dedicated to serving the community and inspiring her students to do the same. She has created a blood pressure clinic for seniors, partnered with the African American Community Advisory Committee in promoting better health through blood pressure screenings and other health-related events. Ms. Wisherop serves with passion as Board Secretary for Heart and Soul, a consumer operated mental health agency in San Mateo County. In addition, Ms. Wisherop is a per diem nurse with Crossroads Home Care and Hospice, serving patients and their families since 2009. This is her first time working as a co-author/co-editor.

PREFACE

WHAT'S NEW AND DIFFERENT IN THE 3RD EDITION

- ***Questions are coded to correspond to the latest NCLEX-RN® TEST PLAN!***
- Compact disk containing 3500 questions and answers, including all the questions in the book and ***1000 new*** questions
- Many more questions in **ALTERNATE-ITEM FORMATS**
- **TWO NEW PRE-TESTS** with 75 questions each (150 total), each with rationales and unique test-taking tips
- Content totally reorganized under the 13 *body systems* (e.g., cardiac, GI, GU, etc.).
- **TWO NEW FINAL TESTS** with 75 questions each (150 total) to aid in identifying topics that need extra study
- A new *comprehensive index* to help quickly locate specific NCLEX-RN® content

We are very pleased that you have selected our book to help you on your path to success on NCLEX-RN®.

Our aim is to lead you all the way, to have PASSING NCLEX-RN® MADE EASY for you—the *first-time test-taker,* the *international nurse,* and the *repeat test-taker.*

With a conceptual framework based on *body systems* as well as on the components of the latest NCLEX-RN® Test Plan (four client needs and their six subcategories), this book differs significantly from other nursing review books. **It is the only nursing review book that thoroughly covers the content in the current NCLEX-RN® Test Plan and has a test-taking tip for each of the more than 3500 questions!**

Each chapter incorporates all the components of the NCLEX-RN® Test Plan. In addition, **Chapter 3** specifically includes content that focuses on **Safe, Effective Care Environment** (with **Management of Care** and **Safety and Infection Control**). **Chapters 4 and 5** emphasize **Health Promotion and Maintenance** (*growth and development, prevention and early detection of disease*). **Chapters 6, 7, 8,** and **9** emphasize **Physiological Integrity** (with **Chapter 6** specifically addressing **Basic Care and Comfort** and **Physiological Adaptation**). **Chapter 8** is devoted to **Pharmacological and Parenteral Therapies; Chapter 9** is on *Nutrition and Diet Therapy.* **Chapter 10** focuses specifically on **Psychosocial Integrity** (*coping and adaptation*), and **Chapter 11** specifically emphasizes **Reduction of Risk Potential.**

In addition, **Chapter 2** is a unique chapter that addresses the needs of **international nurses** and **repeat test-takers;** and **Chapter 7** addresses the special *needs of the geriatric client.*

PROVEN RESULTS

This is the only review book for NCLEX-RN® that has evolved from and been tested with over 300,000 NCLEX-RN® candidates who have taken our national nursing exam review courses over the last **40 years and passed!** The review course content, the framework, the sequence of topics, the test-taking guidelines, and the practice exam questions and answers have been published in this book. **This gives the book an authenticity and relevance that is difficult to attain any other way.**

CONCEPTUAL FRAMEWORK

The conceptual framework of this book concentrates on body systems, as well as on nursing concerns for *client needs* and the essential requirements for safe, effective, competent nursing care. The text emphasizes *practical application* of clinically relevant data. Separate chapters emphasize the content areas of ***nutrition; pharmacology; common diagnostic procedures, treatments, and nursing care;*** and ***management of care,*** including ***ethical and legal aspects in nursing.*** A separate chapter features the *geriatric client.*

SPECIAL FEATURES

There are many special features in this *abundantly illustrated* book (over 205 charts, tables, and illustrations) that make it **stand out from all other nursing review books.** The unique features that help you prepare for exams are: **test-taking tips** for **each of the questions,** lists of common abbreviations and clinical signs **(Appendices C and D),** and a *comprehensive index* to guide you to where in the book you will find the theory (topics) that specifically relate to the official NCLEX-RN® Test Plan. These features provide quick, easy, and interesting ways to review. In the Introduction to NCLEX-RN® section of **Chapter 1,** you'll also find 60 **study tips, anxiety-reducing techniques,** and memorizing ideas.

OTHER FEATURES

- **A practice computer test** (CD-ROM) for self-assessment and familiarization with the NCLEX-RN® computer testing format includes **test-taking tips with each answer.**
- Many **easy-to-find and easy-to-use tables** summarize information for *quick* review and emphasize nursing responsibilities in *a visual way.*
- **Boxed lab data, diagnostic tests, bold-faced hazard alerts and emergencies** visually stand out. **Drug information** is indicated by a , **diets** are indicated by a , **client positioning** is indicated by a to help you focus on important concepts, and **memory tips** are indicated by a .

- Easy-to-find **content divisions** are marked with blue page tabs at the outer margin of each page.
- Emphasis is given to all **five steps of the nursing process,** especially *client teaching* and specific *outcome criteria for evaluation* of the effectiveness of nursing care.
- Current NANDA-approved *nursing diagnoses* are provided as a structure for presenting nursing interventions.
- A thorough **question-and-answer review** at the end of *each chapter,* with a critical thinking focus that also reflects **diverse cultural influences.**

This review book has been updated and revised to incorporate the latest knowledge and current trends in nursing practice and to parallel the **latest NCLEX-RN® Test Plan.** All content has been submitted to outstanding educators and nursing practitioners for their review and critique. We would like to express our appreciation to this editorial review panel for their contributions, which make this book the best to use for complete nursing review.

The book's content includes special topics not commonly covered:

- **Management of care** section including: *delegation,* establishing *priorities, HIPAA* rules, *emergency response plan* (fire safety and preparedness).
- **Infection control:** animal-borne diseases (SARS, West Nile virus, mad cow disease, monkeypox, Lyme disease, rabies, salmonella).
- **Bioterrorism agents and associated syndromes** (anthrax, botulism, plague, smallpox, tularemia, Ebola, Lassa, Hantavirus)
- **Herbal medicines:** dietary supplements and herbal products used for psychiatric conditions; herbs and potential dangers.
- **Complementary** and **alternative therapies**

Chapter 2, Guidelines and Tips for International Nurses and Repeat Test-Takers, is unique. ***No other book*** addresses the special concerns of candidates who have taken the test more than once or who are graduates of nursing programs outside the United States. **Chapter 2** covers:

- **Risk factors** for not passing the first time
- Five steps on **what to do to pass next time**
- **How to know if you are prepared** to take the exam again
- **Sixty test-taking tips and guidelines** to use in answering questions

Chapter 3 has been reorganized, with special focus on Safe and Effective Care Environment: **Management of Care, Cultural Diversity, Ethical and Legal Aspects of Nursing, Nursing Trends,** and **Safety and Infection Control.** Content includes: safe use of equipment, ***delegation,*** establishing ***priorities,*** emergency response plan, **HIPAA** law, *cultural diversity, religious* and *spiritual* influences on health, advance directives, advocacy, organ donation, bioethics and client rights, supervision, disaster planning, and client restraints. Infection control content includes *isolation* precautions, with tables covering *Types of Precautions* and *Illnesses Requiring the Precautions,* and *Infection Control Conditions that Need Additional Precautions.*

Chapter 4, Health Promotion and Maintenance: Nursing Care of the Childbearing Family, is streamlined, visually enhanced, and up-to-date; it contains the most exam-relevant content for both pregnancy and care of the neonate. This chapter includes *detailed* information regarding many important ***diagnostic tests,*** such as chorionic villi sampling and biophysical profile testing, to identify the woman and fetus at risk. ***Numerous illustrations*** are included (e.g., amniocentesis, fetal circulation, and ectopic pregnancy). We include the latest information on ***emergency care*** in labor and birth, perinatal acquired immune deficiency syndrome, sexually transmitted infections, and *preterm labor.* We have *updated* pharmacological information regarding new drug therapies during the perinatal period recommended for the at-risk infant, as well as trends and modes for delivery of *contraceptives* and birth control education. Updated information is included on intrapartum *complications* and *risk factors,* with content on *hepatitis* and *TB* in *pregnancy. Client teaching* and *nursing interventions* are delineated for each of these areas of practice.

Chapter 5, Health Promotion and Maintenance: Nursing Care of the Pediatric Client, has a **new table** with updated immunization information, a pediatric safety and injury prevention chart, coverage of pediatric *emergencies* (revised tables for CPR and foreign body airway obstructive management—previously called Heimlich maneuver), and updated information (nursing care, medications, tests, etc.) concerning all major **physical systems of the body.** Much of this information has been synthesized into table format for *easier reading, recall,* and *application* to client care. **Diagrams** show genetic transmission of sickle cell anemia and hemophilia. **Illustrations** depict five cardiac defects, airway, CPR, TEF and esophageal atresia, developmental dysplasia of the hip, and scoliosis. Coverage is provided for Reye syndrome, Kawasaki disease, and salicylate, acetaminophen, and lead poisoning, as well as appreciation of **cultural diversity** in assessment and nursing interventions.

Chapter 6, Physiological Integrity: Nursing Care of the Adult Client, has been arranged by *head-to-toe body systems,* making it easier to remember important assessment information and to prioritize the plan of care. *Risk factors* have been identified for all conditions, *goals of nursing* are clearly stated, and a brief description of *pathophysiology* is incorporated with each condition. *Nursing interventions* are grouped according to the goal of care and identify appropriate treatments and drug therapies. Handy **tables** include: Factors Affecting Vital

Signs, SIADH Versus Diabetes Insipidus, Bioterrorism, Infectious Diseases (including animal-borne), fluid and electrolyte imbalances, acid-base disorders, assessment differences with valvular defects, hazards of immobility, complications of diabetes, and malignant disorders. The *condensed* and *consolidated* content is supplemented by *many other tables, charts,* and *diagrams,* such as: cardiac dysrhythmias (*new* content on *atrial flutter*), comparison of causes of chest pain, burn care, the Glasgow Coma Scale, chest drainage, comparison of hepatitis types, post-operative complications, enteric and standard precautions, respiratory isolation, care of the adult client with *medical and surgical emergencies,* preventing TPN complications, and TPN dressing changes. **Illustrations** show 12 types of fractures, 8 skin and skeletal tractions, and breast and testicular self-exam. **Special content** covers management of PICC lines, use of metered-dose inhalers, pneumonia severity, pheochromocytoma, Raynaud's disease, SARS, and Guillain-Barré syndrome. The up-to-date content also includes acquired immunodeficiency syndrome, GERD, latex allergies, JCAHO Requirements for Pain Assessment, Lyme disease, compartment syndrome, Crohn's disease, ulcers, external fixation devices for fractures, and lithotripsy.

Chapter 7, Physiological Integrity: Nursing Care of the Geriatric Client, is a concise and highly readable chapter synthesizing 12 key problems associated with care of the older adult. There is a section on *assessment of the older adult* that includes material on normal changes of aging, including a table summarizing common concerns in the older adult. *Five functional rating scales* and *a functional screening* exam are included to make management of care easier:

- Social resources rating scale
- Economic resources rating scale
- Mental health rating scale
- Physical health rating scale
- Performance rating scale for activities of daily living

Chapter 8, Physiological Integrity: Pharmacological and Parenteral Therapies, contains drug classifications and drug treatments with emphasis on **nursing implications.** Content covers *drug conversions* and *calculations,* pediatric medication administration, *fluid and electrolyte therapy,* commonly used *IV fluids,* and obstetric analgesia. Psychotropic and mind-altering substances are included, as well as **tables** on herbal therapies (with potential dangers). **New drugs** have been added for this edition.

Chapter 9, Physiological Integrity: Basic Care and Comfort—Nutrition, contains unique information regarding *ethnic* food patterns, eating problems, nutritional needs of the *elderly, religious* and *ethnic* food preferences, and *cultural* disease treatments involving food. *Special* and *therapeutic diets* are featured, with coverage of medical conditions with dietary management, high-*phosphorus* and *lactose-free* diets, and *anticancer nutrients.*

Chapter 10, Psychosocial Integrity: Behavioral/Mental Health Care Throughout the Life Span, presents psychiatric disorders that have been organized under DSM-IV-TR guidelines. We have included *thorough* coverage of suicide precautions, *midlife* crises, mental health of the *elderly,* substance abuse, post-traumatic stress disorder, amnestic disorders, personality disorders, sleep and eating disturbances, and affective disorders. Content includes a detailed section on psychiatric *emergencies* and therapeutic communication techniques. Also, three developmental sections are included: a table on development of *body image* (includes disturbances and four phases of crises), *human sexuality* throughout the life cycle (with causes of dysfunction and sexual health counseling), and a *table on emotional disturbances in children,* with sections on autistic spectrum disorder, attention deficit-hyperactivity disorder, and child abuse. Nine important sections are: *domestic violence* (abused woman and child; elder abuse/neglect), *diagnostic tests* (for dementia/cognitive disorders and alcohol abuse); mental status assessment (individual, cultural); interviewing; general principles of health teaching; self-concept; coping mechanisms; and treatment modes, with a section on **complementary and alternative methods.** There is also an extensive **glossary.**

Chapter 11, Reduction of Risk Potential: Common Procedures: Diagnostic Tests, Oxygen Therapy, and Hands-on Nursing Care, includes content on commonly used *tubes,* oxygen delivery equipment, and colostomy care, as well as many diagnostic procedures commonly tested on NCLEX-RN®. Also included are diagnostic tests to evaluate *fetal well-being, newborn screening* procedures (with content on Tay-Sachs screening), and *bladder* and *bowel* training. Common client *positions* and *intubation* and *ventilation* are illustrated.

FIVE UNIQUE SELF-EVALUATION TOOLS—OVER 3500 TEST QUESTIONS AND TEST-TAKING TIPS

This book contains four special, *integrated* tests to help you assess your knowledge before taking the NCLEX-RN®. The special **two new** 75-item **Pre-Tests** at the end of **Chapter 1** are intended for students to take *after* reading the **Introduction to NCLEX-RN®** section but *before* reading the rest of this book. It is a pre-assessment tool to let you find your areas of strength and weakness based on the 10 client needs/subneeds of the NCLEX-RN® Test Plan before beginning focused study. The two integrated **Final Tests in Chapter 12** are intended to be taken *after* reviewing each chapter in this book to evaluate your progress. These **two new** 75-item **Final Tests,** the third and fourth integrated exam tools, will assess your readiness to take NCLEX-RN® and identify any last-minute knowledge gaps.

Use the fifth self-evaluation exam tool as a practice **Computer Test** on the CD-ROM anytime in your preparation when you need extra practice or when you want to become familiar with the NCLEX-RN® testing format.

All questions at the *end of chapters* and in the integrated tests have been field-tested for several years with students—a diverse group of candidates who have successfully passed the exam—from all over the United States. These questions have also been reviewed by an editorial panel for appropriateness. The Answers/Rationales/Tips sections in each chapter contain detailed explanations about why a particular answer is *best* and *why the other* options are incorrect, with a **test-taking tip for each question.** We expect that these special integrated tests, end-of-chapter review questions, and corresponding answer sections will prove to be invaluable review tools for each and every student.

In the answers for each of the end-of-chapter review question sections, as well as for the **Pre-Tests, Final Tests,** and **Computer Test,** you will find a four-part code to help you understand exactly what is being tested by each question. The code refers to Integrated Process (e.g., the step of the *nursing process*), the *cognitive level* (level of difficulty of the item), the ***clinical/subject area,*** and the ***client need*** and the ***subcategory of client need*** that applies to that question. The **Computer Test** will track these codes for you to identify your problem areas. Use these codes as a guide for review when you find you did not select the best answer. The **test-taking tips** and **codes are unique to this book;** they are an added study tool to help you assess your strengths and pinpoint problem areas as you prepare for the NCLEX-RN®.

CONTRIBUTORS

Reviewer and Contributing Author to Special Sections in Chapter 6

Estrella Evangelista-Hoffman, RN, CNL, MEd, DNP
Las Vegas, Nevada

Test Item Writers for This Edition

Cheryl Osborne, RN, EdD
Professor, School of Nursing and Director, Gerontology Program
California State University, Sacramento, California

Connie Overman, RN, MS
Former Clinical Faculty, School of Nursing
California State University, Sacramento, California

Carolyn Van Couwenberghe, RN, PhD
Professor, School of Nursing
California State University, Sacramento, California

ACKNOWLEDGMENTS

BONNIE BERGSTROM – YOU are the superstar on my winning team of authors in this 3rd edition. You stepped into the picture at midstream and added your editing expertise and gave of your very special kind of nurturing when we were all under time pressure with manuscript deadlines. You are one-of-a-kind and I'm deeply grateful!

BERTA STEINER and the Bermedica Production, Ltd. staff (including Megan Westerfeld, the copyeditor)—You were invaluable in helping me maintain a vigilant eye for quality control—finding gaps and inconsistencies, and giving shape and form to a complicated manuscript during stops and starts in the editorial process. Above all, you were there for me and my co-authors—we worked as a team.

BOB BUTLER—You were there for me as a conduit in the F.A. Davis communication chain. Your support served as a beacon for decisions in putting my ideas into print.

BOB MARTONE—You contributed important ideas to make this 3rd edition the best yet for visual emphasis, with unique features that are designed to help the user be successful in nursing school exams and NCLEX-RN®.

A special personal thank you also to NEIL KELLY and ROB CRAVEN, whose support for this book over the last eight years and three editions made it a happy "happening." Contacts along the way with each of you went beyond the ordinary and are much appreciated.

Sally

LIST OF TABLES

CHAPTER 10

CHAPTER 11

LIST OF FIGURES

TABLE OF CONTENTS

Chapter 10: Psychosocial Integrity: Behavioral/Mental Health Care Throughout the Life Span 711

Sally Lambert Lagerquist • Janis Ryan Wisherop (Reviewer and Contributor to Selected Sections)

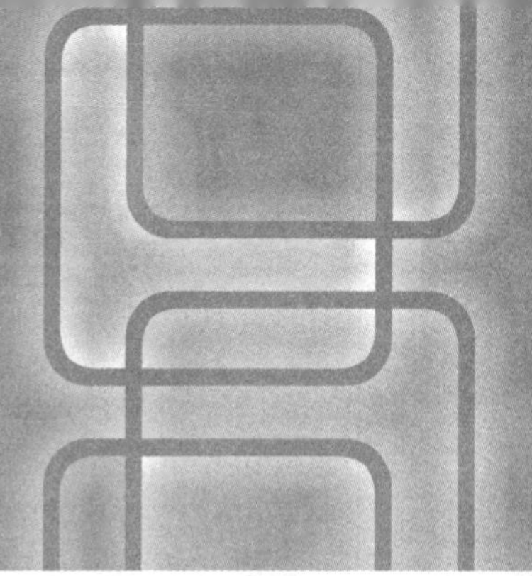

CHAPTER 1

Orientation and Pre-Tests

Sally Lambert Lagerquist • Janice Lloyd McMillin • Robyn Marchal Nelson • Denise Wall Parilo • Kathleen E. Snider • Janis Ryan Wisherop

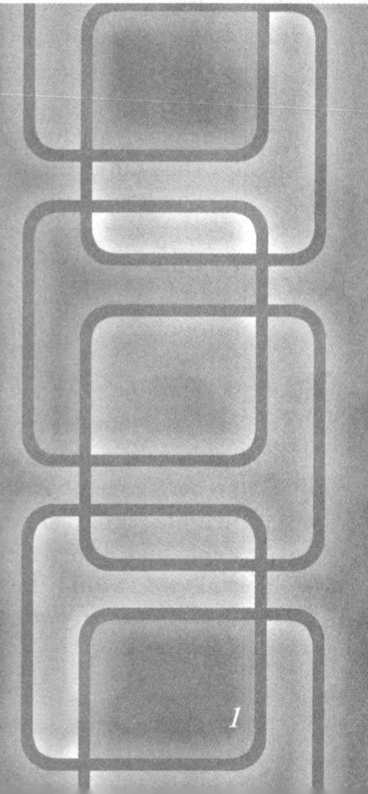

ORIENTATION

How to Use This Review Book as a Study Guide

Although nursing students may know that they are academically prepared to take the computer adaptive National Council Licensure Examination for Registered Nurses (NCLEX-RN)®, many find that reviewing nursing content for the licensure examination itself presents special concerns about *what* and *how* to study.

Some typical concerns about **what to study** are reflected in the following questions:

- Considering that there will be up to 265 questions on the examination, and every candidate gets a different examination, how does one select what is the most important content for review? How does one narrow the focus of study and distinguish the relevant from the irrelevant material?
- What areas should be emphasized?
- How detailed should the review be?
- How does one know what areas to review first?
- Should basic sciences, such as anatomy, physiology, microbiology, and nutrition, be included in the study?

Concerns relating to **how to study** include:

- How does one make the best of limited review time to go over content that may be in lecture and clinical notes compiled during 2 to 4 years of schooling?
- Is it best to review from all the major textbooks used in nursing school?
- Should material be memorized, or should one study from broad principles and concepts?

We have written this nursing review book with the *general* intent of assisting nurses in identifying what they need to study in a format designed to use their study time effectively, productively, and efficiently while preparing for the examination.

The contributing authors have selected content and developed a style of presentation that has been tested by thousands of nursing students attending review courses coordinated by the editor in various cities throughout the United States. This book is the result of this study.

This review book can be used in a variety of ways: (a) as a *starting point* for review of essential content specifically aimed at NCLEX® or Canadian examination preparation, (b) as an *endpoint* of studying for the examinations, (c) as an *anxiety-reduction tool,* (d) as a general guide and *refresher* for nurses not presently in practice, and (e) as a guide for graduates of nursing schools *outside of the United States,* as well as *repeat test-takers* (see **Chapter 2**).

As a Starting Point

This text can be used in early review when a longer study period is needed to *fill in gaps* of knowledge. One cannot remember something if one does not know or understand it. A lengthy review before the examination allows students time to rework and organize notes accumulated during 2 to 4 years of basic nursing education. In addition, an early review allows time for *self-evaluation.* We have provided questions and answers to help students identify areas requiring further study and to help them *integrate* unfamiliar material with what they already know.

As an Endpoint

This text can also be used for a *quick review* (a) to *promote retention and recall* and (b) to aid in determining *nursing actions* appropriate to specific health situations. During the time immediately preceding the examination, the main objective might be to *strengthen previous learning* by refreshing the memory. Or a brief overview may serve to *draw together* the isolated points under key concepts and principles in a way that shows their relationships and relative importance.

As an Anxiety-Reduction Tool

In some students, anxiety related to taking examinations in general may reach such levels that it causes students to be unproductive in study and to function at a lower level during the actual examination. Sections of this chapter are directed toward this problem and provide simple, *practical approaches to the reduction of general anxiety.* For anxiety specifically related to unknown aspects of the licensure examination itself, the section on the *structure, format, and mechanics of the RN examination* might bring relief through its focus on basic examination information (see **pp. 4-11**).

For anxiety related to lack of confidence or skill in test-taking "know-how," the special section on *test-taking techniques* may be helpful (see **Chapter 2**).

As a General Study Guide and as a Refresher for Nurses Not Presently in Practice

Many nursing students will find this review book useful throughout their education as a general study guide as they prepare client care plans and study for midterm and final examinations. It will help them put information into perspective as they learn it. And nurses who have not been in practice for several years will find it a useful reference tool and review device.

Where to Begin

In using this review book to prepare for the licensure examination, the nurse must:

1. Be prepared mentally.
   a. Know the purpose of the examination.
   b. Know the purpose of reviewing.

c. Anticipate what is to come.
d. Decide on a good study method—set a study goal before beginning a particular subject area (number of pages, for example); plan the length of the review period by the amount of material to be covered, not by the clock.

2. Plan the work to be done.
   a. Select one subject at a time for review, and establish and follow a sequence for review of each subject.
      (1) Answer the practice questions following the outline of the selected subject area. (Set a time limit, because pacing is important.)
      (2) Compare your answers with those provided following the questions as a means of evaluating areas of competence.
   b. Identify those subjects that will require additional concentrated study in this review book as well as in basic textbooks.
   c. Study the review text outlines, noting headings, subheadings, and *italics* and **boldface** type for emphasis of relative importance.
   d. Study the content presented in the shaded boxes and chart format to facilitate memorization, understanding, and application.
   e. Repeat the self-evaluation process by taking the test again.
   f. Look up the answers for the correct response to the multiple-choice questions. Do not memorize the answers. Read the rationale explaining *why* it was the correct response. (These explanations serve to correct as well as reinforce. Understanding the underlying principles also serves as an aid in applying the same principles to questions that may be based on similar rationales, but phrased differently on the actual examination.)
   g. If necessary, refer to basic textbooks to relearn any unclear aspects of anatomy, physiology, nutrition, or basic nursing procedures. Look up unfamiliar terminology in a medical dictionary.

While Reviewing

1. Scan the outline for main ideas and topics.
   a. Do not try to remember verbatim what is on each page.
   b. Paraphrase or explain this material to another person.
2. Refer to basic textbooks for details and illustrations as necessary to recall specific information related to basic sciences.
3. Integrate reading with experience.
   a. Think of examples that illustrate the key concepts and principles.
   b. Make meaningful associations.
   c. Look for implications for nursing actions as concepts are reviewed.
4. Take notes on the review outline—use stars and arrows, underscore, highlight with highlighter pens, and write comments in margins, such as "most important" and "memorize," to reinforce the relative importance of points of information.

After Reviewing

1. Repeat the self-evaluation process as often as necessary to gain mastery of content essential to safe nursing practice.
2. Continue to refer to major textbooks to fill in gaps where greater detail or in-depth comprehension is required.
3. Look for patterns in your selection of responses to the multiple-choice practice questions—identify sources of difficulty in choosing the most appropriate answers.
4. Review test-taking strategies (see **Chapter 2, pp. 62-67**).

Key Points to Recall for Better Study

1. *Schedule*—study time should be scheduled so that review begins close to the time at which it will be used. Retention is much better following a well-spaced review. It may be helpful to group material into small learning segments. Study goals should be set before beginning each period of study (number of pages, for example).
2. *Organize*—many students have better retention of material after they have reorganized and relearned it.
3. *Rephrase and explain*—try to rephrase material in your own words or explain it to another person. Reinforce learning through repetition and usage.
4. *Decide on order of importance*—organize study time in terms of importance and familiarity.
5. *Use mechanical memory aids*—mnemonic (memory) devices simplify recall. For example, in "On Old Olympus's Towering Top a Finn and German Viewed Some Hops," the first letter of each word identifies the first letter of a cranial nerve (see **Appendix B**).
6. *Association*—associate new material with related concepts and principles from past experience.
7. *Original learning*—if an unfamiliar topic is presented, do more than review. Seek out sources of additional information.
8. *Make notes*—look for key words, phrases, and sentences in the outlined review material, and mark them for later reference.

9. *Definitions*—look up unfamiliar terms in a dictionary or the glossary of a basic text, or in **Appendix C.**
10. *Additional study*—refer to other textbook references for more detailed information.
11. *Distractors*—keep a pad of paper on hand to jot down extraneous thoughts; get them out of your mind and onto the paper.

Memorization: Purpose and Strategies

You will need to memorize some items before you can rapidly assess or apply that knowledge to a particular situation; for example, you need to be able to recall the standard and lethal doses of a drug before deciding to administer it. Items you should memorize include, but are not limited to:

1. Names of common drugs.
2. Lethal and therapeutic doses.
3. Laboratory norms and values.
4. Growth and development norms.
5. Foods high or low in iron, protein, sodium, potassium, or carbohydrates.
6. Conversion formulas.
7. Anatomical names.
8. List of cranial nerves and their innervations.
9. Definitions of defense mechanisms.

To facilitate memorizing these and other essentials, here are some strategies:

1. Before you work on training your mind to remember, you must *want* to remember the material.
2. You cannot memorize something that you do not understand; therefore, *know* your material.
3. Visualize what you want to memorize; picture it; draw a picture.
4. Use the familiar to provide vivid mental pictures, to peg the unfamiliar.
   a. When needing to remember a *sequence,* use your body to turn material into a picture. Draw a person, then list the first item to be memorized on top of the head, the next item on the forehead, and so on for nose, mouth, neck, chest, abdomen, thighs, knees, and feet.
   b. Use what you already know to tie in with what you want to remember; make it memorable.
   c. Use as pegs the unexpected, the exaggerated. Weird imagery is easiest to recall.
5. Use the blank-paper technique:
   a. Place a large blank sheet on the wall.
   b. After you have studied, draw on the blank paper what you remember.
   c. When you have drawn all that you can recall, check with the book and study what you did correctly and incorrectly.
   d. Take another sheet and do it again. Purpose: to reinforce what you already know and work with what you want to remember.
6. Make up and use mnemonic devices to help you remember the important elements (see **Appendix B**).
7. Repetitively explain to another person the material you want to memorize.
8. Saturate your environment with the material you want to memorize.
   a. Purpose: to overcome the mind's tendency to ignore.
   b. Tape facts, formulas, concepts on walls.
9. Above all, feel confident in your ability to memorize!

The Mechanics of the National Council Licensure Examination for Registered Nurses–Computer Adaptive Test (NCLEX-RN®)

Since 1994, the licensure examination for registered nurses has been administered year-round by computer, in an adaptive format: NCLEX-RN®. Frequently, candidates for the examination have many questions about the structure and format of the test itself and the rules and regulations concerning the examination procedure.

As an aid to reducing apprehension and time spent on speculation, this section is intended to provide information that candidates need, in outline form; the last segment offers a "question-and-answer" format for specific questions frequently asked by nursing students.

This information was verified as correct at the time that it was compiled from information provided by the National Council of State Boards of Nursing, Inc. (NCSBN), and other parties involved in the testing. If you have further questions, contact the board of nursing in your state.

I. WHAT NCLEX® IS

A. National Council Licensure Examination, developed and administered by the National Council of State Boards of Nursing, Inc., with services provided by VUE (Virtual University Enterprises), an NCS (National Computer Systems) Pearson Company.

B. Tests for minimum nursing competence according to a national standard.

C. Pass/fail result; must pass to be issued license from state board of registered nursing.

D. National examination. Application procedure and licensing requirements are determined by each state board and may differ from state to state.

II. CAT: HOW IT WORKS

A. Stands for "computer adaptive testing."

B. "Adaptive" because the computer estimates the candidate's ability after each question; the next question is chosen based on the candidate's estimated ability so far. The test is therefore "adapted" to each candidate; everyone takes a different, "customized" test.

C. Estimated ability is recalculated after each question until it is precise enough to determine whether the candidate is above or below minimum competence level, in all areas of the test plan. The test will stop as soon as this is determined.

D. Example: The first question is at a fairly easy level. The candidate answers correctly, so the computer estimates that the candidate's ability level is above the level of this question and selects a harder question; or if the candidate answers incorrectly, it selects an easier question, to pinpoint where the candidate's ability level lies, in each area of the test plan.

E. After consideration of all available information, the NCSBN determined that safe and effective entry-level RN practice requires a greater level of knowledge, skills, and abilities than was required in 2007 (the date that the NCLEX® was last reviewed/revised). The passing standard was increased in response to changes in U.S. health-care delivery and nursing practice that have resulted in more acutely ill clients being seen by entry-level RNs. An expert panel of nine nurses was convened and performed criterion-referenced standard-setting procedures. The panel's findings supported the creation of a higher passing standard. In addition, the NCSBN considered the results of national surveys of nursing professionals including nursing educators, directors of nursing in acute care settings, and administrators of long-term care facilities. The NCSBN voted on December 10, 2009, to raise the passing standard for the NCLEX® examination. The new passing standard is –0.16 logits on the NCLEX® logistic scale, 0.05 logits higher than the previous standard of –0.21 logits. Logits are usually a foreign concept to the general public. "Logit" is an abbreviation for "log odds unit." Basically, logits are a useful unit of probability. Using the candidate responses, the difficulty of the items relative to each other (not relative to the candidates) is assessed. Once the hierarchy of difficulty for items is established, then the ability of a candidate can be described as the point on this item hierarchy, or continuum, where the candidate has a *50-50* chance of correctly answering an item. When a candidate encounters an item that is lower than his or her ability, then he or she will have a greater than *50-50* chance of answering the item correctly. Conversely, when a candidate encounters an item that is higher than his or her ability, then he or she will have a less than *50-50* chance of answering the question correctly. The deviation from *50-50* is governed by the size of the difference between the person's ability and the item's difficulty. A candidate's ability could be described by illustrating the type of item that he or she finds challenging. The latest passing standard took effect on April 1, 2010, in conjunction with the 2010 NCLEX® Test Plan (see **Section V**).

III. SOME SPECIFICS

A. Format

1. Most questions will be multiple choice, each with four options from which you choose only one option. In addition to multiple-choice items, candidates may be administered items written in alternate formats **(Table 1.1).** The formats may include but are not limited to multiple response (including ordered response), fill-in-the-blank, numerical entry, drag and drop, and/or hot spots. All item types may include multimedia such as charts, tables, graphics, sound, and video.
2. One question at a time appears on screen **(Fig. 1.1)**.
3. Each question stands alone (no "scenarios" with several spin-off questions); no question will relate to information given in *previous* questions.

B. Answering

1. As candidate chooses the answer to each question, he or she will be asked to confirm that answer by pressing the <NEXT> button, *or* can change that answer before confirming.
2. Must answer every question (no penalty for guessing; will simply count as a correct or incorrect answer and adjust difficulty of next question accordingly).
3. Cannot go back to previous questions either to review or change answers (because the level of *subsequent* questions administered is based on *previous* answers).

C. Number of questions

1. 75 to 265, including about 15 "tryout" questions that are not scored (these are questions being field tested for use on future examinations).
2. Depends on number needed to determine whether candidate is definitely above or definitely below minimum competence level.
3. Taking only the minimum can mean **either pass or fail;** it indicates that it took fewer questions to determine whether this candidate is above or below minimum competence, but does not indicate which!

Table 1.1

Description of NCLEX® Question Formats

Multiple Choice

Which clinical feature found on assessment should indicate to a nurse that a client has congestive heart failure? *Select the one best answer.*

1. Fatigue and dyspnea.
2. Cheyne-Stokes breathing and orthostatic hypotension.
3. Liver tenderness and peripheral edema.
4. Pulmonary crackles and weak pulses.

Multiple Response

A client with a history of Graves' disease is admitted for uncontrolled hyperglycemia and a foot ulcer. This client requires close monitoring because of the increased risk of:
Select all that apply.

1. Hypotension.
2. Elevated temperature.
3. Hypothyroidism.
4. Hypoglycemia.
5. Extreme tachycardia.

Fill in the Blank

A child is to receive digoxin 0.07 mg PO twice daily. The label on the bottle of digoxin reads 0.05 mg/mL. A nurse correctly calculates that this client should receive _______ mL of digoxin. Record your answer using one decimal place.

Hot Spot

A client has mitral regurgitation. Where is the best place for a nurse to auscultate the associated murmur?

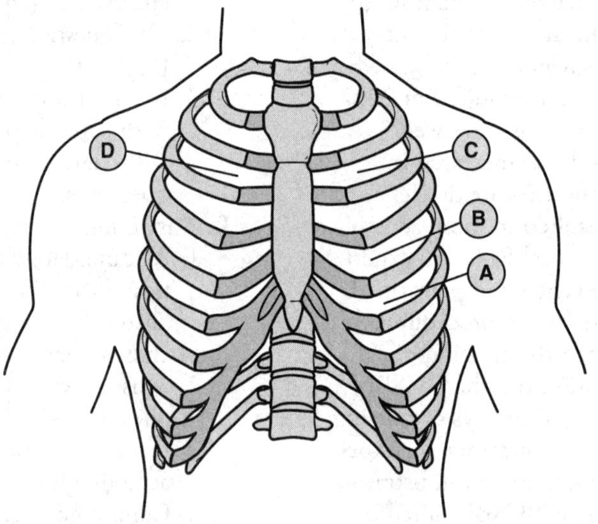

Ordered Response (Prioritization; Drag and Drop)

A nurse prepares to administer a Denver II developmental assessment on a toddler. In which order should the nurse complete the assessment? *Place each action in sequential order.*

_______ Ask child to name doll's body parts.
_______ Ask caregiver if the child uses a spoon and fork.
_______ Ask the child to build a tower of 2 cubes.
_______ Advise parent that the assessment is not an IQ test.
_______ Have child kick ball forward.

Table 1.1

Description of NCLEX® Question Formats—cont'd

Chart or Exhibit
A nurse is caring for a client with a closed chest drainage system. Which area should the nurse identify that regulates the amount of suction? 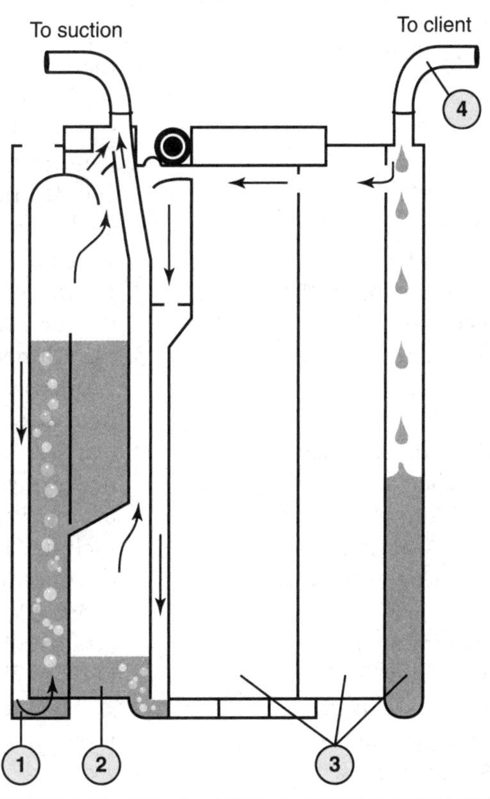

Graphic
When documenting in a client's medical record, which symbol or abbreviation is appropriate for a nurse to use according to the Joint Commission? 1. > 2. @ 3. mL 4. U

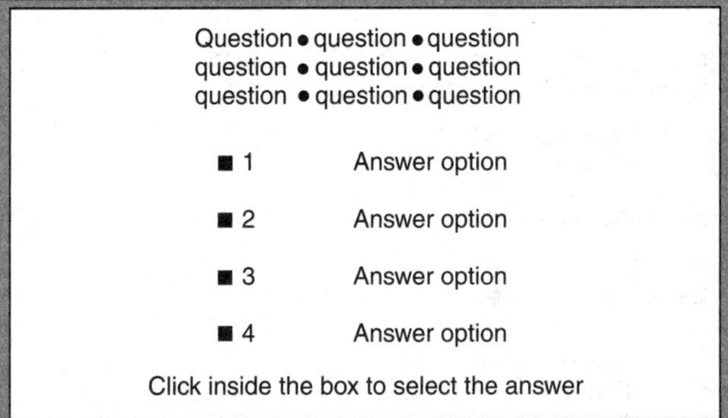

Question • question • question
question • question • question
question • question • question
■ 1 Answer option
■ 2 Answer option
■ 3 Answer option
■ 4 Answer option
Click inside the box to select the answer

Figure 1.1 Sample appearance of NCLEX-RN® question on computer screen.

D. Timing
1. No time limit for each question.
2. Maximum time for test is 6 hours.
3. A preprogrammed optional break is given after 2 hours; a second preprogrammed optional break may be taken after another 1½ hours.

E. The test will stop when any *one* of the following occurs:
1. A "pass" or "fail" determination can be made.
2. The maximum number of questions has been taken (265).
3. The test has lasted for 6 hours, including examination instructions, sample items, and all rest breaks.

F. The computer
1. Computer experience will not be necessary.
2. A mouse is used to move down the list of options and select and confirm answer choice by pressing the <NEXT> button; all keys will be "turned off."
3. An on-screen calculator will be available.
4. Candidate receives a brief orientation in the use of the mouse and on-screen calculator with sample questions before beginning the examination.

IV. ADMINISTRATION

A. Application and scheduling
1. Involves three parties: the state board of nursing, VUE, and Pearson Professional Test Center.
2. Candidate applies to the board of nursing in the state in which licensing is desired; must meet requirements of that state board. (There is a test fee, and some state boards may also require an administrative fee.)
3. After state board determines eligibility and fees are received, candidate will be mailed an *Authorization to Test (ATT)* and information on available Pearson Professional Test Centers, which serve as testing sites (at least one per state; some states have many more).
4. Candidate must schedule an appointment to take the examination by calling NCLEX® Candidate Services or going to the NCLEX® Candidate Web site. (*Note*: These procedures differ in some states, such as Massachusetts. Candidates should follow instructions from state board.)
5. Candidate contacts Pearson Professional Test Center (or other designated test site) to set up testing appointment (5 days/wk, 15 hr/day, in 6-hr time slots). Candidates may test at any test center in any state (they do not have to take the test in the same state to which they have applied for licensure).
6. After testing, results are communicated to state board to which the candidate applied, which mails results to candidate (time frame will differ by state). Candidates who do not pass will receive a Candidate Performance Report, indicating performance in each area of the test plan relative to the passing standard, and information about retesting.

B. Test environment: Pearson Professional Test Center test sites
1. Up to 30 workstations, each with computer terminal, desk lamp, work surface, and scratch paper.
2. Designed for security, monitored by a proctor and by videotape.
3. Candidate must present *Authorization to Test* and two signed pieces of identification, one with picture; candidate must sign in and be fingerprinted and photographed.
4. Lockers or other secured storage provided; personal items restricted in testing room.

V. TEST PLAN, DEVELOPMENT

A. Test plan
1. Bloom's taxonomy for the cognitive domain is used as **a basis for** writing and coding items for the examination. Since the practice of nursing requires application of knowledge, skills, and abilities, the majority of items are written at the application or higher levels of cognitive ability, which requires more complex thought processing.
2. *Client needs* are the bases, or "dimensions," for the test plan **(Table 1.2)**.
3. Health needs of clients: The test plan primarily emphasizes meeting the clients' physical needs in actual or potentially life-threatening, chronic, or recurring *physiological* conditions and the needs of clients who are at risk for complications or untoward effects of treatment. Subneeds include (1) basic care and comfort (6%–12%), (2) pharmacological and parenteral therapies (13%–19%), (3) reduction of risk potential (10%–16%), and (4) physiological adaptation (11%–17%).

The second highest category of emphasis is *safe, effective care environment,* which focuses

Table 1.2

Examination Weight Given to Each Category of Health Needs of Clients Based on Current Practice Analysis Study*

Client Needs/Subneeds	Percentage of Items From Each Category/Subcategory
Safe and Effective Care Environment	
• Management of Care	16%–22%
• Safety and Infection Control	8%–14%
Health Promotion and Maintenance	6%–12%
Psychosocial Integrity	6%–12%
Physiological Integrity	
• Basic Care and Comfort	6%–12%
• Pharmacological and Parenteral Therapies	13%–19%
• Reduction of Risk Potential	10%–16%
• Physiological Adaptation	11%–17%

**Source:* National Council of State Boards of Nursing web site. 2010 NCLEX-RN® Test Plan.

on (1) management of care (16%–22%) and (2) safety and infection control (8%–14%). *Health promotion and maintenance* (6%–12%) covers growth and development throughout the life span and prevention and early detection of disease. *Psychosocial integrity* (6%–12%) concerns coping and adaptation in stress- and crisis-related situations throughout the life cycle.

4. *Nursing process* (nursing behaviors): The examination integrates steps of the nursing process, as applied to client situations from all stages in the life cycle and to common health problems in all the major health areas and based on current morbidity studies. It is a problem-solving approach to client care that includes data collection (assessment, analysis), planning, implementation, and evaluation.
5. Levels of *cognitive ability:* Most items are at the levels of *application* (application of rules, procedures, principles, ideas, and theories, and using a concept in a new situation) and *analysis* (analysis of data to set priorities and see relationships). Some items include knowledge and comprehension (simple recognition or recall of material; restating or reorganizing material to show understanding).
6. Categories of nursing knowledge and other concepts that are commonly tested:
   a. **Caring** ways by which nursing can assist individuals to maintain health and cope with health problems. It involves interaction between nurse and client in a collaborative environment, with mutual respect and trust. The nurse provides hope, support, and compassion to achieve desired outcomes. (See *nursing care plan/implementation* sections in *each* unit.)
   b. **Communication** (see **Chapter 10**).
   c. Effects of age, sex, culture, ethnicity, and religion on health needs (sociocultural components) are integrated into all units; for special emphasis see **Chapters 3** and **9** (dietary implications).
   d. **Documentation;** legal and ethical aspects of nursing, accountability (see **Chapter 3**).
   e. Self-care.
   f. **Teaching-learning;** helping client and significant others to acquire knowledge, skills, and attitudes that facilitate changes in behavior. (See *health teaching* sections [after the conditions] that are part of **Nursing care plan/implementation**.)
   g. Nursing fundamentals (see **Chapter 11**).
   h. Nutrition and diet therapy (see **Chapter 9**).
   i. Pharmacology (see **Chapter 8**).
   j. Communicable diseases (see **Chapters 5** and **6**).
   k. Natural and behavioral sciences (integrated into all units).
   l. Normal growth and development (see **Chapters 4, 5,** and **10**).
   m. Basic human needs (see **Chapter 10**).
   n. Individual coping mechanisms (see **Chapter 10**).
   o. Actual or potential health problems (see **Chapters 4, 5, 6,** and 7).
   p. Life cycle.
   q. Client environment (there is continual reference throughout this book related to protection from harm against airborne irritants, cold, and heat; identification of environmental discomforts such as noise, odors, dust, and poor ventilation; elimination of potential *safety hazards;* maintenance of environmental order; and *cleanliness*).

B. Development

1. The Examination Committee of the National Council prepares the test plan, which is approved by the delegates representing the state boards of nursing. It is designed to reflect the knowledge and skills needed for *minimum competence by a newly licensed nurse to be a safe and effective practitioner in entry-level nursing,* as determined by studies of nursing practice (performed every 3 years to reflect current nursing practice).
2. State boards take turns nominating item writers (faculty, clinical nurse specialists, or beginning practitioners); the Board of Directors of the National Council then selects from this group those who meet the criteria for item writing based on expertise in a particular area of nursing, type of nursing program, credentials, regional balance, etc. The item writers write questions based on common clinical situations and according to the test plan. Then the questions are researched and reviewed by a panel of experts (nominated by the state boards), by those state boards that choose to review, and by the National Council's Examination Committee.
3. Finally, the questions are field tested to eliminate questions that may be ambiguous, irrelevant, or not equally applicable to all regions of the United States. (Each candidate taking the NCLEX® will take 15 of these "tryout" questions, mixed in with the regular questions; they will *not* count toward that candidate's performance.) The data gained through field testing are also used to analyze and determine the difficulty level of a question.

C. Passing standard: The passing standard is *criterion referenced;* this means that there is no fixed percentage of candidates who pass or fail. Passing depends solely on performance in relation to the level of minimum competence. The passing standard is reviewed every 3 years.

VI. FREQUENTLY ASKED QUESTIONS AND ANSWERS ABOUT NCLEX-RN®

A. Test questions, test plan

1. *How many questions will there be?* You will take anywhere from 75 to 265 questions.
2. *Where do the questions come from?* The state boards of nursing nominate item writers, who must meet various criteria (see **V. B. Development, p. 9**).
3. *Will there be questions involving conditions with which I may not have had experience in my nursing program?* Most of the questions are about clients with conditions familiar to you and are representative of common health problems on a national basis. Some questions may relate to nursing problems with which you may not have had prior experience; their purpose is to test your ability to *apply* knowledge of specific principles from the physical, biological, and social sciences to *new* situations.
4. *Can some questions have more than one answer?* Yes. In some questions, only *one* of the four options is the *best* answer. In alternate items, you may be asked to choose more than one option as your answer.
5. *Will I get partial credit for selecting the next-to-the-best answer?* No. Your answer will be treated only as correct or incorrect.
6. *If everyone takes a different test, how can it be fair?* Each candidate is tested according to the *same test plan,* and the *same passing standard.* It may simply require more items to reach a stable pass/fail determination for one candidate, while another may require fewer questions to demonstrate competence level.
7. *Do diploma, associate, and baccalaureate graduates all take the same test? What about graduates from schools outside the United States?* All candidates are held to the *same test plan and passing standard,* and take the "same test." (Of course, due to the nature of CAT, each will receive an "individualized" test, without regard to degree, or to state or country of education.)
8. *Does the examination differ by state?* The examination is a national examination; all candidates are held to the *same test plan and passing standard,* and take questions from the same pool. (Again, through CAT, each candidate receives an "individualized" test, but without regard to state.)

B. Taking the test/after the test

1. *Can I skip questions?* No. You must answer each question in order to move on to the next. You also will not be able to return to previous questions to try them again or change the answer (because the level of *subsequent* questions administered is based on *previous* answers).
2. *What if I just don't know the answer?* Use the tips in **Test-Taking Tips and Guidelines: Sixty Strategies to Use in Answering Questions, Chapter 2, pp. 62-67,** to make your best guess. You will need to answer the question in order to move on to the next question.
3. *When will I know my results? Will the computer tell me?* You will not learn your pass/fail status at the testing center; the results will be communicated directly to your state board of nursing, who will mail the results to you. The time frame may differ from state to state, but most candidates should receive their results within 10 days to 2 weeks after taking the examination. Some states provide a Results-by-Phone Service, where unofficial results are available 3 business days after taking the examination. There is a flat fee for this service. **Note:** Taking only the minimum number of questions, or taking the maximum, is not an indication of whether you have passed or failed. It merely indicates that a lesser, or greater, number of items was required to reach a determination.
4. *What percentage must I answer correctly to pass?* Because of the nature of CAT, a percentage rate is *not* used to determine passing or failure. The test determines whether you are above or below standard competence by determining not the *number* of questions you answer correctly, but rather the *difficulty level* you can *consistently* answer correctly. The process of administering harder or easier questions, as described in **II. CAT: HOW IT WORKS, p. 5,** continues until you reach the level where you answer approximately 50% of the complex questions correctly. **Note:** When practicing with questions of mixed difficulty, such as those in this book, you may wish to use 80% correct as a "benchmark" goal for yourself.
5. *If I do not pass, can I retest only those areas of the test plan in which I tested poorly?* No. The whole examination is on a pass/fail basis.
6. *Can I repeat the examination before I get my results?* No.
7. *How many times can the examination be repeated, and when?* The National Council allows you to repeat the examination not more than once in any 45-day period; however, each state board may set its own, more restrictive time limits and

retake requirements. At present, most states allow the examination to be repeated after 45 days; other states still require a 91-day waiting period before repeating the examination.

8. *Who grants the nursing license?* The license is granted by the state board of nursing to which you applied and for which you took the examination.

C. Testing facilities

1. *Can I bring any materials into the examination room?* There are severe restrictions on personal items allowed in the examination room; you will be provided with a locker or other secure place for your belongings. Do *not* take any study materials (books, notes, calculators, etc.), pens, pencils, candy, chewing gum, drinks, food, watches, pagers, cell phones, note pads or Post-it notes, purses, wallets, or cameras into the examination building.
2. *How many people will take the test at the same time?* Up to 30 people may be at computer workstations in your testing room; however, they may not all be taking the NCLEX®, because Pearson Professional Test Centers also offer other services.
3. *When and where will I take the test?* As soon as you receive your authorization (ATT), you must contact a Pearson Professional Test Center facility to set up your own testing appointment (5 days/wk, 15 hr/day, in 6-hr time slots). There is at least one facility per state, although most states have many more. A candidate must test within the validity dates of the ATT. These dates cannot be extended. If the ATT expires, you may be required to re-register and repay to test.
4. *What accommodations are available for candidates with disabilities?* All test centers are accessible to candidates with disabilities. Other accommodations will be made only with the prior authorization of the board of nursing; contact your state board *before* submitting your application.

How to Prepare for and Score Higher on Examinations

The Psychology of Test-Taking

Many nursing students know the nursing material on which they are being tested, and can demonstrate their nursing skills in practice, but do not know how to prepare themselves for taking and passing examinations.

It is not just a matter of taking examinations but of *knowing how* to take them, taking steps to ensure you can function at full capacity, and using the allotted time in the most productive way. You must learn to use strategy and judgment in answering questions, and to make educated guesses when you are not sure of the right answer.

This section offers practical suggestions to help ensure that you are "at your best" on examination day, and discusses practical strategies for eliminating wrong answers and for increasing your chances of selecting the best ones.

Prepare Physically and Mentally

1. *On the morning of an examination, avoid excessive oral intake of products that act as diuretics for you.* If you know that coffee or cigarettes, for example, increase urgency and frequency, it is best to limit their intake. Undue physiological discomforts can distract your focus from the examination at hand.
2. *Increase your oral intake of foods high in glucose and protein.* These foods reportedly have been helpful to some examinees for keeping up their blood-sugar level. This may enhance your concentration and problem-solving ability at the times when you most need to function at a high level. On the other hand, avoid carbohydrates such as doughnuts, which slow down thinking.
3. *Before examination days, avoid eating exotic or highly seasoned foods to which your system may not be accustomed.* Avoid possible gastrointestinal distress when you least need it!
4. *Use hard candy or something similar* prior to entering the examination room, to help relieve the discomfort of a dry mouth related to a state of anxiety.
5. *Wear comfortable clothes that you have worn before.* The day of an examination is not a good time to wear new footwear or clothes that may prove to be constricting, binding, or uncomfortable, especially at the waistline and shoulder seams.
6. Anxiety states can bring about rapid increases and decreases in body temperature. *Wear clothing that can be shed or added on.* For example, you might bring a sweater that can be put on when you feel chilled or removed when your body temperature fluctuates again.
7. *Women need to be prepared for late, irregular, or unanticipated early onset of menses* on examination day, a time of stress.
8. Examination jitters can elicit anxiety-like reactions, both physiological and emotional. Because anxiety tends to be contagious, *try to limit your contacts with those who are also experiencing examination-related anxiety or who elicit those feelings in you.*
9. *The night before an examination is a good time to engage in a pleasurable activity* as a means of anxiety reduction. You need stamina and endurance for sitting, thinking, and reacting. Give yourself a chance for restful, not energy- or emotion-draining, activities in the days before an examination.

10. *Try a relaxation process* if anxiety reaches an uncomfortable level that cannot be channeled into the service of learning (see **How To Reduce Anxiety, p. 13**).
11. When you arrive home after an examination, *jot down content areas that were unfamiliar to you.* This may serve as a key focus for review.

Tips for NCLEX-RN®

1. Get an early start on the day you take the examination, to avoid raising your anxiety level before the actual examination starts. Allow yourself time for delays in traffic and in public transportation or for finding a parking place. Even allow for a dead battery, flooded engine, flat tire, or bus breakdown. If you are unfamiliar with the area in which the test center is located, find it the day before.
2. Remember that *you do not need to get all the answers right to pass.* The examination is designed to test for *minimum* competence; demonstrating a higher level will not earn a special designation on your license, or any other bonus. Moreover, due to the adaptive nature of the test, you will probably reach a level where you are answering only 50% of the questions correctly; this is *normal* for this test and *should not* in itself be taken as an indication of poor performance (you may be answering 50% of the *very difficult* questions correctly)!
3. Because you cannot skip questions and go back to them, or go back to change answers, it is important that you simply *do the best you can* on a particular question, using the **Test-Taking Tips and Guidelines: Sixty Strategies to Use in Answering Questions, Chapter 2, pp. 62-67,** and *move on.* The adaptive test will give you another chance to show your competence, should you get that question wrong.
4. Remember that, although you cannot change answers you have already "confirmed," you *may change your answer during the selection process.* As you make your answer selection, you will *choose* an answer (by pressing the enter key once) and then *confirm* it (by pressing the <NEXT> key); you will be able to change your mind *before confirming* your answer choice.
5. Although the examination uses different levels of difficulty to estimate your competence level, *do not try to figure out the difficulty level* of each question; likewise, do not try to keep track of the number of questions you are answering. You will only distract yourself and raise your anxiety. Again, simply answer each question to the best of your ability and move on.
6. When taking practice questions, it is a good idea to *aim for an average of 1 minute per question,* so that you will be at a speed to finish the examination even if you *do* need to take the maximum number of questions. For the actual examination, however, the 6-hour time limit is not a problem for most candidates, so go ahead and *take the time to work through a difficult problem,* and make use of the scratch paper provided (but *don't* dwell on a question you "just can't get!").

Tips for Other (Pencil-and-Paper) Tests and Examinations

1. *Answer the easy questions first.* Too often students focus on 1 question for 10 minutes; for example, instead of going on to answer 20 additional questions during this time. The main goal in this type of examination is to answer correctly as many questions as possible.
2. *Your first hunch is usually a good one.* Pay attention to your intuition, which may indicate which answer "feels" best.
3. *Be wise about the timing.* Divide your time. For example, if you have 90 questions and 1½ hours for the test, aim for an average of 1 question per minute. Keep working! Do not lose time looking back at your answers.
4. *If you cannot decide between two multiple-choice answers, make a note of the numbers of the two choices.* This will narrow down your focus when you come back to this question. Leave the question; do not spend much time on those in doubt. When you have completed the test, go back and spend more time on those with which you had trouble.
5. *Exercise care and caution when using electronically scored answer sheets or booklets.* It is essential that you use only the type of pencil or ink specified in the instructions. If erasing is possible, be sure to erase completely; a mere trace might throw out the answer.
6. When using a separate answer sheet or booklet, be especially careful to *mark your answer in the space for the correct question number.* It might be helpful to say to yourself as you answer each question, "Choice No. 4 to question No. 3," to make sure that the right answer goes with each question number.
7. *Stay the entire time allotted.* If you complete the test early, check your answers. On a second look, after you have completed the test, you may find something that you are *now sure* you marked in error the first time. If you were undecided between two possible answers on any questions, use leftover time to reconsider those answers. (Also, look for and erase stray marks, if using electronically scored answer sheets.)

How to Reduce Anxiety

Most people have untapped inner resources for achieving relaxation and tension release in stressful situations (such as during an examination) when they need to function at their highest potential. The goal of this discussion is to help you experience a self-guided approach to reducing your anxiety level to one that is compatible with learning and high performance.

In anxiety-producing settings whenever you feel overwhelmed or blocked, a fantasy experience can be of help in mastering the rising anxiety by promoting a feeling of calm, detached awareness, and a sense of deeper personal coping resources. Through the fantasy you can gain access to a zone of *tranquility* in the center of your being. Guided imagery often carries with it feelings of serenity, warmth, and comfort.

Fantasy experiences are, of course, highly individual. Techniques that help one person experience serenity may frustrate another. Try out the self-guided experiences suggested here, make up your own, and select ones that are best for you. There are endless possibilities for fantasy journeys. The best approach is to work with whatever fantasy occurs to you at the moment. The ideas for a journey presented here are meant to be a springboard for variations of your own.

A fantasy will be more effective if you take as comfortable a physical position as possible, with eyes closed and attention focused on the inner experience. Get in touch with physical sensations, your pattern and rate of breathing, your heartbeat, and pressure points of your body as it comes in contact with the chair and floor.

When you take a fantasy journey by yourself, it is important for you to read over the instructions several times so that you will be able to recall the overall structure of the fantasy. *Then,* close your eyes and take your trip without concern for following the instructions in detail.

Progressive Relaxation

Relaxation approaches are used in a variety of anxiety states whenever stress interferes with the ability to function.

Progressive relaxation training was originated in 1929 by Dr. Edmund Jacobson. It is a technique for attaining self-control over skeletal muscles in order to induce low-level tonus in the major muscle groups. The approach involves learning systematically and sequentially to tense and relax various muscle groups throughout the body.

The *objectives* of this approach are to soothe nerves, combat hypertonus in muscles, and substitute relaxing activities for stressful ones in order to feel comfortable in and more alert to the internal and external environments.

The *theory* behind this method takes as its basis the idea that muscular relaxation and anxiety states produce directly opposite physiological effects and thus cannot coexist. In other words, it is not possible to be tense in any body part that is completely relaxed.

The *physiological changes* during relaxation include decreased oxygen consumption, decreased carbon dioxide elimination, and decreased respiratory rate.

The basic factors vital to eliciting a relaxation response include the following:

1. *Quiet setting*—eliminate unnecessary internal and external stimuli.
2. *Passive, "let-it-happen" attitude*—empty your mind of thoughts and distractions.
3. *Comfortable position*—sit or recline in one position for 20 minutes or so.
4. *Constant stimulus on which to focus*—a repetitive sound, constant gaze on an object or image, or attention to one's own breathing pattern.

Relaxation training is a procedure that can be defined, specified, and memorized until you can go through the exercises mechanically. If you regularly practice relaxation, you will be able to cope more effectively with difficult situations by reaping the physiological and psychological benefits of a balanced and relaxed state.

Instructions

- Sit comfortably in a chair. Shut your eyes and chase your thoughts for a minute; go where your thoughts go.
- Then, let the words go. Become aware of how you *feel,* here and now, not how you would like to feel.
- Shift your awareness to your feet. Do not move them. Become aware of what they are doing.
- Spend 20 to 30 seconds focusing progressively on different parts of your body. Relax each part in turn:

Relax each of your toes; the tops of your feet; the arch of each foot; the insteps, balls, and heels; and your ankles, calves, knees, thighs, and buttocks. Become aware of how your body is contacting the chair in which you are sitting. Let go of your abdominal and chest muscles; relax your back. Release the tension in your shoulders, arms, elbows, forearms, wrists, hands, and each finger in turn; relax the muscles in your throat, lips, and cheeks. Wrinkle your nose; relax your eyelids and eyebrows (first one and then the other); relax the muscles in your forehead and top and back of your head. Relax your whole body.

Concentrate on your breathing; become aware of how you breathe. Allow yourself to inhale and exhale in your usual way. Become aware of the depth of your breathing. Are you expanding the lungs all the way? Or is your breathing shallow? Increase your depth of breathing. Now focus on the rate at which you are breathing. See if you can slow the rate down. When you breathe in, can you feel an inflow of energy that fills your entire body?

- Now concentrate on the sounds in the room.
- Focus on how you feel right now.
- Slowly open your eyes.

Suggestions for Additional Experiential Vignettes

- Imagine yourself leaving the room. In your mind's eye, go through the city and over the fields. Come to a meadow covered with fresh, new grass and flowers. Look out on the meadow and focus on what you see, hear, smell, and feel. Walk through the meadow. See the length and greenness of the grass; see the brilliance and feel the warmth of the sunlight.
- For a more expansive feeling, visualize a mountain in the distance. Fantasize going to the country and slowly ascending a mountain. Walk through a forest. Climb to the top until at last you reach a height where you can see forever. Experience your awareness.
- Focus on a memory of a beautiful place you have been to, enjoyed, and would like to enjoy again. Be there; experience it.
- Imagine that you are floating on your back down a river. It may help at first to breathe deeply and feel yourself sinking. Visualize that you are coming out on a gentle river that is slowly winding its way through a beautiful forest. The sun is out and the rays feel warm on your skin. You pass trees and meadows of beautiful flowers. Smell the grass and flowers. Hear the birds. Look up in the blue sky; see the lazy tufts of clouds floating by. Leave the river and walk across the meadow. Enjoy the grass around your ankles. Come to a large tree . . .

Fill in the rest of the trip—what do you see now? Where do you want to go from here?

Sally L. Lagerquist

PRE-TEST 1 AND 2

Introduction

This **Pre-test** section is unique—it provides you with a special roadmap to your examination success with 150 challenging assessment questions divided into two 75-item examinations.

The **Pre-test 1** is an *initial assessment* tool intended to help you to assess your strengths and weaknesses in your ability to apply the material you have learned in specific clinical areas to any nursing situation. By taking the **Pre-test,** you can focus your subsequent review of content, based on your own analysis of your results.

We suggest that you take the **Pre-test 1** before you read any of the content units in this book. After taking the **Pre-test 1,** you should:

1. Score your answers.
2. Take another look at the questions where your answer was wrong.
3. Identify the **clinical** areas where you need further review (e.g., Child Health, Behavioral and Emotional, Adult Health, Geriatrics, Maternity/Newborn).
4. Read specific *content* chapters **(Chapters 4, 5, 6, 7, and 10)**.
5. Then test yourself again on the **Pre-test 2.**

This time, take all the questions by one **clinical** area at a time (starting with the one you missed the most).

If you are repeating the NCLEX-RN®, also use the **Pre-test 1** and **2** a second time but take questions by client needs/subneeds where you scored **below the passing standard** and/or **near the passing standard.**

Pre-Test 1

Questions

Select the one answer that is best for each question, unless otherwise directed.

1. A 38-year-old client, who is gravida 4, para 2 with gestational diabetes, is scheduled for an amniocentesis at 33 weeks' gestation because of unstable blood sugar. The results of the amniocentesis reveal the lecithin/sphingomyelin ratio (L/S) is 1:1, and the phosphatidylglycerol (PG) is negative. How should a nurse best interpret this data?
   1. The infant is at low risk for congenital anomalies.
   2. The infant is at high risk for intrauterine growth retardation.
   3. The infant is at high risk for respiratory distress syndrome.
   4. The infant is at high risk for birth trauma.

2. A client, who is overweight and has diabetes, has a blood pressure of 148/92 mm Hg. The client's urinalysis reveals microalbuminuria. The client does not want to take drugs despite a family history of brain attack (cerebrovascular accident [CVA]). The correct response by a nurse is:
   1. "Find herbal products to reduce blood pressure and weight."
   2. "Use a drug while lifestyle changes are instituted."
   3. "Evaluate barriers to weight loss and make a plan for exercising and dieting."
   4. "Recheck blood pressure weekly."

3. A school nurse is called to the playground during recess to see a child with hemophilia who has collided with a friend. The child's knee is bruised and swollen and the child reports significant pain. Which actions should the nurse take? *Select all that apply.*
   1. Call emergency medical services (EMS).
   2. Wrap the knee in a compression bandage.
   3. Provide crutches for mobility.
   4. Apply ice packs.
   5. Elevate the injured extremity.
   6. Suggest that the child stay indoors during recess.

4. Which clinical feature found on assessment should indicate to a nurse that a client has congestive heart failure?
   1. Fatigue and dyspnea.
   2. Cheyne-Stokes breathing and orthostatic hypotension.
   3. Liver tenderness and peripheral edema.
   4. Pulmonary crackles and weak pulses.

5. A nurse is caring for a client at 32 weeks' gestation who has been admitted to an obstetrical unit with complete placenta previa. Which symptoms should the nurse identify as being a result of this client's condition? *Select all that apply.*
   1. Painless vaginal bleeding.
   2. Tetanic uterine contractions.
   3. Premature rupture of membranes.
   4. Decreased hemoglobin.
   5. Rigid, boardlike abdomen.

6. A 4-year-old is hospitalized with acute glomerulonephritis. A nurse should feel most confident that the client teaching has been effective and the child has a basic understanding of this condition if the child states:
   1. "I was mean to my sister and now I am sick."
   2. "I have a stomachache but it will get better."
   3. "I don't have much pee pee come out when I use the toilet."
   4. "I have an infection in my stomach."

7. A 34-year-old client, who is gravida 6, para 4, delivered a healthy infant at full term about 18 hours ago. She reports a sharp pain in her left calf while walking to the bathroom. A nurse assesses the client's left calf, which has a confined area of redness, warmth, and tenderness. Which nursing actions are appropriate for this client's nursing care? *Select all that apply.*
   1. Instruct the client to massage the calf to relieve the pain and tenderness.
   2. Encourage the client to ambulate to increase circulation.
   3. Administer anticoagulation therapy as ordered.
   4. Elevate the affected extremity to promote venous blood flow.
   5. Have the client sit up at the side of the bed with affected leg dangling.

8. The nurse is conducting a seminar on sudden infant death syndrome (SIDS) with a group of first-time parents of newborns. The nurse's teaching should emphasize:
   1. Avoiding soft bedding.
   2. Using a pillow.
   3. Using a soft sleep surface.
   4. Promoting co-sleeping with the parents.

9. The laboratory values for an adult client who is NPO are: Na^+ 128, K^+ 3.5, and glucose 130. Which IV solution should a nurse expect will be ordered?
   1. $D_{10}W$ with 40 mEq KCl/L at 150 mL/hr.
   2. ¼NS with 20 mEq KCl/L at 100 mL/hr.
   3. D_5 ¼NS at 50 mL/hr.
   4. D_5NS with 20 mEq KCl/L at 75 mL/hr.

10. A nurse is caring for a teenager immediately following surgical correction of severe scoliosis. Which interventions should the nurse expect to be part of the care plan? *Select all that apply.*
    1. Administer pain medication around the clock.
    2. Check circulation, sensation, and movement (CSM) frequently in extremities.
    3. Monitor urinary catheter output.
    4. Assist child to the chair once per shift.
    5. Assess bowel sounds daily.

11. A client with syndrome of inappropriate antidiuretic hormone (SIADH) secretion has a Na^+ of 128 mEq/L and is confused. A nurse's *primary* goal should be to:
    1. Decrease edema by restricting fluid intake.
    2. Prevent complications of hyponatremia.
    3. Reorient the client to surroundings.
    4. Restore fluid and electrolyte balance.

12. A group of clients who are pregnant are attending a childbirth preparation class. A nurse is discussing the effects of cigarette smoke on fetal development. Which characteristic should the nurse describe as being associated with babies born to mothers who smoked during pregnancy?
    1. Low birth weight.
    2. Large for gestational age.
    3. Preterm birth, but appropriate size for gestation.
    4. Macrosomia.

13. The school nurse inspects the toddlers attending the school's day-care center. Which observation by the nurse is cause for follow-up for pinworms?
    1. All of the toddlers are wearing shoes and socks.
    2. Some of the toddlers are wearing one-piece outfits.
    3. Most of the toddlers have short fingernails.
    4. Most of the toddlers are wearing cloth diapers.

14. A client, who is gravida 4, para 2, is admitted to a labor and delivery unit. A nurse performs a vaginal examination and determines that the client's cervix is 6 cm dilated, 75% effaced, and a +1 station. Based on the nurse's assessment, in which stage of labor is this client?
    1. First phase, latent stage.
    2. First stage, active phase.
    3. First stage, transition phase.
    4. First phase, active stage.

15. A client is admitted with a history of an abdominal aortic aneurysm. A nurse should know that the client has an impending rupture of the aneurysm if the client reports:
    1. Severe right upper quadrant abdominal pain.
    2. Persistent or intermittent lower back pain.
    3. Absent pedal pulses in both extremities.
    4. Chest pain in the epigastric region.

16. A clinic nurse is preparing to administer several scheduled immunizations to a 6-month-old infant. What are the appropriate actions for the nurse to take when preparing and administering immunizations? *Select all that apply.*
1. Draw vaccines into one syringe for injection.
2. Administer injections in either vastus lateralis muscle.
3. Administer injections in either dorsogluteal muscle.
4. Ask the parent to wait outside the exam room.
5. Select a 1-inch needle.
6. Wash hands.

17. A nursing student is assigned to care for a client who is 2 days post–total left hip replacement. Which observation should be reported *immediately* to a staff nurse?
1. Pain rated as 5 on a scale of 0–10.
2. Temperature, 99.6°F; reddened incision.
3. Pain and cramping in the right lower leg.
4. Difficulty tolerating weight-bearing on the left leg.

18. A client, who is gravida 2, para 1, ruptures her membranes spontaneously with a large amount of clear fluid. A nurse performs a vaginal examination and discovers a loop of umbilical cord in the vagina. Which *immediate* action should be taken by the nurse?
1. Place the client on her left side.
2. Attempt to replace the cord.
3. Elevate the client's hips.
4. Cover the cord with a dry, sterile gauze.

19. When assessing a child for symptoms of neurogenic diabetes insipidus, what should a nurse anticipate?
1. Elevated blood glucose.
2. Increased levels of ADH.
3. Increased urine output.
4. Decreased serum sodium.

20. A client, who is gravida 1, para 0, delivered an infant at 39 weeks' gestation this morning. The client tells a nurse that she plans to breastfeed her baby and has taken a class about breastfeeding. The nurse is aware that successful breastfeeding is most dependent on:
1. Mother's educational level.
2. Size of the mother's breast.
3. Mother's desire to breastfeed.
4. Infant's birth weight.

21. Which observation in the newborn of a mother with diabetes would require an *immediate* nursing intervention?
1. Crying.
2. Wakefulness.
3. Jitteriness.
4. Yawning.

22. In teaching a client with vision loss from glaucoma about proper lighting, a nurse knows that:
1. Overhead or ceiling lights are best.
2. Using fluorescent lighting avoids shadows.
3. Brighter lights are needed.
4. Dim lighting is needed.

23. A nursing student is performing an initial newborn assessment. The newborn is observed to have a caput succedaneum. What are likely causes of this condition? *Select all that apply.*
1. Scheduled cesarean delivery.
2. Prolonged active phase of labor.
3. Breech presentation.
4. Vacuum-assisted vaginal delivery.
5. Prolonged second stage of labor.

24. A 65-year-old man with a 45-year history of smoking reports a change in his cough pattern, a nonproductive cough, and generally not feeling well. The chest x-ray reveals an infiltrate. A nurse should suspect:
1. Pneumonia.
2. Chronic obstructive pulmonary disease (COPD).
3. Pulmonary edema.
4. Tuberculosis.

25. A nurse is monitoring the progress of a gravida 3, para 1 client in active labor. Which finding should be reported to a physician *immediately?*
1. Moderate uterine contractions.
2. Frequent urination.
3. The presence of green-tinged amniotic fluid.
4. The presence of scant bloody discharge.

26. The blood pressure of a 28-year-old client who is overweight and does not have diabetes is 136/78 mm Hg. Client education should include:
1. Losing 20 pounds would bring the blood pressure down by as much as 20 points and reduce the risk of stroke.
2. The need to recheck blood pressure weekly so medications can be started as soon as it goes over 140/90 mm Hg.
3. The need for medications in clients who are overweight with a systolic blood pressure over 130/80 mm Hg.
4. Acknowledging that the client has maintained a blood pressure within normal limits.

27. A group of clients is attending a childbirth preparation class. A client asks a nurse how to measure the duration of the uterine contractions. Which is the best description by the nurse about the measurement of the duration of contractions?
1. Duration is measured by timing from the beginning of one contraction to the beginning of the next contraction.
2. Duration is measured by timing from the end of one contraction to the beginning of the next contraction.
3. Duration is measured by timing from the beginning of one contraction to the end of the same contraction.
4. Duration is measured by timing from the peak of one contraction to the end of the same contraction.

28. A client with a history of Graves' disease is admitted for uncontrolled hyperglycemia and a foot ulcer. This client requires close monitoring because of the increased risk of: *Select all that apply.*
   1. Hypotension.
   2. Elevated temperature.
   3. Hypothyroidism.
   4. Hypoglycemia.
   5. Extreme tachycardia.

29. Which order written by a pediatrician for a 2-month-old infant during a well-infant visit should a nurse question?
   1. Administer DTaP (diphtheria, tetanus, and acellular pertussis) vaccine.
   2. Administer Hib (*Haemophilus influenzae* type b) vaccine.
   3. Administer IVP (inactivated poliovirus) vaccine.
   4. Administer MMR (measles, mumps, and rubella) vaccine.

30. Treatment for hypertension is important in the prevention of heart failure. A nurse tells a client that the greatest decrease in blood pressure is most likely to occur with:
   1. Increasing physical activity.
   2. Reducing sodium intake.
   3. Limiting alcohol intake.
   4. Weight loss.

31. A client, who is gravida 3, para 1, is diagnosed with diabetes at 28 weeks' gestation. A nurse is providing instruction about the role of insulin in managing the client's diabetes. Which statement by the nurse is true regarding insulin needs during pregnancy?
   1. Insulin requirements are moderate as the pregnancy progresses.
   2. A decreased need for insulin occurs during the second trimester.
   3. Insulin requirements will increase as the pregnancy progresses.
   4. Elevations in human placental lactogen decrease the need for insulin.

32. A nursing student selects a ½-inch needle with which to administer a DTaP (diphtheria, tetanus, and acellular pertussis) vaccine to a 4-month-old infant. A nursing instructor's best action would be to:
   1. Allow the nursing student to continue preparing the vaccine.
   2. Stop the nursing student from preparing the vaccine.
   3. Question the nursing student regarding the injection route used to administer the vaccine.
   4. Instruct the nursing student to select a shorter needle.

33. A client, who is gravida 1, para 0 at 38 weeks' gestation, is found to have a blood pressure of 170/90 mm Hg. Which action should a nurse take *first?*
   1. Evaluate the urine protein.
   2. Administer an analgesic.
   3. Assess fetal heart tones.
   4. Obtain a diet history.

34. A 12-year-old child is seen in a pediatrician's office for a well-adolescent checkup. The adolescent's *most* important vaccine status for a nurse to assess would be:
   1. Hepatitis B.
   2. Hepatitis A.
   3. MMR (measles, mumps, and rubella).
   4. HPV (human papillomavirus).

35. A client, who fell 10 feet onto a concrete floor, presents to an emergency department. The client does not speak English. The correct action by a nurse to determine the severity of the client's pain would be to:
   1. Call for an interpreter.
   2. Note the client's facial expression.
   3. Observe the client's response to palpation.
   4. Use an illustrative pain scale.

36. The parents of a 6-month-old infant express their concerns regarding the number of vaccines their infant has already received. A nurse's *best* action would be to:
   1. Provide the parents with accurate, user-friendly information regarding vaccines.
   2. Reassure the parents that their concern for their infant's health is appreciated.
   3. Respect the parents' ultimate decision regarding vaccines.
   4. Involve the parents in minimizing potential adverse effects of the vaccines.

37. An undesired consequence of acute pain is the progression to a chronic pain syndrome. The correct approach by a nurse to prevent chronic pain syndrome would be to:
   1. Adequately control acute pain.
   2. Give ordered opiates infrequently.
   3. Give pain medication only when requested by client.
   4. Prevent physical dependence on the prescribed drug.

38. A 42-year-old, who is gravida 1, para 0, has a successful in-vitro fertilization and is 7 weeks pregnant. Based on the client's history, a nurse knows the infant is at risk for:
   1. Respiratory distress syndrome.
   2. Pathological jaundice.
   3. Turner's syndrome.
   4. Down syndrome.

39. A client delivers a 4-pound, 8-ounce neonate at 35 weeks' gestation. A meconium drug screen shows the presence of heroin. The neonate is admitted to the nursery with narcotic abstinence syndrome. Nursing care of the neonate should include:
   1. Teaching the mother to provide tactile stimulation.
   2. Wrapping the neonate snugly in a blanket.
   3. Placing the neonate in the infant car seat.
   4. Initiating an early infant-stimulation program.

40. A client, who is 32 years old, gravida 4, para 1 at 31 weeks' gestation, has been recently diagnosed with gestational diabetes. She has attended a class about managing diabetes during pregnancy. Which statements should indicate to a nurse that the client understands what was taught about gestational diabetes? *Select all that apply.*
   1. "I can't eat any carbohydrates for the rest of my pregnancy."
   2. "I need to keep my blood sugar well controlled so the baby won't grow too large."
   3. "I will have to take insulin for the rest of my life."
   4. "I need to count the grams of carbohydrate for each meal and my snacks."
   5. "I will have to check my blood sugar before I eat in the morning and after each meal."

41. A client with a known history of IV drug use is found to have acute appendicitis with perforation. Following surgery, the client reports severe pain at the surgical incision. There are no signs of abscess formation or other postoperative complications. The correct approach to manage the client's pain would be to:
   1. Give the ordered opioid.
   2. Expect a placebo to be ordered.
   3. Give an NSAID or acetaminophen.
   4. Use nondrug therapies such as visualization.

42. The mother of a school-age child who is isolated at home with chickenpox (varicella) informs a school nurse that, "My child is miserable from the itching. What can I do?" The school nurse's *best* response would be to suggest:
   1. Giving diphenhydramine hydrochloride.
   2. Keeping the child cool.
   3. Changing the linens daily.
   4. Keeping the child's fingernails short and clean.

43. An 84-year-old with diabetes and left leg cellulitis is brought to an emergency department. Vital signs are: BP 132/90 mm Hg, T 99.4°F, P 95, and R 20. Blood glucose is 98. Left leg is red and swollen. The client is admitted to a nursing unit. Which order should be a *priority* for the nurse?
   1. Start ampicillin of 1 gm every 8 hours.
   2. Obtain an ECG.
   3. Administer insulin for elevated blood sugar.
   4. Draw blood cultures.

44. A client, who is gravida 4, para 0 at 39 weeks' gestation, states, "I would like to breastfeed, but my mother-in-law told me my breasts are too small and I won't have enough milk for my baby." Which would be the *best* response by the nurse?
   1. "Your breasts might be small, but if you don't produce enough milk, you can always give the baby some formula."
   2. "You will produce more milk if you use a breast pump and then give it to your baby in a bottle."
   3. "Milk production is increased by the hormone estrogen. You can ask your doctor for a prescription to take."
   4. "The size of the breasts doesn't matter. All women have about the same amount of milk-producing tissue."

45. An African American infant with an umbilical hernia is brought to a well-infant clinic for routine immunizations. During the visit, a nurse notes that the parent has taped the umbilical hernia down on the abdomen to flatten the protrusion. The nurse would be correct in telling the parent that:
   1. Taping is an appropriate practice to follow.
   2. Taping will eliminate the need for a surgical repair because the umbilical hernia will resolve spontaneously with this treatment.
   3. Taping the umbilical hernia down to the abdomen does not help.
   4. Manually reducing the umbilical hernia on a daily basis by the parent will result in resolution of the hernia.

46. A client, who is gravida 3, para 2, is asking a nurse for advice concerning her nightly leg cramps. Which response by the nurse is correct?
   1. "Increase your fluid intake."
   2. "Increase your protein intake."
   3. "Increase your calcium intake."
   4. "Increase your fiber intake."

47. A child hospitalized with measles (rubeola) cries every time a nurse enters the room and turns on the overhead light. The nurse should investigate if the child has:
   1. A fear of bright lights.
   2. An intolerance of light.
   3. Irritated eyes from rubbing.
   4. An enhanced reaction to unanticipated events.

48. A nurse knows that a client with hypercalcemia may experience:
   Select all that apply.
   1. Thirst.
   2. Constipation.
   3. Diarrhea.
   4. Loss of appetite.
   5. Feeling sleepy.
   6. Hyperactivity.

49. A child is hospitalized with scarlet fever. Which food item should the nurse remove from the child's breakfast tray?
   1. Chocolate milk.
   2. Orange juice.
   3. Apple juice.
   4. 2% milk.

50. Positioning to prevent skin breakdown is a nursing concern. Which site is at *greatest risk* for breakdown in this position?

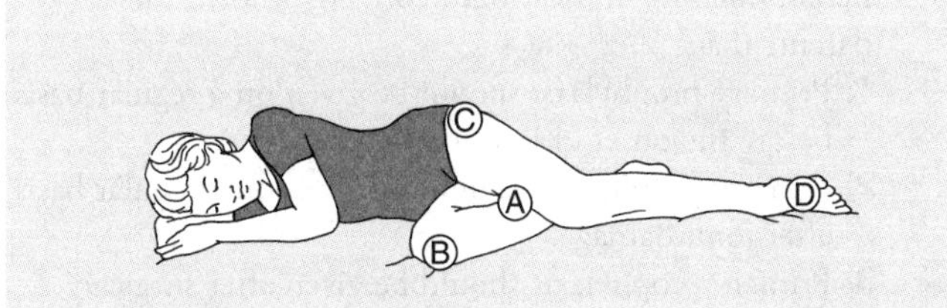

1. A.
2. B.
3. C.
4. D.

51. A client comes to the prenatal clinic to begin care. The nurse would advise her that the routine test(s) during the initial examination is/are:
Select all that apply.
1. Rubella titer.
2. Complete blood count (CBC).
3. Glucose tolerance test.
4. Ultrasound.
5. Blood type and antibody screen.

52. The most appropriate nursing intervention to encourage a child to eat who had a tonsillectomy 24 hours ago is to:
1. Promise the child all the ice cream that the child can eat.
2. Apply an ice collar to the throat 30 minutes prior to the meal.
3. Have the child gargle with mouthwash to relieve any unpleasant taste in the mouth.
4. Tell the child that there will be no television that night if some food is not eaten.

53. With which conditions is a risk of postpartum hemorrhage associated?
Select all that apply.
1. Pregnancy-induced hypertension.
2. The birth of a macrosomatic neonate.
3. Retained placental fragments.
4. Full urinary bladder.
5. Advanced maternal age.

54. A client with Sjögren's syndrome, an autoimmune disorder in women, is scheduled for surgery. The correct nursing action would be:
1. Have a humidifier at the bedside when the client returns from surgery.
2. Lubricate the client's eyes with ointment before surgery.
3. Tell the client that nothing can be taken by mouth for 12 hours.
4. Withhold antidepressant therapy for 6 hours after surgery.

55. A school-age child is hospitalized with mumps (parotitis). Which food item should the nurse remove from the child's lunch tray?
1. Gelatin.
2. Applesauce.
3. An apple.
4. A banana.

56. A client with a history of GI bleeding is admitted with complaints of fatigue, weakness, and shortness of breath. Hgb is 7.4 mg/dL, T 97.8°F, BP 86/45 mm Hg, P 118, and R 22. Two units of packed RBCs are ordered. As a nurse begins the blood transfusion, the client suddenly complains of chills and chest pain. Which actions should be taken by the nurse? *Select all that apply.*
1. Taking the client's vital signs.
2. Giving acetaminophen as ordered.
3. Stopping the blood transfusion.
4. Infusing normal saline to keep vein open.
5. Disposing of blood product in biohazard container.
6. Sending blood product to lab for analysis.

57. A client, who is gravida 5, para 4, delivered a 6-pound, 5-ounce infant 2 hours ago. The client is complaining of severe uterine cramping while breastfeeding. A nurse knows that these symptoms are most likely due to:
1. Mastitis.
2. Uterine involution.
3. Uterine atony.
4. Postpartum endometritis.

58. A child is isolated at home with whooping cough (pertussis). Which parental behavior indicates the need for additional teaching by the nurse?
1. Confining cigarette smoking to the outdoors.
2. Avoiding sudden changes in household temperature.
3. Keeping the child's room well ventilated.
4. Using the fireplace as an additional means of heating the house.

59. A client, who is a 22-year-old primigravida, is at 38 weeks' gestation and 9 cm of dilation. Her contractions are 2 to 4 minutes apart and her uterus palpates soft between very firm contractions. She is very irritable and screaming in pain. A nurse should instruct this client to:
1. Take deep breaths.
2. Practice patterned breathing with deep cleansing breath.
3. Hold her breath and bear down.
4. Do shallow chest breathing.

60. A charge nurse on a pediatric unit is preparing the daily assignment sheet. Which nurse is the *best* choice to care for a child hospitalized with German measles (rubella)?
1. A 25-year-old woman who is a new graduate from nursing school.
2. A 32-year-old woman with 8 years of pediatric nursing experience.
3. A 45-year-old woman who is a new graduate from nursing school.
4. A 50-year-old woman with 25 years of pediatric nursing experience.

61. A client with a brain tumor has been unresponsive to verbal commands and is showing signs of abnormal motor responses. Which motor change should indicate to the nurse that a critical change in the client's condition has occurred?
1. Abnormal flexion of the upper extremities.
2. Extreme extension of arms and legs.
3. Diminished response to painful stimuli.
4. Disappearance of the Babinski response.

62. A 5-year-old child is diagnosed with acute tonsillitis for the third time in a year. The mother asks the nurse, "Can't the pediatrician just take the tonsils out now? Why wait until the infection is over?" The nurse's most accurate response would be:
1. "I agree. Let's talk to the pediatrician about this."
2. "You really shouldn't question the pediatrician's reason for delaying the surgery."
3. "A healthy child is a better candidate for surgery than a sick child."
4. "The inflammation and infection increase the risk of bleeding during the surgery."

63. A 30-year-old man has been recently diagnosed with Cushing's syndrome. He asks a nurse if he will be able to continue riding off-road motorcycles. The correct response by the nurse is:
1. "Continuing important activities will be beneficial to preventing depression."
2. "Because of the potential for obesity of your trunk, a larger bike will be necessary."
3. "Muscle weakness and the increased risk for fractures will require a change in activities."
4. "Visual changes from the disease will prevent you from riding your motorcycles."

64. The care of a client post–traumatic brain injury includes monitoring for signs of brainstem herniation and occlusion of cerebral blood flow. A nurse should recognize a deterioration in the client if which vital sign changes occurred? *Select all that apply.*
1. Tachycardia.
2. Tachypnea.
3. Hypotension.
4. Bradycardia.
5. Hypertension.
6. Bradypnea.

65. When counseling the parents of a child with severe hemophilia, the nurse would correctly inform the parents that:
1. Primary prophylaxis should be given on a regular basis before the onset of joint damage.
2. Primary prophylaxis should be given on a regular basis after joint damage.
3. Primary prophylaxis should be given after surgical procedures.
4. Primary prophylaxis is cost prohibitive.

66. A child is being prepared for a tonsillectomy. The laboratory telephones the pediatric unit and reports that the child's prothrombin time (PT) is 14.1 seconds. The nurse's *first* action should be to:
1. Note the laboratory result in the child's chart.
2. Immediately notify the pediatric surgeon.
3. Call the operating room and cancel the surgery.
4. Release the child to the operating room transporter.

67. Which assessment findings should alert a nurse to the potential of an addisonian crisis in a client? *Select all that apply.*
1. Hyperglycemia and rapid and weak pulse.
2. Hypernatremia and hyperglycemia.
3. Cyanosis and weak pulse.
4. Hypoglycemia and hyponatremia.
5. Hypotension and pallor.

68. A client has mitral regurgitation. Where is the *best* place for a nurse to auscultate the associated murmur?

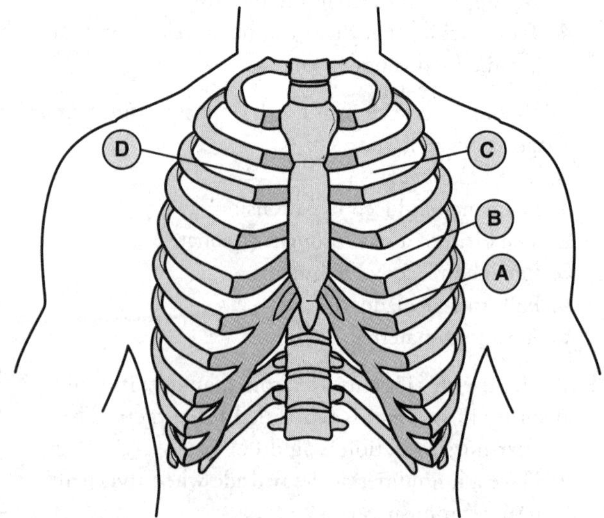

1. A.
2. B.
3. C.
4. D.

69. A 92-year-old client, who recently had a below-the-knee leg amputation, is resisting attempts at rehabilitation. The most likely reason for the resistance is that the client:
1. Has goals that differ from the rehabilitation care plan.
2. Has too many disabilities to realistically plan for rehabilitation.
3. Is too old to undergo rehabilitation.
4. Needs more time to feel comfortable with the dressing change.

70. A nurse prepares to discontinue the IV of a child with a low platelet count. Special precautions taken by the nurse when performing this nursing action should include:
1. Applying a sterile pressure dressing to the IV site.
2. Applying direct pressure to the IV site for 5 minutes.
3. Sending the tip of the IV catheter to the laboratory for a culture.
4. Restraining the child from moving the arm with the IV site for a period of 1 hour.

71. A nursing student is being mentored by a charge nurse on a pediatric unit. The nursing student is assigned to care for a child who has increased intracranial pressure following a head trauma. The charge nurse questions the nursing student regarding positions that would be contraindicated or ineffective when caring for the child. The nursing student should correctly identify:
Select all that apply.
1. Prone position.
2. Supine position.
3. Semi-Fowler's position.
4. Right side-lying position.
5. Left side-lying position.

72. A client is combative and demanding and refuses to swallow any medication following a brain attack (CVA). The correct nursing action is to:
1. Continue to attempt to follow the physician's orders and give the medication anyway.
2. Determine what the client's personality was before the CVA.
3. Apply restraints and request a change in the route of medication.
4. Wait for the client to become more cooperative.

73. A child is to receive digoxin 0.07 mg PO twice daily. The label on the bottle of digoxin reads 0.05 mg/mL. A nurse correctly calculates that this client should receive ______ mL of digoxin. *Fill in the blank.*

74. A nurse is concerned that a client may be at risk for oversedation from opioid therapy using a patient-controlled analgesia (PCA) pump. The most reliable assessment for possible oversedation would be to check:
1. Changes in the level of pain reported by the client.
2. The oxygen saturation level recorded by pulse oximetry.
3. How easily the client can be roused from sleeping.
4. The level of carbon dioxide in the blood using capnography.

75. Physical assessment of a client admitted for a bronchoscopy reveals a thin, muscular man with wheezes in the left lung. Which area should a nurse identify as most likely to be partially obstructed?

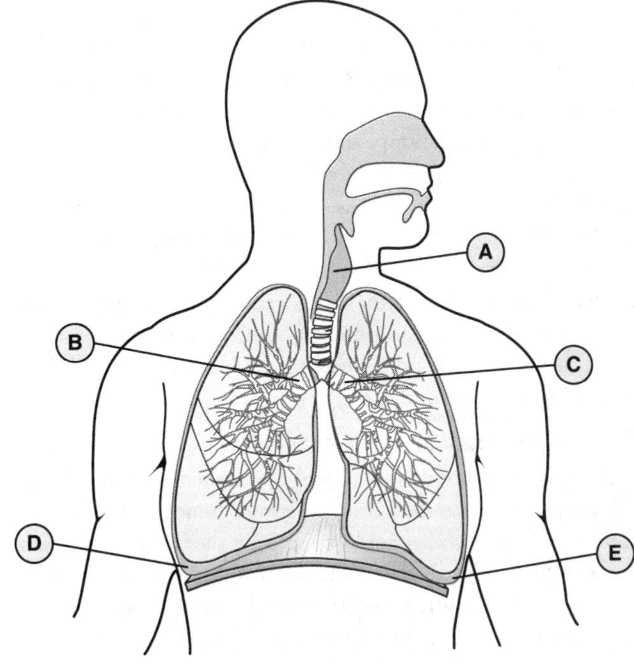

1. A.
2. B.
3. C.
4. D.
5. E.

Answers/Rationales/Tips

1. CORRECT ANSWER: 3. **Answer 1** is incorrect because the *amniocentesis* in this case is *not* used to determine congenital anomalies. **Answer 2** is incorrect because the *amniocentesis* does *not* establish intrauterine growth retardation. **Answer 3 is correct because the test is performed to determine fetal lung maturity. The L/S ratio should be 2:1 with + PG for the infant who would be at low risk for respiratory distress syndrome. Answer 4** is incorrect because the *amniocentesis* is *not* used to test for birth trauma.

■ TEST-TAKING TIP: ***Consider the client's condition; an amniocentesis at 33 weeks' gestation is used to establish lung maturity in an unborn fetus. Eliminate the answers that do not deal directly with this client's condition.***

Content Area: Maternity, Antepartum; ***Integrated Process:*** Nursing Process, Evaluation; ***Cognitive Level:*** Application; ***Client Need/Subneed:*** Physiological Integrity/Reduction of Risk Potential/Diagnostic Tests

2. CORRECT ANSWER: 2. Answer 1 is incorrect because herbs have not been adequately tested for managing a disease this significant. **Answer 2 is correct because this is an impending disaster. The client has genetic risks and risks from hypertension (HTN), obesity, and diabetes. The client already has early renal disease. While losing weight and exercising potentially could bring down the client's BP to under 130/80, the client will be exposed to risks over the months it will take to change. Answer 3** is incorrect because, while losing weight and exercising potentially could bring down the client's BP under 130/80 mm Hg, the client will be exposed to *risks* over the months it will take to change. **Answer 4** is incorrect because this is an impending disaster. A client has genetic risks, and risks from HTN, obesity, and diabetes. A client who already has renal disease needs treatment, *not just assessment.*

■ **TEST-TAKING TIP:** *Only one option will definitely reduce the BP—drug therapy.*

Content Area: Adult Health, Cardiovascular; *Integrated Process:* Communication and Documentation; *Cognitive Level:* Application; *Client Need/Subneed:* Psychosocial Integrity/Therapeutic Communications

3. CORRECT ANSWERS: 2, 4, 5. Answer 1 is incorrect because emergency medical services (EMS) are not required for this joint injury because the condition is not immediately life threatening. The child should be seen by the regular physician. **Answer 2 is correct because the nurse should apply a wrap to the knee for immobility and compression. Answer 3** is incorrect because the child should not continue to ambulate as it could worsen the injury. **Answer 4 is correct because ice should be applied to constrict blood vessels to reduce bleeding, swelling, and pain. Answer 5 is correct because elevating the extremity will help to reduce swelling and bleeding. Answer 6** is incorrect because keeping the child indoors is inappropriate. The child should be permitted to self-limit activities and lead as normal a life as possible.

■ **TEST-TAKING TIP:** *Use the mnemonic RICE (rest, ice, compression, elevation) to remember the treatment for hemophilia.*

Content Area: Child Health, Hematological; *Integrated Process:* Nursing Process, Implementation; *Cognitive Level:* Application; *Client Need/Subneed:* Physiological Integrity/Reduction of Risk Potential/Potential for Complications from Surgical Procedures and Health Alterations

4. CORRECT ANSWER: 1. Answer 1 is correct because congestive heart failure (CHF) or right-sided heart failure reduces cardiac output; and circulating O_2 is reduced, producing fatigue and shortness of breath. Answer 2 is incorrect because Cheyne-Stokes breathing occurs from *neurologic* problems or problems with respiratory gas exchange. **Answer 3** is incorrect because the liver may be enlarged but *not painful.* **Answer 4** is incorrect because crackles would be more consistent with *left*-sided failure, not CHF (right-sided failure).

■ **TEST-TAKING TIP:** *Review the clinical differences between right-sided versus left-sided heart failure.*

Content Area: Adult Health, Cardiovascular; *Integrated Process:* Nursing Process, Analysis; *Cognitive Level:* Application; *Client Need/Subneed:* Physiological Integrity/Physiological Adaptation/Pathophysiology

5. CORRECT ANSWERS: 1, 4. Answer 1 is correct because painless vaginal bleeding is the common symptom of complete placenta previa. Answer 2 is incorrect because tetanic uterine contractions are a symptom of placental abruption, not placenta previa. **Answer 3** is incorrect because premature rupture of membranes is a symptom of placental abruption, not placenta previa. **Answer 4 is correct because the client's hemoglobin level will drop in response to the bleeding caused by a complete placenta previa. It is common to draw serial blood counts to determine when to transfuse the mother or deliver the fetus. Answer 5** is incorrect because a rigid, boardlike abdomen is a symptom of placental abruption, not placenta previa.

■ **TEST-TAKING TIP:** *The important difference between abruption and previa is pain. Abruption is painful with many contractions; previa is painless without contractions.*

Content Area: Maternity, Antepartum; *Integrated Process:* Nursing Process, Analysis; *Cognitive Level:* Application; *Client Need/Subneed:* Physiological Integrity/Physiological Adaptation/Pathophysiology

6. CORRECT ANSWER: 3. Answer 1 is incorrect because the child's statement demonstrates the magical thinking of a preschooler. This child needs additional teaching and reassurance that hospitalization is not a punishment. **Answer 2** is incorrect because, although the child may be experiencing a stomachache, this statement is not the best evidence that the child has a basic understanding of the illness. **Answer 3 is correct because the child's statement demonstrates a basic knowledge that the main reason for hospitalization pertains to a urinary problem. Acute glomerulonephritis involves altered kidney function, resulting in decreased urine output. Answer 4** is incorrect because acute glomerulonephritis is thought to be an immune-complex response to a previous streptococcal illness. Although the child may have a persistent infection and may be receiving antibiotics, **Answer 3** demonstrates greater understanding of the rationale for hospitalization—so that kidney functioning may be monitored and restored.

■ **TEST-TAKING TIP:** *Note that only one answer describes a symptom specific to kidney functioning while the others indicate no understanding (Answer 1) or are too generalized (Answers 2 and 4). Select the option that is specific to the kidneys.*

Content Area: Child Health, Genitourinary; *Integrated Process:* Nursing Process, Evaluation; *Cognitive Level:* Analysis; *Client Need/Subneed:* Physiological Integrity/Physiological Adaptation/Alterations in Body Systems

7. CORRECT ANSWERS: 2, 3, 4. Answer 1 is incorrect because it is contraindicated to massage the site of the deep vein thrombosis (DVT). Massaging the calf can dislodge the clot and lead to an embolism. **Answer 2 is correct because the client should be encouraged to ambulate in addition to receiving anticoagulant therapy, since bedrest itself may**

enhance venous stasis. Answer 3 is correct because the most important goal is to prevent a pulmonary embolism or its recurrence. Incidence of pulmonary embolism depends on whether or not DVT is adequately treated with anticoagulant therapy. Answer 4 is correct because elevation of the affected extremity is important initially because it promotes venous return and decreases edema. **Answer 5** is incorrect because sitting with legs dependent is contraindicated because it increases stasis and edema.

■ TEST-TAKING TIP: *The main goal of DVT treatment is to prevent clots from traveling to major organs and causing mortality and morbidity. Eliminate those options that are not consistent with this goal.*

Content Area: Maternity, Postpartum; ***Integrated Process:*** Nursing Process, Implementation; ***Cognitive Level:*** Application; ***Client Need/Subneed:*** Physiological Integrity/Reduction of Risk Potential/System Specific Assessments

8. CORRECT ANSWER: 1. Answer 1 is correct because the use of soft bedding for a newborn should be avoided. It is believed that newborns sleeping on soft bedding may not be able to move their heads to the side, increasing the risk of suffocation, which may be a cause of SIDS. **Answer 2** is incorrect because the use of a pillow for a newborn should be avoided. It is believed that infants sleeping with a pillow may not be able to move their heads to the side, increasing the risk of suffocation, which may be a cause of SIDS. **Answer 3** is incorrect because the use of a soft sleep surface for a newborn should be avoided. It is believed that infants sleeping on a soft sleep surface may not be able to move their heads to the side, increasing the risk of suffocation, which may be a cause of SIDS. **Answer 4** is incorrect because co-sleeping with parents should be avoided. Studies reveal that bed-sharing has a positive association with SIDS. The leading theory suggests that suffocation is the cause. Parents who wish to share a bed with the newborn are advised to follow the same safeguards in the bed as in the crib (e.g., avoiding soft bedding, pillows, soft sleeping surfaces, and overheating [thermal stress]).

■ TEST-TAKING TIP: *Think "suffocation" when answering this question and eliminate answers that might increase the possibility of this happening. The question asks for what will* prevent *the possibility of suffocation.*

Content Area: Child Health, Respiratory; ***Integrated Process:*** Teaching and Learning; ***Cognitive Level:*** Application; ***Client Need/Subneed:*** Health Promotion and Maintenance/Health Promotion Programs

9. CORRECT ANSWER: 4. **Answer 1** is incorrect because when the sugar of $D_{10}W$ is metabolized, free water remains. At a rate of 150 mL/hr, this would *further decrease* the serum sodium. **Answer 2** is incorrect because, although the fluid rate and potassium in this order are reasonable, the 1/4 normal saline (NS) contains relatively more free water than normal saline does, which would *decrease* the serum sodium further. Clients who are NPO generally need an energy source order as dextrose. **Answer 3** is incorrect because the rate is a *little slow* for normal fluid balance, but could be acceptable if the client was in fluid overload. A client needs potassium, which is not present in this IV. ¼ NS would dilute the serum sodium further. Answer 4 is correct because the client needs potassium, which cannot be replaced with enteral feedings. Fluids are needed when NPO, but the low serum sodium should not be further diluted with rapid administration of hypotonic solutions; thus, normal saline is appropriate. Even though the blood sugar is slightly elevated, it is appropriate to give clients who are NPO some energy source. Dextrose 5% contains only 17 calories/100 mL.

■ TEST-TAKING TIP: *The variables to look at for inclusion are: dextrose, NS, KCl, and at a moderate rate. Consider the effect the solution will have on the laboratory values.*

Content Area: Adult Health, Fluid and Electrolyte Imbalances; ***Integrated Process:*** Nursing Process, Implementation; ***Cognitive Level:*** Analysis; ***Client Need/Subneed:*** Physiological Integrity/Pharmacological and Parenteral Therapies/Parenteral/Intravenous Therapies

10. CORRECT ANSWERS: 1, 2, 3. Answer 1 is correct because the nurse can expect that the child will experience pain related to surgery, and pain medication needs to be provided on a schedule to prevent and treat pain. Answer 2 is correct because circulation, sensation, and movement (CSM) must be assessed often to detect potential neurological complications of spinal surgery. Answer 3 is correct because the child will have a urinary catheter in place and monitoring of the output is essential to protect against the complication of urinary retention. **Answer 4** is incorrect because initial care of this child involves careful logroll turning, not placing the child in a chair as this could injure the surgical area. **Answer 5** is incorrect because bowel sounds should be assessed *frequently* to monitor for possible paralytic ileus after surgery. Monitoring bowel sounds once daily is *not* sufficient.

■ TEST-TAKING TIP: *The key phrase in the stem of the question is "immediately following" surgery. Select priorities that are part of the immediate postsurgical period.*

Content Area: Child Health, Musculoskeletal; ***Integrated Process:*** Nursing Process, Analysis; ***Cognitive Level:*** Analysis; ***Client Need/Subneed:*** Physiological Integrity/Reduction of Risk Potential/Potential for Complications from Surgical Procedures and Health Alterations

11. CORRECT ANSWER: 4. **Answer 1** is incorrect because the client *needs sodium replacement and* fluid restriction. **Answer 2** is incorrect because the client *already* has developed complications. **Answer 3** is incorrect because the confusion is due to *cerebral edema* from the *hyponatremia,* which needs to be corrected. Physiological intervention is needed now, not psychosocial (orientation). Answer 4 is correct because SIADH causes water retention and dilutional hyponatremia.

■ TEST-TAKING TIP: *Only one answer corrects both the fluid and electrolyte problem.*

Content Area: Adult Health, Fluid and Electrolyte Imbalances; ***Integrated Process:*** Nursing Process, Planning; ***Cognitive Level:*** Application; ***Client Need/Subneed:*** Physiological Integrity/Physiological Adaptation/Fluid and Electrolyte Imbalances

12. CORRECT ANSWER: 1. Answer 1 is correct because smoking has a direct association with low birth weight, doubling the risk of an infant who may have a low birth weight. **Answer 2** is incorrect because smoking results in low birth weight, *not large*-for-gestational-age infants. **Answer 3** is incorrect because, although smoking does have an association with preterm birth, the infant would be *low* birth weight, *not* an *appropriate* size for gestation. **Answer 4** is incorrect because smoking results in *low birth* weight, *not macrosomia.*

■ **TEST-TAKING TIP:** *Eliminate macrosomia and large for gestational age because they are essentially the same condition. Smoking causes low-birth-weight, not large infants.*

Content Area: Maternity, Antepartum; ***Integrated Process:*** Teaching and Learning; ***Cognitive Level:*** Application; ***Client Need/Subneed:*** Health Promotion and Maintenance/Ante/Intra/Postpartum and Newborn Care

13. CORRECT ANSWER: 4. Answer 1 is incorrect because the wearing of shoes and socks *is* encouraged to prevent toddlers from acquiring the infestation from contaminated soil. This observation would *not* be cause for follow-up by the school nurse. **Answer 2** is incorrect because the wearing of one-piece outfits prevents the toddlers from touching or scratching their perianal areas and continually reinfecting themselves. This observation would *not* be cause for follow-up by the school nurse. **Answer 3** is incorrect because short fingernails prevent the eggs from being deposited on the hands and under the fingernails of the toddlers, with continual reinfection through scratching their perianal areas. This observation would *not* be cause for follow-up by the school nurse. **Answer 4 is correct because the use of superabsorbent *disposable* diapers, which prevent leakage, are preferred over cloth diapers. Cloth diapers leak, which could result in feces that may be infested with pinworms (enterobiasis) to be spread from toddler to toddler. Cloth diapers would also be taken home to be laundered, which is another way to spread the infestation. The superabsorbent disposable diapers should be disposed of in a closed receptacle as soon as they are soiled.**

■ **TEST-TAKING TIP:** *Ask yourself: What is the relationship between diapers and infestations?*

Picture this: *Diapers cover → Perianal Area ← Infestations occur in*

Remember that diapers *come in direct contact with the toddler's* perianal *area, which is where the* infestation *is located. Superabsorbent disposable diapers would be preferred over cloth diapers because they may prevent leakage of contaminated feces.*

Content Area: Child Health, Gastrointestinal; ***Integrated Process:*** Nursing Process, Analysis; ***Cognitive Level:*** Application; ***Client Need/Subneed:*** Health Promotion and Maintenance/Health Screening

14. CORRECT ANSWER: 2. Answer 1 is incorrect because there is *no first phase* of labor, *only* the *first stage* of labor. **Answer 2 is correct because there are four stages of labor and the first stage covers all phases of cervical dilation. This client is in the first stage, active phase, which is 4 to 8 cm dilation.** **Answer 3** is incorrect because first stage, transition phase would mean the client was *8 to 10 cm* dilated. This client is 6 cm dilated, in the active phase of labor. **Answer 4** is incorrect because there is *no first phase* of labor, *only* the *first stage* of labor.

■ **TEST-TAKING TIP:** ***Eliminate Answers 1 and 4 because there are four stages of labor and* three phases in the first stage *of labor. Eliminate Answer 3 because the woman is* not yet *in transition phase with 6 cm dilation.***

Content Area: Maternity, Intrapartum; ***Integrated Process:*** Nursing Process, Analysis; ***Cognitive Level:*** Application; ***Client Need/Subneed:*** Physiological Integrity/Reduction of Risk Potential/System Specific Assessments

15. CORRECT ANSWER: 2. Answer 1 is incorrect because abdominal pain from an impending rupture is localized in the *middle* or *lower* abdomen to the left of the midline. **Answer 2 is correct because the aneurysm is pressing on the lumbar nerves. Severe back or middle or lower abdominal pain are signs of impending rupture. If the aneurysm ruptures, the back pain will be constant.** **Answer 3** is incorrect because circulation would *not* be impaired before rupture. **Answer 4** is incorrect because the pain is *lower abdomen* or *back.* Epigastric pain is more consistent with *cardiac* or *gastric* problems.

■ **TEST-TAKING TIP:** ***Visualize the location of the abdominal aorta.***

Content Area: Adult Health, Cardiovascular; ***Integrated Process:*** Nursing Process, Analysis; ***Cognitive Level:*** Application; ***Client Need/Subneed:*** Physiological Integrity/Physiological Adaptation/Medical Emergencies

16. CORRECT ANSWERS: 2, 5, 6. Answer 1 is incorrect because the nurse should *not combine* immunizations together in a syringe. **Answer 2 is correct because the appropriate injection site for an infant is the thigh muscle.** **Answer 3** is incorrect because the dorsogluteal muscle is contraindicated for use in infants due to the risk of injury to the sciatic nerve. **Answer 4** is incorrect because parents should be given the option to stay with the child during painful procedures. **Answer 5 is correct since a 1-inch needle is appropriate for infants 4 months of age and older. This length allows the tip of the needle to penetrate deep into the muscle and avoids accidental administration into the subcutaneous tissue. A longer needle (e.g., $1^1/_2$ inch) would be better for adults or older children who are significantly overweight.** **Answer 6 is correct since the nurse should first wash hands prior to any procedure.**

■ **TEST-TAKING TIP:** ***Recall that immunizations are intramuscular injections. The best site for injections in an infant is a well-developed muscle, such as the thigh.***

Content Area: Child Health, Immunizations; ***Integrated Process:*** Nursing Process, Analysis; ***Cognitive Level:*** Application; ***Client Need/Subneed:*** Health Promotion and Maintenance/Immunizations

17. CORRECT ANSWER: 2. Answer 1 is incorrect because this is *not unexpected* following surgery. If the client were unresponsive to pain medication, there might be a greater concern. **Answer 2 is correct because an infection following hip replacement is a**

serious complication that may require removal of the implant. Total joint infections may be disastrous, with prevention of an infection a priority. Usually prophylactic antibiotics are ordered; therefore, the appearance of a wound infection would be a grave concern. **Answer 3** is incorrect because a deep vein thrombosis (DVT) would not be expected until 5 to 7 days after surgery. DVTs do occur in 45% to 70% of clients after hip surgery. Further assessment would be needed, such as the presence of a positive Homans' sign and calf swelling. **Answer 4** is incorrect because the ability to tolerate weight-bearing *varies* with the client's condition, the procedure done, and the type of fixation device used. There is *insufficient* information to know if this is a problem.

■ **TEST-TAKING TIP:** ***When all options are important nursing concerns, look for the one where an immediate response could prevent a serious consequence.***

Content Area: Adult Health, Musculoskeletal; ***Integrated Process:*** Nursing Process, Assessment; ***Cognitive Level:*** Analysis; ***Client Need/Subneed:*** Physiological Integrity/Reduction of Risk Potential/Potential for Complications from Surgical Procedures and Health Alterations

18. CORRECT ANSWER: 3. **Answer 1** is incorrect because placing the client on her left side does not relieve the umbilical cord compression that results in fetal bradycardia. **Answer 2** is incorrect because it is *contraindicated* for the nurse to attempt to replace the cord. Answer 3 is correct because elevating the client's hips is the immediate intervention that helps to release the pressure from the umbilical cord until an emergency cesarean section can be performed. **Answer 4** is incorrect because covering the cord with a dry, sterile gauze does *not* relieve the umbilical cord compression and the fetal bradycardia that results.

■ **TEST-TAKING TIP:** ***The most important intervention is to relieve the umbilical cord compression. Covering the cord with a dry, sterile gauze causes a*** delay ***in relieving the compression. Eliminate the two options (Answers 2 and 4) that specifically focus on the visible cord. Focus on positioning the mother—one position releases cord compression and the other position (Answer 1) does not relieve the compression.***

Content Area: Maternity, Intrapartum; ***Integrated Process:*** Nursing Process, Implementation; ***Cognitive Level:*** Application; ***Client Need/Subneed:*** Physiological Integrity/Physiological Adaptation/Medical Emergencies

19. CORRECT ANSWER: 3. **Answer 1** is incorrect because the child should have a normal blood sugar; the child with *diabetes mellitus* will have elevated blood glucose. **Answer 2** is incorrect because the condition is caused by *decreased* secretion of antidiuretic hormone (ADH). Answer 3 is correct because the child with neurogenic diabetes insipidus (DI) will experience severe diuresis resulting from a decrease in ADH secretion. **Answer 4** is incorrect because the child is likely to have *increased* serum sodium due to massive amounts of fluid loss through the urine.

■ **TEST-TAKING TIP:** ***Recall that neurogenic diabetes insipidus and diabetes mellitus share the common symptom of polyuria.***

Content Area: Child Health, Endocrine; ***Integrated Process:*** Nursing Process, Planning; ***Cognitive Level:*** Application; ***Client Need/Subneed:*** Physiological Integrity/Physiological Adaptation/Fluid and Electrolyte Imbalances

20. CORRECT ANSWER: 3. **Answer 1** is incorrect because successful breastfeeding is *not* necessarily dependent on the mother's educational level. **Answer 2** is incorrect because successful breastfeeding is *not* dependent on the size of the mother's breasts. Answer 3 is correct because successful breastfeeding is most dependent on the mother's desire and commitment to breastfeed. **Answer 4** is incorrect because successful breastfeeding is *not* dependent on the infant's birth weight.

■ **TEST-TAKING TIP:** ***This question is asking about factors that are important for breastfeeding success. The size of the breasts, infant's birth weight, and mother's educational level are not factors in breastfeeding. Select the psychosocial factor ("desire") over physical factors (breast size, weight).***

Content Area: Maternity, Postpartum; ***Integrated Process:*** Nursing Process, Analysis; ***Cognitive Level:*** Comprehension; ***Client Need/Subneed:*** Health Promotion and Maintenance/Ante/Intra/Postpartum and Newborn Care

21. CORRECT ANSWER: 3. **Answer 1** is incorrect because crying is *not* a *specific* finding for immediate nursing intervention. **Answer 2** is incorrect because wakefulness is *not* associated with hypoglycemia, which is the main complication in a newborn of a mother with diabetes. Answer 3 is correct because jitteriness can be indicative of hypoglycemia and the nurse needs to obtain a heel stick blood glucose. **Answer 4** is incorrect because yawning is a *normal* response in a newborn and is *not associated* with hypoglycemia.

■ **TEST-TAKING TIP:** ***Restate the question. This question is asking for the symptoms of hypoglycemia. Examine the answers for the observation that is consistent with hypoglycemia.***

Content Area: Child Health, Newborn; ***Integrated Process:*** Nursing Process, Assessment; ***Cognitive Level:*** Analysis; ***Client Need/Subneed:*** Physiological Integrity/Physiological Adaptation/Alterations in Body Systems

22. CORRECT ANSWER: 2. **Answer 1** is incorrect because overhead or ceiling lights cause *glare or shadows.* Answer 2 is correct because glaucoma causes tunnel vision (loss of peripheral vision) and low vision. The client needs increased light, and sees best in natural lighting (sunlight). Fluorescent lighting does not produce glare and reduces shadows. A task light that can be directed is helpful. **Answer 3** is incorrect because bright lights will *cause glare* and *impair vision.* **Answer 4** is incorrect because the client needs increased lighting and preferably natural light, not dim lighting.

■ **TEST-TAKING TIP:** ***Remember that the client has lost*** peripheral ***vision, so that lighting needs to enhance*** central ***vision without glare or shadows.***

Content Area: Adult Health, Sensory; ***Integrated Process:*** Nursing Process, Analysis; ***Cognitive Level:*** Application; ***Client Need/Subneed:*** Physiological Integrity/Physiological Adaptation/Illness Management

23. CORRECT ANSWERS: 2, 4, 5. **Answer 1** is incorrect because a scheduled cesarean section does *not* increase the pressure on the fetal head or lead to development of caput succedaneum. **Answer 2 is correct because caput succedaneum is a diffuse swelling of the scalp in a newborn caused by pressure from the uterus or vaginal wall during a head-first (vertex) delivery. Prolonged active phase increases the pressure on the fetal head.** **Answer 3** is incorrect because a breech delivery does *not* increase the pressure on the fetal head or lead to development of caput succedaneum. **Answer 4 is correct because vacuum-assisted vaginal delivery increases the pressure on the fetal head and can result in caput succedaneum.** **Answer 5 is correct because caput succedaneum is a diffuse swelling of the scalp in a newborn caused by pressure from the uterus or vaginal wall during a head-first (vertex) delivery. Prolonged second stage increases the pressure on the fetal head.**
■ TEST-TAKING TIP: ***Think about the forces that increase pressure on the fetal head and can cause caput succedaneum.***
Content Area: Child Health, Newborn; *Integrated Process:* Nursing Process, Analysis; *Cognitive Level:* Application; *Client Need/Subneed:* Health Promotion and Maintenance/Ante/Intra/Postpartum and Newborn Care

24. CORRECT ANSWER: 1. **Answer 1 is correct because the symptoms are characteristic of pneumonia.** **Answer 2** is incorrect because the client reports a "*change.*" COPD is a *chronic* condition *with* sputum production. **Answer 3** is incorrect because the development of pulmonary edema includes *frothy* sputum. The client indicates a *nonproductive* cough. **Answer 4** is incorrect because tuberculosis includes a productive cough, fever, sweats, and weight loss.
■ TEST-TAKING TIP: ***Only pneumonia has a nonproductive cough—the others all produce sputum.***
Content Area: Adult Health, Respiratory; *Integrated Process:* Nursing Process, Analysis; *Cognitive Level:* Application; *Client Need/Subneed:* Physiological Integrity/Physiological Adaptation/Pathophysiology

25. CORRECT ANSWER: 3. **Answer 1** is incorrect because *moderate* uterine contractions are a *normal* finding in active labor. **Answer 2** is incorrect because frequent urination is a *normal* finding in active labor as a result of descent of the fetal head and decreased bladder capacity. **Answer 3 is correct because the presence of green-tinged amniotic fluid is not a normal finding and needs to be reported to the physician immediately. Meconium staining can be indicative of fetal distress.** **Answer 4** is incorrect because presence of *scant* bloody discharge is a normal finding in active labor, called bloody show. It is an indicator of cervical *progress.*
■ TEST-TAKING TIP: ***The question is asking about what is not a normal part of active labor. Eliminate the options that are a part of normal labor: moderate contractions, frequent urination, and the presence of scant bloody discharge.***
Content Area: Maternity, Intrapartum; *Integrated Process:* Nursing Process, Assessment; *Cognitive Level:* Analysis; *Client Need/Subneed:* Physiological Integrity/Reduction of Risk Potential/Potential for Complications from Surgical Procedures and Health Alterations

26. CORRECT ANSWER: 1. **Answer 1 is correct because this client has prehypertension without compelling indications for drug treatment. Lifestyle changes are indicated. The client is not recognizing the risk. In one sentence, the risk to the client and how to control the risk were addressed.** **Answer 2** is incorrect because this is prehypertension and should be managed with lifestyle changes to include at least weight loss. **Answer 3** is incorrect because this is prehypertension without compelling indications for drug treatment. **Answer 4** is incorrect because this is prehypertension, *not* a *normal* blood pressure.
■ TEST-TAKING TIP: ***For prehypertension, look for a nondrug option first. Eliminate Answers 2 and 3 with "medications" in the options.***
Content Area: Adult Health, Cardiovascular; *Integrated Process:* Teaching and Learning; *Cognitive Level:* Application; *Client Need/Subneed:* Health Promotion and Maintenance/Lifestyle Choices

27. CORRECT ANSWER: 3. **Answer 1** is incorrect because timing from the beginning of one contraction to the beginning of the next contraction is the correct method for measuring the *frequency* and *not the duration* of a contraction. **Answer 2** is incorrect because timing from the end of one contraction to the beginning of the next contraction is *not* the measurement for the duration of the contraction; it is the *resting* period between contractions. **Answer 3 is correct because duration is measured by timing from the beginning of one contraction to the end of the same contraction.** **Answer 4** is incorrect because timing from the peak of one contraction to the end of the same contraction is *not* the measure of duration or frequency of a contraction.
■ TEST-TAKING TIP: ***There are similar options for answers in this question. Visualize each of the options and try drawing it out if needed. Focus on "beginning . . . end . . ." as the best answer not "beginning . . . beginning . . ." and not "end . . . beginning . . ."***
Content Area: Maternity, Antepartum; *Integrated Process:* Teaching and Learning; *Cognitive Level:* Application; *Client Need/Subneed:* Health Promotion and Maintenance/Ante/Intra/Postpartum and Newborn Care

28. CORRECT ANSWERS: 1, 2, 5. **Answer 1 is correct because the client is at risk for thyroid storm because of a second illness, which can lead to hypotension and if untreated, heart failure.** **Answer 2 is correct because an elevated temperature is a sign of thyroid storm, which is a life-threatening form of hyperthyroidism. When a client with hyperthyroidism suffers a second illness, thyroid storm is a risk.** **Answer 3** is incorrect because Graves' disease is a *hyper*thyroid state. **Answer 4** is incorrect because the added illnesses of hyperglycemia and a foot ulcer may potentiate a thyroid storm. *Hypo*glycemia may be a concern *later* with treatment. **Answer 5 is correct because thyroid storm is an acute episode of thyroid overactivity. The metabolism is markedly increased, and extreme tachycardia occurs.**

■ **TEST-TAKING TIP:** *Focus on the options that would result from a metabolic "storm"—a thyroid storm. Recall that thyroid storm is rare but a* life-threatening *medical emergency.*

Content Area: Adult Health, Endocrine; ***Integrated Process:*** Nursing Process, Analysis; ***Cognitive Level:*** Application; ***Client Need/Subneed:*** Physiological Integrity/Physiological Adaptation/Medical Emergencies

29. CORRECT ANSWER: 4. Answer 1 is incorrect because the DTaP (*diphtheria, tetanus, and acellular pertussis*) vaccine *is* given at 2 months of age. **Answer 2** is incorrect because the Hib (*Haemophilus influenzae type b*) vaccine *is* given at 2 months of age. **Answer 3** is incorrect because IPV (*inactivated poliovirus*) vaccine *is* given at 2 months of age. **Answer 4 is correct because MMR (*measles, mumps, and rubella*) vaccine is not administered until the infant is 12 to 15 months of age. The second dose of this vaccine is given at 4 to 6 years of age.**

■ **TEST-TAKING TIP:** *Select as the "correct" answer the order that is* not *correct.*

Content Area: Child Health, Immunizations; ***Integrated Process:*** Nursing Process, Evaluation; ***Cognitive Level:*** Application; ***Client Need/Subneed:*** Safe and Effective Care Environment/Safety and Infection Control/Error Prevention

30. CORRECT ANSWER: 4. Answer 1 is incorrect because increasing activity may drop the systolic BP up to *9* mm Hg. **Answer 2** is incorrect because limiting sodium only lowers the systolic BP by *8* mm Hg. **Answer 3** is incorrect because limiting alcohol will likely only lower the systolic BP by *2 to 4* mm Hg. **Answer 4 is correct because a weight loss of 10 kg can reduce the systolic BP up to *20* mm Hg.**

■ **TEST-TAKING TIP:** *All options are correct, but weight loss produces the greatest drop. Diagrammatically visualize these measures:*

↑ Physical activity → ↓ weight
↓ Na^+ → ↓ weight
↓ Alcohol intake → ↓ weight

Content Area: Adult Health, Cardiovascular; ***Integrated Process:*** Teaching and Learning; ***Cognitive Level:*** Application; ***Client Need/Subneed:*** Health Promotion and Maintenance/Health and Wellness

31. CORRECT ANSWER: 3. Answer 1 is incorrect because insulin requirements *increase* as the pregnancy progresses. Increasing amounts of human placental lactogen cause the client to be *more insulin resistant,* increasing the need for insulin. **Answer 2** is incorrect because insulin needs decrease during the first trimester, but *steadily increase* as the pregnancy progresses. **Answer 3 is correct because insulin requirements will increase as the pregnancy progresses. The placenta creates increasing amounts of human placental lactogen, causing the client to be more insulin resistant, increasing the need for insulin. Answer 4** is incorrect because elevations in human placental lactogen *increase, not* decrease, the need for insulin.

■ **TEST-TAKING TIP:** *Remember that insulin needs* decrease *during the first trimester, steadily* increase *during the second and third trimesters, then* decrease *after delivery.*

Content Area: Maternity, Antepartum; ***Integrated Process:*** Teaching and Learning; ***Cognitive Level:*** Application; ***Client Need/Subneed:*** Physiological Integrity/Physiological Adaptation/Alterations in Body Systems

32. CORRECT ANSWER: 3. Answer 1 is incorrect because allowing the nursing student to continue would lead to an error that could jeopardize the infant. **Answer 2** is incorrect because just stopping the nursing student is not enough as it will not lead to critical thinking regarding the correct action that needs to be taken. **Answer 3 is correct because it will stimulate the nursing student to think in a critical manner. DTaP (diphtheria, tetanus, and acellular pertussis) vaccine is given intramuscularly and a 1-inch/2.5-cm needle must be used to deposit the vaccine deep in the muscle mass. Answer 4** is incorrect because a *longer*, rather than a shorter needle, is needed for the correct administration of the vaccine (i.e., *deep* in the muscle mass).

■ **TEST-TAKING TIP:** *Choose the "assessment" option (i.e., question the nursing student).*

Content Area: Child Health, Immunizations; ***Integrated Process:*** Teaching and Learning; ***Cognitive Level:*** Application; ***Client Need/Subneed:*** Health Promotion and Maintenance/Principles of Teaching and Learning

33. CORRECT ANSWER: 1. Answer 1 is correct because a high blood pressure (170/90 mm Hg) may be indicative of preeclampsia, or may be due to gestational hypertension, pain, or severe anxiety. The nurse needs to determine if the client has proteinuria. If there is proteinuria, the high blood pressure is suggestive of preeclampsia. Answer 2 is incorrect because administering an analgesic will *not* help to determine the cause of the high blood pressure in this client, and may delay the treatment if the client has preeclampsia. **Answer 3** is incorrect because assessing fetal heart tones is a *general* assessment for *all* clients in the prenatal clinic; it is *not* a *specific* evaluation for the client's high blood pressure. **Answer 4** is incorrect because obtaining a diet history is *not the first* action to take for this client. A diet history is appropriate for a client with *hyperemesis, not* possible preeclampsia.

■ **TEST-TAKING TIP:** *Choose the option that will not delay the evaluation of whether or not this client has preeclampsia. The question only states the client has a* single *high blood pressure, which does not mean that the client* has *preeclampsia.*

Content Area: Maternity, Intrapartum; ***Integrated Process:*** Nursing Process, Implementation; ***Cognitive Level:*** Analysis; ***Client Need/Subneed:*** Physiological Integrity/Physiological Adaptation/Alterations in Body Systems

34. CORRECT ANSWER: 4. **Answer 1** is incorrect because the adolescent would have received the hepatitis B vaccine series in infancy (birth, 1 to 2 months of age, and 6 to 18 months of age). **Answer 2** is incorrect because the adolescent would have received the hepatitis A vaccine series in infancy (2 doses between 12 and 23 months of age). **Answer 3** is incorrect because the adolescent would have received the MMR (measles, mumps, and rubella) vaccine series in infancy/childhood (12 to 15 months of age and 4 to 6 years of age). **Answer 4 is correct because the HPV (human papillomavirus) vaccine is given between 11 and 12 years of age. This would be the most likely vaccine that the adolescent has yet to receive.**

■ **TEST-TAKING TIP:** *Focus on the age-relevant vaccine for a 12-year-old. Vaccines are not limited to infancy/childhood. Knowing the vaccine schedule for 7- to 18-year-olds is critical for correctly answering this question.*

Content Area: Child Health, Immunizations; ***Integrated Process:*** Nursing Process, Assessment; ***Cognitive Level:*** Application; ***Client Need/Subneed:*** Health Promotion and Maintenance/Immunizations

35. CORRECT ANSWER: 4. **Answer 1** is incorrect because this may delay treatment, and the interpreter may not convey the client's pain as accurately as the client with a nonverbal pain scale. **Answer 2** is incorrect because ethnic/cultural groups may "mask" the response to pain (e.g., by denial, rationalization as coping mechanisms). **Answer 3** is incorrect because, depending on the culture, responding to pain may not be acceptable. **Answer 4 is correct because pain scales, like the Oucher Scale, are accurate with many ethnic groups and languages.**

■ **TEST-TAKING TIP:** *Look for an assessment that is the client's own description, even though it is through a projective device.*

Content Area: Adult Health, Pain Control; ***Integrated Process:*** Nursing Process, Assessment; ***Cognitive Level:*** Application; ***Client Need/Subneed:*** Psychosocial Integrity/Cultural Diversity

36. CORRECT ANSWER: 1. **Answer 1 is correct because information is always the best way to reduce parents' anxieties and concerns over vaccines. The information should include the need for each vaccine and what disease each vaccine prevents. Lack of information could needlessly prevent an infant from getting protection against life-threatening diseases.** **Answer 2** is incorrect because, while reassurance of the parents is important, it does *not* replace the need for information. **Answer 3** is incorrect because, while respect for the parents' decisions is important, it does *not* replace the need for information. **Answer 4** is incorrect because, while involving the parents in minimizing potential adverse effects of the vaccine (e.g., administering an age-appropriate dose of acetaminophen prior to the vaccine, etc.) is important, it does *not* replace the need for information.

■ **TEST-TAKING TIP:** *Think "knowledge" as the parents' first need when concerns about their infant arise.*

Content Area: Child Health, Immunizations; ***Integrated Process:*** Nursing Process, Implementation; ***Cognitive Level:*** Application; ***Client Need/Subneed:*** Health Promotion and Maintenance/Immunizations

37. CORRECT ANSWER: 1. **Answer 1 is correct because the most common cause of chronic pain syndrome is failure to control acute pain. Chronic pain syndrome consists of chronic anxiety and depression, anger, and changed lifestyle, all with a variable but significant level of genuine neurologically based pain.** **Answer 2** is incorrect because opiates *are effective* in the treatment of acute pain. **Answer 3** is incorrect because pain medication should be *offered* as ordered. Some clients will not ask. **Answer 4** is incorrect because physical dependence is determined when the drug is *discontinued.* It is expected in all clients who take opioids continuously. It is *not* addiction.

■ **TEST-TAKING TIP:** *Look for the answer that relieves acute pain.*

Content Area: Adult Health, Pain Control; ***Integrated Process:*** Nursing Process, Implementation; ***Cognitive Level:*** Comprehension; ***Client Need/Subneed:*** Physiological Integrity/Pharmacological and Parenteral Therapies/Pharmacological Pain Management

38. CORRECT ANSWER: 4. **Answer 1** is incorrect because respiratory distress syndrome is associated with *preterm* birth, not related to the age of the client at conception. **Answer 2** is incorrect because there are no specific risk factors based on the information given that would put her infant at a higher risk for pathological jaundice. Pathological jaundice usually occurs with an *ABO incompatibility.* **Answer 3** is incorrect because the mutation that causes the missing or altered X chromosome takes place spontaneously. There's *no* evidence that Turner's syndrome is hereditary or is caused by any other environmental or health factors. **Answer 4 is correct because the client's age (42) puts her at a higher risk for an infant with Down syndrome.**

■ **TEST-TAKING TIP:** *The in-vitro fertilization has nothing to do with risk factors that affect an infant. The risk factor is the client's age of 42. Do not let the extraneous information distract from the true risk factor.*

Content Area: Maternity, Antepartum; ***Integrated Process:*** Nursing Process, Analysis; ***Cognitive Level:*** Application; ***Client Need/Subneed:*** Health Promotion and Maintenance/Ante/Intra/Postpartum and Newborn Care

39. CORRECT ANSWER: 2. **Answer 1** is incorrect because tactile stimulation can *increase* the hyperirritability associated with narcotic abstinence syndrome. **Answer 2 is correct because wrapping the newborn snugly in a blanket decreases the hyperirritability and increases feeling of security.** **Answer 3** is incorrect because putting the neonate in the car seat can increase physical and sensory stimulation to the infant. The goal is to *decrease* these effects. **Answer 4** is incorrect because an early stimulation program increases physical and sensory stimulation to the infant. The goal is to *decrease* these effects.

■ TEST-TAKING TIP: *A neonate with narcotic abstinence syndrome needs decreased tactile stimulation. Eliminate the three options that increase stimulation.*
Content Area: Child Health, Newborn; *Integrated Process:* Nursing Process, Implementation; *Cognitive Level:* Analysis; *Client Need/Subneed:* Psychosocial Integrity/Chemical and other Dependencies

40. CORRECT ANSWERS: 2, 4, 5. **Answer 1** is incorrect because the client *will be allowed some* complex carbohydrates, but simple carbohydrates (such as sugar, juice, and cold cereal) are not allowed in a gestational diabetic diet. **Answer 2 is correct because keeping the blood sugar well controlled has a direct relationship to decreasing the risk for macrosomia and hypoglycemia in the neonate.** **Answer 3** is incorrect because many clients with gestational diabetes are diet controlled or controlled with glyburide, and gestational diabetes is resolved after the pregnancy is over. All clients with gestational diabetes have a follow-up glucose tolerance test scheduled about 6 weeks after delivery. **Answer 4 is correct because the diet for gestational diabetes is based on the grams of carbohydrate allowed at each meal and snack. Answer 5 is correct because clients with gestational diabetes are required to test their fasting blood sugar and 1 to 2 hours postprandial.**
■ TEST-TAKING TIP: *Look for phrases like "can't eat any" (meaning none) and "for the rest of my life"; those are both very definitive phrases. Be sure they are totally true before choosing these responses.*
Content Area: Maternity, Antepartum; *Integrated Process:* Nursing Process, Evaluation; *Cognitive Level:* Analysis; *Client Need/Subneed:* Health Promotion and Maintenance/Ante/Intra/Postpartum and Newborn Care

41. CORRECT ANSWER: 1. **Answer 1 is correct because the client must be treated for pain as expressed. The IV drug use may require that a higher dose be given, but the presence of pain as expressed by the client should not be ignored.** **Answer 2** is incorrect because IV drug use may only alter the drug *effectiveness, not* the *feeling* of pain. **Answer 3** is incorrect because these drugs are *not* effective for *moderate to severe* pain. **Answer 4** is incorrect because nondrug therapies *alone* are *not adequate* for pain management.
■ TEST-TAKING TIP: *Remember: pain is what the client says it is—severe. Three of the options involve other measures, but not what was ordered. Select this option that is different.*
Content Area: Adult Health, Pain Control; *Integrated Process:* Nursing Process, Implementation; *Cognitive Level:* Application; *Client Need/Subneed:* Physiological Integrity/Pharmacological and Parenteral Therapies/Pharmacological Pain Management

42. CORRECT ANSWER: 1. **Answer 1 is correct because diphenhydramine hydrochloride (Benadryl) is a nonprescription antihistamine that will safely and effectively reduce the child's itching for up to 4 to 6 hours following a dose of the medication.** **Answer 2** is incorrect because, while keeping the child cool will assist in reducing the child's itching, it is not as effective as diphenhydramine hydrochloride (Benadryl). **Answer 3** is incorrect because, while changing the linens daily will assist in reducing the child's itching, it is not as effective as diphenhydramine hydrochloride (Benadryl). **Answer 4** is incorrect because, while keeping the child's fingernails short and clean will assist in reducing the child's itching, it is not as effective as diphenhydramine hydrochloride (Benadryl).
■ TEST-TAKING TIP: *Choose the direct, most immediate suggestion (Benadryl) rather than the indirect, supportive suggestions (focusing on linens and fingernails). Note that the mother's concern is* **reducing itching.**
Content Area: Child Health, Integumentary; *Integrated Process:* Nursing Process, Implementation; *Cognitive Level:* Application; *Client Need/Subneed:* Physiological Integrity/Physiological Adaptation/Illness Management

43. CORRECT ANSWER: 4. **Answer 1** is incorrect because blood cultures are done *before* treatment. **Answer 2** is incorrect because there is *no* indication of *cardiac* involvement. **Answer 3** is incorrect because blood glucose is not elevated at this time (although diabetes is a risk factor for cellulitis). **Answer 4 is correct because a low-grade temperature and elevated pulse in an older adult are consistent with infection. The specific bacteria causing the infection of the skin and subcutaneous tissue should be identified to prevent sepsis.**
■ TEST-TAKING TIP: *This is a priority question—more data are needed to identify the cause of the infection ("itis").*
Content Area: Adult Health, Integumentary; *Integrated Process:* Nursing Process, Analysis; *Cognitive Level:* Application; *Client Need/Subneed:* Physiological Integrity/Physiological Adaptation/Alterations in Body Systems

44. CORRECT ANSWER: 4. **Answer 1** is incorrect because the volume of breast milk produced is related to *how often* the breasts are emptied of milk. Formula supplementation *decreases* breast milk production since the infant nurses less often. **Answer 2** is incorrect because an *infant is more efficient* at emptying a breast than a breast pump. In addition, oral stimulation of the nipples by the infant stimulates the release of oxytocin, which triggers the let-down reflex. **Answer 3** is incorrect because *estrogen does not* stimulate milk production. *Oxytocin* and *prolactin* are the hormones responsible for breast milk production. **Answer 4 is correct because the amount of milk-producing glandular tissue in all women is approximately the same. The size of large breasts is due to increased fatty tissue.**
■ TEST-TAKING TIP: *Milk production is directly related to the amount of time the infant is nursing. Any other option will lead to decreased milk production.*
Content Area: Maternity, Antepartum; *Integrated Process:* Communication and Documentation; *Cognitive Level:* Application; *Client Need/Subneed:* Health Promotion and Maintenance/Ante/Intra/Postpartum and Newborn Care

45. CORRECT ANSWER: 3. **Answer 1** is incorrect because taping the umbilical hernia down to the abdomen does *not* aid in resolution, and it can produce skin irritation and breakdown. This practice should be discouraged. **Answer 2** is incorrect because taping the umbilical hernia down to the abdomen does *not replace* a surgical repair of the umbilical hernia; it will *not* result in resolution of the umbilical hernia, and it can produce skin irritation and breakdown. Umbilical hernias that do not resolve spontaneously by 3 to 5 years of age should be corrected surgically on an elective basis. **Answer 3 is correct because taping the umbilical hernia down to the abdomen does not aid in resolution of the hernia. It can produce skin irritation and breakdown. This practice should be discouraged.** **Answer 4** is incorrect because manual reduction of the umbilical hernia should *never* be attempted by the parents. This procedure should *only* be done by a pediatrician and/or surgeon.

■ **TEST-TAKING TIP:** *Select the one option that implies "do not do" the taping of the hernia.*

Content Area: Child Health, Gastroenterological; ***Integrated Process:*** Teaching and Learning; ***Cognitive Level:*** Application; ***Client Need/Subneed:*** Psychosocial Integrity/Cultural Diversity

46. CORRECT ANSWER: 3. **Answer 1** is incorrect because increasing fluid intake is good *general* advice for pregnancy, but will *not resolve* the client's concern. **Answer 2** is incorrect because increasing protein intake is a *good* suggestion for clients with *gestational diabetes.* **Answer 3 is correct because leg cramps are caused by low blood calcium levels; increasing calcium intake can decrease leg cramps.** **Answer 4** is incorrect because increasing fiber intake is good *general* advice for pregnancy, but will *not resolve* the client's concern.

■ **TEST-TAKING TIP:** *Eliminate the answers that are good* general *suggestions for pregnancy, but do not address the* specific *concerns of the client.*

Content Area: Maternity, Antepartum; ***Integrated Process:*** Teaching and Learning; ***Cognitive Level:*** Application; ***Client Need/Subneed:*** Health Promotion and Maintenance/Ante/Intra/Postpartum and Newborn Care

47. CORRECT ANSWER: 2. **Answer 1** is incorrect because a fear of bright lights is *not associated* with measles (rubeola) nor is it common in childhood. **Answer 2 is correct because an intolerance of light (photophobia) is a common side effect of measles (rubeola). Dimming lights in the child's room is suggested if photophobia is present.** **Answer 3** is incorrect because, while children with measles (rubeola) frequently rub their eyes, this leads to eye redness and irritation as opposed to intolerance of light (photophobia). **Answer 4** is incorrect because an enhanced reaction to unanticipated events (such as turning on the overhead light) is *not associated with measles* (rubeola), nor is it common in childhood.

■ **TEST-TAKING TIP:** *Focus on the two answers that refer to lights (Answers 1 and 2). Note the word "light" in the stem and in the two answers with the word "light," as opposed to "rubbing" (Answer 3) and "unanticipated events" (Answer 4). Correlate side effects of the disease with the child's behavior.*

Content Area: Child Health, Infectious Disease; ***Integrated Process:*** Nursing Process, Analysis; ***Cognitive Level:*** Analysis; ***Client Need/Subneed:*** Physiological Integrity/Reduction of Risk Potential/Potential for Complications from Surgical Procedures and Health Alterations

48. CORRECT ANSWERS: 1, 2, 4, 5. **Answer 1 is correct because severe thirst may be *secondary* to the polyuria from the high solute (calcium) load.** **Answer 2 is correct because constipation is a common side effect from *decreased tone* in the bowel.** **Answer 3** is incorrect because diarrhea is *not common* with hypercalcemia until levels *above* 17 mg/dL, which is considered a crisis. **Answer 4 is correct because the high calcium increases gastric acid secretion and may intensify gastrointestinal manifestation. Anorexia, nausea, and vomiting are intensified by increased gastric residual volume.** **Answer 5 is correct because high calcium levels depress brain function, leading to ↓ activity.** **Answer 6** is incorrect because hypercalcemia *depresses* neuromuscular excitability, leading to muscle weakness and lethargy.

■ **TEST-TAKING TIP:** *Look at pairs of contradictory options (Answers 2 and 3, and Answers 5 and 6) where both can't be correct answers.* ***Hypercalcemia depresses functions (e.g., bowels and activity).***

Content Area: Adult Health, Fluid and Electrolyte Imbalances; ***Integrated Process:*** Nursing Process, Assessment; ***Cognitive Level:*** Analysis; ***Client Need/Subneed:*** Physiological Integrity/Physiological Adaptation/Fluid and Electrolyte Imbalances

49. CORRECT ANSWER: 2. **Answer 1** is incorrect because chocolate milk is *not* an irritating fluid. **Answer 2 is correct because scarlet fever is associated with an inflamed oral cavity. Because of this, rough foods and irritating fluids are to be avoided. Citrus juices, such as orange juice, would further irritate the inflamed oral cavity.** **Answer 3** is incorrect because apple juice is *not* an irritating fluid. **Answer 4** is incorrect because 2% milk is *not* an irritating fluid.

■ **TEST-TAKING TIP:** *Three of the choices are bland in nature and one choice is irritating in nature. Select the choice that is different from the rest of the choices.*

Content Area: Child Health, Infectious Disease; ***Integrated Process:*** Nursing Process, Implementation; ***Cognitive Level:*** Application; ***Client Need/Subneed:*** Physiological Integrity/Basic Care and Comfort/Nutrition and Oral Hydration

50. CORRECT ANSWER: 1. Right lateral recumbent positioning provides for drainage of oral secretions, which is important with clients who are immobile following a stroke. However, a pillow must be placed between the lower limbs to avoid redness and skin breakdown.

■ **TEST-TAKING TIP:** *Think about what happens when two surfaces rub together.*

Content Area: Adult Health, Integumentary; ***Integrated Process:*** Nursing Process, Implementation; ***Cognitive Level:*** Application; ***Client Need/Subneed:*** Physiological Integrity/Reduction of Risk Potential/Potential for Alterations in Body Systems

51. CORRECT ANSWERS: 1, 2, 5. Answer 1 is correct because rubella titer is part of the initial prenatal laboratory panel. Answer 2 is correct because the CBC is part of the initial prenatal laboratory panel. **Answer 3** is incorrect because the *glucose tolerance test is not* usually part of the initial prenatal panel; it is obtained during the 28th week of pregnancy. **Answer 4** is incorrect because the *ultrasound is not* part of the initial prenatal examination. Answer 5 is correct because blood type and Rh are part of the initial prenatal laboratory panel.

■ TEST-TAKING TIP: *Use the process of elimination to discard the* nonroutine *tests for an* initial *visit (Answers 3 and 4).*

Content Area: Maternity, Antepartum; *Integrated Process:* Nursing Process, Implementation; *Cognitive Level:* Application; *Client Need/Subneed:* Physiological Integrity/Reduction of Risk Potential/Diagnostic Tests

52. CORRECT ANSWER: 2. **Answer 1** is incorrect because milk products, such as ice cream, coat the mouth and throat, causing the child to clear the throat, which may initiate bleeding from the surgical site. Answer 2 is correct because an ice collar applied to the throat 30 minutes prior to the meal will serve as a local anesthetic and reduce the child's oral and throat pain, which will assist in eliciting the child's cooperation with eating. **Answer 3** is incorrect because gargling is to be *avoided* in the *immediate* postoperative period because it can start bleeding from the surgical site. **Answer 4** is incorrect because it is *punitive.* It is not the nurse's role to threaten or punish the child for not eating. It is the nurse's role to find a way to make eating more comfortable for the child.

■ TEST-TAKING TIP: *Think "comfort measures" to encourage the child to eat. Oral and throat pain following a tonsillectomy will prevent a child from eating. Eliminate answers that promise or threaten (Answers 1 and 4).*

Content Area: Child Health, Pediatric Surgery; *Integrated Process:* Nursing Process, Implementation; *Cognitive Level:* Application; *Client Need/Subneed:* Physiological Integrity/Basic Care and Comfort/Non-pharmacological Comfort Interventions

53. CORRECT ANSWERS: 2, 3, 4. **Answer 1** is incorrect because pregnancy-induced hypertension is *not* related to uterine atony or other causes of postpartum hemorrhage. Answer 2 is correct because a macrosomatic (very large) baby can predispose a woman to uterine atony, and thus to hemorrhage. Answer 3 is correct because retained placental fragments *are* a cause of postpartum hemorrhage. Answer 4 is correct because a full urinary bladder *may* result in uterine atony, and thus hemorrhage. **Answer 5** is incorrect because maternal age is *not* a risk factor for hemorrhage. Increased *parity* is related to an increased risk of hemorrhage.

■ TEST-TAKING TIP: *The stem asks for conditions that are associated with a risk for hemorrhage.*

Content Area: Maternity, Postpartum; *Integrated Process:* Nursing Process, Analysis; *Cognitive Level:* Application; *Client Need/Subneed:* Physiological Integrity/Physiological Adaptation/Pathophysiology

54. CORRECT ANSWER: 2. **Answer 1** is incorrect because *pulmonary* dryness is *not* the problem. Answer 2 is correct because, with Sjögren's syndrome, lacrimal glands are destroyed, resulting in dry eyes (keratoconjunctivitis). **Answer 3** is incorrect because *dry mouth* is a *problem.* Twelve hours is *too long.* **Answer 4** is incorrect because antidepressants are *not* a treatment for Sjögren's syndrome.

■ TEST-TAKING TIP: *Note that three options focus on* after *surgery (Answers 1, 3, and 4). Select the option that is "before surgery." Review Sjögren's syndrome—remember dry eyes and mouth.*

Content Area: Adult Health, Immunological; *Integrated Process:* Nursing Process, Implementation; *Cognitive Level:* Application; *Client Need/Subneed:* Physiological Integrity/Reduction of Risk Potential/Therapeutic Procedures

55. CORRECT ANSWER: 3. **Answer 1** is incorrect because eating gelatin would require *no chewing* on the child's part. **Answer 2** is incorrect because eating applesauce would require *no chewing* on the child's part. Answer 3 is correct because mumps (parotitis) is associated with swelling at the jaw line, followed by an earache that is aggravated by chewing. A soft, bland diet is suggested, as well as avoiding foods that require chewing. An apple would require chewing on the child's part. **Answer 4** is incorrect because eating a banana would require *little, if any,* chewing on the child's part.

■ TEST-TAKING TIP: *Think "soft" or "no chewing" in terms of the child's diet. Relate clinical manifestations of the disease to the child's dietary requirements.*

Content Area: Child Health, Infectious Disease; *Integrated Process:* Nursing Process, Implementation; *Cognitive Level:* Application; *Client Need/Subneed:* Physiological Integrity/Basic Care and Comfort/Nutrition and Oral Hydration

56. CORRECT ANSWERS: 1, 3, 4, 6. Answer 1 is correct because a transfusion reaction can lead to *anaphylactic* shock and life-threatening vasodilation and hypotension. **Answer 2** is incorrect because treating pain or a fever is *not* the priority. Answer 3 is correct because the client should *not* receive any more blood, which is the source of the antigen that is causing the allergic response. Answer 4 is correct because a patent IV may be needed for emergency treatment. **Answer 5** is incorrect because the blood needs to be returned to the laboratory, not disposed of. Answer 6 is correct because the *reason* for the allergic reaction needs to be determined.

■ TEST-TAKING TIP: *Note that Answers 5 and 6 are contradictory. Select Answer 6—keep rather than dispose of the blood product. With each option, ask if the statement is a true or false action with a transfusion reaction.*

Content Area: Adult Health, Hematological; *Integrated Process:* Nursing Process, Implementation; *Cognitive Level:* Analysis; *Client Need/Subneed:* Physiological Integrity/Pharmacological and Parenteral Therapies/Blood and Blood Products

57. CORRECT ANSWER: 2. **Answer 1** is incorrect because mastitis is an infection of the breast that occurs postpartum, but is *unrelated to uterine cramping.* **Answer 2 is correct because breastfeeding causes the release of prolactin and oxytocin. Oxytocin is a hormone that causes uterine contractions. The release of oxytocin while breastfeeding speeds uterine involution. This may also cause cramps while breastfeeding in the postpartum period. Cramping is more severe in clients who are multiparous.** **Answer 3** is incorrect because uterine atony is the failure of the uterine muscles to contract normally after the baby and placenta are delivered; there is *no cramping with uterine atony.* **Answer 4** is incorrect because postpartum endometritis is an infection of the endometrium or decidua, extending into the myometrium and parametrial tissues, which is the most common cause of postpartum fever. It does *not cause cramping* during breastfeeding.

■ TEST-TAKING TIP: *Cramping is a sign of contracting of the uterus, not uterine atony, which is the opposite (a lack of cramping). Therefore, eliminate that option.*

Content Area: Maternity, Postpartum; *Integrated Process:* Nursing Process, Analysis; *Cognitive Level:* Application; *Client Need/Subneed:* Health Promotion and Maintenance/Ante/Intra/Postpartum and Newborn Care

58. CORRECT ANSWER: 4. **Answer 1** is incorrect because it is a *desirable* behavior by the parents. Confining cigarette smoke to the outdoors can prevent paroxysms of coughing associated with whooping cough (pertussis). **Answer 2** is incorrect because it is a *desirable* behavior by the parents. Avoiding sudden changes in household temperature can prevent paroxysms of coughing associated with whooping cough (pertussis). **Answer 3** is incorrect because it is a *desirable* behavior by the parents. Keeping the child's room well ventilated can prevent paroxysms of coughing associated with whooping cough (pertussis). **Answer 4 is correct because using the fireplace as an additional means of heating the house creates dust and smoke that may cause paroxysms of coughing associated with whooping cough (pertussis).**

■ TEST-TAKING TIP: *The question asks for the answer that is not a correct action by the parents. Think "triggers" that promote coughing and select the behavior by the parents that may cause paroxysms of coughing.*

Content Area: Child Health, Infectious Disease; *Integrated Process:* Nursing Process, Evaluation; *Cognitive Level:* Application; *Client Need/Subneed:* Physiological Integrity/Physiological Adaptation/Alterations in Body Systems

59. CORRECT ANSWER: 4. **Answer 1** is incorrect because deep breathing is the correct technique for the *latent* phase of the first stage of labor, when the client is trying to relax and allow labor to progress. Taking deep breaths in this phase of labor can lead to hyperventilation. **Answer 2** is incorrect because patterned breathing is the correct technique for the *active* phase of the *first stage* of labor when the client is trying to relieve the pain of labor. Using patterned breathing in this phase of labor can lead to bearing down before complete dilation and hyperventilation. **Answer 3** is incorrect because this client is *not completely dilated* and it is *inappropriate to bear down* with contractions. Pushing before being completely dilated can cause cervical lacerations and edema of the cervix. **Answer 4 is correct because this client is in the transition phase of the first stage of labor. The proper breathing technique is shallow chest breathing, which prevents hyperventilation and bearing down before she is completely dilated.**

■ TEST-TAKING TIP: *Remember the stages and phases of labor and how the client would respond to latent, active, and transition phases of labor. Knowing what could be the client's expected response will guide appropriate coaching for breathing.*

Content Area: Maternity, Intrapartum; *Integrated Process:* Nursing Process, Implementation; *Cognitive Level:* Application; *Client Need/Subneed:* Physiological Integrity/Basic Care and Comfort/Non-pharmacological Comfort Interventions

60. CORRECT ANSWER: 4. **Answer 1** is incorrect because German measles (rubella) has a teratogenic effect on fetuses. At 25 years of age, pregnancy could be a concern for this nurse. **Answer 2** is incorrect because German measles (rubella) has a teratogenic effect on fetuses. At 32 years of age, pregnancy could be a concern for this nurse. **Answer 3** is incorrect because the nurse is a new graduate, and it may be unlikely that she had experience in caring for a child with German measles (rubella). However, at 45 years of age, pregnancy would be an unlikely concern. **Answer 4 is correct because German measles (rubella) has a teratogenic effect on fetuses. At 50 years of age, this likely would not be a concern. And, the nurse's 25 years of pediatric nursing experience would be a plus in caring for the child.**

■ TEST-TAKING TIP: *The clue is in the age of the nurse. Correlate the most severe side effect of this disease (teratogenic) with the childbearing ages of the nurses.*

Content Area: Child Health, Infectious Disease; *Integrated Process:* Nursing Process, Analysis; *Cognitive Level:* Analysis; *Client Need/Subneed:* Safe and Effective Care Environment/Management of Care/Delegation

61. CORRECT ANSWER: 3. **Answer 1** is incorrect because decorticate posturing may result *from painful* stimulation. **Answer 2** is incorrect because decerebrate posturing, a poor prognostic sign, may occur *with painful stimuli.* **Answer 3 is correct because the lack of response to noxious stimuli signals a deepening coma.** **Answer 4** is incorrect because the Babinski reflex is *not* normally present in adults. If present, it is a *pathologic* response.

■ TEST-TAKING TIP: *Remember that a response to pain is desired.*
Content Area: Adult Health, Neurological; *Integrated Process:* Nursing Process, Analysis; *Cognitive Level:* Application; *Client Need/Subneed:* Physiological Integrity/Physiological Adaptation/Alterations in Body Systems

62. CORRECT ANSWER: 4. **Answer 1** is incorrect because the nurse has the necessary knowledge base to correctly answer the parent's question *without* referring to the pediatrician. **Answer 2** is incorrect because the nurse would not want to answer the parent's question with a *closed-ended response.* It does not provide the parent with needed information and tends to abruptly terminate any communication between the nurse and the parent. **Answer 3** is incorrect because, while a healthy child is a better candidate for surgery than a sick child, this is a *general* response rather than a specific response to this parent's question. **Answer 4 is the correct answer because acute inflammation and infection ("itis") of tonsillar tissue increase the risk of bleeding at the time of surgery. The operative site for a tonsillectomy is highly vascular, with the risk of postoperative bleeding already a concern. An active inflammation and infection would increase this concern.**
■ TEST-TAKING TIP: ***The stem in this question asks for the most accurate response. The most specific response is the most accurate response. Choose the specific pathophysiology-based answer.***
Content Area: Child Health, Pediatric Surgery; *Integrated Process:* Nursing Process, Implementation; *Cognitive Level:* Application; *Client Need/Subneed:* Physiological Integrity/Reduction of Risk Potential/Potential for Complications from Surgical Procedures and Health Alterations

63. CORRECT ANSWER: 3. **Answer 1** is incorrect because the clinical manifestations of weakness in Cushing's syndrome *will interfere* with normal activities. There *will be* mood alterations as a result of the hormone imbalance. **Answer 2** is incorrect because continuing the activity will put the client *at risk* for injury (e.g., fractures). **Answer 3 is correct because the overproduction of adrenocortical hormone results in excessive protein breakdown, causing compression fractures and weakness.** **Answer 4** is incorrect because the *risk for falls* is greatest because of *weakness,* not visual problems, although cataracts and glaucoma may result from Cushing's syndrome.
■ TEST-TAKING TIP: ***The "3 Ss" are signs of Cushing's syndrome—too much* sugar, salt, *and* sex hormone, *which* weaken *the client.***
Content Area: Adult Health, Endocrine; *Integrated Process:* Teaching and Learning; *Cognitive Level:* Application; *Client Need/Subneed:* Physiological Integrity/Physiological Adaptation/Pathophysiology

64. CORRECT ANSWERS: 4, 5, 6. **Answer 1** is incorrect because this change is characteristic of *hypovolemic shock.* **Answer 2** is incorrect because respirations would slow with herniation. Rapid respirations would be characteristic of hypovolemic shock. **Answer 3** is incorrect because blood pressure increases, not decreases. **Answer 4 is correct because bradycardia is one of the vital sign changes with Cushing's triad, a grave sign, indicating herniation of the brainstem and occlusion of the cerebral blood flow if treatment is not initiated. Answer 5 is correct because hypertension occurs with brainstem herniation initially (Cushing's triad)—a widening pulse pressure (Cushing's reflex) occurs earlier in an attempt to overcome the increased intracranial pressure (ICP). Answer 6 is correct because bradypnea accompanies bradycardia and hypertension (Cushing's triad) with brainstem herniation.**
■ TEST-TAKING TIP: ***Recognize a widening of the pulse pressure with Cushing's reflex versus hypertension with Cushing's triad.***
Content Area: Adult Health, Neurological; *Integrated Process:* Nursing Process, Analysis; *Cognitive Level:* Application; *Client Need/Subneed:* Physiological Integrity/Physiological Adaptation/Pathophysiology

65. CORRECT ANSWER: 1. **Answer 1 is correct because primary prophylaxis (the infusion of factor VIII concentrate on a regularly scheduled basis *before* the onset of joint damage) has been proven to be effective in preventing arthropathy.** **Answer 2** is incorrect because primary prophylaxis (the infusion of factor VIII concentrate on a regularly scheduled basis before the onset of joint damage) must be given prior to the development of arthropathy. *Secondary,* not primary, prophylaxis involves the infusion of factor VIII concentrate on a regular basis *after* the child experiences a first joint bleed. **Answer 3** is incorrect because primary prophylaxis (the infusion of factor VIII concentrate on a regularly scheduled basis before the onset of joint damage) is *not associated* with special circumstances, such as surgical procedures, which demand additional factor VIII concentrate at unscheduled times. **Answer 4** is incorrect because, while primary prophylaxis is very costly, organizations such as the National Hemophilia Foundation exist to assist in providing resources for this therapy.
■ TEST-TAKING TIP: ***Think of primary prophylaxis as being "before" the problem occurs, and secondary prophylaxis as being "after" the problem occurs. Note that two answers focus on "after" (Answers 2 and 3) and one answer refers to "before" (Answer 1).***
Content Area: Child Health, Hematological; *Integrated Process:* Teaching and Learning; *Cognitive Level:* Application; *Client Need/Subneed:* Safe and Effective Care Environment/Safety and Infection Control/Accident Prevention and Injury Prevention

PRE-TEST

66. CORRECT ANSWER: 1. Answer 1 is correct because a normal prothrombin time (PT) in a child is 11 to 15 seconds. A value of 14.1 seconds is within *normal* limits and the child is a safe candidate for the surgery. Because the tonsillar operative site is highly vascular, bleeding is a concern and coagulation studies are always conducted prior to the surgery. Since other health-care personnel (e.g., the pediatric surgeon, operating room surgical team, etc.) will also need this information before proceeding with the surgery, the nurse's first action should be to note the laboratory result in the child's chart. **Answer 2** is incorrect because the pediatric surgeon will routinely review the child's chart prior to the surgery, and will specifically look for the results of the prothrombin time (PT) before starting the surgery. There is *no need* for the nurse to notify the pediatric surgeon at this time because the prothrombin time is within *normal* limits. **Answer 3** is incorrect because the prothrombin time (PT) is within normal limits and the surgery *can* take place as planned. If the laboratory results were not within normal limits, the nurse would call the operating room and *notify* them. But, it is *not* the nurse's role to cancel the surgery. It is the pediatric surgeon's responsibility to cancel the surgery if needed. **Answer 4** is incorrect because, while it is safe to release the child to the operating room transporter, the nurse should only do so *after* noting the results of the prothrombin time (PT) in the child's chart.

■ **TEST-TAKING TIP:** *The stem asks for a* priority *nursing action. Eliminate the two options that imply that the laboratory result is a problem (Answers 2 and 3).*

Content Area: Child Health, Pediatric Surgery; ***Integrated Process:*** Nursing Process, Analysis; ***Cognitive Level:*** Application; ***Client Need/Subneed:*** Physiological Integrity/Reduction of Risk Potential/Laboratory Values

67. CORRECT ANSWERS: 3, 5. **Answer 1** is incorrect because hyperglycemia would *not* be expected with adrenal hypofunction. **Answer 2** is incorrect because these findings would be seen with *Cushing's* syndrome, not addisonian crisis. **Answer 3 is correct because addisonian crisis is characterized by cyanosis and signs of circulatory collapse.** **Answer 4** is incorrect because this describes Addison's *disease, not* addisonian *crisis.* **Answer 5 is correct because circulatory collapse occurs with addisonian crisis.**

■ **TEST-TAKING TIP:** *Look for the findings that describe the worst clinical picture—circulatory collapse.*

Content Area: Adult Health, Endocrine; ***Integrated Process:*** Nursing Process, Analysis; ***Cognitive Level:*** Analysis; ***Client Need/Subneed:*** Physiological Integrity/Physiological Adaptation/Medical Emergencies

68. CORRECT ANSWER: 1. Answer 1 is correct because the murmur associated with mitral regurgitation would be best heard at the apex, which is the 5th intercostal space, left midclavicular line. **Answer 2** is incorrect because this is the tricuspid area. Although the murmur associated with mitral regurgitation would be audible in this area, it would be best heard at the apex. **Answer 3** is incorrect because it is the pulmonic area: the second intercostal space, left sternal border. Although the murmur associated with mitral regurgitation *may* be audible throughout the precordium, *pulmonic* and *aortic* valve dysfunction would be best heard in this area. **Answer 4** is incorrect because it is the aortic area: the second intercostal space, right sternal border. Although the murmur associated with mitral regurgitation *may* be audible throughout the precordium, aortic valve dysfunction would be best heard in this area.

■ **TEST-TAKING TIP:** *Key words in the question stem are:* **best** *place and* **mitral.**

Content Area: Adult Health, Cardiovascular; ***Integrated Process:*** Nursing Process, Implementation; ***Cognitive Level:*** Application; ***Client Need/Subneed:*** Physiological Integrity/Reduction of Risk Potential/System Specific Assessments

69. CORRECT ANSWER: 1. Answer 1 is correct because resistance or noncompliance is often related to different priorities or goals. **Answer 2** is incorrect because there is *no evidence* to support this choice. **Answer 3** is incorrect because chronological age is *not* the determinant of rehabilitation potential. **Answer 4** is incorrect because rehabilitation plans may actually begin before surgery. It is unnecessary to wait for the client to feel comfortable changing the dressing.

■ **TEST-TAKING TIP:** *Choose the option that requires further assessment of the situation—a review of the goals.*

Content Area: Geriatrics, Musculoskeletal; ***Integrated Process:*** Nursing Process, Analysis; ***Cognitive Level:*** Application; ***Client Need/Subneed:*** Psychosocial Integrity/Coping Mechanisms

70. CORRECT ANSWER: 2. **Answer 1** is incorrect because a sterile pressure dressing is not necessary for the IV site. It would also be unnecessarily restrictive for the child. **Answer 2 is correct because a child with a low platelet count will have bleeding tendencies. When discontinuing the IV, the nurse should treat the IV site as an arterial puncture and apply direct pressure to the site for a minimum of 5 minutes.** **Answer 3** is incorrect because sending the tip of the IV catheter to the laboratory for a culture would only be necessary when sepsis around the IV catheter is suspected. It would also be unnecessarily expensive and would *not* help the child's bleeding tendencies. **Answer 4** is incorrect because it would be unnecessarily restrictive for the child and would *not* help the child's bleeding tendencies.

■ **TEST-TAKING TIP:** *Remember that a decreased platelet count will cause bleeding tendencies.*

Content Area: Child Health, Hematological; ***Integrated Process:*** Nursing Process, Implementation; ***Cognitive Level:*** Application; ***Client Need/Subneed:*** Physiological Integrity/Reduction of Risk Potential/Potential for Complications of Diagnostic Tests/Treatments/Procedures

71. CORRECT ANSWERS: 1, 2, 4, 5. Answer 1 is correct because this position would *not* promote the drainage of cranial fluids that have accumulated due to increased intracranial pressure. In addition, placing the child on the abdomen (prone) could *prevent an adequate airway* from being maintained. Answer 2 is correct because this position would *not* promote the drainage of cranial fluids that have accumulated due to increased intracranial pressure. In addition, placing the child on the back (supine) could increase the possibility of *aspiration*. **Answer 3** is incorrect because this position *would* promote the drainage of cranial fluids that have accumulated due to increased intracranial pressure. Semi-Fowler's is a position in which the child lies on the back with the trunk elevated at approximately a 45-degree angle. **Answer 4 is correct because this position would *not* promote the drainage of cranial fluids that have accumulated due to increased intracranial pressure. (However, right side-lying would *not* prevent an adequate airway from being maintained or *increase* the possibility of aspiration.) Answer 5 is correct because this position would *not* promote the drainage of cranial fluids that have accumulated due to increased intracranial pressure. (However, left side-lying would *not* prevent an adequate airway from being maintained or *increase* the possibility of aspiration.)**

■ **TEST-TAKING TIP:** *Gravity will assist in the drainage of fluids; select the positions that would prevent or are least likely to accomplish this.*

Content Area: Child Health, Neurological; ***Integrated Process:*** Nursing Process, Implementation; ***Cognitive Level:*** Application; ***Client Need/Subneed:*** Safe and Effective Care Environment/Safety and Infection Control/Accident Prevention and Injury Prevention

72. CORRECT ANSWER: 2. **Answer 1** is incorrect because the client *cannot be forced* to take an oral medication. **Answer 2 is correct because the behavior may be a pattern. Family may have suggestions that will help.** **Answer 3** is incorrect because restraints should be a last resort if at all possible. The *route may* need to be changed. **Answer 4** is incorrect because the behavior may be the result of the brain injury and may not change.

■ **TEST-TAKING TIP:** *Choose an option that recognizes the effect of the brain attack on behavior. Select the option for further assessment ("determine personality before . . .") in an attempt to* understand *the behaviors.*

Content Area: Adult Health, Cardiovascular; ***Integrated Process:*** Nursing Process, Implementation; ***Cognitive Level:*** Application; ***Client Need/Subneed:*** Psychosocial Integrity/Behavioral Interventions

73. CORRECT ANSWER: 1.4. Dose desired (0.07 mg) is to dose on hand (0.05 mg) as amount desired (*x*) is to amount on hand (1 mL): 0.07 mg/0.05 mg = *x*/1 mL; *x* = 1.4 mL.

■ **TEST-TAKING TIP:** *Know the standard ratio and proportion calculations and be careful with decimal points.*

Content Area: Child Health, Cardiovascular; ***Integrated Process:*** Nursing Process, Implementation; ***Cognitive Level:*** Analysis; ***Client Need/Subneed:*** Physiological Integrity/Pharmacological and Parenteral Therapies/Dosage Calculation

74. CORRECT ANSWER: 4. **Answer 1** is incorrect because there may be improvement in the client's perception of pain; however, the concern is about oversedation by the drug. There are sedation scales available that do help the nurse identify the onset of sedation in a client. **Answer 2** is incorrect because the client may be receiving supplemental oxygen. **Answer 3** is incorrect because a client who is oversedated can be awakened and will respond to questions appropriately. **Answer 4 is correct because opioids will depress ventilation, causing a buildup of carbon dioxide in the blood. If hypoventilation is present, measuring the level of carbon dioxide is the most reliable indication of possible respiratory depression. Capnography measures breath-by-breath the level of CO_2 and is most often used during anesthesia, in critical care, and in emergency medicine to prevent respiratory depression. If capnography is not available with the client who is on PCA, monitoring the client's respiratory rate and depth and assessing sedation levels are essential.**

■ **TEST-TAKING TIP:** *This question is asking for the "most reliable" indication. If a client is oversedated, ventilation will be affected. Hypoventilation affects CO_2.*

Content Area: Adult Health, Pain Control; ***Integrated Process:*** Nursing Process, Assessment; ***Cognitive Level:*** Application; ***Client Need/Subneed:*** Physiological Integrity/Pharmacological and Parenteral Therapies/Pharmacological Pain Management

75. CORRECT ANSWER: 3. **Answer 1** is incorrect because the trachea is larger and a partial obstruction would most likely produce a crowing sound. **Answer 2** is incorrect because the wheezing was heard in the left lung. **Answer 3, left bronchus, is correct because wheezes occur when there is partial obstruction of the bronchi or bronchioles. The sound is due to increased vibration of air molecules as they pass over the area that is narrowed or partially obstructed. In this client, the wheezing was heard in the left lung.** **Answer 4** is incorrect because the sound produced by the pleura would be a grating sound called a friction rub. **Answer 5** is incorrect because the sound produced by the pleura would be a grating sound called a friction rub.

■ **TEST-TAKING TIP:** *The question is looking for an area of the lung that, when narrowed, would produce a sound. Think "squeeze" with a "wheeze" as the air moves through a narrow tube—the bronchus or bronchioles.*

Content Area: Adult Health, Respiratory; ***Integrated Process:*** Nursing Process, Assessment; ***Cognitive Level:*** Application; ***Client Need/Subneed:*** Physiological Integrity/Reduction of Risk Potential/System Specific Assessments

Pre-Test 2

Questions

Select the one answer that is best for each question, unless otherwise directed.

1. The parents of a 2-year-old child ask a nurse how to best manage their child's temper tantrums. What advice should the nurse give the parents?
   1. The frequency of tantrums can be reduced with a low-sugar diet.
   2. Tantrums may be prevented by alerting the child in advance about a change in activities.
   3. If the child has a tantrum, it is best to hold the child until he/she is calmed.
   4. Spanking is an effective way to eliminate tantrums.

2. A nurse prepares to administer cardiopulmonary resuscitation (CPR). Which actions should the nurse take? *Place in sequential order.*
   ______ 1. Begin chest compressions.
   ______ 2. Open airway.
   ______ 3. Call for help.
   ______ 4. Check for responsiveness and breathing.
   ______ 5. Position flat on back.
   ______ 6. Check pulse.
   ______ 7. Give two breaths.

3. A client, who is a 24-year-old gravida 6, para 5, delivered a 10-pound, 10-ounce baby 6 hours ago, after a 26-hour labor. Upon assessment, an RN finds the client's fundus is 2 fingerbreadths above the umbilicus and slightly deviated to the right. Based on the information provided, for which complication is this client at risk?
   1. Postpartum hemorrhage.
   2. Mastitis.
   3. Endometriosis.
   4. Thrombophlebitis.

4. A client is seen in an emergency department for rotator cuff tendonitis. What is the correct *immediate* treatment?
   1. Hot packs prn.
   2. Muscle relaxant.
   3. A sling for the arm.
   4. ROM every 4 hours.

5. A 3-year-old child is admitted to an emergency department after being struck by an automobile. A nurse's assessment reveals a child with spontaneous eye opening. The child is confused and does not obey commands but is able to localize pain. The nurse correctly calculates a score of ________ on the Glasgow Coma Scale. *Fill in the blank.*

6. The correct nursing action to prevent infection in a client with an external fixation device for an open fracture is to:
   1. Double-glove for dressing changes.
   2. Scrub pin sites with Betadine.
   3. Give prophylactic antibiotics.
   4. Place on contact isolation.

7. During the active phase of labor, a client, who is a gravida 2, para 0, begins to complain of dizziness, tingling in her fingers, and numbness in her lips. The *most* appropriate nursing intervention for this client would be to:
   1. Have her breathe into a paper bag.
   2. Help her assume a left lateral position in bed.
   3. Instruct her in shallow chest breathing.
   4. Notify the physician immediately.

8. A client has been receiving warfarin (Coumadin) and heparin for 2 days following a total knee arthroplasty. Laboratory results show that INR is 1.2, Hct is 34%. A nurse should:
   1. Hold the Coumadin, continue the heparin.
   2. Hold the heparin, continue the Coumadin.
   3. Hold both drugs and call the physician.
   4. Continue both drugs as ordered.

9. Which assessment finding should a nurse most expect in a newborn infant with a cyanotic heart defect?
   1. Clubbing of fingers and toes.
   2. Tachycardia.
   3. Polycythemia.
   4. Distended neck veins.

10. A client will receive a spinal anesthetic for cesarean birth. As the client discusses the surgery, she asks an RN about the possibility of postanesthesia headaches. Which is the most appropriate response by the RN?
    1. "If there is an allergy to the agent used, headaches may occur."
    2. "Headaches should not be a problem with this type of anesthesia."
    3. "This problem may be prevented by keeping the head of the bed flat."
    4. "Medication is available to counteract headaches and is given as needed."

11. A 50-year-old client, who is overweight, is tested at a health fair and the result of a nonfasting blood sugar is 210 mg/dL. A nurse should:
    1. Encourage re-testing in 1 hour.
    2. Encourage re-testing in 1 week.
    3. Tell the client that follow-up is needed later in the week.
    4. Tell the client that the results are normal.

12. A clinic nurse prepares to administer an IM injection to a school-age child. Which pain management technique would be best suited for this child and should be applied during the procedure?
    1. Guided imagery.
    2. Being held by a parent.
    3. Distraction.
    4. Providing oral sucrose.

13. What advice should a nurse give to a person with type 1 diabetes who is beginning a running program in an effort to get in shape?
1. Administer insulin 30 minutes before running.
2. Rotate injection sites from one thigh to the other each day.
3. Carry a sugar source.
4. Avoid running.

14. How should a nurse caring for an elderly client with receptive and expressive aphasia communicate with the client? *Select all that apply.*
1. Speak loudly.
2. Use a picture board or flash cards.
3. Use hands to communicate.
4. Speak slowly.
5. Encourage the client to initiate meaningful communication.
6. Provide support and encouragement.

15. Which client has the *best* control of diabetes?
1. A client who has trouble sticking to diet and exercising but takes meds regularly. FBS is 132 mg/dL, $HgbA_{1c}$ is 11%.
2. A client who has perfect compliance with diet, exercise, and meds. FBS is 96 mg/dL, $HgbA_{1c}$ is 11%.
3. A client whose diabetes is controlled with diet alone. FBS is 452 mg/dL, $HgbA_{1c}$ is 12%.
4. A client who has trouble remembering meds, but good compliance with diet and exercise. FBS is 110 mg/dL, $HgbA_{1c}$ is 7%.

16. A client, who is 17 years old, has delivered a 6-pound, 6-ounce girl at 38 weeks' gestation 3 hours ago. A nurse is completing a routine postpartum assessment. Which assessments should the nurse report to a physician *immediately*? *Select all that apply.*
1. Positive Homans' sign.
2. 2+ deep tendon reflexes.
3. Moderate rubra lochia.
4. Expression of orange-sized clots during fundal massage.
5. Fundus palpable firm at the level of the umbilicus.

17. If a client's blood *sugar* is lowered too rapidly, for what manifestation or dangerous outcome should a nurse observe?
1. Glycosuria.
2. Hyperkalemia.
3. Hypertensive crisis.
4. Confusion from cerebral edema.

18. A nurse assesses a child diagnosed with measles. Which symptom is the nurse *least* likely to observe in a child diagnosed with measles?
1. Slapped cheek appearance.
2. Fever and general malaise.
3. Rash on face, trunk, and limbs.
4. White and red spots on buccal mucosa.

19. Health teaching for a client who is newly diagnosed with diabetes should include:
1. Notify health care provider immediately if the blood sugar is over 150 mg/dL.
2. Call provider if breath smells fruity.
3. Hold insulin if unable to eat.
4. Check blood sugar every hour if sick.

20. A client, who is gravida 3, para 1, is 6 cm dilated, 80% effaced, and a 0 station. The external fetal monitor shows baseline heart rate of 145 bpm, moderate variability, and variable decelerations. What are appropriate nursing interventions for this client? *Select all that apply.*
1. Perform a sterile vaginal exam.
2. Change the client's position.
3. Prepare the client for an emergency cesarean delivery.
4. Administer a fluid bolus.
5. Prepare for a vacuum-assisted delivery.

21. Following a nephrectomy, which complication does a client have the *greatest* risk of developing?
1. Altered nutrition related to NPO status and postoperative ileus.
2. Possible kidney stones related to urinary stasis.
3. Pedal and periorbital edema related to nephrotic syndrome.
4. Possible altered gas exchange related to shallow breathing from pain.

22. An infant is admitted for pyloric stenosis. Which symptoms should a nurse expect to find? *Select all that apply.*
1. Metabolic alkalosis.
2. Olive-shaped mass palpable in the upper right quadrant of abdomen.
3. History of projectile vomiting.
4. Bile-stained vomitus.
5. Decreased urine specific gravity.
6. Small, infrequent stools.

23. A postpartum nurse instructed a client on proper perineal care after delivery of a healthy neonate vaginally after a midline episiotomy. Which client activities should indicate to the nurse that the client has understood the instructions? *Select all that apply.*
1. The client changes her peri pads every 8 hours.
2. The client consistently uses the peri bottle to clean the perineum after each void or bowel movement.
3. The client wipes from back to front after each bowel movement.
4. The client sprays water from the peri bottle directly into the vagina.
5. The client uses the antiseptic spray after rinsing with the peri bottle.

24. Older adults often present with atypical assessment findings. Which symptom will an older adult with a urinary tract infection (UTI) most often develop *first*?
1. Anorexia.
2. Confusion.
3. Fever.
4. Restlessness.

25. While visiting a local park, a nurse witnesses the collapse of a preschool-age child. The nurse assesses the child and finds no pulse and no respirations. The nurse begins compressions. At what rate per minute should the nurse deliver the compressions?
1. 25 compressions per minute.
2. 50 compressions per minute.
3. 75 compressions per minute.
4. 100 compressions per minute.

26. A client reports sharp pain in the calf of the left leg when walking to the bathroom. A nurse notes that the leg has a confined area of warmth, tenderness, and redness. Which nursing action is *most* appropriate for this client?
1. Encouraging the client to ambulate to increase circulation.
2. Instructing the client to massage the affected area to relieve the tenderness.
3. Applying cold packs to the affected area to decrease inflammation.
4. Elevating the affected extremity to promote venous blood flow.

27. A graduate nurse has been working on a medical unit for 3 months. The nurse manager has posted the team leader assignments for the following week. The graduate nurse knows that the major responsibility of the team leader is to:
Select all that apply.
1. Know the condition of the clients on the team.
2. Prioritize the needs of the clients on the team.
3. Supervise the direct care of the nursing assistants.
4. Document the assessments completed by the team members.
5. Make the team assignments for the clients' care.
6. Provide care to the clients who are most acutely ill on the team.

28. A woman has chosen a patch applied to her skin as her method to deliver contraceptive medication. A nurse should instruct the client to call the clinic *immediately* if the client experiences:
Select all that apply.
1. Mild to moderate nausea during the day following the application of the patch.
2. Chloasma.
3. Pain in the legs while walking.
4. Headache unrelieved by acetaminophen.
5. Swelling of the feet and hands.

29. Suddenly, during a labor contraction, a pregnant client experiences a gush of amniotic fluid. Which assessment finding should indicate to a nurse that the client is experiencing a deviation from normal labor patterns?
1. Colored amniotic fluid.
2. Fetal bradycardia with contractions.
3. The client complains of nausea and vomits.
4. The client becomes diaphoretic and irritable.

30. A nurse auscultates the lungs of a client diagnosed with right middle lobe pneumonia. Where should the nurse place the stethoscope where crackles would most likely be heard?

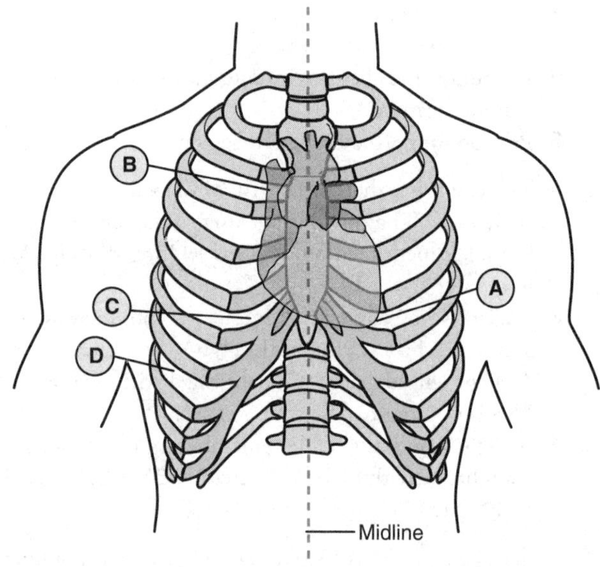

1. A.
2. B.
3. C.
4. D.

31. A nurse provides health teaching to the parents of a school-age child diagnosed with attention deficit-hyperactivity disorder (ADHD). What should the nurse include in the teaching plan?
1. One parent should be responsible for discipline.
2. Prescription bottles should be stored where the child can access for self-care.
3. The home's televisions and radios should be kept at a low to moderate volume.
4. Participation in outdoor sports should be avoided.
5. Medications should be taken daily only as needed.

32. A client with a 6-month history of burning pain and weakness to the thumb and first and middle fingers has a carpal tunnel release done with regional anesthesia. In the PACU, the *priority* nursing assessment should be:
1. Orientation to person, place, time, situation.
2. Brachial pulse.
3. Color, temperature, movement of the fingers.
4. Pupil reaction to light.

33. A client, who is a primigravida, is 6 cm dilated, 100% effaced, and a −3 station. She suddenly has a gush of fluid. Which nursing assessments indicate a complication and should be reported to a physician? *Select all that apply.*

1. Green-tinged fluid.
2. Copious amount of vernix in clear fluid.
3. Decrease in the fetal heart rate baseline from 140 to 100 bpm.
4. Increase in the fetal heart rate baseline to 170 bpm.
5. Small amount of clear fluid.

34. Which conditions would most likely contribute to an increase in a client's need for oxygen (O_2)? *Select all that apply.*

1. Burns over trunk and legs.
2. Hypothermia from environmental exposure.
3. Shivering secondary to an elevated temperature.
4. Agitation associated with anxiety.
5. Neuromuscular blockage during anesthesia.
6. Thyrotoxicosis secondary to Graves' disease.

35. A nurse prepares to administer a Denver II developmental assessment on a toddler. In which order should the nurse complete the assessment? *Place in sequential order.*

________ **1.** Ask child to name doll's body parts.
________ **2.** Ask caregiver if the child uses a spoon and fork.
________ **3.** Ask the child to build a tower of 2 cubes.
________ **4.** Advise caregiver that the assessment is not an IQ test.
________ **5.** Have child kick ball forward.

36. A primigravida presents to a labor and delivery unit at 30 weeks' gestation. Her major complaints are abdominal pain, vaginal bleeding, and dysuria. Which interventions or assessments should a nurse perform when caring for this client? *Select all that apply.*

1. Call the physician for pain medication.
2. Place the client on an external fetal monitor.
3. Obtain a specimen for fern test.
4. Obtain a clean-catch urine specimen.
5. Perform a vaginal exam for cervical dilation.

37. Which conditions would potentially contribute to decreases in cardiac output? *Select all that apply.*

1. Early septic shock.
2. Gastrointestinal bleeding.
3. Congestive heart failure.
4. Use of positive end-expiratory pressure.
5. Regular aerobic exercise.
6. Myocardial infarction.

38. The parents of a child isolated with scarlet fever ask a nurse. "Why didn't our child get a vaccine for this disease?" The nurse's best response is:

1. "The disease is bacterial in nature and responds well to antibiotics."
2. "A vaccine is in development."
3. "Consult your pediatrician as to why the vaccine was not given."
4. "This disease is not communicable; therefore, a vaccine is not necessary."

39. The K^+ level of a client in acute renal failure is 6.8 mEq/L. Which treatments will decrease the potassium level? *Select all that apply.*

1. Rapid infusion of 50% dextrose.
2. Sodium bicarbonate IV.
3. Regular insulin in D_5W.
4. Kayexalate retention enema.
5. Albuterol sulfate (Ventolin) by nebulizer.

40. A client, who is 38 years old, gravida 5, para 0, with type 1 diabetes, is 13 weeks pregnant. Her hemoglobin A_{1c} level is 8.2%. She is attending a prenatal class for clients with high-risk pregnancies. Which possible complications should a nurse anticipate in this client? *Select all that apply.*

1. Oligohydramnios.
2. Polyhydramnios.
3. Macrosomia.
4. Congenital anomalies of the spine.
5. Preeclampsia.

41. A client sustains multiple fractures following a motor vehicle accident. The client is intubated and on a mechanical ventilator. Chest x-ray reveals diffuse bilateral pulmonary infiltrates. The ratio of fractional concentration of inspired oxygen to arterial oxygen concentration (PaO_2/FIO_2 ratio) is 174, central venous pressure (CVP) is 5 mm Hg, and pulmonary capillary wedge pressure (PCWP) is 10 mm Hg. What interventions would be most appropriate for the client? *Select all that apply.*

1. Antibiotic therapy.
2. Addition of positive end-expiratory pressure (PEEP) to ventilator.
3. Prone positioning of client.
4. Inotropic or vasopressor drugs.
5. Heparin drip.
6. Neuromuscular blockade with pancuronium (Pavalon).

42. A client is admitted to labor and delivery with a diagnosis of placental abruption. A nursing priority for this client is to minimize alterations in fetal tissue perfusion. A nurse recognizes that this goal has been met when which finding is noted?

1. Presence of accelerations.
2. Consistent decreased fetal heart rate variability.
3. Evidence of prolonged fetal bradycardia.
4. Presence of consistent late decelerations.

43. Which findings should indicate to a nurse that a traumatic brain injury has resulted in brain death? *Select all that apply.*

1. No response to the cold caloric test.
2. Glasgow Coma Scale (GCS) score of 6.
3. Electroencephalogram (EEG) tracing is flat.
4. Positive gag reflex.
5. No spontaneous respirations.

44. A home health nurse visits a child with hemophilia following a dental extraction. Which medication would the nurse suggest be removed from the family's bathroom medicine cabinet?
1. Acetaminophen.
2. Corticosteroid.
3. Ibuprofen.
4. Epsilon-aminocaproic acid.

45. Following surgery for appendicitis, a client develops peritonitis. Which signs or symptoms should a nurse identify as being consistent with peritonitis? *Select all that apply.*
1. Shallow respirations.
2. Abdominal rigidity.
3. Hyperactive bowel sounds.
4. Abdominal pain.
5. Increased flatus.

46. A nurse is preparing to administer intravenous magnesium sulfate to a client diagnosed with preeclampsia. Which action should the nurse take when administering this medication?
1. Administer a solution of 20 gm magnesium sulfate in 100 mL of lactated Ringer's solution.
2. Monitor maternal VS, FHR, and uterine contractions every hour.
3. Expect the maintenance dose to be approximately 4 gm/hr.
4. Discontinue the infusion and notify the physician of a respiratory rate of <12 breaths/min.

47. When would a client with community-acquired pneumonia be clinically stable enough to change from IV antibiotics to oral antibiotics? When the client has a(n):
1. Temperature of 96.8°F (36°C) or lower.
2. O_2 saturation of at least 80%.
3. Systolic blood pressure that stays at 90 mm Hg or higher.
4. Heart rate that remains at 120 beats/min or lower.

48. An adolescent with hemophilia sustains a bilateral lower extremity injury and is hospitalized. Which selection on the adolescent's lunch menu indicates the need for further dietary counseling by the nurse?
1. A yogurt and fruit plate.
2. A cheeseburger and coleslaw.
3. A slice of cheese pizza and a tossed green salad.
4. A scoop of pasta salad and a cup of vegetable soup.

49. A 44-year-old client has just found out that she is pregnant. The client knows that she is at a higher risk for carrying a fetus with a chromosomal abnormality. Which genetic test for chromosomal abnormalities should a nurse recommend to provide the client with chromosomal results within the first trimester?
1. Genetic karyotyping.
2. Amniocentesis.
3. Chorionic villus sampling (CVS).
4. Ultrasonography.

50. The parents of a baby boy, who is newly diagnosed with hemophilia, state "This can't be true! No one in our family has hemophilia." A nurse's most factual response would be:
1. "You are right. Additional testing is necessary to rule out a diagnostic error."
2. "Difficult as it is, you must try and accept the diagnosis."
3. "Only about 60% of affected children have a positive history for the disease."
4. "Up to one third of all hemophilia cases may be caused by a gene mutation."

51. Which is the most important *initial* nursing action for a client with community-acquired pneumonia?
1. Maintain IV site used for antibiotic therapy.
2. Assess for indications of antibiotic effectiveness.
3. Assist with client mobility.
4. Assess for pain and treat as ordered.

52. A client, who is a primigravida at 39 weeks' gestation, is being instructed on when she should come to the hospital. Which instructions should a nurse include? *Select all that apply.*
1. "Come to the hospital if you are feeling decreased fetal movement."
2. "Come to the hospital when the contractions are regular, about 5 minutes apart, lasting about 60 seconds."
3. "Come to the hospital when you think your amniotic fluid is leaking."
4. "Come to the hospital when you feel increased fetal movement."
5. "Come to the hospital when the contractions are 10–15 minutes apart lasting about 30 seconds."

53. What type of dressing should a nurse use on a stage I pressure ulcer?
1. Wet to dry.
2. Wet.
3. Dry.
4. None.

54. Which pediatrician's orders for a newborn boy with a family history of hemophilia should a nurse question?
1. Administer hepatitis B vaccine.
2. Delay circumcision at this time.
3. Schedule series of well-infant appointments at time of discharge from birth hospital.
4. Finger or heel punctures for blood draws only.

55. A client, who is a primigravida, delivered a healthy neonate by vacuum-assisted vaginal delivery after 24 hours of labor. A nurse is performing a routine postpartum assessment 12 hours later and finds the following vital signs: blood pressure, 118/76 mm Hg; temperature, 100.8°F; pulse, 102; respirations, 20. Which interventions would be appropriate for this client? *Select all that apply.*

1. Call the physician.
2. Encourage her to increase her fluid intake.
3. Assess her fundal height.
4. Assess her lochia.
5. Encourage her to bottle-feed.

56. Causation is an element that must be demonstrated by the plaintiff in a suit against a nurse for professional malpractice. Under what circumstance will the actions of the nurse be determined to be within a legal causal connection? *Select all that apply.*

1. Only if the nurse's action directly causes the harm.
2. If the harm caused was a foreseeable consequence of the nurse's action.
3. If the nurse is named in the lawsuit.
4. If the nurse was involved in any of the client's care.
5. When the nurse did not follow the standards of care and harm was caused.
6. If the nurse performed harmful actions while taking narcotic medications.

57. A toddler, who had a blood lead level (BLL) test result of <10 mcg/dL 1 year ago, presents in the pediatrician's office with a level of 48 mcg/dL. The nurse should anticipate the need for a/an:

1. EEG.
2. CBC.
3. Abdominal x-ray.
4. Chest x-ray.

58. During change of shift, a day shift nurse states that all of a client's urine is to be strained. The evening nurse knows that straining is ordered because:

1. Intake and output will be more accurate.
2. The client has been having difficulty voiding.
3. The composition of renal calculi needs to be identified.
4. Blood clots have been affecting the accuracy of the urinalysis.

59. A 22-year-old client, who is gravida 1, para 0, is attending a routine 38-week prenatal visit. A physician gives the client instructions about when to come to the hospital for evaluation of onset of labor. A nurse evaluates that the client has understood the instructions when she states:

1. "I should go to the hospital when my contractions are less than 2 minutes apart."
2. "I should go to the hospital when I have back pain and an increased vaginal discharge."
3. "I should go to the hospital when I have abdominal pain and painful urination."
4. "I should go to the hospital when my contractions are 5 minutes apart for an hour."

60. A nurse is caring for a client with second-degree burns of both arms. Which care need will be more challenging because of the location of the burn?

1. Reducing risk for immunosuppression and infection.
2. Reducing potential for contractures and deformity.
3. Establishing IV access for administration of fluids.
4. Assessment of vital signs, including blood pressure.

61. A nurse prepares to administer *N*-acetylcysteine (Mucomyst) to a child who ingested a toxic dose of acetaminophen (Tylenol). What equipment will the nurse need to gather in order to administer the medication?

1. An IV setup.
2. An IM setup.
3. A glass of water.
4. A glass of juice.

62. A client, who is gravida 1, para 0 at 35 weeks' gestation, delivered her infant 1 day ago by cesarean section for breech presentation. The infant was admitted to the nursery for unstable blood sugar. Which action by a nurse would be the most appropriate to promote the attachment process between mother and infant?

1. Take pictures of the baby for the mother to see.
2. Take the mother to the nursery and encourage her to participate in his care.
3. Take the mother to the nursery window to see her baby.
4. Tell the mother her baby is very cute and give her an update on his progress.

63. A 3-year-old child has ingested some "pink pills" in an unlabeled bottle found on the floor of the garage. In what order should a nurse correctly perform a gastric lavage and administration of activated charcoal?

1. Perform the gastric lavage and then administer the activated charcoal.
2. Administer the activated charcoal and then perform the gastric lavage.
3. Perform the gastric lavage, leave the saline solution in the stomach, and administer the activated charcoal.
4. Question the order because gastric lavage and activated charcoal are not used together.

64. A client asks a nurse how soon after bowel surgery normal bowel function will return. The best response by the nurse would be:

1. "By 72 hours you should start to pass gas."
2. "Around 48 hours, if there are no complications."
3. "Some function will return by 12 hours."
4. "You'll pass gas by 24 hours."

65. A client is in active labor at 38 weeks' gestation. She requests an epidural for labor pain. Which actions should a nurse take to prepare for this procedure? *Select all that apply.*
1. Sit client upright on the side of the bed.
2. Start a bolus of IV solution.
3. Obtain baseline vital signs.
4. Allow client to empty her bladder.
5. Obtain an informed consent for the procedure.
6. Perform a procedural pause before starting epidural.

66. A teenager with sickle cell anemia tells a clinic nurse that the school has arranged for a nature hike in the nearby mountains. The teen excitedly shows the nurse a new water bottle that has been purchased just for this trip. Which *initial* response by the nurse would be most appropriate?
1. "You realize that this kind of hike might send you into a pain crisis, don't you?"
2. "You should not attend the hike unless you get approval from the physician first."
3. "It's great that you are preparing to hydrate properly on your hike. How else have you planned for the hike?"
4. "That sounds like a lot of fun and is terrific exercise. What do your parents think?"

67. A client, who is diabetic, is scheduled for discharge. A nurse should recognize the need for further teaching if the client states:
1. "I take my oral hypoglycemics during the day because I sleep 8 hours at night."
2. "I've had diabetes for 15 years, and I've never had any problems until now."
3. "I live alone, so I use the microwave often to prepare my meals."
4. "I had been taking a name brand drug, but the generic brand costs less."

68. The lips and oral cavity of a child who ingested a corrosive substance are blistered, peeling, and swollen. The *priority* action for a nurse in the emergency department is to:
1. Keep child NPO.
2. Administer an analgesic.
3. Prepare to induce vomiting.
4. Maintain a patent airway.

69. A client, who is gravida 8, para 7, has saturated three perineal pads with bright red blood during the first hour after delivery. What are appropriate nursing actions for this client? *Select all that apply.*
1. Administer oxytocin.
2. Massage the fundus.
3. Have the client empty her bladder.
4. Administer tocolytics.
5. Check vital signs.

70. Which types of congenital heart disease are characterized by blood flow from right to left? *Select all that apply.*
1. Atrial septal defect.
2. Transposition of the great vessels.
3. Coarctation of the aorta.
4. Tricuspid atresia.
5. Truncus arteriosus.
6. Patent ductus arteriosus.
7. Tetralogy of Fallot.

71. An older client is scheduled to go home following hospitalization for thrombophlebitis. When a nurse offers the client the daily warfarin tablet, the client refuses the medication. The best response by the nurse would be:
1. "You must take the pill as ordered by your doctor."
2. "You have taken this every morning for a week."
3. "Do you want to end up back in the hospital for another week?"
4. "Tell me about your concerns with your medication."

72. A client, who is gravida 7, para 6, delivered an infant at 39 weeks' gestation approximately 14 hours ago. Which assessment finding indicates normal postpartum progression?
1. Firm fundus at the umbilicus and midline with moderate lochia rubra.
2. Firm fundus 1–2 fingerbreadths above the umbilicus and midline with moderate lochia rubra.
3. Firm fundus 1–2 fingerbreadths above the umbilicus and deviated to the right side with large lochia rubra.
4. Firm fundus 3–4 fingerbreadths below the umbilicus and midline with scant lochia rubra.

73. A client has not been following the drug regimen for control of gastroesophageal reflux disease (GERD). The best approach by a nurse to improve compliance would be to:
1. Give the client a choice rather than a directive on when to take the medication.
2. Ensure that the client understands the expected outcome from the drug regimen.
3. Encourage the client to follow the goals set by the physician for optimal management of GERD.
4. Ask the physician or pharmacist to meet with the client prior to discharge.

74. A nurse is performing health teaching with the parents of a 16-month-old child who has tetralogy of Fallot. Which steps should the nurse advise the parents to take to properly respond to a "tet spell"? *Select all that apply.*
1. Call EMS.
2. Sit the child in a chair.
3. Learn CPR.
4. Administer aspirin.
5. Ask the child to cough.
6. Place child on the side with knees to chest.

75. A client, who is 19 years old, gravida 1, para 0, is admitted to labor and delivery at 30 weeks' gestation. The client reports nausea and vomiting, epigastric pain, and a headache. Her vital signs are temperature: 98.8°F, pulse: 78, respirations: 20, and blood pressure: 170/110 mm Hg. Her laboratory values are as follows: WBC: 4.5, hematocrit: 30, platelets: 88,000, AST: 146, ALT: 120. What other assessments should a nurse perform on this client? *Select all that apply.*

1. Deep tendon reflexes.
2. Sterile vaginal exam.
3. Sterile speculum exam.
4. Fern test.
5. Urine protein test.

Answers/Rationales/Tips

1. **CORRECT ANSWER: 2.** **Answer 1** is incorrect because tantrums are related to the child's developmental stage, not his/her diet. **Answer 2 is correct because toddlers may have temper tantrums to express their frustration. Sudden changes in activities should be avoided, and the toddler should be given forewarning about what is coming next.** **Answer 3** is incorrect because tantrums should be ignored. By holding the child, the parents will be providing reinforcement of the tantrum behavior. **Answer 4** is incorrect because even negative reinforcement can reinforce the tantrum behavior. Additionally, spanking should be avoided and it is inappropriate for the nurse to recommend corporal punishment as a behavior modification technique.

■ **TEST-TAKING TIP:** *The key word to the best answer is "prevent." Recall that the toddler needs to be autonomous. By providing the child with information about coming activities, the child will feel more in control and will be less likely to become frustrated.*

Content Area: Child Health, Growth and Development; ***Integrated Process:*** Nursing Process, Implementation; ***Cognitive Level:*** Application; ***Client Need/Subneed:*** Health Promotion and Maintenance/Developmental Stages and Transitions

2. **CORRECT ANSWERS: 4, 3, 6, 5, 1, 2, 7. After determining that the client is nonresponsive and not breathing or is gasping for air, the nurse or someone else calls for help. The pulse is palpated for 10 seconds, and if no pulse is palpated, the client is positioned properly to perform CPR. The order is: 30 chest compressions at 100/min, open the airway, and then 2 breaths. ABC has been changed to CAB; the emphasis is on chest compressions.**

■ **TEST-TAKING TIP:** *Remember: the heart is the first priority.*

Content Area: Adult Health, Cardiovascular; ***Integrated Process:*** Nursing Process, Implementation; ***Cognitive Level:*** Application ***Client Need/Subneed:*** Physiological Integrity/Physiological Adaptation/Medical Emergencies

3. **CORRECT ANSWER: 1. Answer 1 is correct because this client's fundus is higher than expected for this stage after delivery and is deviated to the right, indicating she has a full bladder that can impede the uterus from contracting adequately. This can result in a postpartum hemorrhage.** **Answer 2** is incorrect because this client is not a high risk for mastitis based on the information provided. Mastitis is a breast infection that can result from cracked or sore nipples or failure to fully drain the breast. **Answer 3** is incorrect because endometriosis is a proliferation of endometrial tissue, not related to the delivery of an infant. **Answer 4** is incorrect because thrombophlebitis is a risk factor for *all* women who are pregnant; this client is not at any increased risk because of her history with this delivery.

■ **TEST-TAKING TIP:** *Eliminate complications that are common to* **all** *women who are pregnant, but not directly related to this client's specific risk factors.*

Content Area: Maternity, Postpartum; ***Integrated Process:*** Nursing Process, Analysis; ***Cognitive Level:*** Analysis; ***Client Need/Subneed:*** Physiological Integrity/Reduction of Risk Potential/Potential for Complications from Surgical Procedures and Health Alterations

4. **CORRECT ANSWER: 3.** **Answer 1** is incorrect because heat *increases* swelling. **Answer 2** is incorrect because pain control may be required, but muscle spasm is *not* the source of the pain. **Answer 3 is correct because the injured tissue needs to be immobilized.** **Answer 4** is incorrect because the injured tissue should be *immobilized* and rested.

■ **TEST-TAKING TIP:** *Look for an option that* **rests the extremity.**

Content Area: Adult Health, Musculoskeletal; ***Integrated Process:*** Nursing Process, Implementation; ***Cognitive Level:*** Application; ***Client Need/Subneed:*** Physiological Integrity/Basic Care and Comfort/Assistive Devices

5. **CORRECT ANSWER: 13. To arrive at the correct score on the Glasgow Coma Scale (GCS), recall that the scale is composed of three scoring areas: eye opening (ranges from 1 to 4), best motor response (ranges from 1 to 6), and best auditory/visual response (ranges from 1 to 5). This child receives the maximum score of 4 for spontaneous eye opening, a score of 5 out of 6 for motor response, and 4 out of 5 for auditory/visual response.**

■ **TEST-TAKING TIP:** *Remember that the lowest score an individual can receive on the GCS is 3 (no eye opening and no motor nor auditory/visual response) and the highest is 15.*

Content Area: Child Health, Neurological; ***Integrated Process:*** Nursing Process, Assessment; ***Cognitive Level:*** Analysis; ***Client Need/Subneed:*** Physiological Integrity/Physiological Adaptation/Alterations in Body Systems

6. CORRECT ANSWER: 3. **Answer 1** is incorrect because infections are generally introduced into the wound during the initial trauma and surgery. Although it is possible that infections could be introduced during postoperative wound care, double-gloving would not reduce the risk. **Answer 2** is incorrect because pin site care is controversial. Some surgeons prefer that pins be surrounded with scabs to protect the tissue. Some prefer cleansing with Betadine; however, it is irritating to tissue. **Answer 3 is correct because open fractures create opportunities for microbes to enter the wound. Antibiotics throughout the perioperative period reduce the risk.** **Answer 4** is incorrect because contact isolation is used to prevent transmission of infection to other clients from the client who is isolated. It could not protect the client who is isolated.

■ TEST-TAKING TIP: *Look for clues in the stem, such as "prevent," and a similar word in the options—"prophylactic."*

Content Area: Adult Health, Musculoskeletal; *Integrated Process:* Nursing Process, Planning; *Cognitive Level:* Comprehension; *Client Need/Subneed:* Physiological Integrity/Reduction of Risk Potential/Potential for Complications of Diagnostic Tests/Treatments/Procedures

7. CORRECT ANSWER: 1. **Answer 1 is correct because this client is hyperventilating, resulting in a reduction of carbon dioxide in her blood and causing her symptoms. Having her breathe into a paper bag will increase the carbon dioxide in her blood and alleviate the symptoms.** **Answer 2** is incorrect because helping her to assume a left lateral position in bed will not increase carbon dioxide in her blood. **Answer 3** is incorrect because shallow chest breathing is a form of hyperventilation and will not reverse the imbalance between the oxygen and carbon dioxide levels in the lungs. This imbalance delivers less oxygen to the brain, the heart, and the rest of the body. **Answer 4** is incorrect because this situation can be resolved using nursing interventions that do not require calling the physician.

■ TEST-TAKING TIP: ***When calling the physician is one of the options, consider why you are calling the physician and what assessment information you need before calling. If you cannot identify why you would call the physician and what you want him/her to do about the situation, eliminate the option.***

Content Area: Maternity, Intrapartum; *Integrated Process:* Nursing Process, Implementation; *Cognitive Level:* Analysis; *Client Need/Subneed:* Physiological Integrity/Physiological Adaptation/Alterations in Body Systems

8. CORRECT ANSWER: 4. **Answer 1** is incorrect because the goal is a therapeutic international normalized ratio (INR). Coumadin will be needed to maintain an INR of about 2. **Answer 2** is incorrect because the quick-acting drug, heparin, acts as an anticoagulant "bridge" until the slower onset of Coumadin achieves therapeutic levels. **Answer 3** is incorrect because the client needs anticoagulation, being at high risk for clots. There is no evidence that a contraindication for these drugs exists, such as bleeding. **Answer 4 is correct because clients having knee surgery are at very high risk for thrombus formation and need anticoagulation. Coumadin is convenient because it can be taken for several days of therapy before achieving therapeutic results (an INR level of 2). Until achieved, the quicker acting drug, heparin, is also used.**

■ TEST-TAKING TIP: *Look at the verbs: three "hold" and one "continue." Choose the option that is different in this case.*

Content Area: Adult Health, Musculoskeletal; *Integrated Process:* Nursing Process, Implementation; *Cognitive Level:* Application; *Client Need/Subneed:* Physiological Integrity/Reduction of Risk Potential/Laboratory Values

9. CORRECT ANSWER: 2. **Answer 1** is incorrect because clubbing in fingers and toes will not be evident in an infant. This symptom develops over time and would be expected in an *older* child. **Answer 2 is correct because the newborn with a cyanotic heart defect will most likely experience tachycardia as the heart attempts to improve oxygenation.** **Answer 3** is incorrect because polycythemia *may not* develop *right away,* while tachycardia is present at birth. **Answer 4** is incorrect because distended neck veins are not always present in infants with cyanotic defects even if the infant is in congestive heart failure.

■ TEST-TAKING TIP: *The key word in the stem of the question is "newborn." The correct response should take into account the infant's young age and the fact that the child has not suffered from congenital heart disease for an extended period of time.*

Content Area: Child Health, Cardiovascular; *Integrated Process:* Nursing Process, Assessment; *Cognitive Level:* Analysis; *Client Need/Subneed:* Physiological Integrity/Physiological Adaptation/Pathophysiology

10. CORRECT ANSWER: 3. **Answer 1** is incorrect because, although medication allergies can cause problems, in this case, the headache is due to a spinal needle that creates a passage for the spinal fluid to leak out, changing the fluid pressure around the brain and spinal cord. If enough of the fluid leaks out, a spinal headache may develop. **Answer 2** is incorrect because spinal headaches are one of the common side effects of spinal anesthesia. This answer is inappropriate to tell the client. **Answer 3 is correct because keeping the head of the bed flat can alleviate the headache caused by the difference in pressure. Sitting up can make the headache worse by increasing the pressure difference.** **Answer 4** is incorrect because medication does not provide relief when the origin of the headache is a difference in pressure. A blood patch can be used to stop the leakage of spinal fluid, seal the leak, and alleviate the pressure difference.

■ TEST-TAKING TIP: *Eliminate the answer that provides false information to the client. Choose the one answer that is a specific action that the nurse can take.*

Content Area: Maternity, Intrapartum; *Integrated Process:* Teaching and Learning; *Cognitive Level:* Application; *Client*

Need/Subneed: Physiological Integrity/Reduction of Risk Potential/Potential for Alterations in Body Systems

11. CORRECT ANSWER: 3. **Answer 1** is incorrect because this client's high blood sugar needs *more immediate* follow-up, not just retesting. **Answer 2** is incorrect because this client's high blood sugar needs *more immediate* follow-up by a health-care provider. Answer 3 is correct because this is high, even for a nonfasting sample, and is suggestive of diabetes. The client should be seen soon. **Answer 4** is incorrect because this blood sugar *exceeds* normal limits and is suggestive of diabetes.

■ TEST-TAKING TIP: *By recalling the normal range for non-fasting blood sugar levels, Answer 4 can be eliminated as 210 mg/dL is not normal. Select between: "week," "1 year," or "3 years," and choose the ASAP time frame.*

Content Area: Adult Health, Endocrine; *Integrated Process:* Nursing Process, Implementation; *Cognitive Level:* Application; *Client Need/Subneed:* Physiological Integrity/Reduction of Risk Potential/Laboratory Values

12. CORRECT ANSWER: 1. Answer 1 is correct because the school-age child is old enough to understand and comply with instructions regarding guided imagery, a technique to help the child focus on a pleasant mental image during the procedure. **Answer 2** is incorrect because this technique would most likely be utilized with a *younger* child. **Answer 3** is incorrect because this technique would most likely be utilized with a *younger* child. **Answer 4** is incorrect because this technique would most likely be utilized with an *infant.*

■ TEST-TAKING TIP: *Remember that a school-age child's age range is from 6 to 12 years. If the answer is not suitable for a child up to 12 years of age, it cannot be the correct option.*

Content Area: Child Health, Pain Control; *Integrated Process:* Nursing Process, Implementation; *Cognitive Level:* Application; *Client Need/Subneed:* Physiological Integrity/Basic Care and Comfort/Non-pharmacological Comfort Interventions

13. CORRECT ANSWER: 3. **Answer 1** is incorrect because exercise facilitates glucose uptake into cells independent of insulin. Until the client is able to establish his/her own response, it is advisable to use pre-exercise insulin sparingly, if at all. **Answer 2** is incorrect because, although rotation of insulin sites is important, it is not related to exercise. A person with diabetes should pick one location (such as the right thigh) and rotate injections within that site before switching to another. Answer 3 is correct because people with diabetes should carry a sugar source, especially when beginning an exercise program. Exercise facilitates glucose uptake into cells independent of insulin. If the client took a regular dose of insulin before exercising, the client could become hypoglycemic. **Answer 4** is incorrect because exercise *is* beneficial for diabetes. It should be monitored but *not* prevented.

■ TEST-TAKING TIP: *First, eliminate the two options that focus on* insulin *administration. Next, eliminate the answer that means "do not exercise." Choose a prn option:* carry a sugar *source.*

Content Area: Adult Health, Endocrine; *Integrated Process:* Nursing Process, Implementation; *Cognitive Level:* Application; *Client Need/Subneed:* Physiological Integrity/Physiological Adaptation/Illness Management

14. CORRECT ANSWERS: 2, 3, 4. **Answer 1** is incorrect because the nurse needs to speak distinctly, *not* loudly. Answer 2 is correct because a visual mode is helpful when the client has difficulty hearing (auditory aphasia, receptive) or writing (expressive aphasia, visual). Answer 3 is correct because using gestures such as pointing is one way to establish and encourage communication. Answer 4 is correct because facing the client and speaking slowly allows time to respond. **Answer 5** is incorrect because, with expressive aphasia, the client will have difficulty in initiating speech, but may be able to articulate words that have no meaning. **Answer 6** is incorrect because, although support and encouragement need to be offered, these are general nursing approaches and not specific to this client.

■ TEST-TAKING TIP: *Be aware that the stem asks for specific approaches.*

Content Area: Geriatrics, Sensory; *Integrated Process:* Nursing Process, Implementation; *Cognitive Level:* Application; *Client Need/Subneed:* Psychosocial Integrity/Therapeutic Communications

15. CORRECT ANSWER: 4. **Answer 1** is incorrect because this client has an A_{1c} of 11%, indicating average blood sugars of about 300 mg/dL over the last 3 months. Regardless of client's statement of compliance and the immediate fasting blood sugar of 132, the disease, on average, has been *out of control* for months. **Answer 2** is incorrect because the client claims to be compliant with diet, medications, and exercise, and the normal fasting blood sugar is consistent with this. Looking at the A_{1c} shows that, on average, the client's blood sugar has been about 300 mg/dL over the last 3 months. **Answer 3** is incorrect because this client is only using diet for diabetes management. The *high* fasting blood sugar and A_{1c} indicate that this is clearly *not enough.* Answer 4 is correct because the A_{1c} measures average blood sugar over the previous 3 months. The goal is less than 7%. Short-term compliance can give the client a normal fasting blood sugar, but this is not considered good control of the disease.

■ TEST-TAKING TIP: *$HgbA_{1c}$ is the best indication of compliance. Three of the options are very close in value. Choose the lowest $HgbA_{1c}$ as an example of "best" control.*

Content Area: Adult Health, Endocrine; *Integrated Process:* Nursing Process, Analysis; *Cognitive Level:* Analysis; *Client Need/Subneed:* Physiological Integrity/Reduction of Risk Potential/Laboratory Values

16. CORRECT ANSWERS: 1, 4. **Answer 1 is correct because a positive Homans' sign can be a symptom of deep vein thrombosis and needs to be reported to the physician immediately.** **Answer 2** is incorrect because 2+ deep tendon reflexes are a normal finding, and do not need to be reported to the physician. Deep tendon reflexes that are a 3+ or 4+ may indicate cerebral irritability from preeclampsia and should be reported to the physician. **Answer 3** is incorrect because moderate rubra lochia is a normal finding 3 hours after delivery, and does not need to be reported to the physician. Large rubra lochia or expulsion of blood clots during fundal massage would indicate a postpartum hemorrhage and should be reported to the physician. **Answer 4 is correct because expression of orange-sized clots during fundal massage is a sign of postpartum hemorrhage and should be reported to the physician immediately.** **Answer 5** is incorrect because a fundus that is palpable firm at the level of the umbilicus is a normal finding 3 hours after delivery and does not need to be reported to the physician. A fundus that is deviated from the midline or palpable above the umbilicus is not a normal finding, and should be reported to the physician

■ TEST-TAKING TIP: *When a question asks what should be reported immediately, think of the possible life-threatening client outcome if a situation is not reported to the physician.*

Content Area: Maternity, Postpartum; *Integrated Process:* Nursing Process, Assessment; *Cognitive Level:* Analysis; *Client Need/Subneed:* Physiological Integrity/Physiological Adaptation/Alterations in Body Systems

17. CORRECT ANSWER: 4. **Answer 1** is incorrect because sugar in the urine would *decrease* as the blood sugar came down. **Answer 2** is incorrect because, as insulin takes sugar into the cell, it carries potassium with it. *Hypo*kalemia is a risk of treating high blood sugar. **Answer 3** is incorrect because clients with high blood sugars are generally very dehydrated and require fluids. If blood sugar was reduced too quickly, the blood pressure could potentially *drop* if fluid resuscitation was inadequate. **Answer 4 is correct because sugar adds to the osmolarity of the blood. Lowering the sugar level too fast makes the intracellular osmolarity relatively higher than that in the bloodstream. Water will move from areas of low concentration to areas of high concentration, swelling the cells and resulting in confusion or change in level of consciousness. If this happens in the brain it could have life-threatening consequences.**

■ TEST-TAKING TIP: *Sugar moves back into the cell. Look for an option that involves an effect on the cell (cerebral cells).*

Content Area: Adult Health, Endocrine; *Integrated Process:* Nursing Process, Assessment; *Cognitive Level:* Application; *Client Need/Subneed:* Physiological Integrity/Physiological Adaptation/Pathophysiology

18. CORRECT ANSWER: 1. **Answer 1 is correct because the child with measles is likely to exhibit all of the symptoms listed except for a slapped cheek appearance. The slapped cheek appearance is associated with both fifth disease (erythema infectiosum) and scarlet fever.** **Answer 2** is incorrect since the child with measles may first experience a fever and malaise. **Answer 3** is incorrect because, on or about the third day of infection, the child experiences a generalized rash that spreads from the face to the trunk and limbs. **Answer 4** is incorrect because the child with measles may develop red spots with bluish white centers in the buccal mucosa, known as Koplik's spots.

■ TEST-TAKING TIP: *Answers 2 and 3 are common to many pediatric infectious diseases and can be eliminated since they would not be "least likely" findings. Of the remaining options, recall that Koplik's spots are a hallmark of only one communicable disease (measles) while slapped cheek appearance is common to more than one. Choose the option that is specific to one communicable disease.*

Content Area: Child Health, Infectious Disease; *Integrated Process:* Nursing Process, Assessment; *Cognitive Level:* Application; *Client Need/Subneed:* Physiological Integrity/Physiological Adaptation/Pathophysiology

19. CORRECT ANSWER: 2. **Answer 1** is incorrect because a blood sugar level over 150 mg/dL is *not imminently* dangerous. Changes to diabetic management are better made based on *trends* over days and weeks. **Answer 2 is correct because fruity-smelling breath implies the production of ketones, which would occur with inadequate delivery of glucose to the cells. This can cause a dangerous acidosis and should be corrected immediately.** **Answer 3** is incorrect because clients with diabetes who are unable to eat still need some insulin to handle glucose being made in the liver. The dose will likely need to be reduced, but without insulin the client will become acidotic. **Answer 4** is incorrect because blood sugar should be checked more frequently when ill, but rarely would this need to be done more frequently than every couple of *hours.*

■ TEST-TAKING TIP: *Think about what independent action the client should take—call the provider. Ask which options indicate a* serious change *in the client's condition.*

Content Area: Adult Health, Endocrine; *Integrated Process:* Teaching and Learning; *Cognitive Level:* Application; *Client Need/Subneed:* Physiological Integrity/Physiological Adaptation/Illness Management

20. CORRECT ANSWERS: 1, 2, 4. **Answer 1 is correct because performing a sterile vaginal examination will eliminate the possibility of a prolapsed umbilical cord that may be causing the variable decelerations. Answer 2 is correct because changing the client's position can help alleviate cord compression that could be causing the variable decelerations.** **Answer 3** is incorrect because variable decelerations in the presence of moderate variability and a normal fetal heart rate baseline is *not indicative* of fetal distress, and does not require an emergency cesarean section. **Answer 4 is correct because administering a fluid bolus can increase hydration and decrease the variable decelerations that may be caused by cord compression.** **Answer 5**

is incorrect because the client is *not* completely dilated and is *not ready* for a vacuum-assisted delivery.

■ TEST-TAKING TIP: ***Variable decelerations are caused by umbilical cord compression; think about interventions that can relieve umbilical cord compression. Eliminate the two answers that "prepare" for procedures when the information supplied is not indicative of a problem and/or the client is not ready for the procedure ("vacuum-assisted delivery").***

Content Area: Maternity, Intrapartum; ***Integrated Process:*** Nursing Process, Implementation; ***Cognitive Level:*** Analysis; ***Client Need/Subneed:*** Physiological Integrity/Reduction of Risk Potential/Potential for Complications from Surgical Procedures and Health Alterations

21. CORRECT ANSWER: 4. **Answer 1** is incorrect because postoperative ileus would not be expected to last more than a few days. Most people have nutritional stores to tolerate this early. **Answer 2** is incorrect because one kidney has been removed and therefore could not develop stones. The other kidney has increased flow. Stasis would be unlikely. **Answer 3** is incorrect because nephrotic syndrome occurs when the glomerulus is unable to conserve protein. This could not occur in the removed kidney and is unlikely to occur in the remaining kidney. **Answer 4 is correct because the kidneys are located just under the diaphragm. Postoperative pain, particularly with deep breathing, would be anticipated. The client is therefore likely to do shallow breathing.**

■ TEST-TAKING TIP: *Two options relate to the effects of surgery—decreased peristalsis and pain. Consider the one that all clients will experience—pain.*

Content Area: Adult Health, Renal; ***Integrated Process:*** Nursing Process, Analysis; ***Cognitive Level:*** Application; ***Client Need/Subneed:*** Physiological Integrity/Reduction of Risk Potential/Potential for Complications from Surgical Procedures and Health Alterations

22. CORRECT ANSWERS: 1, 2, 3, 6. **Answer 1 is correct because the infant with pyloric stenosis experiences metabolic alkalosis as a result of excessive vomiting. Answer 2 is correct because this physical assessment (by inspection) is consistent with pyloric stenosis. Answer 3 is correct because this assessment finding is consistent with pyloric stenosis as a result of the pyloric muscle blocking the outflow of stomach contents.** **Answer 4** is incorrect because the infant with pyloric stenosis has *nonbilious* vomiting since the obstruction is *above* the bile duct. **Answer 5** is incorrect because the infant with pyloric stenosis is expected to have some degree of dehydration, which would result in an *increase* in urine specific gravity. **Answer 6 is correct because this assessment finding is consistent with pyloric stenosis as a result of poor intake.**

■ TEST-TAKING TIP: ***Focus on the name of the diagnosis to help identify symptoms. If the pyloric muscle is stenosed, expect the infant to have symptoms resulting from stomach contents and with nutrients not able to progress through the digestive system.***

Content Area: Child Health, Gastrointestinal; ***Integrated Process:*** Nursing Process, Assessment; ***Cognitive Level:*** Application; ***Client Need/Subneed:*** Physiological Integrity/Physiological Adaptation/Pathophysiology

23. CORRECT ANSWERS: 2, 5. **Answer 1** is incorrect because the client needs to change her pads more frequently to stay fresh and help prevent infection. Changing pads about *every 3 to 4* hours is the suggested interval for proper hygiene. **Answer 2 is correct because consistently using the peri bottle to clean the perineum after each void or bowel movement *demonstrates proper* perineal care. The nurse should give instructions to keep the perineum clean to increase comfort and prevent infection. Using a peri bottle and water to rinse after each void or bowel movement helps keep the perineum clean and decreases the chance of infection.** **Answer 3** is incorrect because the client should wipe from *front to back* to decrease chances of infection due to transmitting bacteria from the rectum to the vagina. **Answer 4** is incorrect because the client should spray water *over* the *perineum* and *not directly* into the vagina. **Answer 5 is correct because perineal care should include using antiseptic spray after rinsing. The nurse should give instructions to keep the perineum clean to increase comfort and prevent infection. Using antiseptic spray after rinsing with the peri bottle helps to prevent infection and decreases perineal pain.**

■ TEST-TAKING TIP: *Select the two options that are correct steps when using the peri bottle.*

Content Area: Maternity, Postpartum; ***Integrated Process:*** Nursing Process, Evaluation; ***Cognitive Level:*** Analysis; ***Client Need/Subneed:*** Health Promotion and Maintenance/Ante/Intra/Postpartum and Newborn Care

24. CORRECT ANSWER: 2. **Answer 1** is incorrect because the older adult *frequently* has a poor appetite, so that anorexia would *not* be a change. **Answer 2 is correct because confusion is often the first indication of infection, which progresses rapidly to urosepsis.** **Answer 3** is incorrect because the temperature may *only* be 99°F. **Answer 4** is incorrect because restlessness is a more characteristic finding with *hypoxia.*

■ TEST-TAKING TIP: ***Look for an atypical finding (confusion), something not usually seen with an infection in a younger client.***

Content Area: Adult Health, Renal; ***Integrated Process:*** Nursing Process, Assessment; ***Cognitive Level:*** Application; ***Client Need/Subneed:*** Physiological Integrity/Physiological Adaptation/Alterations in Body Systems

25. CORRECT ANSWER: 4. **The appropriate number of compressions per minute during CPR on a child is 100 per minute.**

■ TEST-TAKING TIP: *Recall that the rate of compressions for CPR is always 100 per minute, regardless of the victim's age.*

Content Area: Child Health, Cardiovascular; ***Integrated Process:*** Nursing Process, Implementation; ***Cognitive Level:*** Application; ***Client Need/Subneed:*** Physiological Integrity/Physiological Adaptation/Medical Emergencies

26. CORRECT ANSWER: 4. **Answer 1** is incorrect because a client with symptoms of thrombophlebitis should be placed on bedrest, *not* encouraged to *ambulate.* **Answer 2** is incorrect because this client has symptoms of thrombophlebitis; massaging the leg can break the thrombus from the venous wall and cause an embolus. **Answer 3** is incorrect because local application *of heat is* one of the treatments for superficial thrombosis, *not ice,* which constricts blood flow. **Answer 4 is correct because this client has a superficial thrombophlebitis. Elevation of the affected extremity, a few days of bedrest, and local application of heat are often all that is needed to treat superficial thrombophlebitis.**

■ TEST-TAKING TIP: *Eliminate the responses that make the condition of thrombophlebitis worse (i.e., massage, Answer 2; ambulate, Answer 1). See key phrase in the correct option: "promote venous blood flow."*

Content Area: Adult Health, Cardiovascular; *Integrated Process:* Nursing Process, Implementation; *Cognitive Level:* Application; *Client Need/Subneed:* Physiological Integrity/Reduction of Risk Potential/Potential for Complications from Surgical Procedures and Health Alterations

27. CORRECT ANSWERS: 1, 2, 5. **Answer 1 is correct because it describes the role of the team leader. Answer 2 is correct because it describes the role of the team leader.** **Answer 3** is incorrect because, even though the team leader may observe specific procedures performed by a nursing assistant, the team leader's role is to *evaluate* care after it is completed. **Answer 4** is incorrect because team members who are qualified to assess are responsible for their *own* documentation. **Answer 5 is correct because it describes the role of the team leader.** **Answer 6** is incorrect because, even though this may be true if qualified personnel are not available, the team leader needs to be available in general as a resource throughout the shift.

■ TEST-TAKING TIP: *Note the key words "major responsibility" in the stem.*

Content Area: Management of Care; *Integrated Process:* Nursing Process, Planning; *Cognitive Level:* Application; *Client Need/Subneed:* Safe and Effective Care Environment/Management of Care/Concepts of Management

28. CORRECT ANSWERS: 3, 4. **Answer 1** is incorrect because nausea may occur as the body adjusts to the increasing hormone levels released by the patch. **Answer 2** is incorrect because chloasma is hyperpigmentation caused by the increased hormone levels. **Answer 3 is correct because pain in the legs while walking can be a sign of thrombophlebitis, a life-threatening complication of hypercoagulability caused by the increased hormone levels. Answer 4 is correct because a headache unrelieved by analgesics can be a symptom of a blood clot in the brain, another life-threatening complication of hypercoagulability caused by the increased hormone levels.** **Answer 5** is incorrect because swelling of the feet and hands is caused by fluid retention, under the influence of increased hormone levels. Do not *confuse* this swelling with symptoms of preeclampsia, which also involves swelling of the extremities, but requires immediate intervention.

■ TEST-TAKING TIP: *The question asks for* **immediate** *notification; think life-threatening complications. Three options (Answers 1, 2, and 5) are annoying, but not life threatening, results of increased hormones. Two options (Answers 3 and 4) are potentially life threatening; choose these options.*

Content Area: Adult Health, Genitourinary; *Integrated Process:* Nursing Process, Implementation; *Cognitive Level:* Analysis; *Client Need/Subneed:* Physiological Integrity/Pharmacological and Parenteral Therapies/Adverse Effects/Contraindications/Interactions

29. CORRECT ANSWER: 1. **Answer 1 is correct because normal amniotic fluid is basically colorless; any color may signify fetal or maternal problems. For example, yellow or green amniotic fluid indicates meconium release due to fetal hypoxia or breech presentation; bloody amniotic fluid may indicate a placental abruption or marginal placenta previa.** **Answer 2** is incorrect because fetal bradycardia *commonly* occurs at the acme of the contraction, due to head compression, which is a benign condition. **Answer 3** is incorrect because nausea with or without emesis is *common* in labor, due to physiological stress. **Answer 4** is incorrect because diaphoresis and irritability *are* signs of transitional phase of labor.

■ TEST-TAKING TIP: *Carefully read the stem of the question; it is asking for the answer that is* **not a normal part of labor.** *Eliminate the answers that are a normal physiological part of labor.*

Content Area: Maternity, Intrapartum; *Integrated Process:* Nursing Process, Assessment; *Cognitive Level:* Analysis; *Client Need/Subneed:* Physiological Integrity/Physiological Adaptation/Alterations in Body Systems

30. CORRECT ANSWER: 3. **Answer 1** is incorrect because the client has pneumonia in the *right* lung, *not* in the *left* lung. **Answer 2** is incorrect because the right *upper* lobe is auscultated here. The client has right *middle* lobe pneumonia. **Answer 3 is correct because this is the area where the right middle lobe is accessible for auscultation.** **Answer 4** is incorrect because the right *lower* lobe is auscultated here. The client has right *middle* lobe pneumonia.

■ TEST-TAKING TIP: *The key words are:* **right, middle** *lobe.*

Content Area: Adult Health, Respiratory; *Integrated Process:* Nursing Process, Implementation; *Cognitive Level:* Application; *Client Need/Subneed:* Physiological Integrity/Reduction of Risk Potential/System Specific Assessments

31. CORRECT ANSWER: 3. **Answer 1** is incorrect because consistency with limit-setting by *both* parents will help the child with ADHD to meet behavioral expectations. **Answer 2** is incorrect because storing ADHD medications puts the child at risk for sharing medications with friends or for potential overdose. The parents can better foster the child's independence in self-care by providing access to the medication in an observed setting, such as at breakfast time.

Answer 3 is correct because excess environmental stimulation can increase the hyperactivity and distractibility of a child with ADHD. **Answer 4** is incorrect because exercise *can* greatly benefit the child with ADHD by providing an outlet for extra energy. **Answer 5** is incorrect because ADHD medications such as Ritalin should be taken *daily* to achieve therapeutic blood levels, not on an "as needed" basis.

■ TEST-TAKING TIP: *When the stem of the question does not ask for a* priority *answer, go through the options and ask whether each statement is a* true *or* false *recommendation. Select all the* true *answers as these should be part of a general teaching plan.*

Content Area: Child Health, Behavioral; ***Integrated Process:*** Teaching and Learning; ***Cognitive Level:*** Application; ***Client Need/Subneed:*** Physiological Integrity/Physiological Adaptation/Alterations in Body Systems

32. CORRECT ANSWER: 3. **Answer 1** is incorrect because this procedure is generally done under regional anesthesia. Priority assessment in the postanesthesia care unit (PACU) would involve evaluating whether anesthesia is wearing off and whether there are complications from surgery, such as damage to nerves or blood vessels. **Answer 2** is incorrect because the brachial pulse is *above* the level of the surgery and would not indicate whether damage had occurred to nerves or blood vessels during the procedure. Answer 3 is correct because checking circulation and sensation in the fingers helps to establish that no damage to blood vessels or nerves occurred during surgery, and that postoperative swelling is not damaging those structures. This procedure is usually done under regional anesthesia; return of sensation and movement indicates anesthesia is wearing off appropriately. **Answer 4** is incorrect because this procedure is usually done under regional anesthesia with sedation, neither of which would create a risk for alteration in pupil response.

■ TEST-TAKING TIP: *Visualize the operative site and choose an option that includes the operative area (*fingers*).*

Content Area: Adult Health, Circulatory; ***Integrated Process:*** Nursing Process, Assessment; ***Cognitive Level:*** Application; ***Client Need/Subneed:*** Physiological Integrity/Reduction of Risk Potential/Potential for Alterations in Body Systems

33. CORRECT ANSWERS: 1, 3, 4. Answer 1 is correct because green-tinged fluid is indicative of meconium staining, a possible indicator of fetal distress, and should be reported to the physician. **Answer 2** is incorrect because vernix in the fluid is a *normal* finding after rupture of membranes, and does *not* need to be reported to the physician. Answer 3 is correct because a decrease in the fetal heart rate baseline to 100 bpm is bradycardia and may indicate umbilical cord prolapse or compression, and should be reported to the physician. Answer 4 is correct because an increase in the baseline fetal heart rate to above 160 bpm can be indicative of an infection, and should be reported to the physician. **Answer 5** is incorrect because a small amount of clear fluid is a *normal* finding after rupture of membranes, and does not need to be reported to the physician.

■ TEST-TAKING TIP: *Eliminate the two options about "clear fluid"; a small amount of fluid may be from rupture of membranes, and a copious amount of vernix is normal.*

Content Area: Maternity, Intrapartum; ***Integrated Process:*** Nursing Process, Analysis; ***Cognitive Level:*** Analysis; ***Client Need/Subneed:*** Physiological Integrity/Physiological Adaptation/Alterations in Body Systems

34. CORRECT ANSWERS: 1, 3, 4, 6. Answer 1 is correct because burns increase cellular metabolism, resulting in an increased oxygen demand. **Answer 2** is incorrect because the metabolic demand and need for oxygen *decrease* with hypothermia. Answer 3 is correct because shivering raises the metabolism and the demand for oxygen. Answer 4 is correct because the energy expended with agitation increases oxygen utilization. **Answer 5** is incorrect because the metabolic demand is *decreased*, and therefore oxygen demand is decreased. Answer 6 is correct because hyperthyroidism increases cellular metabolism and increases oxygen demand.

■ TEST-TAKING TIP: *Eliminate conditions that decrease O_2 demand.*

Content Area: Adult Health, Respiratory; ***Integrated Process:*** Nursing Process, Analysis; ***Cognitive Level:*** Application; ***Client Need/Subneed:*** Physiological Integrity/Physiological Adaptation/Pathophysiology

35. CORRECT ANSWERS: 4, 2, 3, 1, 5. Answer 4. Advising the caregiver is first because the nurse should begin by providing information about this assessment tool. Answer 2. Asking the caregiver about use of spoon and fork is next because the nurse should attempt to score items that can be determined through interview, before asking the child to perform tasks. Answer 3. Asking the child to build a tower is next because the nurse can provide the child with blocks while talking with the caregiver; the child may spontaneously build a tower without prompting. If the nurse has to prompt the child to build a tower, this is best done after the child is given an opportunity to "warm up" during the dialogue between the nurse and caregiver. Answer 1. Asking the child to name body parts is next because language items are best administered following fine motor activities when the child is more comfortable with the nurse. Answer 5. Having the child kick a ball is the last step because gross motor activities should be assessed at the end. Administering gross motor items earlier may be a distraction. The child may then be unwilling to return to the table to perform fine motor activities or engage in an interview.

■ TEST-TAKING TIP: *The approach for the developmental assessment is similar to that of a physical assessment. A nurse should first address the caregiver, and then use a transition object such as a toy for interaction with the child, speaking directly to the child only after trust has been established.*

Content Area: Child Health, Growth and Development; ***Integrated Process:*** Nursing Process, Implementation; ***Cognitive Level:*** Application; ***Client Need/Subneed:*** Health Promotion and Maintenance/Developmental Stages and Transitions

36. CORRECT ANSWERS: 2, 4. Answer 1 is incorrect because the client is probably experiencing preterm labor with a urinary tract infection. Calling the physician to convey information about the client's condition would be important, but *not* specifically for *pain* medication. **Answer 2 is correct because placing the client on an external fetal monitor is standard nursing procedure to evaluate the fetal well-being and the pattern of contractions. With preterm labor, it is important to evaluate uterine activity on the external fetal monitor. Answer 3** is incorrect because the client is not complaining of rupture of membranes. The fern test specifically helps to determine if the amniotic sac is leaking. **Answer 4 is correct because the client is complaining of dysuria. Obtaining a clean-catch urine specimen would be appropriate to evaluate the possibility of a urinary tract infection. Answer 5** is incorrect because the client is preterm and has vaginal bleeding. A vaginal exam is *contraindicated* when the client has vaginal bleeding of unknown origin.

■ **TEST-TAKING TIP:** *The key to this question is* dysuria *and* preterm. *The appropriate interventions for a client who is preterm are different than those for a full-term gestation.*

Content Area: Maternity, Intrapartum; ***Integrated Process:*** Nursing Process, Analysis; ***Cognitive Level:*** Analysis; ***Client Need/Subneed:*** Physiological Integrity/Physiological Adaptation/ Alterations in Body Systems

37. CORRECT ANSWERS: 2, 3, 4, 6. Answer 1 is incorrect because in early septic shock there is actually an *increase* in cardiac output. **Answer 2 is correct because circulating blood volume would be decreased with GI bleeding. Answer 3 is correct because the ventricles are unable to pump the blood efficiently through the heart, so that cardiac output is decreased. Answer 4 is correct because positive end-expiratory pressure (PEEP) increases the intrathoracic pressure; therefore, venous return and cardiac output would be decreased. Answer 5** is incorrect because aerobic exercise *increases* the heart rate and thus cardiac output. **Answer 6 is correct because damage to the myocardium decreases the pumping effectiveness of the heart and impacts cardiac output.**

■ **TEST-TAKING TIP:** *Eliminate the options that increase blood pressure and heart rate.*

Content Area: Adult Health, Cardiovascular; ***Integrated Process:*** Nursing Process, Analysis; ***Cognitive Level:*** Analysis; ***Client Need/Subneed:*** Physiological Integrity/Physiological Adaptation/Pathophysiology

38. CORRECT ANSWER: 1. Answer 1 is correct because scarlet fever is *bacterial* in nature (Group A β-hemolytic streptococci) and responds well to antibiotics (usually penicillin). Vaccines are generally developed for communicable diseases that are *viral* in nature. Answer 2 is incorrect because vaccines are generally developed for communicable diseases that are *viral* in nature as opposed to bacterial. There is no vaccine for scarlet fever in development at the present time. **Answer 3** is incorrect because the nurse has sufficient knowledge about the pathophysiology of scarlet fever to correctly answer the parents' question *without* referring the parents to the pediatrician. **Answer 4** is incorrect because scarlet fever *is* communicable and can be treated with the use of antibiotics (usually penicillin).

■ **TEST-TAKING TIP:** *Eliminate Answers 2, 3, and 4 because they are theoretically incorrect (i.e., there are* no *vaccines for this* bacterial *disease, and scarlet fever* is *communicable).*

Content Area: Child Health, Infectious Disease; ***Integrated Process:*** Teaching and Learning; ***Cognitive Level:*** Application; ***Client Need/Subneed:*** Physiological Integrity/Physiological Adaptation/Alterations in Body Systems

39. CORRECT ANSWERS: 2, 3, 4, 5. Answer 1 is incorrect because dextrose *alone* will *not* directly affect the potassium level. Insulin *also* needs to be given. **Answer 2 is correct because correcting the acidosis with sodium bicarbonate will cause potassium to shift back into the cell. Answer 3 is correct because regular insulin is the first line of treatment for hyperkalemia. Dextrose is used to prevent hypoglycemia, which may occur with the shift of the potassium back into the cell. Answer 4 is correct because Kayexalate is an exchange resin. Potassium is exchanged for Na^+ in the intestines, and potassium is removed via feces. Answer 5 is correct because albuterol has been shown to decrease the potassium level by 0.5 to 1.5 mEq/L.**

■ **TEST-TAKING TIP:** *Review current treatment approaches for hyperkalemia.*

Content Area: Adult Health, Renal; ***Integrated Process:*** Nursing Process, Analysis; ***Cognitive Level:*** Application; ***Client Need/Subneed:*** Physiological Integrity/Pharmacological and Parenteral Therapies/Expected Effects/Outcomes

40. CORRECT ANSWERS: 2, 3, 4, 5. Answer 1 is incorrect because oligohydramnios is *too little* amniotic fluid, and is *not* a complication of type 1 diabetes. **Answer 2 is correct because polyhydramnios, or too much amniotic fluid, is a condition resulting from poor glycemic control during pregnancy, which causes hyperglycemia of the fetus and fetal polyuria (fetal urine is a major source of amniotic fluid). This client's hemoglobin A_{1c} is elevated at 8.2% (the normal is less than 6.0%), indicating poor glycemic control during early pregnancy. Answer 3 is correct because macrosomia, a fetus who is oversized, is a condition resulting from poor glycemic control during pregnancy. The fetus produces too much insulin in response to the maternal hyperglycemia; insulin acts as a growth hormone during fetal development, producing a large fetus. Answer 4 is correct because this client's hemoglobin A_{1c} is elevated at 8.2% (the normal is less than 6.0%), indicating poor glycemic control during early pregnancy, which is highly correlated with spinal anomalies. Answer 5 is correct because preeclampsia is more commonly found in clients with preexisting diabetes. Rates**

of preeclampsia in women with type 1 diabetes are two to four times higher than in normal pregnancies.

■ TEST-TAKING TIP: *Look at two opposite complications (too much . . . too little amniotic fluid) and eliminate one (i.e., too little). Remember that, if the maternal glucose is poorly controlled, the fetus is at greater risk than with well-controlled blood glucose. In this case, the hemoglobin A_{1c} is elevated, meaning the blood sugar has been poorly controlled.*

Content Area: Maternity, Antepartum; *Integrated Process:* Nursing Process, Analysis; *Cognitive Level:* Analysis; *Client Need/Subneed:* Physiological Integrity/Reduction of Risk Potential/Potential for Alterations in Body Systems

41. CORRECT ANSWERS: 2, 3, 4, 6. **Answer 1** is incorrect because the client has acute respiratory distress syndrome (ARDS), *not* an infection, which would call for antibiotic therapy. **Answer 2 is correct because PEEP improves ventilation to the atelectatic alveoli, improving oxygenation. Answer 3 is correct because prone positioning, if not contraindicated, improves oxygenation because more even distribution of ventilation occurs. Answer 4 is correct because these drugs increase contractility of the heart and raise blood pressure, improving perfusion.** **Answer 5** is incorrect because the client has ARDS, not a coagulation problem that would call for anticoagulant therapy. **Answer 6 is correct because neuromuscular blockade decreases oxygen demand.**

■ TEST-TAKING TIP: *Eliminate the options that do not improve oxygenation.*

Content Area: Adult Health, Respiratory; *Integrated Process:* Nursing Process, Analysis; *Cognitive Level:* Analysis; *Client Need/Subneed:* Physiological Integrity/Physiological Adaptation/Medical Emergencies

42. CORRECT ANSWER: 1. **Answer 1 is correct because accelerations are an indication of fetal well-being and a well-oxygenated fetus.** **Answer 2** is incorrect because consistent decreased fetal heart rate variability is an indicator of *decreased* placental perfusion and *poor* oxygenation. **Answer 3** is incorrect because prolonged fetal bradycardia is an indicator of decreased *placental perfusion* and *fetal distress.* **Answer 4** is incorrect because consistent late decelerations are an indicator of poor *uteroplacental perfusion* and fetal distress.

■ TEST-TAKING TIP: *The priority for this client is fetal well-being; consider which of the patterns are indicative of good oxygenation.*

Content Area: Maternity, Intrapartum; *Integrated Process:* Nursing Process, Evaluation; *Cognitive Level:* Analysis; *Client Need/Subneed:* Physiological Integrity/Physiological Adaptation/Medical Emergencies

43. CORRECT ANSWERS: 1, 3, 5. **Answer 1 is correct because the cold caloric test is a test of the oculovestibular reflex, and absence of this reflex indicates severe brainstem injury.** **Answer 2** is incorrect because a GCS of less than 7 indicates *coma,* not *brain* death. **Answer 3 is correct because a flat EEG indicates the absence of electrical activity in the brain.** **Answer 4** is incorrect because a gag reflex *would* indicate brain function. **Answer 5 is correct because the absence of spontaneous respirations indicates the absence of brain function.**

■ TEST-TAKING TIP: *Remember that brain death is an irreversible loss of* all *brain functions.*

Content Area: Adult Health, Neurological; *Integrated Process:* Nursing Process, Analysis; *Cognitive Level:* Application; *Client Need/Subneed:* Physiological Integrity/Physiological Adaptation/Alterations in Body Systems

44. CORRECT ANSWER: 3. **Answer 1** is incorrect because there is *no contraindication* for the use of acetaminophen to control pain in the treatment of hemophilia. **Answer 2** is incorrect because corticosteroids *are* given for the hematuria, acute hemarthrosis, and the chronic synovitis associated with hemophilia. **Answer 3 is correct because, while nonsteroidal anti-inflammatory drugs (NSAIDs), such as ibuprofen, are effective in relieving pain caused by the chronic synovitis associated with hemophilia, they inhibit platelet function, which is essential in controlling bleeding episodes.** **Answer 4** is incorrect because oral use of epsilon-aminocaproic acid (Amicar) prevents clot destruction. Its use is limited to mouth trauma or surgery, and a dose of factor concentrate must be given first. The child may rinse the mouth with this medication and then swallow it.

■ TEST-TAKING TIP: *Select the drug that would be contraindicated. Think "prevent bleeding" in hemophilia, and then select the medication that could cause rather than prevent bleeding.*

Content Area: Child Health, Pharmacology; *Integrated Process:* Teaching and Learning; *Cognitive Level:* Application; *Client Need/Subneed:* Physiological Integrity/Pharmacological and Parenteral Therapies/Adverse Effects/Contraindications/Interactions

45. CORRECT ANSWERS: 1, 2, 4. **Answer 1 is correct because deep breathing causes pressure on the peritoneum from the diaphragm and pain. Expect to see shallow breathing, which causes minimal pressure on the diaphragm. Answer 2 is correct because peritoneal inflammation causes peritoneal contraction and the classic "boardlike abdomen."** **Answer 3** is incorrect because bowel sounds are typically *hypoactive.* **Answer 4 is correct because the inflammation and irritation of the peritoneum cause pain.** **Answer 5** is incorrect because the *decreased* peristalsis will *decrease* flatus.

■ TEST-TAKING TIP: *Eliminate the two options that describe* increased *bowel activity.*

Content Area: Adult Health, Gastrointestinal; *Integrated Process:* Nursing Process, Assessment; *Cognitive Level:* Application; *Client Need/Subneed:* Physiological Integrity/Physiological Adaptation/Pathophysiology

46. CORRECT ANSWER: 4. Answer 1 is incorrect because this is the wrong concentration of magnesium sulfate. The usual concentration is *40* gm of magnesium sulfate in *1,000* mL of lactated Ringer's solution. **Answer 2** is incorrect because, although monitoring vital signs are an important part of every nursing assessment for a client in labor, this client is being treated for preeclampsia, for which the vital signs need to be assessed *more frequently* than every hour. **Answer 3** is incorrect because the maintenance dose should be approximately *2 gm/hr.* The *loading* dose is usually 4 gm over a 30-minute period. **Answer 4 is correct because a respiratory rate of less than 12 breaths/min can be a result of magnesium toxicity. The nurse should discontinue the infusion and notify the physician.**

■ **TEST-TAKING TIP:** *Magnesium is a central nervous system depressant and can cause respiratory failure at a toxic level. Watch the respiratory rate closely.*

Content Area: Maternity, Antepartum; *Integrated Process:* Nursing Process, Implementation; *Cognitive Level:* Application; *Client Need/Subneed:* Physiological Integrity/Pharmacological and Parenteral Therapies/Parenteral/Intravenous Therapies

47. CORRECT ANSWER: 3. Answer 1 is incorrect because a temperature this low is *subnormal* and would not be an accurate indication of antibiotic effectiveness. **Answer 2** is incorrect because the O_2 saturation should be *90% or higher.* **Answer 3 is correct because a systolic BP of 90 mm Hg or higher signals stability of the client.** **Answer 4** is incorrect because a heart rate of 120 is high. A rate of *100 or lower* would indicate client stability.

■ **TEST-TAKING TIP:** *Look for a clinical indicator within normal limits.*

Content Area: Adult Health, Respiratory; *Integrated Process:* Nursing Process, Analysis; *Cognitive Level:* Application; *Client Need/Subneed:* Physiological Integrity/Physiological Adaptation/Alterations in Body Systems

48. CORRECT ANSWER: 2. Answer 1 is incorrect because a yogurt and fruit plate would not be a high-calorie lunch, which could contribute to weight gain while recuperation from the injury takes place. **Answer 2 is correct because diet is an important consideration in the treatment of hemophilia. Excessive body weight can increase the strain on affected joints, especially the knees, and predispose the adolescent to hemarthrosis. Consequently calories need to be supplied in accordance with energy requirements.** **Answer 3** is incorrect because a slice of cheese pizza and a tossed green salad would not be a high-calorie lunch, which could contribute to weight gain while recuperation from the injury takes place. **Answer 4** is incorrect because a scoop of pasta salad and a cup of vegetable soup would not be a high-calorie lunch, which could contribute to weight gain while recuperation from the injury takes place.

■ **TEST-TAKING TIP:** *The correct answer is the "wrong" food choice (i.e., what is not a good choice to eat). Relate calories consumed to potential for additional injury.*

Content Area: Child Health, Hematological; *Integrated Process:* Nursing Process, Evaluation; *Cognitive Level:* Application; *Client Need/Subneed:* Physiological Integrity/Basic Care and Comfort/Nutrition and Oral Hydration

49. CORRECT ANSWER: 3. Answer 1 is incorrect because genetic karyotyping is the name of the *general* test done for analysis of chromosomes; it is *not a specific diagnostic* test. **Answer 2** is incorrect because amniocentesis cannot be performed until *after the first trimester.* **Answer 3 is correct because chorionic villus sampling (CVS) can be performed as early as about 9 weeks' gestation, providing information before the end of the first trimester.** **Answer 4** is incorrect because ultrasonography cannot provide diagnostic chromosomal information; it can *only* provide *general* screening for abnormalities.

■ **TEST-TAKING TIP:** *There is a difference between diagnostic and screening tests. Screening tests are clues to possible problems, but diagnostic tests provide absolute information to make a specific diagnosis. Ultrasound is an example of a screening test, and should be eliminated when the question is asking for a diagnostic test.*

Content Area: Maternity, Antepartum; *Integrated Process:* Nursing Process, Implementation; *Cognitive Level:* Application; *Client Need/Subneed:* Physiological Integrity/Reduction of Risk Potential/Diagnostic Tests

50. CORRECT ANSWER: 4. Answer 1 is incorrect because it supplies the parents with *false hope* that the diagnosis is inaccurate. The diagnosis would not have been presented to the parents without thorough confirmation of the positive diagnostic tests. **Answer 2** is incorrect because it does *not* address the parents' concerns. It is a "closed-ended" response that does not allow for further dialogue between the parents and the nurse. **Answer 3** is incorrect because, while it may be accurate, it does not supply the parents with *why* this happened to their infant. **Answer 4 is correct because it is the response that supplies the parents with the most facts/information. It tells the parents *why* this disease is present in their infant.**

■ **TEST-TAKING TIP:** *Look at the two answers with statistical data (i.e., 60% and ⅓) and choose the lesser percentage.*

Content Area: Child Health, Hematological; *Integrated Process:* Teaching and Learning; *Cognitive Level:* Application; *Client Need/Subneed:* Physiological Integrity/Physiological Adaptation/Pathophysiology

51. CORRECT ANSWER: 1. Answer 1 is correct because antibiotic therapy is the most important aspect of treatment. Maintaining IV site patency and integrity is a key role for the RN and for the client's recovery. **Answer 2** is incorrect because the antibiotics must be administered through a patent site *before* effectiveness can be evaluated. **Answer 3** is incorrect because this is *not the first* action, although mobility is important in improving respiratory function. **Answer 4** is incorrect because IV therapy is the first priority, but the client's comfort is important as pain will affect respiratory status.

■ **TEST-TAKING TIP:** *This is a priority question. All of the options may be correct but one is priority. The sooner the*

antibiotics are started, the sooner the client will be ambulating and breathing comfortably.
Content Area: Adult Health, Respiratory; *Integrated Process:* Nursing Process, Planning; *Cognitive Level:* Analysis; *Client Need/Subneed:* Physiological Integrity/Physiological Adaptation/Illness Management

52. CORRECT ANSWERS: 1, 2, 3. Answer 1 is correct because decreased fetal movement may be an indication of fetal hypoxia, and the fetus should be evaluated using an external fetal monitor. Answer 2 is correct because contractions that are regular, every 5 minutes, and lasting 60 seconds are usually indicative of active labor, and the client should come to the hospital to be evaluated for labor. Answer 3 is correct because, if the client thinks her amniotic fluid is leaking, she should be evaluated for rupture of membranes and labor. **Answer 4** is incorrect because increased fetal movement is a *reassuring* sign, and the client does *not* need to come to the hospital to evaluate the fetal well-being. **Answer 5** is incorrect because contractions that are 10 minutes apart, only lasting for 30 seconds, are usually associated with the *latent* phase of labor, and the client does *not* need to come to the hospital for evaluation of labor.
■ TEST-TAKING TIP: ***Look for pairs of answers that are opposite of each other and eliminate one of them in each "pair." Select Answer 1 and therefore eliminate Answer 4. Select Answer 2 and therefore eliminate Answer 5.***
Content Area: Maternity, Intrapartum; *Integrated Process:* Nursing Process, Implementation; *Cognitive Level:* Analysis; *Client Need/Subneed:* Health Promotion and Maintenance/ Ante/Intra/Postpartum and Newborn Care

53. CORRECT ANSWER: 4. **Answer 1** is incorrect because any dressing that is wet could potentially cause *more damage.* **Answer 2** is incorrect because a wet dressing could macerate the skin. **Answer 3** is incorrect because this probably would *not harm* the area, but observation of the site is easier without a dressing. Answer 4 is correct because no dressing is needed for a stage I pressure ulcer because the skin is intact. Just turn the client frequently and keep pressure off the area.
■ TEST-TAKING TIP: ***Know the depth of tissue involvement with each stage to select the type of dressing.***
Content Area: Adult Health, Integumentary; *Integrated Process:* Nursing Process, Implementation; *Cognitive Level:* Application; *Client Need/Subneed:* Physiological Integrity/ Physiological Adaptation/Illness Management

54. CORRECT ANSWER: 4. **Answer 1** is incorrect because hepatitis B vaccine *should be given* at birth, or definitely prior to discharge from the birth hospital. There is no contraindication in beginning vaccinations for an infant with hemophilia. The nurse does not need to question this order. **Answer 2** is incorrect because a circumcision would involve a small amount of bleeding, which could be difficult to control and might lead to hemorrhage. It *should be delayed* until the disease is confirmed and the severity of the factor deficiency is determined. The nurse does not need to question this order. **Answer 3** is incorrect because s etting up a series of well-infant appointments at the time of discharge from the birth hospital *is a requirement* for all infants and especially those who might have a chronic disease process. The nurse does not need to question this order. Answer 4 is correct because *venipuncture* for blood draws are usually preferred in infants/children with hemophilia. There is usually *less bleeding* after venipuncture than after finger or heel punctures.
■ TEST-TAKING TIP: ***The question calls for an order that is not "OK." Think "prevent blood loss" when answering this question.***
Content Area: Child Health, Hematological; *Integrated Process:* Nursing Process, Evaluation; *Cognitive Level:* Application; *Client Need/Subneed:* Physiological Integrity/Reduction of Risk Potential/Potential for Complications of Diagnostic Tests/ Treatments/Procedures

55. CORRECT ANSWERS: 1, 2, 3, 4. Answer 1 is correct because calling the physician is appropriate when the client's temperature is above 100.4°F. Answer 2 is correct because encouraging her to increase fluids is an appropriate intervention after a long labor and delivery process. Some of the increased temperature may be due to dehydration. Answer 3 is correct because assessing the fundal height is a part of a routine postpartum assessment and should be performed. Answer 4 is correct because assessing the lochia is a part of a routine postpartum assessment and should be performed. **Answer 5** is incorrect because there is no reason given in this scenario for encouraging the client to bottle-feed. Her increased temperature is *not* a reason to choose bottle feeding over breastfeeding.
■ TEST-TAKING TIP: ***This client has a risk factor for postpartum infection, a lengthy labor, and an operative delivery. Her increased temperature may be the* first *sign of infection.***
Content Area: Maternity, Postpartum; *Integrated Process:* Nursing Process, Implementation; *Cognitive Level:* Analysis; *Client Need/Subneed:* Physiological Integrity/Physiological Adaptation/Alterations in Body Systems

56. CORRECT ANSWERS: 2, 5, 6. **Answer 1** is incorrect because the legal causal connection includes *indirect* as well as direct cause. Answer 2 is correct because legal cause includes both harm caused directly by the actions of the nurse and harm caused by others when the actions of the nurse knowingly placed the client at risk of harm. **Answer 3** is incorrect because anyone named in a lawsuit is entitled to a defense that shows that the actions were outside of the legal causal connection. **Answer 4** is incorrect because the involvement of the nurse would have to have some direct or indirect connection to the harm produced. Answer 5 is correct because, if the nurse's actions are outside the standards of care and the actions cause harm to the client, then the nurse's actions are within the legal causal connection. Answer 6 is correct because harm caused by a nurse giving care under the influence of narcotic medications is within the legal causal connection.
■ TEST-TAKING TIP: ***Answers that include absolute words such as "only" (Answer 1) and "any" (Answer 4) are likely to be wrong.***
Content Area: Management of Care, Legal; *Integrated Process:* Nursing Process, Analysis; *Cognitive Level:* Application; *Client Need/Subneed:* Safe and Effective Care Environment/ Management of Care/Legal Rights and Responsibilities

57. CORRECT ANSWER: 3. **Answer 1** is incorrect because an EEG (electroencephalogram) is a study of the electric activity of the brain and would *not detect* lead levels in the toddler's body. **Answer 2** is incorrect because a CBC (complete blood count) is a *general* study of the hematological system, and would *not detect* lead levels in the toddler's body. **Answer 3 is correct because a toddler with a sharp rise in blood lead level (BLL) should have an abdominal x-ray to determine the presence of lead chips, which would be a result of repeated ingestion of lead-based paint chips. If lead chips are discovered in the stomach or small intestine, the bowel is decontaminated using a cathartic before beginning chelation therapy.** **Answer 4** is incorrect because a chest x-ray is a *general* study of the respiratory system, and would *not detect* lead levels in the toddler's body or reveal the presence of lead chips.

■ **TEST-TAKING TIP:** ***Think: Lead poisoning is from ingestion, ingestion is related to the GI system, the GI system fills the abdomen; therefore, select an abdominal x-ray option.***

Content Area: Child Health, Poisoning; ***Integrated Process:*** Nursing Process, Analysis; ***Cognitive Level:*** Application; ***Client Need/Subneed:*** Physiological Integrity/Reduction of Risk Potential/Diagnostic Tests

58. CORRECT ANSWER: 3. **Answer 1** is incorrect because straining does *not* affect intake and output. **Answer 2** is incorrect because the voided urine is strained. Straining does *nothing* to promote voiding. **Answer 3 is correct because straining is done to collect a renal stone for analysis of composition.** **Answer 4** is incorrect because a urinalysis *can* be completed even with blood clots present.

■ **TEST-TAKING TIP:** ***Look for the answer that describes the need to "find" something. Three of the options imply straining will improve urine quantity or quality.***

Content Area: Adult Health, Renal; ***Integrated Process:*** Nursing Process, Analysis; ***Cognitive Level:*** Comprehension; ***Client Need/Subneed:*** Physiological Integrity/Physiological Adaptation/Alterations in Body Systems

59. CORRECT ANSWER: 4. **Answer 1** is incorrect because contractions that are less than 2 minutes apart are *uterine tetany, not* a sign of normal labor. **Answer 2** is incorrect because back pain and increased vaginal discharge are *not* the signs of *normal onset* of labor. **Answer 3** is incorrect because frequent urination is a sign of urinary tract *infection, not* a sign of the normal onset of labor. **Answer 4 is correct because contractions that are 5 minutes apart and regular for an hour are the signs of normal onset of labor.**

■ **TEST-TAKING TIP:** ***Eliminate Answer 3 because it includes painful urination, which is never a sign of normal labor. The other two options are not signs of typical labor.***

Content Area: Maternity, Antepartum; ***Integrated Process:*** Nursing Process, Evaluation; ***Cognitive Level:*** Analysis; ***Client Need/Subneed:*** Health Promotion and Maintenance/Ante/Intra/Postpartum and Newborn Care

60. CORRECT ANSWER: 2. **Answer 1** is incorrect because infection is *not* a greater concern. **Answer 2 is correct because burn wound tissue shortens because of flexion of muscles in wound healing. Contractures will need to be prevented with splints or traction.** **Answer 3** is incorrect because large-bore central line IV catheters via cutdown *can* be placed in any major vessel. **Answer 4** is incorrect because a sterile dressing can be applied under the BP cuff, or a Doppler can be used, or an arterial catheter can be inserted.

■ **TEST-TAKING TIP:** ***Visualize the burn location and how treating the wound would interfere with the care need.***

Content Area: Adult Health, Integumentary; ***Integrated Process:*** Nursing Process, Analysis; ***Cognitive Level:*** Application; ***Client Need/Subneed:*** Physiological Integrity/Physiological Adaptation/Alterations in Body Systems

61. CORRECT ANSWER: 4. **Answer 1** is incorrect because the use of IV *N*-acetylcysteine (Mucomyst) is still investigational. **Answer 2** is incorrect because *N*-acetylcysteine (Mucomyst) is *not* given IM. **Answer 3** is incorrect because the offensive odor of *N*-acetylcysteine (Mucomyst) would *not* be concealed by water. **Answer 4 is correct because *N*-acetylcysteine (Mucomyst) is usually given orally, but is first diluted in fruit juice or soda because of the antidote's offensive odor ("rotten eggs").**

■ **TEST-TAKING TIP:** ***Think of how to best conceal the drug's odor...juice is more effective than water.***

Content Area: Child Health, Poisoning; ***Integrated Process:*** Nursing Process, Implementation; ***Cognitive Level:*** Application; ***Client Need/Subneed:*** Physiological Integrity/Pharmacological and Parenteral Therapies/Medication Administration

62. CORRECT ANSWER: 2. **Answer 1** is incorrect because giving the mother pictures of her baby is appropriate *only* when an infant *is too ill* for physical contact or the mother is too ill to visit in the nursery. **Answer 2 is correct because the combination of direct physical contact between mother and baby and participation in the infant's care helps the mother in recognizing her infant as a distinct individual who is yet a part of her. This process is the beginning of attachment.** **Answer 3** is incorrect because direct physical contact between mother and baby is most likely to promote attachment. Looking through the window doesn't replace *touching and caring for* her infant. **Answer 4** is incorrect because descriptions of the infant *do not* replace physical contact between mother and baby.

■ **TEST-TAKING TIP:** ***Facilitating attachment when an infant is in the nursery is an important part of caring for the mother and helping her to cope with an infant who is ill. Eliminate looking, seeing, and helping. Select direct contact with the baby.***

Content Area: Maternity, Newborn; ***Integrated Process:*** Nursing Process, Implementation; ***Cognitive Level:*** Application; ***Client Need/Subneed:*** Health Promotion and Maintenance/Developmental Stages and Transitions

63. CORRECT ANSWER: 1. **Answer 1 is correct because the ingested toxin is removed by lavage from the stomach, and then the activated charcoal is instilled to aid in the absorption and removal of any medication left after the**

gastric lavage is completed. To "lavage" means to wash the stomach and remove the saline when the lavage is completed. Answer 2 is incorrect because the ingested toxin must be *first removed* by lavage, and then the activated charcoal is instilled to aid in the absorption and removal of any medication left after the gastric lavage is completed. Answer 3 is incorrect because the saline solution contains toxic particles which must be *removed before* the activated charcoal is instilled, which will help to absorb and remove any medication that is left after the gastric lavage is completed. Answer 4 is incorrect because gastric lavage and activated charcoal *are* used together in a sequential pattern when attempting to remove ingested toxins from the stomach.

■ TEST-TAKING TIP: *Focus on the contradictory options here. Since Answer 1 is the opposite of Answer 2, one of them is wrong. Look at the stem that happens to state the correct order: wash and then administer . . . select Answer 1!*

Content Area: Child Health, Poisoning; *Integrated Process:* Nursing Process, Implementation; *Cognitive Level:* Application; *Client Need/Subneed:* Physiological Integrity/Reduction of Risk Potential/Therapeutic Procedures

64. CORRECT ANSWER: 1. **Answer 1 is correct because the bowel should be functioning by 72 hours.** Answer 2 is incorrect because there may be faint bowel sounds, but the bowel will not be fully functional. Answer 3 is incorrect because the effects of general anesthesia on the bowel are still present. Answer 4 is incorrect because the question asks for *full function.* "Gas" is not full function. Some faint bowel sounds may be present.

■ TEST-TAKING TIP: *Think about the magnitude of the surgery. Choose the* longest *time period because the effects of general anesthesia, pain, medications, and immobility will delay the return of peristalsis. After 3 days (72 hours), there would be concern for paralytic ileus if normal bowel function did not return.*

Content Area: Adult Health, Gastrointestinal; *Integrated Process:* Nursing Process, Implementation; *Cognitive Level:* Application; *Client Need/Subneed:* Physiological Integrity/Basic Care and Comfort/Elimination

65. CORRECT ANSWERS: 1, 2, 3, 4, 6. **Answer 1 is correct because the client must be sitting up before beginning the epidural procedure. Answer 2 is correct because an IV bolus must be infused before beginning an epidural procedure. Beginning the infusion is the first step because it takes the longest time and must be completed before the epidural procedure can be started. Answer 3 is correct because baseline vital signs must be recorded before beginning the procedure so that any changes in vital signs can be treated promptly. Answer 4 is correct because allowing a client to empty her bladder will make the procedure more comfortable for the client. In addition, after the epidural procedure, the client will lose sensation to her bladder and may be unable to void.** Answer 5 is incorrect because nurses are not responsible for obtaining an informed consent. It is the responsibility of the physician or anesthesia provider to provide informed consent. **Answer 6, performing a procedural pause, is the final step before beginning the epidural to ensure that this is the correct procedure and the correct client.**

■ TEST-TAKING TIP: *Read the answers carefully. Eliminate Answer 5 completely because an informed consent is not the role of the nurse. The act of* obtaining *a client* signature *on the consent form is* not *the* same *as* informed consent.

Content Area: Maternity, Intrapartum; *Integrated Process:* Nursing Process, Implementation; *Cognitive Level:* Analysis; *Client Need/Subneed:* Physiological Integrity/Reduction of Risk Potential/Potential for Alterations in Body Systems

66. CORRECT ANSWER: 3. Answer 1 is incorrect because it sounds as though the nurse assumes the child has not thought about the potential hazards of the hike. This statement may block effective communication between the nurse and the teenager. Answer 2 is incorrect because the statement implies that the nurse is withholding approval until after a physician's review. This statement prevents effective exchange of communication between the nurse and the teenager. **Answer 3 is correct because the nurse first provides praise for a positive health behavior, then opens up the conversation into a discussion about additional steps that should be taken to promote the child's health.** Answer 4 is incorrect because, although the nurse may want to know how the parents feel about the hike, it is better for the nurse to first explore the teenager's plans and attitudes. If the nurse specifically asks about the parents' thoughts, the teen may feel that the nurse is seeking to block participation in the activity.

■ TEST-TAKING TIP: *Be wary of selecting answers that sound condescending or judgmental. Remember that a teenager with a chronic health condition should have a reasonable sense of possible activity limitations while also having a developmental need to be like peers. The best strategy for the nurse is to explore with the teen the challenges of participating in a mountain hike and to work together to meet mutual health goals.*

Content Area: Child Health, Hematological; *Integrated Process:* Nursing Process, Implementation; *Cognitive Level:* Application; *Client Need/Subneed:* Physiological Integrity/Reduction of Risk Potential/Potential for Alterations in Body Systems

67. CORRECT ANSWER: 4. Answer 1 is incorrect because this *is* an appropriate action. Answer 2 is incorrect because the client recognizes that there has been a problem. Answer 3 is incorrect because this is *not a concern.* **Answer 4 is correct because there may be variations in the *effects* of a name brand versus a generic brand. The physician should be advised.**

■ TEST-TAKING TIP: *The question is asking for the statement that is a problem. When a decision is based on cost, consider the risk to the client.*

Content Area: Adult Health, Endocrine; *Integrated Process:* Nursing Process, Evaluation; *Cognitive Level:* Analysis; *Client Need/Subneed:* Health Promotion and Maintenance/Self-care

68. CORRECT ANSWER: 4. Answer 1 is incorrect because, while the child should be placed on NPO precautions to prevent further damage from the corrosive substance to the esophagus, it is *not* the nurse's *first* priority. **Answer 2** is incorrect because, while the child is undoubtedly experiencing pain and will require an analgesic, it is *not* the nurse's *first* priority. **Answer 3** is incorrect because corrosive substances burn as they go down the esophagus and will burn coming back up the esophagus with vomiting. Inducing vomiting (by any means) is *contraindicated* when dealing with the ingestion of corrosive substances. **Answer 4 is correct because maintaining a patient airway is always the nurse's first priority. In the presence of swelling, the loss of a patent airway is both a real possibility *and* the nurse's first concern.**

■ **TEST-TAKING TIP:** ***When dealing with corrosive substances, remember that they "burn both ways." Select "airway" as first priority in the ABCs (Airway, Breathing, Circulation).***

Content Area: Child Health, Poisoning; ***Integrated Process:*** Nursing Process, Implementation; ***Cognitive Level:*** Application; ***Client Need/Subneed:*** Safe and Effective Care Environment/ Management of Care/Establishing Priorities

69. CORRECT ANSWERS: 1, 2, 3, 5. Answer 1 is correct because administering oxytocin can decrease the bleeding after delivery. Answer 2 is correct because massaging the fundus is the first step to decrease the bleeding. Making sure the fundus is firm and not deviated is an important postpartum assessment. Answer 3 is correct because a full bladder can impede the contraction of the uterus and can cause increased bleeding. Having the client empty her bladder can help decrease uterine bleeding. Answer 4 is incorrect because tocolytics are drugs that reduce contractions in *preterm* labor clients. Tocolytics would be *contraindicated* in a client who is postpartum and actively bleeding. **Answer 5 is correct because vital signs are an important assessment for a client who is postpartum and having a large amount of bleeding. Changes in the heart rate and blood pressure can indicate significant blood loss.**

■ **TEST-TAKING TIP:** ***Remember that tocolytics are used for preterm labor to decrease hyperstimulation in labor, and not used in clients who are postpartum.***

Content Area: Maternity, Postpartum; ***Integrated Process:*** Nursing Process, Implementation; ***Cognitive Level:*** Analysis; ***Client Need/Subneed:*** Physiological Integrity/Physiological Adaptation/Alterations in Body Systems

70. CORRECT ANSWERS: 2, 4, 5, 7. Answer 1 is incorrect because an atrial septal defect causes *left*-to-right blood flow and is a noncyanotic heart defect. **Answer 2 is correct because right-to-left blood flow is found in transposition of the great vessels. Answer 3** is incorrect because coarctation of the aorta causes *left*-to-right blood flow and is a noncyanotic heart defect. **Answer 4 is correct because right-to-left blood flow is found in tricuspid atresia. Answer 5 is correct because right-to-left blood flow is found in truncus arteriosus. Answer 6** is incorrect because a patent ductus arteriosus causes *left*-to-right blood flow and is a noncyanotic heart defect. **Answer 7 is correct because right-to-left blood flow is found in tetralogy of Fallot.**

■ **TEST-TAKING TIP:** ***A helpful mnemonic for remembering cyanotic heart defects is that the most common types begin with the letter "T."***

Content Area: Child Health, Cardiovascular; ***Integrated Process:*** Nursing Process, Analysis; ***Cognitive Level:*** Comprehension; ***Client Need/Subneed:*** Physiological Integrity/Reduction of Risk Potential/Potential for Alterations in Body Systems

71. CORRECT ANSWER: 4. Answer 1 is incorrect because the client has the right to refuse. **Answer 2** is incorrect because this response does not address the reason for refusal. **Answer 3** is incorrect because this is a threatening response and not therapeutic. **Answer 4 is correct because this response attempts to understand the client's actions.**

■ **TEST-TAKING TIP:** ***Choose the option that seeks elaboration.***

Content Area: Geriatrics, Hematological; ***Integrated Process:*** Communication and Documentation; ***Cognitive Level:*** Comprehension; ***Client Need/Subneed:*** Psychosocial Integrity/Therapeutic Communications

72. CORRECT ANSWER: 2. Answer 1 is incorrect because the fundal height is approximately 2 fingerbreadths *below* the umbilicus *immediately after* delivery. The fundal height increases to 1 to 2 fingerbreadths *above* the umbilicus *within 12 hours* after delivery. **Answer 2 is correct because fundal height increases to 1 to 2 fingerbreadths above the umbilicus within 12 hours after delivery. Answer 3** is incorrect because fundal deviation to the right side indicates a *full bladder* and risk for *uterine atony* and *hemorrhage*. **Answer 4** is incorrect because the fundal height is 3 to 4 fingerbreadths below the umbilicus by the *fourth to fifth postpartum day.*

■ **TEST-TAKING TIP:** ***When the options have similarities (in this case, "firm fundus"), ignore that part of the answer and focus on the dissimilarities between the choices.***

Content Area: Maternity, Postpartum; ***Integrated Process:*** Nursing Process, Assessment; ***Cognitive Level:*** Application; ***Client Need/Subneed:*** Health Promotion and Maintenance/ Ante/Intra/Postpartum and Newborn Care

73. CORRECT ANSWER: 2. Answer 1 is incorrect because drug therapy *needs* the directive to take the medication with meals to decrease the release of gastric acid or to accelerate gastric emptying. **Answer 2 is correct because giving the client information also gives the client control over the condition. Answer 3** is incorrect because the client's goals and physician's goals need to be the *same* for the plan of care to be successful. **Answer 4** is incorrect because a referral to the interdisciplinary team may be needed *if* further teaching is needed, or to add reinforcement.

■ **TEST-TAKING TIP:** ***Compliance with treatment requires the client's understanding and agreement.***

Content Area: Adult Health, Gastrointestinal; ***Integrated Process:*** Nursing Process, Implementation; ***Cognitive Level:*** Application; ***Client Need/Subneed:*** Health Promotion and Maintenance/Principles of Teaching and Learning

74. CORRECT ANSWERS: 1, 3, 6. Answer 1 is correct because, after taking action to treat the "tet spell," the parents should activate emergency medical services (EMS). **Answer 2** is incorrect because the child should be placed on the *side, not* upright in a chair. Answer 3 is correct because, before the child might have a "tet spell," parents should first get trained in CPR, in order to be ready should their child need such intervention. **Answer 4** is incorrect because *nothing* should be placed in the child's mouth during a "tet spell." Aspirin is *not* used to treat this condition; it is given for the treatment of heart attack. **Answer 5** is incorrect because coughing will *not* reverse a "tet spell"; it is the treatment for supraventricular tachycardia. Answer 6 is correct because the parents' first response during a "tet spell" should be to place the child in the position that will increase systemic vascular resistance and prevent fainting.

■ TEST-TAKING TIP: ***The best sequence of steps is: CPR training → positioning → calling for help.***

Content Area: Child Health, Cardiovascular; ***Integrated Process:*** Nursing Process, Implementation; ***Cognitive Level:*** Application; ***Client Need/Subneed:*** Physiological Integrity/Physiological Adaptation/Hemodynamics

75. CORRECT ANSWERS: 1, 5. Answer 1 is correct because this client has HELLP syndrome, with a decreased hematocrit, elevated liver function tests, and low platelets. Deep tendon reflexes are an essential part of an assessment for a client with HELLP syndrome. **Answer 2** is incorrect because a sterile vaginal examination is *not* an essential part of assessing a client with HELLP syndrome. The client is *not* complaining of abdominal pain or contractions; therefore, performing a vaginal examination is *not* necessary. **Answer 3** is incorrect because sterile speculum examination is *not* an essential part of assessing a client with HELLP syndrome. The client is *not* complaining of abdominal pain, contractions, or leaking amniotic fluid; therefore, performing a sterile speculum examination is *not* necessary. **Answer 4** is incorrect because a fern test is a test for rupture of amniotic membranes. The client is *not* complaining of *leaking fluid;* therefore, a fern test is *not* necessary. Answer 5 is correct because this client has HELLP syndrome, with a decreased hematocrit, elevated liver function tests, and low platelets. Urine protein is an essential assessment for a client with HELLP syndrome.

■ TEST-TAKING TIP: ***The key to answering this question is to determine what the diagnosis is for this client, which is based on vital signs and laboratory values. Choosing the correct answers depends on recognizing that this client has HELLP syndrome. Remember that HELLP stands for: decreased hematocrit, elevated liver function tests, and low platelets.***

Content Area: Maternity, Antepartum; ***Integrated Process:*** Nursing Process, Assessment; ***Cognitive Level:*** Analysis; ***Client Need/Subneed:*** Physiological Integrity/Physiological Adaptation/Alterations in Body Systems

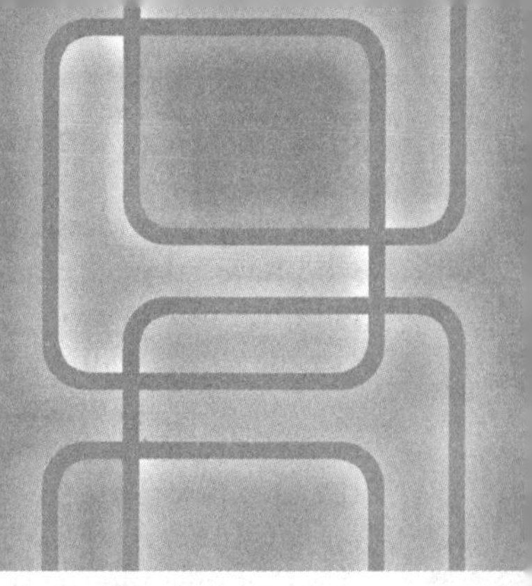

CHAPTER 2

Guidelines and Tips for International Nurses and Repeat Test-Takers

Sally Lambert Lagerquist

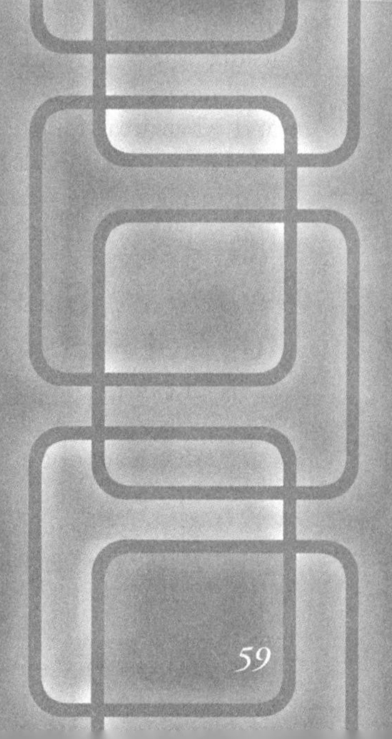

This chapter addresses the special concerns of candidates who have taken the test more than once, as well as international nurses who are graduates of nursing programs outside of the United States.

Since 1977, the authors of this book have had a long history of success in helping repeat test-takers and international nurses to pass because we have developed *an approach that works!* We give you guidelines, strategies, and tips that give *you* the skills and confidence to PASS.

This chapter will help put you in the frame of mind of an examination question writer and an entry-level nurse (which is what is tested on the examination), so that logic, practice, and a systematic approach can lead you to the best answer(s).

Tips for NCLEX-RN® Candidates Who Must Repeat the Examination

Purpose of This Section

Repeat test-takers have somewhat different needs, different starting points, and a different time frame from those who are first-time NCLEX-RN® candidates: that is, figuring out *why* they did not pass, what the Candidate Performance Report (CPR) that they received *means,* and what to do *next.*

Also refer to **Chapter 1—Orientation** in the sections on **How to Use This Review Book as a Study Guide: Where to Begin, While Reviewing, After Reviewing; Key Points to Recall for Better Study; Memorization: Purpose and Strategies;** the section providing information about the structure and format of the computer-adaptive NCLEX-RN®; and the section on how to **Prepare Physically and Mentally.**

What is the Difference Between Taking This Examination for the First Time and Repeating It?

You are "ahead of the game"! You have already received feedback about your examination-related strengths and weaknesses. You know what the examination is really like and what areas to emphasize. You also know what study methods did *not* work for you. Look at the experience you had in taking the examination as a "dry run" for helping you to *pass next time.*

What are Some Risk Factors for Not Passing the First Time?

1. It can readily be *what* you used to study. Often, it is a matter of *what* review materials you used that were not as helpful as other resources could be. Remember, some study aids are better than others. For next time, get a *fresh* start. Use *different* review materials.
2. Using *too many study aids,* from *too many different resources.* You wind up finding that theory and questions in books contradict each other, and there is no one to "referee" as to which books have the right information when books disagree.
3. Reviewing *only with questions and answers* in *books* will not help you to systematically cover *all* the theory that you need to review.
4. Reviewing *primarily with computer tests* is too time-consuming. You can cover more questions in less time by using a book. In addition, when you get through the thousands of questions on the disk or computer test, you cannot be sure that you have reviewed all that you need to know in each subject area, because the material is both limited and fragmented (i.e., it is not organized by concepts or systems). Compare this with a book that has *detailed* explanations for wrong and correct answers, where so much *more* helpful information can be seen at a glance on each page.
5. Taking the examination when you are *not ready, just because* you set an examination date.
6. Going into the examination with little or no review because of life circumstances (e.g., illness, moving, vacations, marriage, baby, job).

It is Not a Matter of How Much You Study for the Test, but *How* You Use the Review Material

At this point in your examination prep, do not start with page 1 and go through page 800+. This is usually overwhelming and not confidence-building. *You* need a *focused* review, starting with your *weakest* area and leaving what you feel most comfortable with toward the end of your reviewing. Discern if you mostly need a review of theory, test-taking strategies, or both. This will determine where you start.

How Do You Know What You Need to Review?

This is based on knowing what the NCLEX-RN® Candidate Performance Report (CPR) means. Look at the client needs/subneeds listed in the CPR that came with your NCLEX® results. Look at the areas where the **boldface** print states that your performance was below the passing standard or near the passing standard (which indicates the amount of improvement you need). This means that these are the areas (#1 through #8) that should be the major focus of your content review to **PASS NEXT TIME** (e.g., *Management of Care, Safety and Infection Control, etc.*).

If the computer stopped when you had taken only 75 to 100 questions, this probably means that you have significant deficiencies and gaps in certain areas of *nursing content.*

If the computer stopped when you had taken more than 100 but less than 200 questions, this usually means that you have *some* identifiable areas where you need to review certain content, as well as to improve your test-taking skills. **Appendix F** will show you where to go in this book to *read* in your areas where improvement is needed.

If the computer stopped when you had taken between 200 and 265 (the maximum number) questions, you were close to passing. Your problem area may very well be a difficulty with or an inconsistency in *answering the questions* when more than one answer could be correct. In this case, help is on the way! Go right to the **Test-Taking Tips and Guidelines: Sixty Strategies to Use in Answering Questions** section in this chapter. These test-taking strategies are designed to help you to pull the question apart to show you:

1. How to choose the best answer when all four options could be right.
2. How to narrow your choices down to two possible answers.
3. How to decide between two options.
4. What to do when you haven't a clue!

You *can learn* our *proven* test-taking techniques for success on the NCLEX-RN®. By following our guidelines before you repeat the examination, you can get quick feedback on your examination-related problem areas in order to better predict your next NCLEX® results *before* you take it (i.e., whether you are at risk for not passing).

What to Do to Pass Next Time

STEP 1: ASSESS yourself. In this book, take the two **Pre-tests** and two **Final tests** all at once. The book questions are also included with additional questions on the CD if you prefer to test electronically.

STEP 2: Score yourself at the end. Determine the percentage of questions that were correct in each of these integrated tests.

STEP 3: In any of the tests where you scored less than 80% correct, tally the **client need subcategories** that your wrong answers represented. Each question is coded by various categories; *you* need to focus primarily on the client subneed category. The codes are found after the rationale paragraph for each question and test-taking tips in the answer section of each test. For example, if most of the questions that you missed were represented by the client need *Management of Care,* **Appendix F** lists the pages in this book where this **content** is covered. You should be sure to review this content before proceeding. Go to **Appendix G** and look up *where* there are specific **questions** in the book that focus on your *most* problematic area(s).

STEP 4: Re-test yourself after reviewing the content areas in which you demonstrated a deficit. *Score* yourself. Try to achieve a correct score of *at least* 80%. You can do it!

How Will You Know That You are Well-Prepared and Ready to Retake the Examination?

When you are getting 80% correct in all of the questions in this book and on the accompanying disk, you are ready!

Most of all, you are ready when you change the "tape recorder" in your mind that keeps saying "I have failed" to "I haven't **PASSED** yet," and from "I hope I pass" to **"I WILL PASS!"**

A Guide for Graduates of Nursing Schools Outside the United States

International nurses who are educated outside the United States can use this book to serve their special needs:

1. To check their experiences, skills, and knowledge for *equivalency* to those of nursing candidates from U.S. programs, in terms of their ability to deliver effective and safe health care as determined by U.S. standards of practice.
2. To identify cultural differences in perception of client needs and nursing responses and actions (see **Chapter 3**).
3. To learn about the structure and format of the examination (see **Chapter 1**).
4. To learn how to prepare for the examination (see **Chapter 1**).
5. To practice taking tests made up of multiple-choice and fill-in-the-blank questions (see questions and test-taking tips in **Chapters 1, 3, 4, 5, 6, 7, 8, 9, 10, 11,** and **12**).
6. To assess the level of language difficulty in reading the examination.
7. To become skilled in test-taking techniques (see following section).

If you are an international nurse and wish to compare your preparation with that of U.S.-educated nurses, you will find that the practice questions with detailed answers and test-taking tips for each question that are included at the end of each major content chapter can serve as an effective **self-assessment** guide. If you find that you need further in-depth study after taking the practice tests and reviewing the essential content presented in outline format and in tables and figures throughout the book, you may wish to seek assistance from online or mobile review courses for self-paced review on DVD, CD-ROM, or mobile device. In addition, **Chapter 8** may help you review **drugs** used in the United States that may be called by other names outside the United States.

Cultural differences may be one cause of incorrect answers stemming from your different perception of clients' needs or nursing action. In addition, **Chapter 3** contains the code of ethics and standards of nursing practice and legal aspects that pertain to nursing *in the United States.* We suggest that the international nurse become familiar with these sections to determine what is *emphasized* in this country.

The **Orientation** section (see **Chapter 1**) is designed to help the international nurse know **what to expect during the examination,** what the **examination structure and format** will be like, **what content will be covered,** and how it will be **scored.** It will also help the examination candidate learn **how to study** for the test, **how to take a multiple-choice test,** and **how to reduce test-taking anxiety.**

If you are concerned about your ability to read and comprehend English as it might be used in the examination, first check yourself by looking at the examination questions in this book. The terms used here are those used in the health care field and are considered to be those a nurse needs to know and use. If the vocabulary is different from yours or is difficult, look at the list of common terms in **Appendix C.** You may also want to consult local colleges for courses in *English as a second language (ESL courses).*

If you are not familiar with or proficient in taking examinations with multiple-choice questions when more than one answer looks good, the approximately 3530 test questions in this book and the accompanying disk will provide you with sufficient practice for taking such a test. The following section on test-taking tips was specifically included to help you choose the best answer(s) by *narrowing* your choices to *increase* your chances of selecting the best answer(s).

Test-Taking Tips and Guidelines: Sixty Strategies to Use in Answering Questions

In a standard *four-answer multiple-choice* question, if you can systematically eliminate false answers, you can reduce the four-answer question to a two-answer one and thereby make your chances as good as those in the true-false type of question; that is, the odds will favor your guessing half of the answers correctly. Other questions will ask you to "select all that apply" from five to seven options by clicking in the correct boxes to select the answers (*multiple-response* questions).

In the **alternate** items, you may see charts and tables, or you may find pictures and graphs requiring identification of a correct location (*"hot spot"*) by either **point-and-click** or **fill-in-the-blank.** In the items requiring a *calculation,* determine which numbers are needed to figure out the correct numerical answer and use the drop-down calculator to fill in the blank. Another alternate item is the "*drag and drop*–ordered" response, in which you are asked to arrange all the correct responses in priority order: identify action or factor that you think should be *first,* then identify which should be *last.*

We think that the following pointers will assist you to narrow down your choices systematically and intelligently.

1. *Always, all, everyone, never, none, only, every, must.* Answers that include *global* words such as these should be viewed with caution because they imply that there are no exceptions. There are very few instances in which a correct answer is that absolute.

   Example: **Nurses should exercise caution in interviewing clients who have an alcohol use/dependency problem because:**
   1. These clients *always* exaggerate.
   2. These clients are *never* consistent.

   Any such suggested answer should be looked at with care because any exception will make that a false response. A more reasonable answer to the preceding might be "Clients who have an alcohol use/dependency problem may not be reliable historians."

2. *Broadest, most comprehensive answers.* Choose the answer that includes all the others, which is referred to here as the *"umbrella effect."*

   Example: **A main nursing function in group therapy is to:**
   1. Help clients give and receive feedback in the group.
   2. Encourage clients to bring up their concerns.
   3. Facilitate group interaction among the members.
   4. Remind clients to address their comments to the group.

   Number 3 is the best choice because all the other choices fall under it.

3. Test how *reasonable* the answer is by posing a specific situation to yourself. For example, the question might read, "The best approach when interviewing children who have irrational fears is to: (1) Help them analyze why they feel this way." Ask yourself if it is reasonable to use Freudian analysis with 2-year-old children.
4. *Focus on the client.* Usually the reason for doing something with a client is *not* to preserve the good reputation of the *doctor, hospital,* or *nurse,* or to enforce *rules.* Wrong choices would focus on enlisting the client's cooperation for the purpose of fulfilling orders or because it is the rule. On seeing a client out of bed against orders, instead of just saying, "It's against doctor's orders for you to get up," you might better respond by focusing on how the client is reacting to the restriction on mobility, by saying, for example, "I can see that you want to get up and that it is upsetting to you to be in bed now. Let me help you get back

to bed safely and see what I can do for you." Examples of client-centered options are: *acknowledging,* offering a *choice,* and determining *preferences.*

5. *Eliminate any answer that takes for granted that anyone is unworthy or ignorant.* For example, in the question, "The client should not be told the full extent of her condition because . . .," a poor response would be, ". . . she would not understand." Choose an answer that focuses on the client as a worthy human being.
6. When you do *not* know the best answer, and need to guess, *look for the answer that may be different from the others.* For example, if all choices but one are stated in milligrams and the exception reads "1 g," that choice may be a *distractor* or the *best choice.*
7. Read the question carefully to see if a *negative* modifier is used. If the question asks, "Which of the following is least helpful," be sure to gear your thinking accordingly. Emphasize a key word such as *least, contraindicated,* or *avoid* as you read the questions. In this type of question, a correct answer may reflect something that is false.
8. *Do not look for a pattern* in the correct answers. If you have already selected option 3 for several questions in a row, do not be reluctant to choose option 3 again, if you think that it is the correct response.
9. *Look for the choices that you* ***know*** *either* ***are*** *correct or* ***may be*** *incorrect.* You can save time and narrow your selection by using this strategy. This strategy is also useful when the question requires you to select *all options that apply.* Read each option and determine if it is correct or not; if correct, click on the box to the left of the option. There is no partial credit if you select some but not all that apply.
10. In eliminating potentially wrong psychosocial answers, remember to look for examples of what has been included in the *nontherapeutic responses* list in **Chapter 10** (e.g., denying feelings, false reassurance, changing the subject).
11. Wrong choices tend to be either *very brief* or *very long and involved.*
12. Better psychosocial nursing responses to select are those responses that (a) focus on *feelings* (unless safety is at stake!): "How did that make you feel?" (b) *reflect* the client's comments: "You say that made you angry"; (c) communicate *acceptance* of the client by the nurse rather than criticism or a value judgment; (d) *acknowledge* the client: "I see that you are wincing"; and (e) stay in the *here-and-now:* "What will help now?" Examples of better choices can be found in the *therapeutic responses* list in **Chapter 10.**
13. Look for the *average, acceptable, safe, common, typical, "garden variety"* responses, not the "exception to the rule," esoteric, or controversial responses.
14. Eliminate the response that may be the best for a *physician* to make. Look for an *RN role-appropriate psychosocial response;* for example, *psychiatrists* analyze the *past,* and *nurses* in general focus on *present* feelings and situations.
15. *Look for similarities and groupings* in responses and the one-of-a-kind key idea in multiple-choice responses.

   Example: **At which activity would it be important to protect the client who is on phenothiazines from the side effects of this drug?**
   1. Sunday church services.
   2. A twilight concert.
   3. A midday movie in the theater.
   4. A luncheon picnic on the hospital grounds.

   Choices 1, 2, and 3 all involve indoor activities. Choice 4 involves outdoor exposure during the height of the sun's rays. Clients need to be protected against photosensitivity and burns when on phenothiazines.

16. Be sure to note whether the question asks for what is the *first* or *initial* response to be made or action to be taken by the nurse. The choices listed may all be correct, but in this situation selecting the response with the *highest priority* is important. If the question asks for an *immediate* action, probably all answers are correct and you need to choose the *priority* answer. Identify words that set a priority: *best, main, primary, greatest, most.*
17. When you do not know the specific facts called for in a question, use your *skills of reasoning;* for example, when an answer involves amounts or time (mainly *numbers*) and you do not know the answer and cannot find any basis for reasoning (all else being equal), *avoid the extreme* responses (the highest or lowest numerical values).
18. *Give special attention to questions in which each word counts.* The purpose of this type of question may be not only to test your knowledge but also to see if you can read accurately and find the main point (e.g., early vs. late sign of shock). In such questions, each answer may be a profusion of words, but there may be one or two words that make the critical difference. If the option has several aspects, *all* the parts must be correct for that answer to be correct. If you can eliminate one aspect in an answer, you can eliminate the other options with that aspect.
19. All else being equal, select the response that you best *understand.* Long-winded statements are likely to be included as distractors and may be a

lot of words signifying little or nothing, such as "criteria involved in implementing conceptual referents for standardizing protocol." You may want to eliminate *unusual* or *highly technical* language. Relate the situation to something that is *familiar* to you.

20. *"Select all that apply"* questions require that all correct responses must be selected to get credit. First pick out *key* words (write them down, if that is helpful to you). Translate, into *your own* words, the gist of what is asked in the question. You might close your eyes at this point and see if the answer "pops" into mind. *Then,* skim the answer choices, looking for the response that corresponds to what first came into your mind. Key ideas or themes to look for in psychosocial responses have been covered in this section—for example, look for a "feeling" response, acceptance, acknowledgment of the client, and reflection.
21. Look for the *best* answer, not the right answer; for example, *incorrect* action may be the *best* answer *if* the stem asks for an action that is *not appropriate* (e.g., "Which of the following is an inappropriate action?" can be rephrased to say "Which action is wrong?").
22. To narrow down the choices, first find two *contradictory* options; for example, hypo–hyper, flex–extend, give–withhold, dilate–constrict, increase–decrease, bradycardia–tachycardia; then focus on which one may be the correct or best choice.
23. Focus on the *age-appropriate* answer (e.g., "When caring for a *toddler,* with what safety issue should the nurse be concerned?").
24. *Time* sequence points to the best choice. For example, ask yourself *when* is this taking place (e.g., prenatal or postpartum; preoperative or postoperative; before, during, or after; early or late; immediately?).
25. In medication administration questions, apply the *5 rights:*
    - Right Medication
    - Right Route
    - Right Client
    - Right Dosage
    - Right Time
26. When more than one answer looks right, choose the *first step* of the nursing process (*"assess"* before "implement"). Assessment words and phrases indicate priority:
    - Ascertain
    - Assess
    - Check
    - Collect
    - Detect
    - Determine
    - Find out
    - Identify
    - Look
    - Monitor
    - Observe
    - Obtain information
    - Recognize
27. Isolate the *verbs* from the rest of the question (e.g., *ask* is better than *tell, give,* or *ignore*).
28. Do not overlook the obvious answer: **KIS** (**K**eep **I**t **S**imple). For example, the best answer for what to do when there is a malodor in the room of a client with a colostomy is to "check the stoma for fecal leakage." If it smells like feces, check for feces.
29. As you read what is given for assessment findings (e.g., signs and symptoms) ask yourself: Is this *OK?* or is it *not OK?*
30. When two options are correct, choose the one that covers them *both* (i.e., *incorporates* the other, like a telescope).

    Example: **Two hours after a liver biopsy, the nurse finds the client lying on the left side. What is the best nursing action at this time?**
    1. Check for bleeding.
    2. Turn the client onto the right side.

    Both options are correct, but choose option 2 because it incorporates option 1; it is possible to *check for bleeding* while *turning* the client over onto the right side (where the liver is), to put pressure on the site (as a *preventive* measure when postbiopsy bleeding is possible).
31. Look at *root* words to give you a clue: for example, hemi = one half (hemianopsia = "half without vision"). Break down unfamiliar words in the stem.
32. Remember *Maslow*—"soma before psyche"—physiological needs are *before* psychosocial needs (i.e., physical needs first). Use Maslow's hierarchy to establish *priorities* when more than one answer looks correct.

    Example: **What is the priority nursing care for a client after ECT?**
    1. Reorient to time and place.
    2. Put the side rails up.
    3. Explain that memory loss is an expected outcome.

    When all three options are good (as in this case), select the *physical* aspect of care first (option 2) rather than either of the two psychosocial options.
33. Think *safety* as the best choice when more than one answer could be right. Safety is a *priority.* See the preceding example, where putting side rails up is a "safety" action.

34. *Visualize the condition, behavior, situation,* and the options to help you choose the best answer. Form a *mental image* (e.g., what *flexion* looks like versus *extension*); *visualize and sound out the answers* (e.g., to eliminate trite clichés or "authoritarian-sounding" responses such as "That's not allowed here").
35. "Would that you could that the *ideal* be possible." Choose an answer for the "ideal," not real, world. Do not rely solely on real-world experiences to answer NCLEX® questions (i.e., on the examination, answer as if you *have* all the time, all the staff, and all the equipment).
36. When in doubt as to which answer is best, use the *process of elimination* first (e.g., eliminate what you know is incorrect) to narrow your choice to two options. The best choice will provide an answer to what the question is *asking.*
37. Apply the *ABCS* when the question calls for priorities:
    - **A**irway
    - **B**reathing
    - **C**irculation
    - **S**afety
38. An important goal is to *maximize* client actions. For example, choose options that have indicator words for "encourage":
    - Reinforce
    - Support
    - Facilitate
    - Assist
    - Help
    - Aid
    - Foster
39. Try to turn options into *true-or-false responses* if possible in order to narrow down to two possible options. For example, when a question asks about adjusting insulin dosage, ask yourself, "What is true about adjusting the dose?" "Is it true or false that dosage is increased when the client has an infection?" (True). "Is it true or false that dosage is decreased when blood glucose level increases?" (False). If you find no "true" answers, look at the choices for a "maybe" answer.
40. Use *acronyms* and memory aids to help remember theory in selecting an answer (see **Appendix B**).

    SWISS—management of Cushing's syndrome:
    - **S**ugar (hyperglycemia)
    - **W**ater (fluid retention)
    - **I**nfection (prone to ...)
    - **S**odium (retention)
    - **S**ex changes (no menses)

    Five "*Ps*" of assessing fracture:
    - **P**ain
    - **P**allor
    - **P**ulselessness
    - **P**aresthesia
    - **P**aralysis

    WOUND[2] healing—affected by:
    - **W**ound dimensions
    - **O**verweight
    - **U**ndiagnosed infections
    - **N**utritional deficiencies
    - **D**iabetes, **D**isabilities (e.g., immunosuppressed)
41. *Reword* the question if the stem says "further teaching is necessary" (e.g., the *best* answer will have an *incorrect* statement).
42. Recognize what is *normal.* For example, are the data presented normal, or is the sign/symptom presented an "*Uh-oh!*" (meaning that a problem exists)?
43. Do *not delegate* functions of assessment, evaluation, and nursing judgment to a Licensed Vocational/Practical Nurse (LVN/LPN) or CNA (Certified Nursing Assistant) (e.g., do *not* delegate: admitting a client from the OR to the unit; establishing a plan of care; teaching or giving telephone advice; handling invasive lines).
44. *Do delegate* activities to an LVN/LPN or CNA for clients who are *stable* with *predictable* outcomes (e.g., help ambulate a client who is 2 days postsurgery). *Do delegate* to an LVN/LPN or CNA activities that involve *standard,* unchanging procedures (e.g., take vital signs after ambulation, *do clean* catheterizations, *simple* dressing changes, suction chronic tracheostomies using *clean* technique).
45. In *positioning* a client, decide what you are trying to *prevent* (e.g., contractures) or *promote* (e.g., venous return).
46. To help decide in which position to place a client, form a *mental image of each position* in the options (e.g., picture supine, high Fowler's, semi-Fowler's, Sims', prone, Trendelenburg, lithotomy, dorsal recumbent).
47. When none of the options looks good, identify the nursing *concept* implied in the *options* given (e.g., risk factors for infection).
48. When in doubt, first reread the *question stem* to obtain clues, then reread the options. When you come across a question that is about unfamiliar nursing content (e.g., paracentesis), first ask yourself, "What is the topic of the question?", then "What do the *answer choices mean?*", and then reword the question using the clues from the *options.*

    Example: **What is most important for the nurse to ask a client immediately after a paracentesis?**
    1. **"Are you in pain?"**
    2. **"Do you feel dizzy?"**

3. **"Does your underwear fit better around the belt line?"**
4. **"Do you need to urinate?"**

The first clue is in the question stem: *most important, immediately after.* Then, based on rereading the options, you can reword the question to, "What is an untoward reaction (complication) after this procedure?" The answer choices relate to *expected* outcomes (1, 3), a question that is not relevant to ask *after* the procedure (4), and a *complication* (2), which is the correct option.

49. Recognize *expected* outcomes of drugs and treatments/procedures.

Example: What will indicate improvement in the condition of the client who has anorexia nervosa?
1. **The client has gained weight.**
2. **The client weighs herself every day.**
3. **The client eats all the foods served to her.**
4. **The client asks the parents to bring her favorite foods.**

Choose the option that shows progress toward the goal (in this condition, it is weight gain that is expected).

50. When you do *not* know the answer, choose what will cause the *least harm.*

Example: The nurse suspects abdominal wound dehiscence when lifting the edges of the client's dressings. What should the nurse do next?
1. **Tell the client to remain quiet and not cough.**
2. **Offer a warm drink to help relax the client.**
3. **Place the client with feet elevated.**
4. **Change the dressing.**

Option 1 is the best answer, because it will not *add* damage that could happen with changing the position or the dressing.

51. Take care of the *client first,* not the equipment or the family (unless a family member is the focus of the question).

52. If one option has *generally, usually, tends to* but other options do not have these qualifiers, use the one option that does have the qualifier as the best answer.

53. Identify clues in the stem, that is, look for a *similar* word or phrase used in the stem and in one of the options. For example, if the question states that the client is on an *intermediate*-acting insulin (NPH), and the stem asks for its peak action, look for a *middle* time. Among choices of 4, 6 to 12, 12 to 14, or 15 to 18 hours after the injection, choose 6 to 12 hours (as the midpoint).

54. If two options are similar, *neither* can be the answer because both are distractors.

Example: What might the nurse expect to see when a client with cirrhosis is hospitalized with ascites?
1. **Client is likely to be anorexic.**
2. **Client's intake will be poor, especially if served large portions.**

You can eliminate both of these options because they are saying the same thing in different words: the client is likely to not be interested in eating.

55. Don't "pass the buck"—think what is a *nursing action* that an RN can do *before* calling the MD.

Example: After surgery, a client with diabetes complains of nausea, and appears lethargic and flushed, with BP 108/78, P 100, R 24 and deep. What is the next action?
1. **Call the MD.**
2. **Check the client's glucose.**
3. **Give an antiemetic.**
4. **Change the IV infusion rate.**

The nurse should *assess* (option 2) *before* calling the MD (who may *then* order an antiemetic, option 3, and alter the IV infusion rate, option 4).

56. Focus on key words in the *stem* of the question as your clue:

- Best
- Essential
- Highest
- Immediate
- Least likely
- Most
- Most appropriate
- Most likely
- Vital

57. "Action" does not always mean choose an "implementation" type of answer. The question may ask: "What is the best nursing action?" However, the answer may be an "assessment" option.

Example: What is the best action for the nurse to take when a mother at the clinic reports that her child who has diabetes is hyperglycemic in the morning (215 mg/dL), although the child has been well controlled with NPH and regular insulin before breakfast and dinner?
1. **Suggest that the mother give the bedtime snack earlier.**
2. **Suggest that the insulin be given later in the evening.**

3. **Suggest that they continue with the same regimen.**
4. **Check the blood sugar now, and suggest that the mother check it during the night.**

Choose "check," which is an "assessment" response (option 4), although the question (the stem) is phrased as an implementation ("best action" is an implementation).

58. Remember the *nursing hierarchy.* Go to the next line of *nursing* authority (e.g., staff → charge nurse; LPN/LVN → staff nurse) when the question asks to whom to report a situation. For example, if the question is about an LVN/LPN, the best answer is to report to the staff nurse.
59. When the question includes laboratory values, ask yourself whether the given value is "Uh-oh!" (meaning too high or too low), or "Uh-huh" (meaning not a particular problem). For example, a serum K^+ of 8.5 is "Uh-oh!" (too high).
60. *Prevention* is a key concept (e.g., when the question deals with infection control, and in health teaching).

Example: **The primary objective in ileostomy teaching with a client during the early postoperative period is to:**
1. **Facilitate maintenance of intake and output records.**
2. **Control unpleasant odors.**
3. **Prevent skin excoriation around the stoma.**
4. **Reduce the risk of postoperative wound infection.**

Choose "prevention" (option 3), which in turn may prevent contamination of the abdominal incision (option 4). Options 1 and 2 are *secondary* objectives.

Confidence, Performance, Pass!

Chapter 2 is aimed at helping you to take the NCLEX-RN® with more and improved test-taking skills.

THINK: ↑ confidence
THINK: ↑ performance
THINK: Pass NCLEX-RN®

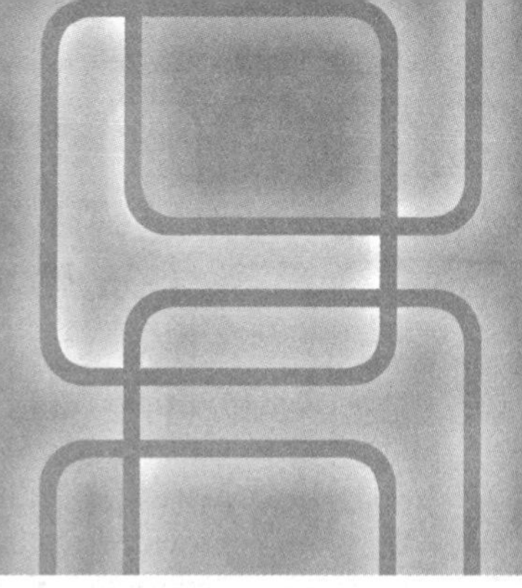

CHAPTER 3

Safe, Effective Care Environment

Management of Care, Cultural Diversity, Ethical and Legal Aspects of Nursing, Nursing Trends, and Safety and Infection Control

Sally Lambert Lagerquist • Janice Lloyd McMillin • Robyn Marchal Nelson • Denise Wall Parilo • Kathleen E. Snider

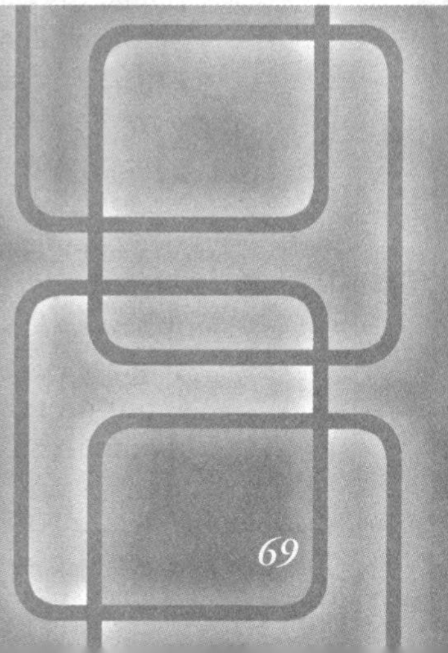

MANAGEMENT

MANAGEMENT OF CARE

I. CONCEPTS OF MANAGEMENT

A. *Definitions*

1. *Case management*—process that involves comprehensive coordination of activities and services provided to the client throughout the continuum of care or episode. *Activities* include: case finding, screening, intake, assessment, problem identification, **prioritization** of client's problems and needs, planning, reassessment, evaluation, documentation, designing and monitoring clinical pathways, and identification of variances.
2. *Continuous quality improvement*—process used to make improvements in client care; indicators of excellence are identified and process involves actively including input from and **collaboration** with the client (whose needs are at the center of the process), the family, and all health-care team members.
3. *Incidents/variance reports*—part of quality improvement, where occurrences take place in a health-care agency that are not typical according to medical orders, may be an accident, or may be a violation of policy and procedures (e.g., wrong medication dose, a client or visitor falls, needle stick by nurse). These are considered unexpected incidents, exceptions that happen during client care.
4. *Quality assurance*—activities that evaluate the quality of care provided to clients to ensure that it meets predetermined standards of excellence.
5. *Resource management*—providing appropriate number and type of resources needed by clients to achieve desired outcomes.
6. *Supervision*—process of guiding, encouraging, and assessing the work of others to whom tasks were delegated.
7. *Delegate responsibility and direct nursing care provided by others*—based on particular client/family needs and on job description, roles, functions, and skills of other nursing personnel: client's condition (stable or medically fragile), *complexity* of required care, *potential risks for harm* to client, degree of needed *problem-solving* expertise, *predictability* of outcome, type and *level of client interaction* required. *Important:* The person who delegated the task has the responsibility and final accountability for effective completion of the task.

B. *Management theories*

1. *Microlevel* theories: clarify and predict behavior (e.g., motivation) of the individual, with input on the group/organization (e.g., group dynamics).
2. *Macrolevel* theories: focus on best ways to make changes within an organization, organizing projects, obtaining resources, attaining goals.
3. *Intrapersonal/interpersonal* theories:
   a. *Cognitive:* belief—a person's motivation is based on expectations about what will happen as a result of own behavior; involves goal setting, with regular feedback to increase motivation to achieve.
   b. *Scientific management:* belief—repetition of task will result in expertise.
   c. *Neoclassical management:* based on Maslow (i.e., person continuously strives to meet higher level needs); **ERG** (**E**xistence, **R**elatedness, **G**rowth); job redesign (i.e., ensures that task has validity, significance, autonomy, and feedback).
   d. *Social/reinforcement:* belief—motivation comes from learning from those with whom a person identifies; conditioned by reinforcement.

C. *Management behaviors*

1. *Decision maker*
   a. Initiator of new projects.
   b. Crisis handler (e.g., interpersonal conflicts among staff).
   c. Resource allocator (people, physical, financial).
   d. Negotiator.
2. *Communicator*
   a. Monitor of data collection and processing.
   b. Dissemination of collected information.
   c. Speaker on behalf of agency.
3. *Representative*
   a. Institutional figurehead.
   b. Group leader.
   c. Liaison between agency and community.

II. ESTABLISHING PRIORITIES

A. When managing a number of clients at the same time, the nurse needs to set priorities by *assessing types of care* needed:

1. Decide on the *most important nursing activity* (giving a medication? performing a treatment? taking vital signs? providing nutrition? measuring I&O? etc.).
2. Identify the *first* action the nurse needs to take.
3. Select the *best* nursing action.
4. Determine which client needs *immediate* care.

B. Determine priorities with the guidance of:

1. **Maslow's hierarchy of needs** (see **Fig. 10.1, p. 715**)
   a. Choose *physiological* needs (survival) as the highest level of priority.
   b. Followed by *safety* needs.
   c. Then *psychological* needs (care and belonging).
   d. Lastly, *self-actualization* needs.

2. **Steps of the Nursing Process (A²DPIE)**
   a. First is *assessment (data collection).*
   b. Next, *analyze* the data (*nursing diagnoses*).
   c. Then, *plan* (goals).
   d. Followed by *implementation* (actions).
   e. Finally, *evaluation* (outcome).
3. **ABCS**
   a. Airway (e.g., patent airway)
   b. Breathing
   c. Circulation
   d. Safety
4. **RACE** (e.g., in event of fire)
   a. *Remove* the client.
   b. Then sound the *alarm.*
   c. *Call* the fire department.
   d. *Extinguish* the fire.

III. DISASTER PLANNING

A. *Definition:* any man-made (e.g., toxic material spill, riot, explosion, structural collapse) or naturally occurring (e.g., communicable disease epidemic, flood, hurricane, earthquake) event that results in destruction or devastation that causes suffering, creates human needs, and cannot be alleviated without support

B. *Goal:* reduce vulnerability to prevent recurrence

C. *Benefits* of a disaster plan:
1. Decrease in costs of damage control.
2. Decreased extent and duration of injury.
3. Decreased loss of life.
4. Increased ability to respond to unforeseen disasters.

D. *Health-care components*
1. Early warning signals, with *realistic* expectations.
2. Brief and succinct assessment of those at risk.
3. Simple, flexible rescue chains that unfold in organized stages/steps.

E. *Nursing responsibilities*
1. *Nurses at the scene:* assisting with rescue, evacuation, and first aid.
2. *Nurses at the hospital:* triaging victims and providing acute care.
   a. *Triage:* a system of client evaluation to set up priorities, assign appropriate staff, and start treatment.
      (1) *In emergencies:* greatest risk receives priority.
      (2) *In major disasters:* selection is based on doing what can be done to benefit the *largest* number; those needing highly specialized care may be given minimal or no care. First, take care of those needing *minimal* care to save their lives, and who in turn can be available to help others.
3. *Nurses at community shelters or health clinics:* assessing, planning, implementing, and evaluating ongoing health-care needs of victims.

F. *Level of prevention*
1. *Primary prevention:* prevention of disaster and limiting consequences when cannot be prevented.
   a. *Nursing activities:* identification of factors that pose actual or potential problem.
2. *Secondary prevention:* responding to the disaster, halting it, and resolving problems caused by it.
   a. *Nursing activities:* assessment of extent of injuries; tagging victims for treatments and evaluation; providing first aid; identifying complications; coordinating activities of shelter workers.
3. *Tertiary prevention:* recovery and prevention of recurrence.
   a. *Nursing activities:* implementing community's disaster plan; providing continuous assessment, planning, implementation, and evaluation; providing counseling as needed to victims and coworkers; educating the public about disaster preparedness.

IV. EMERGENCY RESPONSE PLAN: FIRE SAFETY AND PREPAREDNESS

A. Know location of:
1. Escape routes, escape doors. Keep fire exits clear.
2. Available equipment.
   a. Fire alarms.
   b. Fire sprinkler controls.
   c. Fire extinguishers.

B. Identify fire hazards.
1. Faulty electrical equipment and wiring.
2. Overloaded circuits.
3. Plugs not properly grounded.
4. Smoking.
5. Combustible substances → spontaneous combustion.

C. Prevention.
1. Report frayed or exposed electrical wires.
2. *Avoid* overloaded circuits.
3. *Don't* use extension cords.
4. Use only three-pronged grounded plugs.
5. *Avoid* clutter.
6. Remove cigarettes and matches from room; control smoking according to institutional policy; limit smoking to designated areas.
7. Immediately report smoke odors and burning.

D. Action to take in event of fire in immediate vicinity:
1. Move clients to safety (triage those who are not ambulatory or are otherwise incapacitated).
2. Sound alarm.
3. Close all windows and doors.
4. Shut off valves for O_2.
5. Follow agency policy about *announcing* fire and location, *notifying* fire company, and evacuation plan.
6. *Avoid* using elevators.

V. SAFE USE OF EQUIPMENT (see also **p. 84**)

A. Suspect malfunction in equipment when it:
1. Does not work consistently or correctly.
2. Makes unusual noise.
3. Gives off unusual odor.
4. Produces extreme temperature.
5. Produces sparks.

B. Replace immediately; don't repair it.

C. Call maintenance department to check for safety and repair.

D. When O_2 is in use:
1. Secure the O_2 according to institutional policy.
2. Remove flammable liquids from the area.
3. Put up "oxygen in use" signs.

CULTURAL

CULTURAL DIVERSITY IN NURSING PRACTICE*

With increasing ethnocultural diversity among health-care clients and staff, health-care providers must increase their sensitivity to and knowledge of cultural concepts, be aware of both similarities and differences in values and beliefs that exist across cultures, and know how this may affect health-care delivery. Important objectives are to increase respect and sensitivity for diversity in order to minimize potential for transgressing cultural norms, and to provide culturally conscious health-care and working relationships among clients and staff from dissimilar cultures.

The purpose of this section is to provide a framework/structure for assessing, planning, and implementing culturally conscious interventions.

We have selected 10 essential areas as guidelines for assessing cultural characteristics that have implications for health and health care: **communication, family roles, biocultural ecology, high-risk health behaviors, nutrition, pregnancy and childbearing practices, death rituals, spirituality, health-care practices,** and **health-care practitioners.**

I. COMMUNICATION

A. *Language*
1. What is the usual *volume* and *tone* of speech?
   a. *Guidelines:* use interpreters (to provide meaning behind words) rather than translators (who just restate words); *avoid* use of relatives and children; use interpreters of same age and gender when possible. Select the words you use carefully, *avoiding* buzz words and jargon. Speak clearly, pacing yourself to be neither too fast nor too slow. Words that are slurred, have many syllables in them, or are too technical make communication more difficult. Speaking too fast may overload the client and make it difficult for the client to follow. Speaking too slowly may lose the client's attention.
      (1) Select the gestures you use with care, using your nonverbal behavior to underscore your words and your actions. The proper use of gestures can clarify a message, and drawings can sometimes be helpful. Be careful, however; not all gestures mean the same thing in all cultures.

B. *Cultural communication patterns (see **Table 3.1**)*
1. Willingness to share their *thoughts and feelings.*
2. Use and meaning of *touch* between family, friends, same sex, opposite sex, with health-care provider.
3. *Personal space:* meaning of distance and physical proximity.
4. *Eye contact:* special meaning for staring (rude, "evil eye"); for avoidance of eye contact (e.g., not caring, not listening, not trustworthy); variation of eye contact among family, friends, strangers, and socioeconomic groups.
5. *Facial* expression: how emotions are shown (or not) in facial expressions; use and meaning of smiles.
6. *Standing, greeting* strangers: what is acceptable.

C. *Concept of time:* past, present, or future oriented; social time vs. clock time

D. *Names:* expected greetings by health-care providers

II. FAMILY ROLES

A. *Gender roles:* patriarchal or egalitarian; change in perceived head of household during different life stages; male/female norms (e.g., stoic, modest)

B. *Prescriptive* (*should* do), *restrictive* (should *not* do), *taboo* behaviors for children and adolescents
1. *Prescriptive* (e.g., "Fat children are healthy").
2. *Restrictive* practices (e.g., silence, not anger, at parents).
3. *Taboo* (e.g., discussion of sexuality).

C. *Family roles and priorities*
1. Family goals and priorities (family needs may have priority over individual health needs).
2. Developmental tasks.
3. Aged: status and role.
4. Extended family (biological and nonbiological): role and importance.
5. How social status is gained: through heritage? Educational accomplishments?

D. *Alternative lifestyles*
1. Nontraditional families: single parents, blended families, communal families, same-sex families.

III. BIOCULTURAL ECOLOGY

A. *Variations in color of skin* and *biological variations*
1. ***Skin color:*** special problems/concerns: assessment of jaundice, "mongolian" spots, and

*Sally Lagerquist (was in *Addison-Wesley's Nursing Examination* Review ed. 2, Unit 7, p. 633 [out of print]).

blood/oxygenation levels in *dark skin.*
Considerations for health care:
   a. Assessment of *anemia:* examine oral mucosa and nailbed capillary refill.
   b. Assessment of *jaundice* (e.g., in Asian people): look at sclera.
   c. Assessment of rashes: palpate.
   d. Get a baseline of skin color from family.
   e. Use direct sunlight.
   f. Look at areas with least amount of pigmentation.
   g. Compare skin in corresponding areas.
2. *Biological* variations in ***body, size, shape, and structure:*** long bones, width of hips and shoulders, flat nose bridges (relevance for fitting eyeglasses), shorter builds (at variance with normative growth curves); mandibular and palatine dimensions (relevance for fitting dentures); teeth (peg, extra, natal, large size); ears (free, floppy, attached); eyelids (epicanthic folds).
3. *Diseases and health conditions:*
   a. Specific risk factors related to **climate, topography** (e.g., air pollution, mosquito-infested tropical areas).
   b. ***At-risk groups for endemic*** **diseases** (those that occur continuously in a specific ethnic group): e.g., malaria, liver and renal impairment, infectious blindness and scleral infections, otitis media, respiratory diseases (e.g., tuberculosis, coccidioidomycosis).
   c. Increased **genetic *susceptibility*** for diseases and health conditions (e.g., diabetes, dwarfism, muscular dystrophy, cystic fibrosis, myopia, keloid formation, gout, cancer of stomach is more prevalent in blood type O, sickle cell anemia, Tay-Sachs disease).
4. Variations in ***drug metabolism*** (e.g., cardiovascular effects of propranolol in Chinese; peripheral neuropathy in Native Americans on isoniazid).
5. Variations in ***blood groups*** (e.g., Native Americans usually are type O and no type B; Rh-negative nonexistent in Eskimos, more often in Caucasians); twinning (dizygote) is highest among African Americans.

IV. HIGH-RISK HEALTH BEHAVIORS

A. Use of alcohol, tobacco, recreational drugs
B. Level of physical activity; increased calorie consumption
C. Use of safety measures (e.g., seat belts and helmets and safe-driving practices)
D. Self-care using folk and magicoreligious practices before seeking professional care

V. NUTRITION: See also **Chapter 9, Cultural Food Patterns.**

A. *Meaning* of food: symbolic, socialization role; denotes caring and closeness and kinship, and expression of love and anger
B. Common foods and rituals
   1. Major ingredients commonly used (high sodium, fat, spices).
   2. Preparation practices (e.g., kosher does not mix meat with dairy in cooking, eating, serving).
   3. Afternoon tea (British), morning coffee (American).
   4. Fasting (e.g., Muslims, Catholics, Jews).
   5. Foods not allowed (e.g., no shellfish or pork in kosher diet).
C. Nutritional deficiencies and food limitations
   1. Enzyme deficiencies (e.g., in *glucose*-6-phosphate dehydrogenase deficiency, *fava bean* can cause hemolysis and acute anemic crisis).
   2. Food intolerances (e.g., *lactose deficiency*).
   3. Significant nutritional deficiencies, such as *calcium* (Southeast Asian immigrants).
   4. Native food limitations that may cause special health difficulties, such as *poor intake of lysine and other amino acids* (Hindu).
D. Use of food for health promotion, to treat illness, and in disease prevention
   1. "Hot and cold" theories.

VI. PREGNANCY AND CHILDBEARING PRACTICES

A. *Fertility* and views toward pregnancy, contraception, and abortion
B. *Prescriptive, restrictive, and taboo* practices related to *pregnancy, birthing* practices, and *postpartum period*
   1. *Pregnancy:* foods, exercise, intercourse, and avoiding weather-related conditions.
   2. *Birthing process:* reactions during labor, presence of men, position for delivery, preferred types of health-care practitioners, place for delivery.
   3. *Postpartum* period: bathing, cord care, exercise, foods, role of men.

VII. DEATH RITUALS

A. Death rituals and expectations
   1. Cultural expectations of response to death and grief.
   2. Meaning of death, dying, and afterlife.
      a. Euthanasia.
      b. Autopsies.
B. Purpose of death rituals and mourning practices
C. Specific burial practices (e.g., cremation)

VIII. SPIRITUALITY

A. Use of prayer, meditation, or symbols
B. Meaning of life and individual sources of strength
C. Relationship between spiritual beliefs and health practices

CULTURAL

IX. HEALTH-CARE PRACTICES

A. *Health-seeking beliefs and behaviors*
1. Beliefs that influence health-care practices.
   a. Perception of illness (e.g., punishment for sin, work of persons who are malevolent).
2. Health promotion and prevention practices.
   a. Acupuncture.
   b. Yin and yang:
      (1) Increased yin results in nervous, digestive disorders.
      (2) Increased yang results in dehydration, fever, irritability.

B. *Responsibility* for health care
1. Acute care: curative or fatalistic.
2. Who assumes responsibility for health care?
3. Role of health insurance.
4. Use of over-the-counter medications.

C. *Folklore practices*
1. Combination of folklore, magicoreligious beliefs, and traditional beliefs that influence health-care behaviors.

D. *Barriers to health care* (e.g., language, economics, geography)

E. *Cultural responses to health and illness*
1. Beliefs and responses *to pain* that influence interventions.
   a. Special meaning of pain.
2. Beliefs and views about *mental illness/mental health care.*
   a. Therapies must include *extended* families as opposed to individuals or nuclear families.
   b. Cultural and racial as well as individual components must be considered when assessing precipitating or predisposing causes of illness (e.g., need to atone for sins).
   c. Values may conflict: for example, individualism versus concern for family or social interactions; self-actualization versus survival needs.
   d. Some ethnic groups *do not value or possess* qualities required for some psychiatric therapies, such as verbal skills, introspection, ability to delay gratification, and ability to discuss personal problems with strangers.
   e. Therapy resources *may not be accessible or considered useful or relevant* for members of some ethnic groups.
   f. Common feelings and behavior patterns may be shared by many "minority" groups:
      (1) Feelings of *inferiority and inadequacy,* often a result of prejudice and racism.
      (2) *Incompetent* behavior as an outcome of feeling inferior and inadequate.
      (3) *Suppressed anger,* resulting in displaced hostility and paranoid ideas.
      (4) *Withholding and withdrawal;* not comfortable with sharing feelings or experiences.
      (5) *Selective inattention;* may block out or deny frustration or insults.
      (6) *Overcompensation* in some areas to make up for denied opportunities in other areas.
3. Different perception of *mentally and physically* handicapped.
4. Beliefs and practices related to *chronic* illness and *rehabilitation.*
5. Cultural perceptions of the *sick role.*

F. *Acceptance of blood transfusions and organ donation*

X. HEALTH-CARE PRACTITIONERS

A. Traditional vs. biomedical care
1. Does the *age* of practitioner matter?
2. Does the *gender* of practitioner matter?

B. Status of health-care provider
1. How different members of health-care practice see each other.

XI. ADDITIONAL CULTURAL CONSIDERATIONS—for other cultural influences related to children and families, refer to **Table 3.1.**

Table 3.1

Cultural Influences on Health-Care Practices with Children and Adults

Cultural Group	Belief	Practice
African Americans (numerous groups from varying locales)	***Health*** is viewed as harmony with nature ***Illness*** may be viewed as "will of God" or a "punishment" (especially in children); illness can be caused by "natural" (polluted food/water) as well as "unnatural" (hex) sources • May distrust health-care practitioner who is from the majority group (shown by silence) • Reluctant to give permission for organ donation	• Self-care and folk medicine prevalent • Try home remedies first or consult with an "old woman" in the community (especially for children) • May make use of root doctors, spiritualist, voodoo priests • May seek opinion of black minister, who is highly influential in health-care decisions • Prefer use of last name (upon greeting)

Table 3.1

Cultural Influences on Health-Care Practices with Children and Adults—cont'd

Cultural Group	Belief	Practice
Americans (usually of Caucasian, European descent)	***Health*** is viewed as a combination of physical and emotional well-being ***Illness*** may be viewed in rational/scientific terms; believe in germ and stress theories • Increasing interest in health promotion as reflected in lifestyle • May view alternative health care as possibility/valuable, either independently or in conjunction with Western medicine	• Believe that infant can "tell" mother its health-care needs • Early/routine prenatal and well baby/child care and immunizations • Increasing reliance on/demand for "specialists" in child health care
Asian Americans (numerous groups from varying locales)	***Health*** is viewed as a balance between energy forces of yin (cold) and yang (hot); harmony with universal order; pleasing good spirits/avoiding evil spirits ***Illness*** may be viewed as an "imbalance" • Child's good health reflects well upon the parent/family • Honor and "face" important • Suppress emotions	• Goal of health-care therapy: restore balance of yin and yang • Restoration of health with: tai chi, acupressure/acupuncture, diet, folk healers, herbs, massage, moxibustion (heat applied to skin over specific areas) 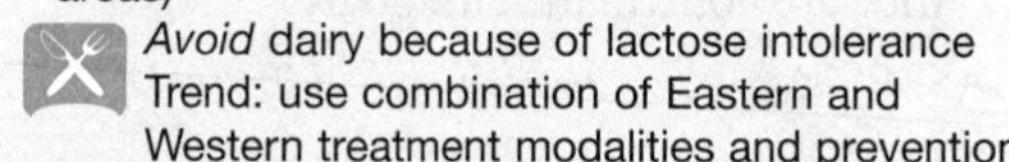 *Avoid* dairy because of lactose intolerance Trend: use combination of Eastern and Western treatment modalities and prevention • Elderly treated with respect • Close, extended families; father/eldest son are primary decision makers • Direct eye contact may show disrespect
Hispanic and Mexican Americans (numerous groups from varying locales)	***Health*** is viewed as a reward/"good luck" ***Illness*** may be viewed as punishment or an imbalance between hot and cold • Individual is passive recipient of disease, which is caused by external forces (supernatural)	• "Curandero" (folk healer) may be consulted about *mal de ojo* (evil eye) and *susto* (fright) before a health-care practitioner from the majority group • "Hot" diseases are treated with "cold" remedies (does not refer to temperature) • Use: herbs, prayers, religious artifacts/rituals; visits to shrines (strong association between religion and health) • Children highly valued/desired and taken everywhere with family, which can lead to interruptions when consulting with health-care practitioner • Family support during labor • Elderly treated with respect • Men make key decisions in matters outside of the home • Silence may indicate disapproval of plan of care • Very emotionally expressive when grieving
Native Americans/American Indians (numerous tribes from varying locales)	***Health*** is viewed as a state of harmony with nature and the universe ***Illness*** may be viewed as a price to be paid for past/future deeds • All disorders believed to have *supernatural* aspects/influences	• Going to the physician/hospital is associated with illness/disease; may delay seeking care as health state is viewed as part of a "natural process" (example: adolescent becomes pregnant) • Reliance on: diviners/diagnosticians, herbs, medicine man, rituals, singers; may carry objects to protect self against witchcraft; full family involvement • Children who are obstinate are respected, while children who are docile are considered weak; can lead to conflict with health-care practitioner from majority group • Elderly treated with respect • Blood and organ donation generally not accepted • Handshake, light touch OK, but maintain respectful distance while interacting

Adapted from Hockenberry, M, & Wilson, D: *Wong's Nursing Care of Infants and Children,* ed 8. Mosby, St. Louis, 2007.

RELIGIOUS AND SPIRITUAL INFLUENCES ON HEALTH

Religious and spiritual beliefs can have a major impact on health and illness. Each religion has its own rituals and traditions that must be observed, with the belief that if these are not followed, the outcomes may negatively affect the client's well-being or their family.

I. DEFINITION OF TERMS

A. *Religion*—an organized belief system in God or supernatural, using prayer, meditation, or symbols

B. *Spirituality*—encompasses more than religious beliefs; includes values, meaning, and purpose in life; can provide inspiration and sustain a person or group during crisis

C. *Values clarification*—aligns values and beliefs so that they are consistent with goals

II. ASSESSMENT *OF RELIGIOUS AND SPIRITUAL BELIEFS*

A. Beliefs about birth and what follows death

B. Code of ethics about right and wrong

C. View of health, causes of illness, or what may be the cure for the problem

D. Dietary laws

E. Relationship of mind, body, and spirit

F. Importance of work and money as they relate to religion

G. Pain: purpose of, response to, treatment for

H. Importance of family

I. Meaning of life, individual sources of hope and strength

J. Religious practices that conflict with health practices and use of health services

III. ANALYSIS/NURSING DIAGNOSIS

A. *Risk for spiritual distress* related to prolonged pain; health-care choices that are in conflict with religious practices; anxiety and guilt due to violating religious beliefs; lashing out against the religion

IV. NURSING CARE PLAN/IMPLEMENTATION

A. Acknowledge client's beliefs

1. Provide contact with clergy of choice.
2. Provide opportunity to carry out practices not detrimental to client's health.

B. Do *not* impose beliefs and values of health-care system

V. EVALUATION/OUTCOME CRITERIA

A. Increased satisfaction related to medical care decision

B. Decrease in feelings of stress, guilt, depression, anger

NURSING ETHICS

Nursing ethics involves rules and principles to guide right conduct in terms of moral duties and obligations to protect the rights of human beings. In nursing, ethical codes provide professional standards and formal guidelines for nursing activities to protect both the nurse and the client.

I. CODE OF ETHICS—serves as a frame of reference when judging priorities or possible courses of action. *Purposes:*

A. To provide a basis for regulating relationships between nurse, client, coworkers, society, and profession.

B. To provide a standard for excluding unscrupulous nursing practitioners and for defending nurses unjustly accused.

C. To serve as a basis for nursing curricula.

D. To orient new nurses and the public to ethical professional conduct.

II. ANA CODE OF ETHICS FOR NURSES incorporates the following key elements of what the nurse needs to do*:

A. Demonstrate respect for *human dignity* and *uniqueness* of individual regardless of health problem or socioeconomic level

B. Maintain client's *right to privacy* and *confidentiality*

C. Protect the client from *incompetent, unethical,* or *illegal* behavior of others

D. Accept *responsibility* for informed individual nursing judgment and behavior

E. Maintain *competence* through ongoing professional development and *consultation*

F. Maintain responsibility when *delegating* nursing care, based on competence/qualification criteria

G. Work on maintaining/improving standards of care in employment setting

H. Protect consumer from misinformation/misrepresentation

III. BIOETHICS—a philosophical field that applies ethical reasoning process for achieving clear and convincing resolutions to issues and dilemmas (conflicts between two obligations) in health care.†

A. Purpose of applying ethical reflection to nursing concerns:

1. Improve quality of professional nursing decisions.
2. Increase sensitivity to others.
3. Offer a sense of moral clarity and enlightenment.

---

*Adapted from recording at JONA and Nurse Educator's Joint Leadership Conference, 1981, A. J. Davis, "Ethical Dilemmas in Nursing."

†Adapted from AAA Code of Ethics on Nurses, Washington, DC.

B. Framework for analyzing an ethical issue:
1. Who are the relevant participants in the situation?
2. What is the required action?
3. What are the probable and possible benefits and consequences of the action?
4. What is the range of alternative actions or choices?
5. What is the intent or purpose of the action?
6. What is the context of the action?

C. Principles of bioethics:
1. *Autonomy*—the right to make one's own decisions.
2. *Nonmalfeasance*—the intention to do no harm.
3. *Beneficence*—the principle of attempting to do things that benefit others.
4. *Justice*—the distribution, as fairly as possible, of benefits, resources, and burdens.
5. *Veracity*—the intention to tell the truth.
6. *Confidentiality*—the social contract guaranteeing another's privacy.
7. *Respect*—acknowledge the rights of others.
8. *Fidelity*—keep promises and commitments.

IV. CLIENT'S BILL OF RIGHTS†

A. Right to appropriate treatment that is most supportive and least restrictive to personal freedom.

B. Right to individualized treatment plan, subject to review and reassessment.

C. Right to active participation in treatment, with the risk, side effects, and benefits of all medication and treatment (and alternatives) to be discussed.

D. Right to give and withhold consent (exceptions: emergencies and when under conservatorship).
1. *Advance directives:* legal, written, or oral statements made by a person who is mentally competent about treatment preferences. In the event the person is unable to make these determinations, a designated surrogate decision maker can do so. Each state has own specific laws with restrictions.
   a. **Living will:** legal document that specifically identifies treatment desires and states that the person does not wish to have extraordinary lifesaving measures (e.g., DNR) when not able to make decisions about own care.
   b. **Durable power of attorney (health care proxy):** legal document giving designated person authority to make health-care decisions on client's behalf when client is unable to do so.

E. Right to be free of experimentation unless following recommendations of the National Commission on Protection of Human Subjects (with informed, voluntary, written consent).

F. Right to be free of restraints and seclusion except in an emergency.

G. Right to humane environment with reasonable protection from harm and appropriate privacy.

H. Right to confidentiality of medical records.

I. Right of access to personal treatment record.

J. Right to as much freedom as possible to exercise constitutional rights of association (e.g., use of telephone, personal mail, having visitors) and expression.

K. Right to information about these rights in both written and oral form, presented in an understandable manner at outset and periodically thereafter.

L. Right to assert grievances through a grievance mechanism that includes the power to go to court.

M. Right to obtain *advocacy* assistance.
1. *Definition:* an *advocate* is a person who pleads for a cause or who acts on a client's behalf.
2. *Goals:* help client gain greater self-determination and encourage freedom of choices; increase sensitivity and responsiveness of the health-care, social, political systems to the needs of the client.
3. *Characteristics:* assertiveness; willingness to speak out for or in support of client; ability to negotiate and obtain resources for positive outcomes; willingness to take risks, and take necessary measures in instances of incompetent, unethical, or illegal practice by others that may jeopardize client's rights.

N. Right to criticize or complain about conditions or services without fear of retaliatory punishment or other reprisals.

O. Right to referral to complement the discharge plan.

V. CONFLICTS AND PROBLEMS—ETHICAL DILEMMAS

A. *Personal values versus professional duty*—nurses have the right to refuse to participate in those areas of nursing practice that are against their personal values, as long as a client's welfare is not jeopardized. *Example:* therapeutic abortions.

B. *Nurse versus agency*—conflict may arise regarding whether or not to give out needed information to a client or to follow agency policy, which does not allow it. *Example:* a teenager who is emotionally upset asks a nurse about how to get an abortion, a discussion that is against agency policy.

C. *Nurse versus colleagues*—conflict may arise when determining whether to ignore or report others' behavior. *Examples:* you see another nurse steal medications; you know that a peer is giving a false reason when requesting time off; or you observe a colleague who is intoxicated.

ETHICS/LEGAL

---

†Adapted from AAA Code of Ethics on Nurses, Washington, DC.

D. *Nurse versus client/family*—conflict may stem from knowledge of confidential information. Should you tell? *Example:* client or family member relates a vital secret to the nurse.

E. *Conflicting responsibilities*—to whom is the nurse primarily responsible when needs of the agency and the client differ? *Example:* a physician asks a nurse not to list all supplies used for client care, because the client cannot afford to pay the bill.

F. *Ethical dilemmas*—stigma of diagnostic label (e.g., AIDS, schizophrenia, addict); involuntary psychiatric confinement; right to control individual freedom; right to suicide; right to privacy and confidentiality.

LEGAL ASPECTS OF NURSING

I. DEFINITION OF TERMS

A. *Common law:* accumulation of law as a result of judicial court decisions.

B. *Civil law* (private law): law that derives from legislative codes and deals with relations between private parties.

C. *Public law:* concerns relationships between an individual and the state. The thrust of public law is to attain what are deemed valid public goals, such as reporting child abuse.

D. *Criminal law:* concerns actions against the safety and welfare of the public, such as robbery. It is part of the public law.

E. *Informed consent:* implies that significant benefits and risks of any procedure, as well as alternative methods of treatment, have been *explained;* person has had *time* to ask questions and have these answered; person has agreed to the treatment *voluntarily* and is legally competent to give consent; and communication is in a *language known to the client.*

F. *Reasonably prudent nurse:* nurse must react as a reasonably prudent nurse trained in that specialty area would react. For example, if a nurse works with fetal monitors, she must know how to use the monitors, know how to read the strips, and know what actions to take based on the findings.

II. NURSING LICENSURE—mandatory licensure required in order to practice nursing.

A. *Nurse Practice Act:* each state has one to protect nurses' professional capacity, to set educational requirements, to distinguish between nursing and medical practice, to define scope of nursing practice, to legally control nursing through licensing, and to define standards of professional nursing.

B. *American Nurses Association:* "The practice of nursing means the performance for compensation of professional services requiring substantial specialized knowledge of the biological, physical, behavioral, psychological, and sociological sciences and of nursing theory as the basis for assessment, diagnosis, planning, intervention, and evaluation in the promotion and maintenance of health; the casefinding and management of illness, injury, or infirmity; the restoration of optimum function; or the achievement of a dignified death. Nursing practice includes but is not limited to: administration, teaching, counseling, supervision, delegation, and evaluation of practice and execution of the medical regimen, including the administration of medications and treatments prescribed by any person authorized by state law to prescribe. Each registered nurse is directly accountable and responsible to the consumer for the quality of nursing care rendered." (American Nurses Association: *Nursing: Scope and Standards of Practice.* American Nurses Association, Washington, DC, 2004).

C. *Revoking a license:* Board of Examiners in each state in the United States and each province in Canada has the power to revoke licenses for just cause, such as incompetence in nursing practice, conviction of crime, drug addiction, obtaining license through fraud, or hiding criminal history (see **Section XI. A., B., C., p. 83**).

III. CRIMES AND TORTS

A. *Crime:* an act committed in violation of societal law and punishable by fine or imprisonment. A crime does not have to be intended (as in giving a client an accidental overdose that proves to be lethal).

1. *Felonies:* crimes of a serious nature (e.g., murder) punishable by imprisonment of longer than 6 months.
2. *Misdemeanors:* crimes of a less serious nature (e.g., shoplifting), usually punishable by fines or short prison term or both.

B. *Tort:* a wrong committed by one individual against another or another's property. Fraud, negligence, and malpractice are torts (e.g., losing a client's hearing aid, or bathing the client in water that causes burns).

1. *Fraud:* misrepresentation of fact with intentions for it to be acted on by another person (e.g., falsifying college transcripts when applying for a graduate nursing program).
2. *Negligence:* "Omission to do something that a reasonable person, guided by those *ordinary* considerations which ordinarily regulate human affairs would *do;* or doing something which a reasonable and prudent person would *not* do" (Brent N: *Nurses and the Law.* Saunders,

Philadelphia, 1997). Types of negligent acts related to:

a. Sponge counts: incorrect counts or failure to count.
b. Burns: heating pads, solutions, steam vaporizers.
c. Falls: side rails left down, infant left unattended.
d. Failure to observe and take appropriate action—forgetting to take vital signs and check dressing in a client who is newly postoperative.
e. Wrong medicine, wrong dose and concentration, wrong route, wrong client.
f. Mistaken identity—wrong client for surgery.
g. Failure to communicate—ignore, forget, fail to monitor, report, or document client's status or to report complaints of client or family.
h. Loss of or damage to client's property—dentures, jewelry, money.
i. Inappropriate use of equipment (e.g., excessive IV fluids via pump).

3. *Malpractice:* part of the law of negligence as applied to the *professional* person; any professional misconduct, unreasonable lack of skill, or lack of fidelity in professional duties, such as accidentally giving wrong medication or forgetting to give correct medication or instilling wrong strength of eyedrops into the client's eyes. Proof of intent to do harm is not required in acts of commission or omission.

IV. INVASION OF PRIVACY—compromising a person's right to withhold self and own life from public scrutiny. *Implications for nursing—avoid* unnecessary discussion of client's medical condition; client has a right to refuse to participate in clinical teaching; obtain consent before teaching conference.

V. LIBEL AND SLANDER—wrongful action of communication that damages person's reputation by print, writing, or pictures (libel), or by spoken word using false words (slander). *Implications for nursing*—make comments about client only to another health team member caring for that client.

VI. PRIVILEGED COMMUNICATIONS—information relating to condition and treatment of client requires confidentiality and protection against invasion of privacy. This applies only to court proceedings. Selected person does not have to reveal in court a client's communication to him or her. The purpose of privileged communication is to encourage the client to communicate honestly with the treating practitioner. It is the client's privilege at any time to permit the professional to release information. Therefore, if the client asks the nurse to testify, the nurse must truthfully give all information. However, if the nurse is a witness against the client, without the client's permission to release information, the nurse must keep the information confidential by invoking the privileged communication rule if the state law recognizes it and if it applies to the nurse.

VII. ASSAULT AND BATTERY—violating a person's right to refuse physical contact with another.

A. Definitions

1. *Assault*—the attempt to touch another or the threat to do so and person fears and believes harm will result.
2. *Battery*—physical harm through willful touching of person or clothing, without consent.

B. *Implications for nursing*—need to obtain consent to treat, with special provisions when clients are underage, unconscious, or mentally ill.

VIII. GOOD SAMARITAN ACT—protects health practitioners against malpractice claims resulting from assistance provided at scene of an emergency (unless there was willful wrongdoing) as long as the level of care provided is the same as any other reasonably prudent person would give under similar circumstances (see also **Section VII, p. 82**).

IX. NURSES' RESPONSIBILITIES TO THE LAW

A. A nurse is liable for nursing acts, even if directed to do something by a physician.

B. A nurse is *not* responsible for the negligence of the employer (hospital).

C. A nurse is responsible for refusing to carry out an order for an activity believed to be injurious to the client.

D. A nurse cannot legally diagnose illness or prescribe treatment for a client. (This is the physician's responsibility.)

E. A nurse is legally responsible when participating in a criminal act (such as assisting with criminal abortions or taking medications from client's supply for own use).

F. A nurse should reveal client's confidential information only to appropriate health-care team members.

G. A nurse is responsible for explaining nursing activities but not for commenting on medical activities in a way that may distress the client or the physician.

H. A nurse is responsible for recognizing and protecting the rights of clients to refuse treatment or medication, and for reporting their concerns and refusals to the physician or appropriate agency people.

I. A nurse must respect the dignity of each client and family.

X. ORGAN DONATION

A. Legal aspects to protect potential donors and to expedite acquisition
1. Prohibits selling of organs (National Organ Transplant Act).
2. Guidelines regarding who can donate, how donations are to be made, and who can receive donated organs (Uniform Anatomical Gift Act).
3. Legal definition of brain death (Uniform Determination of Death Act)—*absence of: breathing movement, cranial nerve reflex, response to any level of painful stimuli, and cerebral blood flow;* and *flat EEG.*

B. Donor criteria
1. Contraindications for being organ donator: *HIV-positive* status and *metastatic cancer.*
2. Prospective donors of both organs and tissues: those with no neurological functions, but have cardiopulmonary functions.
3. Prospective donors of only tissues: those with no cardiopulmonary function (e.g., can donate corneas, eyes, saphenous veins, cartilage, bones, skin, heart valves).

C. Management of donor
1. Maintain body temperature at greater than 96.8°F with room temperature at 70° to 80°F, warming blankets, warmer for intravenous fluids.
2. Maintain greater than 100% Pao_2 and suction/turn and use positive end-expiratory pressure (PEEP) to prevent *hypoxemia* caused by airway obstruction, *pulmonary edema.*
3. Maintain central venous pressure at 8 to 10 mm Hg and systolic blood pressure at greater than 90 mm Hg to prevent *hypotension* caused by complete dilation of systemic vasculature due to destruction of brain's vasomotor center, cessation of antidiuretic hormone production, and decreased cardiac output. Give fluid bolus and vasopressors, and monitor sodium levels.
4. Maintain fluid and electrolyte balance due to volume depletion. Monitor for *hyponatremia, hyperkalemia,* and *hypokalemia,* and intake and output.
5. Prevent infections due to invasive procedures (e.g., tubes, catheters) by using *aseptic* technique.

Questions Most Frequently Asked by Nurses About Nursing and the Law

I. TAKING ORDERS

A. *Should I accept verbal phone orders from a physician?* Generally, no. Specifically, follow your hospital's bylaws, regulations, and policies regarding this. Failure to follow the hospital's rules could be considered negligence.

B. *Should I follow a physician's orders if (a) I know it is wrong, or (b) I disagree with his or her judgment?* Regarding (a)—no, if you think a reasonable, prudent nurse would not follow it; but first inform the physician and record your decision. Report it to your supervisor. Regarding (b)—yes, because the law does not allow you to substitute your nursing judgment for a doctor's medical judgment. Do record that you questioned the order and that the doctor confirmed it before you carried it out.

C. *What can I do if the physician delegates a task to me for which I am not prepared?* Inform the physician of your lack of education and experience in performing the task. Refuse to do it. If you inform the physician and still carry out the task, both you and the physician could be considered negligent if the client is harmed by it. If you do not tell the physician and carry out the task, you are solely liable.

II. OBTAINING CLIENT'S CONSENT FOR MEDICAL AND SURGICAL PROCEDURES: *Is a nurse responsible for getting a consent for medical-surgical treatment?* Obtaining consent requires explaining the procedure and risks involved, which is the physician's responsibility. A nurse may accept responsibility for *witnessing* a consent. This carries with it little legal liability other than obtaining the correct signature and describing the client's condition at time of signing.

III. CLIENT'S RECORDS (DOCUMENTATION)

A. *What should be written in the nurse's notes?* All facts and information regarding a person's condition, treatment, care, progress, and response to illness and treatment. Document consent or refusal of treatment. Purpose of record: factual documentation of care given to meet legal standards; used to refute unwarranted claims of negligence or malpractice.

B. *How should data be recorded?* Entries should:
1. State date and time given.
2. Be written, signed, and titled by caregiver or supervisor who observed action.
3. Follow chronological sequence.
4. Be accurate, factual, objective, complete, precise, and clear.
5. Be legible; use black pen.
6. Use universal abbreviations.
7. Have all spaces filled in on documentation forms; leave no blank spaces.

IV. CONFIDENTIAL INFORMATION

A. *If called on the witness stand in court, do I have to reveal confidential information?* It depends on your state, because each state has its own laws pertaining

ETHICS/LEGAL

to this. Consult a lawyer. Inform the judge and ask for specific directions before relating in court information that was given to you within a confidential, professional relationship.

B. *Am I justified in refusing (on the basis of "invasion of privacy") to give information about the client to another health agency to which a client is being transferred?* No. You are responsible for providing continuity of care when the client is moved from one facility to another. Necessary and adequate information should be transferred between professional health-care workers. The client's consent for this exchange of information should be obtained. Circumstances under which confidential information can be released include:

1. By authorization and consent of the client.
2. By order of the court.
3. By statutory mandate, as in reporting cases of communicable diseases or child, elder, or dependent adult abuse.

V. WHAT IS THE HEALTH INSURANCE PORTABILITY AND ACCOUNTABILITY ACT (HIPAA)?

A. Importance of this act for nurses: nurses need to be able to answer client questions regarding the national privacy standards. The principles of the law reinforce professional responsibility to avoid unintentional disclosure of information (e.g., in elevators and hallways).

B. Overview of HIPAA: The first-ever federal privacy standards to protect clients' medical records and other health information provided to health plans, doctors, hospitals, clinics, nursing homes, pharmacies, and other health-care providers took effect on April 14, 2003. Developed by the Department of Health and Human Services (HHS), these new standards provide clients with **access** to their medical records and **more control** over how their personal health information is used and disclosed. The standards represent a uniform, federal floor of privacy protections for consumers across the country. State laws providing additional protections to consumers are not affected by this new rule.

C. Client protections: The new privacy regulations ensure a national floor of privacy protections for clients by limiting the ways that health plans, pharmacies, hospitals, and other covered entities can use clients' personal medical information. The regulations protect medical records and other individually identifiable health information, whether it is on paper, in computers, or communicated orally. Key provisions and points related to these new standards include:

1. **Access to medical records.** Clients generally should be able to see and obtain copies of their medical records within 30 days of request, and to request corrections if they identify errors and mistakes. The covered entities must consider the changes, but do not have to agree to the changes, and they may charge clients for the cost of copying and sending the records.
2. **Notice of privacy practices.** Covered entities must provide a notice to their clients stating how they may use personal medical information and their rights under the new privacy regulation. Clients also may ask covered entities to restrict the use or disclosure of their information beyond the practices included in the notice, as long as the restriction does not interfere with activities related to treatment, payment, or operations (e.g., family members may not be given information about a diagnosis without client permission).
3. **Limits on use of personal medical information.** The privacy rule sets limits on how covered entities may use individually identifiable health information. The client has a right to have access to accounting (i.e., the right to know *who* has been given access to their protected health information). The health-care facility must be able to produce a *list* describing people, companies, or agencies who have received protected information. In addition, clients must sign a specific authorization before a covered entity can release their medical information to a life insurer, a bank, or another outside business for purposes not related to their health care.
4. **Prohibition on marketing.** HIPAA sets new restrictions and limits on the use of client information for *marketing* purposes. Covered entities must first obtain an individual's specific authorization before disclosing their client information for marketing. At the same time, the rule permits doctors and other covered entities to communicate freely with clients about treatment options and other health-related information, including disease-management programs.
5. **Stronger state laws may remain in effect.** The new federal privacy standards do not affect state laws that provide additional privacy protections for clients. The privacy rule sets a national "floor" of privacy standards that protect all Americans, but any state law that provides additional protections would continue to apply. When a state law requires a certain disclosure—such as reporting an infectious disease outbreak to the public health authorities—the federal privacy regulations would not preempt the state law.

6. **Confidential communications.** Under the privacy rule, a client can request that covered entities take reasonable steps to ensure that communications with the client are confidential. The client has the right to request that communications about protected health information remain anonymous if mailed.
7. **"Minimum necessary" rule.** It guides the provider to use only the minimum amount of information necessary to meet the client care needs. The actual diagnosis may not be needed. This would relate to the use of e-mail or faxes to communicate client information.
8. **Telephone requests for personal health information.** Inpatient confidentiality must be protected. The nurse may be able to verify whether a client is in the hospital, but only if the caller asks for the client by name; otherwise the caller should be directed to the client or family.
9. **Complaints about violations of privacy.** A health-care facility must identify the privacy officer and state how to contact the officer.

D. There are additional situations where medical information may be disclosed without authorization, such as:

1. For workers' compensation or similar programs.
2. For public health activities (e.g., reporting births or deaths; injury or disability; abuse or neglect of children, elders and dependent adults; or reactions to medications), to prevent or control disease or injury.
3. To a health oversight agency, such as the State Department of Health Services.
4. In response to a court or administrative order, subpoena, warrant, or similar process.
5. To law enforcement officials in certain limited circumstances.
6. To a coroner, medical examiner, or funeral director.
7. To organizations that handle organ, eye, or tissue procurement or transplantation.
8. Public health: information may be used or disclosed to avert a serious threat to health or safety of an individual or the public (**Tarasoff Principle/Duty to Warn**).
9. Food and Drug Administration (FDA): health information relating to adverse events with respect to immunizations and/or health screening tests may be disclosed.
10. For members of the armed forces, health information may be disclosed as required by military command authorities.
11. To notify a person who may have been exposed to a disease or may be at risk for contracting or spreading a disease or condition.

VI. LIABILITY FOR MISTAKES—yours and others.

A. *Is the hospital or the nurse liable for mistakes made by the nurse while following orders?* Both the hospital and the nurse can be sued for damage if a mistake made by the nurse injures the client. The nurse is responsible for own actions. The hospital would be liable, based on the doctrine of *respondeat superior.*

B. *Who is responsible if a nursing student or another staff nurse makes a mistake? The supervisor? The instructor?* Ordinarily the instructor and/or supervisor would not be responsible unless the court thought the instructor and/or supervisor was negligent in supervising or in assigning a task beyond the capability of the person in question. No one is responsible for another's negligence unless he or she contributed to or participated in that negligence. Each person is personally liable for his or her own negligent actions and failure to act as a reasonably prudent nurse.

C. *Am I responsible for injury to a client by a staff member who was observed (but not reported) by me to be intoxicated while giving care?* Yes, you may be responsible. You have a duty to take reasonable action to prevent a client's injury.

VII. GOOD SAMARITAN ACT: *For what would I be liable if I voluntarily stopped to give care at the scene of an accident?* You would be protected under the Good Samaritan Act and required to live up to reasonable and prudent nursing standards in those specific circumstances. You would not be treated by the law as if you were performing under professional standards of properly sterile conditions, with proper technical equipment (see also **Section VIII, p. 79**).

VIII. LEAVING AGAINST MEDICAL ADVICE (AMA): *Would I or the hospital be liable if a client left "AMA," refusing to sign the appropriate hospital forms?* None of the involved parties would ordinarily be liable in this case as long as (a) the medical risks were explained, recorded, and witnessed, and (b) the client is a competent adult. The law permits clients to make decisions that may not be in their own best health interest. You cannot interfere with the right and exercise of the decision to accept or reject treatment.

IX. RESTRAINTS: *Can I put restraints on a client who is combative even if there is no order for this?* Only in an emergency, for a limited time (not longer than 24 hours), for the limited purpose of protecting the client from injury—*not* for convenience of personnel. Notify attending physician immediately. Consult with another staff member, obtain client's consent if possible, and get coworker to witness the record. Check frequently to ensure restraints do not impair circulation, cause pressure sores, or other

ETHICS/LEGAL

injury. Remove restraints at the first opportunity, and use them only as a last resort after other reasonable means have not been effective ("right to least restrictive environment"). Restraints of any degree may constitute *false imprisonment.* Freedom from unlawful restraint is a basic human right protected by law. In July 1992, the Food and Drug Administration (FDA) issued a warning that use of restraints "no longer represents responsible, primary management of a client's behavioral problem." It is necessary to advise the client and family of decision to restrain, explain risks and benefits, and obtain informed consent.

The Joint Commission (formerly known as the Joint Commission on Accreditation of Healthcare Organizations [JCAHO]) has published standards to minimize injury and complications from the use of restraints:

- Use *alternatives* to physical restraints whenever possible (e.g., offer explanations; ask someone to stay with client; use clocks, calendars, TV, and radio).
- Use only under supervision of *licensed* health-care provider.
- Use according to manufacturer's direction to avoid strangulation or circulation impairment.
- Provide frequent monitoring of client in restraints and allow regular, supervised restraint-free periods to prevent injury.
- Obtain written order promptly from practitioner upon initiation of restraints and throughout duration of use.
- Documentation must include: time applied and removed; type; medical reason (description of dangerous behavior) and alternatives tried before application of restraints; response.

A. *Nursing responsibilities*

1. Provide padding to protect skin, bony prominences, and intravenous lines.
2. Secure restraints to parts of bed or chair that will move with the client and not constrict movement. *Never* secure restraints to bed rails or mattress.
3. Use knots with hitches for easy removal, as required.
4. Maintain proper body alignment when securing restraints.
5. Remove restraints at least every 2 hours to allow for activities of daily living.

X. WILLS: *What do I do when a client asks me to be a witness to her or his will?* There is no legal obligation to participate as a witness, but there is a moral and ethical obligation to do so. You should not, however, help draw up a will because this could be considered practicing law without a license. You would be witnessing that (a) the client is signing the document as her or his last will and testament; (b) at that time, to the best of your knowledge, the client (testator) was of sound mind, was lucid, and understood what the client was doing (i.e., the client must not be under the influence of drugs or alcohol or otherwise unable to know what she or he is doing); and (c) the testator was under no overt coercion, as far as you could tell, but was acting freely, willingly, and under own impetus.

XI. DISCIPLINARY ACTION

A. *For what reasons may the RN license be suspended or revoked?*

1. Obtaining license by fraud (omission of information, false information).
2. Negligence and incompetence; assuming duties without adequate preparation.
3. Substance abuse.
4. Conviction of crime (state or federal).
5. Practicing medicine without a license.
6. Practicing nursing without a license (expired, suspended).
7. Allowing unlicensed person to practice nursing or medicine that places the client at risk.
8. Giving client care while under the influence of alcohol or other drugs.
9. Habitually using drugs.
10. Discriminatory and prejudicial practices in giving client care (pertaining to race, skin color, religion, sex, age, or ethnic origin).
11. Falsifying a client's record; failure to maintain a record for each client.
12. Breach in client confidentiality.
13. Physically or verbally abusing a client.
14. Abandoning a client.

B. *What could happen to me if I am proven guilty of professional misconduct?*

1. License may be revoked.
2. License may be suspended.
3. Behavior may be censured and reprimanded.
4. You may be placed on probation.

C. *Who has the authority to carry out any of the aforementioned penalties?* The State Board of Registered Nursing that granted your license.

D. *I am the head nurse. One of my nursing aides has a history of failing to appear to work and not giving notice of or reason for absence. How should I handle this?* An employee has the right to know hospital policies, what is expected of an employee, and what will happen if an employee does not meet the expectations stated in his or her job description or in hospital policies and procedures. As a head nurse, you must document behavior factually, clearly, and concisely, as well as any discussion and decision about future course of action. The employee must have the chance to read and sign this documentation. The head nurse then sends a copy to her or his supervisor.

XII. FLOATING: *Is a nurse hired to work in psychiatry obligated to cover in the intensive care unit (ICU) when the latter is understaffed?* The issue is the hiring contract (implied or expressed). The contract is a composite of the mutual understanding by involved parties of rights and responsibilities, any written documents, and hospital policies. If the nurse was hired as a psychiatric nurse, he or she could legally refuse to go to the ICU. If the hospital intends to float personnel, such a policy should be clearly stated during the hiring process. Also at this time, the employer should determine the employee's education, skills, and experience. On the other hand, if emergency staffing problems exist, a nurse should go to the ICU regardless of personal preference, but should request orientation and not assume responsibility beyond level of experience or education.

XIII. DISPENSING MEDICATION: *Can a nurse legally remove a drug from a pharmacy when the pharmacy is closed (during the night) if the physician insists that the nurse go to the pharmacy to get the specifically prescribed medication immediately?* Within the legal boundaries of the Pharmacy Act, a nurse may remove one dose of a particular drug from the pharmacy for a particular client during an unanticipated emergency within a limited time and availability of resources. However, the hospital should have a written policy for the nurse to follow and should authorize a specific person to use the services of the pharmacy under certain circumstances.

XIV. ILLEGIBLE ORDERS: *What should I do if I cannot decipher the physician's handwriting when she or he persists in leaving illegible orders?* Talk to the physician regarding the dangers of your giving the wrong amount of the wrong medication via the wrong route at the wrong time. If that does not help, follow appropriate channels. Do **not** follow an order you cannot read. You will be liable for following orders you thought were written.

XV. HEROIC MEASURES: *The wife of a client who is terminally ill approaches me with the request that heroic measures not be used on her husband. She has not discussed this with him but knows that he feels the same way. Can I act on this request?* No. The client is the only one who can legally make the decision as long as he or she is mentally competent.

XVI. MEDICATION: *A physician orders pain medication prn for a client. The client asks for the medication, but when I question her she says the pain "isn't so bad." If in my judgment the client's pain is not severe, am I legally covered if I give half of the pain medication dosage ordered by the physician?* A nurse cannot substitute his or her judgment for the physician's judgment. If you alter the amount of medication prescribed by the physician without a specific order to do so, you may be liable for practicing medicine without a license.

XVII. MALFUNCTIONING EQUIPMENT: *At the end-of-shift report, the nurse going off duty tells me that the tracheal suctioning machine is malfunctioning and describes how she got it to work. Should I plan to use the machine in the evening shift and follow her suggestions about how to make it work?* Do not plan to use equipment that you know is not functioning properly. You could be held liable because you could reasonably foresee that proper functioning of equipment would be needed for your client. You have been put on notice that there are defects. Report this to the supervisor or person responsible for maintaining equipment in proper working order. (Also see **p. 72: Safe Use of Equipment.**)

Ethical and Legal Considerations in Intensive Care of the *Acutely Ill* Neonate

I. RESPONSIBILITIES OF THE HEALTH AGENCY

A. Provide a neonatal intensive care unit (NICU) or transfer to another hospital.

B. *Personnel—adequate number trained in neonate diseases, special treatment, and equipment.*

C. Equipment—adequate supply on hand, functioning properly (especially temperature regulator in incubator, oxygen analyzer, blood-gas machine).

II. INFANTS WHO ARE DYING

A. Decision regarding resuscitation in cardiac arrest, with brain damage from cerebral anoxia. It is difficult to predict the effect of anoxia in infancy on the child's later life.

B. Decision to continue supportive measures.

C. Issue of euthanasia, such as in severe myelomeningocele at birth.

1. Active euthanasia (giving overdose).
2. Passive euthanasia (not placing on respirator).

III. EXTENDED ROLE OF NURSE IN NICU—may raise issues of nursing practice versus medical practice, as when a nurse draws blood samples for blood gas determinations without prior order. To be legally covered:

A. The nurse must be trained to perform specialized functions.

B. The functions must be written into the nurse's job description.

ETHICS/LEGAL

IV. ISSUE OF NEGLIGENCE—such as cross-contamination in nursery.

V. ISSUE OF MALPRACTICE—such as assigning care of an infant who is critically ill on respirator to a student or aide who is untrained.

A. May be liable for inaccurate bilirubin studies for neonatal jaundice; may be legally responsible if brain damage occurs in absence of accurate laboratory tests.

B. May be liable for brain damage in an infant due to respiratory or cardiac distress. Nurse must make sure that there are frequent blood gas determinations to ensure adequate oxygen to prevent brain damage. Nurse also must make sure that the infant is not receiving too high a concentration of oxygen, which may lead to retrolental fibroplasia.

Legal Aspects of Psychiatric Care

I. FOUR SETS OF CRITERIA TO DETERMINE CRIMINAL RESPONSIBILITY AT TIME OF ALLEGED OFFENSE

A. *M'Naghten Rule* (1832)—a person is not guilty if:
1. Person did not know the *nature and quality* of the act.
2. Person could not distinguish right from wrong—if person did not know what he or she was doing, person did not know it was wrong.

B. *The Irresistible Impulse Test* (used together with M'Naghten Rule)—person knows right from wrong, but:
1. Driven by *impulse* to commit criminal acts regardless of consequences.
2. Lacked premeditation in sudden violent behavior.

C. *American Law Institute's Model Penal Code (1955) Test*
1. Not responsible for criminal act if person lacks capacity to "appreciate" the wrongfulness of it or to "conform" conduct to requirements of law.
2. Excludes "an abnormality manifested only by repeated criminal or antisocial conduct"—namely, psychopathology.
3. Includes "knowledge" and "control" criteria.

D. *Durham Test* (Product Rule—1954): accused is not criminally responsible if act was a "product of mental disease." Discarded in 1972.

II. TYPES OF ADMISSIONS

A. *Voluntary:* person, parent, or legal guardian applies for admission; person agrees to receive treatment and to follow hospital rules; civil rights are retained.

B. *Involuntary:* process and criteria vary among states **(Fig. 3.1)**.

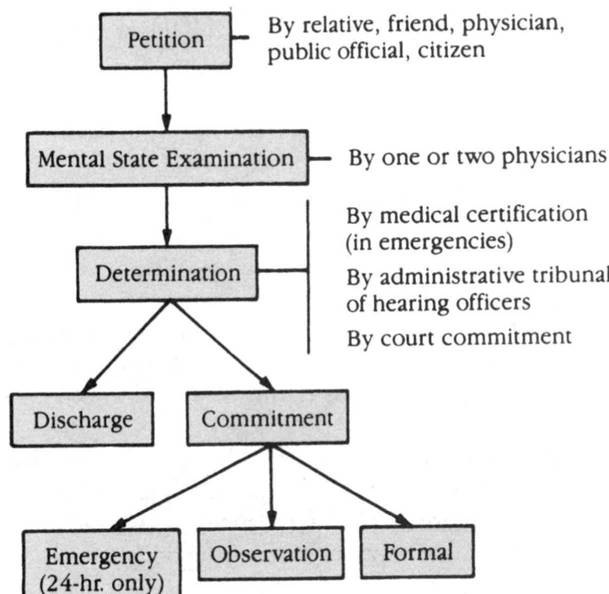

Figure 3.1 Typical procedure for involuntary commitment.

III. LEGAL AND CIVIL RIGHTS OF CLIENTS WHO ARE HOSPITALIZED—the right to:

A. Wear own clothes, keep and use personal possessions and reasonable sum of money for small purchases.

B. Have individual storage space for private use.

C. See visitors daily.

D. Have reasonable access to confidential phone conversations.

E. Receive unopened correspondence and have access to stationery, stamps, and a mailbox.

F. Refuse shock treatments, lobotomy.

IV. CONCEPTS CENTRAL TO COMMUNITY MENTAL HEALTH (COMMUNITY MENTAL HEALTH ACT, 1980)

A. *Systems* perspective: scope of care moves beyond the individual to the community, with influences from biological, psychological, and sociocultural forces.

B. Emphasis on *prevention: primary* (reduce incidents by preventing harmful social conditions); *secondary* (early identification and treatment of disorders to reduce duration); *tertiary* (early rehabilitation to reduce impairment from disorders).

C. *Interdisciplinary collaboration:* flexible roles based on unique areas of expertise.

D. *Consumer participation and control.*

E. *Comprehensive services:* ambulatory care, partial hospitalization, 24-hour hospitalization and emergency care; consultation and education; screening services.

F. *Continuity of care.*

Legal Aspects of Preparing a Client for Surgery

I. NO SURGICAL PROCEDURE, HOWEVER MINOR, CAN PROCEED WITHOUT THE VOLUNTARY, INFORMED, AND WRITTEN CONSENT OF THE CLIENT.

A. Surgical permits are witnessed by the physician, nurse, or other authorized person.

B. Surgical permits protect the client against unsanctioned surgery and also protect the surgeon and hospital staff against claims of unauthorized operations.

C. *Informed consent* means that the operation has been fully explained to the client, including possible complications and disfigurements, as well as whether any organ or parts of the body are to be removed.

D. Adults and emancipated minors may sign their own operative permits if they are mentally competent; permission for surgery of minor children and adults who are incompetent or unconscious must be obtained from a responsible family member or guardian.

E. The signed operative permit is placed in a prominent place on the client's chart and accompanies the client to the operating room.

F. *Legal issues in the emergency department: recordkeeping* plays an essential role in both the prevention and defense of malpractice suits. Detailed documentation not only provides for continuity of care but also perpetuates evidence that care was appropriately given. Records should:

1. Be written legibly.
2. Clearly note events and time of occurrence.
3. Contain all laboratory slips and results of other tests.
4. Describe events and clients objectively.
5. Clearly note physician's parting instructions to the client.
6. Be signed where appropriate, such as with doctor's orders.
7. Contain descriptions of every event that might lead to a lawsuit, such as fights, injuries, equipment failures.

G. *Consent*—although there is no law requiring written consent before performing medical treatment, all elective procedures can only be performed if the client has been fully informed and voluntarily consents to the procedure.

1. If informed consent cannot be obtained because of the client's condition and immediate treatment is necessary to save life or safeguard health, the emergency rule can be applied. This rule implies consent. However, if time allows, it is advisable to obtain either oral or written informed consent from someone who has authority to act for the client.
2. Verbal consents should be recorded in detail, witnessed and signed by *two* individuals.
3. Written or verbal consent can be given by alert, coherent, or otherwise competent adults, by parents, legal guardian, or person in *loco parentis* (one standing in for the parent with the parent's rights, duties, and responsibilities) of minors or adults who are incompetent.
4. If the minor is 14 years old or older, consent must be acquired from the minor as well as from the parent or legal guardian. *Emancipated minors* can consent for themselves.

TRENDS IN NURSING PRACTICE

I. OVERALL CHARACTERISTICS

A. Some trends are subtle and slow to emerge; others are obvious and quickly emerge.

B. Trends may conflict; some will prevail, others get modified by social forces.

II. GENERAL TRENDS

A. *Broadened focus of care*—from care of ill to care of sick and healthy, from care of individual to care of family. Focus on prevention of illness, promotion of optimum level of health, holism.

B. *Increasing scientific base*—in biological-social-physical sciences, not mere reliance on intuition, experience, and observation.

C. *Increasingly complex technical skills* and use of *technologically advanced equipment,* such as monitors and computers.

D. *Increased independence* in use of judgment, such as teaching nutrition in pregnancy and providing primary prenatal care.

E. *New roles,* such as *nurse clinician,* require advanced skills in a particular area of practice. *Examples:* psychiatric nurse consults with staff about problems; *primary care* nurse takes medical histories and does physical assessment; one nurse coordinates 24-hour care during hospital stay; *independent nurse practitioner* has her or his own office in community where clients come for care; case management.

F. *Community nursing services* rather than hospital-based; needs of the healthy are served as well as those of the ill.

G. *Development of nursing standards* to reflect specific nursing functions and activities.

1. Ensure *safe* standard of care to clients and families.
2. Provide criteria to measure *excellence* and *effectiveness* of care.

ETHICS/LEGAL

III. TRENDS IN CARE OF CHILDBEARING FAMILY

A. *Consumerism:*
1. Consumer push for humanization and individualization of health care during the childbearing cycle to reflect client's role in decision making, preferences, and cultural diversity.
2. Emphasis on family-centered care (including father, siblings, grandparents).
3. Increase in options available for conduct of birth experience and setting for birth: birthing homes, alternative birth center (ABC) in hospitals; birthing chairs; side-lying position for birth; family-centered cesarean birth; health-care provider (MD, RN, lay midwife); length of postpartum stay.
4. Increased consumer awareness of legal issues, client's rights.
5. Major nursing role: client advocate.

B. *Social trends:*
1. Alternative lifestyles of families—single parenthood, communal living, surrogate motherhood, marriages without children.
2. Earlier sexual experimentation—availability of assistance to emancipated minors.
3. Increase in number of older (>38 years) primiparas.
4. Legalization of abortion; availability to emancipated minors.
5. Smaller families.
6. Rising divorce rates.

C. *Technologies:*
1. Development of genetic and bioengineering techniques.
2. Development of prenatal diagnostic techniques, with options for management of each pregnancy.
3. In vitro fertilization and embryo transplantation.

IV. TRENDS IN COMMUNITY MENTAL HEALTH (1960s–1990s)

A. Shift from institutional to community-based care.

B. Preventive services.

C. Consumer participation in planning and delivery of services.

D. Original 12 essential services (1975) reduced to 5 (indicated by asterisk [*]) (1981).

*1. 24-hour inpatient care.
*2. Ambulatory care.
*3. Partial hospitalization (day or night).
4. Emergency care.
*5. Consultation and education.
6. Follow-up care.
7. Transitional services.
8. Services for children and adolescents.
9. Services for elderly.
*10. Screening services (courts).
11. Alcohol abuse services.
12. Drug abuse services.

E. Protecting human rights of persons in need of mental health care.

F. Developing an advocacy program for those who are chronically mentally ill.

G. Improving delivery of services to underserved and high-risk populations (e.g., minorities).

V. ANA STANDARDS OF CLINICAL NURSING PRACTICE*

A. Use of *nursing process:* assessment, nursing diagnosis, planning, implementation, evaluation, outcome identification.

B. Performance appraisal review.

C. Continuing education.

D. Collegiality; *peer review.*

E. Ethics.

F. Interdisciplinary collaboration.

G. Research.

H. Resource utilization—utilization of community health systems.

VI. *FOUR LEVELS* OF NURSING PRACTICE

A. *Promotion of health* to increase level of wellness. *Example:* provide dietary information to reduce risks of coronary artery diseases.

B. *Prevention of illness or injury. Example:* immunizations.

C. *Restoration of health. Example:* teach how to change dressing, care for wound.

D. *Consolation of dying*—assist person to attain peaceful death.

VII. *FOUR COMPONENTS* OF NURSING CARE

A. *Nursing care activities*—assist with basic needs, give medications and treatments; observe response and adaptation to illness and treatments; teach self-care; guide rehabilitation activities for daily living.

B. *Case management—a process that includes coordination of total client care*—all health team members should work together toward common goals.

C. *Continuity of care*—process of ensuring that ongoing physical, medical, and emotional health-care needs are assessed, planned for, and coordinated with all providers, for desired outcomes, without interruption of service when the location of care is transferred.

D. *Evaluation of care*—flexibility and responsiveness to changing needs: clients' reactions and perceptions of their needs.

---

*Adapted from the complete description in American Nurses Association: *2004 Nursing: Scope and Standards of Practice.* Washington, DC, American Nurses Association, 2004. Reprinted with permission. (Rationale and assessment factors for the Standards of Clinical Nursing Practice are available from the American Nurses Association.)

ETHICS/LEGAL

VIII. THREE MAIN NURSING ROLES in relation to care of clients and their families (emphasis of each role varies with the situation, with adaptation of skills and modes of care as necessary)

A. *Therapeutic role* (instrumental). *Function:* work toward "cure" in acute setting.

B. *Caring role* (expressive). *Function:* provide support through human relations, show concern, demonstrate acceptance of differences.

C. *Socializing role. Function:* offer distractions and respite from focus on illness.

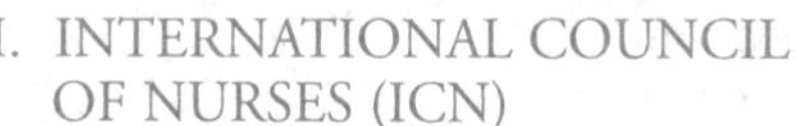

NURSING ORGANIZATIONS

I. INTERNATIONAL COUNCIL OF NURSES (ICN)

A. *Purpose:* to provide a medium through which national nursing associations can work together and share common interests; formed in 1899

B. *Functions*

1. Serves as representatives of and spokespersons for nurses at international level.
2. Promotes organization of national nurses' associations.
3. Assists national organizations to develop and improve services for public health practice of nursing and social/economic welfare of nurses.

II. WORLD HEALTH ORGANIZATION (WHO)—special intergovernmental agency of the United Nations, formed in 1948

A. *Purpose:* to bring all people to the highest possible level of health

B. *Functions:* provides assistance in the form of education, training, improving health standards, fighting disease, and reducing water pollution in member countries

III. AMERICAN NURSES ASSOCIATION (ANA)—national professional association in the United States, composed of the nurses' associations of the 50 states, Guam, Virgin Islands, Puerto Rico, and Washington, DC

A. *Purpose:* to foster high standards of nursing practice and promote the education and welfare of nurses

B. *Functions:* officially represents professional nurses in the United States and internationally; defines practice of nursing; lobbies and promotes legislation affecting nurses' welfare and practice

IV. NATIONAL LEAGUE FOR NURSING (NLN)—composed of both individuals and agencies

A. *Purpose:* to foster the development and improvement of all nursing services and nursing education

B. *Functions*

1. Provides educational workshops.
2. Assists in recruitment for nursing programs.
3. Provides testing services for both RN and LPN (LVN) nursing programs.

SAFETY AND INFECTION CONTROL: GUIDELINES FOR ISOLATION AND STANDARD PRECAUTIONS

A key component of the NCLEX-RN® test plan is injury prevention in the provision of a safe environment. This section also identifies potential risks to child safety with recommendations for a child-safe environment.

I. GUIDELINES FOR ISOLATION AND INFECTION CONTROL

A. Guidelines for Isolation Precautions (**Table 3.2**)

B. Contact Precautions—Summary (**Table 3.3**)

(text continues on page 91)

Table 3.2

Guidelines for Isolation Precautions

The Hospital Infection Control Advisory Committee and the Centers for Disease Control and Prevention have concluded that some fluids, secretions, and excretions not covered under Universal Precautions (UP) represent a potential source of nosocomial and community-acquired infections. The term *Universal Precautions* has been replaced in the hospital setting by a two-tiered system of isolation: **Standard Precautions** for control of nosocomial infections; and **Transmission-based Precautions** for clients known or suspected to be infected with highly transmissible pathogens. ***Standard Precautions*** incorporate the major components of blood and body fluid precautions from *Universal Precautions.* ***Transmission-based Precautions*** may be combined for diseases that have multiple routes of transmission and are used in addition to ***Standard Precautions.***

Standard Precautions

Use **Standard Precautions**, or the equivalent, for the care of all clients.

1. *Handwashing.*
   a. Wash hands **after touching:** blood, body fluids, secretions, excretions, and contaminated items, whether or not gloves are worn. Wash hands **immediately:** after gloves are removed, between client contacts, and when otherwise indicated to avoid transfer of microorganisms to other clients or environments. It may be necessary to wash hands between tasks and procedures on the same client to prevent cross-contamination of different body sites.

Table 3.2

Guidelines for Isolation Precautions—cont'd

b. Use a plain (non-antimicrobial) soap for routine hand washing.

c. Use an antimicrobial agent or a waterless antiseptic agent for specific circumstances (e.g., control of outbreaks or hyperendemic infections), as defined by the infection control program (see *Contact Precautions* for additional recommendations on using antimicrobial and antiseptic agents).

2. *Gloves.* Wear gloves (clean, nonsterile gloves are adequate) **when touching:** blood, body fluids, secretions, excretions, and contaminated items. Put on clean gloves just before touching *mucous membranes* and *nonintact skin.* Change gloves between tasks and procedures on the same client after contact with material that may contain a high concentration of microorganisms. Remove gloves promptly after use, before touching noncontaminated items and environmental surfaces, and before going to another client; wash hands **immediately** to avoid transfer of microorganisms to other clients or environments.
3. *Mask, eye protection, face shield.* Wear a mask and eye protection or a face shield to protect mucous membranes of the eyes, nose, and mouth during procedures and client care activities that are likely to generate splashes or sprays of blood, body fluids, secretions, and excretions.
4. *Gown.* Wear a gown (a clean, nonsterile gown is adequate) to protect skin and to prevent soiling of clothing during procedures and client care activities that are likely to generate splashes or sprays of blood, body fluids, secretions, or excretions. Select a gown that is appropriate for the activity and amount of fluid likely to be encountered. Remove a soiled gown as promptly as possible, and wash hands to avoid transfer of microorganisms to other clients or environments.
5. *Client care equipment.* Handle used client care equipment soiled with blood, body fluids, secretions, and excretions in a manner that prevents skin and mucous membrane exposures, contamination of clothing, and transfer of microorganisms to other clients and environments. Ensure that reusable equipment is not used for the care of another client until it has been cleaned and reprocessed appropriately. Ensure that single-use items are discarded properly.
6. *Environmental control.* Ensure that the hospital has adequate procedures for the routine care, cleaning, and disinfection of environmental surfaces, beds, bed rails, bedside equipment, and other frequently touched surfaces, and ensure that these procedures are being followed.
7. *Linens.* Handle, transport, and process used linens soiled with blood, body fluids, secretions, and excretions in a manner that prevents skin and mucous membrane exposures and contamination of clothing, and that avoids transfer of microorganisms to other clients and environments.
8. *Occupational health and blood-borne pathogens.*
   a. Take care to prevent injuries when using needles, scalpels, and sharp instruments or devices; when handling sharp instruments after procedures; when cleaning used instruments; and when disposing of used needles. ***Never*** recap used needles, or otherwise manipulate them using both hands, or use any other technique that involves directing the point of a needle toward any part of the body; rather, use either a one-handed "scoop" technique or a mechanical device designed for holding the needle sheath. Do ***not*** remove used needles from disposable syringes by hand, and do ***not*** bend, break, or otherwise manipulate used needles by hand. Place used disposable syringes and needles, scalpel blades, and other sharp items in appropriate puncture-resistant containers that are located as close as practical to the area in which the items were used, and place reusable syringes and needles in a puncture-resistant container for transport to the reprocessing area.
   b. Use mouthpieces, resuscitation bags, or other ventilation devices as an alternative to mouth-to-mouth resuscitation methods in areas where the need for resuscitation is predictable.
9. *Client placement.* Place a client who contaminates the environment or who does not (or cannot be expected to) assist in maintaining appropriate hygiene or environmental control in a private room. If a private room is not available, consult with infection control professionals regarding client placement or other alternatives.

Transmission-Based Precautions

Airborne Precautions

In addition to **Standard Precautions**, use ***Airborne Precautions,*** or the equivalent, for clients known or suspected to be infected with microorganisms transmitted by airborne droplet nuclei (small-particle residue [5 microns or smaller in size] of evaporated droplets containing microorganisms that remain suspended in the air and that can be dispersed widely by air currents within a room or over a long distance).

1. ***Client placement.*** Place the client in a private room that has (1) monitored negative air pressure in relation to the surrounding area, (2) 6–12 air changes per hour, and (3) appropriate discharge of air outdoors or monitored high-efficiency filtration of room air before the air is circulated to other areas in the hospital. Keep the room door closed and the client in the room. *When a private room is not available,* place the client in a room with a client who has active infection with the same microorganism, unless otherwise recommended, but with no other infection (cohorting). When a private room is not available and cohorting is not desirable, consultation with infection control professionals is advised before client placement.
2. ***Respiratory protection.*** Wear respiratory protection when entering the room of a client with known or suspected infectious pulmonary tuberculosis. People who are susceptible should not enter the room of clients known or suspected to have *measles* (rubeola) or *varicella* (chickenpox) if other caregivers who are immune are available. If persons who are susceptible must enter the room of a client known or suspected to have measles (rubeola) or varicella, they should wear respiratory protection. Persons immune to measles (rubeola) or varicella need not wear respiratory protection.
3. ***Client transport.*** Limit the movement and transport of the client from the room to essential purposes only. If transport or movement is necessary, minimize client dispersal of droplet nuclei by placing a *surgical mask* on the client, if possible.
4. ***Additional precautions for preventing transmission of tuberculosis.*** Consult CDC "Guidelines for Preventing the Transmission of Tuberculosis in Health-Care Facilities" for additional prevention strategies.

Continued

Table 3.2

Guidelines for Isolation Precautions—cont'd

Droplet Precautions

In addition to **Standard Precautions,** use **Droplet Precautions,** or the equivalent, for a client known or suspected to be infected with microorganisms transmitted by droplets (large-particle droplets [larger than 5 microns in size] that can be generated by the client during coughing, sneezing, talking, or the performance of procedures).

1. ***Client placement.*** Place the client in a private room. When a private room is not available, place the client in a room with a client who has active infection with the same microorganism but with no other infection (cohorting). When a private room is not available and cohorting is not achievable, maintain spatial separation of at least 3 ft between the client who is infected and other clients and visitors. Special air handling and ventilation are not necessary, and the door may remain open.
2. ***Mask.*** In addition to standard precautions, wear a mask when working within 3 ft of the client. (Logistically, some hospitals may want to implement the wearing of a mask to enter the room.)
3. ***Client transport.*** Limit the movement and transport of the client from the room to essential purposes only. If transport or movement is necessary, minimize client dispersal of droplets by masking the client, if possible.

Contact Precautions

In addition to **Standard Precautions,** use **Contact Precautions,** or the equivalent, for specified clients known or suspected to be infected or colonized with epidemiologically important microorganisms that can be transmitted by direct contact with the client (hand or skin-to-skin contact) that occurs when performing client care activities that require touching the client's dry skin or indirect contact (touching) with environmental surfaces or client care items in the client's environment.

1. ***Client placement.*** Place the client in a private room. When a private room is not available, place the client in a room with a client who has active infection with the same microorganism but with no other infection (cohorting). When a private room is not available and cohorting is not achievable, consider the epidemiology of the microorganism and the client population when determining client placement. Consultation with infection control professionals is advised before client placement.
2. ***Gloves and handwashing.*** In addition to wearing gloves as outlined under **Standard Precautions,** wear gloves (clean, nonsterile gloves are adequate) when entering the room. During the course of providing care for a client, change gloves after having contact with infective material that may contain high concentrations of microorganisms (fecal material and wound drainage). Remove gloves before leaving the client's environment and wash hands **immediately** with an antimicrobial agent or a waterless antiseptic agent. After glove removal and hand washing, ensure that hands do *not* touch potentially contaminated environmental surfaces or items in the client's room to avoid transfer of microorganisms to other clients or environments.
3. ***Gown.*** In addition to wearing a gown as outlined under **Standard Precautions**, wear a gown (a clean, nonsterile gown is adequate) when entering the room if you anticipate that your clothing will have substantial contact with the client, environmental surfaces, or items in the client's room; or if the client is *incontinent* or has *diarrhea*, an *ileostomy*, a *colostomy*, or *wound drainage* not contained by a dressing. Remove the gown before leaving the client's environment. After gown removal, ensure that clothing does *not* contact potentially contaminated environmental surfaces to avoid transfer of microorganisms to other clients or environments.
4. ***Client transport.*** Limit the movement and transport of the client from the room to essential purposes only. If the client is transported out of the room, ensure that precautions are maintained to minimize the risk of transmission of microorganisms to other clients and contamination of environmental surfaces or equipment.
5. ***Client care equipment.*** When possible, dedicate the use of noncritical client care equipment to a single client (or cohort of clients infected or colonized with the pathogen requiring precautions) to avoid sharing between clients. If use of common equipment or items is unavoidable, adequately clean and disinfect them before use for another client.

Source: Centers for Disease Control and Prevention and Hospital Infection Control Practices Advisory Committee.

Table 3.3

Contact Precautions—Summary

1. Private room if the client's hygiene is poor. In general, clients with the same infection *may share* a room.
2. Masks are *not* indicated.
3. Gowns are indicated if soiling is likely.
4. Gloves are indicated for touching infective material.
5. Hands must be washed before and after touching the client or potentially contaminated articles.
6. Contaminated articles should be discarded or bagged and labeled.

C. Standard Precautions—Summary (**Table 3.4**)
D. Airborne and Droplet Precautions—Summary (**Table 3.5**)
E. Infection Control by Clinical Syndrome/Condition (**Table 3.6**)
F. Infection Control When Caring for Infants, Children, and Adolescents (**Table 3.7**)
G. Summary: Types of Precautions and Illnesses Requiring the Precautions (**Table 3.8**)

II. GUIDELINES FOR ENVIRONMENTAL SAFETY
A. Safety Considerations When Caring for Hospitalized Infants, Children, and Adolescents (**Table 3.9**)
B. Safety and Injury Prevention—Home Safety (**Table 3.10**)

INFECTION CONTROL

Table 3.4

Standard Precautions—Summary

- **Wash your hands** and any other skin surfaces immediately and thoroughly if they become contaminated with blood or other body fluids. Use lots of soap and hot water.
- **Wear clean gloves** whenever there is potential exposure to blood or other body fluids except sweat. Wear surgical gloves for performing venipunctures, for touching mucous membranes or nonintact skin, or whenever there is a possibility of exposure to blood or body fluids. **Remove gloves** after contact with each client. **Discard used gloves** immediately after use in an appropriate receptacle (e.g., a plastic bag with a "biohazard" label). **Wash your hands** immediately after removing gloves.
- Use *mask, protective eyewear, face shield, gown* during any procedure that is likely to generate splashes of blood or other body fluids.
- Handle all **needles, intravenous equipment,** and **sharp instruments** with extreme care:
  1. *Never* recap, remove, bend, or break needles after use or manipulate them in any other way by hand.
  2. Dispose of syringes, needles, scalpel blades, and other sharp items in a puncture-resistant container kept within easy reach.

Table 3.5

Airborne and Droplet Precautions—Summary

When Used

For infectious diseases that are transmitted through inhalation of airborne particles (e.g., tuberculosis) or infected microorganisms in droplets (e.g., *Haemophilus influenzae,* pertussis)

Precautions

Isolate in private room (clients infected with same disease can be placed in same room)
Client should wear mask if out of room for testing, etc.
Masks to be worn by personnel when working within 3 ft of client
Gowns *not* necessary
Contaminated articles need to be labeled before being sent for decontamination
Provide adequate ventilation in client's room
Careful hand washing

Table 3.6

Infection Control
Conditions That Need Additional Precautions

Clinical Syndrome or Condition	Potential Pathogens	Empirical Precautions
Diarrhea		
• Acute diarrhea with a likely infectious cause in a client who is incontinent or is in diapers	Enteric pathogens	Contact
• Diarrhea in an adult with a history of recent antibiotic use	*Clostridium difficile*	Contact
Meningitis		
Rash or exanthems, generalized, etiology unknown		
• Petechial/ecchymotic with fever	*Neisseria meningitidis*	Droplet
• Vesicular	Varicella	Airborne and Contact
• Maculopapular with coryza and fever	Rubeola (measles)	Airborne

Continued

Table 3.6

Infection Control—cont'd

Conditions That Need Additional Precautions

Clinical Syndrome or Condition	Potential Pathogens	Empirical Precautions
Respiratory Infections		
• Cough/fever/upper lobe pulmonary infiltrate in a client who is *HIV negative* or a client at *low risk* for HIV infection	• *Mycobacterium tuberculosis*	Airborne
• Cough/fever/pulmonary infiltrate in any lung location in a client who is *HIV infected* or a client at *high risk* for HIV infection	• *Mycobacterium tuberculosis*	Airborne
• Paroxysmal or severe persistent cough during periods of *pertussis* activity	• *Bordetella pertussis*	Droplet
• Respiratory infections, particularly *bronchiolitis* and *croup*, in infants and young children	• Respiratory syncytial or parainfluenza virus	Contact
Risk of Multidrug-Resistant Microorganisms		
• *History of infection* or colonization with multidrug-resistant organisms	Resistant bacteria	Contact
• *Skin, wound, or urinary tract infection* in a client with a *recent* hospital or nursing home stay in a facility where multidrug-resistant organisms are prevalent	Resistant bacteria	Contact
Skin or Wound Infection		
• *Abscess* or draining wound that cannot be covered	*Staphylococcus aureus*, group A streptococcus	Contact

Adapted from CDC Healthcare Infection Control Practices Advisory Committee, from www.cdc.gov/ncidod/hip/ISOLAT/isopart2.htm.

Table 3.7

Infection Control When Caring for Infants, Children, and Adolescents

Type	Definition	Equipment	Clinical Applications
Standard precautions	Reduce the risk of transmission of infection from all recognized and unrecognized sources of infection (formerly termed *universal precautions*)	• Gloves • Protective eyewear • Gown • Mask	• Blood • Body fluids • Secretions • Excretions • Any break in skin or mucous membranes
Airborne precautions	Reduce the risk of airborne transmission of infectious agents transmitted by airborne droplet nuclei	• Special air handling systems • Ventilation systems: HEPA filter masks, N95 respirator	• Measles • Varicella • Tuberculosis
Droplet precautions	Reduce the risk of airborne transmission of infectious agents transmitted by large-particle droplets	• Surgical mask	• *Haemophilus influenzae* type b • Meningitis • Pertussis • Streptococcal pharyngitis • Scarlet fever
Contact precautions	Reduce the risk of transmission of infectious agents by direct client contact or indirect contact with contaminated items in the client's environment	• Gloves • Gown	• Enteric infections • Skin/wound infections • Respiratory syncytial virus (RSV) • Herpes simplex • Impetigo • Viral hemorrhagic conjunctivitis

Table 3.8

Summary: Types of Precautions and Illnesses Requiring the Precautions

Standard Precautions

Use *Standard Precautions* for the care of all clients.

Airborne Precautions

In addition to *Standard Precautions,* use *Airborne Precautions* for clients known or suspected to have serious illnesses transmitted by airborne droplet *nuclei.*

Examples of such illnesses include:
- Measles
- Varicella (including disseminated zoster)
- Tuberculosis

Droplet Precautions

In addition to *Standard Precautions,* use *Droplet Precautions* for clients known or suspected to have serious illnesses transmitted by *large*-particle droplets.

Examples of such illnesses include:
- Invasive *Haemophilus influenzae* type b disease, including meningitis, pneumonia, epiglottitis, and sepsis
- Invasive *Neisseria meningitidis* disease, including meningitis, pneumonia, and sepsis

Other serious bacterial respiratory infections spread by droplet transmission, including:
- Diphtheria (pharyngeal)
- *Mycoplasma* pneumonia
- Pertussis
- Pneumonic plague
- Streptococcal (group A) pharyngitis, pneumonia, or scarlet fever in infants and young children

Serious viral infections spread by droplet transmission, including:
- Adenovirus
- Influenza
- Mumps
- Parvovirus B19
- Rubella

Contact Precautions

In addition to *Standard Precautions,* use *Contact Precautions* for clients known or suspected to have serious illnesses easily transmitted by *direct* client contact or by contact with items in the client's environment.

Examples of such illnesses include:
Gastrointestinal, respiratory, skin, or wound infections or colonization with multidrug-resistant bacteria judged by the infection control program, based on current state, regional, or national recommendations, to be of special clinical and epidemiologic significance

Enteric infections with a low infectious dose or prolonged environmental survival, including:
- *Clostridium difficile*
- For clients who are in diapers or incontinent: enterohemorrhagic *Escherichia coli* O157:H7, *Shigella,* hepatitis A, or rotavirus

Respiratory syncytial virus, parainfluenza virus, or enteroviral infections in infants and young children

Skin infections that are highly contagious or that may occur on dry skin, including:
- Diphtheria (cutaneous)
- Herpes simplex virus (neonatal or mucocutaneous)
- Impetigo
- Major (noncontained) abscesses, cellulitis, or decubiti
- Pediculosis
- Scabies
- Staphylococcal furunculosis in infants and young children
- Zoster (disseminated or in the host who is immunocompromised)
- Viral/hemorrhagic *conjunctivitis*
- Viral hemorrhagic infections (*Ebola, Lassa,* or *Marburg*)

Adapted from Fundamentals of Isolation Precautions, CDC Healthcare Infection Control Practices Advisory Committee, from www.cdc.gov/ncidod/hip/ISOLAT/isopart2.htm.

Table 3.9

Safety Considerations When Caring for Hospitalized Infants, Children, and Adolescents

Area of Concern	Safety Interventions
Security	• Be alert to all visitors; restrict prn • Monitor/report suspicious visitors • Assess high-risk children (e.g., custody disputes) • Identify person to whom child is discharged • All staff to wear photo ID, especially when transporting child • Transport one child at a time; *never* leave child unattended during transport • Do *not* allow visitors to borrow scrubs or lab coat • Infants placed near nurses' station, in direct line of vision • Access to pediatrics unit limited; doors alarmed to indicate when someone enters or leaves the unit
Electrical equipment (e.g., apnea monitor, ECG monitor, respirator)	• Maintain all equipment in good working order • Remove leads when not attached to monitor • Unplug power cord when not connected to equipment • Keep equipment away from moisture (e.g., puddle of water, tub) • Do *not* turn off alarm for any reason • Always check the child when an alarm sounds; *never* ignore the alarm • Teach other children *not* to touch or play with the equipment **Home care:** • CPR guidelines posted near bed • Emergency numbers posted near phone • Notify electric company, get on priority service list in case of power outage • Use intercom or monitoring system
Environment	• Keep unused electrical outlets covered with childproof caps • Secure screens on all windows • Strap infant securely into infant seat, high chair, stroller • Discourage use of walkers • Crib rails up at all times when infant or young child is alone • When a crib rail is down, keep one hand on the infant or young child at all times • Keep plants or flowers out of the reach of infants or young children • *No* small or sharp objects within reach of infants or young children; no pins on diapers • *No* small or removable parts of toys of infants or young children • Keep all medications out of the reach of infants or young children • *Never* leave an infant or young child alone in a bath or near water

Table 3.10

Safety and Injury Prevention—Home Safety

These safety measures should be used in homes where children live and in homes they frequently visit, e.g., grandparents or babysitters.

Burns, Electrical, and Fire	Falls
• Guards in front of or around heating appliances, fireplace, furnace (including floor furnace) • Electrical wires in good repair and out of reach • Electrical outlets "capped" • Smoke detectors operational • Matches out of reach • All heated appliances/objects placed out of child's reach and disconnected when not in use • Hot water heater set at 49°C (120°F) or lower • Pot handles turned toward back of stove or toward center of table • Cool, *not* hot, mist vaporizer used • Fire extinguisher(s) available and operational • Family escape plan (in case of fire) current • "9-1-1" and address of home with nearest cross street posted near phone	• Exits, halls, stairs free of obstructions and well lighted • Nonskid mats and safety strips in tubs and showers and on stairs • Decals on glass doors/walls • Safety glass in doors/walls/windows • Gates at doors/stairwells • Guard rails on upstairs windows • Safety locks/latches that prevent/limit opening in use on doors/windows • Crib rails raised to full height and mattress kept in low position • Restraints used in high chairs and other infant/child furniture • Pediatrician's phone number posted near phone

Table 3.10

Safety and Injury Prevention—Home Safety—cont'd

Aspiration and Suffocation	Bodily Injury
• Small objects stored out of reach and hanging objects (e.g., mobile) placed out of reach • Toys inspected for broken or removable parts • Plastic bags and plastic-covered pillow/mattress not accessible or in use • Cribs with slats meet federal regulations (slats <2⅜ inches [6 cm] apart with snug fitted mattress) • Bathroom and kitchen faucets firmly turned off • Toilet seats in down position or latched shut • Locked gates by fenced-in pools, spas, etc. • Proper safety equipment by pools, spas, etc. • Wading pools kept empty when not in use • Doors to dishwashers, refrigerators, washing machines, and dryers kept closed • Food cut into "sticks" rather than "coins" • Adult family member trained in CPR and first aid for choking	• Knives, unloaded firearms, power tools stored in locked cabinet • Pets properly restrained and immunized for rabies • Outdoor play equipment kept in safe, working condition • Yard free of glass, nails, litter, etc. • Nearest emergency department's phone number posted near phone
Poisoning	
• Toxic substances placed on high shelf in locked cabinet • "Extra" quantities of toxic substances *not* stored in the house • Used containers of poisonous substances *not* accessible by the child • Household cleaners/disinfectants kept in original containers, separate from food and out of reach • Medications clearly labeled in childproof containers and stored out of reach • Poison Control Center phone number and address of home with nearest cross street posted near phone	

Adapted from Hockenberry, M, & Wilson, D: *Wong's Nursing Care of Infants and Children.* ed 8. Mosby, St. Louis, 2007.

Questions

Select the one answer that is best for each question, unless otherwise directed.

1. An RN would be judged negligent if which event occurred during client care?
   1. Speaking harshly to a client.
   2. Refusing a care assignment.
   3. Making a medication error resulting in injury.
   4. Delegating a dressing change to an LPN/LVN.

2. Which client is most appropriate for an RN to delegate to a CNA?
   1. A client who is 3 days post–abdominal surgery with decreased breath sounds.
   2. A client who is 8 hours postop thyroidectomy with decreased blood pressure.
   3. A client who is stable, 4 days post–gunshot wound with abdominal wound dehiscence.
   4. A client who is 2 days post-thoracotomy on an epidural fentanyl drip.

3. Which client would be appropriate for the RN to delegate to the LVN/LPN?
   1. A client who needs IV antibiotics and a central line dressing change.
   2. A client in liver failure who needs a blood transfusion.
   3. A client who is postop and needs IV pain medication.
   4. A client with GI bleeding who needs procedural sedation for a CT scan.

4. A client dies in the hospital. The driver's license indicates that the client wanted to be an organ donor. The family is refusing organ donation. What is the correct action by an RN?
   1. Discuss with the family the legality of the driver's license indicating organ donation.
   2. Respect the family's wishes.
   3. Seek legal advice to carry out client's wishes.
   4. Activate the donor team to go forward with the organ donation process.

5. A client is admitted with an existing advance directive that states "Do Not Resuscitate" (DNR). The client goes into cardiac arrest. How should a nurse respond?
   1. Do not resuscitate the client as detailed in the advance directive.
   2. If the client is admitted to the hospital, a new advance directive is needed; therefore, resuscitate the client.
   3. Start chest compressions, but do not intubate.
   4. Intubate only to secure an airway.

QUESTIONS

6. When assessing a client with peripheral neuropathy, which question is *most* important for a nurse to ask?
   1. "Do you have to turn your head to obtain lateral vision?"
   2. "Can you feel me touching your feet?"
   3. "At what time of day are the tremors at their worst?"
   4. "Is the hearing loss worse on one side or the other?"

7. What isolation precautions are necessary for a client with a history of hepatitis C who is "anti-HCV positive?"
   1. Enteric precautions.
   2. Resistant-organism contact precautions.
   3. Reverse isolation.
   4. Standard precautions.

8. A charge nurse on a medical-surgical floor observes a certified nursing assistant (CNA) taking care of a client with impaired vascular circulation. What behavior by the aide requires *immediate* action by the RN?
   1. Aide places client's feet in warm water.
   2. Aide elevates client's legs.
   3. Aide places sheepskin between overlapped toes.
   4. Aide applies lanolin to client's legs.

9. During hospital orientation for new graduates, an instructor covers health-care–associated infections (HAI), formerly referred to as nosocomial infections. Which infections are known to be spread to the client by health-care providers during care? *Select all that apply.*
   1. *Clostridium difficile.*
   2. *Pseudomonas.*
   3. Methicillin-resistant *Staphylococcus aureus* (MRSA).
   4. Vancomycin-resistant enterococcus (VRE).
   5. Human immunodeficiency virus (HIV).
   6. *Helicobacter pylori.*

10. A client in rehabilitation following a brain attack is receiving tube feedings at 75 mL/hr, Na^+ is 148, K^+ is 4.2, creatinine is 1.2, glucose is 145. What should a nurse ask a physician, as part of the SBAR (Situation, Background, Action, Recommendation) communication?
    1. "Do you want to turn the feeding rate down?"
    2. "Do you want to start D_5W IV?"
    3. "Do you want to give intermittent tap water through the feeding tube?"
    4. "Do you want to give a more concentrated formula?"

11. The most effective intervention to help a client quit smoking, that a nurse could suggest, is:
    1. Acupuncture.
    2. Tapering off the number of cigarettes smoked.
    3. Counseling.
    4. Selective serotonin reuptake inhibitors.

12. When an RN returns from dinner break, which client should be assessed *first?*
    1. 82-year-old, 2 days post–total hip replacement with a platelet count of 98,000.
    2. 28-year-old, IV drug abuser who is 3 days post–aortic valve replacement, with a central line and triple antibiotics due.
    3. 76-year-old, 1 day post–abdominal aortic aneurysm repair.
    4. 46-year-old, stable, 4 hours after cardiac catheterization.

13. A client with MRSA is transferred to a nursing unit. A charge nurse should place the client in a room with:
    1. A client who is HIV +.
    2. A client who is under treatment for Crohn's disease.
    3. Another client with MRSA.
    4. A client with a leg fracture.

14. Under which circumstance can an RN safely delegate tasks to unlicensed assistive personnel (UAP)?
    1. The assignment is given in writing.
    2. Supervision is given to complete the tasks that have been provided.
    3. Task competency was verified during orientation.
    4. The RN provides verbal instructions for the tasks.

15. A client is prepared for a bronchoscopic examination. The RN gives an IV sedative. Which activity could be delegated to an LPN/LVN?
    1. Teaching the client about the procedure.
    2. Giving the client smalls sips of water for dry mouth.
    3. Walking with the client to the bathroom before the procedure.
    4. Checking the client's blood pressure and pulse.

16. Four clients walked into an ambulatory clinic at the same time. Which client should a nurse assess *first?*
    1. A 45-year-old client with a swollen, bruised ankle, who is limping.
    2. A 30-year-old client with a temperature of 102°F, vomiting, and diarrhea.
    3. A 40-year-old client with a sore throat, temperature 101°F, swollen lymph glands.
    4. A 35-year-old client complaining of a severe headache, vomiting, and stiff neck.

17. Which client should an RN direct an LPN/LVN to check on *first?*
    1. A client with rheumatoid arthritis who needs splints reapplied.
    2. A client with diabetes with a blood sugar of 75, who finished breakfast and needs a snack.
    3. A client with GI bleeding who was up to use the bedside commode.
    4. A client with COPD on O_2 at 2 L who needs vital signs and pulse oximetry checked.

QUESTIONS

18. When relocating an older client from a family home to an assisted-living community, the correct action by a nursing case manager is to:
   1. Maintain the client's level of economic independence.
   2. Ensure the client's perceived control with the move to an assisted-living setting.
   3. Select a facility close to remaining family.
   4. Assess availability of culturally appropriate meals.

19. Following report on four clients, which client should a nurse assess *first?*
   1. A client with a chest tube inserted for a spontaneous pneumothorax, with respirations of 18.
   2. A client with possible acute pyelonephritis. Urine output is 25 mL in the past 2 hours.
   3. A client 2 days post–radical mastectomy, who is crying and upset.
   4. A client on reverse isolation who needs pain medication.

20. Which finding should a nurse report *immediately* to a physician?
   1. After 2 days of IV penicillin, client has developed a rash around neck and face.
   2. Client has only eaten 20% of the meals for 2 days.
   3. Client who has a pulse of 100 and irregular; who was previously 80 and regular.
   4. No bowel movement for 4 days, and a firm abdomen.

21. An RN delegates the administration of a nasogastric tube feeding to a licensed practical/vocational nurse (LPN/LVN). Which statement about responsibility in this situation is most accurate?
   1. The RN is responsible for delegated care.
   2. This task should not be delegated.
   3. The LPN/LVN is responsible for own actions.
   4. The LPN/LVN should respectfully refuse to initiate this care.

22. Following antibiotic therapy, a client develops bloody diarrhea. A nurse suspects *Clostridium difficile,* which often occurs when antibiotics disrupt the normal intestinal flora and injure the lumen of the bowel. Control of this infection will include:
   Select all that apply.
   1. Nurse wearing mask at all times.
   2. Hand hygiene and wearing gloves.
   3. Keeping client's room door closed.
   4. Cleaning over-the-bed table and side rails daily.
   5. Drug treatment with metronidazole (Flagyl).

23. A hospital client with cancer has a low white blood cell (WBC) count (<1,000/mm^3). Preventing infection is a high priority. Measures to minimize infection include:
   Select all that apply.
   1. A private room if possible.
   2. Measuring temperature rectally for greater accuracy.
   3. Request that family bring fresh fruits from home.
   4. Shave with an electric razor if needed.
   5. Give stool softeners to prevent constipation.
   6. Change IV solution every 24 hours.

24. After receiving an end-of-shift report on four clients, a nurse plans client care. Which client should the nurse assess *first?*
   1. Client admitted through the emergency department 3 hours ago with acute abdominal pain.
   2. Client awaiting discharge and the spouse is at the bedside.
   3. Client in wrist restraints who has a sitter in the room.
   4. Client who had a chest tube inserted 24 hours ago for a pneumothorax.

25. Which client should a nurse assess *first?*
   1. Client with pancreatitis complaining of jaw pain, 4 on a scale of 10.
   2. Client dependent on insulin who complains of feeling shaky and hungry.
   3. Client who is confused, who has activated the bed alarm used to prevent falls.
   4. Client with "red-colored urine" drainage in Foley bag following TURP surgery.

26. Following a major earthquake, clients begin to arrive in an emergency department. Using the disaster triage system, which client should be treated *first?*
   1. Client with an open pneumothorax and severe dyspnea.
   2. Client with major head trauma; pupils fixed and dilated.
   3. Client with a closed fracture of the femur.
   4. Client with multiple abrasions and contusions.

27. Which activities could an RN delegate to a certified nursing assistant (CNA)? *Select all that apply.*
   1. Taking routine vital signs.
   2. NG tube irrigation for a client who is postoperative.
   3. Feeding a client for the first time who had a stroke.
   4. Colostomy irrigation for a client who is comatose.
   5. Walking with a client who has aphasia.
   6. Shaving a client with a tracheostomy.

28. Medicare has enacted a new policy that states that, if a client develops certain conditions while in the hospital, the hospital will not be reimbursed for the care of the client. Which condition does a nurse know that quality care can prevent?
   1. Yeast infections.
   2. Poor blood sugar control.
   3. Unexpected weight loss.
   4. Unexpected surgery.

29. To ensure that the hospital is delivering quality care, a nurse participates in collecting data for core measures, which are:
   1. Measurements that are taken on a client when first admitted to the hospital.
   2. Standardized, evidence-based performance measures needed for hospital accreditation.
   3. Measurements taken for the infection control nurse.
   4. Standardized forms that are used by clients to evaluate hospitals.

30. One of the hospital-acquired conditions that Medicare will not pay for is falls. The nursing staff is responsible for fall prevention. The best predictor of the likelihood of a client falling while hospitalized is:

1. The need to urinate during the night.
2. A history of falling before admission.
3. Presence of morning stiffness and muscle rigidity.
4. Change in medications since admitted.

31. A client is very agitated and needs to have soft restraints applied. To ensure the safety of the client, the nurse should:

1. Tie restraints to the side rails.
2. Keep the head of the bed elevated 30 degrees to keep tension on the restraints.
3. Inspect the client's skin under the restraints every 2 hours.
4. Turn on the lights in the room to see the client.

32. A nurse returns to work after vacation and the clients are all new to the RN. National Patient Safety Goals require that at least two pieces of identification must be used to establish client identity. The best approach to identifying the clients before giving medications would be to:

1. Have the client spell name and give date of birth.
2. Check the room number and bracelet.
3. Ask the family and client to verify the name.
4. Check the client's Medication Administration Record (MAR) and chart.

33. To prevent a catheter-associated bloodstream infection, when would hand washing be required? *Select all that apply.*

1. Before and after palpating around the site.
2. Before and after a dressing change.
3. When touching the administration set.
4. Only when not wearing gloves.
5. Before and after insertion of the catheter.

34. An RN observes the hand hygiene routine of a nursing assistant. Additional teaching will be needed if the RN observes that:

1. Hands were rubbed together for 10 seconds.
2. Soap lather dripped off hands.
3. Water was only lukewarm.
4. Hands were not dried thoroughly.

35. A nurse in an emergency department performs triage of clients in the waiting room. Which child should the nurse send for *immediate* examination?

1. A 1-month-old infant crying vigorously with a history of frequent sneezing.
2. A 2-year-old child with fever and urinary frequency.
3. A 6-month-old infant with a sunken fontanel and history of poor feeding.
4. A 9-year-old with complaints of pain and a possible arm fracture.

36. A nurse prepares to admit a child diagnosed with respiratory syncytial virus (RSV). Which infection control measure would be most appropriate for this child?

1. Place child in a negative pressure room.
2. Place child on contact precautions.
3. Place child on airborne precautions.
4. Place child in a positive pressure room.

37. A nurse is caring for an infant with acute gastroenteritis with an estimated 10% weight loss. Which actions should the nurse take when caring for this infant? *Select all that apply.*

1. Administer IV fluid bolus of 5 mL/kg.
2. Apply antibacterial hand foam.
3. Put on gloves and gown.
4. Administer IV antibiotic.
5. Monitor hourly urine output.
6. Initiate IV therapy.

38. A school nurse receives a call from the parent of a child diagnosed with chickenpox. The parent asks when the child may return to school. What is the best information that the nurse should provide to this parent?

1. Children with chickenpox may return to school once all of the lesions have scabbed over.
2. The child may attend classes after being on antibiotics for 24 hours.
3. It is recommended that the child remain home until the fever has subsided.
4. Once the child has a positive varicella titer, school attendance may resume.

39. A nurse receives morning report on today's client assignments. In which order should the nurse assess these children? Place each client *in order of priority from first to last.*

________ **1.** A 4-year-old with encopresis and a parent at bedside.
________ **2.** An 8-year-old in traction for fractured femur, with no parent at bedside.
________ **3.** A 5-year-old who has just returned from bronchoscopy, with parents at bedside.
________ **4.** A 12-year-old scheduled today for appendectomy, with no parent at bedside.

40. A 4-year-old child is being discharged from a hospital following treatment for Kawasaki disease. Before the child is discharged, the parents should be taught to:

1. Auscultate the heart.
2. Administer antibiotics prior to dental work.
3. Return to the clinic for repeat doses of immunoglobulin.
4. Discuss the postponement of immunizations with the primary care practitioner.

41. A nurse is counseling the parent of a young child with HIV. What information is essential for the nurse to convey during the first meeting?
1. Children with HIV have shorter life expectancies than adults with HIV.
2. Growth may be inhibited in the child with HIV.
3. Adherence to antiretroviral therapy is critical for the child's health.
4. Immunizations should be delayed until the child enters preschool.

42. A nurse is assigned to care for multiple clients who had surgery 2 days ago. Following the 7 a.m. shift report, which client should the nurse assess *first?*
1. A 59-year-old, after a knee arthroplasty, with a WBC of 12,000.
2. An 88-year-old, with CHF and post–hip pinning, who was medicated for pain at 0600.
3. A 24-year-old, who had a splenectomy at age 18, with a temperature of 38.8°C.
4. A 67-year-old, with an abscess post–femur fracture, with a platelet count of 100,000.

43. A nurse is caring for a postoperative client. Which nursing action will prevent infection?
1. Swab IV access port with Betadine for 60 seconds before injecting through it.
2. Maintain perineal skin integrity by inserting an indwelling bladder catheter.
3. Keep skinfolds moist to prevent breakdown.
4. Remove dressing to assess wound only during needed dressing changes.

44. Which nursing action is appropriate in the care of a client admitted with pneumonia who had a right mastectomy 3 years ago?
1. Check right radial pulse every 4 hours.
2. Start an IV on the left forearm.
3. Keep the right arm below heart level.
4. Avoid range of motion on right arm.

45. A drop of a client's blood splashes on a nurse's skin in an area where the nurse had a small, dried scab. The appropriate nursing action is to:
1. Cover the scab with a dry gauze.
2. Apply ointment to keep scab moist.
3. Wash the site without disrupting the scab.
4. Scrub scab with Betadine for 5 minutes.

46. A nurse has received an end-of-shift report on four clients. Which client should the nurse see *first?*
1. A client who is a stockbroker, admitted with GERD, with BP of 160/90.
2. A client who is an athlete, admitted with a torn ACL, whose pulse is 57.
3. A client who is 78 years old with a temperature of 101°F (38.3°C).
4. A client who is post–laparoscopic cholecystectomy, with shoulder pain.

47. The parents of a child with sickle cell anemia ask for information about heredity. What information should a nurse provide? *Select all that apply.*
1. If both parents have sickle cell trait, there is a 25% chance their offspring will have sickle cell anemia.
2. If one parent has sickle cell anemia and the other does not, their offspring will have a 50% chance of having sickle cell trait.
3. If both parents carry sickle cell trait, there is a 50% chance their offspring will have sickle cell trait.
4. If one parent has sickle cell anemia and the other carries trait, their offspring will have a 50% chance of having sickle cell anemia.
5. If one parent has sickle cell anemia and the other does not, their offspring will have a 25% chance of having sickle cell anemia.

48. A client, who is a 19-year-old gravida 2, para 1, delivers a 10-pound neonate by cesarean section after 36 hours of labor and failure to progress. The client has developed abdominal tenderness, a fever of 102.2°F (39°C), and foul-smelling lochia. A nurse should recognize that the most likely reason for the client's condition is:
1. Endometriosis.
2. Postoperative wound infection.
3. Pelvic thrombophlebitis.
4. Endometritis.

49. A nurse tells a client that a positive reaction to a tuberculosis (TB) test will be determined by:
1. The appearance of redness after 24 hours.
2. The size of the induration 48 hours after the test.
3. The diameter of the reddened area at the site.
4. The length of time it takes before redness or induration appears.

50. In making room in a hospital for emergency admission of clients who were in a disaster, which client can be discharged?
1. Client with a fractured femur complaining of calf pain.
2. Client with bronchial asthma with 95% oxygen saturation on room air.
3. An elderly client with temperature of 101°F (38.3°C).
4. Client experiencing rebound abdominal pain with palpation.

51. In prioritizing care, to which client should a nurse respond *first?*
1. Client on NG bolus feeding, with NG medication due and tube is pulled out.
2. Client with IV chemotherapy and the infusion pump is alarming.
3. Client who is incontinent and lying in feces.
4. Client is yelling, "I want to go home" and pressing the call button.

52. An HIV-positive client with type 1 diabetes gives birth at 28 weeks' gestation because of severe preeclampsia. She is asking a nurse about breastfeeding her infant in the neonatal intensive care unit. The nurse should explain to the client that that breastfeeding is contraindicated in the client with:
  1. Diabetes.
  2. Positive HIV.
  3. Hypertension.
  4. Thyroid disease.

53. In what position should a client in a wheelchair be placed to facilitate a safe transfer to bed, if the client has had a right-sided brain attack (stroke)?
  1. Weakened (R) side of the client next to the bed.
  2. Weakened (R) side of the client away from the bed.
  3. Weakened (L) side of the client next to the bed.
  4. Weakened (L) side of the client away from the bed.

54. Where should a nurse place the call light for a client with a right-sided brain attack and left homonymous hemianopsia?
  1. On the client's right side.
  2. On the client's left side.
  3. Directly in front of the client.
  4. Where the client prefers.

55. A client has a colostomy following surgery for colon cancer. Which assessment finding would require *immediate* action by a nurse?
  1. Stoma is raised 2 cm from the abdominal wall.
  2. Bleeding was noted from the stoma during care.
  3. Complaint of pain with light touch.
  4. Stoma was pinkish-red in color.

56. A nurse prepares a hospital room for the pending admission of a 1-week-old infant with hyperbilirubinemia. Which piece of equipment would be best suited for this infant?
  1. Isolette.
  2. Open crib.
  3. Hospital bed with side rails up.
  4. Bassinette.

57. Following report on four clients, the *priority* intervention for a nurse should be to:
  1. Request an antiemetic for a client who has been vomiting during the night.
  2. Report a K^+ level of 5.9 in a client receiving Kayexalate.
  3. Complete the assessment of the four clients.
  4. Notify the family that the client with chest pain was now in ICU.

58. A client, who is gravida 1, para 0, is attending a prenatal visit. She asks about water aerobic exercise class. A nurse gives the client instructions about swimming and bathing during pregnancy. Which client statement indicates that health teaching has *not* been effective?
  1. "I can continue to swim as long as my membranes aren't ruptured."
  2. "I can relax in a hot tub for 30 minutes after swimming."
  3. "I can take a warm bath everyday."
  4. "I should avoid sitting in the sauna for prolonged periods."

59. A client, who is a 28-year-old gravida 4, para 3, presents to labor and delivery with the fetal head crowning. A physician is called for an emergent delivery, but has not yet arrived. After the neonate's head is delivered, which nursing intervention would be the most appropriate?
  1. Check for a nuchal cord.
  2. Place antibiotic ointment in the infant's eyes.
  3. Use a DeLee suction to remove secretions.
  4. Assess the neonate for heart rate and respirations.

60. A family lives in an apartment building built in the 1950s, which has lead pipes. The family cannot afford to move. To prevent exposure to lead through the water, a nurse should instruct the family to:
  1. Boil all water and use it immediately.
  2. Use hot water from the tap for cooking purposes.
  3. Use cold water from the tap for cooking purposes.
  4. Buy bottled water for cooking purposes.

61. What would the appropriate infection control technique be for changing a leg dressing on a client who has *Pneumocystis jiroveci* (formerly *carinii*) pneumonia (PCP)?
  1. Double-bag all contaminated dressings.
  2. Wear a mask during the dressing change.
  3. Wash hands after removing gloves.
  4. Place the client in protective isolation.

62. The *first* nursing concern for a client following bronchoscopy should be to:
  1. Ambulate as soon as sedation wears off.
  2. Check for the return of the gag reflex.
  3. Teach how to use the incentive spirometer.
  4. Position the client on the unaffected side.

63. While a client is getting out of bed, the chest tube catches on the night stand and is pulled out. What should a nurse do *first?*
  1. Cover the opening with sterile gauze.
  2. Hold client's gown over opening.
  3. Put the client back to bed.
  4. Call the MD for help.

64. Which person should be restricted from visiting a client with TB until at least 2 weeks of drug therapy has been completed?
  1. The client's 25-year-old son.
  2. The client's 3-year-old granddaughter.
  3. The client's 74-year-old mother.
  4. The client's middle-aged neighbor.

65. Client teaching on how long the medication for TB should be taken would include:
1. Until the client feels better.
2. Daily for at least 9 months.
3. Until the sputum culture is negative.
4. For the rest of the client's life.

66. When a client's family members come to visit, they would be adhering to respiratory isolation precautions when they:
1. Put on gowns, gloves, and masks.
2. Keep the door to the client's room open.
3. Wash their hands when leaving.
4. Avoid contact with the client's roommate.

67. Which task should a nurse delegate to a certified nursing assistant (CNA)?
1. Irrigation of a nasogastric tube.
2. Walking with a client who is postoperative.
3. Administering a pain medication.
4. Feeding a client for the first time following a brain attack.

68. A nurse notices that a client's signed consent form states "amputation of the right leg," although it is the left leg that is to be amputated. The client has already received preoperative medications. What should the nurse do?
1. Call the nearest relative to come in to sign a new form.
2. Have the client sign another form.
3. Cross out the error and initial the form.
4. Call the MD to reschedule the surgery.

69. What should be the *first* nursing actions for a client admitted to an emergency department following an accident?
1. Check respirations, circulation, neurological response.
2. Align the spine, check pupils, check for hemorrhage.
3. Check respirations, stabilize spine, check circulation.
4. Assess level of consciousness, circulation.

70. A staff RN and a nurse's aide are caring for six clients. The RN delegates the following assignments to the nurse's aide: vital signs, baths, and intake and output for all clients. What is the RN's accountability for the delegated work?
1. Assume that the nurse's aide has completed the assignment.
2. Communicate with the nurse's aide every hour as to the status of the assignment.
3. Ask the clients if they have received appropriate care from the nurse's aide.
4. Define client parameters to the nurse's aide that must be reported to the RN.

71. On a skilled nursing unit, an LVN/LPN reports to a staff nurse that a client is short of breath. What is the most important *initial* response by the RN?
1. Ask the LVN/LPN if this is a new symptom.
2. Do an independent nursing assessment of the client.
3. Ask the LVN/LPN to describe what is meant by shortness of breath.
4. Check the client's chart for a current x-ray report.

72. A night RN reports that a client, admitted with a diagnosis of gastric ulcer, is reporting syncope and dizziness. What should be the *initial* nursing intervention by the RN?
1. Keep the client on bedrest.
2. Call for a STAT Hgb and Hct.
3. Give a STAT dose of sucralfate (Carafate).
4. Check the client's vital signs.

73. A client, admitted to the emergency department with a myocardial infarction (MI), is experiencing chest pain and becomes profusely diaphoretic and apprehensive. What should be the *initial* intervention by the RN?
1. Increase the nasal oxygen from 2 L/min to 6 L/min.
2. Check the troponin and myoglobin levels on the chart.
3. Give the prn dose of morphine sulfate 3 mg IV push.
4. Get a 12-lead ECG.

74. An RN observes another RN speaking harshly and reprimanding a client for being incontinent. What action should be taken?
1. Intervene and tell the RN that a report on client abuse will be made.
2. Document the incident on the client's chart.
3. Advise the supervisor by writing an objective account of the incident.
4. Discuss the incident with the RN, and the nurses can then change the assignment between themselves.

75. Which nursing intervention should be implemented before the deflation of a tracheostomy cuff?
1. Have the obturator available.
2. Take a pulse oximetry reading.
3. Suction the trachea and mouth.
4. Encourage deep breathing and coughing.

Answers/Rationales/Tips

1. CORRECT ANSWER: 3. **Answer 1** is incorrect because speaking harshly or yelling at a client is *unprofessional* conduct. **Answer 2** is incorrect because an RN *can* refuse an assignment for *personal ethical* reasons or if unqualified to give care. **Answer 3 is correct because an action that results in an injury can be judged as negligent.** **Answer 4** is incorrect because a dressing change *is* within the scope of practice for the LPN/LVN.

■ TEST-TAKING TIP: ***Review the definitions of negligence as compared to unethical or unprofessional behavior.***

Content Area: Management of Care, Legal; ***Integrated Process:*** Communication and Documentation; ***Cognitive Level:*** Comprehension; ***Client Need/Subneed:*** Safe and Effective Care Environment/Management of Care/Legal Rights and Responsibilities

2. CORRECT ANSWER: 1. Answer 1 is correct because the CNA could encourage use of the incentive spirometer and ambulate the client as ordered in a client who is postoperative *GI* surgery and needs routine help with postoperative self-care (breathing exercises). **Answer 2** is incorrect because this client is *unstable.* Hemorrhage is a risk. **Answer 3** is incorrect because dehiscence may be followed by *evisceration. Close* assessment is needed. **Answer 4** is incorrect because the RN must assess and monitor epidural analgesia.

■ **TEST-TAKING TIP:** *Choose the client who is most stable—a client who needs assistance, but not assessment and monitoring.*
Content Area: Management of Care, Delegation; ***Integrated Process:*** Nursing Process, Analysis; ***Cognitive Level:*** Application; ***Client Need/Subneed:*** Safe and Effective Care Environment/ Management of Care/Delegation

3. CORRECT ANSWER: 2. Answer 1 is incorrect because central lines are *not routinely* part of the LVN/LPN scope of practice. **Answer 2 is correct because the client's condition is not going to change suddenly.** **Answer 3** is incorrect because pain management and assessment of the drug response is done by the *RN.* **Answer 4** is incorrect because this client is *unstable* and will need close assessment of sedation for the computed tomography (CT) scan.

■ **TEST-TAKING TIP:** *Look for the option that is different from the others. The correct option is the client who is the most stable, and within the scope of practice for the LVN/LPN.*
Content Area: Management of Care, Delegation; ***Integrated Process:*** Nursing Process, Analysis; ***Cognitive Level:*** Application; ***Client Need/Subneed:*** Safe and Effective Care Environment/ Management of Care/Delegation

4. CORRECT ANSWER: 2. Answer 1 is incorrect because the driver's license "dot" is *not* a legally binding document of client wishes. **Answer 2 is correct because the family's wishes must be followed. If the client had an advance directive, this may not have been an issue.** **Answer 3** is incorrect because, *without* a legally executed advance directive on file, there is no use in pursuing the issue. **Answer 4** is incorrect because no donor procurement agency will go against the family.

■ **TEST-TAKING TIP:** *Look for the option that is different from the others. Three of the choices continue the question of donation. Only one acknowledges the wishes of the family in the absence of a health care agent for this client.*
Content Area: Management of Care, Legal; ***Integrated Process:*** Nursing Process, Implementation; ***Cognitive Level:*** Application; ***Client Need/Subneed:*** Safe and Effective Care Environment/ Management of Care/Legal Rights and Responsibilities

5. CORRECT ANSWER: 1. Answer 1 is correct because the advance directive is an expression of the client's wishes. **Answer 2** is incorrect because, as long as the advance directive is current, it covers this admission. **Answer 3** is incorrect because the client's wishes are clear—do not resuscitate. **Answer 4** is incorrect because *no action* is to be taken if the client has a DNR.

■ **TEST-TAKING TIP:** *The stem and correct option includes the same phrase—do not resuscitate. Know the legality of the advance directive.*
Content Area: Management of Care, Legal; ***Integrated Process:*** Nursing Process, Implementation; ***Cognitive Level:*** Application; ***Client Need/Subneed:*** Safe and Effective Care Environment/ Management of Care/Advance Directives

6. CORRECT ANSWER: 2. Answer 1 is incorrect because peripheral neuropathy is a condition caused by nerve damage, generally in the feet. It does *not affect vision.* **Answer 2 is correct because peripheral neuropathy is a condition caused by nerve damage in the feet, sometimes also in the legs and upper extremities. Clients have either decreased sensation or neuropathic pain from the condition. Clients with this condition need extra assessments and care to protect the affected extremities from injury. They may require seizure or psychiatric drugs to assist with the pain. If a client has diabetes, avoidance of high blood sugar levels is also important.** **Answer 3** is incorrect because peripheral neuropathy is a condition caused by nerve damage, generally in the feet. It does *not cause tremors.* **Answer 4** is incorrect because peripheral neuropathy is a condition caused by nerve damage, generally in the feet. It does *not cause hearing loss.*

■ **TEST-TAKING TIP:** *Look for a clue in the stem, "neuro." Think of nerves, sensations, and feelings.*
Content Area: Adult Health, Neurological; ***Integrated Process:*** Nursing Process, Assessment; ***Cognitive Level:*** Application; ***Client Need/Subneed:*** Safe and Effective Care Environment/ Safety and Infection Control/Accident Prevention and Injury Prevention

7. CORRECT ANSWER: 4. Answer 1 is incorrect because the presence of antibodies against the hepatitis C virus (HCV) means that the client has had hepatitis C in the past but is not necessarily still infected. This is a *blood-borne* infection; therefore, enteric precautions are *not* required. **Answer 2** is incorrect because resistant-organisms contact precautions are used for *bacterial* infections that are not easily treated with standard antibiotics. Hepatitis C is a *viral* infection. **Answer 3** is incorrect because "reverse isolation" is an outdated term describing practices that had been designed to protect clients who are vulnerable to infection. **Answer 4 is correct because the presence of antibodies against the hepatitis C virus (HCV) means that the client has had hepatitis C in the past, but is not necessarily still infected. Management of this potential blood-borne infection involves standard precautions.**

■ **TEST-TAKING TIP:** *Know the indications for the different approaches to infection control.* Without *evidence of active disease, standard precautions are used with* all *clients.*
Content Area: Adult Health, Infectious Disease; ***Integrated Process:*** Nursing Process, Planning; ***Cognitive Level:***

Application; ***Client Need/Subneed:*** Safe and Effective Care Environment/Safety and Infection Control/Standard/Transmission-based/Other Precautions

8. CORRECT ANSWER: 1. Answer 1 is correct because heat is contraindicated since the client has reduced sensation from impaired vascular circulation. Injury may result. Answer 2 is incorrect because elevation *will* improve *circulation* and venous return. **Answer 3** is incorrect because this action *will* prevent *breakdown.* **Answer 4** is incorrect because this action is appropriate dry skin care in impaired vascular circulation.

■ **TEST-TAKING TIP:** *Eliminate the options that are familiar and effective strategies to improve venous return (Answer 2) and prevent skin breakdown (Answers 3 and 4).*

Content Area: Adult Health, Vascular; ***Integrated Process:*** Nursing Process, Analysis; ***Cognitive Level:*** Application; ***Client Need/Subneed:*** Safe and Effective Care Environment/Management of Care/Supervision

9. CORRECT ANSWERS: 1, 3, 4. Answer 1 is correct because poor hand hygiene spreads this infection. Answer 2 is incorrect because this organism *occurs naturally* in the client. **Answer 3 is correct because poor hand hygiene spreads this infection. Answer 4 is correct because poor hand hygiene spreads this infection. Answer 5** is incorrect because spread of this organism is through *direct contact* with a client who is infected. **Answer 6** is incorrect because the organism is found in the *stomach* and associated with *ulcer disease.*

■ **TEST-TAKING TIP:** *Consider the* mode *of transmission. Look for organisms that are controlled by the* hand hygiene *of the health-care provider.*

Content Area: Adult Health, Infectious Diseases; ***Integrated Process:*** Nursing Process, Analysis; ***Cognitive Level:*** Comprehension; ***Client Need/Subneed:*** Safe and Effective Care Environment/Safety and Infection Control/Standard/Transmission-based/Other Precautions

10. CORRECT ANSWER: 3. Answer 1 is incorrect because there is *no reason to slow* the feedings down. **Answer 2** is incorrect because, although D_5W IV would help keep the sodium down, it is *not* necessary to use the *IV* route when the gut is working. **Answer 3 is correct because full-strength tube feedings can cause hypernatremia. This is generally managed with enteral electrolyte-free water. Tap water is appropriate directly into the GI system; it does not need to be sterile. Answer 4** is incorrect because a more concentrated formula would *further increase* the serum sodium.

■ **TEST-TAKING TIP:** *Interpret the laboratory data. Consider how a concentrated tube feeding will affect fluid and electrolyte levels. Use SBAR to meet client needs. Eliminate the option pertaining to rate (Answer 1). Focus on route: IV (Answer 2) vs. feeding tube (Answer 3).*

Content Area: Adult Health, Gastrointestinal; ***Integrated Process:*** Nursing Process, Implementation; ***Cognitive Level:*** Analysis; ***Client Need/Subneed:*** Safe and Effective Care Environment/Management of Care/Collaboration with Interdisciplinary Team

11. CORRECT ANSWER: 3. Answer 1 is incorrect because there are *no data* supporting the efficacy of acupuncture as a quitting strategy. However, it may create another opportunity to quit, so it should not be discouraged if the client is interested. **Answer 2** is incorrect because tapering has been associated with nicotine *withdrawal* symptoms and subsequent failure to quit. Setting a "quit" day is currently the preferred strategy. **Answer 3 is correct because the 1-year quit rate for a person completing a group counseling program is 20%. Individual counseling has a small but significant impact on quitting. Answer 4** is incorrect because there is an antidepressant approved for use with smoking cessation (Wellbutrin), but it is *not* a selective serotonin reuptake inhibitor.

■ **TEST-TAKING TIP:** *Quitting smoking, like losing weight, is best accomplished in a supportive environment.*

Content Area: Adult Health, Substance Abuse; ***Integrated Process:*** Caring; ***Cognitive Level:*** Application; ***Client Need/Subneed:*** Safe and Effective Care Environment/Management of Care/Referrals

12. CORRECT ANSWER: 4. Answer 1 is incorrect because there is *not an immediate* risk to the client from the low platelets. **Answer 2** is incorrect because this client is likely stable. Drug withdrawal would have been a concern in the *early* postoperative period. **Answer 3** is incorrect because this client is not in the immediate postoperative period (*first 24 hours*). This client should be seen second. **Answer 4 is correct because there is a risk of bleeding at the insertion site and other postcatheterization complications. Stability of vital signs and ECG need to be assessed.**

■ **TEST-TAKING TIP:** *Select the earlier time frame here—hours, not days. Also, look for the client who is most unstable, as indicated by the* greatest likelihood *of a* change *in condition.*

Content Area: Adult Health, Triage; ***Integrated Process:*** Nursing Process, Analysis; ***Cognitive Level:*** Analysis; ***Client Need/Subneed:*** Safe and Effective Care Environment/Management of Care/Establishing Priorities

13. CORRECT ANSWER: 3. Answer 1 is incorrect because this client is at risk for *opportunistic* infections. **Answer 2** is incorrect because this client is at risk for a compromised immune system from treatment and a potential infection. **Answer 3 is correct because all other choices are vulnerable to infection. Answer 4** is incorrect because this client is at risk of developing an infection in the *bone.*

■ **TEST-TAKING TIP:** *Choose the option that is different from the others. Three of the clients are vulnerable to infection.*

Content Area: Adult Health, Infectious Disease; ***Integrated Process:*** Nursing Process, Implementation; ***Cognitive Level:*** Analysis; ***Client Need/Subneed:*** Safe and Effective Care Environment/Safety and Infection Control/Standard/Transmission-based/Other Precautions

14. CORRECT ANSWER: 3. **Answer 1** is incorrect because competency needs to be demonstrated before delegating. **Answer 2** is incorrect because the UAP needs to demonstrate competency before performing a task. **Answer 3 is correct because, when delegating, the RN needs to confirm that the UAP has met the task competencies. If delegating to a licensed staff (LPN/LVN), the assignment must be within the scope of practice.** **Answer 4** is incorrect because the UAP needs to demonstrate competency before the task is delegated.

■ **TEST-TAKING TIP:** *Choose the one option that has "verify" in the option, to ensure that the tasks will be performed safely.*

Content Area: Management of Care, Delegation; *Integrated Process:* Nursing Process, Implementation; *Cognitive Level:* Comprehension; *Client Need/Subneed:* Safe and Effective Care Environment/Management of Care/Delegation

15. CORRECT ANSWER: 4. **Answer 1** is incorrect because teaching is done *before* sedation by the RN. **Answer 2** is incorrect because the client could be *NPO.* **Answer 3** is incorrect because the client has received sedation and would *not* be *ambulatory.* **Answer 4 is correct because the client has been given IV sedation. Vital signs (VS) need to be checked after receiving sedation. The LVN/LPN can take the VS, but the RN must assess the findings.**

■ **TEST-TAKING TIP:** *There is only one safe choice. Three of the options would* not *be done* after *giving sedation.*

Content Area: Adult Health, Respiratory; *Integrated Process:* Nursing Process, Implementation; *Cognitive Level:* Application; *Client Need/Subneed:* Safe and Effective Care Environment/Management of Care/Delegation

16. CORRECT ANSWER: 4. **Answer 1** is incorrect because the signs are consistent with a *soft tissue* injury, which is *not* immediately life threatening. **Answer 2** is incorrect because the signs and symptoms are *not imminently* life threatening. The risk of dehydration would be a *greater* concern in a *very young* child or an *older* adult. **Answer 3** is incorrect because the signs and symptoms are *not imminently* life threatening. A throat culture would be indicated to determine if the cause is *viral* or *bacterial.* **Answer 4 is correct because the classic signs and symptoms of bacterial meningitis in an adult are severe headache and neck stiffness (nuchal rigidity). This is a serious condition because of the proximity to the brain and spinal cord and the possibility of sepsis.**

■ **TEST-TAKING TIP:** *Rule out the conditions that are not life threatening in a young adult or middle-aged adult.*

Content Area: Adult Health, Triage; *Integrated Process:* Nursing Process, Analysis; *Cognitive Level:* Analysis; *Client Need/Subneed:* Safe and Effective Care Environment/Management of Care/Establishing Priorities

17. CORRECT ANSWER: 3. **Answer 1** is incorrect because the client has a *chronic* condition that is not life threatening. **Answer 2** is incorrect because the blood sugar is *not* dangerously low. **Answer 3 is correct because it is important to determine if the client is actively bleeding. Since this client is the most unstable, the RN needs to ask the LPN/LVN to check on this client first.** **Answer 4** is incorrect because the client has a *chronic* condition and any changes would develop gradually.

■ **TEST-TAKING TIP:** *Consider which client is* most unstable *and the condition that could change suddenly.*

Content Area: Management of Care, Delegation; *Integrated Process:* Nursing Process, Analysis; *Cognitive Level:* Analysis; *Client Need/Subneed:* Safe and Effective Care Environment/Management of Care/Establishing Priorities

18. CORRECT ANSWER: 2. **Answer 1** is incorrect because this is *only part* of the desired control the client will hopefully retain. **Answer 2 is correct because preserving the client's control over the decision is important to a successful adjustment.** **Answer 3** is incorrect because this is *not* an *essential* criterion for placement; however, it would be *beneficial* to the family and client. **Answer 4** is incorrect because meals may be important, but are *not most important* to adjustment.

■ **TEST-TAKING TIP:** *Choose the option that* encompasses *the other options. If the client is involved with food choices, finances, and location, the client retains perceived control.*

Content Area: Management of Care, Case Management; *Integrated Process:* Nursing Process, Implementation; *Cognitive Level:* Application; *Client Need/Subneed:* Safe and Effective Care Environment/Management of Care/Case Management

19. CORRECT ANSWER: 2. **Answer 1** is incorrect because there is *no indication* that the client is unstable or experiencing respiratory difficulty. **Answer 2 is correct because pyelonephritis is an infectious process that can lead to acute renal failure. If kidney function is inadequate, the client may develop a life-threatening condition, such as hyperkalemia.** **Answer 3** is incorrect because this response by the client would be a *normal* reaction to the change in body image. **Answer 4** is incorrect because there is *no indication* that the client is unstable. Pain management is important. However, the client with the inadequate urine output needs further assessment *first.*

■ **TEST-TAKING TIP:** *Look for the client who is most unstable.*

Content Area: Adult Health, Triage; *Integrated Process:* Nursing Process, Analysis; *Cognitive Level:* Analysis; *Client Need/Subneed:* Safe and Effective Care Environment/Management of Care/Establishing Priorities

20. CORRECT ANSWER: 3. **Answer 1** is incorrect because, if a rash develops after several days of therapy, it is not an emergency situation. The rash *may or may not* be related to the drug. **Answer 2** is incorrect because there are *independent nursing actions* that need to be considered *before* contacting the physician. Answer 3 is correct because a change in cardiac status is a priority and potentially life threatening, which requires the nurse to collaborate with the physician on the appropriate action. **Answer 4** is incorrect because there are additional actions by the *nurse* that can be done *before* contacting the physician—checking for bowel sounds, a review of the client's dietary intake, activity status, and checking for impaction.

■ TEST-TAKING TIP: *Consider which situation requires the nurse to collaborate with the physician to meet the client's needs.*

Content Area: Adult Health, Triage; *Integrated Process:* Communication and Documentation; *Cognitive Level:* Analysis; *Client Need/Subneed:* Safe and Effective Care Environment/ Management of Care/Collaboration with Interdisciplinary Team

21. CORRECT ANSWER: 1. Answer 1 is correct because the RN can never delegate the ultimate responsibility for the client. Before delegating, the RN needs to determine that the LPN/LVN is competent. **Answer 2** is incorrect because tube feedings *are* within the scope of LPN/LVN practice, and *can* be delegated. **Answer 3** is incorrect because, even though the LPN/LVN *has* accountability, the RN can *never delegate* responsibility. **Answer 4** is incorrect because this *is* a task appropriate for the LPN/LVN, assuming that the LPN/LVN has shown competency in the procedure.

■ TEST-TAKING TIP: *Remember that only the* authority *to do something is delegated—not the responsibility.*

Content Area: Management of Care, Legal; *Integrated Process:* Nursing Process, Analysis; *Cognitive Level:* Comprehension; *Client Need/Subneed:* Safe and Effective Care Environment/ Management of Care/Delegation

22. CORRECT ANSWERS: 2, 4, 5. **Answer 1** is incorrect because the bacterium is *not* spread by *air or droplets.* Answer 2 is correct because the bacterium can be spread on *the hands* of health care providers. **Answer 3** is incorrect because the bacterium is *not airborne.* Answer 4 is correct because *C. difficile* is relatively *resistant* to disinfectants. Therefore, items that are close to the client should be cleaned daily with a bleach-and-water solution. Answer 5 is correct because metronidazole and vancomycin are the drugs of choice.

■ TEST-TAKING TIP: *Know that* C. difficile *is transmitted by direct contact with infected clients.*

Content Area: Adult Health, Infectious Disease; *Integrated Process:* Nursing Process, Planning; *Cognitive Level:* Application; *Client Need/Subneed:* Safe and Effective Care Environment/Safety and Infection Control/Standard/ Transmission-based/Other Precautions

23. CORRECT ANSWERS: 1, 4, 5, 6. Answer 1 is correct because a private room would reduce exposure of the client to other organisms transmitted by close contact with other clients. **Answer 2** is incorrect because rectal temperatures are to be avoided because rectal trauma may occur. **Answer 3** is incorrect because fresh fruits do not minimize susceptibility to infection, and unless peeled before given to the client, may be a source of bacteria. Answer 4 is correct because an electric razor avoids the risk of cuts. Answer 5 is correct because constipation and straining at stool may cause rectal tears. Answer 6 is correct because the chance of infection increases after 24 hours for IV solutions, and 72 hours with IV tubing.

■ TEST-TAKING TIP: *Choose options that reduce exposure to or risk from organisms.*

Content Area: Adult Health, Oncological; *Integrated Process:* Nursing Process, Analysis; *Cognitive Level:* Application; *Client Need/Subneed:* Safe and Effective Care Environment/Safety and Infection Control/Standard/Transmission-based/Other Precautions

24. CORRECT ANSWER: 1. Answer 1 is correct because a newly admitted client with abdominal pain is not stable and is first priority. The cause of the pain is unknown and vital signs should be assessed. **Answer 2** is incorrect because the client is going home (fourth priority). **Answer 3** is incorrect because the client is being observed by *someone* and would be third priority. **Answer 4** is incorrect because it is important to assess the *respiratory* status and chest tube functioning soon (second priority).

■ TEST-TAKING TIP: *Start with the client who is most unstable or critical.*

Content Area: Adult Health, Triage; *Integrated Process:* Nursing Process, Analysis; *Cognitive Level:* Analysis; *Client Need/Subneed:* Safe and Effective Care Environment/ Management of Care/Establishing Priorities

25. CORRECT ANSWER: 1. Answer 1 is correct because jaw pain is *not* a typical pain pattern for pancreatitis; therefore, the client needs to be assessed for myocardial ischemia. **Answer 2** is incorrect because this client would be seen *third.* The client is able to recognize and verbalize symptoms of hypoglycemia and the need to eat. The client could call the nurse if symptoms were increasing. **Answer 3** is incorrect because this client would be seen *second.* This client is at high risk for falling. The reason for the alarm needs to be assessed. **Answer 4** is incorrect because this client would be assessed *last.* Red-colored urine is *normal* after a transurethral resection of the prostate (TURP), and the presence of urine in the bag indicates the urine *is* flowing.

■ TEST-TAKING TIP: *Top priority in this situation is a client with a potentially life-threatening condition (cardiac).*

Content Area: Adult Health, Triage; *Integrated Process:* Nursing Process, Analysis; *Cognitive Level:* Analysis; *Client Need/Subneed:* Safe and Effective Care Environment/ Management of Care/Establishing Priorities

26. CORRECT ANSWER: 1. Answer 1 is correct because a client color-coded *red* (emergency) is the first priority. This client has a life-threatening problem that needs immediate action. **Answer 2** is incorrect because this client would be color-coded *black* (dead) and is nonsalvageable. **Answer 3** is incorrect because this client would be color-coded *yellow* (caution), and is the *second priority* level because the fracture is *closed.* **Answer 4** is incorrect because this client would be color-coded *green* (walking wounded) and would be the *third priority.* Evaluation would be delayed.

■ **TEST-TAKING TIP:** ***Memorize the color-coded disaster triage system: black = dead; red = emergency; yellow = caution; and green = go.***

Content Area: Adult Health, Triage; ***Integrated Process:*** Nursing Process, Analysis; ***Cognitive Level:*** Analysis; ***Client Need/Subneed:*** Safe and Effective Care Environment/Safety and Infection Control/Emergency Response Plan

ANSWERS

27. CORRECT ANSWERS: 1, 5. Answer 1 is correct because the activity is technical, and there is no potential for harm to the client. The RN would need to evaluate the findings. **Answer 2** is incorrect because the need for a nasogastric (NG) tube may indicate that the client is *not stable.* The outcome is *not predictable* from client to client. **Answer 3** is incorrect because the RN needs to *assess* the client's ability to *swallow,* to *prevent* aspiration of food. **Answer 4** is incorrect because the procedure requires *assessment* and *judgment* regarding how much to instill to irrigate and *evaluation* of the results. **Answer 5 is correct because it is routine and not complex. The client's condition is not life threatening.** **Answer 6** is incorrect because special precautions are needed to ensure that hair particles do not enter the tracheostomy. This procedure requires assessment, which needs to be done by a licensed staff member.

■ **TEST-TAKING TIP:** ***Only the RN can assess the condition and evaluate the response of clients who are unstable.***

Content Area: Management of Care, Delegation; ***Integrated Process:*** Nursing Process, Analysis; ***Cognitive Level:*** Analysis; ***Client Need/Subneed:*** Safe and Effective Care Environment/Management of Care/Delegation

28. CORRECT ANSWER: 2. **Answer 1** is incorrect because yeast is present on the *skin normally, not* transmitted because of poor hand hygiene. **Answer 2 is correct because poor blood sugar control is related to the quality of care received while hospitalized.** **Answer 3** is incorrect because weight loss is a result of *illness, not care.* **Answer 4** is incorrect because the need for surgery is determined by *diagnosis, not* quality of care.

■ **TEST-TAKING TIP:** ***Look for an option that is most influenced by quality of care.***

Content Area: Management of Care, Quality Improvement; ***Integrated Process:*** Nursing Process, Analysis; ***Cognitive Level:*** Application; ***Client Need/Subneed:*** Safe and Effective Care Environment/Management of Care/Performance Improvement (Quality Improvement)

29. CORRECT ANSWER: 2. **Answer 1** is incorrect because core measures data are collected *during* the hospital experience on admission. **Answer 2 is correct because these measures or standards of care are required by the Joint Commission to ensure that the best practices are being used in the hospital. An example of a core measure is the standard of care for a client admitted with heart failure.** **Answer 3** is incorrect because core measures are documentations of the standard of care for *certain* categories of clients or services, not a specific nurse's role. **Answer 4** is incorrect because the *hospital* collects and submits the data to JCAHO, *not* the client.

■ **TEST-TAKING TIP:** ***"Core" is central to the operation of the hospital—quality performance is the objective of care.***

Content Area: Management of Care, Quality Improvement; ***Integrated Process:*** Nursing Process, Implementation; ***Cognitive Level:*** Comprehension; ***Client Need/Subneed:*** Safe and Effective Care Environment/Management of Care/Performance Improvement (Quality Improvement)

30. CORRECT ANSWER: 2. **Answer 1** is incorrect because there is *no history* stated in the stem of the question that the client is unable to get to the bathroom. *In* the hospital, this would increase the risk. **Answer 2 is correct because the circumstances of a previous fall can be used to plan specific interventions to prevent a fall.** **Answer 3** is incorrect because there is an increased risk, but *no history* here, that the client is unable to ambulate safely. **Answer 4** is incorrect because the drug effects are *not known,* although medications are a cause of falls.

■ **TEST-TAKING TIP:** ***All of the options are risk factors, but a*** prior ***history and the cause of the falls is the best predictor.***

Content Area: Management of Care, Safety; ***Integrated Process:*** Nursing Process, Analysis; ***Cognitive Level:*** Application; ***Client Need/Subneed:*** Safe and Effective Care Environment/Safety and Infection Control/Accident Prevention and Injury Prevention

31. CORRECT ANSWER: 3. **Answer 1** is incorrect because restraints are *never* tied to the side rails. This increases the chance of injury. **Answer 2** is incorrect because ideally there should be *no tension* on the restraints. **Answer 3 is correct because the tightness of the restraints and the effects on client's skin must be frequently assessed.** **Answer 4** is incorrect because usually the lights should *be dimmed* to decrease stimuli when a person is agitated.

■ **TEST-TAKING TIP:** ***Choose an option that*** directly ***relates to the client; side rails, head of bed, or lights*** indirectly ***affect the client.***

Content Area: Adult Health, Integumentary; ***Integrated Process:*** Nursing Process, Implementation; ***Cognitive Level:*** Application; ***Client Need/Subneed:*** Safe and Effective Care Environment/Safety and Infection Control/Use of Restraints/Safety Devices

32. CORRECT ANSWER: 1. Answer 1 is correct because spelling the name and stating birth date would only be possible by the actual client. **Answer 2** is incorrect because clients can *wander* in and out of rooms. **Answer 3** is incorrect because client misidentification has been reported with *verbal* affirmation of name. **Answer 4** is incorrect because there is no assurance that the client who is receiving the medication is the client on the MAR.

■ **TEST-TAKING TIP:** *Look for the most reliable form of identity verification.*

Content Area: Management of Care, Error Prevention; ***Integrated Process:*** Nursing Process, Implementation; ***Cognitive Level:*** Comprehension; ***Client Need/Subneed:*** Safe and Effective Care Environment/Safety and Infection Control/Error Prevention

33. CORRECT ANSWERS: 1, 2, 3, 5. Answer 1 is correct because hand washing is the most important technique to reduce the risk of infections. Answer 2 is correct because hand washing is the most important technique to reduce the risk of infections. Answer 3 is correct because hand washing is the most important technique to reduce the risk of infections. **Answer 4** is incorrect because gloves *do not replace* the need for frequent hand washing. **Answer 5 is correct because hand washing is the most important technique to reduce the risk of infections.**

■ **TEST-TAKING TIP:** *Choose every opportunity to wash hands.*

Content Area: Adult Health, Integumentary; ***Integrated Process:*** Nursing Process, Analysis; ***Cognitive Level:*** Application; ***Client Need/Subneed:*** Safe and Effective Care Environment/Safety and Infection Control/Standard/Transmission-based/Other Precautions

34. CORRECT ANSWER: 1. Answer 1 is correct because hands should be vigorously rubbed together for at least 15 seconds, not 10 seconds. **Answer 2** is incorrect because the lather is *not* a contaminant if dripped in the sink. **Answer 3** is incorrect because the friction of rubbing is most important, *not* the temperature of the H_2O. **Answer 4** is incorrect because inadequate drying is *not* an immediate problem with regard to transmission of organisms from client to client.

■ **TEST-TAKING TIP:** *The stem asks for what is not "OK." The most important part of effective hand washing is friction.*

Content Area: Adult Health, Integumentary; ***Integrated Process:*** Nursing Process, Evaluation; ***Cognitive Level:*** Application; ***Client Need/Subneed:*** Safe and Effective Care Environment/Safety and Infection Control/Standard/Transmission-based/Other Precautions

35. CORRECT ANSWER: 3. **Answer 1** is incorrect because frequent sneezing is a normal finding in young infants when they attempt to clear the airway of secretions. Since the child is crying vigorously, oxygenation appears satisfactory at this time. **Answer 2** is incorrect because, although the child is at risk for dehydration due to frequent voiding and fever, a 2-year-old child is better able to compensate for dehydration than an infant, and the child may also have adequate oral intake. **Answer 3 is correct because the infant's history and assessment findings are suggestive of moderate to severe dehydration, which should be addressed quickly.** **Answer 4** is incorrect because, although the child's pain control is a concern, dehydration is the top priority.

■ **TEST-TAKING TIP:** *Follow the ABCs for prioritization. If all of the children have stable airways, look for the child that is at risk of circulatory collapse. In this case, the 6-month-old infant is at greatest risk due to age and history.*

Content Area: Child Health, Fluid and Electrolyte Imbalances; ***Integrated Process:*** Nursing Process, Assessment; ***Cognitive Level:*** Application; ***Client Need/Subneed:*** Safe and Effective Care Environment/Management of Care/Establishing Priorities

36. CORRECT ANSWER: 2. **Answer 1** is incorrect since a negative pressure room should only be used for controlling the spread of an infectious agent that can remain suspended in the air, such as tuberculosis. **Answer 2 is correct because RSV is transmitted by contact. The child diagnosed with RSV should be placed on contact precautions (gown, gloves) with strict emphasis on hand washing.** **Answer 3** is incorrect because RSV is *not* an airborne infectious agent. **Answer 4** is incorrect since the child with RSV does *not* need a positive pressure room. Positive pressure rooms keep outside air from entering the client's space and are designed specifically to protect clients who are severely immunocompromised from acquiring infections while hospitalized.

■ **TEST-TAKING TIP:** *Airborne precautions and negative pressure rooms are similar responses and can be eliminated.*

Content Area: Child Health, Respiratory; ***Integrated Process:*** Nursing Process, Analysis; ***Cognitive Level:*** Application; ***Client Need/Subneed:*** Safe and Effective Care Environment/Safety and Infection Control/Standard/Transmission-based/Other Precautions

37. CORRECT ANSWERS: 2, 3, 5, 6. **Answer 1** is incorrect because an appropriate fluid bolus for a child with severe dehydration is 20 mL/kg. **Answer 2 is correct because the nurse should first clean the hands for infection prevention. Answer 3 is correct because the nurse should wear personal protective equipment for enteric precautions after cleaning hands.** **Answer 4** is incorrect because acute gastroenteritis is typically caused by a *viral* illness such as rotavirus, not bacterial illness. Antibiotics would be administered for *bacterial,* not *viral,* infection. **Answer 5 is correct because the child's urinary output should be monitored frequently to determine the response to treatment. Answer 6 is correct because, once the nurse is protected, IV fluids should be administered to correct the severe dehydration.**

■ **TEST-TAKING TIP:** *Answers 2 and 3 go together (nurse's self-protection). Answers 5 and 6 go together (give fluid, monitor output).*

Content Area: Child Health, Gastrointestinal; ***Integrated Process:*** Nursing Process, Implementation; ***Cognitive Level:*** Application; ***Client Need/Subneed:*** Safe and Effective Care Environment/Safety and Infection Control/Standard/Transmission-based/Other Precautions

38. CORRECT ANSWER: 1. **Answer 1 is correct because the child is not considered contagious once all of the chickenpox (varicella) lesions have crusted.** **Answer 2** is incorrect because antibiotics are not effective against chickenpox as it is a viral infection. **Answer 3** is incorrect because a child with or without fever but who has open lesions is still considered infectious. **Answer 4** is incorrect because a positive varicella titer indicates that the child has been exposed to varicella, not that the child is no longer contagious to others.

■ **TEST-TAKING TIP:** *Look for answer options to eliminate when you know that they cannot be correct. If you know that chickenpox is caused by a virus, you can eliminate Answer 2. Answer 4 can be crossed out if you recall that a titer only provides information about the child's exposure,* not *a risk to others. Of the remaining two choices, you can eliminate Answer 3 since many illnesses are contagious during the prodromal period when fever may or may not be present. Therefore, fever is not related to communicability, and the best answer is Answer 1.*

Content Area: Child Health, Infectious Disease; *Integrated Process:* Nursing Process, Implementation; *Cognitive Level:* Application; *Client Need/Subneed:* Safe and Effective Care Environment/Safety and Infection Control/Standard/Transmission-based/Other Precautions

39. CORRECT ANSWERS: 3, 2, 4, 1. **Answer 3. The third client would be seen first because this child has been under recent sedation and has had the airway manipulated. A nurse should assess this child for high risk for respiratory complications. Answer 2. The second client would be seen second because the child should be assessed for potential complications of traction. Additionally, this is a younger school-age child who is in the room alone, needing the nurse's attention to make sure toys, food, etc. are within the child's reach. Answer 4. The fourth client would be seen third because the child has an unstable condition, at risk for rupture of the appendix. The child also needs to be assessed, with documentation done and a presurgical checklist completed, before the child can be transported to surgery as soon as the operating room is ready. This child is usually ambulatory and is old enough to call the nurse for urgent needs; therefore, this child is a lower priority than the child immobilized by traction. Answer 1. The first client would be seen last because the child with encopresis has a condition associated with constipation and fecal retention in which watery colonic contents bypass hard fecal masses and pass through the rectum. This is the lowest priority because this condition does not have the potential for acute complications, and the child's parent is at the bedside.**

■ **TEST-TAKING TIP:** *Children with the potential for airway complications (the third client) and hazards of immobility (the second client) should be the nurse's highest priority. Younger children (the third client) and those without a parent (the second client) at the bedside should also be a top priority.*

Content Area: Child Health, Hospitalization; *Integrated Process:* Nursing Process, Implementation; *Cognitive Level:* Analysis; *Client Need/Subneed:* Safe and Effective Care Environment/Management of Care/Establishing Priorities

40. CORRECT ANSWER: 4. **Answer 1** is incorrect because having the parents learn to auscultate the heart is not the best way to assist them in monitoring for cardiac complications. Rather, the parents should be taught to look for symptoms of impaired circulation, such as fatigue and pallor. **Answer 2** is incorrect because it is not recommended that children with a history of Kawasaki disease receive prophylactic antibiotics prior to dental work. Kawasaki disease affects the coronary arteries, not the endocardium, so the risk of bacterial endocarditis is not increased. **Answer 3** is incorrect because repeat doses of immunoglobulin are not indicated for this condition. **Answer 4 is correct because a key component in the treatment of Kawasaki disease is the administration of intravenous immune globulin (IVIG). Parents should be advised that immunizations, such as the MMR (measles-mumps-rubella), may be delayed for some months since IVIG could render the vaccinations ineffective.**

■ **TEST-TAKING TIP:** *The answer options should help you recall that immunoglobulin is a cornerstone of treatment for Kawasaki disease. Since this treatment modulates the immune system, select the answer option that addresses a potential effect of the treatment.*

Content Area: Child Health, Infectious Disease; *Integrated Process:* Teaching and Learning; *Cognitive Level:* Application; *Client Need/Subneed:* Safe and Effective Care Environment/Safety and Infection Control/Standard/Transmission-based/Other Precautions

41. CORRECT ANSWER: 3. **Answer 1** is incorrect because, although the younger the child is when the diagnosis of HIV is made, the lower the life expectancy, this information is best discussed when the parent has questions regarding prognosis. This *should not* be the nurse's main focus during an *initial* counseling session. **Answer 2** is incorrect because, although children with HIV are at risk for developing failure to thrive, nutrition is *not* the most important topic of an *initial* meeting. **Answer 3 is correct because it is essential that the parent recognize the importance of following through with the medication regimen prescribed by the practitioner. Failure to do so could quickly lead to resistant HIV and opportunistic infection.** **Answer 4** is incorrect because immunization is one of the keys to infection prevention in the child with HIV and should *not be delayed.*

■ **TEST-TAKING TIP:** *Note the time frame given in the stem of the question:* "during the first meeting." *Initial counseling sessions regarding chronic illnesses should stress those self-care topics that have the greatest potential for harm, especially in the short term.*

ANSWERS

Content Area: Child Health, Infectious Disease; *Integrated Process:* Teaching and Learning; *Cognitive Level:* Application; *Client Need/Subneed:* Safe and Effective Care Environment/ Safety and Infection Control/Standard/Transmission-based/ Other Precautions

42. CORRECT ANSWER: 3. **Answer 1** is incorrect because a *slight* elevation in WBC count is common with the normal inflammation accompanying surgery. No postoperative risks are identified in these data and thus no immediate treatment is required. **Answer 2** is incorrect because an elderly client who is postoperative with a history of congestive heart failure (CHF) should be evaluated for response to pain medications and respiratory status, but is not the most critical of the clients described. **Answer 3 is correct because bloodstream infections are of great concern in clients without the normal filter of the spleen. The high temperature indicates this client could be septic and will require immediate care with fluids and antibiotics.** **Answer 4** is incorrect because a platelet count of 100,000, although low, does not put this client at a clinically significant risk of bleeding. Assessment and care of more critical clients should take priority.

■ TEST-TAKING TIP: *Three of the clients have orthopedic conditions. Choose the only option that concerns a vital organ (spleen). Who is at imminent risk? Think about the stability of the clients. Select the most unstable.*

Content Area: Adult Health, Infection Control; *Integrated Process:* Nursing Process, Assessment; *Cognitive Level:* Analysis; *Client Need/Subneed:* Safe and Effective Care Environment/ Management of Care/Establishing Priorities

43. CORRECT ANSWER: 4. **Answer 1** is incorrect because Betadine (an iodine solution) might be introduced into the IV. If the port requires cleaning, use an alcohol swab. **Answer 2** is incorrect because indwelling bladder catheters are associated with infections. If there were a perineal wound, a bladder catheter might help to protect the wound from infection, but when perineal tissue is intact it should be maintained that way with normal skin cleaning. **Answer 3** is incorrect because moisture promotes growth of skin organisms such as yeast. Skinfolds should be kept *dry.* **Answer 4 is correct because wounds that require dressings should be covered. Frequent removal for wound assessments increases infection risk and reduces optimal presence of healing fluids and substances in wound bed.**

■ TEST-TAKING TIP: *Look for the option that provides the* greatest *protection or reduces risk.*

Content Area: Adult Health, Infection Control; *Integrated Process:* Nursing Process, Implementation; *Cognitive Level:* Application; *Client Need/Subneed:* Safe and Effective Care Environment/Safety and Infection Control/Standard/ Transmission-based/Other Precautions

44. CORRECT ANSWER: 2. **Answer 1** is incorrect because neither the mastectomy nor the pneumonia puts the client at risk for problems with arterial circulation. It is not necessary to do frequent pulse checks. **Answer 2 is correct because, during breast surgery, lymph nodes are removed to rid the body of spreading cancer. This leaves the distal tissue at risk for swelling and infections. IV catheters, carrying a risk of infection, should be placed in the opposite arm.** **Answer 3** is incorrect because lymph nodes may have been removed from the right auxiliary area with the mastectomy; the client is at risk for arm swelling. *Raising* the arm is permitted and may help minimize swelling. **Answer 4** is incorrect because *movement* of the right arm will help promote venous return in this arm with limited lymphatic damage.

■ TEST-TAKING TIP: *Three of the choices relate to the right arm, only one the left arm. Choose the option, in this case, that is* different.

Content Area: Adult Health, Respiratory; *Integrated Process:* Nursing Process, Implementation; *Cognitive Level:* Application; *Client Need/Subneed:* Physiological Integrity/Reduction of Risk Potential/Potential for Alterations in Body Systems

45. CORRECT ANSWER: 3. **Answer 1** is incorrect because the immediate goal is to remove the potentially infectious material. Covering the scab will *not* accomplish this. **Answer 2** is incorrect because ice will *not* help remove the blood from the nurse's skin. **Answer 3 is correct because washing is the most effective way of removing potentially infectious material. Avoid disrupting the scab, which is providing a microbial barrier.** **Answer 4** is incorrect because scrubbing the scab may remove the barrier that prevents blood from entering the nurse's body.

■ TEST-TAKING TIP: *Washing the area is the* first *action for controlling the spread of infection.*

Content Area: Adult Health, Infection Control; *Integrated Process:* Nursing Process, Implementation; *Cognitive Level:* Application; *Client Need/Subneed:* Safe and Effective Care Environment/Safety and Infection Control/Standard/ Transmission-based/Other Precautions

46. CORRECT ANSWER: 1. **Answer 1 is correct because the elevated blood pressure may indicate stress or pain, and further assessment is needed to establish why the blood pressure is elevated.** **Answer 2** is incorrect because a low pulse is common in athletes. **Answer 3** is incorrect because this client would not be the first priority. The nurse should see this client *second,* as the temperature in the older adult may not be an accurate indicator of the client's condition. **Answer 4** is incorrect because right shoulder pain or pain in the scapular area are *normal* and result from the *gas* used to insufflate the abdominal cavity during the procedure.

■ TEST-TAKING TIP: *Look at the vital signs; select the* elevated BP. *Choose the client who is most unstable, or the condition that puts the client at greater risk.*

Content Area: Adult Health, Triage; *Integrated Process:* Nursing Process, Analysis; *Cognitive Level:* Analysis; *Client Need/ Subneed:* Safe and Effective Care Environment/Management of Care/Establishing Priorities

47. CORRECT ANSWERS: 1, 3, 4. Answer 1 is correct because this is the probability for these parents to have a child with sickle cell anemia. **Answer 2** is incorrect because the probability for these parents to have a child with sickle cell trait is 100%. **Answer 3 is correct because this is the probability for these parents to have a child with sickle cell trait. Answer 4 is correct because this is the probability for these parents to have a child with sickle cell anemia.** **Answer 5** is incorrect because the probability for these parents to have a child with sickle cell anemia is zero.

■ **TEST-TAKING TIP:** *Write out a mendelian square when considering heredity. See the table below, which uses the letter "S" to represent sickle cell trait and "s" to represent no trait, with "SS" indicating an individual with sickle cell disease. In the example, a parent with sickle cell disease is paired with a parent who carries the trait, with a resulting 50% chance that their offspring will have the disease or carry the trait.*

	S	S
S	SS	SS
s	Ss	Ss

Content Area: Child Health, Hematological; ***Integrated Process:*** Nursing Process, Analysis; ***Cognitive Level:*** Application; ***Client Need/Subneed:*** Safe and Effective Care Environment/ Management of Care/Case Management

48. CORRECT ANSWER: 4. Answer 1 is incorrect because endometriosis is a condition where tissue similar to the lining of the uterus (the endometrial stroma and glands, which should only be located inside the uterus) is found *elsewhere* in the body. It is *not* an infection and does *not* cause fever, abdominal tenderness, or foul-smelling lochia. **Answer 2** is incorrect because, even though this client is at risk for postoperative wound infection, a postoperative wound *infection does not cause foul-smelling* lochia. **Answer 3** is incorrect because, although this client is at risk for pelvic thrombophlebitis, which causes fever, it does not have foul-smelling lochia or abdominal tenderness. **Answer 4 is correct because the most common reason for postpartum fever is endometritis. Other symptoms include abdominal tenderness and foul-smelling lochia. Postpartum endometritis occurs in 15% to 20% of unscheduled cesarean deliveries after a prolonged labor.**

■ **TEST-TAKING TIP:** *Endometriosis and endometritis sound similar; the ending "itis" usually indicates infection.*

Content Area: Maternity, Intrapartum; ***Integrated Process:*** Nursing Process, Analysis; ***Cognitive Level:*** Analysis; ***Client Need/Subneed:*** Safe and Effective Care Environment/Safety and Infection Control/Standard/Transmission-based/Other Precautions

49. CORRECT ANSWER: 2. Answer 1 is incorrect because redness alone is not an indication of a positive test. Also, the reaction is assessed at 48 hours after testing, not after 24 hours. **Answer 2 is correct because the presence of a positive TB test is determined by the size of the induration. Induration of 10 mm or more is a positive reaction.** **Answer 3** is incorrect because redness is not the indicator of a reaction. The diameter of the induration (raised area) is important. **Answer 4** is incorrect because the test is not read before 48 hours regardless of when redness or induration appears.

■ **TEST-TAKING TIP:** *Select the only option that just addresses* induration. *The other three all include redness.*

Content Area: Adult Health, Infectious Disease; ***Integrated Process:*** Nursing Process, Assessment; ***Cognitive Level:*** Application; ***Client Need/Subneed:*** Safe and Effective Care Environment/Safety and Infection Control/Standard/ Transmission-based/Other Precautions

50. CORRECT ANSWER: 2. Answer 1 is incorrect because calf pain may indicate an embolus, which can be fatal. **Answer 2 is correct because the oxygen saturation is normal. The asthma is being controlled.** **Answer 3** is incorrect because older adults have subnormal temperatures, so the cause of the elevated temperature has not been resolved. **Answer 4** is incorrect because rebound abdominal pain may indicate appendicitis. Rupture may occur if untreated.

■ **TEST-TAKING TIP:** *Look for the client whose condition is most stable. Determine if the clinical situation is a* normal *state and choose that option.*

Content Area: Adult Health, Triage; ***Integrated Process:*** Nursing Process, Analysis; ***Cognitive Level:*** Analysis; ***Client Need/Subneed:*** Safe and Effective Care Environment/ Management of Care/Establishing Priorities

51. CORRECT ANSWER: 2. Answer 1 is incorrect because there is *no immediate* risk to the client. **Answer 2 is correct because chemotherapy drugs are toxic and can cause tissue destruction if infiltrated, and maintaining the access port is vital to therapy.** **Answer 3** is incorrect because there is *no immediate* risk to the client. **Answer 4** is incorrect because there is *no immediate* risk to the client.

■ **TEST-TAKING TIP:** *Look for the client who is most vulnerable to a* serious *consequence. Eliminate those answers that focus on GI feeding (Answer 1), elimination (Answer 3), and psychosocial need (Answer 4).*

Content Area: Adult Health, Triage; ***Integrated Process:*** Nursing Process, Analysis; ***Cognitive Level:*** Analysis; ***Client Need/Subneed:*** Safe and Effective Care Environment/ Management of Care/Establishing Priorities

52. CORRECT ANSWER: 2. Answer 1 is incorrect because diabetes is *not* a contraindication for breastfeeding. **Answer 2 is correct because HIV can be transmitted through breast milk.** **Answer 3** is incorrect because hypertension is *not* a contraindication for breastfeeding. **Answer 4** is incorrect because thyroid disease is *not* a contraindication for breastfeeding.

■ **TEST-TAKING TIP:** *Consider the risk and benefit of breastfeeding. The transmission of HIV is a* bigger *risk to the neonate than the benefit of breastfeeding.*

Content Area: Maternity, Postpartum; ***Integrated Process:*** Teaching and Learning; ***Cognitive Level:*** Application; ***Client Need/Subneed:*** Safe and Effective Care Environment/ Safety and Infection Control/Standard/Transmission-based/ Other Precautions

53. CORRECT ANSWER: 4. **Answer 1** is incorrect because the right side would *not* be weakened. **Answer 2** is incorrect because the right side would *not* be weakened. **Answer 3** is incorrect because the unaffected *right* side should be next to the bed. **Answer 4 is correct because, with a right-sided brain attack, the client would have *left*-sided hemiplegia or weakness. The client's unaffected side should be closest to the bed to facilitate the transfer.**

■ TEST-TAKING TIP: *Visualize the client with weakness on the* **opposite** *side of the brain attack.*

Content Area: Adult Health, Cardiovascular; ***Integrated Process:*** Nursing Process, Implementation; ***Cognitive Level:*** Application; ***Client Need/Subneed:*** Safe and Effective Care Environment/ Safety and Infection Control/Accident Prevention and Injury Prevention

54. CORRECT ANSWER: 1. **Answer 1 is correct because the client has left visual field blindness. The client will see *only* from the *right* side.** **Answer 2** is incorrect because the client would not see the call light on the left side. **Answer 3** is incorrect because the client only sees from the nasal portion of the left eye and the temporal area of the right eye. Directly in front is better than the left side, but *not the best* choice. **Answer 4** is incorrect because the nurse must ensure client safety by placing the call light where it will be seen.

■ TEST-TAKING TIP: *Requires knowledge of visual fields and optic nerve structure.*

Content Area: Adult Health, Neurological; ***Integrated Process:*** Nursing Process, Implementation; ***Cognitive Level:*** Application; ***Client Need/Subneed:*** Safe and Effective Care Environment/ Safety and Infection Control/Accident Prevention and Injury Prevention

55. CORRECT ANSWER: 3. **Answer 1** is incorrect because the stoma *will* be 1 to 2 cm above the skin. Because the stoma is swollen after surgery, the size will change. **Answer 2** is incorrect because *some* bleeding is *normal.* If it bleeds *too often,* the physician should be notified. **Answer 3 is correct because, since there are no nerves in the mucous membranes, there should be no pain when touching. Pain would possibly indicate a problem internally.** **Answer 4** is incorrect because this is a *normal* appearance. If the stoma becomes *dusky* in color, this could need *immediate* action.

■ TEST-TAKING TIP: *Pain is not normal and indicates a problem for any client situation.*

Content Area: Adult Health, Gastrointestinal; ***Integrated Process:*** Nursing Process, Analysis; ***Cognitive Level:*** Application; ***Client Need/Subneed:*** Safe and Effective Care Environment/ Management of Care/Establishing Priorities

56. CORRECT ANSWER: 1. **Answer 1 is correct because the infant will likely be receiving phototherapy, which requires the baby to be unclothed. The isolette allows the baby to be in a closed, temperature-regulated environment.** **Answer 2** is incorrect because the open crib will put the infant at risk for alterations in body temperature, and the phototherapy should be applied through a shield such as plastic to minimize ultraviolet radiation exposure. **Answer 3** is incorrect because a hospital bed is unsafe for an infant. **Answer 4** is incorrect because the bassinette will put the infant at risk for alterations in body temperature, and the phototherapy should be applied through a shield such as plastic to minimize ultraviolet radiation exposure.

■ TEST-TAKING TIP: *Think about the possible treatments for a child with hyperbilirubinemia. Since the child will likely receive phototherapy, the equipment must be suited for this treatment.*

Content Area: Child Health, Hematological; ***Integrated Process:*** Nursing Process, Implementation; ***Cognitive Level:*** Application; ***Client Need/Subneed:*** Safe and Effective Care Environment/ Safety and Infection Control/Safe Use of Equipment

57. CORRECT ANSWER: 2. **Answer 1** is incorrect because there is *no indication* that this client is the most unstable of the four clients. **Answer 2 is correct because the K^+ level is above the normal high of 5.5 mEq/L. An elevated K^+ can have serious effects on the heart and affect the stability of the client. The physician needs to be called regarding the report so that changes in treatment can be made to manage the elevated K^+.** **Answer 3** is incorrect because it is the client with the *elevated* K^+ who is at risk for *life-threatening arrhythmias,* and the K^+ level needs to be reported right away. **Answer 4** is incorrect because the client sent to ICU is receiving close observation. The family of this client definitely needs to be contacted *after* reporting the client with the elevated K^+ level.

■ TEST-TAKING TIP: *Consider which client is at* greatest risk *for a life-threatening consequence.*

Content Area: Adult Health, Triage; ***Integrated Process:*** Nursing Process, Analysis; ***Cognitive Level:*** Analysis; ***Client Need/Subneed:*** Safe and Effective Care Environment/ Management of Care/Establishing Priorities

58. CORRECT ANSWER: 2. **Answer 1** is incorrect because swimming *is* a suggested exercise for pregnancy and is safe *unless* the amniotic membranes have ruptured. **Answer 2 is correct because women who are pregnant should not sit in hot tubs for *longer than 10* minutes. Becoming overheated in a hot tub is not recommended during pregnancy. The American College of Obstetricians and Gynecologists (ACOG) also recommends that women who are pregnant should never let their core body temperature rise above 102.2°F. Women who choose to use a hot tub should monitor their temperature to avoid overheating.** **Answer 3** is incorrect because a warm bath, which is not uncomfortable or scalding, *is* a safer way to relax. In a bath, much of the upper body will remain out of the water, making it less likely to overheat. Additionally, the water in a bath begins to cool off, as opposed to a hot tub, which further reduces a risk of overheating. **Answer 4** is incorrect because a sauna, like a hot tub, can lead to overheating and should be used with *caution in short periods* of time.

■ TEST-TAKING TIP: *This question is asking which statement is* **not** *a safe action by the client and therefore requires further health teaching.*

Content Area: Maternity, Antepartum; ***Integrated Process:*** Nursing Process, Evaluation; ***Cognitive Level:*** Analysis; ***Client Need/Subneed:*** Safe and Effective Care Environment/Safety and Infection Control/Accident Prevention and Injury Prevention

59. CORRECT ANSWER: 1. Answer 1 is correct because, before delivery of the neonate's body, it is important to check for a cord around the neonate's neck. It is the first action after delivery of the head and before the shoulders are delivered. **Answer 2** is incorrect because antibiotic ointment in the infant's eyes can *wait* for up to *an hour.* It is *not a priority* after the delivery of the head. **Answer 3** is incorrect because the DeLee suction is *no longer used* to remove secretions; a *bulb syringe* should be used to remove secretions prior to delivery of the neonate's body. **Answer 4** is incorrect because the body needs to be delivered before the heart rate and respirations can be evaluated. This is *not the first* action after delivery of the neonate's head.

■ **TEST-TAKING TIP:** *Think "cord" as the first action* after *delivery of the head and* before *the shoulders and body. Picture the cardinal movements and the process of delivery.*

Content Area: Maternity, Intrapartum; ***Integrated Process:*** Nursing Process, Implementation; ***Cognitive Level:*** Application; ***Client Need/Subneed:*** Safe and Effective Care Environment/Safety and Infection Control/Accident Prevention and Injury Prevention

60. CORRECT ANSWER: 3. **Answer 1** is incorrect because *hot* water can cause leakage of lead from old pipes. Cold water should be used for drinking, cooking, and preparation of infant formula. Cold water reduces the leakage of lead from old pipes. **Answer 2** is incorrect because hot water can cause leakage of lead from old pipes. The family should use cold water for drinking, cooking, and preparation of infant formula. Cold water reduces the leakage of lead from old pipes. **Answer 3 is correct because hot water can cause leakage of lead from old pipes. The family should use cold water for drinking, cooking, and preparation of infant formula. Cold water reduces the leakage of lead from old pipes.** **Answer 4** is incorrect because buying bottled water may *not* be financially realistic or possible for this family. The family should instead use the available cold water in their apartment building for drinking, cooking, and preparation of infant formula. Cold water reduces the leakage of lead from old pipes.

■ **TEST-TAKING TIP:** *Hot causes "dilation," whereas cold causes "constriction." This is true in pipes as well as in the human body. "Dilation" will lead to the release of lead particles.*

Content Area: Child Health, Poisoning; ***Integrated Process:*** Teaching and Learning; ***Cognitive Level:*** Application; ***Client Need/Subneed:*** Safe and Effective Care Environment/Safety and Infection Control/Handling Hazardous and Infectious Materials

61. CORRECT ANSWER: 3. **Answer 1** is incorrect because the nurse is not responsible for double-bagging the soiled dressing, which would be placed in the contaminated receptacle. **Answer 2** is incorrect because PCP is *not* transmitted through droplets. Masks and eyewear are only indicated when the procedure may produce splashes of blood or body fluids. A routine dressing change of a leg wound should not require a mask. **Answer 3 is correct because standard (universal) precautions should be used, and washing hands is the most important technique for preventing disease transmission.** **Answer 4** is incorrect because reverse (protective) isolation would usually be indicated for a client with AIDS with a very low WBC count. There is no information indicating that that is the status.

■ **TEST-TAKING TIP:** *Look for hand washing and gloves first.*

Content Area: Adult Health, Infectious Disease; ***Integrated Process:*** Nursing Process, Implementation; ***Cognitive Level:*** Application; ***Client Need/Subneed:*** Safe and Effective Care Environment/Safety and Infection Control/Standard/Transmission-based/Other Precautions

62. CORRECT ANSWER: 2. **Answer 1** is incorrect because this is a priority question. Ambulating *after* the sedation wears off is not wrong; it just is *not the first* concern. **Answer 2 is correct because the throat will have been anesthetized to facilitate passage of the tube. If the gag reflex has not returned before food or fluid is given, the client may aspirate.** **Answer 3** is incorrect because teaching should have been done *before* the procedure. It is also *not the first* concern. **Answer 4** is incorrect because *no particular* positioning is indicated following a diagnostic bronchoscopy.

■ **TEST-TAKING TIP:** Priority: *Which option, if not done, would cause* greatest harm *to the client?*

Content Area: Adult Health, Respiratory; ***Integrated Process:*** Nursing Process, Implementation; ***Cognitive Level:*** Analysis; ***Client Need/Subneed:*** Safe and Effective Care Environment/Management of Care/Establishing Priorities

63. CORRECT ANSWER: 2. **Answer 1** is incorrect because, although plausible, gauze is *not occlusive* and may not be readily available. **Answer 2 is correct because the priority is to prevent air from entering the chest cavity with the most occlusive method. (Gloves might be available, but time is critical.)** **Answer 3** is incorrect because it would take too much time to reposition the client in bed. Cover the opening immediately, *then* put the client to bed. **Answer 4** is incorrect because the best answer requires action by the nurse, *not* the physician.

■ **TEST-TAKING TIP:** Priority: *Do something to reduce* immediate *risk to the client—a sucking hole. Consider the two options that include "cover" and choose the one with the most available resource.*

Content Area: Adult Health, Respiratory; ***Integrated Process:*** Nursing Process, Implementation; ***Cognitive Level:*** Analysis; ***Client Need/Subneed:*** Safe and Effective Care Environment/Management of Care/Establishing Priorities

64. CORRECT ANSWER: 2. **Answer 1** is incorrect because, unless the person is debilitated, is taking steroids, or is immunosuppressed, there is no restriction. **Answer 2 is correct because infants and children under age 5 are susceptible to TB.** **Answer 3** is incorrect because, unless the person is debilitated, is taking steroids, or is immunosuppressed, there is no restriction. **Answer 4** is incorrect because, unless the person is debilitated, is taking steroids, or is immunosuppressed, there is no restriction.

■ TEST-TAKING TIP: *Identify the nursing concept being tested—low immunity.*

Content Area: Adult Health, Infectious Disease; *Integrated Process:* Nursing Process, Planning; *Cognitive Level:* Analysis; *Client Need/Subneed:* Safe and Effective Care Environment/ Safety and Infection Control/Standard/Transmission-based/ Other Precautions

65. CORRECT ANSWER: 2. **Answer 1** is incorrect because the client will feel better soon after drug therapy is started, but must take the drug long after physical improvement results. **Answer 2 is correct because total destruction of the infection takes at least 9 months, if not longer.** **Answer 3** is incorrect because a negative culture occurs in 2 months; however, the disease process can reactivate if drug therapy is stopped prematurely. **Answer 4** is incorrect because, although some pathologic changes with TB may be difficult to treat, lifelong therapy is *not* required.

■ TEST-TAKING TIP: *Choose the only specific time element listed (9 months). Know the expected outcome of treatment.*

Content Area: Adult Health, Infectious Disease; *Integrated Process:* Teaching and Learning; *Cognitive Level:* Application; *Client Need/Subneed:* Physiological Integrity/Physiological Adaptation/Illness Management

66. CORRECT ANSWER: 3. **Answer 1** is incorrect because respiratory isolation guidelines do *not* require gowns and gloves for visitors or for staff during *casual* contact. Masks would be worn by the client (if alert) or by family and staff if in *close* contact. TB is transmitted by airborne droplets. **Answer 2** is incorrect because the door should *not* be open to the hallway. Ventilation is important, but is handled through the facility's ventilation system. **Answer 3 is correct because hand washing is the best method for reducing cross-contamination. Gowns and gloves are not always required when entering a client's room.** **Answer 4** is incorrect because it is not part of respiratory isolation requirements. (Usually the client will be in a private room, but the isolation precautions do not stipulate this.)

■ TEST-TAKING TIP: *The most important action for infection control is hand washing.*

Content Area: Adult Health, Infectious Disease; *Integrated Process:* Nursing Process, Evaluation; *Cognitive Level:* Application; *Client Need/Subneed:* Safe and Effective Care Environment/Safety and Infection Control/Standard/ Transmission-based/Other Precautions

67. CORRECT ANSWER: 2. **Answer 1** is incorrect because the nasogastric tube may not be correctly positioned. **Answer 2 is correct because nursing assistants can walk clients (or feed them, *if* there is no risk of aspiration). If assessment is required, the task cannot be delegated.** **Answer 3** is incorrect because nursing assistants cannot administer medications. **Answer 4** is incorrect because the client's ability to swallow must be assessed before the client is fed by a nursing assistant.

■ TEST-TAKING TIP: *Do not delegate functions of assessment, evaluation, and nursing judgment.*

Content Area: Management of Care, Delegation; *Integrated Process:* Nursing Process, Planning; *Cognitive Level:* Application; *Client Need/Subneed:* Safe and Effective Care Environment/Management of Care/Delegation

68. CORRECT ANSWER: 4. **Answer 1** is incorrect because a competent client, not a relative, gives consent. There is no indication of an emergency. **Answer 2** is incorrect because the client has received the preoperative medication, so he or she cannot sign a consent form. **Answer 3** is incorrect because the responsibility for a correct consent form is the MD's, not the nurse's. **Answer 4 is correct because the responsibility for an accurate informed consent is the physician's. An exception to this answer would be a life-threatening emergency, but there are no data to support another response.**

■ TEST-TAKING TIP: *Know the legal responsibility for informed consent. There is potential for risk in this situation.*

Content Area: Management of Care, Informed Consent; *Integrated Process:* Nursing Process, Implementation; *Cognitive Level:* Analysis; *Client Need/Subneed:* Safe and Effective Care Environment/Management of Care/Informed Consent

69. CORRECT ANSWER: 3. **Answer 1** is incorrect because *preventing* damage, if the neck was broken, would be a priority over neurological checks. **Answer 2** is incorrect because checking the airway is not included. **Answer 3 is correct because checking the airway would be a priority, and a neck injury should be suspected.** **Answer 4** is incorrect because checking the airway and stabilizing the neck and spine are not included.

■ TEST-TAKING TIP: *When appropriate for the injury, remember "ABCs" as priorities.*

Content Area: Adult Health, Trauma; *Integrated Process:* Nursing Process, Implementation; *Cognitive Level:* Analysis; *Client Need/Subneed:* Safe Effective Care Environment/ Management of Care/Establishing Priorities

70. CORRECT ANSWER: 4. **Answer 1** is incorrect because the nurse's aide may not communicate the status of the assignment to the RN, or may be hesitant to report uncompleted work. The RN *cannot* assume. **Answer 2** is incorrect because, depending on the condition of the clients, the time interval between communications may *vary.* **Answer 3** is incorrect because the clients may not be aware of the care needed. **Answer 4 is correct because setting definite parameters will guide the nurse's aide as to the priorities and what should be reported to the RN.**

■ TEST-TAKING TIP: *Three of the options are inappropriate (Answers 1 and 3) or unrealistic (Answer 2). Look at the* verbs *to help select the best option for the concept of accountability; "assume" (no!); "communicate" and "ask" (too similar); "define" (yes!).*

Content Area: Management of Care, Delegation; *Integrated Process:* Nursing Process, Implementation; *Cognitive Level:* Analysis; *Client Need/Subneed:* Safe and Effective Care Environment/Management of Care/Delegation

ANSWERS

71. CORRECT ANSWER: 3. **Answer 1** is incorrect because it will not provide enough data to make a decision. It may yield only a "yes" or "no" reply. **Answer 2** is incorrect because there are insufficient data to warrant this action as a priority for RN intervention. **Answer 3 is correct because more information is necessary in order to *clarify* the urgency of the situation. This information will help delineate and prioritize nursing interventions.** **Answer 4** is incorrect because, although this is valuable information, it is *not* the best *initial* response by the RN.

■ **TEST-TAKING TIP:** *Key word: "initial." Note that two options (Answers 1 and 3) focus on asking for more data from the LVN/LPN; choose the one that is likely to provide* **more information** *(i.e., "describe").*

Content Area: Adult Health, Respiratory; ***Integrated Process:*** Nursing Process, Implementation; ***Cognitive Level:*** Analysis; ***Client Need/Subneed:*** Safe and Effective Care Environment/ Management of Care/Establishing Priorities

72. CORRECT ANSWER: 1. Answer 1 is correct because the priority is to maintain client safety. With syncope and dizziness, the client is at high risk for falling. **Answer 2** is incorrect because, although a current hemoglobin (Hgb) and hematocrit (Hct) would be important data to assess for bleeding, these tests are *not* the highest priority. **Answer 3** is incorrect because sucralfate (Carafate) is primarily prescribed for the short-term management of duodenal, *not* gastric, ulcers. **Answer 4** is incorrect because, although vital signs are an important assessment, especially with syncope and dizziness, safety is the priority in this situation, followed by further assessment.

■ **TEST-TAKING TIP:** *The key word is "initial"; safety is the priority with a client complaining of syncope and vertigo.*

Content Area: Adult Health, Gastrointestinal; ***Integrated Process:*** Nursing Process, Implementation; ***Cognitive Level:*** Analysis; ***Client Need/Subneed:*** Safe and Effective Care Environment/Management of Care/Establishing Priorities

73. CORRECT ANSWER: 3. **Answer 1** is incorrect because increasing the oxygen to 6 L/min is unnecessary. The usual rate of oxygen is 2 to 4 L/min to maintain the pulse oximeter reading at 96% to 98%. **Answer 2** is incorrect because, although these levels are important data, the urgency of the client's situation is comfort and pain management while increasing coronary artery perfusion. **Answer 3 is correct because morphine sulfate is given for chest pain at a rate of 1 mg/min repeated every 5 minutes as needed to block pain perception. However, in myocardial ischemia it decreases anxiety and oxygen demand as it promotes vasodilation.** **Answer 4** is incorrect because it is not the priority. However, this test will probably be ordered if the client's symptoms suggest an extension of the infarction.

■ **TEST-TAKING TIP:** *Look at the symptom in the stem (pain); choose an option (analgesic) that relates to* pain *management.*

Content Area: Adult Health, Cardiovascular; ***Integrated Process:*** Nursing Process, Implementation; ***Cognitive Level:*** Analysis; ***Client Need/Subneed:*** Safe and Effective Care Environment/ Management of Care/Establishing Priorities

74. CORRECT ANSWER: 3. **Answer 1** is incorrect because confronting the RN may escalate the situation and result in conflict. This choice does *not* resolve the basic issue of client abuse by the staff member. **Answer 2** is incorrect because documentation may compound the situation, creating legal ramifications. **Answer 3 is correct. *Objective* reporting allows for client advocacy while maintaining anonymity for the staff. It allows the supervisor to initiate *corrective and therapeutic action* with the person who is abusive, while protecting clients from such abuse in the future. Appropriate action is objective reporting and following the agency's chain of command.** **Answer 4** is incorrect because it is a temporary measure and does not address the basic problem.

■ **TEST-TAKING TIP:** *Look for the most comprehensive action that ensures client safety and protects all clients. The key word in Answer 3 is "objective."*

Content Area: Management of Care, Advocacy; ***Integrated Process:*** Communication and Documentation; ***Cognitive Level:*** Analysis; ***Client Need/Subneed:*** Safe and Effective Care Environment/Safety and Infection Control/Reporting of Incident/Event/Irregular Occurrence/Variance

75. CORRECT ANSWER: 3. **Answer 1** is incorrect because the tracheostomy should not become dislodged if it is secured with appropriately fitting tracheostomy ties. The obturator should *always* be at the bedside. **Answer 2** is incorrect because the purpose of deflating a tracheostomy cuff is to alleviate pressure and wean the client from the tube. This assessment would be essential if the tracheostomy tube were being *removed.* **Answer 3 is correct because secretions may have pooled above the tracheostomy cuff. If these are not suctioned before deflation, the secretions may be aspirated.** **Answer 4** is incorrect because, although it is an important intervention for any client with respiratory difficulties, deep breathing and coughing at this time may precipitate additional movement of the tracheostomy tube and bronchospasm.

■ **TEST-TAKING TIP:** *Identify the nursing concept (i.e., to prevent aspiration). Oxygenation (Answers 2 and 4) and replacement of the tracheostomy tube (Answer 1) do not address this concept. All air passages should be free of secretions before deflating a tracheostomy cuff.*

Content Area: Adult Health, Respiratory; ***Integrated Process:*** Nursing Process, Implementation; ***Cognitive Level:*** Application; ***Client Need/Subneed:*** Safe and Effective Care Environment/ Safety and Infection Control/Safe Use of Equipment

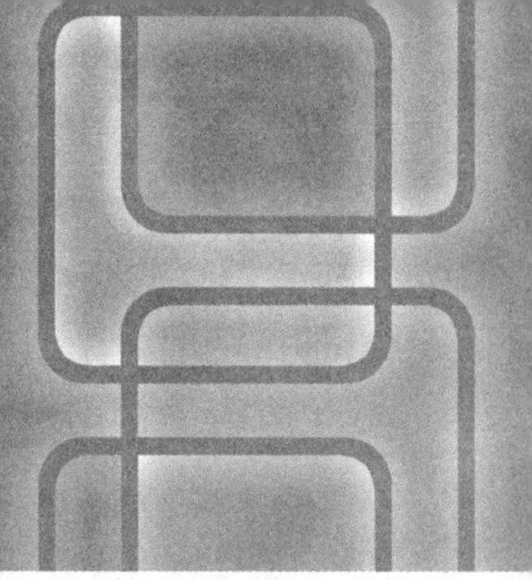

CHAPTER 4

Health Promotion and Maintenance

Nursing Care of the Childbearing Family

Janice Lloyd McMillin

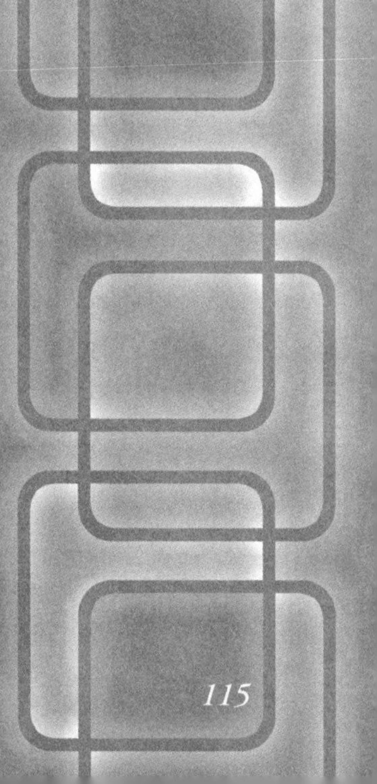

GROWTH AND DEVELOPMENT

Biological Foundations of Reproduction

General overview: This review of the structures, functions, and important assessment characteristics of the reproductive system provides essential components of the database required for accurate nursing judgments. Comparing normal characteristics and established patterns with nursing assessment findings assists in identifying client needs and in planning, implementing, and evaluating appropriate goal-directed nursing interventions.

Female Reproductive Anatomy and Physiology

I. THE FEMALE PELVIS (FIG. 4.1)

A. Two hip bones (right and left innominate: sacrum, coccyx).

B. False pelvis—upper portion above brim, supportive structure for uterus during last half of pregnancy.

C. True pelvis—below brim; pelvic inlet, midplane, pelvic outlet. Fetus passes through during birth.

II. PELVIC MEASUREMENTS

A. Diagonal conjugate—12.5 cm or greater is adequate size; evaluated by examiner.

B. Conjugate vera—11 cm is adequate size; can be measured by x-ray (not commonly performed).

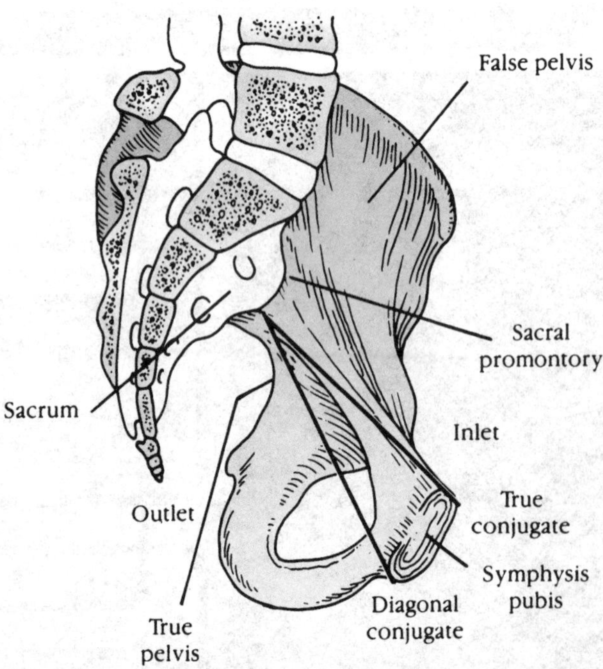

Figure 4.1 The female pelvis.

C. Obstetric conjugate—measured by x-ray (not commonly performed).

D. Tuber-ischial diameter—9 to 11 cm indicates adequate size; evaluated by examiner.

III. FEMALE EXTERNAL ORGANS

A. Mons veneris—protects symphysis.

B. Labia majora—covers, protects labia minora.

C. Labia minora—two located within labia majora.

D. Clitoris—small erectile tissue.

E. Hymen—thin membrane at opening of vagina.

F. Urinary meatus—opening of urethra.

G. Bartholin glands—producers of alkaline secretions that enhance sperm motility, viability.

IV. FEMALE INTERNAL REPRODUCTIVE ORGANS (FIG. 4.2)

A. Vagina—outlet for menstrual flow, depository of semen, lower birth canal.

B. Cervix—cone-shaped neck of the uterus that protrudes into the vagina.

C. Uterus—muscular organ that houses fetus during gestation.

D. Fallopian tubes—two tubes stretching from cornua of uterus to ovaries; transport ovum.

E. Ovaries—two oval-shaped structures that produce ovum and hormones (estrogen and progesterone).

F. Breasts—two mammary glands capable of secreting milk for infant nourishment.

V. MENSTRUAL CYCLE (FIG. 4.3)

A. Reproductive hormones

1. *Follicle-stimulating hormone (FSH)*—secreted during the first half of cycle; stimulates development of graafian follicle; secreted by anterior pituitary.
2. *Interstitial cell-stimulating hormone, luteinizing hormone (ICSH, LH)*—stimulates ovulation and development of corpus luteum; secreted by pituitary.
3. *Estrogen*—assists in ovarian follicle maturation; stimulates endometrial thickening; responsible for development of secondary sex characteristics; maintains endometrium during pregnancy. Secreted by ovaries and adrenal cortex during cycle and by placenta during pregnancy.
4. *Progesterone*—aids in endometrial thickening; facilitates secretory changes; maintains uterine lining for implantation and early pregnancy; relaxes smooth muscle. Secreted by corpus luteum and placenta.
5. *Prostaglandins*—substances produced by various body organs that act hormonally on the endometrium to influence the onset and continuation of labor. A medication that may be used to facilitate onset of second-trimester abortion; also used to efface the cervix before induction of labor in term pregnancies.

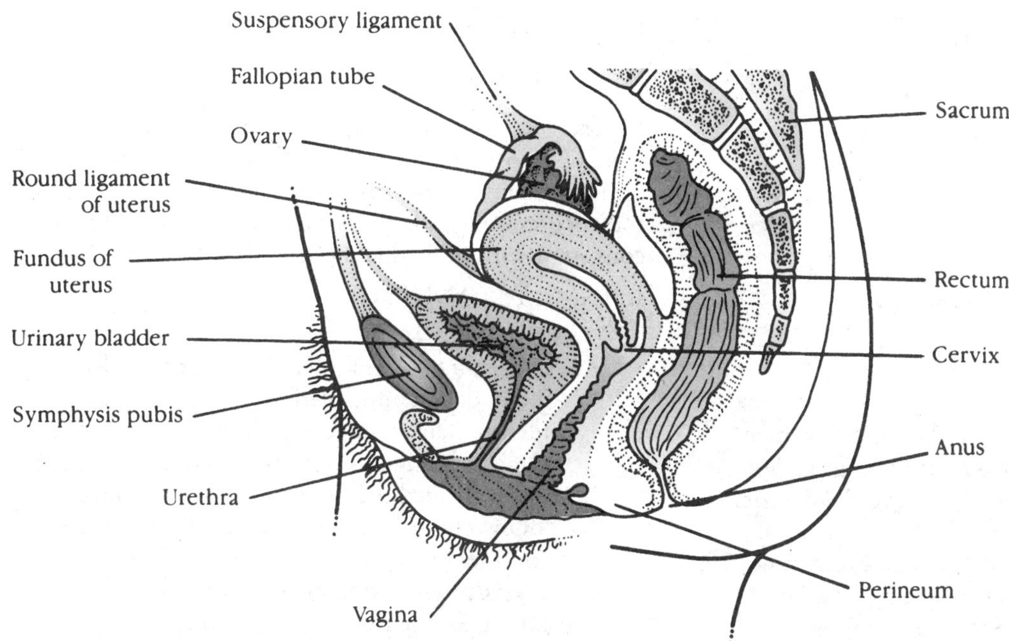

Figure 4.2 Female internal reproductive organs.

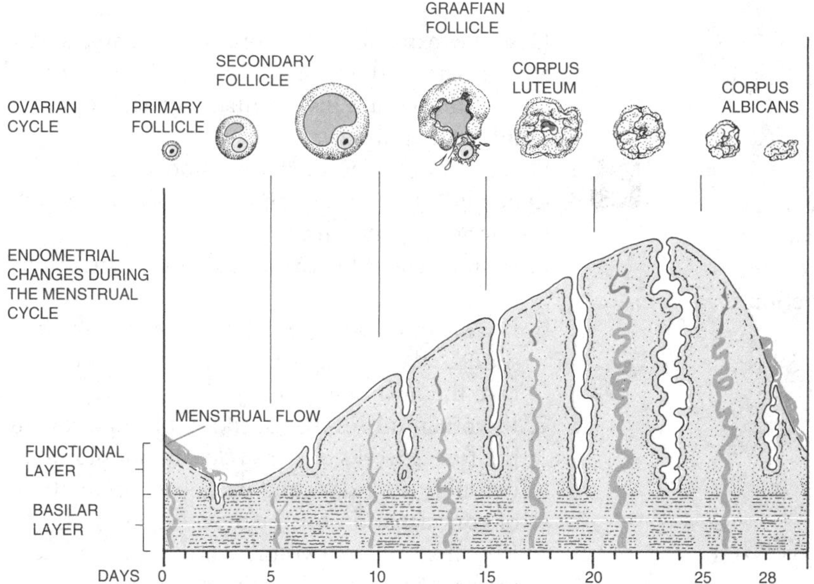

Figure 4.3 The menstrual cycle. (From Venes, D [ed]: *Taber's Cyclopedic Medical Dictionary,* ed 20. FA Davis, Philadelphia, 2005, p 1341.)

B. **Ovulation**—maturation and release of egg from ovary; generally occurs 14 days *before* beginning of next menses.

C. **Menstruation**—vaginal discharge of blood and fragments of the endometrium; cyclic; occurs in response to dropping levels of estrogen and progesterone.

D. **Fertilization**—impregnation of ovum by sperm.

E. **Implantation**—fertilized ovum attaches to uterine wall for growth.

F. **Menopause**—normally occurring cessation of menses with gradual decrease in amount of flow and increase in the time between periods at end of fertility cycle; average age is 51 to 52. Early menopause rare but may be influenced by hypothyroidism, surgical ovarian removal, overexposure to radiation. *Treatments* during menopause for symptom relief: hormone replacement therapy, isoflavanoids, vitamins B and E for hot flashes, vaginal creams for dyspareunia (painful intercourse), and calcium for osteoporosis. Alternative treatments include herbal supplements and soy.

G. **Spinnbarkeit**—stretchable, thin cervical mucus present at ovulation.

VI. ASSESSMENT OF REPRODUCTIVE TRACT/REPRODUCTIVE HEALTH:

A. Health history
1. Menarche: onset and duration.
2. Menstrual problems.
3. Contraceptive use.
4. Pregnancy history.
5. Fertility problems.
6. Lifestyle choices that may have an impact on health and reproductive decision making.

B. Physical examination
1. External, internal reproductive organs.
2. Breast examination.
3. *Mammography*—every 1 to 2 years for women beginning age 40; annually beginning age 50; earlier and more frequently if have **risk factors for breast cancer:**
   a. Mother, daughter, or sister had breast cancer.
   b. Menses before age 11, or menopause before age 45 or after age 55.
   c. Previous benign needle biopsies.
   d. Birth of first child greater than 30 years old.
   e. High-fat diet, obesity.
   f. Obesity after menopause.
   g. Alcohol intake of 2 to 5 drinks per day.
   h. Nulliparous.
   i. Personal history of cancer.
   j. Defects in certain genes (*BRCA1, BRCA2, HER*).
4. Pap smear—First Papanicolaou (Pap) smear at age 18 or earlier if sexually active; then annually until three consecutive normal Paps. After three consecutive normal Paps, physician discretion is recommended.
5. Tests for sexually transmitted infections (STIs).

VII. ANALYSIS/NURSING DIAGNOSIS:

A. *Health-seeking behaviors* related to health promotion.

B. *Health-seeking behaviors* related to menopause.

VIII. NURSING CARE PLAN/IMPLEMENTATION:

A. Discuss anatomy and physiology of reproductive tract.

B. Review menstruation, ovulation, fertilization.

C. Explain need for periodic Pap smears, annual gynecological examinations, including mammography.

D. Discuss lifestyle choices and sexuality issues that might affect health.

IX. EVALUATION/OUTCOME CRITERIA:

A. Woman displays basic understanding of anatomy and physiology.

B. Woman understands cycle and contraception.

C. Woman regularly seeks preventive care and performs monthly breast self-examination (BSE).

MATERNAL/INFANT

Decision Making Regarding Reproduction

General overview: During the reproductive years, the woman who is sexually active often faces the decision to postpone, prevent, or terminate a pregnancy. The nursing role focuses on assisting her to make an informed decision consistent with individual needs.

I. FAMILY PLANNING

A. Assessment:
1. Determine interest in and present knowledge of methods of family planning.
2. Identify factors affecting choice of method: cultural and religious objections, contraindications for individual methods, motivation/ability to follow chosen method successfully, financial considerations, and sexual orientations.

B. Analysis/nursing diagnosis: *knowledge deficit* regarding family planning methods/options.

C. Nursing care plan/implementation: Goal: *health teaching* to facilitate informed decision making, selection of option appropriate to individual needs, desires.
1. Describe, explain, discuss options available and appropriate to the woman. Include information on advantages and disadvantages of each option (**Tables 4.1** and **4.2**).
2. Demonstrate, as necessary, method selected.
3. Quick health teaching reminders for missed oral hormone preparations:
   a. Woman should take one pill at the same time every day for 21 (or 28) days.
   b. If woman misses one pill, she should take it as soon as she remembers it; she should then take the next one at the usual time.
   c. If woman misses two or more pills in a row in the first 2 weeks of her cycle, she should take two pills for 2 days and use a backup method of contraception for the next 7 days.
   d. If woman misses two pills in the third week, or three or more pills anytime:
      (1) A *Sunday starter* should keep taking pills until the next Sunday, then start a new pack that Sunday. She should use a backup method of contraception for the next 7 days.
      (2) A *day 1 starter* should throw out the rest of the pack and start a new pack that day. She should use a backup method of contraception for the next 7 days.
   e. *28-day pill pack:* If woman misses any of the seven pills that do not have any hormones, she should throw out the pills missed and

(text continues on page 122)

Table 4.1

Contraception

Method	Action/Effectiveness	Advantages	Disadvantages and Side Effects
Hormonal Contraceptives			
Pill—combination of estrogen and progesterone	• Suppresses ovulation by suppressing production of FSH and LH	• Convenient; easy to take • Withdrawal bleeding cycles are predictable	• *Absolute contraindications* (e.g., thromboembolic or coronary artery disease; some cancers or liver disease)
Oral contraceptives (daily)	• *Most efficient* form of contraception (99.7%) if used consistently	• Not related to sex act • Safe for older nonsmoking women until menopause • Many noncontraceptive health benefits (oral)	• *Relative contraindications* (e.g., migraines, hypertension, immobility 4 weeks or more, abnormal genital bleeding) • Some decrease in glucose tolerance • Effectiveness decreased if taken during use of barbiturates, phenytoin, antibiotics • **No protection against STIs**
Contraceptive patch—combination of estrogen and progesterone (change q wk)	• Suppresses ovulation • Thickens cervical mucus • Decreases sperm penetration • 99% effective in women <198 lb; 92% effective in women >198 lb	• Convenient • Patch applies to abdomen, buttocks, upper arm, or upper torso • Changed once/week	• *Absolute contraindications* (e.g., thromboembolic or coronary artery disease, some cancers or liver disease) • *Relative contraindications* (e.g., migraines, hypertension, immobility 4 weeks or more, allergic reaction to patch) • **No protection against STIs**
Mini-pill—progestin only (PO daily)	• Impairs fertility • Thickens cervical mucus • Decreases sperm penetration • Alters endometrial maturation • *Effectiveness:* undetermined; can reach 100% reliability if used exactly as prescribed	• Convenient, easy to take	• Ovulation may occur • Irregular bleeding, mood changes, weight gain • May change glucose and insulin values • **No protection against STIs**
Depo-Provera—synthetic progesterone (IM q 3 mo)	• Suppresses ovulation • Thickens cervical mucus • Changes the uterine lining, making it harder for sperm to enter or survive in the uterus • *Effectiveness:* 99.7%	• Private • Effective after 24 hours • Does not require regular attention • Does not interrupt sex play • Has no estrogen • May decrease risk for ovarian and uterine cancers	• Requires injections every 3 months • Delay of return to fertility • Possible weight gain and irregular bleeding • **No protection against STIs**
Emergency Postcoital Contraception			
Estradiol (100 mcg) and levonorgestrel (0.5 mg)	• Antifertility; taken within 72 hours of unprotected sex • Take as soon as possible; repeat 12 hours later • *Effectiveness:* 75%–85%	• Available prn	• Nausea, headache, dizziness
Intrauterine Devices (IUDs)			
Small, T-shaped, medicated device inserted into uterine cavity	• Prevents fertility	• Can be used by women who cannot use hormonal contraception; no disruption of ovulation pattern	• *Contraindications:* history of PID, pregnancy, undiagnosed genital bleeding, genital malignancy, abnormal uterine cavity, severe cervicitis, HIV/AIDS, history of ectopic pregnancy, history of toxic shock

Continued

MATERNAL/INFANT

Table 4.1

Contraception—cont'd

Method	Action/Effectiveness	Advantages	Disadvantages and Side Effects
• Copper (Paragard)	• Recommended for women who have had at least one child • Damages sperm in transit to fallopian tube	• Can be used effectively for 10 years	• *Risks:* uterine perforation, infection (may be followed by PID) in the first 3 months of insertion; unnoticed expulsion • *Side effects* (especially with Paragard): heavy flow, spotting between periods, and cramping within first few months of insertion • Must check for string after each menses and before intercourse
• Progesterone (Mirena)	• Alters cervical mucus and endometrial maturation • *Effectiveness:* 90%–99%	• Not necessary to change every year. Can be used up to 5 years. • Less blood loss during menses and decreases primary dysmenorrhea	• **No protection against STIs**
Mechanical Barriers			
Diaphragm: shallow rubber device that fits over cervix	• Barrier preventing sperm from entering cervix (**if** it is correct size, undamaged, correctly placed, and used with spermicide) • *Effectiveness:* 83%–90%; 99% in highly motivated women	• Does not interrupt sex act, except to add spermicide just before act* • Insert up to 6 hours before intercourse and leave in place for 6 hours after last intercourse, but not longer than 24 hours • Safe: no side effects from well-fitted device if woman is not allergic to diaphragm or spermicide • Decreased incidence of vaginitis, cervicitis, PID	• Requires careful cleansing with warm water and mild soap; powder with cornstarch, and store away from heat. • Use might be associated with TSS† • Size/fit must be checked after birth, second/third-trimester abortion, weight gain or loss of 15–20 lb or more, or every 2 years • Spermicide must be reinserted for additional acts that may follow after initial intercourse
Cervical cap: 1¼–1½-inch soft natural rubber dome with a firm but pliable rim	• Physical barrier to sperm • Spermicide inside cap adds a chemical barrier • *Effectiveness* depends on its fit. • 80%–91% effective for nulliparas • 60%–74% effective in multiparas	• Worn for 8 hours but not longer than 48 hours • No need to add spermicide for repeated acts of intercourse	• Need a Pap smear every year: higher rate of conversion from class I to class III‡ • If in place over 48 hours, it produces an odor and might be associated with TSS† • Cannot be worn during menstrual flow (menses) or up to at least 6 weeks postpartum • *Contraindications:* abnormal Pap smear, hard to fit, history of TSS or genital infection, allergy • Change after genital surgery, abortion or birth, major change in weight • Must be checked each year • **Does not protect against STIs**
Female condom: vaginal sheath of natural latex rubber with flexible rings at both the closed and the open ends	• Barrier preventing sperm from entering vagina • *Effectiveness* similar to other mechanical methods used with spermicide (79%–95%) *Note:* Male and female condoms should not be used at the same time	• Apply up to 8 hours in advance of intercourse; spermicide added just before intercourse • Heightens sensation for man • About as satisfying for both woman and man as intercourse without it • **Provides protection from STIs**	• Cost • A new one must be used for every act of intercourse

Table 4.1

Contraception—cont'd

Method	Action/Effectiveness	Advantages	Disadvantages and Side Effects
Condom: thin, stretchable latex sheath to cover penis	• Barrier preventing sperm from entering vagina, applied over erect penis before loss of pre-ejaculatory drops and is held in place as penis is withdrawn  • Spermicidal foam, jelly, or cream is also used* • *Effectiveness* rate: 64%–98% when used with spermicide	• Safety—no side effects • **Provides protection from spread of STIs**  With spermicide (0.5 gm of nonoxynol-9) added to interior or exterior surface, provides protection from STIs, including HIV	• Check expiration date • Requires high motivation to use correctly/consistently • Must be properly applied and removed • Sheath may tear during intercourse • Can have small undetectable holes
Chemical Barriers			
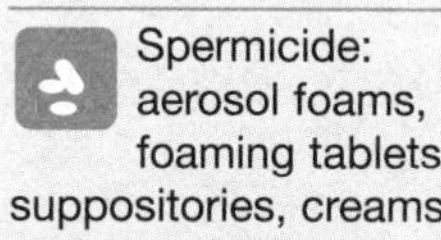 Spermicide: aerosol foams, foaming tablets, suppositories, creams, and films (VCF)	• Physical barrier to sperm penetration • Chemical action on sperm (kills sperm) • Nonoxynol-9 has a bacteriostatic action • *Effectiveness* rate: 70%–98% when used with diaphragm or condoms	• Increases effectiveness of mechanical barriers • Ease of application. Aids lubrication of vagina* • Requires no medical examination or prescription • May be used during lactation • Backup for missed oral contraceptive pills	• Messy • Some people are allergic to preparations • Tabs or suppositories take 10–15 minutes to dissolve • If it is only method being used, each intercourse should be preceded (by 30 minutes) by a fresh application; may be allergenic
Other Methods			
• Natural family planning: basal body temperature (BBT) each morning before any physical activity • Symptothermal variation: BBT plus cervical mucus changes • Calendar method • Predictor test for ovulation	• Requires sexual abstinence during woman's fertile period (4 days before ovulation), and for 3 or 4 days after ovulation • *Effectiveness:* about 80%	• Physically safe to use—no drugs or appliances are used; meets requirements of most religions	• Effectiveness depends on high level of motivation and diligence • Requires fairly predictable menstrual cycle

*Spermicide provides lubrication, but if additional lubrication is needed, use water-based products only (e.g., K-Y Jelly).
†TSS: toxic shock syndrome. Although there is no direct link between TSS and use of the diaphragm or cervical cap, a possible association remains (see **p. 122**).
‡Class I Pap smear: no abnormal cells; class III Pap smear: suspicious abnormal cells present.

Table 4.2

Sterilization

Method	Advantages	Disadvantages and Side Effects
Men		
Vas deferens is occluded (ligated and severed; bands; clips) to prevent passage of sperm	• Relatively simple surgical procedure	• Sterility is not immediate; sperm are cleared from vas after about 15 ejaculations; need to have follow-up semen analysis to confirm sterility • Antibody produced to own sperm
	• Does not affect endocrine function, production of testosterone • Does not alter volume of ejaculate	• Some men become impotent due to psychological response to procedure
	• Tubal reconstruction usually possible (90%)	• Fertility after tubal reconstruction (30%–85%)
		• **Does not protect against STIs**

Continued

Table 4.2

Sterilization—cont'd

Method *Women*	Advantages	Disadvantages and Side Effects
Both fallopian tubes are ligated and severed, or occluded with bands or clips to prevent passage of eggs; fulguration of the tubes at the cornu is most effective	• Abdominal surgery utilizing 1-inch incision and laparoscopy • Greater than 99.5% effective	• Major surgery (if done by laparotomy) with possible complications of anesthesia, infection, hemorrhage, and trauma to other organs; psychological trauma in some • Success rate for pregnancy after tubal reversal using microsurgical techniques: 40%–75%
Hysterectomy or oophorectomy or both	• Abdominal or vaginal surgery • Absolute sterility	

keep taking one pill a day until the pack is empty. She does not need a backup method of contraception.

4. Alert woman to discontinue use of *oral hormone contraceptive* preparations and report any of the following signs of potential problems to the physician **STAT: "ACHES"***
   A—Abdominal pain: possible problem with the liver or gallbladder.
   C—Chest pain or shortness of breath: possible clot within lungs or heart.
   H—Headaches (sudden or persistent): possibly caused by stroke (brain attack) or hypertension.
   E—Eye problems: possible vascular incident or hypertension.
   S—Severe leg pain: possible thromboembolic process.
5. Signs of *potential problems* related to IUD use: **"PAINS"***
   P—Period (menstrual) late, abnormal spotting or bleeding.
   A—Abdominal pain, pain during coitus (dyspareunia).
   I—Infection, abnormal vaginal discharge.
   N—Not feeling well; fever or chills.
   S—String missing (nonpalpable on vaginal self-examination, or not seen on speculum examination).
6. **Toxic Shock Syndrome** (TSS)
   a. Signs/symptoms:
      (1) Fever of sudden onset—over 102°F (38.9°C).
      (2) Hypotension—systolic pressure 90 mm Hg; orthostatic dizziness; disorientation.
      (3) Rash—diffuse, macular erythroderma (resembling sunburn).
      (4) Sore throat; severe nausea, vomiting.
      (5) Copious vaginal discharge.
   b. Instructions for prevention:
      (1) General
         (a) Avoid use of tampons, cervical caps, and diaphragms during the postpartum period (6 weeks).
         (b) Do not use any of the above if you have a history of TSS.
         (c) Call physician if you experience sudden onset of a high fever, vomiting, diarrhea, or skin rash.
         (d) Insert clean tampons and contraceptive devices with clean hands.
         (e) Remove within prescribed time limits.
      (2) Tampons
         (a) Change tampons every 3 to 6 hours.
         (b) Do not use superabsorbent tampons.
         (c) For overnight protection, substitute other products such as sanitary napkins or minipads.
      (3) Diaphragm or cervical cap
         (a) Avoid use during your menstrual period.
         (b) Remove within 8 hours after intercourse (diaphragm must be removed no later than 24 hours; the cap, no later than 48 hours).

D. Evaluation/outcome criteria:
1. Woman avoids or achieves a pregnancy as desired.
2. Woman expresses comfort and satisfaction with method selected.

II. INFERTILITY

A. Definition: inability to conceive after 1 year of unprotected intercourse.

B. Pathophysiology: contributing factors—hormonal deficiencies, reproductive system disorders, congenital anomalies, male impotence, sexual knowledge deficit, debilitating disease.

*Source: Hatcher, R, et al: Contraceptive Technology, ed. 16. Irving, New York.

C. Assessment:
1. History—general health, reproduction, social history.
2. Maternal diagnosis
   a. Basal body temperature (BBT) (**Fig. 4.4**).
   b. Endocrine studies.
   c. Huhner test (postcoital).
   d. Rubin's test (tubal patency).
   e. Hysterosalpingogram (tubal patency).
3. Male diagnosis—history, physical examination, laboratory studies (e.g., semen analysis).

D. Analysis/nursing diagnosis: *altered sexuality, altered family process* related to infertility.

E. Nursing care plan/implementation:
1. Provide emotional support.
2. Explain testing procedures for diagnosis.
3. Assist with referral process.

F. Evaluation/outcome criteria:
1. The couple conceives, *or,*
2. If the couple does not conceive, they accept referral for help with adoption, other reproductive alternatives, or childlessness.

III. INTERRUPTION OF PREGNANCY—also known as elective, voluntary, or therapeutic abortion. Once the diagnosis of pregnancy and the length of gestation are established, the woman faces the decision to interrupt or to maintain the pregnancy (**Table 4.3**).

A. Decision-making stage:
1. **Assessment:**
   a. Health history:
      (1) Determine woman's feelings about the pregnancy, reasons for considering abortion, level of maturity; if decision was

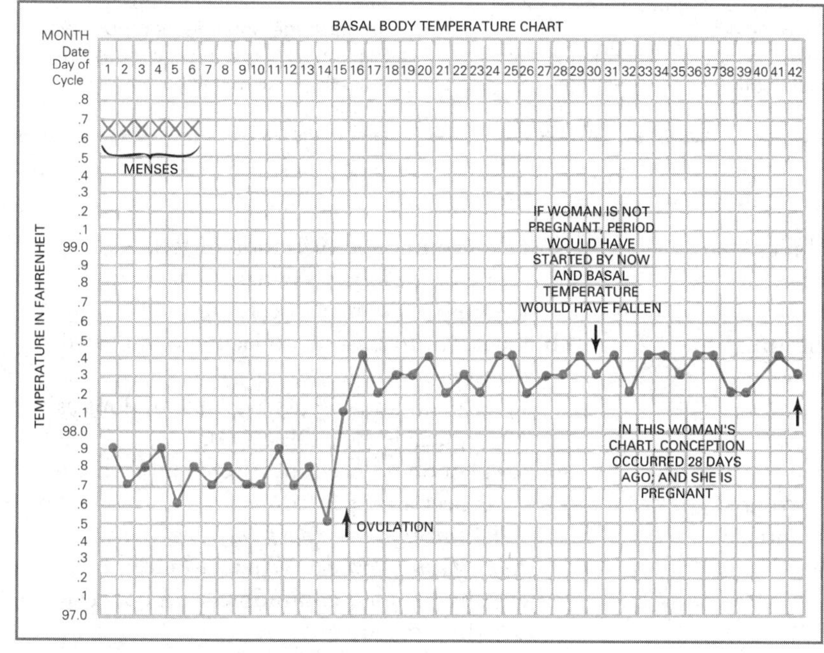

Figure 4.4 Basal body temperature chart. (From Venes, D [ed]: *Taber's Cyclopedic Medical Dictionary,* ed 20. FA Davis, Philadelphia, 2005.)

Table 4.3

Interruption of Pregnancy (Elective/Voluntary Abortion)

Method	Advantages	Disadvantages and Side Effects
First-Trimester Procedures		
Early uterine evacuation (EUE)—aspiration of endometrium through undilated cervix	• Performed for women who have not yet missed a menstrual period • 100% effective if implantation site is not missed	• Cervical trauma may occur and may lead to incompetent cervix • Hemorrhage
RU 486 (mifepristone)—a progesterone antagonist; taken up to 7 weeks' gestation (56 days LMP); taken orally	• Prevents implantation of fertilized egg • Most effective in early gestation, during luteal phase, within 10 days of first missed period	• Slight nausea and fatigue during period of bleeding • Uterine aspiration may be needed if RU 486 does not work
Misoprostol (Cytotec)—initiates uterine contractions; given intravaginally	• Softens cervix and aids in expelling products of conception	

Continued

Table 4.3

Interruption of Pregnancy (Elective/Voluntary Abortion)—cont'd

Method	Advantages	Disadvantages and Side Effects
Uterine aspiration (vacuum or suction curettage)—cannula suction under local anesthesia, following cervical dilatation, usually with laminaria tent	• Relatively few complications—minimal bleeding, minimal discomfort • Outpatient procedure	• Performed after one or two missed menstrual periods • Cervical or endometrial trauma possible
Surgical dilation and curettage (D & C)—cervix dilated with laminaria tents; endometrium scraped with metal curette or flexible aspiration tip, under local anesthesia (paracervical block)	• After cervix is dilated, procedure takes about 15 minutes • Outpatient procedure • Relatively few complications (≤1%): bleeding like a heavy period, some cramping	• Performed after one or two missed periods • Possible but rare; cervical trauma, uterine perforation infection, hemorrhage
Second-Trimester Procedures		
D & E (dilation and evacuation)—extends D & C and vacuum curettage up to 20 weeks' gestation	Woman does not experience labor	Requires 3 days for laminaria to dilate cervix; procedure done on third day
Second- and Third-Trimester Procedures		
Hysterotomy—cesarean delivery	• Available for gestations more than 14–16 weeks • Preferred method if woman wishes a tubal ligation or hysterectomy to follow	• *After:* major surgery complications—hemorrhage and infection possible • Fetus may be born alive, causing ethical, moral, religious, and legal problems

MATERNAL/INFANT

already made before she came to clinic, how was decision made? Does she have a support system?

(2) Identify factors influencing/complicating her decisions (religious beliefs, cultural mores, peer and family pressures).

(3) Information needs.

b. Physical examination.

c. *Laboratory tests:* blood type, Rh, hemoglobin, hematocrit, urinalysis, pregnancy test, antibody titer, other tests dependent on her health status.

2. **Analysis/nursing diagnosis:**

a. *Ineffective coping* related to emotional conflicts associated with need for decision to continue/terminate pregnancy.

b. *Altered family* process related to intrafamily conflict associated with need for/decision to continue/terminate pregnancy.

c. *Anticipatory grieving* related to loss of pregnancy/child.

d. *Altered self-concept, self-esteem disturbance* related to possible guilt feelings associated with pregnancy/termination.

e. *Knowledge deficit* related to available options.

3. **Nursing care plan/implementation:**

a. Goal: *emotional support* to minimize impact on self-image and self-esteem.

(1) Maintain accepting, nonjudgmental attitude.

(2) Encourage verbalization of feelings, perceptions, and values.

(3) Support woman's decision.

b. Goal: *health teaching* to facilitate informed decision making.

(1) Explain and discuss available options as applicable (see **Table 4.3**).

(2) Describe procedure selected and what to expect after procedure.

c. Goal: *minimize impact on intrafamily relations, family process.* Where applicable, encourage open communication between deciding partners.

4. **Evaluation/outcome criteria:**

a. Woman states she understands all information necessary to give consent.

b. Woman expresses comfort and satisfaction with the decision.

B. Preoperative period

1. **Assessment:**

a. Reassess woman's emotional and physical status and current feelings regarding decision.

b. Determine woman's current knowledge/understanding of authorization form, anticipated procedure, and consequences (informed consent).

c. Monitor woman's physiological and (if awake) psychological response to procedure.

2. **Analysis/nursing diagnosis:**
   a. *Anxiety/fear* related to procedure, potential complications.
   b. *Knowledge deficit* related to ongoing procedure, sights, sounds, and sensations experienced.
3. **Nursing care plan/implementation:**
   a. Goal: *provide opportunity to reconsider decision regarding termination of pregnancy.*
      (1) Check to ensure all required permission (informed consent) forms have been signed/filed.
      (2) Refer to physician if woman is ambivalent or insecure in decision.
   b. Goal: *reduce anxiety/fear related to procedure.*
      (1) Explain all anticipated preoperative, operative, and postoperative care.
      (2) Assist with procedure; if woman is awake, explain what is happening and what she may be experiencing.
   c. Goal: *emotional support* to facilitate effective coping.
      (1) Encourage verbalization of feelings, fears, concerns.
      (2) Support woman's decision.
4. **Evaluation/outcome criteria:** woman does not experience physiological or psychological problems during procedure.

C. Postoperative period

1. **Assessment:**
   a. Monitor *physiological* response to procedure (vital signs, blood loss, uterine cramping).
   b. Determine *psychological* response (happy, relieved; guilt feelings, lowered self-esteem).
   c. Determine desire for family planning information.
   d. Determine need for Rh_0(D) immune globulin, *rubella* vaccination
2. **Analysis/nursing diagnosis:**
   a. *Pain* related to procedure.
   b. *High risk for infection* related to lack of knowledge of postabortal self-care.
3. **Nursing care plan/implementation:**
   a. Goal: *provide and explain postoperative care.*
      (1) Administer intravenous (IV) fluids.
      (2) Administer medications prn for discomfort.
      (3) Administer oxytocic medications for uterine atony, prn.
      (4) If mother is *Rh-negative*, 8 or more weeks of gestation, and laboratory tests indicate no current sensitization (i.e., she is Coombs' negative):
         (a) Explain rationale for postabortion administration of Rh_0 (D antigen) immune globulin (RhoGAM).
         (b) Administer RhoGAM, as ordered.
      (5) Provide and explain perineal care.
   b. Goal: *health teaching* to facilitate active participation in own health maintenance, informed decision making, provide predischarge anticipatory guidance (also provide in written form with attention to woman's level of reading skill and understanding, and in her native language whenever possible):
      (1) Immediately report any cramping, excessive bleeding, signs of infection.
      (2) Provide name and telephone number of person to call if she has questions.
      (3) Schedule a postabortal checkup.
      (4) Discuss contraception, if woman indicates interest; or give her place and name to call for information later.
      (5) Discuss resumption of tampon use (3 days to 3 weeks as ordered) and sexual intercourse (1 to 3 weeks as ordered).
      (6) Discuss need to *avoid* douching.
4. **Evaluation/outcome criteria:**
   a. Woman returns for postabortal appointment.
   b. Woman suffers no adverse physical sequelae to the procedure.
   c. Woman suffers no adverse psychological sequelae to the procedure.
   d. Woman is successful in achieving her goal of either contraception or conception at the time she desires.
5. Postabortion psychological impact:
   a. Majority—relieved and happy.
   b. Small number (5% to 10%)—negative feelings, such as guilt or low self-esteem.

CHILDBEARING: PREGNANCY BY TRIMESTER

General overview: This review of the normal physiological and psychosocial changes occurring during each trimester of pregnancy provides essential components of the database for accurate nursing judgments and anticipatory guidance during the prenatal period. Complications of pregnancy are correlated with the trimester of common occurrence; relationships with other NCLEX® categories of human function are described.

I. GENERAL ASPECTS OF NURSING CARE

A. Assessment—based on nursing knowledge of the following:

1. Biophysical and psychosocial aspects of conception and gestation.
2. Parameters of normal pregnancy.
3. Risk factors, signs, symptoms, and implications of deviations from normal patterns of maternal and fetal health.

B. Analysis/nursing diagnosis:

1. *Knowledge deficit* related to normal pregnancy-related alterations (physiological and emotional alterations per trimester).
2. *Pain* related to normal physiological alterations in pregnancy.
3. *Altered elimination* related to normal physiological changes during pregnancy (polyuria, constipation).
4. *Altered nutrition* related to increased metabolic needs due to pregnancy.
5. *Impaired adjustment* related to altered self-image; anticipated role change; resurgence of old, unresolved conflicts.

C. Nursing care plan/implementation:

1. Goal: *emotional support.*
   a. Encourage verbalization of feelings, fears, concerns.
   b. Validate normalcy of behavioral response to pregnancy.
2. Goal: *anticipatory guidance.*
   a. Facilitate achievement of developmental tasks.
   b. Strengthen coping techniques for pregnancy, labor, birth. Suggest appropriate resources (preparation for childbirth classes).
3. Goal: *health teaching.* Describe, explain, discuss:
   a. Normal physiological alterations during pregnancy.
   b. Common discomforts of pregnancy, management.

MATERNAL/INFANT

D. Evaluation/outcome criteria:

1. Woman takes an active, informed part in her pregnancy-related care.
2. Woman copes effectively with common alterations associated with pregnancy (physiological, psychological, role change).
3. Woman successfully carries an uneventful pregnancy to term.

II. BIOLOGICAL FOUNDATIONS OF PREGNANCY

A. Conception

1. *Egg*—life span, approximately 24 hours after ovulation.
2. *Sperm*—life span, approximately 72 hours after ejaculation into female reproductive tract.
3. *Conception* (fertilization)—usually occurs 12 to 24 hours after ovulation, within fallopian tube.
4. *Implantation* (nidation)—usually occurs within 7 to 9 days of conception, or about day 21 to 23 of a 28-day menstrual cycle.
5. *Ovum*—period of conception until primary villi have appeared; usually about 12 to 14 days.
6. *Embryo*—period from end of ovum stage until measurement reaches approximately 3 cm; 54 to 56 days.
7. *Fetus*—period from end of embryo stage until birth.

First Trimester
Susceptible to teratogens
Heart functions at 3–4 wk
Eye formation at 4–5 wk
Arm and leg buds at 4–5 wk
Recognizable face at 8 wk
Brain: rapid growth
External genitalia at 8 wk
Placenta formed at 12 wk
Bone ossification at 12 wk

Second Trimester
Less danger from teratogens after 12 wk
Facial features formed at 16 wk
Fetal heartbeat heard by 18–20 wk; with a fetoscope/Doppler at 10–12 wk
Quickening at 18–20 wk
Length: 10 inches, weight: 8–10 oz
Vernix: present

Third Trimester
Iron stored
Surfactant production begins in increasing amounts
Size: 15 inches, 2–3 lb
Calcium stored at 28–32 wk
Reflexes present at 28–32 wk
Subcutaneous fat deposits at 36 wk
Lanugo shedding at 38–40 wk
Average size: 18–22 inches, 7.5–8.5 lb at 38–40 wk

B. Anatomical and physiological modifications

1. *Bases of functional alterations*
   a. *Hormonal*—**Table 4.4** discusses the effects of estrogen and progesterone during pregnancy. Nursing implications provide the knowledge base for the following:
      (1) Anticipatory guidance regarding normal maternal adaptations.
      (2) Early identification of deviations from normal patterns.
   b. *Mechanical*—enlarging uterus → displacement and pressure; increased weight of uterus and breasts → changes in posture and pressure.
2. *Breasts*—enlarged darkened areolae; secrete colostrum.
3. *Reproductive organs*
   a. *Uterus*
      (1) Amenorrhea. Occasional spotting common, especially at time of first missed menstrual period.
      (2) Increased vascularity adds to increase in size and softening of the lower uterine segment (*Hegar's sign*).

Table 4.4

Hormones of Pregnancy

Primary Effects	Clinical Implications for Nursing Actions
Estrogen	
Level rises in serum and urine	Basis of test for maternal/placental/fetal well-being
Uterine enlargement	Probable sign of pregnancy
Breast enlargement	Probable sign of pregnancy; increased tingling, tenderness
Genital enlargement: increased vascularization, hyperplasia	Vaginal growth facilitates vaginal birth
Softens connective tissue	Results in backache and leg ache; relaxes joints to increase size of birth canal and rib cage
Alters nutrient metabolism:	*Gastrointestinal and metabolic changes:*
Decreases HCl and pepsin	Digestive upsets
Antagonist to insulin—makes glucose available to fetus	Anti-insulin effect challenges maternal pancreas to produce more insulin; failure of beta cells to respond leads to "gestational" diabetes. For the woman who is insulin dependent, insulin requirements increase by an average of 67% during the second half of pregnancy
Supports fat deposition	Protect source of energy for fetus
Sodium and water retention; edema of lower extremities (nonpitting)	Meet increased plasma volume needs and maintain fluid reserve
Hematological changes:	
Increased coagulability	Increased tendency to thrombosis
Increased sedimentation rate (SR)	SR loses diagnostic value for heart disease
Vasodilation: spider nevi; palmar erythema	Resolves spontaneously after birth
Increased production of melanin-stimulating hormone	Resolves spontaneously after birth; causes chloasma and linea nigra
Progesterone	
Development of decidua	High levels result in tiredness, listlessness, and sleepiness
Reduces uterine excitability	Protection against abortion/early birth (i.e., *maintains pregnancy*)
Development of mammary glands	Prepares breasts for lactation
Alters nutrient metabolism:	*Nutritional significance:*
Antagonist to insulin	Diabetogenic
Favors fat deposition	Energy reserve
Decreases gastric motility and relaxes sphincters	Favors heartburn and constipation
Increased sensitivity of respiratory center to CO_2	Increased depth, some dyspnea, increased sighing
Decreased smooth-muscle tone:	*Decreased tone can lead to:*
Colon	Constipation
Bladder, ureters	Stasis of urine with ↑ chance of infection
Veins	Dependent edema; varicosities
Gallbladder	Gallbladder disease
Increased basal body temperature (BBT) by 0.5°C	Discomfort from hot flashes and perspiration
Human Chorionic Gonadotropin	
Maintains corpus luteum during early pregnancy	Placenta must "take over" after a few weeks
Stimulates male testes	Increased testosterone in male fetuses
May suppress immune response	May inhibit response to foreign protein (e.g., fetal portion of placenta) *Diagnostic value:* Basis for pregnancy test *Decreased* level with threatened abortion *Increased* level with multiple pregnancy *Very high* level with hydatidiform mole

Continued

MATERNAL/INFANT

Table 4.4

Hormones of Pregnancy—cont'd

Primary Effects	Clinical Implications for Nursing Actions
Human Placental Lactogen	
Antagonizes insulin	Diabetogenic; may → gestational diabetes or complicate management of existing diabetes
Mobilizes maternal free fatty acids	Increased tendency of ketoacidosis in pregnant diabetic
Prolactin	
Suppressed by estrogen and progesterone	No milk produced before birth
Increased level after placenta is delivered	**Milk production** (lactation) 2–3 days after birth
Follicle-Stimulating Hormone	
Production suppressed during pregnancy; level returns to prepregnant levels within 3 weeks after birth	No ovulation during pregnancy; ovulation usually returns within 6 weeks for 15%, within 12 weeks for 30%
Oxytocin	
Causes uterus to contract when the oxytocin levels exceed those of estrogen and progesterone	Labor induction or augmentation; treatment for postpartum uterine atony

MATERNAL/INFANT

(3) Growth is due to hypertrophy and hyperplasia of existing muscle cells and connective tissue.
(4) Fundal height measurement landmarks:

Uterus	Nonpregnant	Pregnant (at Term)
Length	6.5 cm	32 cm
Width	4 cm	24 cm
Depth	2.5 cm	22 cm
Weight	50 gm	1000 gm

b. *Cervix*
(1) Increased vascularity → softening (*Goodell's sign*) and deepened blue-purple coloration (*Chadwick's sign*).
(2) Edema, hyperplasia, thickening of mucous lining, and increased mucus production; formation of mucous plug by end of second month.
(3) Becomes shorter, thicker, and more elastic.

c. *Vagina*
(1) Hyperemia deepens color (*Chadwick's sign*).
(2) Hypertrophy and hyperplasia thicken vaginal mucosa.
(3) Relaxation of connective tissue.
(4) pH acidic (4.0–6.0).
(5) Leukorrhea—nonirritating.

d. *Perineum*
(1) Increases in size—hypertrophy of muscle cells, edema, and relaxation of elastic tissue.
(2) Deepened color—increased vascularization/hyperemia.

e. *Ovaries*
(1) Ovum production ceases.
(2) Corpus luteum persists; produces hormones to weeks 10 to 12 until placenta "takes over."

C. Alterations affecting fluid-gas transport

1. *Cardiovascular system* (**Table 4.5**)
a. **Physiological changes**
(1) Heart displaced upward and to the left.
(2) Circulation:
(a) Cardiac volume increases by 20% to 30%.
(b) Labor—cardiac output increases by 20% to 30%.
(3) Hemoglobin and hematocrit values remain between 10 and 14 gm and 35% and 42%; normal drop is 10% during second trimester.
(4) Hypercoagulability—increased levels of blood factors VII, VIII, IX, and X.
(5) Nonpathological increased sedimentation rate—due to 50% increase in fibrinogen level.
(6) Blood pressure should remain stable with drop in second trimester.
(7) Heart rate often increases 10 to 15 beats/min at term.
(8) Compression of pelvic veins → stasis of blood in lower extremities.
(9) Compression of inferior vena cava when supine → bradycardia → reduced cardiac output, faintness, sweating, nausea (*supine hypotension*). *Fetal response:* marked bradycardia due to hypoxia secondary to decreased placental perfusion.

Table 4.5

Blood Values

Component	Prepregnant	Pregnant	Postpartum*
WBC	4000–11,000	9000–16,000 (↑); 25,000—labor	20,000–25,000 within 10–12 days of birth, then returns to normal
RBC volume	1600 mL	1900 mL	Prepregnant level of 1600 mL
Plasma volume	2400 mL	3700 mL	Prepregnant level of 2400 mL
Hct (PCV)	37%–47%	32%–42% (↓)	At 72°, returns to prepregnant level of 37%–47%
Hgb (at sea level)	12–16 g/dL	10–14 g/dL	At 72°, returns to prepregnant level of 12–16 g/dL
Fibrinogen	250 mg/dL	400 mg/dL	At 72°, returns to prepregnant level of 250 mg/dL

*Postpartum values depend on factors of amount of blood loss, mobilization, and physiological edema (excretion of extravascular water). Normal blood loss for vaginal birth is 300 to 400 mL.

b. **Assessment:**
   (1) Apical systolic murmur.
   (2) Exaggerated splitting of first heart sound.
   (3) Physiological anemia.
   (4) Dependent edema in third trimester (**Table 4.6**).
   (5) *Vena cava syndrome* (supine hypotension)—drop in systolic blood pressure may occur due to compression of descending aorta and inferior vena cava when supine.
   (6) Varicosities (vulvar, anal, leg).

c. **Nursing care plan/implementation:** Goal: *health teaching.*
   (1) *Elevate* lower extremities frequently.
   (2) Apply support hose.
   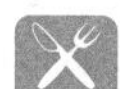
   (3) *Avoid* excess intake of sodium.
   (4) Assume *side-lying* position at rest.
   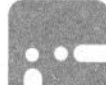
   (5) Learn signs and symptoms of pregnancy-induced hypertension.

2. *Respiratory system*
   a. **Physiological changes:**
      (1) Increased: tidal volume, vital capacity, respiratory reserve, oxygen consumption, production of CO_2.
      (2) Diaphragm elevated, increased substernal angle → flaring of rib cage.
      (3) Uterine enlargement prevents maximum lung expansion in third trimester.
   b. **Assessment:**
      (1) Shortness of breath or dyspnea on exertion and when lying flat in third trimester.
      (2) Nasal stuffiness due to estrogen-induced edema (see **Table 4.6**).
      (3) Deeper respiratory excursion.
   c. **Nursing care plan/implementation:** Goal: *health teaching.*
      (1) Sit and stand with good posture.

Table 4.6

Common Discomforts During Pregnancy

Discomfort and Cause	Health Teaching
Morning sickness—first 3 months; nausea and vomiting; may occur anytime, day or night; *cause:* hormonal, psychological, and empty stomach	 Alternate dry carbohydrates and fluids hourly; take dry carbohydrates before rising, stay in bed 15 more minutes; *avoid* empty stomach, offending odors, and food difficult to digest (e.g., food high in fat); *avoid* acidic foods (e.g., citrus)
Fatigue (sleep hunger)—first 3 months; *cause:* possibly hormones; often returns in late pregnancy when physical load is great	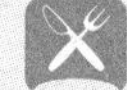 Iron supplement if anemic—foods high in *iron, folic acid,* and *protein*; adequate rest
Fainting (syncope)—early pregnancy, due to slightly decreased arterial blood pressure; late pregnancy, due to venous stasis in lower extremities	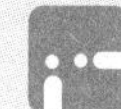 *Elevate feet;* sit down when necessary; when standing, do not lock knees; *avoid* prolonged standing, fasting
Urinary frequency—enlarging uterus presses on bladder, turgescence of structures from hormone stimulation; relieved somewhat as uterus rises from pelvis; recurs with lightening	*Kegel exercises; limit fluids* just before bedtime to ensure rest; rule out urinary tract infection

Continued

MATERNAL/INFANT

Table 4.6

Common Discomforts During Pregnancy—cont'd

Discomfort and Cause	Health Teaching
Vaginal discharge—months 2–9; mucus less acidic, and increases in amount (leukorrhea)	Cleanliness important; treat only if infection sets in; douche **contraindicated** in pregnancy
Hot flashes—heat intolerance, due to increased metabolism → diaphoresis	Alter clothing, bathing, and environmental temperature prn
Headache—cause unknown; possibly blood pressure change, nutritional, tension (unless associated with preeclampsia)	If pain relief needed, consult physician (*avoid* over-the-counter drugs without prescription); reduce tension
Nasal stuffiness—due to increased vascularization; allergic rhinitis of pregnancy	Antihistamines and nasal sprays by *prescription only*
Heartburn—enlarging uterus and hormones slow digestion; progesterone → reverse peristaltic waves → reflux of stomach contents into esophagus	Physician may prescribe an antacid; *avoid* use of antacids containing sodium; instead of leaning over, bend at the knees, keeping torso straight; sit on firm chairs; *limit fatty and fried* foods; small, frequent meals
Flatulence—altered digestion from enlarging uterus and hormones	Maintain regular bowel habits, *avoid* gas-forming foods; antiflatulent may be prescribed
Insomnia—fetal movements, fears or concerns, and general body discomfort from heavy uterus	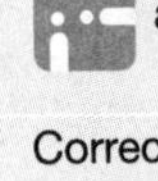 Medication by prescription only; exercise; side-lying *positions* with pillow supports; change position often; back rubs, ventilate feelings
Shortness of breath—enlarging uterus limits expansion of diaphragm	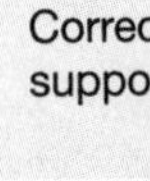 Good posture; cut down/stop smoking; *position*—supine and upright
Backache—increased elasticity of connective tissue, increased weight of uterus, and increased lumbar curvature	Correct posture, low-heeled, wide-base shoes, and abdominal support (binders); do pelvic rock often; *avoid* fatigue
Pelvic joint pain—hormones relax connective tissue and joints and allow movement within joints	Rest; good posture; will go away after giving birth, in 6–8 weeks; *avoid* prolonged standing/walking
Leg cramps—pressure of enlarging uterus on nerve supplying legs; possible causes: lack of calcium, fatigue, chilling, and tension	Stretch affected muscle and hold until it subsides; *do not rub* (may release a blood clot, if present); ↑ calcium intake
Constipation—decreased motility (hormones, enlarging uterus) and increased reabsorption of water; iron therapy (oral)	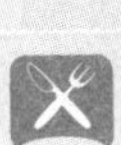 *Diet*—prunes, fruits, vegetables, roughage, and fluids; regular habits; exercise; sit on toilet with knees up; *avoid* enemas, mineral oil, laxatives
Hemorrhoids—varicosities around anus; aggravated by pushing with stool and by uterus pressing on blood vessels supplying lower body	As above, *avoid* constipation; pure Vaseline or Desitin is mild and sometimes soothing; use any other preparation with prescription only
Ankle edema—normal and nonpitting; gravity	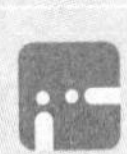 Rest legs often during day with legs and hips raised
Varicose veins—lower legs, vulva, pelvis; pressure of heavy uterus; relaxation of connective tissue in vein walls; hereditary	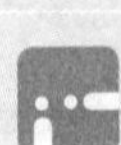 Progressively worse with subsequent pregnancies and obesity; *elevate* legs above level of heart; support hose may help
Cramp in side or groin—round ligament pain; stretching of round ligament with cramping	To get out of bed, turn to side, use arm and upper body and push up to sitting position

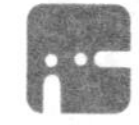

(2) When resting, assume *semi-Fowler's position.*
(3) *Avoid* overdistention of stomach.

D. Alterations affecting elimination

1. *Urinary system*
   a. **Physiological changes:**
      (1) Relaxation of smooth muscle results in conditions that can persist 4 to 6 weeks after birth:
         (a) Dilatation of ureters.
         (b) *Decreased* bladder tone.
         (c) Increased potential for urinary stasis and urinary tract *infection* (UTI).
      (2) *Increased* glomerular filtration rate (50%) during last two trimesters.
      (3) *Increased* renal plasma flow (25%–50%) during first two trimesters; returns to near-normal levels by end of last trimester.
      (4) *Increased* renal-tubular reabsorption rate—compensates for increased glomerular activity.
      (5) Glycosuria—reflects kidney's inability to reabsorb all glucose filtered by glomeruli (may be normal or may indicate gestational diabetes; glycosuria always warrants further testing).
      (6) *Increased* renal clearance of urea and creatinine (creatinine clearance used as test of renal function during pregnancy).
      (7) Hormone-induced turgescence of bladder and pressure on bladder from gravid uterus (see **Table 4.5**).
   b. **Assessment:**
      (1) Urinary frequency, first and third trimesters (see **Table 4.6**).
      (2) Nocturia.
      (3) Stress incontinence in third trimester.
   c. **Nursing care plan/implementation:** Goal: *health teaching.*
      (1) Void with urge, to prevent bladder distention.
      (2) Learn signs and symptoms of UTI.
      (3) Decrease fluid intake in late evening.
      (4) Perform *Kegel* exercises to reduce incontinence.
2. *Gastrointestinal system* (see **Table 4.6**)
   a. **Physiological changes:**
      (1) General decrease in smooth-muscle tone and motility due to actions of progesterone.
      (2) *Intestines:* slowed peristalsis, increased water reabsorption in bowel.
      (3) *Stomach*
         (a) Gastric emptying time is delayed (e.g., 3 hours vs. 1½ hours).
         (b) Gastric secretion of HCl and pepsin decreases.
         (c) Decreased motility delays emptying; increased acidity.
      (4) *Cardiac sphincter* relaxes.
      (5) Increasing size of *uterus* and displacement of *intra-abdominal organs.*
      (6) *Gallbladder:* decreased emptying.
   b. **Assessment:**
      (1) Nausea and vomiting in first trimester.
      (2) Constipation and flatulence.
      (3) Hemorrhoids.
      (4) Heartburn, reflux esophagitis, indigestion.
      (5) Hiatal hernia.
      (6) Epulis—edema and bleeding of gums.
      (7) Ptyalism—excessive salivation.
      (8) Jaundice.
      (9) Gallstones.
      (10) Pruritus due to increased retention of bile salts.

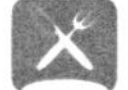

   c. **Nursing care plan/implementation:** Goal: *health teaching: dietary.*
      (1) Nausea and vomiting
         (a) *Avoid* fatty food; increase carbohydrates.
         (b) Eat small, frequent meals.
         (c) Eat dry crackers in morning.
         (d) *Decrease* liquids with meals.
         (e) *Avoid* odors that predispose to nausea.
         (f) *Avoid* acidic foods (e.g., citrus, tomatoes).
      (2) Constipation and flatulence
         (a) *Increase* fluids (6–8 glasses/day).
         (b) Maintain exercise regimen.
         (c) Add *fiber* to diet.
         (d) *Avoid* mineral oil laxatives.
         (e) *Avoid* gas-producing foods (e.g., beans, cabbage).
      (3) Heartburn and indigestion
         (a) *Eliminate* fatty, spicy, or acidic foods.
         (b) Eat small, frequent meals (6/day).
         (c) Eat slowly.
         (d) *Avoid* gastric irritants (e.g., alcohol, coffee).

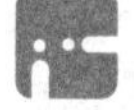

         (e) *Avoid* lying flat.
         (f) Take antacids without sodium or phosphorus.
         (g) Try chewing gum to increase the secretion of alkaline saliva.
         (h) Wait 2 to 3 hours after meals before lying down.
         (i) Wear loose-fitting clothes.
      (4) Hemorrhoids

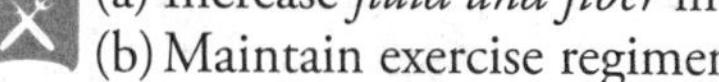

         (a) Increase *fluid and fiber* intake.
         (b) Maintain exercise regimen.

(c) *Avoid* constipation and straining to defecate.
(d) Take warm sitz baths.
(e) Apply witch hazel pads.
(f) *Elevate* hips and legs frequently.
(g) Use hemorrhoidal ointments only with advice of health-care provider.

E. Alterations affecting nutrition

1. **Physiological changes:**
   a. *Gastrointestinal system*
      (1) Gingivae soften and enlarge due to increased vascularity.
      (2) Increased saliva production.
   b. *Endocrine system*
      (1) *Increased* size and activity of pituitary, parathyroids, adrenals.
      (2) *Increased* vascularity and hyperplasia of thyroid.
      (3) Pancreas—*increased* insulin production during second half of pregnancy, needed to meet rising maternal needs; human placental lactogen (HPL) and insulinase deactivate maternal insulin; may precipitate *gestational diabetes* in women who are susceptible.
   c. *Metabolism*
      (1) Basal metabolic rate (BMR)—*increases* 25% as pregnancy progresses, due to increasing oxygen consumption; protein-bound iodine (PBI) *increases* to 7 to 10 mcg/dL; metabolism returns to normal by sixth postpartum week.
      (2) Protein—need *increased* for fetal and uterine growth, maternal blood formation.
      (3) Water retention—*increased.*
      (4) Carbohydrates—need *increases* to spare protein stores.
         (a) *First half of pregnancy*—glucose rapidly and continuously siphoned across placenta to meet fetal growth needs; may lead to hypoglycemia and faintness.
         (b) *Second half of pregnancy*—placental production of anti-insulin hormones; normal maternal hyperglycemia; affects coexisting diabetes.
      (5) Fat—*increased* plasma lipid levels.
      (6) Iron—supplements recommended to meet *increased* need for red blood cells (RBCs) by maternal/placental/fetal unit.
2. **Assessment:**
   a. Weight gain: 20 to 35 lb (11.5–16 kg); depends on body mass index (BMI) and prepregnant nutritional status.
   b. Normal pattern: first trimester, 2 to 5 lb (1–2.3 kg); remainder of gestation, approximately 1 lb/wk (0.4–0.5 kg/wk).
3. **Nursing care plan/implementation:** Goal: *health teaching.*
   a. Evaluate diet for adequacy of nutrient and caloric intake.
   b. Evaluate cultural, religious, and economic influences on diet.
   c. Review dietary recommendation for pregnancy with woman.
   d. *Avoid* dieting in pregnancy (even if obese).
   e. Supplement diet with *vitamins, iron,* or *folic acid* on advice of health provider.
   f. *Ptyalism:*
      (1) Suck hard candies.
      (2) Perform frequent oral hygiene.
      (3) Maintain adequate oral intake (6–8 glasses/day).
      (4) Use lip balm to prevent chapping.
   g. *Epulis:*
      (1) Frequent oral hygiene.
      (2) Use soft toothbrush.
      (3) Floss gently.
      (4) See dentist regularly.

F. Alterations affecting protective functions— *integumentary system*

1. **Physiological changes**—estrogen-induced vascular and pigment changes.
2. **Assessment:**
   a. Increased pigmentation (chloasma and linea nigra).
   b. Striae gravidarum (stretch marks).
   c. Increased sebaceous and sweat gland activity.
   d. Palmar erythema.
   e. Angiomas—vascular "spiders."
3. **Nursing care plan/implementation:** Goal: *health teaching.*
   a. Bathe or shower daily.
   b. Reassure woman that skin changes decrease after pregnancy.

G. Alterations affecting comfort, rest, mobility— *musculoskeletal system*

1. **Physiological changes**
   a. Progesterone, estrogen, and relaxin-induced relaxation of joints, cartilage, and ligaments.
   b. Function in childbearing—increases anteroposterior diameter of rib cage and enlarges birth canal.
2. **Assessment:**
   a. Complaint of pelvic "looseness."
   b. Duck-waddle walk.
   c. Tenderness of symphysis pubis.
   d. Lordosis (exaggerated lumbar curve)—*increased* weight of pelvis tilts pelvis forward; to compensate, woman throws head and shoulders backward; complaint of leg and back strain and fatigue (see **Table 4.6**).
   e. Feet often increase by half a shoe size or more.

3. **Nursing care plan/implementation:** Goal: *health teaching.*
   a. Good body alignment—tuck pelvis under; tighten abdominal muscles.
   b. Pelvic-rock exercises.
   c. Squat; bend at knees, ***not*** at waist.
   d. Wear low-heeled, sturdy shoes.
   e. *Avoid* tight-fitting clothing that interferes with circulatory return in legs.

III. PSYCHOSOCIAL-CULTURAL ALTERATIONS

A. *Emotional changes*—affected by: age, maturity, support system, amount of current stresses, coping abilities, physical and mental health status. *Developmental tasks of pregnancy:*
1. Accept the pregnancy as real: "I am pregnant"; progress from symbiotic relationship with the fetus to perceiving the child as an individual.
2. Seek and ensure acceptance of child by others.
3. Seek protection for self and fetus through pregnancy and labor ("safe passage").
4. Prepare realistically for the coming child and for necessary role change: "I am going to be a parent."

B. *Physical bases of changes*
1. *Increased* metabolic demands may result in anemia and fatigue.
2. *Increased* hormone levels (steroids, estrogen, progesterone)—affect mood as well as physiology.

C. *Characteristic behaviors*—**Table 4.7** describes behaviors commonly exhibited in each trimester.

D. *Sexuality and sexual expression*—feelings and expressions of sexuality may vary during pregnancy due to maternal adaptations and physiological changes.

E. *Intrafamily relationships*
1. Pregnancy is a maturational crisis for the family.

MATERNAL/INFANT

Table 4.7

Behavioral Changes in Pregnancy

Assessment/Characteristics	Nursing Care Plan/Implementation
First Trimester	
Emotional lability (mood swings)	Encourage verbalization of feelings, concerns
Displeasure with subjective symptoms of early pregnancy (nausea, fatigue, etc.)	*Health teaching:* diet, rest, relaxation, diversion
Feelings of ambivalence	Validate normalcy of feelings, behaviors
Second Trimester	
Accepts pregnancy (usually coincides with awareness of fetal movement [i.e., "quickening"])	Encourage exploration of feelings of dependency, introspection, mood swings
Becomes introspective: resolves old conflicts (feelings toward mother, sexual intimacy, masturbation)	Discuss childbirth preparation and preparation-for-parenthood classes; refer, as necessary
Reevaluates self, lifestyle, marriage	
Daydreams, fantasizes self as "mother"	
Seeks out other women who are pregnant and new mothers	
Third Trimester	
Altered body image	Encourage verbalization of concerns, discomforts of late pregnancy
Fears body mutilation (stretching of body tissues, episiotomy, cesarean birth)	Help meet dependency needs; offer reassurance, as possible
Distress over loss of control over body functions (ptyalism, colostrum leakage, leukorrhea, urinary frequency, constipation, stress incontinence)	*Health teaching:* Kegel exercises; preparation for labor. Anticipatory guidance and planning for needs of self, baby, and family in early postpartum
Anxiety for baby (deformity, death)	
Fears pain, loss of control in labor	
Acceptance of impending labor during last 2 weeks (ready to "move on")	

2. Requires changes in lifestyle and interactions:
   a. Increased financial demands.
   b. Changing family and social relationships.
   c. Adapting communication patterns.
   d. Adapting sexual patterns.
   e. Anticipating new responsibilities and needs.
   f. Responding to reactions of others.

Prenatal Management

I. INITIAL ASSESSMENT: Goal: *establish baseline for health supervision, teaching, emotional support, or referral.*

II. OBJECTIVES:

A. Determine woman's present health status and validate pregnancy.
B. Identify factors affecting or affected by pregnancy.
C. Determine current gravidity and parity.
D. Identify present length of gestation.
E. Establish an estimated date of delivery (EDD). Nägele's determination of EDD—*subtract 3 months, add 7 days* to last menstrual period (LMP).
F. Determine relevant knowledge deficit.

MATERNAL/INFANT

III. ASSESSMENT: *history*

A. *Family*—inheritable diseases, reproductive problems.
B. *Personal*—medical, surgical, gynecological, past obstetric, average nonpregnant weight.
1. *Gravida*—a pregnant woman.
   a. *Nulligravida*—woman who has *never* been pregnant.
   b. *Primigravida*—woman with a *first* pregnancy.
   c. *Multigravida*—woman with a *second or later* pregnancy.
2. *Para*—refers to *past pregnancies* (not number of babies) that reached viability (20–22 weeks whether or not born alive).
   a. *Nullipara*—woman who has *not* carried a pregnancy to viability (e.g., may have had one or more abortions).
   b. *Primipara*—woman who has carried *one* pregnancy to viability.
   c. *Multipara*—woman who had *two or more* pregnancies that reached viability.
   d. *Grandmultipara*—woman who has had *six or more* viable pregnancies.
3. *Examples of gravidity/parity.* Several methods of describing gravidity and parity are in common use. One method **(GTPAL)** describes number of "**G**ravida" (pregnancies), **T**erm (or full-term) infants, **P**reterm infants, **A**bortions, and number of **L**iving children.
   a. A woman who is pregnant for the *first* time and is currently *undelivered* is designated as 1-0-0-0-0. *After* giving birth to a full-term living neonate, she becomes 1-1-0-0-1.
   b. If a woman's second pregnancy ends in abortion and she has a living child from a previous pregnancy, born at term, she is designated as 2-1-0-1-1.
   c. A woman who is pregnant for the fourth time and whose previous pregnancies yielded one full-term neonate, premature twins, and one abortion (spontaneous or induced), and who now has three living children, may be designated as 4-1-1-1-3.
   d. Others record as follows: number gravida/number para. Applying this system to the examples given above, those mothers would be designated as follows: a—G1P1; b—G2P1; c—G4P2.
   e. Others include recording of abortions:
      G1P1 Ab0
      G2P1 Ab1
      G4P2 Ab1

IV. ASSESSMENT: ***initial physical aspects:***

A. Height and weight.
B. Vital signs.
C. Blood work—hematocrit and hemoglobin for anemia; type and Rh factor; tests for sickle cell trait, syphilis, rubella antibody titer, and hepatitis B screen.
D. Urinalysis—glucose, protein, ketones, signs of infection, and pregnancy test (human chorionic gonadotropin [HCG]).
E. Breast examination.
F. Pelvic examination.
1. Signs of pregnancy.
2. Adequacy of pelvis and pelvic structures.
3. Size and position of uterus.
4. Papanicolau smear.
5. Smears for monilial and trichomonal infections.
6. Signs of pelvic inflammatory disease.
7. Tests for STIs: Gonorrhea (gonococcus [GC]), chlamydia.

G. *Validation of pregnancy*—physician or midwife makes differential diagnosis between presumptive/probable signs/symptoms of early pregnancy and other signs.
1. *Presumptive symptoms*—subjective experiences.
   a. Amenorrhea—more than 10 days past missed menstrual period.
   b. Breast tenderness, enlargement.
   c. Nausea and vomiting.
   d. Quickening (weeks 16–18).
   e. Urinary frequency.
   f. Fatigue.
   g. Constipation (50% of women).

2. *Presumptive signs*
   a. Striae gravidarum, linea nigra, chloasma (after week 16).
   b. Increased basal body temperature (BBT)
3. *Probable signs*—examiner's objective findings.
   a. Positive pregnancy test.
   b. Enlargement of abdomen/uterus.
   c. Reproductive organ changes (after sixth week):
      (1) *Goodell's sign*—cervical softening.
      (2) *Hegar's sign*—softening of lower uterine segment.
      (3) Vaginal changes (*Chadwick's sign*): purple hue in vulvar/vaginal area.
   d. Ballottement (after 16–20 weeks).
   e. *Braxton Hicks* contractions.
4. *Positive signs of pregnancy:*
   a. Fetal heart tones.
      (1) Doptone: weeks 10 to 12.
      (2) Fetoscope: week 20.
   b. Examiner visualizes and feels fetal movements (usually after week 24).
   c. Sonographic examination (after week 14) when fetal head is sufficiently developed for accurate determination of gestational age. Pregnancy may be detected as early as fifth or sixth week after LMP.

V. ASSESSMENT: ***nutritional status:***

A. Physical findings suggesting poor nutritional status:
   1. Skin: rough, dry, scaly.
   2. Lips: lesions in corners.
   3. Hair: dull, brittle.
   4. Mucous membranes: pale.
   5. Dental caries.

B. Height, weight, age—average weight gain approximately 24 lb. Range 24 to 32 lb is best for mother and neonate.

C. Laboratory values—Hemoglobin (Hgb): less than 10.5/100 mg; hematocrit (Hct): less than 32% indicates anemia.

D. Nutrition history.

E. Analysis/nursing diagnosis:
   1. *Altered nutrition: less than body requirements* related to anemia, vitamin/mineral deficit.
   2. *Altered nutrition: more than body requirements* related to obesity.

F. Nursing care plan/implementation: Goal: *health teaching.*
   1. Nutritional counseling for diet in pregnancy and/or lactation.

G. Evaluation/outcome criteria:
   1. If *underweight* at conception: should gain 28 to 42 lb (12.5–18 kg).
   2. If *overweight at conception:* 15 to 25 lb (7–11.5 kg).
   3. If *obese at conception:* 15 lb (7 kg) or more.

VI. ASSESSMENT: ***psychosocial aspects:***

A. Pregnancy: planned or not; desired or not.

B. Present plans:
   1. Carry pregnancy, keep baby.
   2. Carry pregnancy, adoption.
   3. Abortion.

C. Cultural, ethnic influences on decisions: will influence range of activities, types of safeguarding actions, diet, and health-promotion behaviors.

D. Parenting potential: actively seeking medical care and information about pregnancy, childbirth, parenthood.

E. Family readiness for childbearing and child rearing:
   1. Physical maintenance.
   2. Allocation of resources: identify support system.
   3. Division of labor.
   4. Socialization of family members.
   5. Reproduction, recruitment, launching of family members into society.
   6. Maintenance of order (relationships within family).

F. Perceptions of present and projected family relationships.

G. Review lifestyle for smoking, drugs, alcohol (ETOH), attitudes about pregnancy, health-care practices, and risks for hepatitis and human immunodeficiency virus (HIV).

VII. ANALYSIS/NURSING DIAGNOSIS:

A. *Altered role performance* related to stress imposed by developmental tasks.

B. *Ineffective coping: individual, family* related to stress caused by developmental tasks/crises.

C. *Altered family process* related to developmental tasks. First baby may precipitate individual or family developmental crisis.

VIII. NURSING CARE PLAN/IMPLEMENTATION:

A. Goal: *anticipatory guidance/support.*
   1. Discuss mood swings, ambivalent feelings, negative feelings.
   2. Reinforce "normalcy" of such feelings.

B. Goal: *increase individual/family coping skills, reduce intrafamily stress.*
   1. Reinforce family strengths (both partners), sense of family identity.
      a. Encourage open communication between partners; share feelings and concerns.
      b. Increase understanding of mutual needs, encourage mutuality of support.
      c. Increase tendency of mother to turn to partner as most significant person (as opposed to physician).
      d. Enhance bond, success of childbirth preparation classes.

2. Promote understanding/acceptance of role change.
   a. Facilitate/support achievement of developmental tasks.
   b. Reduce probability of postpartum psychological problems.
   c. Promote family bonding.

C. Goal: *health teaching.*
1. *Siblings:*
   a. Alert parents to sibling needs for security, love.
   b. Include sibling in pregnancy experience.
   c. Provide clear, simple explanations of happenings.
   d. Continue demonstrations of love.
   e. Describe increased status ("big sister/brother").
   f. Discuss possible misbehavior to gain attention.
2. *Relatives:* alert parents to possible negative feelings of in-laws.
3. Referral to childbirth preparation/parenting classes.
4. Appropriate community referrals for financial relief to decrease stress and provide aid.

IX. EVALUATION/OUTCOME CRITERIA:

A. Actively participates in pregnancy-related decision making.
B. Expresses satisfaction with decisions made.
C. Demonstrates growth and development in parenting role.
D. Prepared for the birth and for early parenthood.

Antepartum

I. NURSING CARE AND OBSTETRIC SUPPORT

A. General aspects of prenatal management
1. *Scheduled visits:*
   a. Once monthly—until week 28.
   b. Every 2 weeks—weeks 28 to 36.
   c. Weekly—week 36 until labor.
2. **Assessment:**
   a. General well-being, signs of deviations, concerns, questions.
   b. Weight gain pattern.
   c. Blood pressure (sitting).
   d. Abdominal palpation:
      (1) Fundal height; tenderness, masses, hernia.
      (2) Fetal heart rate (FHR).
      (3) Leopold's maneuver for presentation (after week 32).
   e. Laboratory tests:
      (1) Urinalysis—for protein, sugar, signs of asymptomatic infection; drug screen for high-risk groups.
      (2) Venous blood—Hgb, Hct; blood type and Rh factor; rapid plasma reagin (RPR); rubella titer, antibody titer, sickle cell. HIV and hepatitis antigen recommended for all pregnant clients.
      (3) Cultures (vaginal discharge; cervical scrapings, for *Chlamydia trachomatis, Neisseria gonorrhoeae*).
      (4) Tuberculosis (TB) screening in high-risk areas.
      (5) Multiple marker screen, 16 to 18 weeks optimum time.
      (6) Serum glucose screen, 24 to 28 weeks; 1-hour glucose tolerance test.
   f. Follow up on medications (vitamins, iron) and nutrition.
   g. If TB positive during pregnancy, isoniazid (INH) and rifampin given daily. INH is associated with increase in fetal malformations, particularly neurotoxicity. Pyridoxine administered simultaneously to prevent their development.

B. Common minor discomforts during pregnancy (for **Assessment,** see **Table 4.6**).
1. **Etiology:** normal maternal physiological/psychological alterations in pregnancy.
2. **Nursing care plan/implementation:**
   a. Goal: *anticipatory guidance.* Discuss the importance of adequate rest, exercise, diet, and hydration in minimizing symptoms.
   b. Goal: *health teaching* (see **Table 4.6**).
3. **Evaluation/outcome criteria:** woman avoids, minimizes, or copes effectively with minor usual discomforts of pregnancy.

C. Danger signs:
1. **Etiology:** Specific disease processes are discussed under **Complications.**
2. **Nursing care plan/implementation:** Goal: *health teaching*—to safeguard status. Signs to report *immediately:*
   a. **Persistent vomiting** beyond first trimester or severe vomiting at any time. *Possible cause:* Hyperemesis gravidarum.
   b. Fluid discharge from vagina—**bleeding or amniotic fluid** (anything other than leukorrhea). *Possible causes:* Placental problem, rupture of membranes (ROM).
   c. Severe or unusual **pain:** abdominal. *Possible cause:* Abruptio placentae.
   d. Chills or **fever** (if lasts over 24 hours, or over 102°F). *Possible cause:* Infection.
   e. Urinary frequency or **burning on urination.** *Possible cause:* UTI.
   f. **Absence of fetal movements** after quickening, lasting more than 24 hours. *Possible cause:* Intrauterine fetal death.

g. Visual disturbances—**blurring, double vision,** "spots before eyes." *Possible cause:* Preeclampsia.
h. **Swelling** of fingers, ankles, hands, feet, or face. *Possible cause:* Preeclampsia.
i. Severe, frequent, or continual **headache.** *Possible cause:* Preeclampsia.
j. Muscle irritability or **convulsions.** *Possible cause:* Preeclampsia.
k. **Rapid weight gain** not associated with eating. *Possible cause:* Preeclampsia.
l. **More than four uterine contractions** per hour (before 38 weeks). *Possible cause:* Preterm labor.

3. **Evaluation/outcome criteria:**
   a. Actively participates in own health maintenance/pregnancy management.
   b. Identifies early signs of potentially serious complications during the antepartal period.
   c. Promptly reports and seeks medical attention.

II. COMPLICATIONS DURING THE ANTEPARTUM

A. General aspects:

1. **Etiology:**
   a. Normal alterations and increasing physiological stress of pregnancy affect status of coexisting medical disorders.
   b. Conditions affecting mother's general health also affect ability to adapt successfully to normal physiological stress of pregnancy.
   c. Aberrations of normal pregnancy.
2. Goal: *reduce incidence of health problems affecting maternal/fetal health and pregnancy outcome.*
   a. Identify presence of risk factors and signs and symptoms of complications early.
   b. Treat emerging complications promptly and effectively.
   c. Minimize effects of complications on pregnancy outcome.
3. **Assessment:** risk factors:
   a. Age:
      (1) Adolescent.
      (2) Primigravida, age 35 or older.
      (3) Multigravida, age 40 or older.
   b. Socioeconomic level: lower.
   c. Ethnic group.
   d. Previous pregnancy history:
      (1) Habitual abortion.
      (2) Multiparity greater than 5.
      (3) Previous stillbirths.
      (4) Previous cesarean birth.
      (5) Previous preterm labor or delivery.
   e. Multifetal pregnancy.
   f. Prenatal care:
      (1) Enters health-care system late in pregnancy.
      (2) Irregular/episodic prenatal care visits.
      (3) Noncompliance with medical/nursing recommendations.
   g. Preexisting or coexisting medical disorders:
      (1) Cardiovascular: hypertension, heart disease.
      (2) Diabetes.
      (3) Other: renal, respiratory, infections, acquired immunodeficiency syndrome (AIDS).
   h. Substance abuse.
4. **Nursing care plan/implementation:**
   a. Goal: *health teaching* (discussed under specific health problem).
   b. Goal: *early identification/treatment of emerging health problems* (if any).
      (1) Monitor status and progress of pregnancy.
      (2) Refer for medical management, as necessary.
   c. Goal: *emotional support.*
5. **Evaluation/outcome criteria:**
   a. Understands present health status, interactions of coexisting disorder and pregnancy.
   b. Accepts responsibility for own health maintenance.
   c. Makes informed decisions regarding pregnancy.
   d. Minimizes potential for complications of coexisting disorder/pregnancy.
      (1) Avoids factors predisposing to health problems.
      (2) Understands and implements therapeutic management of coexisting disorder/pregnancy.
      (3) Increases compliance with medical/nursing recommendations.
   e. Carries uneventful pregnancy to term.

B. Disorders affecting fluid-gas transport: cardiac disease

1. **Pathophysiology:** cardiac overload → cardiac decompensation → right-sided heart failure → systemic edema.
2. **Etiology:**
   a. Congenital heart defects.
   b. Valvular damage—due to rheumatic fever (most common lesion is mitral stenosis, which can lead to pulmonary edema and emboli).
   c. Increased circulating blood volume and cardiac output—exceeds cardiac reserve. Greatest risk: *after 28 weeks of gestation*—reaches maximum (30%–50%) volume increase; *postpartum*—due to diuresis.
   d. Secondary to treatment (e.g., tocolysis and steroids).
   e. Pregnancy after valve replacement.

3. Normal physiological alterations during pregnancy that *mimic cardiac disorders:*
   a. Systolic murmurs, palpitations, tachycardia, and hyperventilation with some dyspnea on normal moderate exertion.
   b. Edema of lower extremities.
   c. Cardiac enlargement.
   d. Elevated sedimentation rate near term.
4. **Assessment:**
   a. Medical evaluation of cardiac status. Classification of severity of cardiac involvement:
      (1) *Class I*—least affected; asymptomatic with ordinary activity.
      (2) *Class II*—activities somewhat limited; ordinary activities cause fatigue, dyspnea, angina.
      (3) *Class III*—moderate/marked limitation of activity; common activities result in severe symptoms of fatigue, etc.
      (4) *Class IV*—most affected; symptomatic (dyspnea, angina) at rest; should *avoid* pregnancy.
   b. **Cardiac decompensation:**
      (1) *Subjective symptoms*
         (a) Palpitations; feeling that the heart is "racing."
         (b) Increasing fatigue or difficulty breathing, or both, with the usual activities.
         (c) Feeling of smothering and/or frequent cough.
         (d) Periorbital edema; edema of face, fingers (e.g., rings do not fit anymore), feet, legs.
      (2) *Objective signs*
         (a) Irregular weak, rapid pulse (≥100 beats/min).
         (b) Rapid respirations (≥25 breaths/min).
         (c) Progressive, generalized edema.
         (d) Crackles (rales) at base of lungs, after two inspirations and exhalations.
         (e) Orthopnea; increasing dyspnea on minimal physical activity.
         (f) Moist, frequent cough.
         (g) Cyanosis of lips and nailbeds.
5. **Analysis/nursing diagnosis:**
   a. *Fluid volume excess* related to inability of compromised heart to handle increased workload (decreased cardiac reserve → congestive heart failure).
   b. *Impaired gas exchange* related to pulmonary edema secondary to congestive heart failure.
6. **Nursing care plan/implementation:**
   a. *Medical management:*
      (1) Diuretics, electrolyte supplements.
      (2) Digitalis (dose may need to be higher because of dilution in the increased blood volume of pregnancy).
      (3) Antibiotics—prophylaxis against rheumatic fever; treatment of bacterial infections during pregnancy.
      (4) Anticoagulants. Heparin is preferred because its large molecule cannot easily cross placenta. Occasionally, sequelae may include maternal hemorrhage, preterm birth, stillbirth.
      (5) Oxygen, as needed.
      (6) Mitral valvotomy for mitral stenosis often brings dramatic relief.
   b. Goal: *health teaching.*
      (1) Need for compliance with therapeutic regimen, medical/nursing recommendations.
      (2) Drug actions, dosage, necessary actions (how to take own pulse, reportable signs/symptoms).
      (3) Methods for *decreasing work of heart:*
         (a) Adequate *rest*—minimum 10 hours sleep each night; 30-minute nap after each meal.
         (b) *Avoid* heavy physical *activity* (including housework), fatigue, excessive weight gain, emotional stress, infection.
         (c) *Avoid situations* of reduced ambient O_2, such as smoking, exposure to pollutants, flight in unpressurized small planes.
   c. Goal: *nutritional counseling.*
      (1) Well-balanced *diet;* adequate protein, fresh fruits and vegetables, water.
      (2) *Avoid* "junk food," stimulants (caffeine), excessive salt intake.
   d. Goal: *anticipatory planning:* management of **labor.**
      (1) Goal: *minimize physiological and psychological stress.*
      (2) *Medical management:*
         (a) Reevaluation of cardiac status before EDD and labor.
         (b) Regional anesthesia for labor/birth.
         (c) Low-outlet forceps or vacuum extraction birth; episiotomy.
         (d) Continuous hemodynamic monitoring.
      (3) **Assessment:** continuous.
         (a) Physiological response to labor stimuli—*frequent vital signs* (pulse rate most sensitive and reliable indicator of impending congestive heart failure).
         (b) Color, respiratory effort, diaphoresis.
         (c) Contractions, etc.—same as for any mother in labor.

MATERNAL/INFANT

(4) **Nursing care plan/implementation:** *labor.*
 (a) Goal: *safeguard status.*
  (i) Report *promptly:* pulse rate over 100; respirations more than 24 between contractions.
  (ii) Oxygen at 6 liters, as needed.
 (b) Goal: *emotional support*—to reduce anxiety, facilitate cooperation.
  (i) Encourage verbalization of feelings, fears, concerns.
  (ii) Explain all procedures.
 (c) Goal: *promote cardiac function. Position*—semirecumbent; support arms and legs.
 (d) Goal: *promote relaxation/control over labor discomfort.* Encourage Lamaze (or other) breathing/relaxation techniques.
 (e) Goal: *reduce stress on cardiopulmonary system.* Discourage bearing-down efforts.
 (f) Goal: *relieve stress of pain, eliminate bearing-down.* Prepare for regional anesthesia.
 (g) Goal: *maintain effective cardiac function.* Administer medications, as ordered (e.g., digitalis, diuretics, antibiotics).

e. Goal: *anticipatory planning:* **postpartum** management.
 (1) Factors increasing risk of cardiac decompensation:
  (a) Delivery → rapid, decreased intra-abdominal pressure → vasocongestion and rapid rise in cardiac output.
  (b) Loss of placental circulation.
  (c) Normal diuresis increases circulating blood volume.
 (2) **Assessment:**
  (a) Observe for tachycardia or respiratory distress.
  (b) Monitor blood loss, I&O—potential hypovolemic shock, cardiac overload due to diuresis.
  (c) Pain level—potential neurogenic shock.
  (d) Same as for any woman who is postpartum (fundus, signs of infection, etc.).
 (3) **Nursing care plan/implementation:** *postpartum.*
  (a) Goal: *minimize stress on cardiopulmonary system.*
   (i) Rest, dangle, ambulate with assistance.
   (ii) Gradual increase in activity—as tolerated without symptoms.
   (iii) *Position:* semi-Fowler's if needed.
   (iv) Extra help with newborn care.

7. **Evaluation/outcome criteria:**
 a. Successfully carries uneventful pregnancy to term.
 b. Experiences no cardiopulmonary decompensation during labor, birth, or postpartum.

C. Disorders affecting fluid-gas transport in fetus: Rh incompatibility

1. **Pathophysiology**—in a mother who is Rh negative: Rh-positive fetal red blood cells enter the maternal circulation → maternal antibody formation → antibodies cross placenta and enter fetal bloodstream → attack fetal red blood cells → hemolysis → anemia, hypoxia.
 a. The mother who is pregnant and Rh positive carries her infant (Rh negative *or* positive) without incident.
 b. The mother who is pregnant and Rh positive carries an Rh-negative infant without incident.
 c. The mother who is pregnant and Rh negative *usually* carries her first Rh-positive child without problems *unless* she has been sensitized by inadvertent transfusion with Rh-positive blood. *Note:* Fetal cells do not usually enter the maternal bloodstream until placental separation (at abortion, abruptio placentae, amniocentesis, or birth).
2. **Etiology:**
 a. The Rh factor is an antigen on the red blood cells of some people (these people are Rh positive); the Rh factor is dominant; a person may be homozygous or heterozygous for Rh factor.
 b. A person who is Rh negative is homozygous for this recessive trait—does *not* carry the antigen; develops antibodies when exposed to Rh-positive red blood cells (isoimmunization) through transplacental (or other) transfusion.
 c. Following birth of an infant who is Rh positive, if fetal cells enter the mother's bloodstream, maternal antibody formation begins; antibodies remain in the maternal circulation.
 d. At time of next pregnancy with fetus who is Rh positive, antibodies cross placenta → hemolysis. *Note: Degree* of hemolysis depends on amount (titer) of maternal antibodies present.
3. Possible serious complication (fetal)—rare today. *Hydrops fetalis*—most severe hemolytic reaction: severe anemia, cardiac decompensation, hypoxia, edema, ascites, hydrothorax; may be stillborn.
4. **Assessment:**
 a. *Prenatal*—diagnostic procedures:
  (1) Maternal blood type and Rh factor.
  (2) Indirect Coombs' test—to determine presence of Rh sensitization (titer indicates amount of maternal antibodies).

(3) Amniocentesis—as early as 26 weeks of gestation—amount of bilirubin by-products indicates severity of hemolytic activity.

b. *Intrapartum* observation of amniotic fluid (after membrane rupture).
   (1) Straw-colored fluid—mild disease.
   (2) Golden fluid—severe fetal disease.

c. *Postnatal* (see **III. A. Rh incompatibility, p. 215**).

5. **Nursing care plan/implementation:**
   a. Goal: *prevent isoimmunization in women who are Coombs' negative*
      (1) *Postabortion*—if no evidence of Rh sensitization (antibody formation) in the mother who is Rh negative, administer RhoGAM.
      (2) *Prenatal*—if no evidence of sensitization, administer RhoGAM at 28 weeks of gestation, as ordered, to all women who are Rh negative.
      (3) *Postpartum*—if no evidence of sensitization, administer RhoGAM within 72 hours of birth to women who are Rh negative and who gave birth to a baby who is Rh positive.

Give RhoGAM to:
1. Mother who is Rh negative who gives birth to neonate who is Rh positive.
2. Mother who is Rh negative after spontaneous or induced abortion (>8 weeks).
3. Mother who is Rh negative after amniocentesis or chorionic villus sampling (CVS).
4. Mother who is Rh negative between 28 and 32 weeks of gestation.

   b. Goal: *health teaching.*
      (1) Explain, discuss that RhoGAM suppresses antibody formation in susceptible woman who is Rh negative carrying fetus that is Rh positive. *Note:* Cannot reverse sensitization if already present.
      (2) Required during and after each pregnancy with fetus who is Rh positive.

6. **Evaluation/outcome criteria:**
   a. Successfully carries pregnancy to term.
   b. No evidence of Rh isoimmunization.
   c. Birth of viable infant.

D. Disorders affecting fluid-gas transport in fetus: tuberculosis

1. **Pathophysiology:** *Mycobacterium tuberculosis* primarily is spread as an airborne aerosol from infected → noninfected individuals, through the lung. Initial TB infection usually → latent or dormant infection in hosts with normally functioning immune systems. *M. tuberculosis* is a slow-growing obligate aerobe and a facultative intracellular parasite.

2. **Etiology**:
   a. Symptoms of tuberculosis in pregnancy are vague and nonspecific. Fatigue, shortness of breath, sweating, and tiredness can all be attributed to the pregnancy.
   b. Reluctance of health-care professionals to perform a chest x-ray on a woman who is pregnant due to fear of harming the fetus → delay in diagnosis.

3. **Assessment:**
   a. Heaf and Mantoux skin tests (as reliable as in women who are nonpregnant).
   b. Same as for women who are nonpregnant: sputum examination, and culture and scans.

4. **Nursing care plan/implementation**:
   a. Goal: *prevent spread of disease.*
      (1) Initial treatment regimen: isoniazid (INH), rifampin (RIF), and ethambutol (EMB).
      (2) Pyridoxine (vitamin B_6) recommended for women who are pregnant and taking INH.
      (3) Routine use of pyrazinamide (PZA) should be *avoided* because of inadequate teratogenicity data.
      (4) *Avoid:* streptomycin (which interferes with development of the ear; may cause congenital deafness).
   b. Goal: *health teaching.*
      (1) Explain, discuss transmission of disease, importance of completion of medication regimen.
      (2) Because small concentration of antituberculosis drugs in breast milk do not produce toxicity in the newborn who is nursing, breastfeeding should *not* be discouraged for a woman who is HIV seronegative and is planning to take (or is taking) INH or other anti-TB medications.
   c. Goal: *TB treatment for women who are HIV infected and pregnant.*
      (1) If have a positive *M. tuberculosis* culture or suspected TB disease, treat *without delay.*
      (2) Rifamycin.
      (3) Although routine use of pyrazinamide not recommended if pregnant (due to inadequate teratogenicity data), benefits for women who are HIV infected and pregnant outweigh potential pyrazinamide-related risks to fetus.

E. Disorders affecting fluid-gas transport in fetus: hepatitis B (HBV)

1. **Pathophysiology:** Hepatitis B is one of the most highly transmitted forms of hepatitis from mother to child around the world, especially in developing countries. Hepatitis B virus (HBV) is highly contagious; the risk that newborn infant will develop hepatitis B is 10% to 20% if the mother is positive for the hepatitis B surface antigen (HBsAg); and as high as 90% if she is also positive for the HBeAg (hepatitis Be antigen).
2. **Etiology:** Usually, hepatitis B is passed on during delivery with exposure to the blood and fluids during the birth process.
3. **Assessment:**
   a. Blood: highest concentration.
   b. Semen, vaginal secretions, wound exudates: lower concentration.
   c. Hepatitis B surface antigen = active infection.
4. **Nursing care plan/implementation**:
   a. Goal: *prevent spread of disease.*
      (1) Hepatitis B immune globulin (HBIG) to infant at birth.
      (2) Hepatitis B vaccine at 1 week, 1 month, 6 months after birth.
   b. Goal: *health teaching.*
      (1) Explain, discuss transmission of disease, importance of completion of vaccination regimen.
      (2) Centers for Disease Control and Prevention (CDC) has recommended that all newborn infants be vaccinated for hepatitis B.
      (3) The risk of HBV infection in children is not only from perinatal transmission from mothers who are HBV infected, but also from close contact with household members and caregivers who have acute or chronic HBV infection.
      (4) Ensure that all infants born to mothers who are HBsAg positive receive timely and appropriate immunoprophylaxis with HBIG and hepatitis B vaccine.
      (5) Discontinue interferon therapy during pregnancy (effect on fetus is unknown).

F. Disorders affecting nutrition: diabetes mellitus

1. **Pathophysiology:** increased demand for insulin exceeds pancreatic reserve → inadequate insulin production; enzyme (insulinase) activity breaks down circulating insulin → further reduction in available insulin; increased tissue resistance to insulin; glycogenolysis/gluconeogenesis → ketosis.
2. **Etiology:** increased metabolic rate; action of placental hormones (see following), enzyme (insulinase) activity.
3. *Normal physiological* alterations during pregnancy that may *affect* management of the woman who is *diabetic,* or *precipitate gestational diabetes* in women who are susceptible:
   a. Hormone production:
      (1) Human placental lactogen (HPL).
      (2) Progesterone.
      (3) Estrogen.
      (4) Cortisol.
   b. *Effects of hormones:*
      (1) Decreased glucose tolerance.
      (2) Increased metabolic rate.
      (3) Increased production of adrenocortical and pituitary hormones.
      (4) Decreased effectiveness of insulin (increased resistance to insulin by peripheral tissues).
      (5) Increased gluconeogenesis.
      (6) Increased size and number of islets of Langerhans to meet increased maternal needs.
      (7) Increased mobilization of free fatty acids.
      (8) Decreased renal threshold, increased glomerular filtration rate; glycosuria common.
      (9) Decreased CO_2-combining power of blood; higher metabolic rate increases tendency to acidosis.
   c. *Effect of pregnancy on diabetes:*
      (1) Nausea and vomiting—predispose to ketoacidosis.
      (2) Insulin requirements—relatively stable or may decrease in first trimester; rapid *increase* during second and third trimesters; rapid *decrease* after birth to prepregnant level.
      (3) Pathophysiological progression (nephropathy, retinopathy, and arteriosclerotic changes) may appear; existing pathology may worsen.
4. *Effect of poorly controlled diabetes on pregnancy*—increased incidence of:
   a. Infertility.
   b. UTI.
   c. Vaginal infections (moniliasis).
   d. Spontaneous abortion.
   e. Congenital anomalies (three times as prevalent).
   f. Preeclampsia/eclampsia.
   g. Polyhydramnios.
   h. Preterm labor and birth.
   i. Fetal macrosomia—cephalopelvic disproportion (CPD).
   j. Stillbirth.
5. **Assessment:** *gestational diabetes (mellitus)*
   a. History:
      (1) Family history.
      (2) Previous infant 9 lb or more.

(3) Unexplained fetal wastage—abortion, stillbirth, or early neonatal death.
(4) Obesity with very rapid weight gain.
(5) Polyhydramnios (excessive amniotic fluid).
(6) Previous infant with congenital anomalies.
(7) Increased tendency for intense vaginal or urinary tract infections.
(8) Previous history of gestational diabetes.

b. Symptoms: **"3 Ps"**—**p***olydipsia,* **p***olyphagia,* **p***olyuria*—and weight loss.

c. *Abdominal assessment:*
(1) Fetal heart rate.
(2) Excessive fundal height.
(a) Polyhydramnios.
(b) Large-for-gestational-age (LGA) fetus. *Note:* With vascular pathology, small-for-gestational-age (SGA) fetus.

d. *Medical diagnosis*—procedures:
(1) 50-gm oral glucose tolerance test (GTT): woman ingests 50 gm oral glucose solution; 1 hour later plasma glucose obtained. If 140 mg/dL, 3-hour oral GTT ordered.
(2) Abnormal 3-hour GTT: two or more of the following findings are diagnostic of gestational diabetes:
(a) Fasting blood sugar (FBS) ≥95 mg/dL.
(b) One hour ≥180 mg/dL.
(c) Two hours ≥155 mg/dL.
(d) Three hours ≥140 mg/dL.
(3) *Diabetic classification criteria:*
(a) *Type 1*—autoimmune disease in which the body's immune system destroys pancreatic beta cells; ↓ production of insulin; need additional insulin. About 10% with diabetes are type 1.
(b) *Type 2*— ↑ insulin resistance despite adequate insulin production; *treatment* may include: diet, exercise, weight loss, oral drugs to stimulate release of insulin; or insulin injections. About 90% with diabetes are type 2.
(c) *Gestational*—occurs in about 3% of all pregnancies. GTT administered at 24 to 28 weeks' gestation; two abnormal values indicate diagnosis of gestational diabetes. About 40% of women with gestational diabetes will develop type 2 diabetes within 5 years.

e. Woman with known diabetes—all classes.
(1) Knowledge and acceptance of disease and its management:
(a) Signs and symptoms of hyperglycemia/hypoglycemia (see **Table 6.28**).
(b) Appropriate behaviors (e.g., skim milk for symptoms of hypoglycemia).
(2) Skill and accuracy in monitoring serum glucose (dextrometer use).
(3) Skill and accuracy in preparing and administering insulin dosage; site rotation; subcutaneous injection in abdomen.
(4) Close monitoring—prenatal status assessment every 2 weeks until 30 weeks, then weekly until birth. Alert to signs of emerging problems (need for insulin adjustment, polyhydramnios, macrosomia).
(5) Other—as for any woman who is pregnant.

6. **Analysis/nursing diagnosis:**
a. *Knowledge deficit* related to pathophysiology, interactions with pregnancy, management (e.g., insulin administration).
b. *Altered nutrition, more or less than body requirements,* related to weight gain.
c. High-risk pregnancy: high risk for infection, ketosis, fetal demise, fetal macrosomia, cephalopelvic disproportion, polyhydramnios, preterm labor and birth, congenital anomalies.

7. **Nursing care plan/implementation:**
a. Goal: *health teaching.*
(1) Pathophysiology of diabetes, as necessary; effect of pregnancy on management.
(2) Signs and symptoms of hyperglycemia, hypoglycemia; appropriate management of symptoms.
(3) Hygiene—to reduce probability of infection.
(4) Exercise—needed to control serum glucose levels, to regulate weight gain, and for feeling of well-being.
(5) Need for close monitoring during pregnancy.
(6) Insulin regulation:
(a) Requirements vary through pregnancy: *first trimester*—may decrease with some periods of hypoglycemia due to fetal drain; *second trimester*—increased need for insulin; *third trimester*—needs may be triple prepregnant dose; acidosis more common in late pregnancy (precipitated by emotional stress, infection).
(b) Serum glucose testing—dextrometer, blood glucose, or other.
(c) Preparation and self-administration of insulin injection, as necessary.
(d) Prompt reporting of fluctuating serum glucose levels.
(7) Diagnostic testing/hospitalization:
(a) Nonstress test.
(b) Sonography.
(c) Amniocentesis.

b. Goal: *dietary counseling.*
   (1) Optimal weight gain—about 24 lb.
   (2) Needs 25 to 35 calories/kg of ideal body weight (1800–2600 calories).
   (3) Protein—18% to 25% (2 gm/kg, or about 70 gm daily).
   (4) Carbohydrates: 50% to 60% in complex form (milk, bread).
   (5) Fats—25% to 30% unsaturated.
   (6) *No* fruit juice; *no* cold cereal; carbohydrates limited.

c. *Medical management:* hospitalize woman for:
   (1) Regulation of insulin (oral hypoglycemics **contraindicated** in early pregnancy, due to teratogenicity; cross placental barrier).
   (2) Control of infection.
   (3) Determination of fetal jeopardy or indications for early termination of pregnancy.

8. **Evaluation/outcome criteria:**
   a. Understands and accepts diagnosis of diabetes.
   b. Actively participates in effective management of diabetes and pregnancy.
   c. Maintains serum glucose levels within acceptable parameters (e.g., 70–120 mg/dL).
      (1) Monitors serum glucose levels accurately (dextrometer, blood glucose).
      (2) Prepares and self-administers insulin appropriately.
      (3) Complies with dietary regimen.

9. **Antepartal** *hospitalization*
   a. **Assessment:**
      (1) *Medical evaluation*—procedures:
         (a) Serum glucose levels (↓ 120 mg/dL).
         (b) Sonography for fetal growth: biophysical profile (BPP) evaluates fetal physical well-being and volume of amniotic fluid.
         (c) Nonstress testing/contraction stress testing.
         (d) Amniocentesis for fetal maturity. *Note:* Lecithin/sphingomyelin (L/S) ratio may be elevated in women who are diabetic; *phosphatidylglycerol* [*PG*] more accurate for women who are diabetic.
      (2) **Nursing assessment:**
         (a) Daily weight, vital signs, FHR q4h, I&O.
         (b) Fundal height and Leopold's maneuver on admission.
   b. **Nursing care plan/implementation:** Goal: *emotional support* to reduce anxiety and tension, which contribute to insulin imbalance.
      (1) Explain all procedures.
      (2) Assist with tests for fetal status.
      (3) Prepare for possibility of preterm or cesarean birth.

10. *Anticipatory planning*—management of **labor**
   a. **Assessment:** continuous.
      (1) Signs and symptoms of hyperglycemia, hypoglycemia (see **Table 6.28**). Hourly blood sugar measurements.
      (2) Electronic fetal monitoring—to identify signs of fetal distress.
      (3) Other—as for any woman in labor.
   b. **Nursing care plan/implementation:** Goal: *safeguard maternal/fetal status.*
      (1) *Position:* lateral Sims'—to reduce compression of inferior vena cava and aorta due to polyhydramnios or LGA baby. (*Supine hypotensive syndrome* results from compression; reduced placental perfusion increases incidence of fetal hypoxia/anoxia.)
      (2) *Medical management*—varies widely.
         (a) Timing—amniocentesis to determine PG and *phosphatidylinositol* levels (estimate fetal pulmonary surfactant).
         (b) Insulin added to intravenous infusion of 0.9 NaCl and titrated to maintain serum glucose approximately 100 mg/dL. 5% to 10% D/W IV needed to prevent hypoglycemia that may lead to maternal ketoacidosis; hyperglycemia may result in newborn hypoglycemia.
         (c) Ultrasound to identify macrosomia >4050 gm.

11. *Anticipatory planning*—management of **postpartum**
   a. Factors influencing serum glucose levels:
      (1) Loss of placental hormones that degrade insulin.
      (2) Lower metabolic rate. Woman requiring large doses of insulin may need to triple caloric intake and decrease insulin by one-half.
   b. **Assessment:**
      (1) Observe for:
         (a) Hypoglycemia.
         (b) Infection.
         (c) Preeclampsia/eclampsia (higher incidence in women who are diabetic).
         (d) Hemorrhage (associated with polyhydramnios, macrosomia, induction of labor, forceps birth, or cesarean birth).
      (2) Monitor healing of episiotomy/abdominal incision.
   c. **Nursing care plan/implementation:**
      (1) *Medical management:* insulin calibration—requirement may drop to one-half or two-thirds pregnant dosage on first postpartum day if woman is on full diet (due to loss of human placental lactogen and conversion of serum glucose to lactose).

(2) *Nursing management*
(a) Goal: *euglycemia.* Blood glucose, insulin as ordered.
(b) Goal: *avoid trauma, reduce risk of UTI. Avoid* catheterization, where possible.
(c) Goal: *health teaching.* Nipple care—to prevent fissures and possible mastitis.
(d) Goal: *reduce serum glucose and insulin needs.* Encourage/support breastfeeding → antidiabetogenic effect. *Note:* If *acetonuria* occurs, stop breastfeeding while physician readjusts diet/insulin balance; may pump breasts to maintain lactation. If *hypoglycemic,* adrenalin level rises → decreased milk supply and let-down reflex.

12. *Anticipatory guidance*—**discharge plan/implementation**
a. Goal: *counseling.* Reinforce recommendations of physicians/genetic counselors.
(1) Risk of infant inheriting gene for diabetes is greater if mother has early-onset, insulin-dependent disease.
(2) Increased risk of congenital disorders.
b. Goal: *family planning.*
(1) Oral contraceptives are controversial because they decrease carbohydrate tolerance; may be cautiously prescribed for women with no vascular disease and who are nonsmokers. Intrauterine device (IUD) **contraindicated** because of impaired response to infection. Barrier contraceptives (diaphragm or condoms with spermicides) recommended.
(2) Tubal ligation: if mother has vascular involvement (i.e., retinopathy or nephropathy), increased risk with later pregnancies.
c. Goal: *health teaching.*
(1) Self-care measures.
(2) Importance of eating on time, even if infant must wait to breastfeed or bottle feed.
(3) Importance of adequate rest and exercise to maintain insulin/glucose balance.
(4) Organize schedule to care for infant, other children, and her diabetes. Allow time for self.
d. **Evaluation/outcome criteria:**
(1) Successfully completes an uneventful pregnancy, labor, and birth of a newborn who is normal and healthy.
(2) Makes informed judgments regarding parenting, family planning, management of her diabetes.

MATERNAL/INFANT

G. Disorders affecting psychosocial-cultural behaviors: substance abuse

1. **Assessment:** woman who is pregnant and abuses substances
a. *Medical history*
(1) Infections: HIV-positive status, AIDS, STIs, hepatitis, cirrhosis, cellulitis, endocarditis, pancreatitis, pneumonia.
(2) Psychiatric illness: depression, paranoia, irritability.
(3) Trauma related to violence.
b. *Obstetric history*
(1) Spontaneous abortions.
(2) History of abruptio placentae.
(3) Preterm labor.
(4) Preterm rupture of membranes.
(5) Fetal death.
(6) Low-birth-weight (LBW) infants.
(7) Tremors/seizures.
c. *Current pregnancy*
(1) Preterm labor contractions.
(2) Hypoactivity or hyperactivity in fetus.
(3) Poor or decreased weight gain.
(4) STI.
(5) Undiagnosed vaginal bleeding.
(6) Drugs being used and methods of self-administration.
d. *Psychosocial history*
(1) Attitudes re: pregnancy.
(2) Current support system: lacking.
(3) Current living arrangements; lifestyle.
(4) History of psychiatric illness.
(5) History of physical, sexual abuse.
(6) Involvement with legal system.
e. *Physical examination*
f. *Commonly abused substances*
(1) Nicotine.
(2) Alcohol (fetal alcohol syndrome [FAS] or fetal alcohol effects [FAE]).
(3) Marijuana.
(4) Stimulants—cocaine, crack, ice, methamphetamine.
(5) Opiates—heroin, methadone, Darvon, codeine, Vicodin, OxyContin.
(6) Sedatives, hypnotics.
(7) Caffeine.
(8) Ecstasy.
g. *Neonatal outcomes*
(1) LBW, small heads.
(2) Irritable, difficult to console.
(3) Disorganized suck-swallow reflex.
(4) Impaired motor development.
(5) Congenital anomalies: genitourinary, gastrointestinal, limb anomalies.
(6) Cerebral infarctions.

(7) Breastfeeding allowed; thought to ease infant withdrawal.
(8) Poor, slow weight gain; failure to thrive.

2. **Analysis/nursing diagnosis:**
   a. *Altered nutrition: less than body requirements*—poor weight gain related to poor nutrition.
   b. *Altered nutrition: less than body requirements*—slow fetal growth related to slow gain in weight.
   c. *Altered placental function* related to high risk for abruptio placentae.
   d. *Noncompliance* with health-care protocols related to persistent drug use.
   e. *Altered parenting* related to psychological illness (substance dependence).
3. **Nursing care plan/implementation:**
   a. Early identification of substance abuse.
   b. Stabilize physiological status.
   c. Fetal surveillance.
   d. Urge consistent obstetric care.
   e. Refer for social services.
4. **Evaluation/outcome criteria:**
   a. Seeks out and uses social services and drug treatment program.
   b. Abstains from illicit substances during pregnancy.
   c. Successfully completes an uneventful pregnancy, labor, and birth of normal healthy infant.

Lifestyle Choices and Influences That Impact Health in Pregnancy, Intrapartum, Postpartum, and Newborn **(see also STIs, pp. 146–148, pp. 153–157, and substance abuse, pp. 144–145)**

I. OTHER HIGH-RISK WOMEN

A. An adolescent who is pregnant

1. **General aspects:**
   a. Pregnancy in women between 12 and 17 years old.
   b. Incidence has started to ↓; approximately one third of all births are to adolescents.
   c. *Predisposing factors:* early menarche, early experimentation with sex, poor family relationships, poverty, late or no prenatal care, cultural influence.
   d. *Associated health problems:* preeclampsia, preterm labor, SGA infants, anemia, bleeding disorders, infections, CPD.
   e. *Social problems:* mothers who are poorly educated, child abuse, single-parent families, mothers who are unemployed or working at minimum wage or who lack support system.
2. **Assessment:**
   a. Present physical/health status.
   b. Feelings toward pregnancy.
   c. Plans for the future.
   d. Factors influencing decisions related to self, pregnancy, baby.
   e. Signs and symptoms of complications of pregnancy (see **A. 1. d.** *Associated health problems*).
   f. Need/desire for health maintenance information (family planning).
3. **Analysis/nursing diagnosis:**
   a. *Ineffective coping, individual/family,* related to need to alter lifestyle, plans, expectations.
   b. *Altered family processes* related to unexpected/unwanted pregnancy.
   c. *Altered parenting* related to intrafamily stress secondary to unexpected pregnancy, developmental tasks.
   d. *Self-esteem disturbance* related to altered self-concept, body image, role performance, personal identity.
   e. *Knowledge deficit* related to family planning, health maintenance, risk factors, pregnancy options.
   f. *Altered nutrition* related to lifestyle.
4. **Nursing care plan/implementation:**
   a. Goal: *emotional support.*
      (1) Ensure confidentiality.
      (2) Establish acceptant, supportive environment.
      (3) Encourage verbalization of feelings, concerns, fears, desires, etc.
      (4) Maintain continuity of care—consistency of nursing approach, to establish trust, confidentiality.
   b. Goal: *facilitate informed decision making.* Discuss available options; aid in exploring implications of possible decisions.
   c. Goal: *nutritional counseling* (anemia).
      (1) Needs for own growth and that of fetus.
      (2) High-quality diet—value for character of skin, return to prepregnant figure.
      (3) Include pizza, hamburgers, milkshakes as acceptable—to minimize anger at being "different."
   d. Goal: *health teaching.*
      (1) Rest, exercise, hygiene—as for other women.
      (2) Prevention of infection—STI, UTI, etc.
      (3) Breast self-examination; Pap smear.
      (4) Future family planning options (see **Table 4.1**).

e. Goal: *assist in achievement of normal developmental tasks.* Encourage exploration of new role and responsibilities.
f. Goal: *referral to appropriate resources.*
(1) Abortion; adoption resources.
(2) Preparation for childbirth and parenting classes.
(3) Family counseling.
(4) Social services.
g. Goal: *assist in facilitating/continuing/completing basic education.*
(1) Communicate with school nurse.
(2) Explore other options available in community.

5. **Evaluation/outcome criteria:**
a. Makes informed decisions appropriate to individual and family needs, desires.
b. Actively participates in own health maintenance.
(1) Complies with medical/nursing recommendations.
(2) Minimizes potential for complications of pregnancy.
c. Copes effectively with normal physiological and psychosocial alterations of pregnancy.
d. Both woman and baby's father express satisfaction with decision and management of this pregnancy. If parenthood is chosen and pregnancy is successful, accepts parenting role.

B. Older mother: primigravida over age 35

1. **General aspects**—higher incidence of congenital anomalies (e.g., Down syndrome), increased possibility of complications of pregnancy. However, generally it is a conscious decision to have postponed childbearing. Individuals are usually used to making own decisions regarding career and health care.
2. **Assessment:**
a. Same as for other women who are pregnant.
b. Reaction to reality of pregnancy.
c. Family response to pregnancy.
3. **Analysis/nursing diagnosis:**
a. *Fear* related to threat to pregnancy.
b. *Knowledge deficit* related to aspects of pregnancy care.
4. **Nursing care plan/implementation:**
a. Goal: *anticipatory guidance.* Preparation for parenthood, altered lifestyle, potential change of career. Assist with realistic expectations. Refer to "over 30" parents' support group.
b. Goal: *health teaching.* Explain, discuss special diagnostic procedures (**Fig. 4.5**) (**Amniocentesis**).
c. Other—same as for other women who are pregnant.
5. **Evaluation/outcome criteria:**
a. Experiences normal, uncomplicated pregnancy, labor, and birth of a newborn who is normal and healthy.
b. Expresses satisfaction with decision and outcome of this pregnancy.

C. Older mother: multipara over age 40

1. **General aspects**
a. Increased incidence of preexisting and coexisting medical disorders (hypertension, diabetes, arthritis).
b. Increased incidence of complications of pregnancy (preeclampsia/eclampsia, hemorrhage).
c. Smoking is major risk factor.
2. **Assessment:**
a. Same as for other women who are pregnant.
b. Reaction to pregnancy (varies from pleasure at still being "young enough," to despair, if facing decision to abort).
c. History, signs and symptoms of coexisting disorders.
d. Indications of reduced physical ability to cope with normal physiological alterations of pregnancy.
e. Family constellation: stage of family developmental cycle, responses to this pregnancy (especially adolescents' reaction to parents' pregnancy).
3. **Analysis/nursing diagnosis:** same as for over-35 age group.
4. **Nursing care plan/implementation:**
a. Goal: *emotional support.* Encourage verbalization of feelings, fears, concerns.
b. Goal: *referral to appropriate resource.*
(1) Genetic counseling.
(2) Abortion/support groups.
(3) Preparation for childbirth and parenthood classes.
c. Goal: *facilitate/support effective family process.* Involve family in preparation for birth and integration of newborn into family unit.
d. Other—same as for other women who are pregnant.
5. **Evaluation/outcome criteria:**
a. Makes informed decisions related to pregnancy.
b. Expresses satisfaction with decision and outcome of this pregnancy.
c. Experiences uncomplicated pregnancy, labor, and birth of a newborn who is normal and healthy.

D. AIDS

1. **General aspects**—AIDS is a serious condition affecting the immune system. Heterosexual

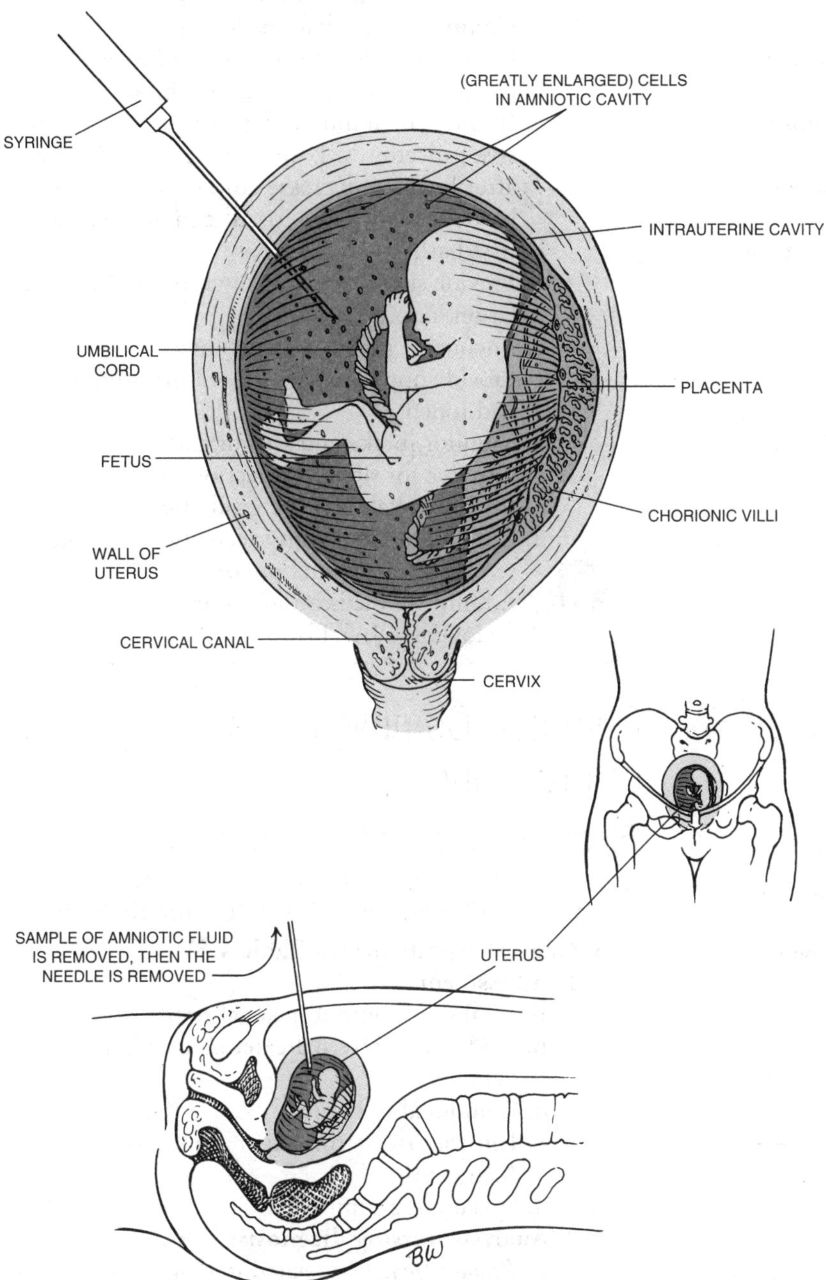

Figure 4.5 Amniocentesis. (From Venes, D [ed]: *Taber's Cyclopedic Medical Dictionary,* ed 20. FA Davis, Philadelphia, 2005, p 92.)

women are considered at risk if they or their sexual partners:
   a. Are HIV positive.
   b. Use IV drugs (50%).
   c. Received blood between 1977 and 1985 (9%).
   d. Are homosexual or bisexual men (39%).
   e. Have hemophilia.
2. **Assessment**—general symptoms:
   a. Malaise.
   b. Chronic cough; possible tuberculosis.
   c. Chronic diarrhea.
   d. HIV positive.
   e. Weight loss: 10 lb in 2 months.
   f. Night sweats; lymphadenopathy.
   g. Skin lesions; thrush.
   h. Pelvic inflammatory disease (PID); STIs; vulvovaginitis (usually, yeast [*Candidiasis*]), often refractory and severe.
   i. Cervical cytologic abnormalities; often infected with human papillomavirus (HPV).

3. **Analysis/nursing diagnosis:**
   a. *Altered nutrition, less than body requirements,* related to general malaise.
   b. *Fatigue,* related to altered health status, weight loss.
   c. *Fear* related to progressively debilitating disease.
   d. *Knowledge deficit* related to disease progression, treatment, life expectancy.
   e. *Ineffective individual coping* related to disease progression.
4. **Nursing care plan/implementation:**
   a. Identify women at risk.
   b. Protect confidentiality.
   c. Implement standard precautions.
   d. Use proper gloves, gown, hand washing.
   e. Use protective eyewear and mask during labor, birth.
5. **Evaluation/outcome criteria:**
   a. No further transmission of virus.
   b. Woman's confidentiality maintained.
   c. Standard precautions implemented.
   d. Emotional support implemented.
   e. Supportive groups contacted.
6. **Women who are HIV positive**—*pregnancy management:*
   a. *Antepartum*
      (1) Increased incidence of other STIs (gonorrhea, syphilis, herpes, HPV).
      (2) Increased incidence of cytomegalovirus (CMV).
      (3) Differential diagnosis for all pregnancy-induced complaints.
      (4) Counsel regarding nutrition.
      (5) Advise about risk to infant.
      (6) Counsel regarding safer sex.
   b. *Intrapartum*
      (1) Focus on prevention of transmission.
      (2) Mode of birth not based on disease.
      (3) External electronic fetal monitoring (EFM) preferred.
      (4) *Avoid* use of fetal scalp electrodes or fetal scalp sampling.
   c. *Postpartum*
      (1) No remarkable alteration in disease progression.
      (2) Breastfeeding **contraindicated.**
      (3) Implement standard precautions for mother and infant.
      (4) Refer to specialists in AIDS care and treatment.
7. **Newborn or neonate:**
   a. **General aspects:** Neonatal AIDS—transmission may be transplacental, contact with maternal blood at birth, or postnatal exposure to parent who is infected (i.e., breastfeeding). Classic signs evident in adult often not present. Common signs: lymphadenopathy, hepatosplenomegaly, oral *candidiasis,* bacterial infections, failure to thrive.
   b. Implement standard precautions for all invasive procedures. Bathe infant immediately after birth to decrease contact with mother's blood. Wear gloves for all contact before first bath.
   c. Provide supportive nursing care (thermoregulation, respiratory).
   d. Encourage parent-infant contact.
   e. Provide opportunities for sensory stimuli and touch.
   f. Monitor intake and weight gain.
   g. Observe for signs of infection.
   h. Initiate social service consultation.
   i. Counsel family about vaccinations (should receive all *except* oral polio).
   j. Administer medications as ordered (zidovudine [AZT]).

Common Complications of Pregnancy

First-Trimester Complications

I. COMPLICATIONS AFFECTING FLUID-GAS TRANSPORT: HEMORRHAGIC DISORDERS

A. General aspects (review **Table 4.8**)
1. **Assessment:**
   a. Vital signs, output, general status.
   b. Evidence of internal/external bleeding.
   c. Pain.
   d. Emotional response.
   e. Perineal pads saturated and number (pad count).
   f. Speculum examination.
2. **Analysis/nursing diagnosis:**
   a. *Knowledge deficit* related to diagnosis, prognosis, treatment, sequelae.
   b. *Anxiety/fear* related to loss of pregnancy, surgery.
   c. *Fluid volume deficit, potential/actual,* related to excessive blood loss.
   d. *Pain.*
   e. *Ineffective coping, individual/family,* related to knowledge deficit and fear.
   f. *Anticipatory/dysfunctional grieving,* related to loss of pregnancy.
   g. *Disturbance in self-esteem, body image, role performance,* related to threat to self-image as woman and childbearer.

Table 4.8

Emergency Conditions

Assessment/Observations	Possible Problem	Nursing Care Plan/Implementation
First Trimester		
Fluid-Gas Transport		
a. *Cramping*—with or without bleeding or passage of tissue	• Abortion (before 24 weeks): threatened, imminent, incomplete, septic	• Bedrest, sedation, *avoid* coitus—if threatened; bedrest, start IV fluids and draw blood for laboratory work: CBC, type/crossmatch, electrolytes, platelets, HCG levels
b. *Passage of tissue* (products of conception; grapelike vesicles) or *brown spotting;* fundus too high for gestational age; *blood pressure* elevated. Often associated with hyperemesis gravidarum and preeclampsia	• Hydatidiform mole (trophoblastic disease)	• Vital signs q5–15 min, prn
c. Severe *pain, shock* out of proportion to amount of overt blood; shoulder-strap pain (*Kehr's sign*), a "referred pain" that indicates intra-abdominal bleeding (or rupture of ovarian cyst); amenorrhea of 6–12 weeks	• Ectopic pregnancy	• Save all pads or tissue passed through vagina for physician evaluation **No** rectal or vaginal examination until physician is present
d. Malodorous *discharge; hyperthermia and chills;* tender abdomen	• Septic abortion (self-induced or "criminal")	• Take complete history, if possible Convulsion precautions if hypertensive
e. *Ecchymosis or bleeding*—with a history that includes any or all of the following: had symptoms of pregnancy, but they subsided; pregnancy test negative; uterine size diminishing; no FHR	• Missed abortion with possible DIC (retained dead fetus syndrome)	• Emotional support for loss of pregnancy (through nurse's manner, tone of voice, touch, use of woman's name; keep her informed of what is happening); oxygen, prn
Second Trimester		
Assessment/Observations	**Possible Problem**	**Nursing Care Plan/Implementation**
Fluid-Gas Transport		
a. Cramping; passage of products of conception	• Late abortion	• Same as for first trimester
b. Labor—cervical changes, "show"	• Incompetent cervical os	• See physician immediately for possible cerclage
c. *Prolonged* nausea and vomiting; unexplained *hypertension* or *preeclampsia;* passage of dark blood or grapelike vesicles; *absent FHRs;* excessive fundal height for gestation	• Hydatidiform mole	• Maintain hydration; assess for dehydration; refer to physician
Sensory-Perceptual		
a. *Preeclampsia/eclampsia*	With increased severity: renal failure, circulatory collapse, stroke, coagulation defects (DIC); abruptio placentae; convulsions	Pharmacological management of hypertension (see **Chapter 6**)
Assessment: hypertension first noted after 24 weeks; followed by increased proteinuria *Symptoms:* blurred or double vision; pain: headache, epigastric (late sign) *Signs:* BP ≥ 160/110; 3+ proteinuria Edema: facial, digital; pulmonary Oliguria Hyperreflexia		**Convulsion precautions:** 1. Emergency tray at bedside 2. Oxygen/suction 3. Start IV 4. Padded siderails 5. Limit environmental stimulation 6. Constant observation 7. Deep tendon reflexes 8. Daily weight 9. I&O—strict 10. Note any complaints and changes 11. Prepare for lab work (type and crossmatch, CBC, platelets, BUN and creatinine, uric acid, SGOT, SGPT)

Continued

Table 4.8

Emergency Conditions—cont'd

Assessment/Observations	Possible Problem	Nursing Care Plan/Implementation
Second Trimester		
Fluid-Gas Transport		
b. *Convulsions* in absence of hypertension, proteinuria, or facial edema	Stroke, epilepsy, drug toxicity; intracranial injury; diabetic complications; encephalopathy	**Convulsion care:** 1. Oxygen/mask; drugs (Valium, magnesium sulfate IV) 2. Observe: a. Uterine tone, FHR, fetal activity b. Signs of labor 3. Emotional support for woman and family
Third Trimester		
Fluid-Gas Transport		
a. *Bleeding: painless, bright red*, vaginal Contractions or uterine tone normal	Placenta previa	**No vaginal examination** Apply fetal monitor; assess for labor *Position:* semi- to high Fowler's Ultrasound to verify placental location
b. *Pain:* abdomen rigid and tender to touch Increased uterine tone; signs of shock disproportionate to visible blood loss; may have loss of FHTs; associated with: preeclampsia, multiparity, precipitous labor, oxytocin induction, trauma, cocaine use	Abruptio placentae	As for placenta previa; *position:* Sims' Prepare for possible emergency cesarean delivery

3. **Nursing care plan/implementation:**
   a. Goal: *minimize blood loss, stabilize physiological status.*
      (1) Facilitate prompt medical management.
      (2) Administer IV fluids, blood, as ordered.
      (3) Administer analgesics, as needed.
   b. Goal: *prevent infection.* Strict aseptic technique.
   c. Goal: *emotional support.*
      (1) Encourage verbalization of anxiety, fears, concerns.
      (2) Supportive care for grief reaction (see **pp. 730–732**).
4. **Evaluation/outcome criteria:**
   a. Blood loss minimized; physiological status stable.
   b. Copes effectively with loss of pregnancy.

B. Spontaneous abortion: *before viable age of 20 to 22 weeks*

1. **Etiology:**
   a. Defective products of conception.
   b. Insufficient production of progesterone.
   c. Acute infections.
   d. Reproductive system abnormalities (e.g., incompetent cervical os).
   e. Trauma (physical or emotional).
   f. Rh incompatibility.
2. **Assessment:** types
   a. *Threatened*—mild bleeding, spotting, cramping; cervix closed.
   b. *Inevitable*—moderate bleeding, painful cramping; cervix dilated, positive nitrazine test (membranes ruptured).
   c. *Imminent*—profuse bleeding, severe cramping, urge to bear down.
   d. *Incomplete*—fetal parts or fetus expelled; placenta and membranes retained.
   e. *Complete*—all products of conception expelled; minimal vaginal bleeding.
   f. *Habitual/recurrent*—history of spontaneous loss of three or more successive pregnancies.
   g. *Missed*—fetal death with no spontaneous expulsion within 4 weeks.
      (1) Anorexia, malaise, headache.
      (2) Fundal height—inconsistent with gestational estimate.
      (3) Laboratory—prolonged clotting time, due to resultant concurrent hypofibrinogenemia (disseminated intravascular coagulation [DIC], a major threat to mother).
   h. *Elective abortions* (intentionally induced loss of pregnancy).

3. **Analysis/nursing diagnosis:**
   a. *Altered family processes* related to pregnancy, circumstances surrounding abortion.
   b. *Sexual dysfunction* related to compromised self-image, altered interpersonal relationship, guilt feelings.
4. **Nursing care plan/implementation:**
   a. *Threatened*—Goal: *health teaching.* Suggest: *avoid* coitus and orgasm, especially around normal time for menstrual period.
   b. *Incomplete, inevitable, imminent.*
      (1) Goal: *safeguard status.*
         (a) Save all pads, clots, tissue for expert diagnosis.
         (b) Report immediately any change in status, excessive bleeding, signs of infection, shock.
         (c) Prepare for surgery.
      (2) Goal: *comfort measures.*
         (a) Administer analgesics, as necessary.
         (b) Bedrest, quiet diversional activities.
      (3) Goal: *emotional support.*
         (a) Encourage verbalization of fear, concerns.
         (b) Reduce anxiety, as possible.
         (c) If pregnancy terminates, facilitate grieving process; assist in working through guilt feelings (see **pp. 183–184**).
         (d) Supportive care for grief reaction (see **pp. 730–732**).
      (4) Goal: *prevent isoimmunization* (see **II. C. 5. Rh incompatibility, p. 140**).
      (5) *Medical management:*
         (a) Laboratory—blood type and Rh factor, indirect Coombs' test, platelets, serum fibrinogen, clotting time.
         (b) Replace blood loss; maintain fluid levels with IV.
         (c) Dilation and curettage or dilation and evacuation.
         (d) *Habitual*—determine etiology.
5. **Evaluation/outcome criteria:**
   a. *Threatened*—responds to medical/nursing regimen; abortion avoided, successfully carries pregnancy to term.
   b. *Spontaneous abortion*—after uterus emptied.
      (1) Bleeding is controlled.
      (2) Vital signs are stable.
      (3) Copes effectively with loss of pregnancy.
      (4) Expresses satisfaction with care.
   c. *Habitual abortion*—cause identified and corrected; carries subsequent pregnancy to successful termination.

C. Hydatidiform mole (complete)

1. **Pathophysiology**—chorionic villi degenerate into grapelike cluster of vesicles; may be antecedent to choriocarcinoma.
2. **Etiology**—genetic base of complete mole (sperm enters empty egg and its chromosomes replicate; 23 pairs of chromosomes are all paternal); rare complication; more common in women over 45 years of age and women who are Asian.
3. **Assessment:**
   a. Uterus—rapid enlargement; fundal height inconsistent with gestational estimate.
   b. Brownish discharge—beginning about week 12; may contain vesicles.
   c. Signs and symptoms of preeclampsia/eclampsia (before third trimester), increased incidence of hyperemesis gravidarum.
   d. *Medical evaluation*—procedures:
      (1) Sonography, x-ray, amniography—no fetal parts present; "snowstorm."
      (2) Laboratory test—for elevated human chorionic gonadotropin (HCG) levels.
      (3) Follow-up surveillance of HCG levels for at least 1 year; persistent HCG level is consistent with choriocarcinoma; x-ray.
4. **Analysis/nursing diagnosis:**
   a. *Anxiety/fear* related to treatment, possible sequelae of hydatidiform mole (choriocarcinoma).
   b. *Potential for injury* related to hemorrhage, perforation of uterine wall, preeclampsia/eclampsia.
   c. *Fluid volume deficit* related to hemorrhage.
5. **Nursing care plan/implementation:**
   a. *Medical management*
      (1) Monitor for preeclampsia.
      (2) Evacuate the uterus—hysterectomy may be necessary.
      (3) Strict contraception for at least 1 year to enable accurate assessment of status.
      (4) Choriocarcinoma—chemotherapy (methotrexate plus dactinomycin) or radiation therapy, or both.
   b. *Nursing management*
      (1) Goal: *safeguard status.* Observe for hemorrhage, passage of retained vesicles and abdominal pain, or signs of infection (because woman is at risk for perforation of uterine wall).
      (2) Goal: *health teaching.*
         (a) Explain, discuss diagnostic tests; prepare for tests.
         (b) Discuss contraceptive options.
         (c) Importance of follow-up.
      (3) Goal: *preoperative and postoperative care.*
      (4) Goal: *emotional support.* Facilitate grieving.
6. **Evaluation/outcome criteria:**
   a. Verbalizes understanding of diagnosis, tests, and treatment.
   b. Complies with medical/nursing recommendations.

c. Tolerates surgical procedure well.
   (1) Bleeding controlled.
   (2) Vital signs stable.
   (3) Urinary output adequate.
d. Copes effectively with loss of pregnancy.
e. Returns for follow-up care/surveillance.
f. Selects and effectively implements method of contraception; avoids pregnancy for 1 year or more.
g. Tests for HCG remain negative for 1 year; no evidence of malignancy.
h. Achieves a pregnancy when desired.
i. Successfully carries pregnancy to term; normal, uncomplicated birth of viable infant.

D. Ectopic pregnancy (Fig. 4.6)

1. **Pathophysiology**—implantation outside of uterine cavity.
2. Types:
   a. Tubal (most common).
   b. Cervical.
   c. Abdominal.
   d. Ovarian.
3. **Etiology:**
   a. PID—pelvic salpingitis and endometritis.
   b. 43% caused by STI-related factors: 25%, chlamydial; 20%, previous STI.
   c. Tubal or uterine anomalies, tubal spasm.
   d. Adhesions from PID or past surgeries.
   e. Presence of IUD.
4. **Assessment:** dependent on implantation site.
   a. *Early signs*—abnormal menstrual period (usually following a missed menstrual period), spotting, some symptoms of pregnancy; possible dull pain on affected side.
   b. *Impending or posttubal rupture*—sudden, acute, lower abdominal pain; nausea and vomiting; signs of shock; referred shoulder pain (*Kehr's sign*) or neck pain—due to blood in peritoneal cavity; blood in cul-de-sac may → rectal pressure.
   c. Sharp, localized pain when cervix is touched during vaginal examination; shock and circulatory collapse in some, usually following vaginal examination.
   d. Positive pregnancy test in many women.
5. **Analysis/nursing diagnosis:**
   a. *Fear* related to abdominal pain and pregnancy status.
   b. *Grief* related to pregnancy loss.
6. **Nursing care plan/implementation:**
   a. *Medical management:* Methotrexate, a folic acid antagonist, which acts by inhibiting cell division (may be used in early ectopic pregnancy).
   b. Surgical removal/repair.
   c. *Nursing management:*
      (1) Goal: *preoperative and postoperative care, health teaching.*
      (2) Goal: *supportive care for grief reaction;* encourage verbalization of anxiety and concerns of further pregnancies.
7. **Evaluation/outcome criteria:**
   a. Woman experiences uncomplicated postoperative course.
   b. Woman copes effectively with loss of pregnancy.

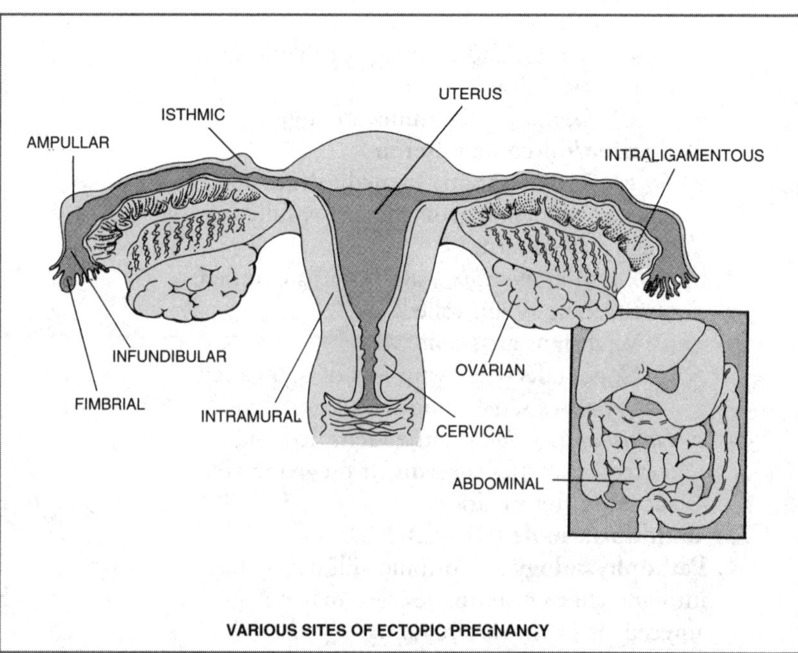

Figure 4.6 Ectopic pregnancy. (From Venes, D [ed]: *Taber's Cyclopedic Medical Dictionary,* ed 19. FA Davis, Philadelphia, 2001.)

MATERNAL/INFANT

II. COMPLICATIONS AFFECTING NUTRITION/ELIMINATION: HYPEREMESIS GRAVIDARUM

A. Pathophysiology—pernicious vomiting during first 14 to 16 weeks (peak incidence around 10 weeks of gestation); excessive vomiting at any time during pregnancy. Potential hazards include the following:
1. Dehydration with fluid and electrolyte imbalance.
2. Starvation, with loss of 5% or more of body weight; protein and vitamin deficiencies.
3. Metabolic acidosis—due to breakdown of fat stores to meet metabolic needs.
4. Hypovolemia and hemoconcentration; *increased* blood urea nitrogen (BUN); *decreased* urinary output.
5. Embryonic or fetal death may result, and the woman may suffer irreversible metabolic changes or death.

B. Etiology:
1. Physiological—secretion of HCG, decrease in free gastric HCl, decreased gastrointestinal motility. Increased incidence in hydatidiform mole and multifetal pregnancy (due to high levels of HCG).
2. Psychological—thought to be related to rejection of pregnancy or sexual relations.

C. Assessment:
1. Intractable vomiting.
2. Abdominal pain.
3. Hiccups.
4. Marked weight loss.
5. Dehydration—thirst, tachycardia, skin turgor.
6. Increased respiratory rate (metabolic acidosis).
7. Laboratory—*elevated* BUN.
8. *Medical evaluation:* rule out other causes (infection, tumors).

D. Analysis/nursing diagnosis:
1. *Altered nutrition, less than body requirements,* related to inability to retain oral feedings.
2. *Fluid volume deficit* related to dehydration.
3. *Ineffective individual coping* related to symptoms, insecurity in role, psychological stress of unwanted pregnancy.
4. *Personal identity disturbance* related to symptoms or perception of self as inadequate in role, sick, socially unpresentable.

E. Nursing care plan/implementation:
1. Goal: *physiological stability.*
   a. Rest GI tract (keep NPO) (e.g., maintain IV fluids, parenteral nutrition).
   b. Progress diet, as ordered; present small feedings attractively; ↑ carbohydrates, ↓ fat, ↓ acidic foods.
   c. Weigh daily, assess hydration; note weight gain.
   d. Antiemetics (IV, suppository).
2. Goal: *minimize environmental stimuli.*
   a. Limit visitors and phone calls.
   b. Bedrest with bathroom privileges.
3. Goal: *emotional support.*
   a. Establish accepting, supportive environment.
   b. Encourage verbalization of anxiety, fears, concerns.
   c. Support positive self-image.

F. Evaluation/outcome criteria:
1. Woman's signs and symptoms subside; she takes oral nourishment and gains weight.
2. Woman's pregnancy continues to term without recurrence of hyperemesis.

III. COMPLICATIONS AFFECTING PROTECTIVE FUNCTION: SEXUALLY-TRANSMITTED INFECTIONS (STIS).

This category measures applications of knowledge about conditions related to client's capacity to maintain defenses and prevent physical and chemical trauma, injury, *infection,* and threats to health status.

A. Vaginitis—inflammation of vagina.
1. **Pathophysiology**—local inflammatory reaction (redness, heat, irritation/tenderness, pain). May cause preterm labor in pregnancy.
2. **Etiology:**
   a. Common causative organisms:
      (1) Bacteria—streptococci, *Escherichia coli,* gonococci, *Chlamydia,* bacterial vaginosis.
      (2) *Viruses*—herpes simplex virus type 2, CMV, HPV
      (3) Protozoa—*Trichomonas vaginalis.*
      (4) Fungi—*Candida albicans.*
   b. Atrophic changes—due to declining hormone level (women who are postmenopausal).
3. **Assessment:** differentiate among common vaginal infections:
   a. Vulvovaginal erythema.
   b. Pruritus, dysuria, dyspareunia.
   c. Vaginal discharge—color, consistency.
4. **Analysis/nursing diagnosis:** *pain* related to inflammation, discharge.
5. **Nursing care plan/implementation:**
   a. Goal: *emotional support.*
   b. Goal: *health teaching.* Instruct woman in self-care measures to promote comfort and healing:
      (1) Perineal care.
      (2) Sitz baths.
      (3) Douching (as ordered). *Not* recommended during pregnancy.
      (4) Exposing vulva to air.
      (5) Cotton briefs.
      (6) Proper insertion of vaginal suppository.
      (7) Antibiotic use, as ordered.

c. Goal: *prevent reinfection.*
   (1) Suggest sexual partner use condom until infection is eliminated—or abstain from intercourse.
   (2) Recommend sexual partner seek examination and treatment.
d. Goal: *medical consultation/treatment.* Refer for diagnosis and treatment.

6. **Evaluation/outcome criteria:**
   a. Woman is asymptomatic; unable to recover organism from body fluids or tissue.
   b. Woman avoids reinfection.
   c. Woman carries pregnancy to term without complications.

B. Gonorrhea

1. **Pathophysiology:**
   a. *Men*—early infection usually confined to urethra, vestibular glands, anus, or pharynx. Untreated: ascending infection may involve testes, causing sterility.
   b. *Women*—early infection usually confined to vestibular glands, endocervix, urethra, anus (vagina is resistant). May ascend to involve pelvic structures (e.g., PID: fallopian tubes, ovaries); scarring may cause sterility.
   c. *Women* who are pregnant—may result in preterm rupture of membranes, amnionitis, preterm labor, postpartum salpingitis.
   d. Sequelae (untreated):
      (1) May develop carrier state (asymptomatic; organism resident in vestibular glands).
      (2) Systemic spread may result in gonococcal:
         (a) Arthritis.
         (b) Endocarditis.
         (c) Meningitis.
         (d) Septicemia.
   e. *Newborn*—ophthalmia neonatorum (gonococcal conjunctivitis). Untreated sequela: blindness.
2. **Etiology:** gram-negative diplococcus (*Neisseria gonorrhoeae*).
3. **Epidemiology:**
   a. Portal of entry—oral or genitourinary mucous membranes.
   b. Mode of transmission—usually sexual contact.
   c. Incubation period: 2 to 5 days; may be asymptomatic.
   d. Communicable period—as long as organisms are present; to 4 days after antibiotic therapy begun.
4. **Assessment:**
   a. History of known (or suspected) contact.
   b. *Men:*
      (1) Complaint of mucoid or mucopurulent discharge.
      (2) *Medical diagnosis*—procedure: urethral discharge Gram stain.
   c. *Women:*
      (1) Often asymptomatic; acute infection: severe vulvovaginal inflammation, venereal warts, greenish-yellow vaginal discharge.
      (2) *Medical diagnosis*—procedure: endocervical culture.
   d. Gonococcal urethritis (men and women)—sudden severe dysuria, frequency, burning, edema.
   e. Salpingitis/oophoritis—severe, sudden abdominal pain, fever (with or without vaginal discharge).
5. **Analysis/nursing diagnosis:** *impaired tissue integrity* related to tissue inflammation.
6. **Nursing care plan/implementation:**
   a. Goal: *emotional support.*
   b. Goal: *health teaching* to prevent transmission, sequelae, reinfection.
      (1) Need for accurate diagnosis and effective treatment, follow-up examination in 7 to 14 days, and culture.
      (2) All sexual partners need examination, treatment.
      (3) Possible sequelae/complications (sterility, carrier state).
   c. Goal: *medical consultation/treatment.*
      (1) Determine allergy to antibiotics.
      (2) Refer for diagnosis and treatment.
         (a) Diagnosis: culture.
         (b) Treatment—ceftriaxone IM, plus doxycycline PO. May use erythromycin or spectinomycin in pregnancy.
         (c) Follow-up culture before birth.
         (d) Notification of sexual partners.
7. **Evaluation/outcome criteria:**
   a. Verbalizes understanding of mode of transmission, prevention, importance of examination, treatment of sexual contacts.
   b. Informs sexual contacts of need for examination.
   c. Returns for follow-up examinations.
   d. Successfully treated; weekly follow-up cultures: negative on two successive visits.
   e. Avoids reinfection.

C. *Chlamydia trachomatis*

1. **Pathophysiology:**
   a. Most common sexually transmitted infection in United States.
   b. Initial infection mild in women; inflammation of cervix with discharge.
   c. If untreated, may lead to urethritis, dysuria, PID, tubal occlusion, infertility.

MATERNAL/INFANT

2. **Etiology:**
   a. *Chlamydia trachomatis* has maternal-fetal effects.
   b. Bacteria can exist only within living cells.
   c. Transmission is by direct contact from one person to another.
3. **Assessment—maternal:**
   a. Inflamed cervix (may be asymptomatic).
   b. Cervical congestion, edema.
   c. Mucopurulent discharge.
4. **Assessment—fetal-neonatal:**
   a. Increased incidence of stillbirth.
   b. Preterm birth may result.
   c. Contact with infected mucus occurs during birth.
   d. Newborn may be asymptomatic.
   e. Conjunctivitis; may lead to scarring.
   f. *Chlamydial* pneumonia.
5. **Analysis/nursing diagnosis:**
   a. *Pain* related to inflamed reproductive organs.
   b. *Fatigue* related to inflammation.
   c. *Knowledge deficit* related to mode of treatment, disease transmission.
6. **Nursing care plan/implementation:**

   a. Treatment with antibiotics, generally doxycycline or azithromycin. Erythromycin in pregnancy.

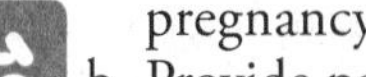

   b. Provide pain relief, analgesics.
   c. Counsel regarding use of condoms, spermicidal agents (containing nonoxynol-9) to prevent reinfection.
7. **Evaluation/outcome criteria:**
   a. Woman understands treatment and shows compliance.
   b. Woman understands portal of entry and risk for reinfection.

D. Herpes genitalis

1. **Pathophysiology**—initial infection: varies in severity of symptoms, may be local or systemic; duration: prolonged; morbidity: severe.
2. **Etiology**—Herpes simplex virus type 2.
3. **Epidemiology:**
   a. Portal of entry—skin, mucous membranes.
   b. Mode of transmission—usually sexual.
   c. Incubation: 3 to 14 days.
   d. Communicable period—while organisms are present.
4. **Assessment:**
   a. Lesions—painful, red papules; pustular vesicles that break and form wet ulcers that later crust; self-limiting (3 weeks).
   b. Severe itching, tingling, or pain.
   c. Discharge—copious; foul smelling.
   d. Dysuria.
   e. Lymph nodes—enlarged, inflammatory, inguinal.
   f. Woman who is pregnant—vaginal bleeding, spontaneous abortion, fetal death.
   g. May shed virus for 7 weeks.
   h. *Medical diagnosis:* multinucleated giant cells in microscopic examination of lesion exudate; culture for herpes simplex virus (HSV).
5. **Analysis/nursing diagnosis:**
   a. *Pain* related to inflammation process.
   b. *Fear* related to longevity of disease.
   c. *Fear* related to no cure for disease.
   d. *Knowledge deficit* related to transmission to future partners, suppressive treatment.
6. **Nursing care plan/implementation:**
   a. Goal: *emotional support.*
   b. Goal: *health teaching.*
      (1) Virus remains in body for life (dormant, noninfectious) in 25% to 30% of population; small percentage have symptoms.
      (2) Recurrence probable; usually shorter and milder.
      (3) Need for close surveillance during pregnancy; cesarean birth may be indicated if woman has active genital lesions or positive culture.
   c. Goal: *promote comfort.*
   d. Goal: *accurate definitive treatment.* Refer for diagnosis and treatment.
      (1) Diagnosis—cervical smears, labial and vaginal smears.
      (2) Treatment—acyclovir; used for suppressive treatment only.
7. **Evaluation/outcome criteria:**
   a. Woman remains asymptomatic.
   b. Pregnancy continues to term with no newborn effects.

E. Syphilis

1. **Pathophysiology:**
   a. *Primary stage:* nonreactive RPR.
      (1) *Men:* 3 to 4 weeks after contact, painless, localized penile/anal ulcer (chancre); lymph nodes—enlarged, regional.
      (2) *Women:* often asymptomatic; labial, vaginal, or cervical chancre.
      (3) *Medical diagnosis*—procedure: dark-field microscopic examination of lesion exudate.
   b. *Secondary stage:* reactive Venereal Disease Research Laboratories (VDRL).
      (1) 6 to 8 weeks after infection.
      (2) Rash—macular, papular; on trunk, palms, soles.
      (3) Malaise, headache, sore throat, weight loss, low-grade temperature.
   c. *Latent stage:* reactive serologic test for syphilis (STS). Asymptomatic; noninfectious.

d. *Tertiary stage:*
(1) Gumma formation in skin, cardiovascular system, or central nervous system.
(2) Psychosis.

2. **Etiology:** *Treponema pallidum* (spirochete).
3. **Epidemiology:**
a. Portal of entry—skin, mucous membranes.
b. Mode of transmission—usually sexual.
c. Incubation period—9 days to 3 months.
d. Communicable period—primary and secondary stages.
4. **Assessment:**
a. *Primary*—chancre, when detectable.
(1) *Medical diagnosis*—procedure: dark-field examination of lesion exudate.
b. *Secondary:*
(1) Malaise, lymphadenopathy, headache, elevated temperature.
(2) Macular, papular rash on palms and soles; may be disseminated.
(3) *Medical diagnosis*—(see **d.**, following).
c. *Tertiary:*
(1) Subcutaneous nodules (gumma).
(2) *Note:* Gumma formation may affect any body system; symptoms associated with area of involvement.
d. *Medical diagnosis*—procedures: stages other than primary—STS: VDRL, RPR, *T. pallidum* immobilization (TPI), fluorescent treponemal antibody absorption (FTA). *False-positive STS* in: collagen diseases, infectious mononucleosis, malaria, systemic tuberculosis.
5. **Analysis/nursing diagnosis:**
a. *Pain* related to inflammation process.
b. *Knowledge deficit* related to treatment and transmission of the disease.
6. **Nursing care plan/implementation:**
a. Goal: *emotional support*
(1) Nonjudgmental.
(2) Caring, supportive manner.
b. Goal: *health teaching.*
(1) Need for accurate diagnosis and treatment, follow-up examinations.
(2) All sexual partners need examination and treatment.
c. Goal: *medical consultation/treatment.*
(1) Refer for diagnosis and treatment. *Note:* In pregnancy—treatment by 18th gestational week prevents congenital syphilis in neonate; however, treat at time of diagnosis.
(2) Treatment:
(a) Primary, secondary—benzathine penicillin G, 2.4 million units.
(b) Other stages—7.2 million units over 3-week period.
(c) Erythromycin or doxycycline for clients who are allergic to penicillin.
7. **Evaluation/outcome criteria:**
a. If treated by 18th week of pregnancy, congenital syphilis is prevented.
b. Appropriate treatment after 18th week cures both mother and fetus; however, any fetal damage occurring before treatment is irreversible.
c. Follow-up VDRL: nonreactive at 1, 3, 6, 9, and 12 months.
d. *Tertiary*—cerebrospinal fluid examination negative at 6 months and 1 year following treatment.
e. Verbalizes understanding of mode of transmission, potential sequelae without treatment, importance of examination/treatment of sexual contacts, preventive techniques.
f. Informs contacts of need for examination.
g. Returns for follow-up visit.
h. Avoids reinfection.

F. Pelvic inflammatory disease (PID)

1. **Pathophysiology**—ascending pelvic infection; may involve fallopian tubes (salpingitis), ovaries (oophoritis); may develop pelvic abscess (most common complication), pelvic cellulitis, pelvic thrombophlebitis, peritonitis.
2. **Etiology:**
a. *Chlamydia trachomatis.*
b. Gonococci.
c. Streptococci.
d. Staphylococci.
3. **Assessment:**
a. Pain: acute, abdominal.
b. Vaginal discharge: foul smelling.
c. Fever, chills, malaise.
d. *Elevated* white blood cell (WBC) count.
4. **Analysis/nursing diagnosis:**
a. *Pain* related to occluded tubules.
b. *Infertility* related to permanent block of tubes.
c. *Knowledge deficit* related to transmission of disease.
d. *Altered urinary elimination* related to dysuria.
5. **Nursing care plan/implementation**—for **woman who is hospitalized:**
a. Goal: *emotional support.*
b. Goal: *limit extension of infection.*
(1) Bedrest—*position:* semi-Fowler's, to promote drainage.
(2) *Force fluids* to 3000 mL/day.
(3) Administer antibiotics, as ordered.

c. Goal: *prevent autoinocculation/transmission.*
 (1) Strict aseptic technique (hand washing, perineal care).
 (2) Contact-item isolation.

d. Goal: *Health teaching:* if untreated: high risk of tubal scarring, sterility, or ectopic pregnancy; pelvic adhesions; transmission of disease.

e. Goal: *promote comfort.*
 (1) Analgesics, as ordered.
 (2) External heat, as ordered.

6. **Evaluation/outcome criteria:**
 a. Woman responds to therapy; uneventful recovery.
 b. Woman avoids reinfection.

Second-Trimester Complications (see Table 4.8)

I. COMPLICATIONS AFFECTING COMFORT, REST, MOBILITY: INCOMPETENT CERVIX

A. Pathophysiology—inability of cervix to support growing weight of pregnancy; associated with repeated spontaneous second trimester abortion.

B. Etiology:
1. Unknown.
2. Congenital defect in cervical musculature (exposure to diethylstilbestrol [DES]).
3. Cervical trauma during previous birth, abortion; aggressive, deep, or repeated dilation and curettage.

C. Assessment:
1. History of habitual, second-trimester abortions.
2. Painless, progressive cervical effacement and dilation during second trimester.
3. Signs of threatened abortion or (early third-trimester) preterm labor.

D. Analysis/nursing diagnosis:
1. *Pain* related to early dilation.
2. *Fear* related to possible pregnancy loss.

E. Nursing care plan/implementation:
1. *Medical management*
 a. Cerclage surgical procedure (*Shirodkar, McDonald*).
2. *Preoperative nursing management*
 a. Goal: *reduce physical stress on incompetent cervix.* Bedrest, supportive care.
 b. Goal: *emotional support.* Encourage verbalization of anxiety, fear, concerns.
 c. Goal: *health (preoperative) teaching.* Explain procedure—purse-string suture encircles cervix and reinforces musculature.
 d. Goal: *preparation for surgery.*
3. *Postoperative nursing management*
 a. Goal: *maximize surgical result.* Bedrest, supportive care.
 b. Goal: *health teaching.*
  (1) *Avoid:* strenuous physical activity; straining, infection.
  (2) Report promptly: signs of labor (vaginal bleeding, cramping).
  (3) Need for continued, close health surveillance.

F. Evaluation/outcome criterion: woman carries pregnancy to successful termination.

II. COMPLICATIONS AFFECTING SENSORY/PERCEPTUAL FUNCTIONS: PREGNANCY-INDUCED HYPERTENSION (PIH); PREECLAMPSIA/ECLAMPSIA

A. Pathophysiology:
1. Generalized arteriospasm → increased peripheral resistance, decreased tissue perfusion, and hypertension.
2. *Kidney:*
 a. Reduced renal perfusion and vasospasm → glomerular lesions.
 b. Damage to membrane → loss of serum protein (albuminuria). *Note:* Reduced serum albumin/globulin (A/G) ratio alters blood osmolarity → edema.
 c. Increased tubular reabsorption of sodium → increased water retention (edema).
 d. Release of angiotensin contributes to vasospasm and hypertension.
3. *Brain:* decreased oxygenation, cerebral edema, and vasospasm → visual disturbances and hyperirritability, convulsions, and coma.
4. *Uterus:* decreased placental perfusion → increased risk of SGA baby, abruptio placentae, oligohydramnios.

B. Etiology: unknown. *Risk factors:*
1. Pregnancy—occurs only when a functioning trophoblast is present; more common in *first* pregnancies. Onset: develops after week 20 of gestation, through labor, and up to 48 hours postpartum.
2. Coexisting conditions—diabetes, multifetal gestation, polyhydramnios, renal disease.
3. Angiotensin gene T235.

C. Assessment—types:
1. *Preeclampsia—mild*
 a. **Hypertension**—systolic increase of 30 mm Hg or more over baseline; diastolic rise of 15 mm Hg or more.
 b. **Proteinuria**—1 gm/day.
 c. Edema—digital and periorbital; **weight gain** over 0.45 kg (1 lb)/wk.
2. *Preeclampsia—severe*
 a. Increasing hypertension—systolic at or above 160 mm Hg or more than 50 mm Hg over baseline; diastolic, 110 mm Hg or more.

MATERNAL/INFANT

b. Urine: *proteinuria* (5 gm or more in 24 hours); *oliguria* (400 mL or less in 24 hours).
c. Hemoconcentration, hypoproteinemia, hypernatremia, hypovolemic condition.
d. Nausea and vomiting.
e. Epigastric pain—due to edema of liver capsule.
f. Cerebral or visual disturbances (before convulsive state):
(1) Disorientation and somnolence.
(2) Severe frontal **headache.**
(3) Increased irritability; **hyperreflexia.**
(4) **Visual disturbance:** blurred vision, halo vision, dimness, blind spots.
g. **HELLP** syndrome (**H**emolysis, **E**levated **L**iver enzymes, and **L**ow **P**latelets).

3. *Eclampsia*
a. Tonic and clonic convulsions; coma.
b. Renal shutdown—oliguria, anuria.

D. Assessment—woman who is hospitalized:
1. Vital signs (blood pressure in side-lying position, pulse, respirations)—q2–4h, while awake (if mild to moderate preeclampsia) or as necessary. *Note:* Record, report persistent *hypertension.*
2. Fetal heart tones at time of vital signs.
3. Deep tendon reflexes (DTRs) and clonus—to identify/monitor CNS hyperirritability.
4. I&O—to identify diuresis. (*Note:* Oliguria indicates pathologic progression.)
5. Urinalysis (clean-catch specimen) for protein, daily or after each voiding, as necessary.
6. Signs of pathologic progression (see **II. C. Assessment**—types).
7. Signs of labor, abruptio placentae (*Note:* high blood pressure, or a rapid drop, may initiate abruptio), DIC.
8. Emotional status.
9. Daily weight, amount/distribution of *edema* (pitting; pedal, digital, periorbital)—to identify signs of mobilization of tissue fluid, diuresis.

E. Analysis/nursing diagnosis:
1. *Fluid volume excess:* hemoconcentration, edema related to altered blood osmolarity and sodium/water retention.
2. *Altered nutrition, less than body requirements:* protein deficiency related to loss through damaged renal membrane.
3. *Altered tissue perfusion* related to increased peripheral resistance and vasospasm in renal, cardiovascular system.
4. *Altered urinary elimination:* oliguria, anuria related to hypovolemia, vasospasm.
5. *Sensory/perceptual alterations:* visual disturbances, hyperirritability related to cerebral edema, decreased oxygenation to brain.
6. *Anxiety* related to symptoms, implications of pathophysiology.
7. *Diversional activity deficit* related to need for reduced environmental stimuli, bedrest.
8. *Risk for injury* related to seizure.

F. Prognosis:
1. *Good*—symptoms mild, respond to treatment.
2. *Poor*—convulsions (number and duration); persistent coma; hyperthermia, tachycardia (≥120 beats/min); cyanosis, and liver damage.
3. *Terminal*—pulmonary edema, congestive heart failure (CHF), acute renal failure, cerebral hemorrhage. The earlier the symptoms appear, the poorer the outcome for the pregnancy.

G. Nursing care plan/implementation: Goal: *health teaching.*
1. *Rest*—frequent naps in *lateral Sims' position.*
2. Immediate report of **danger signs:**
a. Digital and periorbital edema.
b. Severe headache, irritability.
c. Visual disturbances.
d. Epigastric pain.
3. *Do roll-over* test (blood pressure while on back and lateral positions).
4. Importance of regular prenatal visits.
5. Monitoring own blood pressure between prenatal visits.

H. Nursing care plan/implementation—woman who is hospitalized:
1. Goal: *reduce environmental stimuli,* to minimize stimulation of hyperirritable CNS. Limit visitors and phone calls.
2. Goal: *emotional support.*
a. Encourage verbalization of anxiety, fears, concerns.
b. Explain all procedures, seizure precautions.
3. Goal: *supportive care.*
a. Encourage bedrest—to increase tissue perfusion, promote diuresis.
b. *Position:* lateral Sims'—to reduce risk of supine hypotensive syndrome.
4. Goal: *health teaching.* Rest with reduced stimuli.
5. Goal: *monitor and administer drugs as ordered.*
a. Anticonvulsants (especially magnesium sulfate).
b. Antihypertensives.
c. Diuretics (used rarely, and only in presence of CHF).
d. Blood volume expanders.
6. Goal: *seizure precautions.* To safeguard maternal/fetal status:
a. Observe for signs and symptoms of *impending* convulsion:

(1) Frontal headache.
(2) Epigastric pain.
(3) Sharp cry.
(4) Eyes: fixed, unresponsive.
(5) Facial twitching.

MATERNAL/INFANT

b. Emergency items (suction equipment, airway, drugs, IV fluids) immediately available.

7. Goal: *convulsion care* (woman with eclampsia).
   a. Maintain patent *airway;* administer oxygen.
   b. *Safety*—padded bed rails.
   c. Reduce environmental stimuli: dim lights, quiet.
   d. Observe, report, and record:
      (1) Onset and progression of convulsion.
      (2) If followed by coma or incontinence.
   e. Prepare for immediate cesarean delivery; check FHR. Close observation for 48 hours postpartum, even if no further convulsions.

I. Evaluation/outcome criteria:

1. Woman complies with medical/nursing plan of care.
2. Woman's symptoms respond to treatment; progression halted.
3. Woman carries uneventful pregnancy to successful termination.

Third-Trimester Complications (see Table 4.8)

I. COMPLICATIONS AFFECTING FLUID-GAS TRANSPORT

A. Placenta previa—abnormal implantation; near or over internal cervical os. Increased incidence with multiparas, multiple gestation, previous uterine surgery.

1. **Assessment:**
   a. *Painless, bright red vaginal bleeding* (may be intermittent); absence of contractions, abdomen soft.
   b. If in labor, contractions usually normal.
   c. Boggy lower uterine segment—palpated on vaginal examination. (*Note:* If placenta previa is suspected, internal examinations are **contraindicated.**)
   d. *Medical diagnosis—procedure:* sonography—to determine placental site.
2. **Analysis/nursing diagnosis:**
   a. *Anxiety* related to bleeding, outcome.
   b. *Fluid volume deficit* related to excessive blood loss.
   c. *Altered tissue perfusion* related to blood loss.
   d. *Altered urinary elimination* related to hypovolemia.
   e. *Fear* related to fetal injury or loss.
3. **Nursing care plan/implementation:**
   a. *Medical management*
      (1) Sterile vaginal examination under double setup.
      (2) Vaginal birth possible if bleeding minimal, marginal implantation; if fetal vertex is presenting so that presenting part acts as tamponade.
      (3) Cesarean birth for complete previa.
   b. *Nursing management.* Goal: *safeguard status.*
4. **Evaluation/outcome criteria: (Table 4.9)** (see following section on abruptio placentae).

B. Abruptio placentae—premature separation of normally implanted placenta from uterine wall.

1. **Assessment:**
   a. Sudden-onset, *severe* abdominal pain.
   b. Increased uterine tone—may contract unevenly, fails to relax between contractions; very tender.
   c. Shock usually more profound than expected on basis of external bleeding or internal bleeding.

MATERNAL/INFANT

Table 4.9

Comparison of Placenta Previa and Abruptio Placenta

Pathology *Placenta Previa*	Etiology	Assessment	Nursing Care Plan/Implementation
Types:	More common with multiparity, advanced maternal age	**Painless,** *bright red* vaginal bleeding	**No** vaginal or rectal examinations or enemas
Marginal—low-lying	Fibroid tumors	Usually manifests in 8th month	Bedrest (*high Fowler's* if marginal previa)
Partial—partly covers internal cervical os	Endometriosis	*Postpartum:* signs of hemorrhage, infection	• Continuous fetal monitor
Complete—covers internal cervical os	Old uterine scars Multiple gestation		• Maternal vital signs q4h, or prn • Note character and amount of bleeding Emotional support

Continued

Table 4.9

Comparison of Placenta Previa and Abruptio Placenta—cont'd

Pathology *Abruptio Placenta*	Etiology	Assessment	Nursing Care Plan/Implementation
Types:	Preeclampsia/eclampsia	**Pain: sudden, severe**	*Position:* supine; elevate (right) hip
Partial—small part separates from uterine wall	• Before birth of second twin • Traction on cord	• Abdomen: rigid • Uterus: very tender to touch	• Monitor: vital signs, blood loss, fetus
Complete—total placenta separates from uterine wall	• Rupture of membranes • High parity	• Fetal hyperactivity; bradycardia, death	• I&O (anuria, oliguria; hematuria)
Retroplacental—bleeding (concealed)	• Chronic renal hypertension	• Shock: rapid, profound • Port-wine amniotic fluid	Prepare for surgery Emotional support
Marginal—occurs at edges; external bleeding	• Oxytocin induction/augmentation of labor • Cocaine use • Trauma	• Signs of DIC • *Postpartum:* signs of atony, infection, pulmonary emboli	• Fluid, blood replacement

MATERNAL/INFANT

d. *Medical evaluation—procedures:* DIC screening (bleeding time, platelet count, prothrombin time, activated partial thromboplastin time, fibrinogen); sonogram to see placental hemoseparation.

2. **Analysis/nursing diagnosis:**
   a. *Fluid volume deficit* related to bleeding.
   b. *Potential for fetal injury* related to uteroplacental insufficiency.
   c. *Fear* related to unknown outcome.
3. **Potential complications:**
   a. Afibrinogenemia and DIC.
   b. Couvelaire uterus—bleeding into uterine muscle.
   c. Amniotic fluid embolus.
   d. Hypovolemic shock.
   e. Renal failure.
   f. Uterine atony, hemorrhage, infection in postpartum.
4. **Nursing care plan/implementation:**
   a. *Medical management*
      (1) Control: hemorrhage, hypovolemic shock; replace blood loss.
      (2) Cesarean birth.
      (3) Fibrinogen, crystalloids, blood replacement.
      (4) IV heparin—by infusion pump—to reduce coagulation and fibrinolysis.
   b. *Nursing management.* Goal: *safeguard status.*
5. **Evaluation/outcome criteria:**
   a. Experiences successful termination of pregnancy.
      (1) Woman gives birth to viable newborn (by vaginal or cesarean method).
      (2) Woman has minimal blood loss.
      (3) Woman's assessment findings within normal limits.
      (4) Woman retains capacity for further childbearing.
   b. No evidence of complications (anemia, hypotonia, DIC) during postpartum period.

II. COMPLICATIONS AFFECTING COMFORT, REST, MOBILITY

A. Polyhydramnios—amniotic fluid over 2000 mL (normal volume: 500–1200 mL).

1. **Etiology:** unknown. *Risk factors:*
   a. Maternal diabetes.
   b. Multifetal gestation.
   c. Erythroblastosis fetalis.
   d. Preeclampsia/eclampsia.
   e. Congenital anomalies (e.g., anencephaly, upper-GI anomalies, such as esophageal atresia).
2. **Assessment:**
   a. Fundal height: excessive for gestational estimate.
   b. Fetal parts: difficult to palpate, small in proportion to uterine size.
   c. Increased discomfort—due to large, heavy uterus.
   d. Increased edema in vulva and legs.
   e. Shortness of breath.
   f. GI discomfort—heartburn, constipation.
   g. Susceptibility to *supine hypotensive syndrome*—due to compression of inferior vena cava and descending aorta while in supine position.

h. *Medical diagnosis—procedures:*
   (1) Sonography—to diagnose multifetal pregnancy, gross fetal anomaly, locate placental site.
   (2) Amniocentesis—to diagnose anomalies, erythroblastosis.
3. **Potential complications:**
   a. Maternal respiratory impairment.
   b. Premature rupture of membranes (PROM) with prolapsed cord or amnionitis.
   c. Preterm labor.
   d. Postpartum hemorrhage—due to overdistention and uterine atony.
4. **Analysis/nursing diagnosis:**
   a. *Pain* related to excessive size of uterus impinging on diaphragm, stomach, bladder.
   b. *Impaired physical mobility* related to increased lordotic curvature of back, increased weight on legs.
   c. *Altered tissue perfusion* related to decreased venous return from lower extremities, compression of body structures by overdistended uterus.
   d. *Potential fluid volume deficit* related to potential uterine atony in immediate postpartum, secondary to loss of contractility due to overdistention.
   e. *Sleep pattern disturbance* related to respiratory impairment and discomfort in side-lying position.
   f. *Anxiety* related to discomfort, potential for complications associated with congenital anomalies.
   g. *Altered urinary elimination* (frequency) related to pressure of overdistended uterus on bladder.
5. **Nursing care plan/implementation:**
   a. *Medical management*
      (1) Amniocentesis—remove excess fluid very slowly, to prevent abruptio placentae.
      (2) Termination of pregnancy—if fetal abnormality present *and* woman desires.
   b. *Nursing management*
      (1) Goal: *health teaching.*
         (a) Need for *lateral Sims' position* during resting; semi-Fowler's may alleviate respiratory embarrassment.
         (b) Explain diagnostic or treatment procedures.
         (c) Signs and symptoms to be ***reported immediately:*** bleeding, loss of fluid through vagina, cramping.
      (2) Goal: *prepare for diagnostic and/or treatment procedures.*
         (a) Permission for amniocentesis.
      (3) Goal: *emotional support for loss of pregnancy* (if applicable).
         (a) Encourage verbalization of feelings.
         (b) Facilitate grieving: permit parents to see, hold infant; if desired, take photograph, footprints for them.
6. **Evaluation/outcome criteria:**
   a. Woman complies with medical/nursing management.
   b. Woman's symptoms of respiratory impairment, etc., reduced; comfort promoted.
   c. Woman experiences normal, uncomplicated pregnancy, labor, birth, and postpartum.

III. DIAGNOSTIC TESTS TO EVALUATE FETAL GROWTH AND WELL-BEING

A. Daily fetal movement count (DFMC)
1. Assesses fetal activity.
2. Noninvasive test done by woman who is pregnant.
3. Five to 10 movements per hour: normal activity.
4. Five movements or less per hour may indicate fetal jeopardy or sudden change in movement pattern.
5. Assess for fetal sleep patterns.

B. Nonstress test (NST)
1. Correlates fetal movement with FHR. Requires electronic monitoring.
2. *Reactive test*—three accelerations of FHR to 15 beats/min above baseline FHR, lasting for 15 seconds or more, over 20-minute time period.
3. *Nonreactive test*—no accelerations or acceleration less than 15 beats/min above baseline FHR. May indicate fetal jeopardy. Vibroacoustic simulator (VAS) to differentiate hypoxia from fetal sleep.
4. Unsatisfactory test—data that cannot be interpreted or inadequate fetal activity; repeat.

C. Contraction stress test (CST); oxytocin challenge test (OCT)
1. Correlates fetal heart rate response to spontaneous or induced uterine contractions.
2. Requires electronic monitoring.
3. Indicator of uteroplacental sufficiency.
4. Identifies pregnancies at risk for fetal compromise from uteroplacental insufficiency.
5. Increasing doses of oxytocin are administered to stimulate uterine contractions until three in 10-minute period.
6. Interpretation: *negative* results indicate absence of late decelerations with all contractions.
7. *Positive* results indicate late FHR decelerations with contractions.
8. Nipple stimulation (breast self-stimulation test) may also release enough systemic oxytocin to contract uterus to obtain CST. Instruct *not* to do at home.

D. Biophysical profile (BPP)
1. Observation by ultrasound of four variables for 30 minutes and results of nonstress testing:
   a. Fetal body movements.
   b. Fetal tone.
   c. Amniotic fluid volume.
   d. Fetal breathing movements.
2. Variables are scored at 2 for each variable if present, score of 0 if not present; score of less than 6 is associated with perinatal mortality.

E. Ultrasound
1. Noninvasive procedure involving passage of high-frequency sound waves through uterus to obtain data regarding fetal growth, placental positioning, and the uterine cavity.
2. Purpose may include:
   a. Pregnancy confirmation.
   b. Fetal viability.
   c. Estimation of fetal age.
   d. Biparietal diameter (BPD) measurement.
   e. Placenta location.
   f. Detection of fetal abnormalities.
   g. Confirmation of fetal death.
   h. Identification of multifetal gestations.
   i. Amniotic fluid index.
3. No risk to mother with infrequent use. Fetal risk not determined on long-term basis.

MATERNAL/INFANT

F. Amniocentesis (see **Fig. 4.5**)
1. Invasive procedure for amniotic fluid analysis to assess fetal lung maturity or disease; done after 14 weeks of gestation.
2. Needle placed through abdominal-uterine wall; designated amount of fluid is withdrawn for examination.
3. Empty bladder if gestation greater than 20 weeks.
4. Risk of complications less than 1%. Ultrasound *always* precedes this procedure.
5. *Possible complications:* onset of contractions; infections (probably amnionitis); placental punctures; cord puncture; bladder or fetal puncture.
6. Advise women to observe and report the following to physician: fetal hypoactivity or hyperactivity, vaginal bleeding, vaginal discharge (clear or colored), signs of labor, signs of infection.

G. Analysis of amniotic fluid
1. Chromosomal studies to detect genetic aberrations.
2. Biochemical analysis of fetal cells to detect inborn errors of metabolism.
3. Determination of fetal lung maturity by assessing *lecithin/sphingomyelin* ratio.
4. Evaluation of *phospholipids;* aids in determining lung maturity.
5. Determination of *creatinine* levels; aids in determining fetal age. (*Greater than 1.8* mg/dL indicates fetal maturity and the fetal age.)
6. Assesses isoimmune disease.
7. Presence of meconium may indicate fetal hypoxia.

H. Chorionic villus sampling (CVS)
1. Cervically invasive procedure.
2. Advantage—results can be obtained after 10 weeks of gestation due to fast-growing fetal cells.
3. Procedure—removal of small piece of tissue (chorionic villus) from fetal portion of placenta. Tissue reflects genetic makeup of fetus.
4. Determines some genetic aberrations and allows for earlier decision for induced abortion (if desired) from abnormal results. Does not diagnose neural tube defects; clients who have CVS need further diagnoses with ultrasound.
5. Protects "pregnancy privacy" because results can be obtained before the pregnancy is apparent and decisions can be made regarding abortion or continuation of gestation.
6. Risks involve: spontaneous abortion, infection, hematoma, intrauterine death, Rh isoimmunization, and fetal limb defects, if done before 9 weeks of gestation.

THE INTRAPARTUM EXPERIENCE

General overview: This review of the anatomical and physiological determinants of successful labor provides baseline data against which the nurse compares findings of an ongoing assessment of the woman in labor. Nursing actions are planned and implemented to meet the present and emerging needs of the woman in labor.

I. BIOLOGICAL FOUNDATIONS OF LABOR

A. Premonitory signs
1. *Lightening*—process in which the fetus "drops" into the pelvic inlet.
   a. *Characteristics*
      (1) Nullipara—usually occurs 2 to 3 weeks before onset of labor.
      (2) Multipara—commonly occurs with onset of labor.
   b. *Effects*
      (1) Relieves pressure on diaphragm—breathing is easier.
      (2) Increases pelvic pressure.
         (a) Urinary frequency returns.

(b) Increased pressure on thighs.
(c) Increased tendency to vulvar, vaginal, perianal, and leg varicosities.

2. *Braxton Hicks contractions*—may become more uncomfortable.

B. Etiology: unknown. *Theories* include:
1. Uterine overdistention.
2. Placental aging—*declining* estrogen/progesterone levels.
3. *Rising* prostaglandin level.
4. Fetal cortisol secretion.
5. Maternal/fetal oxytocin secretion.

C. Overview of labor process—forces of labor (involuntary uterine contractions) overcome cervical resistance; cervix thins *(effacement)* and opens (0–10 cm *dilation*) (**Table 4.10**). Voluntary contraction of secondary abdominal muscles during the second stage (e.g., pushing, bearing-down) forces fetal descent. Changing pelvic dimensions force fetal head to accommodate to the birth canal by molding (cranial bones overlap to decrease head size).

Stages of labor:
1. *First*—begins with establishment of regular, rhythmic contractions; ends with complete effacement and dilation (10 cm); divided into three phases:
   a. Latent and early active.
   b. Active.
   c. Transitional.

Table 4.10

First Stage of Labor

Phases of First Stage	Assessment: Expected Maternal Behaviors	Nursing Care Plan/Implementation
0–4 cm: Latent Phase and Early Active Phase		
1. *Time:* multipara 5–6 hours; nullipara 8–10 hours, average	1. Usually comfortable, euphoric, excited, talkative, and energetic, but may be fearful and withdrawn	1. Provide encouragement, feedback for relaxation, companionship, hydration, nutrition
2. *Contractions:* regular, mild, 5–10 minutes apart, 20–30 seconds' duration	2. Relieved or apprehensive that labor has begun	2. Coach during contractions: signal beginning of contraction, mark the seconds, signal end of contraction; "Follow my breathing," "Watch my lips," etc.
3. Low-back pain and abdominal discomfort with contractions	3. Alert, usually receptive to teaching, coaching, diversion, and anticipatory guidance	3. Comfort measures: position change for comfort; praise; keep aware of progress; maintain hydration
4. Cervix thins: some bloody show		
5. *Station:* Multipara −2 to +1; nullipara 0.		
4–8 cm: Midactive Phase, Phase of Most Rapid Dilation		
1. Average *time:* nullipara 1–2 hours; multipara 1½–2 hours	1. Tired, less talkative, and less energetic	1. Coach during contractions; partner (coach) may need some relief
2. *Contractions:* 2–5 minutes apart, 30–40 seconds' duration, intensity increasing	2. More serious, malar flush between 5 and 6 cm, tendency to hyperventilate, may need analgesia, needs constant coaching	2. *Comfort measures* (to partner too—as needed): position for comfort while preventing hypotensive syndrome; encourage relaxation, focusing her on areas of tension; provide counterpressure to sacrococcygeal area, prn; praise; keep aware of progress; minimize distractions from surrounding environment (loud talking, other noises); offer analgesics and anesthetics, as appropriate; provide hygiene: mouth care, ice chips, clean perineum; warmth, as needed
3. Membranes may rupture now		3. Monitor progress of labor and maternal/fetal response, color of fluid, time of rupture of membranes (ROM)
4. Increased bloody show		4. If monitors are in use, attention on mother; periodically check accuracy of monitor readouts
5. *Station:* −1 to 0		

Continued

Table 4.10

First Stage of Labor—cont'd

Phases of First Stage	Assessment: Expected Maternal Behaviors	Nursing Care Plan/Implementation
8–10 cm: Transition, Deceleration Period of Active Phase		
1. Average *time:* nullipara 40 minutes–1 hour; multipara 20 minutes 2. *Contractions:* 1½–2 minutes apart, 60–90 seconds' duration, strong intensity	1. If not under regional anesthesia, more introverted; may be amnesic between contractions 2. Feeling she cannot make it; increased irritability, crying, nausea, vomiting, and belching; increased perspiration over upper lip and between breasts; leg tremors; and shaking	1. Stay with woman (couple) and provide constant support 2. Continue to coach with contractions: may need to remind, reassure, and encourage her to reestablish breathing techniques and concentration with each contraction; coach panting or "he-he" respirations to prevent pushing
3. Increased vaginal show; rectal pressure with beginning urge to bear down	3. May have uncontrollable urge to push at this time	3. Comfort measures; remind her and partner her behavior is normal and "OK"; coach breathing to quell nausea; offer ice chips
4. *Station*: +13 to +14		4. Assist with countertension techniques woman requested 5. Monitor contractions, FHR (after each contraction), vaginal discharge, perineal bulging, maternal vital signs; record every 15 minutes 6. Assess for bladder filling 7. Keep mother (couple) aware of progress 8. Prepare partner for birth (scrub, gown, etc.)

MATERNAL/INFANT

2. *Second*—begins with complete dilation and ends with birth of infant.
3. *Third*—begins with birth of infant and ends with expulsion of placenta.
4. *Fourth*—begins with expulsion of placenta; ends when maternal status is stable (usually 1–2 hours postpartum).

D. Anatomical/physiological determinants

1. **Maternal**
   a. *Uterine contractions*—involuntary; birth; begin process of involution.
      (1) *Characteristics:* rhythmic; increasing tone (*increment*), peak (*acme*), relaxation (*decrement*).
      (2) *Effects:*
         (a) Decreases blood flow to uterus and placenta.
         (b) Dilates cervix during first stage of labor.
         (c) Raises maternal blood pressure during contractions.
         (d) With voluntary bearing-down efforts (abdominal muscles), expels fetus (second stage) and placenta (third stage).
         (e) Begins involution.
      (3) **Assessment:**
         (a) Frequency—time from beginning of one contraction to beginning of the next.
         (b) Duration—time from beginning of contraction to its relaxation.
         (c) Strength (intensity)—resistance to indentation.
         (d) False/true labor—differentiation (**Table 4.11**).
         (e) Signs of dystocia (dysfunctional labor) (see **pp. 184–186**).
   b. *Pelvic structures and configuration:*
      (1) *False pelvis*—above linea terminalis (line travels across top of symphysis pubis around to sacral promontory); supports gravid uterus during pregnancy.
      (2) *True pelvis*—below linea terminalis; divided into:
         (a) Inlet—"brim," demarcated by linea terminalis.
            (i) Widest diameter: transverse.
            (ii) Narrowest diameter: anterior-posterior (true conjugate).
         (b) Midplane—pelvic cavity.
         (c) Outlet.
            (i) Widest diameter: anterior-posterior (requires internal rotation of fetal head for entry).
            (ii) Narrowest diameter: transverse (intertuberous); facilitates birth in occipitoanterior (OA) position.

Table 4.11

Assessment: Differentiation of False/True Labor

False Labor	True Labor
Contractions: Braxton Hicks intensify (more noticeable at night); short, *irregular,* little change	*Contractions:* begin in lower back, radiate to abdomen ("girdling"), become *regular,* rhythmic; *frequency, duration, intensity increase*
Discomfort: mostly abdominal and groin	*Discomfort:* mostly low back
Relieved by change of position or activity (e.g., walking)	*Unaffected* by change of position, activity, drinking two glasses of water, or moderate analgesia
Cervical changes—none; *no* effacement or dilation progress	*Cervical changes—progressive* effacement and dilation

(3) *Classifications*
 (a) Gynecoid—normal female pelvis; rounded oval.
 (b) Android—normal male pelvis; funnel shaped.
 (c) Anthropoid—oval.
 (d) Platypelloid—flattened, transverse oval.

2. **Fetal**
 a. *Fetal head* (**Fig. 4.7**).
 (1) Bones—one occipital, two frontal, two parietals, two temporals.
 (2) Suture—line of junction or closure between bones; sagittal (longitudinal), coronal (anterior), and lambdoid (posterior, frontal); permit molding to accommodate head to birth canal.
 (3) Fontanels—membranous space between cranial bones during fetal life and infancy.
 (a) *Anterior* "soft spot"—diamond shaped; junction of coronal and sagittal sutures; closes (ossifies) by *18 months.*
 (b) *Posterior*—triangular; junction of sagittal and lambdoid sutures; closes by *4 months of age.*
 b. *Fetal lie*—relationship of fetal long axis to maternal long axis (spine).
 (1) Transverse—shoulder presents.
 (2) Longitudinal—vertex or breech presents.
 c. *Presentation*—fetal part entering inlet first (**Fig. 4.8**).
 (1) *Cephalic*—vertex (most common); face, brow.
 (2) *Breech*
 (a) *Complete*—feet and legs flexed on thighs; buttocks and feet presenting.
 (b) *Frank*—legs extended on torso, feet up by shoulders; buttocks presenting.
 (c) *Footling*—single (one foot), double (both feet) presenting.
 d. *Attitude*—relationship of fetal parts to one another (e.g., head flexed on chest).
 e. *Position*—relationship of presenting fetal part to quadrants of maternal pelvis; vertex most common, occiput anterior on maternal left side (LOA) (see **Fig. 4.8**).

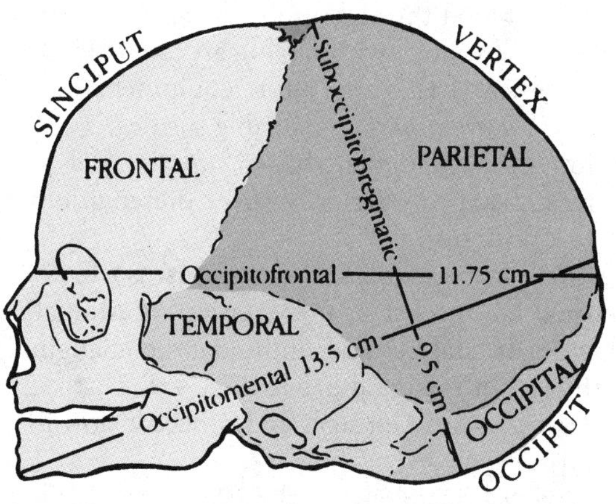

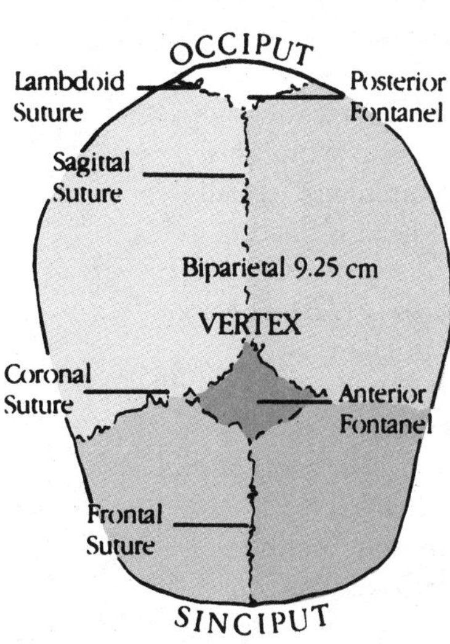

Figure 4.7 The fetal head. *Bones:* two frontal, two temporal, one occipital, two parietal. *Sutures:* sagittal, frontal, coronal, lambdoid. *Fontanels:* anterior, posterior. (From Clinical Education Aid No. 13. Used with permission of Ross Products Division, Abbott Laboratories, Inc., Columbus, OH 43216.)

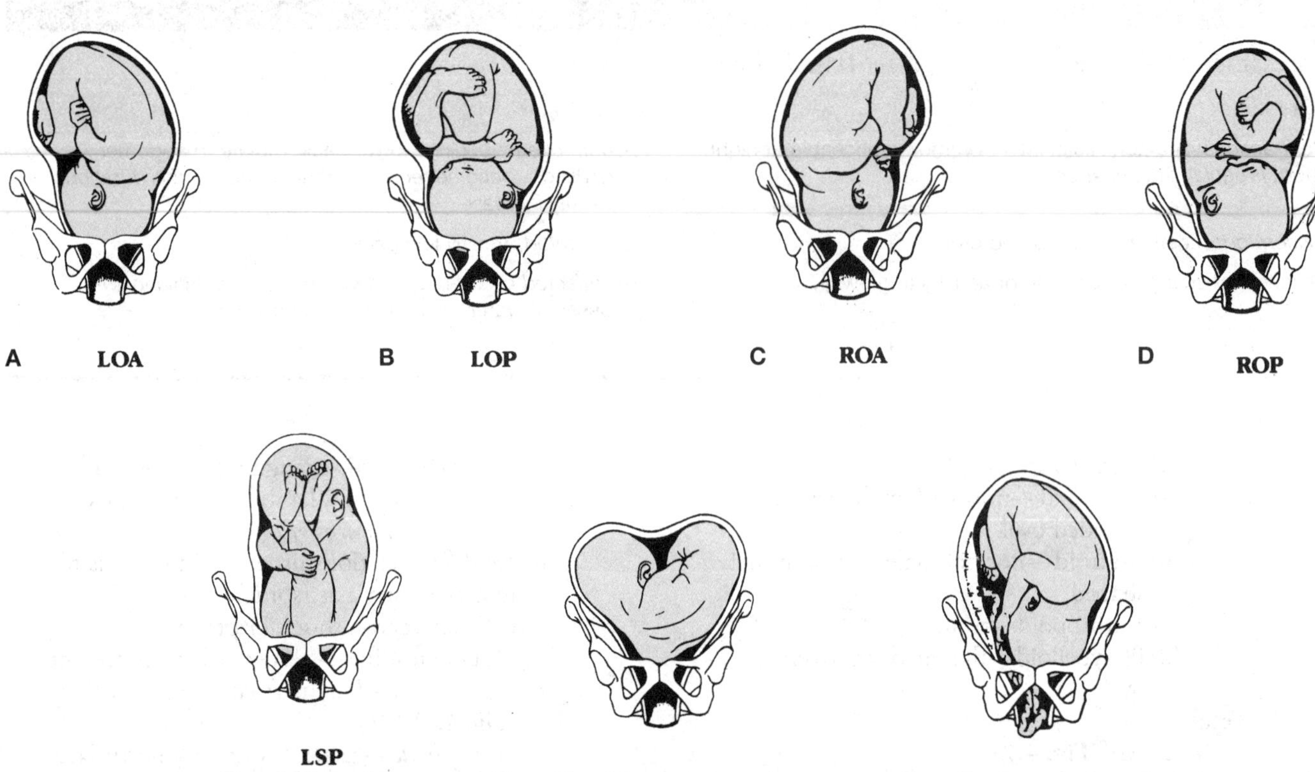

Figure 4.8 **Categories of fetal presentation.** (A) Left occipitoanterior (**LOA**): fetal occiput is in left anterior quadrant of maternal pelvis. (B) Left occipitoposterior (**LOP**): fetal occiput is in left posterior quadrant of maternal pelvis. (C) Right occipitoanterior (**ROA**): fetal occiput is in right anterior quadrant of maternal pelvis. (D) Right occipitoposterior (**ROP**): fetal occiput is in right posterior quadrant of maternal pelvis. (E) Left sacroposterior (**LSP**): fetal sacrum is in left posterior quadrant of maternal pelvis. (F) **Shoulder presentation with fetus in transverse lie.** (G) **Prolapse of umbilical cord** with fetus in LOA position. (From Clinical Education Aid No. 18. Used with permission of Ross Products Division, Abbott Laboratories, Inc., Columbus, OH 43216.)

3. **Assessment:** determine presentation and position.
   a. *Leopold's maneuver*—abdominal palpation.
      (1) *First*—palms over fundus, breech feels softer, not as round as head would be.
      (2) *Second*—palms on either side of abdomen, locates fetal back and small parts.
      (3) *Third*—fingers just above pubic symphysis, grasp lower abdomen; if unengaged, presenting part is mobile.
      (4) *Fourth*—facing mother's feet, run palms down sides of abdomen to symphysis; check for cephalic prominence (usually on right side), and if head is floating or engaged.
   b. *Location of fetal heart tones (FHTs)*—heard best through fetal back or chest.
      (1) *Breech* presentation—usually most audible *above* maternal umbilicus.
      (2) *Vertex* presentation—usually most audible *below* maternal umbilicus.
      (3) Changing location of most audible FHTs—useful indicator of fetal descent.
      (4) Factors affecting audibility:
         (a) Obesity.
         (b) Maternal position.
         (c) Polyhydramnios.
         (d) Maternal gastrointestinal activity.
         (e) Loud uterine bruit—origin: hissing of blood through maternal uterine arteries; synchronous with maternal pulse.
         (f) Loud funic souffle—origin: hissing of blood through umbilical arteries; synchronous with fetal heart rate (FHR).
         (g) External noise, faulty equipment.
   c. *Vaginal examination:* palpable sutures, fontanels (triangular-shaped superior, diamond-shaped inferior = vertex presentation, OA position).
4. *Cardinal movements of the* **mechanisms of normal labor**—vertex presentation, positional changes of fetal head accommodate to changing diameters of maternal pelvis (**Fig. 4.9**).
   a. *Descent*—head engages and proceeds down birth canal.
   b. *Flexion*—head bent to chest; presents smallest diameter of vertex (suboccipital-bregmatic).

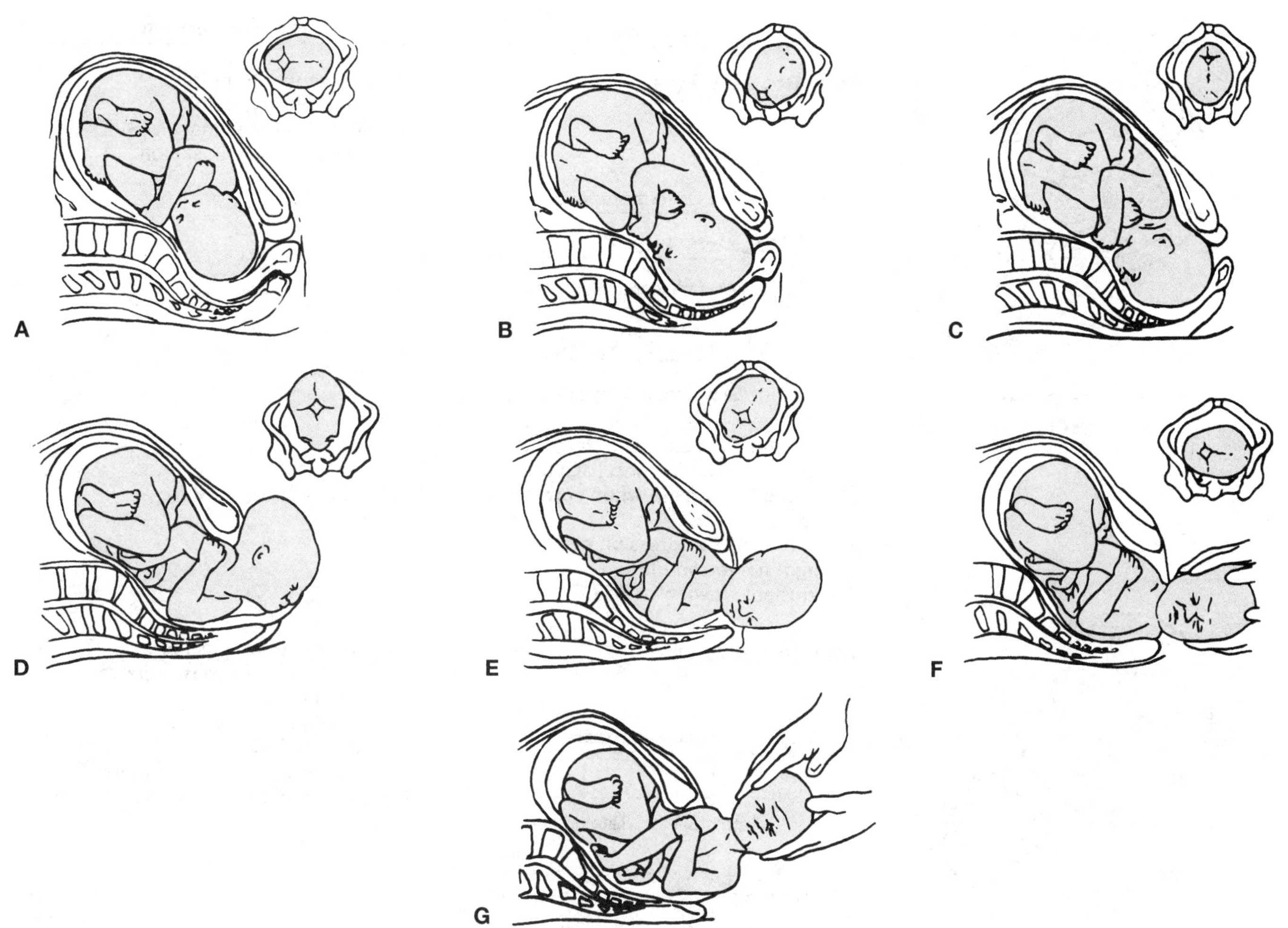

Figure 4.9 **Cardinal movements in the mechanism of labor with the fetus in vertex presentation.** (A) Engagement, descent, flexion. (B) Internal rotation. (C) Extension beginning (rotation complete). (D) Extension complete. (E) External rotation (restitution). (F) External rotation (shoulder rotation). (G) Expulsion. (From Clinical Education Aid No. 13. Used with permission of Ross Products Division, Abbott Laboratories, Inc., Columbus, OH 43216.)

c. *Internal rotation*—during second stage of labor, transverse diameter of fetal head enters pelvis; occiput rotates 90 degrees to bring back of neck under symphysis (e.g., left occipitotransverse [LOT] to LOA to OA); presents smallest diameter (biparietal) to smallest diameter of outlet (intertuberous).
d. *Extension*—back of neck pivots under symphysis, allows head to be born by extension.
e. *Restitution*—head returns to normal alignment with shoulders (with LOA, results in head facing right thigh), presents smallest diameter of shoulders to outlet.
f. *Delivery of head*—shoulders in anterior-posterior position.
g. *Expulsion*—birth of neonate completed.

5. **Assessment:** relationship of fetal head to ischial spines (**degree of descent**).
   a. *Engagement*—widest diameter of presenting part has passed through pelvic inlet (e.g., biparietal diameter of fetal head).
   b. *Station*—relationship of presenting part to ischial spines (IS).
      (1) *Floating*—presenting part above inlet, in false pelvis.
      (2) Station –5 is at inlet (presenting part well above IS).
      (3) Station 0—presenting part at IS (engaged).
      (4) Station +4—presenting part at the outlet.

E. Warning signs during labor

1. *Contraction*—hypertonic, poor relaxation, or tetanic (greater than 90 seconds long and ≤2 minutes apart).
2. *Abdominal pain*—sharp, rigid abdomen.
3. *Vaginal bleeding*—profuse.
4. *FHR*—late decelerations, prolonged variable decelerations, bradycardia, tachycardia (**Fig. 4.10**), decreased variability.
5. *Maternal hypertension.*
6. *Meconium-stained amniotic fluid (MSAF).*
7. *Prolonged ROM.*

Pattern	Description	Nursing Intervention
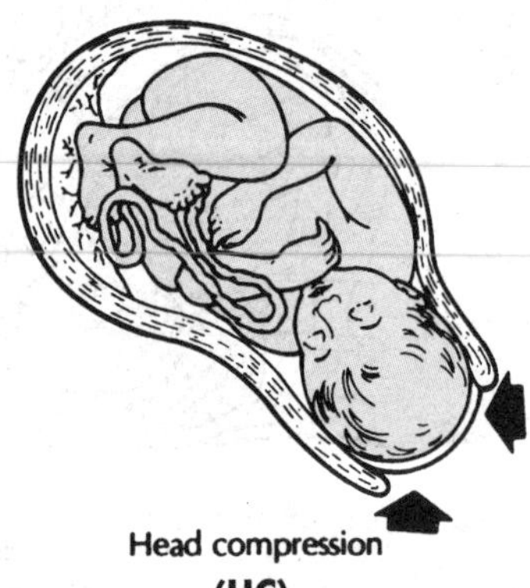 Head compression (HC)	**Early Decelerations** 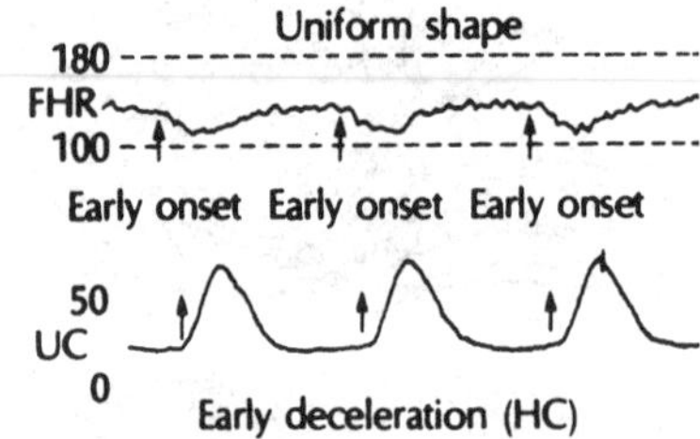 1. FHR begins to slow with the onset of the uterine contraction (UC) and returns to baseline when contraction is over. 2. Fetal head compression occurs. 3. Vagal nerve stimulation. 4. Transient slowing of FHR.	No intervention required. Continue observation. Sterile vaginal examination (SVE) to check for dilation, station.
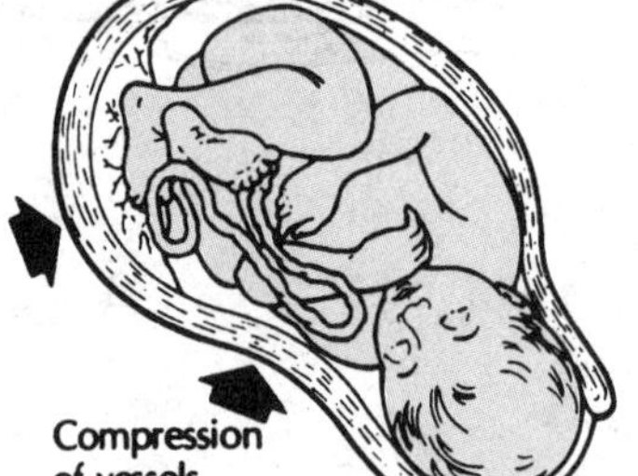 Uteroplacental insufficiency (UPI)	**Late Decelerations** 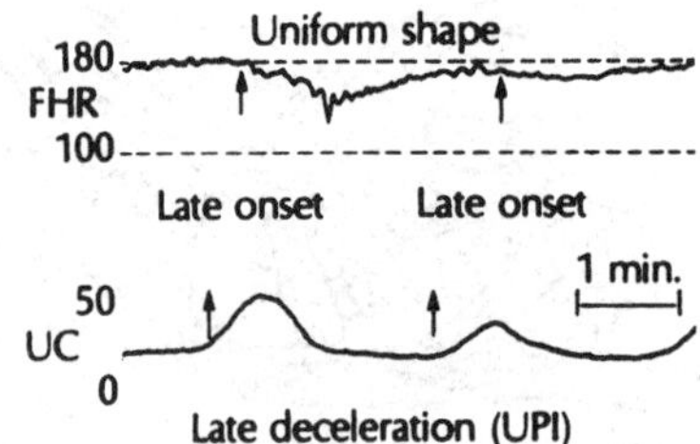 1. FHR begins to fall at height of the UC and returns to baseline after contraction has ceased. 2. FHR usually remains within normal range. 3. Indicates some degree of uteroplacental insufficiency. 4. Baseline variability.	Change maternal position. Turn off Pitocin; increase rate of maintenance IV. Begin oxygen by face mask Notify physician. Check blood pressure and pulse rate. Possible candidate for cesarean birth.
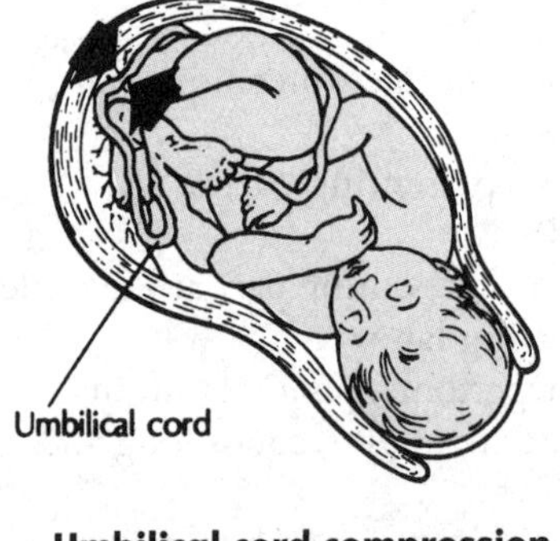 Umbilical cord compression (CC)	**Variable Decelerations** 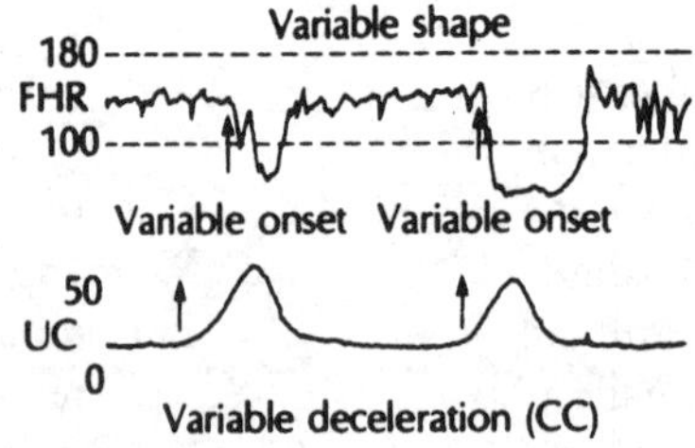 1. Slowing of FHR either with a contraction or in between contractions. Unrelated pattern of FHR and uterine contraction. 2. Pattern may be U shaped or V shaped. Transitory acceleration may precede or follow the deceleration. 3. FHR may fall below 100 beats/min; then returns immediately to baseline. 4. Usually indicates cord compression.	Change maternal position to alleviate cord pressure. Turn off Pitocin; increase rate of maintenance IV. Begin oxygen by face mask. Notify physician. Check blood pressure and pulse rate. Possible candidate for cesarean birth. Possible candidate for amnio infusion.

Figure 4.10 Fetal heart rate (FHR) decelerations and nursing interventions.

II. PARTICIPATORY CHILDBIRTH TECHNIQUES

A. Psychoprophylaxis—Lamaze method

1. Premise—conditioned responses to stimuli occupy nerve pathways, reducing perception of pain. Emphasis is on childbirth as a natural event, with a woman who is informed as the active participant. The ability to relax effectively reduces the perception of pain, and the involvement of the coach fosters the family concept.
2. Childbirth partners are taught:
   a. Anatomy and physiology of labor.
   b. Psychology of man and woman.
   c. What to expect in the birthing setting.
   d. Conditioned responses to labor stimuli.
      (1) Concentration on focal point.
      (2) Breathing techniques.
      (3) Need for active coaching to enable woman to:
         (a) Use techniques appropriate to present stage of labor.
         (b) Avoid hyperventilation.
   e. Specific stage—appropriate techniques:
      (1) *First stage of labor—early:* slow, deep chest breathing; *active:* patterned breathing.
      (2) *Transition* (8–10 cm)—rapid, shallow breathing pattern, to prevent pushing prematurely.
         (a) Panting.
         (b) Pant-blow.
         (c) "He-he" pattern.
      (3) *Second stage of labor*
         (a) Pushing (or bearing-down)—aids fetal descent through birth canal.
         (b) Panting—aids relaxation between contractions; prevents explosive birth of head.
   f. Effects on labor behaviors/coping:
      (1) Helps mother cope with and assist contractions.
      (2) Prevents premature bearing-down efforts; reduces possibility of cervical lacerations, edema due to pushing on incompletely dilated cervix.
      (3) When appropriate, improves efficiency of bearing-down efforts.

B. Other methods—include parent classes, classes for siblings, multiparas, and those who plan cesarean birth.

III. NURSING ACTIONS DURING FIRST STAGE OF LABOR

A. Assessment: careful evaluation of:

1. *Antepartal history*
   a. EDD
   b. Genetic and familial problems.
   c. Preexisting and coexisting medical disorders, allergies.
   d. Pregnancy-related health problems (hyperemesis, bleeding, etc.).
   e. Infectious diseases (past and present herpes, etc.).
   f. Past obstetric history, if any.
   g. Pelvic size estimation.
   h. Height.
   i. Weight gain.
   j. Laboratory results:
      (1) Blood type and Rh factor.
      (2) Serology.
      (3) Urinalysis.
      (4) Hepatitis.
      (5) Rubella.
   k. Prenatal care history.
   l. Use of medications.
2. *Admission findings*
   a. Emotional status.
   b. Vital signs.
   c. Present weight.
   d. Fundal height.
   e. Estimated fetal weight.
   f. Edema.
   g. Urinalysis (for protein and glucose).
3. *FHR*—normal, 110 to 160 beats/min (see **Fig. 4.10**).
   a. Check and record every 15 to 30 minutes—monitor fetal response to physiological stress of labor.
   b. *Bradycardia* (mild, 100–110 beats/min, or 30 beats/min lower than baseline reading).
   c. *Tachycardia* (moderate, 160–179 beats/min, or 30 beats/min above baseline reading lasting 5 or more minutes).
4. *Contractions*—every 15 to 30 minutes.
   a. Place fingertips over fundus, use gentle pressure; contraction felt as hardening or tensing.
   b. Time: frequency and duration.
   c. Intensity/strength at acme:
      (1) Weak—easily indent fundus with fingers.
      (2) Moderate—some tension felt, fundus indents slightly with finger pressure.
      (3) Strong—unable to indent fundus.
5. *Maternal response to labor*—assess for effective coping, cooperation, and using effective breathing techniques.
6. *Maternal vital signs*—between contractions.
   a. Response to pain or use of special breathing techniques alters pulse and respirations.
   b. BP, P, RR—if normotensive: on admission, and then every hour and prn; after regional anesthesia: every 30 minutes (every 5 minutes first 20 minutes).

MATERNAL/INFANT

c. Temperature—if within normal range: on admission, and then every 4 hours and prn. Every 2 hours after rupture of membranes.
d. Before and after analgesia/anesthesia.
e. After rupture of membranes (see **Amniotic fluid embolus, pp. 186–187**).

7. Character and amount of *bloody show.*
8. *Bladder* status: encourage voiding every 1 to 2 hours, monitor output.
   a. Determine bladder distention—palpate just above symphysis (full bladder may impede labor progress or result in trauma to bladder).
   b. Admission urinalysis—check for protein and glucose.
9. Signs of deviations from normal patterns.
10. *Status of membranes:*
    a. Intact.
    b. Ruptured (nitrazine paper turns blue on contact with alkaline amniotic fluid). Fluid may be placed on a glass slide to dry; a fernlike crystallization of sodium chloride will appear. Note, record, and report:
       (1) Time—danger of *infection* if ruptured more than 24 hours.
       (2) FHR stat and 10 minutes later—to check for *prolapsed cord.*
       (3) Character and color of fluid (see **11.b.** and **c.**).
11. Amniotic fluid.
    a. Amount—polyhydramnios (>2000 mL)—associated with *congenital anomalies/poorly controlled diabetes.*
    b. Character—thick consistency or odor associated with *infection.*
    c. Color—normally clear with white specks.
       (1) Yellow—presence of bilirubin; *Rh* or *ABO incompatibility.*
       (2) Green or meconium stained; if fetus in vertex position, indicates recent *fetal hypoxia* secondary to respiratory distress in fetus.
       (3) Port wine—may indicate *abruptio placentae.*
12. *Labor progress:*
    a. Effacement.
    b. Dilation.
    c. Station.
    d. Bulging membranes.
    e. Molding of fetal head.
13. *Perineum*—observe for bulging.

B. Analysis/nursing diagnosis:

1. *Anxiety, fear* related to uncertain outcome, pain.
2. *Ineffective individual coping* related to lack of preparation for childbirth or poor support from coach.
3. *Altered nutrition: less than body requirements* related to physiological stress of labor.
4. *Altered urinary elimination* related to pressure of presenting part.
5. *Altered thought processes* related to sleep deprivation, transition, analgesia.
6. *Fluid volume deficit* related to anemia, excessive blood loss.
7. *Impaired (fetal) gas exchange* related to impaired placental perfusion.

C. Nursing care plan/implementation:

1. Goal: *comfort measures.*
   a. Maintain hydration of oral mucosa. Encourage sucking on cool washcloth, ice chips, lollipops, clear liquids (if ordered).
   b. Reduce dryness of lips. Apply lip balm.
   c. Relieve backache. Apply sacral counterpressure (particularly with occipitoposterior [OP] presentation).
   d. Encourage significant other to participate.
   e. Encourage ambulation when presenting part engaged.
2. Goal: *management of physical needs.*
   a. Encourage frequent voiding to prevent full bladder from impeding oncoming head.
   b. Encourage ambulation throughout labor; *lateral Sims' position with head elevated to:*
      (1) Encourage relaxation.
      (2) Allow gravity to assist in anterior rotation of fetal head.
      (3) Prevent compression of inferior vena cava and descending aorta (*supine hypotensive syndrome*).
      (4) Promote placental perfusion.
   c. Perineal prep, if ordered to promote cleanliness.
   d. Fleet's enema, if ordered—to stimulate peristalsis, evacuate lower bowel. *Note:* **contraindicated** if:
      (1) Cervical dilation (4 cm or more) with unengaged head—due to possibility of cord prolapse.
      (2) Fetal malpresentation/malposition—due to possible fetal distress.
      (3) Preterm labor—may stimulate contractions.
      (4) Painless vaginal bleeding—due to possible placenta previa.
3. Goal: *management of psychosocial needs. Emotional support:*
   a. Encourage verbalization of feelings, fears, concerns.
   b. Explain all procedures.
   c. Reinforce self-concept ("You're doing well!").

4. Goal: *management of discomfort.*
   a. Analgesia or anesthesia—may be required or desired—to facilitate safe, comfortable birth.
   b. Support/enhance/teach childbirth techniques.
      (1) Reinforce appropriate *breathing techniques* for current labor status.
         (a) If woman is **hyperventilating,** to increase $Paco_2$, minimize fetal acidosis, and relieve symptoms of vertigo and syncope, suggest:
            (i) Breathe into paper bag.
            (ii) Breathe into cupped hands.
         (b) Demonstrate appropriate breathing for several contractions—to reestablish rate and rhythm.
5. Goal: *sustain motivation.*
   a. Offer support, encouragement, and praise, as appropriate.
   b. Keep informed of status and progress.
   c. Reassure that irritability is normal.
   d. Serve as surrogate coach when necessary (if no partner, before partner arrives, while partner changes clothes, during needed breaks); assist with effleurage, breathing, focusing.
   e. Discourage bearing-down efforts by pant-blow until complete (10-cm) dilation to avoid cervical edema/laceration.
   f. Facilitate informed decision making regarding medication for relaxation or pain relief.
   g. Minimize distractions: quiet, relaxed environment; privacy.

D. Evaluation/outcome criteria:

1. Woman manages own labor discomfort effectively.
2. Woman maintains control over own behavior.
3. Woman successfully completes first stage of labor without incident.

IV. NURSING ACTIONS DURING SECOND STAGE OF LABOR

A. Assessment:

1. Maternal (or couple's) response to labor.
2. FHR—continuous electronic monitoring, or after each contraction with fetoscope, Doppler.
3. Vital signs.
4. Time elapsed—average: 2 minutes to 1 hour; prolonged second stage increases risk of: fetal distress, maternal exhaustion, psychological stress, intrauterine infection.
5. Contraction pattern—average every 1½ to 3 minutes, lasting 60 to 90 seconds.
6. Vaginal discharge—increases.
7. Nausea, vomiting, disorientation, tremors, amnesia between contractions, panic.
8. Response to regional anesthesia, if administered.
   a. Signs of hypotension—reduces placental perfusion, increases risk of fetal hypoxia.
   b. Effect on contractions—note and report any slowing of labor progress.
9. Efforts to bear down—increases expulsive effects of uterine contractions.
10. Perineal bulging with contractions—fetal head distends perineum, crowns; head born by extension.

B. Analysis/nursing diagnosis:

1. *Pain* related to strong uterine contractions, pressure of fetal descent, stretching of perineum.
2. *High risk for injury:*
   a. Infection related to ruptured membranes, repeated vaginal examinations.
   b. Laceration related to pressure of fetal head exceeding perineal elasticity.
3. *Impaired skin integrity* related to laceration, episiotomy.
4. *Fluid volume deficit* related to hypotension secondary to regional anesthesia.
5. *Anxiety* related to imminent birth of fetus.
6. *Ineffective individual coping* related to prolonged sensory stimulation (contractions) and anxiety.
7. *Altered urinary elimination* related to anesthesia and contractions, descent of fetal head.
8. *Sleep pattern disturbance.*

C. Nursing care plan/implementation:

1. Goal: *emotional support.*
   a. To sustain motivation/control:
      (1) Never leave mother and significant other alone during second stage.
      (2) Keep informed of progress.
      (3) Direct bearing-down efforts (pushing) without holding breath* while pushing. Encourage pushing "out through vagina" and encourage mother to touch crowning head; position mirror so woman can see perineal bulging with effective efforts; minimize distractions.
   b. To allay significant other's anxiety: reassure regarding mother's behavior if she is not anesthetized.
   c. Support family choices.
2. Goal: *safeguard status.*
   a. Precautions when putting legs in stirrups:
      (1) If varicosities, **do not put legs in stirrups.**

*The woman must be discouraged from using the **Valsalva maneuver** (holding one's breath and tightening abdominal muscles) for pushing during the second stage. This activity increases intrathoracic pressure, reduces venous return, and increases venous pressure. Cardiac output and blood pressure increase, and pulse slows temporarily. During the Valsalva maneuver, fetal hypoxia may occur. The process is reversed when the woman takes a breath.

(2) *Avoid* pressure to popliteal veins; pad stirrups.
(3) Ensure proper, even alignment by adjusting stirrups.
(4) Move legs simultaneously into or out of stirrups—to *avoid* nerve, ligament, and muscle strain.
(5) Provide proper support to woman not using stirrups. Do **not** hold legs (can cause back injury).

b. Support woman in whatever position selected for birth (e.g., side-lying position).
c. Cleanse perineum, thighs as ordered.

3. Goal: *maintain a comfortable environment.*
   a. Free of unnecessary noise, light.
   b. Comfortable temperature (warm).
4. *Medical management:*
   a. Episiotomy may be performed to facilitate birth.
   b. Forceps may be applied to exert traction and expedite birth.
   c. Vacuum extraction also used to assist birth.
5. Birthing room birth with alternative positions (squat).

D. Evaluation/outcome criteria:
1. Cooperative, actively participates in birth; maintains control over own behavior.
2. Successful, uncomplicated birth of viable infant.
3. All assessment findings within normal limits (vital signs, emotional status, response to birth).
4. Presence of significant other.

V. NURSING ACTIONS DURING THIRD STAGE OF LABOR

A. Assessment:
1. Time elapsed—average: 5 minutes; prolonged third stage (greater than 25 minutes) may indicate complications (placenta accreta).
2. Signs of *placental separation:*
   a. Increase in bleeding from the vagina.
   b. Cord lengthens.
   c. Uterus rises in abdomen, assumes globular shape.
3. Assess mother's level of consciousness.
4. Examine placenta for intactness and number of vessels in umbilical cord (normal: three. *Note:* two vessels only—associated with increased incidence of congenital anomalies); condition of placenta for calcification, infarcts, etc.

B. Analysis/nursing diagnosis:
1. *Family coping: potential for growth* related to bonding, beginning achievement of developmental tasks.
2. *Fluid volume deficit* related to blood loss during third stage.

C. Nursing care plan/implementation:

1. Goal: *prevent uterine atony.* Administer oxytocin, as ordered.
2. Goal: *facilitate parent-child bonding.*
   a. While protecting neonate from cold stress, encourage parents to see, hold, touch neonate.
   b. Comment about neonate's individuality, characteristics, and behaviors.
   c. After neonate is assessed for congenital anomalies (e.g., cleft palate, esophageal atresia), encourage breastfeeding, if desired.
3. Goal: *health teaching.*
   a. Describe, discuss common neonatal behavior in transitional period (periods of reactivity, sleep, hyperactivity).
   b. Demonstrate removal of mucus by aspiration with bulb syringe.
   c. Demonstrate ways of facilitating breastfeeding.

D. Evaluation/outcome criteria:
1. Woman has a successful, uneventful completion of labor.
   a. Minimal blood loss.
   b. Vital signs within normal limits.
   c. Fundus well contracted at level of umbilicus.
2. Parents express satisfaction with outcome, demonstrate infant attachment.

VI. NURSING ACTIONS DURING THE FOURTH STAGE OF LABOR—1 TO 2 HOURS POSTPARTUM

A. Assessment—every 15 minutes four times; then, every 30 minutes two times—or until stable—to monitor response to physiological stress of labor/birth.
1. Vital signs:
   a. *Temperature* taken once; if elevated, requires follow-up—may indicate infection, dehydration, excessive blood loss. Note, record, report temperature of 100.4°F (38°C).
   b. *Blood pressure*—every 15 minutes × 4.
      (1) Returns to prelabor level—due to loss of placental circulation and increased circulating blood volume.
      (2) Elevation may be in response to use of oxytocic drugs or preeclampsia (first 48 hours).
      (3) Lowered blood pressure—may reflect significant blood loss during labor/birth, or occult bleeding.
   c. Pulse—every 15 minutes × 4.
      (1) Physiological bradycardia—due to normal vagal response.
      (2) Tachycardia—may indicate excessive blood loss during labor/birth, dehydration, exhaustion, maternal fever, or occult bleeding.

2. Location and tone of fundus—every 15 minutes × 4 to ensure continuing contraction; prevent blood loss due to uterine relaxation.
   a. Fundus—firm; at or slightly lower than the umbilicus; in midline.
   b. May be displaced by distended bladder—due to normal diuresis; common cause of bleeding in immediate postpartum, uterine atony.
3. Character and amount of vaginal flow.
   a. Moderate lochia rubra.
   b. Excessive loss: if perineal pad saturated in 15 minutes, or blood pools under buttocks.
   c. Bright red bleeding may indicate cervical or vaginal laceration.
4. Perineum.
   a. Edema.
   b. Bruising—due to trauma.
   c. Distention/hematoma, rectal pain.
5. Bladder fullness/voiding—to prevent distention.
6. Rate of IV, if present; response to added medication, if any.
7. Intake and output—to evaluate hydration.
8. Recovery from analgesia/anesthesia.
9. Energy level.
10. Verbal, nonverbal interaction between woman and significant other.
    a. Dialogue.
    b. Posture.
    c. Facial expressions.
    d. Touching.
11. Interactions between parent(s) and newborn; signs of bonding (culturally appropriate).
    a. Eye contact with newborn.
    b. Calls by name.
    c. Explores with fingertips, strokes, cuddles.
12. Signs of **postpartum emergencies:**
    a. Uterine atony, hemorrhage.
    b. Vaginal hematoma.

B. Analysis/nursing diagnosis:

1. *Fluid volume deficit* related to excessive intrapartum blood loss, dehydration.
2. *Altered urinary elimination* related to intrapartum bladder trauma, dehydration, blood loss.
3. *Impaired skin integrity* related to episiotomy, lacerations, cesarean birth.
4. *Altered family processes* related to role change.
5. *Altered parenting* related to interruption in bonding secondary to:
   a. Compromised maternal status.
   b. Compromised neonatal status.
6. *Knowledge deficit* related to self-care procedures, infant care.
7. *Fatigue* related to sleep disturbances and anxiety.
8. *Anxiety* regarding status of self and infant.
9. *Altered nutrition, less than body requirements,* related to decreased food and fluid intake during labor.

C. Nursing care plan/implementation:

1. Goal: *comfort measures.*
   a. Position, pad change.
   b. Perineal care—to promote healing; to reduce possibility of infection.
   c. Ice pack to perineum; as ordered—to reduce edema, discomfort, and pain related to hemorrhoids.
2. Goal: *nutrition/hydration.* Offer fluids, foods as tolerated.
3. Goal: *urinary elimination.*
   a. Encourage voiding—to *avoid* bladder distention.
   b. Record: time, amount, character.
   c. Anticipatory guidance related to nocturnal diuresis and increased output.
4. Goal: *promote bonding.*
   a. Provide privacy, quiet; encourage sustained contact with newborn.
   b. Encourage: touching, holding baby; breastfeeding (also promotes involution).
5. Goal: *health teaching.*
   a. Perineal care—front to back, labia closed (after *each* void/bowel movement).
   b. Hand washing—before and after each pad change; after voiding, defecating; before and after baby care.
   c. Signs to report:
      (1) Uterine cramping/ ↑ pain.
      (2) Increased vaginal bleeding, passage of large clots.
      (3) Nausea, dizziness.

D. Evaluation/outcome criteria:

1. Expresses comfort, satisfaction in fourth stage.
2. Vital signs stable, fundus contracted, moderate lochia rubra, perineum undistended.
3. Tolerates food and fluids well.
4. Voids an adequate amount.
5. Demonstrates culturally appropriate contact with infant.
6. Verbalizes abnormal signs to report to physician.
7. Returns demonstration of appropriate perineal care.
8. Ambulates without pain, dizziness, numbness of legs.

VII. NURSING MANAGEMENT OF THE NEWBORN IMMEDIATELY AFTER BIRTH

A. Assessment:

1. Mucus in nasopharynx, oropharynx.
2. *Apgar score:* note and record—at 1 and 5 minutes of age (**Table 4.12**).
   a. Score of 7–10: *good* condition.
   b. Score of 4–6: *fair* condition; assess for CNS depression.
   c. Score of 0–3: *poor* condition; requires immediate intervention. *Asphyxia neonatorum*—fails to breathe spontaneously within 30–60 seconds after birth; heart rate (HR) <100.
3. Number of vessels in umbilical stump.
4. Passage of meconium stool, urine.
5. General physical appearance/status.
   a. Signs of respiratory distress (nasal flaring, grunting, sternal retraction, cyanosis, tachypnea).
   b. Skin condition (meconium stained, cyanosis, jaundice, lesions).
   c. Cry—presence, pitch, quality.
   d. Signs of birth trauma (lacerations, dislocations, fractures).
   e. Symmetry (absent parts, extra digits, gross malformations, ears, palm creases, sacral dimples).
   f. Molding, caput succedaneum, cephalohematoma.
   g. Assess gestational age.
6. Identify high-risk infant.

B. Analysis/nursing diagnosis:

1. *Ineffective airway clearance* related to excessive nasopharyngeal mucus.
2. *Ineffective breathing pattern* related to CNS depression secondary to intrauterine hypoxia narcosis, prematurity, and lack of pulmonary surfactant.
3. *Impaired gas exchange* related to respiratory distress.
4. *Fluid volume deficit* related to birth trauma; hemolytic jaundice.
5. *Impaired skin integrity* related to cord stump.
6. *High risk for injury* (biochemical, metabolic) related to impaired thermoregulation.
7. *Ineffective thermoregulation* related to environmental conditions/prematurity.

C. Nursing care plan/implementation:

1. Goal: *ensure patent airway.*
   a. Suction mouth first, then nose; when stimulated, sensitive receptors around entrance to nares initiate gasp, causing aspiration of mucus present in mouth.
   b. Suction with bulb syringe.
      (1) If deeper suctioning necessary, use DeLee Mucus Trap attached to suction. Oral use of DeLee is contraindicated due to risk of contact with baby's secretions (new DeLee now available that has no such risk).
      (2) *Avoid* prolonged, vigorous suctioning.
         (a) Reduces oxygenation.
         (b) May traumatize tissue, cause edema, bleeding, laryngospasm, and cardiac arrhythmia.
   c. Assist gravity drainage of fluids. *Position:* head dependent (Trendelenburg) and side-lying position.
2. Goal: *maintain body temperature*—to conserve energy, preserve store of brown fat, decrease oxygen needs; prevent acidosis. Prevent chilling:
   a. Minimize exposure; dry quickly.
   b. Keep warm; apply hat.
   c. Take temperature hourly until stable.
3. Goal: *identify infant:*
   a. Apply Identiband.
   b. Take infant's footprints and maternal fingerprints.
4. Goal: *prevent eye infection* (gonorrheal and *chlamydial ophthalmia neonatorum*). Within 1 hour of birth, apply antibiotic ointment in each eye.
5. Goal: *facilitate prompt identification/vigilance for potential neonatal complications.*
   a. Record significant data from mother's chart:
      (1) History of: pregnancy, diabetes, hypertension, current drug abuse, excessive caffeine, medications, alcohol, malnutrition.

Table 4.12

Apgar Score

Sign	0	1	2
Heart rate	Absent	<100	>100
Respiratory effort	Absent	Slow and irregular	Good and strong, loud crying
Activity: muscle tone	Flaccid	Some flexion or extremities	Active motions, general flexion
Reflex irritability	No response to stimuli	Weak cry or grimace	Cry: vigorous
Appearance: color	Blue, pale	Body pink, extremities blue	Completely pink

MATERNAL/INFANT

(2) Course of labor, evidence of fetal distress, medications received in labor.
(3) Birth history of anesthesia.
(4) Apgar score; resuscitative efforts.

6. Goal: *facilitate prompt identification/intervention in hemolytic problems of the newborn.*
   a. Collect and send cord blood for appropriate tests:
      (1) Blood type and Rh factor.
      (2) Coombs' test.
   b. Give vitamin K to facilitate clotting.

D. Evaluation/outcome criteria: successful transition to extrauterine life.
1. Status satisfactory; all assessment findings within normal limits.
2. Responsive in bonding process with parents.

VIII. NURSE-ATTENDED EMERGENCY BIRTH (PRECIPITATE BIRTH)

—When woman presents without prenatal care (to emergency department), may represent drug abuse.

IMMINENT BIRTH

A. Assessment: identify signs of *imminent birth:*
1. Strong contractions.
2. Bearing-down efforts.
3. Perineal bulging; crowning.
4. Mother states, "It's coming."

B. Analysis/nursing diagnosis:
1. *Pain* related to:
   a. Strong, sustained contractions.
   b. Descent of fetal head.
   c. Stretching of perineum.
2. *Anxiety/fear* related to imminent birth.
3. *Ineffective individual coping* related to circumstances surrounding birth; anxiety, fear for self and infant.
4. *Injury* (mother) related to lacerations (vaginal, perineal).
5. *Fluid volume deficit* related to:
   a. Lacerations.
   b. Uterine atony.
   c. Retained placental fragments.
6. *Impaired gas exchange* (infant) related to intact membranes after birth.
7. *Risk for injury* (infant) related to:
   a. Precipitate birth.
   b. Trauma.
   c. Hypoxia.

C. Nursing care plan/implementation:
1. Goal: *reduce anxiety/fear*—reassure mother.
2. Goal: *delay birth,* as possible.
   a. Discourage bearing-down efforts.
   b. Encourage panting.
   c. *Side-lying position* to slow descent and allow for more controlled birth.
3. Goal: *prevent infection.*
   a. Provide clean field for birth.
   b. *Avoid* touching birth canal without gloved hands.
   c. Support perineum (and advancing head) with sterile (or clean) towel.
4. Goal: *prevent, or minimize, infant hypoxia* and perineal lacerations.
   a. If membranes intact as head emerges, tear at neck to facilitate first breath.
   b. Feel for cord around neck (if present, and if possible, slip cord over head; if tight, *and* sterile equipment at hand, clamp cord in two places, cut between clamps, unwrap cord). If unsterile environment, keep fetus and placenta attached—do not cut cord.
5. Goal: *facilitate/assist birth.*
   a. Hold head in both hands.
   b. Apply gentle downward pressure to bring anterior shoulder under pubic symphysis.
   c. Gently lift head to ease birth of posterior shoulder.
   d. Support infant as body slips free of mother's body.
6. Goal: *facilitate drainage of mucus and fluid →* patent airway.
   a. Hold infant in head-dependent *position.*
   b. Clear mucus with bulb syringe (if available), or use fingertip, wipe with towel.
7. Goal: *prevent placental transfusion*—hold infant level with placenta until cord stops pulsating; clamp and cut.
8. Goal: *prevent chilling.*
   a. Wrap infant in towel or other clean material.
   b. Place infant on *side, head dependent,* on mother's abdomen.
   c. Dry head, cover with cap or material.
9. Goal: *stimulate respiration.* If neonate *fails to breathe* spontaneously:
   a. Maintain body temperature—dry and cover.
   b. Clear airway

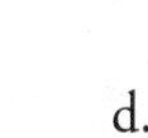

      (1) *Position:* head *down.*
      (2) Turn head to *side.*
   c. Stimulate.
      (1) Rub back gently.
      (2) Flick soles of feet.
   d. If no response to stimulation:
      (1) Slightly extend neck to "sniffing" *position* (head tilt–chin lift method).
      (2) Place mouth over newborn's nose and mouth and exhale air in cheeks, saying "ho" (prevents excessive pressure).

10. Goal: begin *cardiopulmonary resuscitation (CPR)* if heart rate <60 beats/min.
    a. Place infant on firm, flat surface.
    b. With two fingers placed ½ to ¾ of an inch above the xyphoid process, depress ⅓ to ½ depth of anterior-posterior chest.
    c. Assist ventilation on upstroke of every third compression (3:1 ratio).
    d. Go immediately to emergency department.
11. Goal: *maintain infant's body temperature.*
    a. Wrap placenta with baby, if cord intact.
    b. Place infant in mother's arms.

PLACENTAL SEPARATION

A. Assessment—*third stage:* identify signs of *placental separation.*

B. Nursing care plan/implementation:

1. Goal: *avoid/minimize potential for complications* (everted uterus, tearing of placenta with fragments remaining, separation of cord from placenta).
    a. *Avoid* traction (pulling) on cord.
    b. *Avoid* vigorous fundal massage.
    c. Discourage maternal bearing-down efforts unless placenta visible at introitus.
    d. With fundus well contracted, and placenta visible at introitus, encourage mother to bear down to expel placenta.
2. Goal: *prevent maternal hemorrhage* (uterine atony).
    a. Encourage breastfeeding, or stimulate nipple.
    b. Gently massage fundus, support lower part of uterus, and express clots when uterus is contracted.
    c. Encourage voiding if bladder is full.
    d. Get to a medical facility.
3. Goal: *encourage bonding/stimulate uterine contractions.* Encourage breastfeeding.
4. Goal: *legal accountability* as birth attendant. Record date, time, birth events, maternal and fetal status.

C. Evaluation/outcome criteria:

1. Experiences normal spontaneous birth of viable infant over intact perineum.
2. Uncomplicated fourth stage—status satisfactory for both mother and infant.
3. Expresses satisfaction in management and result.

IX. ALTERATIONS AFFECTING PROTECTIVE FUNCTION

A. Induction of labor—deliberate initiation of uterine contractions.

1. Indications for:
    a. History of rapid or silent labors, precipitate birth.
    b. Woman resides some distance from hospital (controversial).
    c. Coexisting medical disorders:
        (1) Uncontrolled diabetes.
        (2) Progressive preeclampsia.
        (3) Severe renal disease.
        (4) Cardiac disease.
    d. PROM—spontaneous rupture of membranes before onset of labor and less than 37 weeks from last menstrual period. **Hazards:**
        (1) Maternal—intrauterine infection (chorioamnionitis, endometritis).
        (2) Fetal—sepsis; prolapsed cord.
    e. Rh or ABO incompatibility, fetal hemolytic disease.
    f. Congenital anomaly (e.g., anencephaly).
    g. Postterm pregnancy with nonreactive nonstress test (NST), or oligohydramnios.
    h. Intrauterine fetal demise.
2. *Criteria for induction:*
    a. Absence of CPD, malpresentation, or malposition.
    b. Engaged vertex of single gestation.
    c. Nearing, or at term.
    d. Fetal lung maturity.
        (1) Survival rate—better at 32 weeks or more.
        (2) *Lecithin/sphingomyelin* ratio greater than 2:1.
        (3) Mother who is diabetic—PG is present in amniotic fluid.
    e. "Ripe" cervix—softening, partially effaced, or ready for effacement/dilation (if not already present). *Note:* Intravaginal or paracervical application of prostaglandin gel, or misoprostol may be used to prepare cervix for labor.
3. *Methods:*
    a. Amniotomy—artificial rupture of membranes with fetal head engaged and dilation of cervix.
    b. Intravenous oxytocin infusion.
4. *Potential complications:*
    a. *Amniotomy*—irrevocably committed to birth. **Hazards:**
        (1) Prolapsed cord.
        (2) Infection.
    b. *IV oxytocin infusion:*
        (1) Overstimulation of uterus.
        (2) Decreased placental perfusion/fetal distress, neonatal jaundice.
        (3) Precipitate labor and birth.
        (4) Cervical/perineal lacerations.
        (5) Uterine rupture.
        (6) Postpartum hemorrhage.
        (7) Water intoxication—if large doses given in D/W over prolonged period (antidiuretic effect increases water reabsorption).
        (8) Hypertensive crisis.

BEFORE INDUCTION

5. **Assessment**—*before induction:*
   a. Estimate of gestation (EDD, fundal height, cervical status).
   b. *Bishop's score:* evaluation of cervical inducibility.
   c. General health status:
      (1) Weight, vital signs, FHR, edema.
      (2) Status of membranes.
      (3) Vaginal bleeding.
      (4) Coexisting disorders.
   d. History of previous labors, if any.
   e. Emotional status.
   f. Knowledge/understanding of anticipated procedures:
      (1) Amniotomy (artificial rupture of membranes).
      (2) Cervical ripening (prostaglandin gel, Cervidil, Cytotec).
      (3) IV oxytocin infusion.
      (4) Fetal monitoring
   g. Preparation for childbirth (Lamaze method, etc.); coping strategies. Identify support person.
6. **Analysis/nursing diagnosis:**
   a. *Knowledge deficit* related to process of induction.
   b. *Anxiety/fear* related to need for induction of labor.
   c. *Ineffective individual coping* related to psychological stress.
   d. *Pain* related to uterine contractions.
7. **Nursing care plan/implementation:**
   a. Goal: *health teaching.*
      (1) Explain rationale for procedures:
         (a) *Amniotomy.*
            (i) Induces labor.
            (ii) Relieves uterine overdistention.
            (iii) Increases efficiency of contractions, shortening labor.
         (b) *Oxytocin infusion.*
            (i) Induces labor.
            (ii) Stimulates uterine contractions.
         (c) *Internal fetal monitor.*
            (i) Provides continuous assessment of uterine response to oxytocin stimulation.
            (ii) Provides continuous assessment of fetal response to physiological stress of labor.
      (2) *Describe procedure*—to reduce anxiety and increase cooperation.
      (3) *Explain advantages/disadvantages*—to ensure "informed consent."
   b. Goal: *emotional support*—encourage verbalization of concerns; reassure, as possible.
8. **Evaluation/outcome criterion:** woman verbalizes understanding of process, rationale, procedures, and alternatives.

DURING INDUCTION AND LABOR

9. **Assessment**—*during induction and labor:*
   a. *Amniotomy*—same as for spontaneous rupture of membranes:
      (1) Observe fluid—note color, amount.
      (2) Monitor FHR; assess for fetal distress.
      (3) Observe for signs of prolapsed cord.
      (4) Assess fetal activity.
         (a) *Excessive* activity may indicate distress.
         (b) *Absence* of activity may indicate distress or demise.
   b. *IV oxytocin infusion:*
      (1) Continually assess response to oxytocin stimulation/flow rate; always given by controlled infusion.
         (a) Uterine contractions.
         (b) Maternal vital signs, FHR.
      (2) Identify signs of:
         (a) *Deviation* from normal patterns:
            (i) Lack of response to increasing flow rate.
            (ii) Uterine hyperstimulation (contractions—less than 2 minutes apart).
            (iii) Lack of adequate uterine relaxation between contractions.
         (b) *Side effects* of oxytocin: diminished output—potential water intoxication.
         (c) **Hazards** to mother or fetus:
            (i) Sustained (over 90-second) or tetanic (strong, spasmlike) contractions—potential abruptio placentae, uterine rupture, fetal hypoxia/anoxia/death.
            (ii) *Fetal* arrhythmias, decelerations.
            (iii) *Maternal* hypertension—potential for hypertensive crisis, cerebral hemorrhage.
10. **Nursing care plan/implementation:**
   a. Same as for other women in labor.
   b. If indications of deviations from normal patterns:

      (1) Change maternal position.
      (2) Stop oxytocin infusion, maintain IV with Ringer's lactate, etc.
      (3) Begin oxygen per mask; up to 8 to 10 L/min.
      (4) Notify physician promptly.
      (5) Check maternal blood pressure and pulse rate.
   c. Anticipatory guidance: may or may not have strong contractions soon after induction starts.

11. **Evaluation/outcome criteria:**
    a. Demonstrates response to oxytocin stimulation.
        (1) Establishes desired contraction pattern, not hyperstimulated.
        (2) Progresses through labor—within normal limits:
            (a) Normotensive.
            (b) Voids in adequate amounts.
            (c) No evidence of deviation from normal contraction patterns.
    b. No evidence of fetal distress.
    c. Experiences normal vaginal birth of viable infant.

B. Operative obstetrics—procedures used to prevent trauma/reduce hazard to mother or infant during the birth process.

1. **Episiotomy**—incision of perineum to facilitate infant's birth.
    a. Rationale:
        (1) Surgical incision reduces possibility of laceration.
        (2) Protects infant's head from pressure exerted by resistant perineum.
        (3) Shortens second stage of labor.
    b. Types:
        (1) Midline—chance of extension into anal sphincter greater than with mediolateral.
        (2) Mediolateral—healing is more painful than midline.
    c. **Assessment:**

        (1) **REEDA:**
            (a) ***R***edness
            (b) ***E***dema
            (c) ***E***cchymosis
            (d) ***D***ischarge
            (e) ***A***pproximation (suture line intact, separated)
        (2) Healing.
        (3) Bruised; hematoma.
        (4) Tenderness; pain. *Note:* Evaluate complaints of pain carefully. If intense, and unrelieved by usual measures, report promptly. May indicate vulvar, paravaginal, or ischiorectal abscess or hematoma.
    d. **Analysis/nursing diagnosis:**
        (1) *Pain* related to labor process.
        (2) *Impaired skin integrity* related to surgical incision.
        (3) *Fluid volume deficit* related to hematoma.
        (4) *Sexual dysfunction* related to discomfort.
    e. **Nursing care plan/implementation:**
        (1) Goal: *prevent/reduce edema, promote comfort and healing.*
            (a) Place covered ice pack during immediate postpartum.
            (b) Administer analgesics, topical sprays, ointments, witch hazel pads, hydrocortisone.
            (c) Encourage use of sitz bath or rubber ring.
            (d) Encourage Kegel exercises.
            (e) Do *health teaching:*
                (i) Instruct in tightening gluteal muscles before sitting.
                (ii) Instruct to *avoid* sitting on one hip.
        (2) Goal: *minimize potential for infection.*
            (a) Teach/provide perineal care during fourth stage of labor.
            (b) *Health teaching:* instruct in self-perineal care after voiding, defecation, and with each pad change.
    f. **Evaluation/outcome criteria:**
        (1) Woman's incision heals by primary intention.
        (2) Woman demonstrates appropriate self-perineal care.
        (3) Woman evidences no signs of hematoma, infection, or separation of suture line.
        (4) Woman experiences minimal discomfort.
2. **Forceps-assisted birth**—use of instruments to assist birth of infant.
    a. Indications:
        (1) Fetal distress.
        (2) Maternal need:
            (a) Exhaustion.
            (b) Coexisting disease, such as cardiac disorder.
            (c) Poor progress in second stage.
            (d) Persistent fetal occipitotransverse (OT) or occipitoposterior (OP) position.
    b. *Criteria* for forceps application:
        (1) Engaged fetal head.
        (2) Ruptured membranes.
        (3) Full dilation.
        (4) Absence of CPD.
        (5) Some anesthesia has been given; usually, episiotomy has been performed.
        (6) Empty bladder.
    c. *Types:*
        (1) Low—outlet forceps.
        (2) Mid—applied after head is engaged (rarely used).
        (3) Piper forceps—applied to after-coming head in selected breech births (rarely done).
    d. *Potential complications:*
        (1) *Maternal:*
            (a) Lacerations of birth canal, rectum, bladder.
            (b) Uterine rupture/hemorrhage.

(2) *Neonatal:*
(a) Cephalohematoma.
(b) Skull fracture.
(c) Intracranial hemorrhage, brain damage.
(d) Facial paralysis.
(e) Direct tissue trauma (abrasions, ecchymosis).
(f) Umbilical cord compression.

e. **Assessment:**
(1) FHR immediately before—and after—forceps application (forceps blade may compress umbilical cord).
(2) Observe mother/newborn for injury or signs of complications.

f. **Analysis/nursing diagnosis:**
(1) *Self-esteem disturbance* related to inability to give birth without surgical assistance.
(2) *Anxiety/fear* related to infant's appearance (forceps marks) or awareness of potential complications.

g. **Nursing care plan/implementation:**
(1) Goal: *minimize feelings of failure due to inability to give birth "naturally."*
(a) Explain, discuss reasons/indications for forceps-assisted birth.
(b) Emphasize no maternal control over circumstances.
(2) Goal: *reduce parental anxiety, maternal guilt over infant bruising/forceps marks.* Explain condition is temporary and has no lasting effects on child's appearance.

h. **Evaluation/outcome criteria:**
(1) Woman verbalizes understanding of reasons for forceps-assisted birth.
(2) Woman evidences no interruption in bonding with infant.
(3) Woman experiences uncomplicated recovery.

3. **Vacuum extraction** (soft plastic cup with vacuum from a handheld suction pump). Used to assist in rotation or delivery of the fetal head.
a. Risks may include caput succedaneum and cephalohematoma.
b. Causes neonatal jaundice; intraventricular hemorrhage can result in death.

4. **Cesarean birth**—incision through abdominal wall and uterus to give birth.
a. Indications for *elective* cesarean birth:
(1) Known CPD.
(2) Previous uterine surgery (e.g., myomectomy), repeated cesarean births (depends on type of incision done).
(3) Active maternal genital herpes type 2 infection; human papillomavirus (HPV).
(4) Breech presentation. *Note:* To reduce infant morbidity/mortality, elective cesarean birth is common method of choice.
(5) Neoplasms of cervix, uterus, or birth canal.
(6) Maternal diabetes with placental aging; fetal macrosomia (CPD); >4050 gm.

b. *Criterion* for elective cesarean birth:
L/S ratio greater than 2:1—indicates presence of pulmonary surfactant; less risk of respiratory distress syndrome.

c. *Indications for emergency cesarean birth:*
(1) **Fetal:**
(a) *Fetal distress:* prolapsed cord, repetitive late decelerations, prolonged bradycardia.
(b) *Fetal jeopardy:* Rh or ABO incompatibility.
(c) *Fetal malposition*/malpresentation.
(2) **Maternal:**
(a) *Uterine* dysfunction; rupture.
(b) *Placental* disorders:
(i) Placenta previa.
(ii) Abruptio placentae, with Couvelaire uterus.
(c) Severe maternal preeclampsia/eclampsia.
(d) Fetopelvic disproportion.
(e) Sudden maternal death.
(f) Carcinoma.
(g) Failed induction.

d. *Types:*
(1) Low segment—method of choice:
(a) Transverse incision through abdominal wall and lower uterine segment.
(b) Transverse incision through abdominal wall, with vertical incision of lower uterine segment.
(c) Advantages—fewer complications:
(i) Less blood loss.
(ii) More comfortable convalescence.
(iii) Less adhesion formation.
(iv) Lower risk of uterine rupture in subsequent pregnancy/labor and birth.
(v) Cosmetically more acceptable.
(2) Classical—vertical incision through abdominal wall and uterus. May be necessary for anterior placenta previa and transverse lie, less than 28 weeks' prematurity.
(3) Porro's—hysterotomy followed by hysterectomy. Necessary in presence of:
(a) Hemorrhage from uterine atony.
(b) Placenta accreta/percreta.
(c) Large uterine myomas.
(d) Ruptured uterus.
(e) Cancer of uterus or ovary.

e. **Assessment:**
(1) Maternal physical status.
(a) Vital signs.
(b) Labor status, if any.
(c) Contractions (if any).
(d) Membranes (intact; ruptured).
(e) Bleeding.
(2) Fetal status.
(a) FHR pattern.
(b) Color and amount of amniotic fluid.
(c) Biophysical profile (BPP), if performed.
(3) Maternal emotional status.
(4) Understanding of procedure, indications for, implications.
(5) Other—as for any abdominal surgery (see **Chapter 6**).

f. **Analysis/nursing diagnosis:**
(1) *Self-esteem disturbance* related to perceived failure to give birth vaginally.
(2) *Anxiety/fear* related to impending surgery and/or reasons for cesarean birth.
(3) *Ineffective individual coping* related to anxiety and fear for self, infant.
(4) *Fluid volume deficit* related to abdominal surgery or reason for cesarean birth.
(5) *Pain* related to abdominal surgery.
(6) *Constipation* related to decreased bowel activity.
(7) *Altered urinary elimination* related to fluid volume deficit.

g. **Nursing care plan/implementation:**
(1) *Preoperative:*
(a) Goal: *safeguard fetal status.*
(i) Monitor fetal heart rate continually.
(ii) Notify neonatology and neonatal intensive care unit (NICU) of scheduled surgical birth, if suspect complications.
(b) Goal: *health teaching.*
(i) Describe, discuss anticipated anesthesia.
(ii) Explain rationale for preoperative antacids to minimize effects of aspiration: cimetidine, Bicitra, histamine blocker to decrease production of gastric acid; Reglan (metoclopramide), to hasten gastric emptying.
(iii) Describe, explain anticipated procedures—abdominal shave, indwelling catheter, intravenous fluids—to woman and support person.
(c) Other—as for any abdominal surgery.
(d) Prepare for cesarean birth.
(2) *Postoperative:*
(a) Same as for other clients having abdominal surgery (see **Chapter 6**).
(b) Same as for other women who are postpartum.

h. **Evaluation/outcome criteria:**
(1) Verbalizes understanding of reasons for cesarean birth.
(2) Successful birth of viable infant.
(3) Evidences no surgical/birth complications.
(4) Evidences no interference with bonding.
(5) Expresses satisfaction with procedure and result.

5. **Trial of labor after cesarean (TOLAC)**
a. Candidates for TOLAC.
(1) Previous low transverse cesarean birth.
(2) Fetal head well engaged in pelvis (vertex presentation).
(3) Soft, anterior cervix.
(4) Preexisting reason for repeat cesarean birth not apparent.
b. **Assessment:**
(1) Monitor FHR carefully during trial of labor.
(2) Monitor contractions carefully for adequate progress of labor.
(3) Observe mother for signs of complications/uterine rupture.
c. **Analysis/nursing diagnosis:**
(1) *Knowledge deficit* related to trial of labor.
(2) *Fear* related to outcome for fetus.
(3) *Ineffective individual coping* related to labor progress and outcome.

Complications During the Intrapartum Period

I. GENERAL ASPECTS

A. Pathophysiology—interference with normal processes and patterns of labor/birth result in maternal or fetal jeopardy (e.g., **preterm** labor, **dysfunctional** labor patterns; **prolonged** [over 24 hours] labor; **hemorrhage: uterine rupture**/inversion, **amniotic fluid embolus**).

B. Etiology:
1. **Preterm labor**—unknown.
2. **Dysfunctional labor** (**dystocia:** see **p. 184**):
a. Physiological response to anxiety/fear/pain—results in release of catecholamines, increasing physical/psychological stress → myometrial dysfunction; painful and ineffectual labor.
b. Iatrogenic factors: premature or excessive analgesia, particularly during latent phase.

MATERNAL/INFANT

c. *Maternal factors:*
   (1) Pelvic contractures.
   (2) Uterine tumors (e.g., myomas, carcinoma).
   (3) Congenital uterine anomalies (e.g., bicornate uterus).
   (4) Pathological contraction ring (*Bandl's* ring).
   (5) Rigid cervix, cervical stenosis/stricture.
   (6) Hypertonic/hypotonic contractions.
   (7) Prolonged rupture of membranes. *Note:* Intrauterine infection may have caused rupture of membranes or may follow rupture.
   (8) Prolonged first or second stage.
   (9) Medical conditions: diabetes, hypertension.

d. *Fetal factors:*
   (1) Macrosomia (LGA).
   (2) Malposition/malpresentation.
   (3) Congenital anomaly (e.g., hydrocephalus, anencephaly).
   (4) Multifetal gestation (e.g., interlocking twins).
   (5) Prolapsed cord.
   (6) Postterm.

e. *Placental factors:*
   (1) Placenta previa.
   (2) Inadequate placental function with contractions.
   (3) Abruptio placentae.
   (4) Placenta accreta.

f. Physical restrictions: when confined to bed, *flat position,* etc.

C. Assessment:
1. Antepartal history.
2. Emotional status.
3. Vital signs, FHR.
4. Contraction pattern (frequency, duration, intensity).
5. Vaginal discharge.

D. Analysis/nursing diagnosis:
1. *Anxiety/fear* for self and infant related to implications of prolonged or complicated labor/birth.
2. *Pain* related to hypertonic contractions/dysfunctional labor.
3. *Ineffective individual coping* related to physical/psychological stress of complicated labor/birth, lowered pain threshold secondary to fatigue.
4. *High risk for injury* related to prolonged rupture of membranes, infection.
5. *Fluid volume deficit* related to excessive blood loss secondary to placenta previa, abruptio placentae, Couvelaire uterus, DIC.

E. Nursing care plan/implementation:
1. Goal: *minimize physical/psychological stress during labor/birth.* Assist woman in coping effectively:
   a. Reinforce relaxation techniques.
   b. Support couple's effective coping techniques/mechanisms.
2. Goal: *emotional support.*
   a. Encourage verbalization of anxiety/fear/concerns.
   b. Explain all procedures—to minimize anxiety/fear, encourage cooperation/participation in care.
   c. Provide quiet environment conducive to rest.
3. Goal: *continuous monitoring of maternal/fetal status and progress through labor*—to identify early signs of dysfunctional labor, fetal distress; facilitate prompt, effective treatment of emerging complications.
4. Goal: *minimize effects of complicated labor on mother, fetus.*
   a. *Position* change: lateral Sims'—to reduce compression of inferior vena cava.
   b. Oxygen per mask, as indicated.
   c. Institute interventions appropriate to emerging problems (see specific disorder).

F. Evaluation/outcome criteria:
1. Woman has successful birth of viable infant.
2. Maternal/infant status stable, satisfactory.

II. DISORDERS AFFECTING PROTECTIVE FUNCTIONS: **Preterm labor**—occurs after 20 weeks of gestation and before beginning of week 38.

A. Pathophysiology—physiological events of labor (i.e., contractions, spontaneous rupture of membranes, cervical effacement/dilation) occur before completion of normal, term gestation.

B. Etiology—causes may be from maternal, fetal, or placental factors.

C. *Coexisting disorders:*
1. Infections that may cause PROM.
2. PROM of unknown etiology.
3. PIH (preeclampsia/eclampsia).
4. Uterine overdistention.
   a. Polyhydramnios.
   b. Multifetal gestation.
5. Maternal diabetes, renal or cardiovascular disorder, UTI.
6. Severe maternal illness (e.g., pneumonia, acute pyelonephritis).
7. Abnormal placentation.
   a. Placenta previa.
   b. Abruptio placentae.
8. Iatrogenic: miscalculated EDD for repeat cesarean birth (rare).
9. Fetal death.

10. Incompetent cervical os (small percentage).
11. Uterine anomalies (rare).
    a. Intrauterine septum.
    b. Bicornate uterus.
12. Uterine fibroids.
13. Positive fetal fibronectin assay (protein found in fetal tissue, membranes, amniotic fluid, and the decidua) found in cervical/vaginal fluid first half of pregnancy and normally absent through mid to late pregnancy (↑ risk of preterm labor by 20%).

D. *Prevention:*
1. *Primary*—close obstetric supervision; education in signs/symptoms of labor.
2. *Secondary*—prompt, effective treatment of associated disorders (see **II. C., pp. 181–182**).
3. *Tertiary*—suppression of preterm labor.
    a. Bedrest.
    b. *Position:* side-lying—to promote placental perfusion.
    c. Hydration.
    d. Pharmacological (may require "informed consent"; follow hospital protocol). Beta-adrenergic agents, $MgSO_4$ (recent studies show poor results with $MgSO_4$), Procardia to reduce sensitivity of uterine myometrium to oxytocic and prostaglandin stimulation; increase blood flow to uterus.
    e. May be maintained at home with adequate follow-up and health teaching.

E. Contraindications for suppression: Labor is not suppressed in presence of:
1. Placenta previa or abruptio placentae with hemorrhage.
2. Chorioamnionitis.
3. Erythroblastosis fetalis.
4. Severe preeclampsia.
5. Severe diabetes (e.g., "brittle").
6. Increasing placental insufficiency.
7. Progressive cervical dilation of 4 cm or more.
8. Ruptured membranes (with maternal fever).

F. Assessment:
1. Maternal vital signs. Response to medication:
    a. Hypotension.
    b. Tachycardia, arrhythmia.
    c. Dyspnea, chest pain.
    d. Nausea and vomiting.
2. Signs of infection:
    a. Increased temperature.
    b. Tachycardia.
    c. Diaphoresis.
    d. Malaise.
    e. Increased baseline fetal heart rate; ↓ variability.
3. Contractions: frequency, duration, strength.
4. Emotional status—signs of denial, guilt, anxiety, exhaustion.
5. Signs of continuing and progressing labor. *Note:* Vaginal examination *only* if indicated by other signs of continuing labor progress:
    a. Effacement.
    b. Dilation.
    c. Station.
6. Status of membranes.
7. Fetal heart rate, activity (continuous monitoring).

G. Analysis/nursing diagnosis:
1. *Anxiety/fear* related to possible outcome.
2. *Self-esteem disturbance* related to feelings of guilt, failure.
3. *Impaired physical mobility* related to imposed bedrest.
4. *Knowledge deficit* related to medication side effects.
5. *Ineffective individual coping* related to possible outcome.
6. *Impaired gas exchange* related to side effects of medication (circulatory overload; pulmonary edema).
7. *Diversional activity deficit* related to imposed bedrest, decreased environmental stimuli.
8. *Altered urinary elimination* related to bedrest.
9. *Constipation* related to bedrest.

H. Nursing care plan/implementation:
1. Goal: *inhibit uterine activity.* Administer medications as ordered—terbutaline, magnesium sulfate, Procardia, Indocin.
2. Goal: *safeguard status.*
    a. Continuous maternal/fetal monitoring.
    b. I&O—to identify early signs of possible circulatory overload.

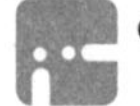

    c. *Position:* side-lying—to increase placental perfusion, prevent supine hypotension.
    d. Report **promptly** to physician:
        (1) Maternal pulse of 110 or more.
        (2) Diastolic pressure of 60 mm Hg or less.
        (3) Respirations of 24 or more; crackles (rales).
        (4) Complaint of dyspnea.
        (5) Contractions: increasing frequency, strength, duration, or cessation of contractions.
        (6) Intermittent back and thigh pain.
        (7) Rupture of membranes.
        (8) Vaginal bleeding.
        (9) Fetal distress.
3. Goal: *comfort measures.*
    a. Basic hygienic care—bath, mouth care, cold washcloth to face, perineal care.
    b. Back rub, linen change—to promote relaxation.
4. Goal: *emotional support.*
    a. Encourage verbalization of guilt feelings, anxiety, fear, concerns; provide factual information.
    b. Support positive self-concept.
    c. Keep informed of progress.

5. Goal: *provide quiet diversion.* Television, reading materials, handicrafts (may not be able to focus well if on magnesium therapy).
6. Goal: *health teaching.*
   a. Explain, discuss proposed management to suppress preterm labor.
   b. Describe, discuss side effects of medication.
   c. Explain rationale for bedrest, position.

I. If labor continues to progress:

1. Goal: *facilitate infant survival.*
   a. Administer betamethasone, as ordered, 24 to 48 hours before birth—to increase/stimulate production of pulmonary surfactant.
   b. Give antibiotic to mother to ↓ chance of neonatal sepsis.
   c. Notify NICU—to increase chances for fetal survival; ensure prompt, expert management of neonate; and provide information and support to parents.
   d. Monitor progress of labor to identify signs of impending birth. *Note:* May give birth before complete (10-cm) dilation.
   e. Consider transfer to high-risk facility.
   f. Prepare for birth, or cesarean birth if infant less than 34 to 36 weeks of gestation.
2. Goal: *emotional support.*
   a. Do *not* leave woman (or couple) alone.
   b. Encourage verbalization of anxiety, fear, concern.
   c. Explain all procedures.
3. Goal: *comfort measures. Note:* Analgesics used conservatively—to prevent depression of fetus/neonate.
4. Goal: *support effective coping techniques.* Encourage/support Lamaze (or other) techniques—coach, as necessary; discourage hyperventilation.
5. Goal: *health teaching*—for severe preterm birth.
   a. Discuss need for episiotomy, possibility of outlet forceps–assisted birth—to reduce stress on fetal head, or
   b. Prepare for cesarean birth—to reduce possibility of fetal intraventricular hemorrhage.
   c. Give rationale for avoiding use of medications to reduce contraction pain.

J. Immediate care of neonate:

1. Goal: *safeguard status.*
   a. Stabilize environmental temperature—to prevent chilling (isolette or other controlled-temperature bed).
   b. Suction, oxygen, as needed; may need intubation.
   c. Parenteral fluids, as ordered—to support normal acid-base balance, pH; administer antibiotics, as necessary.
   d. Arrange transport to high-risk facility, as necessary.
2. Goal: *continuous monitoring of status.*
   a. Electronic monitors—to observe respiratory and cardiac functions.
   b. Blood samples—to monitor blood gases, pH, hypoglycemia.

K. Postpartum care: Goal: *emotional support.*

1. Facilitate attachment—photos, if baby transferred or mother unable to visit.
2. If couple, foster sense of mutual experience and closeness.
3. Help her/them maintain a positive self-image.
4. Encourage touching of infant before transport to nursery or high-risk facility; father/partner may accompany infant and report back to mother.
5. Encourage early contact—to facilitate mother's need to ventilate her feelings.
6. Assist parent(s) with grieving process, if necessary.
7. Refer to support group if necessary.

L. *Other*—as for any woman who is postpartum.

M. Evaluation/outcome criteria:

1. Woman verbalizes understanding of medical/nursing recommendations and treatments.
2. Woman complies with medical/nursing regimen.
3. Woman experiences no discomfort from side effects of therapy.
4. Woman experiences successful outcome—labor inhibited.
5. Woman carries pregnancy to successful termination.
6. If preterm birth occurs, woman copes effectively with outcome (physiologically compromised neonate, neonatal death).

III. GRIEF AND CHILDBEARING EXPERIENCE.

The loss of a pregnancy or a newborn, or the birth of a child who is physiologically compromised (preterm, congenital disorder) is a crisis situation. The unexpected outcome can cause the parent(s) to suffer a sense of loss of self-esteem, self-concept, positive body image, feelings of worth (see **Postpartum depression/psychosis, p. 199**).

A. Assessment:

1. Response to loss of the "fantasy child"/real child.
   a. Behavioral—anger, hostility, depression, disinterest in activities of daily living, withdrawal.
   b. Biophysical—somatic complaints (stomach pain, malaise, anorexia, nausea).
   c. Cognitive—feelings of guilt.
2. Knowledge/understanding/perception of situation.
3. Coping abilities, mechanisms.
4. Support system.

B. Analysis/nursing diagnosis:

1. *Ineffective family coping: compromised* related to psychological stress due to fear for infant, guilt feelings, impact on self-image.
2. *Ineffective individual coping* related to anxiety, stress.

MATERNAL/INFANT

3. *Ineffective family coping: disabling* related to disturbance in intrafamily relations secondary to individual coping deficits, recriminations.
4. *Altered parenting* related to lack of effective bonding secondary to emotional separation from infant, feelings of guilt.
5. *Dysfunctional grieving* related to guilt feelings, impact of loss on self-concept.
6. *Disturbance in body image, self-esteem, role performance* related to perceived failure to complete gestational task, produce perfect, healthy infant; associated with sleep deprivation.
7. *Social isolation* related to severe coping deficit, dysfunctional grieving, disturbance in self-esteem.

C. Nursing care plan/implementation:

1. Goal: *emotional support.*
   a. Provide privacy; encourage open expression/verbalization of feelings, fears, concerns, perceptions.
   b. Crisis intervention techniques.
2. Goal: *facilitate bonding, effective coping, or anticipatory grieving processes.*
   a. Encourage contact and participation in care of premature or compromised infant.
   b. Keep informed of infant's status.
   c. Provide realistic data.
3. Goal: *health teaching.*
   a. Clarify misperceptions, as appropriate.
   b. Discuss, demonstrate infant care techniques (e.g., feeding infant who has cleft lip or palate).
   c. Refer to appropriate community resources.

D. Evaluation/outcome criteria:

1. Woman verbalizes recognition and acceptance of diagnosis.
2. Woman verbalizes understanding of relevant information regarding treatment, prognosis.
3. Woman makes informed decision regarding infant care.
4. Woman demonstrates comfort and increasing participation in care of neonate.
5. Woman shows evidence of culturally appropriate bonding (eye contact, cuddles, calls infant by name).

IV. DISORDERS AFFECTING COMFORT, REST, MOBILITY: DYSTOCIA

A. Definition—difficult labor.

B. *General aspects*—there are **6 Ps** that affect the progress of labor: *Mother—"3 Ps": **p**sych, **p**lacenta, **p**osition* and *Fetus—"3 Ps": **p**ower, **p**assageway, **p**assenger*

1. **Pathophysiology**—see specific disorders.
2. **Etiology**—due to effects of three other factors that affect the **FETUS:**
   a. ***POWER:*** forces of labor (uterine contractions, use of abdominal muscles).
      (1) Premature analgesia/anesthesia.
      (2) Uterine overdistention (multifetal pregnancy, fetal macrosomia).
      (3) Uterine myomas.
      (4) Grandmultipara.
   b. ***PASSAGEWAY:*** resistance of cervix, pelvic structures.
      (1) Rigid cervix.
      (2) Distended bladder.
      (3) Distended rectum.
      (4) Dimensions of the bony pelvis: pelvic contractures.
   c. ***PASSENGER:*** accommodation of the presenting part to pelvic diameters.
      (1) Fetal malposition/malpresentation.
         (a) Transverse lie.
         (b) Face, brow presentation.
         (c) Breech presentation.
         (d) Persistent occipitoposterior position.
         (e) CPD.
      (2) Fetal anomalies.
         (a) Hydrocephalus.
         (b) Conjoined ("Siamese") twins.
         (c) Meningomyelocele.
      (3) Fetal size: macrosomia.
3. **Hazards:**
   a. *Maternal:*
      (1) Fatigue, exhaustion, dehydration—due to prolonged labor.
      (2) Lowered pain threshold, loss of control—due to prolonged labor, continued uterine contractions, anxiety, fatigue, lack of sleep.
      (3) Intrauterine infection—due to prolonged rupture of membranes and frequent vaginal examinations.
      (4) Uterine rupture—due to obstructed labor, hyperstimulation of uterus.
      (5) Cervical, vaginal, perineal lacerations—due to obstetric interventions.
      (6) Postpartum hemorrhage—due to uterine atony or trauma.
   b. *Fetal:*
      (1) Hypoxia, anoxia, demise—due to decreased O_2 concentration in cord blood.
      (2) Intracranial hemorrhage—due to changing intracranial pressure.

C. Hypertonic dysfunction

1. **Pathophysiology**—increased resting tone of uterine myometrium; diminished refractory period; prolonged latent phase:
   a. *Nullipara*—more than 20 hours.
   b. *Multipara*—more than 14 hours.
2. **Etiology**—unknown. Theory—ectopic initiation of incoordinate uterine contractions.
3. **Assessment:**
   a. Onset—early labor (latent phase).

b. Contractions:
   (1) Continuous fundal tension, incomplete relaxation.
   (2) Painful.
   (3) Ineffectual—no effacement or dilation.
c. Signs of fetal distress:
   (1) Meconium-stained amniotic fluid.
   (2) FHR irregularities.
d. Maternal vital signs.
e. Emotional status.
f. *Medical evaluation:* vaginal examination, x-ray pelvimetry, ultrasonography—to rule out CPD (rarely used).

4. **Analysis/nursing diagnosis:**
   a. *Pain* related to hypertonic contractions, incomplete uterine relaxation.
   b. *Anxiety/fear* for self and infant related to strong, painful contractions without evidence of progress.
   c. *Ineffective individual coping* related to fatigue, exhaustion, anxiety, tension, fear.
   d. *Impaired gas exchange (fetal)* related to incomplete relaxation of uterus.
   e. *Sleep pattern disturbance* related to prolonged ineffectual labor.
5. **Nursing care plan/implementation:**
   a. *Medical management:*

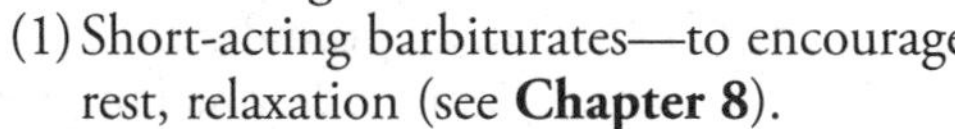

      (1) Short-acting barbiturates—to encourage rest, relaxation (see **Chapter 8**).
      (2) Intravenous fluids—to restore/maintain hydration and fluid-electrolyte balance.
      (3) If CPD, cesarean birth.
   b. *Nursing management:*
      (1) Goal: *emotional support*—assist coping with fear, pain, discouragement.
         (a) Encourage verbalization of anxiety, fear, concerns.
         (b) Explain all procedures.
         (c) Reassure. Keep couple informed of progress.
      (2) Goal: *comfort measures.*

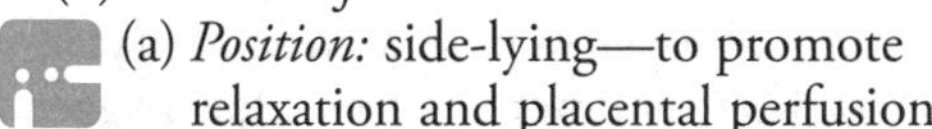

         (a) *Position:* side-lying—to promote relaxation and placental perfusion.
         (b) Bath, back rub, linen change, clean environment.
         (c) Environment: quiet, darkened room—to minimize stimuli and encourage relaxation, warmth.
         (d) Encourage voiding—to relieve bladder distention; to test urine for ketones.
      (3) Goal: *prevent infection.* Strict aseptic technique.
      (4) Goal: *prepare for cesarean birth* if necessary.
6. **Evaluation/outcome criteria:**
   a. Relaxes, sleeps, establishes normal labor pattern.
   b. Demonstrates no signs of fetal distress.
   c. Successfully completes uneventful labor.

D. Hypotonic dysfunction during labor

1. **Pathophysiology**—after normal labor at onset, contractions diminish in frequency, duration and strength; lowered uterine resting tone; cervical effacement and dilation slow/cease.
2. **Etiology:**
   a. Premature or excessive analgesia/anesthesia (epidural block or spinal block).
   b. CPD.
   c. Overdistention (polyhydramnios, fetal macrosomia, multifetal pregnancy).
   d. Fetal malposition/malpresentation.
   e. Maternal fear/anxiety.
3. **Assessment:**
   a. Onset—may occur in latent phase; most common during active phase.
   b. Contractions: normal previously, demonstrate:
      (1) Decreased frequency.
      (2) Shorter duration.
      (3) Diminished intensity (mild to moderate).
      (4) Less uncomfortable.
   c. Cervical changes—slow or cease.
   d. Signs of fetal distress—rare.
      (1) Usually occur late in labor due to infection secondary to prolonged rupture of membranes.
      (2) Tachycardia.
   e. Maternal vital signs may indicate infection (↑ temperature).
   f. *Medical diagnosis*—procedures: vaginal examination.
4. **Analysis/nursing diagnosis:**
   a. *Knowledge deficit* related to limited exposure to information.
   b. *Anxiety/fear* related to failure to progress as anticipated; fear for fetus.
   c. *High risk for injury* (infection) related to prolonged labor or ruptured membranes.
5. **Nursing care plan/implementation:**
   a. *Medical management:*
      (1) Amniotomy—artificial rupture of membranes.
      (2) Oxytocin augmentation of labor—intravenous infusion of oxytocin to increase frequency, duration, strength, and efficiency of uterine contractions (see **Induction of labor, p. 176**).
      (3) If CPD, cesarean birth.
   b. *Nursing management:*
      (1) Goals: *emotional support, comfort measures, prevent infection*—same as for ***Hypertonic dysfunction*** (see **pp. 184–185**).
      (2) Other (see **Induction of labor, p. 176**).

6. **Evaluation/outcome criteria:**
   a. Reestablishes normal labor pattern.
   b. Experiences successful birth of viable infant.

V. DISORDERS AFFECTING FLUID-GAS TRANSPORT: *maternal*

A. Uterine rupture

1. **Pathophysiology**—stress on uterine muscle exceeds its ability to stretch.
2. **Etiology:**
   a. Overdistention—due to large baby, multifetal gestation.
   b. Old scars—due to previous cesarean births or uterine surgery.
   c. Contractions against CPD, fetal malpresentation, pathological retraction ring (*Bandl's*).
   d. Injudicious obstetrics—malapplication of forceps (or application without full effacement/dilation).
   e. Tetanic contraction—due to hypersensitivity to oxytocin (or excessive dosage) during induction/augmentation of labor.
3. **Assessment:**
   a. Identify predisposing factors early.
   b. *Complete rupture*
      (1) Pain: sudden, sharp, abdominal; followed by cessation of contractions; tender abdomen.
      (2) Signs of shock; vaginal bleeding.
      (3) Fetal heart tones—absent.
      (4) Presenting part—not palpable on vaginal examination.
   c. *Incomplete rupture*
      (1) Contractions: continue, accompanied by abdominal pain and failure to dilate; may become dystonic.
      (2) Signs of shock.
      (3) May demonstrate vaginal bleeding.
      (4) Fetal heart tones—absent/bradycardia.
4. **Prognosis**
   a. Maternal—guarded.
   b. Fetal—grave.
5. **Analysis/nursing diagnosis:**
   a. *Pain* related to rupture of uterine muscle.
   b. *Fluid volume deficit* related to massive blood loss secondary to uterine rupture.
   c. *Anxiety/fear* related to concern for self, fetus.
   d. *Altered tissue perfusion* related to blood loss secondary to uterine rupture.
   e. *Altered urinary elimination* related to necessary conservation of intravascular fluid secondary to blood loss.
   f. *Anticipatory grieving* related to expected loss of fetus; inability to have more children.

6. **Nursing care plan/implementation:**
   a. *Medical management:*
      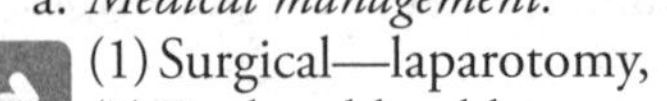
      (1) Surgical—laparotomy, hysterectomy.
      (2) Replace blood loss—transfusion, packed cells.

      (3) Reduce possibility of infection—antibiotics.
   b. *Nursing management:*
      (1) Goal: *safeguard status.*
         (a) Report *immediately;* mobilize staff.
         (b) Prepare for immediate laparotomy.
         (c) Oxygen per mask—to increase circulating oxygen level.
         (d) Order STAT type and crossmatch for blood—to replace blood loss.
         (e) Establish IV line—to infuse fluids, blood, medications.
         (f) Insert indwelling catheter—to deflate bladder.
         (g) Abdominal prep—to remove hair, bacteria.
         (h) Surgical permit (informed consent) for hysterectomy.
      (2) Goal: *emotional support*—to allay anxiety (woman and family).
         (a) Encourage verbalization of fears, anxiety, concerns.
         (b) Explain all procedures.
         (c) Keep family informed of progress.
7. **Evaluation/outcome criteria:**
   a. Experiences successful termination of emergency; minimal blood loss.
   b. Postoperative status stable.

B. Amniotic fluid embolus (anaphylactoid syndrome)

1. **Pathophysiology:** acute cor pulmonale—due to embolus blocking vessels in pulmonary circulation; massive hemorrhage—due to DIC resulting from entrance of thromboplastin-like material into bloodstream.
2. **Etiology**—amniotic fluid (with any meconium, lanugo, or vernix) enters maternal circulation through open venous sinuses at placental site; travels to pulmonary arterioles. Triggers cardiogenic shock and anaphylactoid reaction.
   a. Rare.
   b. Associated with: tumultuous labor, abruptio placentae, artificial ROM, placement of intrauterine catheter.
3. **Prognosis**—poor; often fatal to mother.
4. **Assessment:**
   a. May occur during labor, at time of rupture of membranes, or immediately postpartum.
   b. Sudden dyspnea and cyanosis.
   c. Chest pain.
   d. Hypotension, tachycardia.
   e. Frothy sputum.

f. **Signs of DIC:**
(1) Purpura—local hemorrhage.
(2) Increased vaginal bleeding—massive.
(3) Rapid onset of shock.

5. **Analysis/nursing diagnosis:**
a. *Impaired gas exchange* related to pulmonary edema.
b. *Risk for fluid volume deficit* related to DIC.
c. *Anxiety/fear* for self and fetus related to severity of symptoms, perception of jeopardy.

6. **Nursing care plan/implementation:**
a. *Medical management:*
(1) IV heparin, whole blood.
(2) Birth: immediate, by forceps, if possible; or cesarean birth.
(3) Digitalize, as necessary.
b. *Nursing management:*
(1) Goal: *assist ventilation.*
(a) *Position:* semi-Fowler's.
(b) Oxygen under positive pressure.
(c) Suction prn.
(2) Goal: *facilitate/expedite administration of fluids, medications, blood.*
(a) Establish intravenous line with large-bore needle.
(b) Administer heparin, fluids, as ordered.
(3) Goal: *restore cardiopulmonary functions, if needed.* Cardiopulmonary resuscitation techniques.
(4) Goal: *emotional support* of woman, family.
(a) Allay anxiety, as possible.
(b) Explain all procedures.
(c) Keep informed of status.

7. **Evaluation/outcome criteria:**
a. Dyspnea relieved.
b. Bleeding controlled.
c. Successful birth of viable infant.
d. Uneventful postpartum course.

VI. DISORDERS AFFECTING FLUID-GAS TRANSPORT: *fetal*

A. Fetus in jeopardy—general aspects:

1. **Pathophysiology**—maternal hypoxemia, anemia, ketoacidosis, Rh isoimmunization, or decreased uteroplacental perfusion.

2. **Etiology**—*maternal:*
a. Preeclampsia/eclampsia, PIH.
b. Heart disease.
c. Diabetes.
d. Rh or ABO incompatibility.
e. Insufficient uteroplacental/cord circulation due to:
(1) Maternal hypotension/hypertension.
(2) Cord compression:
(a) Prolapsed.
(b) Knotted.
(c) Nuchal.
(3) Hemorrhage; anemia.
(4) Placental problem:
(a) Malformation of the placenta/cord.
(b) Premature "aging" of placenta.
(c) Placental infarcts.
(d) Abruptio placentae.
(e) Placenta previa.
(5) Postterm gestation.
(6) Maternal infection.
(7) Polyhydramnios.
(8) Hypertonic uterine contractions.
f. Premature rupture of membranes (PROM) with chorioamnionitis.
g. Dystocia (e.g., from CPD).

3. **Assessment**—intrapartum:
a. Amniotic fluid examination—at or after rupture of membranes. *Signs of fetal distress:* meconium stained, vertex presentation—due to relaxation of fetal anal sphincter secondary to hypoxia/anoxia. *Note:* Fetus "gasps" in utero—may aspirate meconium and amniotic fluid.
b. Fetal activity:
(1) Hyperactivity—due to hypoxemia, elevated CO_2.
(2) Cessation—possible fetal death.
c. Methods of monitoring FHR:
(1) Fetoscope.
(2) Phonocardiography with microphone application.
(3) Internal fetal electrode—attached directly to fetus through dilated cervix after membranes ruptured.
(4) Doppler probe using ultrasound flow.
(5) Cardiotocograph—transducer on maternal abdomen transmits sound.
d. Abnormal FHR patterns (see **Fig. 4.10**).
(1) Persistent arrhythmia.
(2) Persistent tachycardia of 160 or more beats/min.
(3) Persistent bradycardia of 100 or fewer beats/min.
(4) *Early deceleration*—due to vagal response to head compression.
(5) *Late deceleration*—due to uteroplacental insufficiency.
(6) *Variable deceleration*—due to cord compression.
(7) Decreased or loss of variability in FHR pattern.
e. *Medical evaluation*—procedures: fetal blood gases, pH (rarely performed).
(1) Purpose—to identify fetal acid-base status.
(2) Requirements for:
(a) Ruptured membranes.
(b) Cervical dilation.
(c) Engaged head.

MATERNAL/INFANT

(3) Procedure—under sterile condition, sample of fetal scalp blood obtained for analysis.
(4) Signs of fetal distress:
(a) pH less than 7.20 (normal range is 7.3–7.4).
(b) *Increased* CO_2
(c) *Decreased* PO_2

4. **Analysis/nursing diagnosis:**
a. *Impaired gas exchange, fetal,* related to decreased placental perfusion/insufficient cord circulation.
b. *Altered tissue perfusion* related to hemolytic anemia.
c. *High risk for fetal injury* related to hypoxia.

B. Prolapsed umbilical cord

1. **Pathophysiology**—cord descent in advance of presenting part; compression interrupts blood flow, exchange of fetal/maternal gases → fetal hypoxia, anoxia, death (if unrelieved).
2. **Etiology:**
a. Spontaneous or artificial rupture of membranes before presenting part is engaged.
b. Excessive force of escaping fluid, as in polyhydramnios.
c. Malposition—breech, compound presentation, transverse lie.
d. Preterm or fetus who is SGA—allows space for cord descent.
3. **Assessment:**
a. Visualization of cord outside (or inside) vagina.
b. Palpation of pulsating mass on vaginal examination.
c. Fetal distress—variable deceleration and persistent bradycardia.
4. **Analysis/nursing diagnosis:**
a. *Impaired gas exchange, fetal,* related to interruption of blood flow from placenta/fetus.
b. *Anxiety/fear, maternal,* related to knowledge of fetal jeopardy.
5. **Nursing care plan/implementation:**
a. Goal: *reduce pressure on cord.*
(1) *Position:* knee to chest; lateral modified Sims' with hips elevated; modified Trendelenburg.
(2) With gloved hand, support fetal presenting part.
b. Goal: *increase maternal/fetal oxygenation:* oxygen per mask (8–10 L/min).
c. Goal: *protect exposed cord:* continuous pressure on the presenting part to keep pressure off cord.
d. Goal: *identify fetal response* to above measures, reduce threat to fetal survival: monitor FHR continuously.
e. Goal: *expedite termination of threat to fetus:* prepare for immediate cesarean birth.
f. Goal: *support mother and significant other* by staying with them and explaining.
6. **Evaluation/outcome criteria:**
a. FHR returns to normal rate and pattern.
b. Uncomplicated birth of viable infant.

VII. SUMMARY OF DANGER SIGNS DURING LABOR

A. Contractions—strong, every 2 minutes or less, lasting 90 seconds or more; poor relaxation between contractions.
B. Sudden sharp abdominal pain followed by board-like abdomen and shock—abruptio placentae or uterine rupture.
C. Marked vaginal bleeding.
D. **FHR** periodic pattern decelerations—late; variable; absent variability (see **Fig. 4.10**).
E. Baseline.
1. Bradycardia (<100 beats/min).
2. Tachycardia (>160 beats/min).
F. Amniotic fluid.
1. Amount: excessive; diminished.
2. Odor.
3. Color: meconium stained; port-wine; yellow.
4. 24 hours or more since rupture of membranes.
G. Maternal hypotension, or hypertension.

THE POSTPARTUM PERIOD

General overview: This review of the normal physiological and psychological changes occurring during the postpartum period (birth to 6 weeks after) provides the database necessary for assessing the woman's progress through involution, planning and implementing care, anticipatory guidance, health teaching, and evaluating the results. Emerging problems are identified by comparing the woman's status against established standards.

I. BIOLOGICAL FOUNDATIONS OF THE POSTPARTUM PERIOD

A. Uterine involution—integrated processes by which the uterus returns to nonpregnant size, shape, and consistency.
1. **Assessment:**
a. Contractions ("afterpains")—shorten muscles, close venous sinuses, restore normal tone.
(1) Frequency, intensity, and discomfort decrease after first 24 hours.
(2) More common in multiparas and after birth of a large baby; primiparous uterus remains contracted.
(3) Increased by breastfeeding.
b. Autolysis—breakdown and excretion of muscle protein (decreasing size of myometrial

MATERNAL/INFANT

cells). Lochia—sloughing of decidua and blood.

c. Formation of *new endometrium*—4 to 6 weeks until placental site healed.

d. *Cervix*

(1) *Immediately following* birth—bruised, small tears; admits one hand.

(2) *Eighteen hours* after birth—becomes shorter, firmer; regains normal shape.

(3) *One week* postpartum—admits two fingers.

(4) Never returns fully to prepregnant state.

(a) Parous os is wider and not perfectly round.

(b) Lacerations heal as scars radiating out from the os.

e. *Fundal height and consistency*

(1) After birth—at umbilicus; size and consistency of firm grapefruit.

(2) Day 1 (first 12 hours)—one finger above umbilicus.

(3) Descends by one fingerbreadth daily until day 10.

(4) Day 10—behind symphysis pubis, nonpalpable.

f. *Lochia*

(1) Character:

(a) Days 1 to 3: rubra (red).

(b) Days 3 to 7: serosa (pink to brown).

(c) Day 10: alba (creamy white).

(2) Amount:

(a) Moderate: 4 to 8 pads/day (average 6 pads/day).

(b) Following cesarean birth: less lochia—due to manipulation during surgery.

(3) Odor: normal lochia has characteristic "fleshy" odor; foul odor is characteristic of infection.

(4) Clots: normal: a few small clots, most commonly on arising—due to pooling. *Note:* Large clots and *heavy* bleeding are associated with uterine atony, retained placental fragments.

B. Birth canal

1. *Vagina*—never returns fully to prepregnant state.

a. First few weeks postpartum—thin walled, due to lack of estrogen; few rugae.

b. Week 3: rugae may reappear.

2. *Pelvic floor*

a. Immediately after birth—infiltrated with blood, stretched, torn.

b. Month 6: considerable tone regained.

3. *Perineum*

a. Immediately following birth—edematous; may have episiotomy (or repaired lacerations); hemorrhoids.

b. Healing, incisional line clean; no separation.

c. Hematoma—blood in connective tissue beneath skin; complains of pain, unrelieved by mild analgesia or heat; perineal distention; painful, tense, fluctuant mass.

C. Abdominal wall

1. Overdistention during pregnancy may → rupture of elastic fibers, persistent striae, and diastasis of the rectus muscles.

2. Usually takes 6 to 8 weeks to retrogress, depending on previous muscle tone, obesity, and amount of distention during pregnancy.

3. Strenuous exercises discouraged until 8 weeks postpartum.

D. Cardiovascular system—characteristic changes:

1. Immediately after birth—*increased* cardiac load, due to:

a. Return of uterine blood flow to general circulation.

b. Diuresis of excess interstitial fluid.

2. Volume—returns to prepregnant state (4 L) in about 3 weeks. Major reduction—during first week, due to diuresis and diaphoresis.

3. Blood values (see **Table 4.5**).

a. High WBC during labor (25,000–30,000/mm^3), drops to normal level in first few days.

b. Week 1—Hgb, RBC, Hct, elevated fibrinogen return to normal.

4. Blood coagulation

a. During labor: rapid consumption of clotting factors.

b. During postpartum: increased consumption of clotting factors. Hypercoagulability maintained during first few days postpartum; predisposes to thrombophlebitis, pulmonary embolism.

5. **Assessment: potential complications**—vital signs:

a. *Temperature*—elevated in:

(1) Excessive blood loss, dehydration, exhaustion, infection.

(2) Elevation: 100.4°F (38°C) after first day postpartum suggests puerperal infection.

b. *Pulse*—physiological bradycardia (50–70 beats/min) common through second day postpartum; may persist 7 to 10 days; etiology: unknown. *Tachycardia*—associated with: excessive blood loss, dehydration, exhaustion, infection.

c. *Blood pressure*—generally unchanged. *Elevation*—associated with: preeclampsia, essential hypertension.

E. Urinary tract—characteristic changes:

1. Output—increased due to: diuresis (12 hours to 5 days postpartum); daily output to 3000 mL.

2. Urine constituents:
   a. Sugar—primarily lactose, usually not detected by conventional dipstick.
   b. Acetonuria—after prolonged labor; dehydration.
   c. Proteinuria—first 3 days in response to the catalytic process of involution ≤1+.
3. Dilation of ureters—subsides in first few weeks.
4. **Assessment: potential complications**—measure first few voidings, palpate bladder to determine emptying.
   a. Edema, trauma, or anesthesia may → retention with overflow.
   b. Overdistended bladder—common cause of excessive bleeding in immediate postpartum.

F. Integument (skin)—characteristic changes:
1. Striae—persist as silvery or brownish lines.
2. Diastasis recti abdominis—some midline separation may persist.
3. Diaphoresis—excessive perspiration for first few (approximately 5) days.
4. Breast changes (see **II. A. 3. Breasts,** below).
5. Linea nigra and darkened areolae fade.

G. Legs
1. Should have no redness, tenderness, local areas of increased skin temperature, or edema.
2. May have some soreness from birth position.
3. *Homans' sign* should be negative (no calf pain when knee is extended and gentle pressure applied to dorsiflex the foot).

H. Weight—characteristic changes:
1. Initial weight loss—fetus, placenta, amniotic fluid, excess tissue fluid.
2. Weighs more than in prepregnant state (weight maintained in breasts).
3. Week 6—weight loss is individualized.

I. Menstruation and ovarian function—first menstrual cycle may be anovulatory.
1. *Nonnursing*—ovulation at 4 to 6 weeks; menstruation at 6 to 8 weeks.
2. *Nursing*—anovulatory period varies (39 days to 6 months or more); some for duration of lactation; contraceptive value: *very unreliable.*

II. NURSING MANAGEMENT DURING THE POSTPARTUM PERIOD

A. Assessment—minimum of twice daily.
1. Vital signs.
2. Emotional status, response to baby.
3. *Breasts*
   a. Observe: size, symmetry, placement and condition of nipples, leakage of colostrum. Normal: although one breast is usually larger than the other, breasts are essentially symmetrical in shape; nipples: in breast midline, erectile, intact (no signs of fissure); bilateral leakage of colostrum is common.
   b. *Note:* reddened areas, elevations, supernumerary nipples, inverted nipples, cracks.
   c. Observe for signs of (normal) engorgement (i.e., tenderness, distention, prominent veins). Transient; normally occurs shortly before lactation is established—due to venous and lymphatic stasis.
   d. Palpate for: local heat, edema, tenderness, swelling (signs of localized infection).
4. Fundus, lochia, perineum.
5. Voiding and bowel function.
6. Legs (see **I. G.**).
7. Signs of complications.

B. Analysis/nursing diagnosis (see **VI. NURSING ACTIONS DURING THE FOURTH STAGE OF LABOR, pp. 172–173**).

C. Nursing care plan/implementation:
1. Goal: *comfort measures.*
   a. Perineal care—to promote healing, prevent infection.
   b. Sitz baths—to promote healing.
   c. Apply topical anesthetics, witch hazel to episiotomy area, hemorrhoids.
   d. Administer mild analgesia, as ordered.
   e. Instruct in tensing buttocks on position change—to reduce stress on suture line, discomfort.
   f. Breast care: mother who *is bottle-feeding*
      (1) Wash daily with clear water and mild soap.
      (2) Support with well-fitting brassiere.
      (3) For engorgement:
         (a) Prevent with tight binder.
         (b) Treat with ice pack and mild analgesic.
         (c) *Avoid* nipple stimulation.
      (4) See also **Breastfeeding and lactation (pp. 192–193)**.
2. Goal: *encourage normal bowel function.* (Normal to take 1 to 3 days for function to resume.)
   a. Administer stool softeners, as ordered.
   b. Encourage ambulation.
   c. Increase *dietary fiber* (salads, fresh fruit, vegetables, bran cereals).
   d. Provide adequate fluid intake.
3. Goal: *health teaching and discharge planning.*
   a. Reinforce appropriate perineal self-care.
   b. Reinforce hand washing (see **VI. NURSING ACTIONS DURING THE FOURTH STAGE OF LABOR, pp. 172–173**).
   c. *Infant care*
      (1) Bathing, cord care, circumcision care, diapering.
      (2) Feeding, burping, scheduling.
      (3) Assessment—temperature, skin color, newborn rash, jaundice.

(4) Normal stool cycle and voiding pattern.
(5) Common sleep/activity patterns.
(6) Signs to report **immediately:**
(a) Fever, vomiting, diarrhea.
(b) Signs of inflammation or infection at cord stump.
(c) Bleeding from circumcision site.
(d) Lethargy, irritability.

d. *Self-care*
(1) Adequate rest, nutrition, hydration.
(2) Breast self-examination; wear bra to support breasts and promote comfort.
(3) Normal process of involution; lochial patterns.

e. Resumption of intercourse approximately 4 weeks postpartum (wait until lochia stops).
(1) Explain that time interval varies as to first postpartum ovulation.
(2) Family planning options may resume if desired:
(a) If not breastfeeding, oral contraceptives (estrogen and progesterone); low-dose progesterone given to mothers who are breastfeeding (see **Table 4.1**).
(b) Long-acting progestins (subcutaneous implants or injectable). Safe to use during lactation.
(c) Use of IUD or diaphragm decided at postpartum checkup.
(d) Emphasize need to recheck size and fit of diaphragm.
(e) Other options: condom plus spermicides.

f. Exercises—to restore muscle tone, relieve tension.
(1) Mild exercise during first few weeks.
(a) Deep abdominal breathing.
(b) Supine head-raising.
(c) Stretching from head to toe.
(d) Pelvic tilt.
(e) Kegel—to regain perineal muscle tone.
(2) Strenuous exercises (sit-ups, leg lifts)—deferred until later in postpartum.

g. Maternal signs to report **immediately:**
(1) Prolonged lochia rubra.
(2) Cramping.
(3) Signs of infection.
(4) Excessive fatigue, depression.
(5) Dysuria.

4. Goal: *anticipatory guidance*—discharge planning: mothers are discharged earlier in their postpartum recovery today—(6–48 hours after birth if asymptomatic).
a. Discuss, assist in organizing time schedule. Nap, when possible, when infant asleep—to minimize fatigue.
b. Common maternal emotional/behavior changes, feelings:
(1) Jealous of infant; guilt feelings.
(2) "Baby blues"—due to hormonal fluctuations, fatigue, change of lifestyle.
(3) Feelings of inadequacy.
c. Discuss support groups, aid in identifying supportive people.

D. Evaluation/outcome criteria:
1. Woman experiences normal, uncomplicated postpartum period. All assessment findings within normal limits.
2. Woman returns demonstrations of appropriate self-care measures/techniques:
a. Perineal care, pad change, hand washing.
b. Breast care, breast self-examination.
3. Woman verbalizes understanding of:
a. Need for adequate rest and diversion.
b. Appropriate time for resumption of intercourse and exercise.
c. Appropriate nutritional intake to meet needs (own and, if breastfeeding, infant's).
d. Signs to be reported immediately.
e. Returns demonstration of appropriate infant care measures.
f. Evidences beginning comfort and increasing confidence in parenting role.

E. Postpartum assessment—6 or less weeks after birth:
1. Weight, vital signs, urine for protein, complete blood count (CBC).
2. Breast examination lactating or not.
3. Pelvic examination—involution and position of uterus; perineal healing; tone of pelvic floor.
4. Desire for selection of method of contraception.

III. PSYCHOLOGICAL/BEHAVIORAL CHANGES.

Achievement of developmental tasks—progress in assuming maternal role.

A. Assessment:
1. *Taking-in* phase—1 to 3 days following birth.
a. Talkative; verbally relives labor/birth experience.
b. Passive, dependent, concerned with own needs (eating, sleeping, elimination).
2. *Taking-hold* phase—day 3 to 2 weeks.
a. Impatient to control own bodily functions, care for self.
b. Expresses interest/concern in learning how to care for baby (desire to assume "mothering" role).
c. Responds to positive reinforcement.
3. *Letting-go* phase—mother "lets go" of former self-concept, role, lifestyle; begins to integrate new role and self-concept as "mother."
a. Feelings of insecurity, inadequacy.
b. Hesitancy in approaching infant care tasks.

4. "Baby blues"—may appear on day 4 or 5. *Note:* Often, father/partner experiences same feelings.
   a. Thought to result from fatigue (sleep deprivation), realization of need for role change, recognition of new responsibilities, hormonal change.
   b. Mild depression, cries without provocation.
   c. Frightened—intimidated by own perceptions of responsibilities, hormonal changes.
5. Lag in experiencing "maternal feelings"—usually resolved within 6 weeks.
   a. May contribute to "baby blues."
   b. Guilt regarding lack of "maternal feelings."
   c. Diminished by prompt bonding experience.

B. Analysis/nursing diagnosis:

1. *Ineffective family coping: compromised,* related to achieving developmental tasks.
2. *Situational low self-esteem* related to perceived inadequacy in acceptance of maternal role.
3. *Ineffective individual coping* related to "baby blues," lag in experiencing maternal feelings.

C. Nursing care plan/implementation:

1. *Taking-in.* Goal: *emotional support.*
   a. Encourage verbalization of labor/birth experiences; compliment parents on "how well" they did.
   b. Explore feelings of disappointment, if any.
   c. Meet dependency needs; comment on appearance, hair, personal gowns.
   d. Encourage rooming in.
2. *Taking-hold.* Goal: *health teaching.*
   a. Discuss self-care, postpartum physiological/psychological changes.
   b. Demonstrate infant care; mother returns demonstration.

D. Evaluation/outcome criteria:

1. Woman demonstrates beginning comfort in maternal role.
2. Woman develops confidence and competence in infant care.
3. Woman expresses satisfaction with self, infant; eager to return home.
4. Woman succeeds in breastfeeding. (Tension inhibits let-down reflex; baby nurses poorly.)

IV. BREASTFEEDING AND LACTATION

A. Biological foundations:

1. *Antepartal* alterations:
   a. High estrogen/progesterone levels—stimulate proliferation and development of breast ducts.
   b. High progesterone levels—also → development of mammary lobules and alveoli.
2. *Postpartum* alterations:
   a. Rapid drop in estrogen/progesterone levels.
   b. Increased secretion of prolactin—stimulates alveolar cells → milk.
   c. Suckling—stimulates release of oxytocin → contraction of ducts → milk ejection (let-down reflex).
   d. Engorgement—due to venous and lymphatic stasis.
      (1) Immediately precedes lactation.
      (2) Lasts about 24 hours.
      (3) Frequent feeding reduces engorgement.

B. Assessment:

1. Colostrum (yellowish fluid)—continues for first 2 to 3 days; has some antibiotic, immunologic, and nutritive value.
2. Milk (bluish-white, thin)—secreted on about third day.

C. Analysis/nursing diagnosis:

1. *Knowledge deficit* related to breastfeeding techniques.
2. *Pain* related to engorgement.
3. *Personal identity disturbance* related to problems in breastfeeding.
4. *Sleep pattern disturbance* related to discomfort or infant care needs.

D. Nursing care plan/implementation:

1. Goal: *promote successful breastfeeding.*
   a. Encourage first feeding within 1 hour after giving birth.
   b. Encourage emptying both breasts at each feeding and before engorgement to stimulate milk production, prevent mastitis.
   c. Encourage rest, relaxation, fluids.
   d. *Nutritional* counseling (see **Chapter 9**).
      (1) Additional 500 calories daily—may be supplied by one extra pint of milk, one extra egg, and one extra serving of meat, citrus fruit, and vegetable.
      (2) Increase fluid intake to 3000 mL daily.
2. Goal: *prevent or relieve engorgement.*
   a. Pain: relieved by warm packs, emptying breasts.
   b. Wear good, supportive bra.
   c. Administer analgesics, as ordered/necessary.
3. Goal: *health teaching.*
   a. Instruct, demonstrate *rooting reflex* and putting infant to breast. Infant must grasp nipple and areola over location of milk sinuses.
   b. Demonstrate burping techniques, what to do if infant chokes; removing infant from breast.
   c. Instruct in *basic nipple care.*
      (1) Teach good hand washing.
      (2) Nurse on each breast, making sure areola is in mouth, alternating position of infant.

(3) Alternate "beginning" breast.
(4) Break suction before removing infant from breast.
(5) Air-dry nipples after each feeding and apply lanolin if abraded. *Note:* Creams, lotions, or ointments block secretion of a natural bacteriostatic oil by Montgomery glands—and infant may refuse breast until it is washed. Instead: expressed milk may be massaged gently around nipple.
(6) Teach daily hygiene of breasts.

d. Instruct in care of cracked or *fissured nipples.*
(1) Encourage and support mothers.
(2) Air-dry nipples after each feeding.
(3) Use nipple shield if nipples extremely sore.
(4) Discontinue nursing for 48 hours; maintain milk supply by expressing milk with pump.

e. Discuss avoiding use of any drugs except under medical supervision—may affect infant or suppress lactation.

f. Discuss possibility of sexual stimulation during breastfeeding.
(1) Validate normalcy and acceptability.
(2) *Note:* During orgasm, milk may squirt from nipples.

g. Explain that contraceptive value of nursing is unpredictable; the time that ovulation is inhibited varies widely.

h. Explain *contraindications to breastfeeding:*
(1) Active tuberculosis.
(2) Severe chronic maternal disease.
(3) Mastitis (temporary interruption may be necessary).
(4) Some therapeutic drugs.
(5) Severe cleft lip or palate in newborn (may pump and give in special bottles).
(6) HIV-positive status; AIDS.

E. Evaluation/outcome criteria:

1. Woman verbalizes understanding of breastfeeding techniques, nutritional requirements for successful lactation.
2. Woman successfully demonstrates breastfeeding; infant nurses well.
3. Woman demonstrates appropriate burping techniques; clears excessive mucus from infant's mouth without incident.
4. Woman verbalizes understanding of basic breast care techniques:
   a. Self-examination.
   b. Clear water bath.
   c. Drying nipples after bathing, feeding.
   d. Care of cracked or irritated nipples.
   e. Correct infant positioning for feeding.

Complications During the Postpartum Period

I. DISORDERS AFFECTING FLUID-GAS TRANSPORT

A. Postpartum hemorrhage

1. Definition—loss of 500 mL of blood or more during first 24 hours postpartum in vaginal birth; 1000 mL in cesarean birth.
2. **Pathophysiology**—excessive loss of blood secondary to trauma, decreased uterine contractility; results in hypovolemia.
3. **Etiology** (in decreasing order of frequency):
   a. Uterine atony
   (1) Uterine overdistention (multipregnancy, polyhydramnios, fetal macrosomia).
   (2) Multiparity.
   (3) Prolonged or precipitous labor.
   (4) Anesthesia—deep inhalation or regional (particularly saddle block).
   (5) Myomata (fibroids).
   (6) Oxytocin induction of labor.
   (7) Overmassage of uterus in postpartum.
   (8) Distended bladder.
   b. Lacerations—cervix, vagina, perineum.
   c. Retained placental fragments—usually delayed postpartum hemorrhage.
   d. Hematoma—deep pelvic, vaginal, or episiotomy site.
4. **Assessment:**
   a. Uterus—boggy, flaccid; excessive vaginal bleeding (dark; seepage, large clots)—due to uterine atony, retained placental fragments.
   b. Late signs of shock—air hunger; anxiety/apprehension, tachycardia, tachypnea, hypotension.
   c. Blood values (admission and postpartum)—hemoglobin (Hgb), hematocrit (Hct), clotting time.
   d. Estimated blood loss: during labor/birth; in early postpartum.
   e. Pain: vulvar, vaginal, perineal.
   f. Perineum: distended—due to edema; discoloration—due to hematoma. May complain of rectal pressure.
   g. Lacerations—bright red vaginal bleeding with firm fundus.
5. **Analysis/nursing diagnosis:**
   a. *Fluid volume deficit* related to excessive blood loss secondary to uterine atony, retained placental fragments.
   b. *Anxiety/fear* related to unexpected complication.
   c. *Altered tissue perfusion* related to decreased oxygenation secondary to blood loss.
   d. *Activity intolerance* related to fatigue.

MATERNAL/INFANT

6. **Nursing care plan/implementation:**
   a. *Medical management:*
      (1) IV oxytocin infusion; IV or oral ergot preparations (ergonovine [Ergotrate Maleate]; methylergonovine [Methergine]; carboprost (Prostin/M15), an oxytocic; prostaglandin.
      (2) Order blood work: clotting time, platelet count, fibrinogen level, Hgb, Hct, CBC.
      (3) Type and crossmatch for blood replacement.
      (4) Surgical:
         (a) Repair of lacerations.
         (b) Evacuation, ligation of hematoma.
         (c) Curettage—retained placental fragments.
   b. *Nursing management:*
      (1) Goal: *minimize blood loss.*
         (a) Notify physician promptly of abnormal assessment findings.
         (b) Order lab work STAT, as directed—to determine blood loss and etiology.
         (c) Fundal massage.
         (d) Administer medications to stimulate uterine tone. For ergot products and carboprost, monitor blood pressure (**contraindicated** in PIH).
      (2) Goal: *stabilize status.*
         (a) Establish IV line—to enable administration of medications and rapid absorption/action. Administer whole blood (with larger catheter).
         (b) Administer medications, as ordered to control bleeding, combat shock.
         (c) Prepare for surgery, as ordered.
      (3) Goal: *prevent infection.* Strict aseptic technique.
      (4) Goal: *continual monitoring.* Vital signs, bleeding (do pad count or weigh pads), fundal status.
      (5) Goal: *prevent sequelae* (*Sheehan's* syndrome).
      (6) Goal: *health teaching*—after episode: Reinforce appropriate perineal care and hand-washing techniques.
7. **Evaluation/outcome criteria:**
   a. Maternal vital signs stable.
   b. Bleeding diminished or absent.
   c. Assessment findings within normal limits.

B. Subinvolution—delayed return of uterus to normal size, shape, position.

1. **Pathophysiology**—inability of inflamed uterus (endometritis) to contract effectively → incomplete uterine involution; failure of contractions to effect closure of vessels in site of placental attachment → bleeding.
2. **Etiology:**
   a. PROM with secondary amnionitis, endometritis.
   b. Retained placental fragments.
   c. Oxytocin stimulation or augmentation of labor of overdistended uterine muscle may interfere with involution.
3. **Assessment:**
   a. Uterus: large, boggy; lack of uterine tone; failure to shrink progressively.
   b. Discharge: persistent lochia; painless fresh bleeding, hemorrhagic episodes.
4. **Analysis/nursing diagnosis:**
   a. *Pain* related to tender, inflamed uterus secondary to endometritis.
   b. *Anxiety/fear* related to change in physical status.
   c. *Knowledge deficit* related to diagnosis, treatment, prognosis.
   d. *High risk for injury* related to infection.
   e. *Fluid volume deficit* related to excessive bleeding.
5. **Nursing care plan/implementation:**
   a. *Medical management:*
      (1) Have woman void or catheterize; massage fundus.
      (2) Surgical (curettage)—to remove placental fragments.
      (3) Antibiotic therapy—to treat intrauterine infection.
      (4) Oxytocics—to stimulate/enhance uterine contractions.
   b. *Nursing management:*
      (1) Goal: *health teaching.*
         (a) Explain condition and treatment.
         (b) Describe, demonstrate perineal care, pad change, hand washing.
      (2) Goal: *emotional support.* Encourage verbalization of anxiety regarding recovery, separation from newborn.
      (3) Goal: *promote healing.*
         (a) Encourage rest, compliance with medical/nursing regimen.
         (b) Administer oxytocics, antibiotics, as ordered.
6. **Evaluation/outcome criteria:**
   a. Verbalizes understanding of condition and treatment.
   b. Complies with medical/nursing regimen.
   c. Demonstrates normal involutional progress.
   d. All assessment findings (vital signs, fundal height, consistency, lochial discharge) within normal limits.
   e. Expresses satisfaction with care.

C. Hypofibrinogenemia

1. **Pathophysiology**—decreased clotting factors, fibrinogen; may be accompanied by DIC.

2. **Etiology:**
   a. Missed abortion (retained dead fetus syndrome).
   b. Fetal death, delayed emptying of uterine contents.
   c. Abruptio placentae; Couvelaire uterus.
   d. Amniotic fluid embolism.
   e. Hypertension.
3. **Assessment:**
   a. Observe for bleeding from injection sites, epistaxis, purpura.
   b. See **DIC assessment, p. 429** in **Chapter 6.**
   c. Maternal vital signs, color.
   d. I&O.
   e. *Medical evaluation*—procedures.
      (1) Thrombin clot test—important: size and persistence of clot.
      (2) Prothrombin time—*prolonged.*
      (3) Bleeding time—*prolonged.*
      (4) Platelet count—*decreased.*
      (5) Activated partial thromboplastin time—*prolonged.*
      (6) Fibrinogen (factor I concentration)—*decreased.*
      (7) Fibrin degradation products—present.
4. **Analysis/nursing diagnosis:**
   a. *Fluid volume deficit* related to uncontrolled bleeding secondary to coagulopathy.
   b. *Anxiety/fear* related to unexpected critical emergency.
   c. *Altered tissue perfusion* related to decreased oxygenation secondary to blood loss.
5. **Nursing care plan/implementation:**
   a. *Medical management:*
      (1) Replace platelets.
      (2) Replace blood loss.
      (3) IV heparin—to inhibit conversion of fibrinogen to fibrin.
   b. *Nursing management:*
      (1) Goal: *continuous monitoring.*
         (a) Vital signs.
         (b) I&O hourly.
         (c) Skin: color, emergence of petechiae.
         (d) Note, measure (as possible), record, and report blood loss.
      (2) Goal: *control blood loss.*

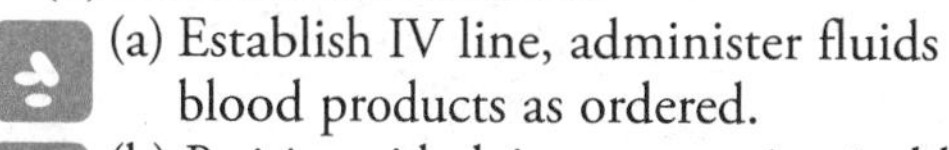

         (a) Establish IV line, administer fluids or blood products as ordered.

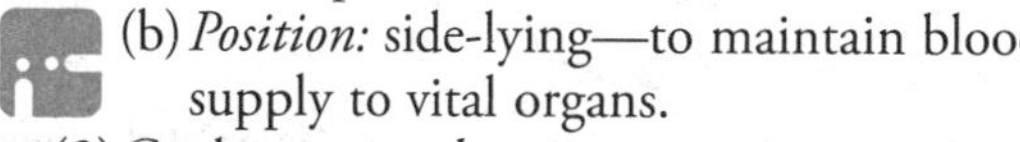

         (b) *Position:* side-lying—to maintain blood supply to vital organs.
      (3) Goal: *emotional support.*
         (a) Encourage verbalization of anxiety, fear, concerns.
         (b) Explain all procedures.
         (c) Remain with woman continuously.
         (d) Keep woman and family informed.
6. **Evaluation/outcome criteria:**
   a. Bleeding controlled.
   b. Laboratory studies—returning to normal values.
   c. Status stable.

II. DISORDERS AFFECTING PROTECTIVE FUNCTIONS: postpartum infection **(Table 4.13).**

A. General aspects

1. Definition—reproductive system infection occurring during the postpartum period.
2. **Pathophysiology**—bacterial invasion of birth canal; most common: localized infection of the lining of the uterus (endometritis).
3. **Etiology:**
   a. Anaerobic nonhemolytic streptococci.
   b. *E. coli.*
   c. *C. trachomatis* (bacteroides).
   d. Staphylococci.

Table 4.13

Postpartum Infections

Condition/Etiology *Postpartum Infection*	Assessment: Signs/Symptoms	Nursing Interventions
Traumatic labor and birth and postpartum hemorrhage make woman more vulnerable to infection by such bacteria as nonhemolytic streptococci, *Escherichia coli,* and *Staphylococcus* species	• Depends on location and severity of infection; usually include fever, pain, swelling, and tenderness • Temperature of 100.4°F (38°C) or more after first 24 hours after birth on two or more occasions indicates puerperal infection ("childbed fever")	1. Monitor: Signs and symptoms, drainage (e.g., uterine) 2. Obtain culture and sensitivity 3. Administer *antimicrobial* agents and *analgesic* agents 4. Ensure comfort; encourage rest 5. Use standard precautions 6. *Force fluids* and provide *high*-calorie diet 7. Keep family informed of mother's and newborn's progress 8. Promote maternal-infant contact as soon as possible 9. Plan and implement discharge and follow-up care

Continued

Table 4.13

Postpartum Infections—cont'd

Condition/Etiology	Assessment: Signs/Symptoms	Nursing Interventions
Endometritis		
Microorganisms invade placental site and may spread to entire endometrium	Temperature, chills, anorexia, malaise, boggy uterus, foul-smelling lochia, and cramps	1. Administer *antimicrobial* agents and *analgesic* agents 2. Encourage *Fowler's position* to promote drainage 3. *Force fluids* 4. Take standard precautions
Pelvic Cellulitis or Parametritis		
Microorganisms spread through lymphatics and invade tissues surrounding uterus	Fever, chills, lower abdominal pain, and tenderness	1. Administer *antimicrobial* agents and *analgesic* agents 2. Encourage bedrest 3. *Force fluids*
Perineal Infection		
Trauma to perineum makes woman more vulnerable to infection	Localized pain, fever, swelling, redness, and seropurulent drainage	1. Administer *antimicrobial* agents and *analgesic* agents 2. Provide sitz baths or heat/cold applications 3. Take standard precautions
Mastitis		
Lesions or fissure on nipples allow entry of microorganisms (e.g., *Staphylococcus aureus*) from infant's nose/mouth or mother's unwashed hands (Breastmilk is a good medium for growth of organism)	• Marked engorgement, pain, chills, fever, tachycardia • If untreated, single or multiple breast abscesses may form	1. Order culture and sensitivity studies of mother's milk 2. Administer *antimicrobial* agents and *analgesic* agents 3. Apply heat or cold therapy 4. Assist with incising and draining abscesses 5. Use standard precautions and perform meticulous hand washing
Thrombophlebitis		
Infected pelvic or femoral thrombi Increased tendency to clot formation during pregnancy, trauma to tissues, and hemorrhage decrease new mother's resistance to infection	• Pain, chills, and fever • *Femoral:* stiffness of affected area or part and positive *Homans'* sign • *Pelvic:* severe chills and wide fluctuations in temperature	*Femoral:* 1. Rest and *elevate* leg 2. Administer *antimicrobial* agents, *analgesic* agents, and *anticoagulants* *Pelvic:* 1. Encourage bedrest 2. Force fluids 3. Administer *antimicrobial* agents and *anticoagulants*

4. Predisposing conditions:
   a. Anemia.
   b. PROM.
   c. Prolonged labor.
   d. Repeated vaginal examinations during labor.
   e. Intrauterine manipulation (e.g., manual extraction of placenta).
   f. Retained placental fragments.
   g. Postpartum hemorrhage.
5. **Assessment:**
   a. Fever 38°C (100.4°F) or more on two or more occasions, after first 24 hours postpartum.
   b. Other signs of infection: pain, malaise, dysuria, subinvolution, foul lochial odor.
6. **Analysis/nursing diagnosis:**
   a. *Fluid volume deficit* related to excessive blood loss, anemia.
   b. *Knowledge deficit* related to danger signs of postpartum period.
   c. *High risk for injury* related to infection.
7. **Nursing care plan/implementation:** prevention
   a. Goal: *prevent anemia.*
      (1) Minimize blood loss—accurate postpartum assessment and management of bleeding.

      (2) *Diet: high protein, high vitamin.*

      (3) Vitamins, iron—suggest continuing prenatal pattern until postpartum checkup.

MATERNAL/INFANT

b. Goal: *prevent entrance/transport of microorganisms.*
   (1) *Strict aseptic technique* during labor, birth, and postpartum (standard precautions).
   (2) Minimize vaginal examinations during labor.
   (3) Perineal care.

c. Goal: *health teaching.*
   (1) Hand washing—before and after each pad change, after voiding or defecating.
   (2) Perineal care—from front to back; use clear, warm water or mild antiseptic solution as a cascade; do *not* separate labia.
   (3) Maintain sterility of pads; apply from front to back.
   (4) *Avoid* use of tampons until normal menstrual cycle resumes.

8. **Evaluation/outcome criteria:**
   a. Woman has assessment findings within normal limits:
      (1) Vital signs.
      (2) Rate of involution (fundal height, consistency).
      (3) Lochia: character, amount, odor.
   b. Woman avoids infection.

B. Endometritis—infection of lining of uterus.

1. **Pathophysiology** (see **II. A. General aspects, p. 195**).
2. **Etiology**—most common: invasion by normal body flora (e.g., anaerobic streptococci).
3. Characteristics:
   a. Mild, localized—asymptomatic, or low-grade fever.
   b. Severe—may lead to ascending infection, parametritis, pelvic abscess, pelvic thrombophlebitis.
   c. If remains localized, self-limiting; usually resolves within 10 days.
4. **Assessment:**
   a. Signs of infection: fever, chills, malaise, anorexia, headache, backache.
   b. Uterus: large, boggy, extremely tender.
      (1) Subinvolution.
      (2) Lochia: dark brown; foul odor.
5. **Analysis/nursing diagnosis:**
   a. *Anxiety/fear* related to effects on self and newborn.
   b. *Self-esteem disturbance and altered role performance* related to inability to meet own expectations regarding parenting, secondary to unexpected hospitalization.
   c. *Pain* related to inflammation/infection.
   d. *Ineffective individual coping* related to physical discomfort and psychological stress associated with self-concept disturbance; worry, guilt, concern regarding newborn at home.
   e. *Altered family processes*—interruption of adjustment to altered life pattern related to postpartum infection/hospitalization.
6. **Nursing care plan/implementation:**
   a. Goal: *prevent cross-contamination.* Contact-item isolation.

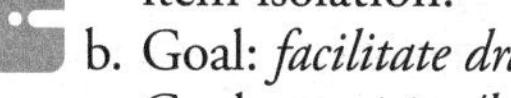

   b. Goal: *facilitate drainage. Position:* semi-Fowler's.
   c. Goal: *nutrition/hydration.*
      (1) *Diet: high calorie, high protein, high vitamin.*
      (2) Push *fluids* to 4000 mL/day (oral or IV, or both, as ordered).
      (3) I&O.
   d. Goal: *increase uterine tone/facilitate involution.* Administer medications, as ordered (e.g., oxytocics, antibiotics).
   e. Goal: *minimize energy expenditure,* as possible.
      (1) Bedrest.
      (2) Maximize rest, comfort.
   f. Goal: *emotional support.*
      (1) Encourage verbalization of anxiety, concerns.
      (2) Keep informed of progress.
7. **Evaluation/outcome criteria:**
   a. Vital signs stable, within normal limits.
   b. All assessment findings within normal limits.
   c. Unable to recover organism from discharge.

C. Urinary tract infections

1. **Pathophysiology**—normal physiological changes associated with pregnancy (e.g., ureteral dilation) and the postpartum period (e.g., diuresis, increased bladder capacity with diminished sensitivity of stretch receptors) → increased susceptibility to bacterial invasion and growth → ascending infections (cystitis, pyelonephritis).
2. **Etiology:** usually bacterial.
3. Predisposing factors:
   a. Birth trauma to bladder, urethra, or meatus.
   b. Bladder hypotonia with retention (due to intrapartum anesthesia or trauma).
   c. Repeated or prolonged catheterization, or poor technique.
   d. Weakening of immune response secondary to anemia, hemorrhage.
4. **Assessment:**
   a. Maternal vital signs (fever, tachycardia).
   b. Dysuria, frequency (flank pain—with pyelonephritis).
   c. Feeling of "not emptying" bladder.
   d. Cloudy urine; frank pus.
5. **Analysis/nursing diagnosis:**
   a. *Altered urinary elimination* related to diuresis, dysuria, inflammation/infection.
   b. *Pain* related to dysuria secondary to cystitis.
   c. *Knowledge deficit* related to self-care (perineal care).

6. **Nursing care plan/implementation:**
   a. Goal: *minimize perineal edema.* Perineal ice pack in fourth stage—to limit swelling secondary to trauma, facilitate voiding.
   b. Goal: *prevent overdistention of bladder.*
      (1) Monitor level of fundus, lochia, bladder distention. (*Note:* Distended bladder displaces uterus, limits its ability to contract → boggy fundus, increases its vaginal bleeding.)
      (2) Encourage *fluids* and voiding; I&O.
      (3) Aseptic technique for catheterization.
      (4) Slow emptying of bladder on catheterization—to maintain tone.
   c. Goal: *identification of causative organism*—to facilitate appropriate medication (antibiotics). Obtain clean-catch (or catheterized) specimen for culture and sensitivity.
   d. Goal: *health teaching.* See previous discussion of fluids, general hygiene, diet, and medications.
7. **Evaluation/outcome criteria:**
   a. Voiding: quantity sufficient (although small, frequent output may mean overflow with retention).
   b. Urine character: clear, amber, or straw colored.
   c. Vital signs: within normal limits.
   d. No complaints of frequency, urgency, burning on urination, flank pain.

D. Mastitis—inflammation of breast tissue:
1. **Pathophysiology**—local inflammatory response to bacterial invasion; suppuration may occur; organism can be recovered from breast milk.
2. **Etiology**—most common: *Staphylococcus aureus;* source—most common: infant's nose, throat.
3. **Assessment:**
   a. Signs of infection (may occur several weeks in postpartum).
      (1) Fever.
      (2) Chills.
      (3) Tachycardia.
      (4) Malaise.
      (5) Abdominal pain.
   b. Breast
      (1) Reddened area(s).
      (2) Localized/generalized swelling.
      (3) Heat, tenderness, palpable mass.
4. **Analysis/nursing diagnosis:**
   a. *Impaired skin integrity* related to nipple fissures, cracks.
   b. *Pain* related to tender, inflamed tissue secondary to infection.
   c. *Disturbance in body image, self-esteem* related to association of breastfeeding with female identity and role.
   d. *Anxiety/fear* related to sexuality; impact on breastfeeding, if any.
5. **Nursing care plan/implementation:**
   a. Goal: *prevent infection. Health teaching* in early postpartum:
      (1) Hand washing.
      (2) Breast care—wash with warm water only (*no* soap)—to prevent removing protective body oils.
      (3) Let breast milk dry on nipples to prevent drying of tissue.
      (4) Clean bra (with no plastic pads or liners) to support breasts, reduce friction, minimize exposure to microorganisms.
      (5) Good breastfeeding techniques (see **pp. 192–193**).
      (6) Alternate position of infant for nursing to change pressure areas.
   b. Goal: *comfort measures.*
      (1) Encourage bra or binder—to support breasts, reduce pain from motion.
      (2) Local heat or ice packs as ordered—to reduce engorgement, pain.
      (3) Administer analgesics, as necessary.
   c. Goal: *emotional support.*
      (1) Encourage verbalization of feelings, concerns.
      (2) If breastfeeding is discontinued, reassure woman she will be able to resume breastfeeding.
   d. Goal: *promote healing.*
      (1) Maintain lactation (if desired) by manual expression or breast pump, q4h.
      (2) Administer antibiotics as ordered.
6. **Evaluation/outcome criteria:**
   a. Woman promptly responds to medical/nursing regimen.
      (1) Symptoms subside.
      (2) Assessment findings within normal limits.
   b. Woman successfully returns to breastfeeding.

E. Thrombophlebitis
1. **Pathophysiology**—inflammation of a vein secondary to lodging of a clot.
2. **Etiology:**
   a. Extension of endometritis with involvement of pelvic and femoral veins.
   b. Clot formation in pelvic veins following cesarean birth.
   c. Clot formation in femoral (or other) veins secondary to poor circulation, compression, and venous stasis.
3. **Assessment:**
   a. Pelvic—pain: abdominal or pelvic tenderness.
   b. Calf—pain: positive *Homans'* sign (pain elicited by flexion of foot with knee extended).
   c. Femoral
      (1) Pain.
      (2) Malaise, fever, chills.
      (3) Swelling—"milk leg."

4. **Analysis/nursing diagnosis:**
   a. *Pain* in affected region related to local inflammatory response.
   b. *Anxiety/fear* related to outcome.
   c. *Ineffective individual coping* related to unexpected postpartum complications, hospitalization, separation from newborn.
   d. *Impaired physical mobility* related to imposed bedrest to prevent emboli formation and dislodging clot (embolus).
5. **Nursing care plan/implementation:**
   a. Goal: *prevent clot formation.*
      (1) Encourage early ambulation.
      (2) *Position: avoid* prolonged compression of popliteal space, use of knee gatch.
      (3) Apply thromboembolic disease (TED) hose, or sequential compression device, as ordered, preoperatively or postoperatively, or both, for cesarean birth.
   b. Goal: *reduce threat of emboli.*
      (1) Bedrest, with cradle to support bedding.
      (2) Discourage massaging "leg cramps."
   c. Goal: *prevent further clot formation.* Administer anticoagulants, as ordered.
   d. Goal: *prevent infection.*
      (1) Administer antibiotics, as ordered.
      (2) Push *fluids.*
   e. Goal: *facilitate clot resolution.* Heat therapy, as ordered.
6. **Evaluation/outcome criteria:**
   a. Symptoms subside; all assessment findings within normal limits.
   b. No evidence of further clot formation.

III. DISORDERS AFFECTING PSYCHOSOCIAL-CULTURAL FUNCTIONS—postpartum depression/psychosis

A. General aspects
1. Can occur in both new parents and experienced parents.
2. Usually occurs within 2 weeks of birth.
3. Increased incidence among single parents
4. Increased incidence among women with history of clinical depression.
5. Most common symptomatology: affective disorders.
6. Psychiatric intervention required if prolonged or severe; if underlying cause unresolved; increased risk in subsequent pregnancies.

B. Etiology—theory: birth of child may emphasize:
1. Unresolved role conflicts.
2. Unachieved normal development tasks.

C. Assessment:
1. Withdrawal.
2. Paranoia.
3. Anorexia, sleep disturbance, mood swings.
4. Depression—may alternate with manic behavior.
5. Potential for self-injury or child abuse/neglect.

D. Analysis/nursing diagnosis:
1. *Ineffective individual coping* related to perceived inability to meet role expectations ("mother") and ambivalence related to dependence/independence.
2. *Self-esteem disturbance and altered role performance* related to "femaleness" and reaction to responsibility for care of newborn.
3. *High risk for violence,* self-directed or directed at newborn, related to anger or depression.
4. *Ineffective family coping* related to lack of support system in early postpartum.
5. *Altered family processes* related to psychological stress, interruption of bonding.
6. *Altered parenting* related to hormonal changes and stress.

E. Nursing care plan/implementation:
1. Goal: *emotional support.*
   a. Encourage verbalization of feelings, fears, anxiety, concerns.
   b. Support positive self-image, feelings of adequacy, self-worth.
      (1) Reinforce appropriate comments and behaviors.
      (2) Encourage active participation in self-care, comment on accomplishments.
      (3) Reduce threat to self-image, fear of failure. Maintain support, gradually increase tasks.
2. Goal: *safeguard status of mother/newborn.*
   a. Unobtrusive, protective environment.
   b. Stay with woman when she is with infant.
3. Goal: *nutrition/hydration.*
   a. Encourage selection of favorite foods—to aid security in decision making; counteract anorexia (refusal to eat) by tempting appetite.
   b. Push *fluids* (juices, soft drinks, milkshakes)—to maintain hydration.
4. Goal: *minimize stress, facilitate effective coping.* Administer therapeutic medications, as ordered.
   a. Schizophrenia—phenothiazines.
   b. Depression—mood elevators.
   c. Manic behaviors—sedatives, tranquilizers.

F. Evaluation/outcome criteria:
1. Woman increases interaction with infant.
2. Woman expresses interest in learning how to care for infant.
3. Woman evidences no agitation, depression.
4. Woman actively participates in caring for self and infant.
5. Woman demonstrates increasing comfort in mothering role.
6. Woman has positive family interactions.

THE NEWBORN INFANT

General overview: Effective nursing care of the newborn infant is based on: (1) knowledge of the conditions present during fetal life; (2) requirements for independent extrauterine life; and (3) alterations needed for successful transition. *The first 24 hours are the most hazardous.*

I. BIOLOGICAL FOUNDATIONS OF NEONATAL ADAPTATION—*General aspects:*

A. *Fetal anatomy and physiology*

1. *Fetal circulation*—five intrauterine structures that differ from extrauterine structures (**Fig. 4.11**):
   a. *Umbilical vein*—carries oxygen and nutrient-enriched blood from placenta to ductus venosus and liver.
   b. *Ductus venosus*—connects to inferior vena cava; allows most blood to bypass liver.
   c. *Foramen ovale*—allows fetal blood to bypass fetal lungs by shunting it from right atrium into left atrium.
   d. *Ductus arteriosus*—allows fetal blood to bypass fetal lungs by shunting it from pulmonary artery into aorta.
   e. *Umbilical arteries* (two)—allow return of deoxygenated blood to the placenta.
2. *Umbilical cord*—extends from fetus to center of placenta: usually 50 cm (18–22 inches) long and 1 to 2 cm (½–1 inch) in diameter. Contains:
   a. *Wharton's jelly*—protects umbilical vessels from pressure, cord "kinking," and interference with fetal-placental circulation.
   b. Umbilical vein—carries oxygen and nutrients from placenta to fetus.
   c. Two umbilical arteries—carry deoxygenated blood and fetal wastes from fetus to placenta. *Note:* Absence of one artery indicates need to rule out intra-abdominal anomalies.
3. *Characteristics of fetal blood*
   a. Fetal hemoglobin (HbF)
      (1) Higher oxygen-carrying capacity than adult hemoglobin.
      (2) Releases oxygen easily to fetal tissues.
      (3) Ensures high fetal oxygenation.
      (4) Normal range at term: 12 to 22 g/dL; average: 15 to 20 g/dL.
   b. Total blood volume at term: 85 mL/kg body weight; Hct: 38% to 62%, average 53%; RBCs: 3 to 7 million, average 4.9 million/unit.

B. *Extrauterine adaptation: tasks*

1. Establish and maintain ventilation, successful gas transfer—requires patent airway and adequate pulmonary surfactant.

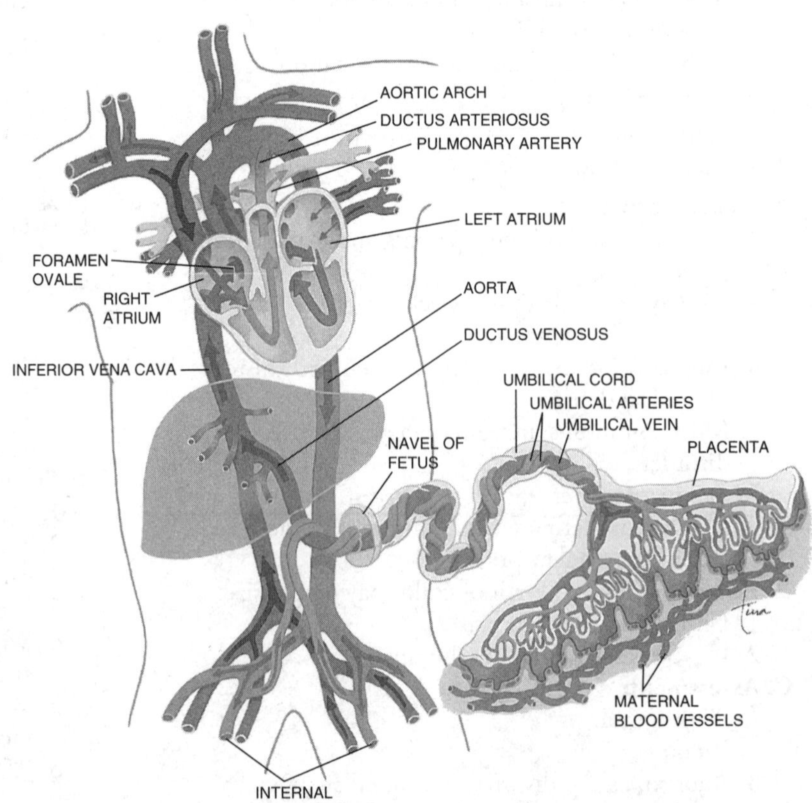

Figure 4.11 Fetal circulation. (From Venes, D [ed]: *Taber's Cyclopedic Medical Dictionary,* ed 20. FA Davis, Philadelphia, 2005, p 422.)

2. Modify circulatory patterns—requires closure of fetal structures.
3. Absorb and utilize fluids and nutrients.
4. Excrete body wastes.
5. Establish and maintain thermal stability.

C. Nursing care plan/implementation:

1. Facilitate successful transition to independent life.
2. Protect infant from physiological stress and environmental hazards.
3. Encourage development of a strong family unit.

II. ADMISSION/ASSESSMENT: 1 TO 4 HOURS AFTER BIRTH

A. Admission assessment of normal, term neonate

1. Color and reactivity.
2. General appearance, symmetry.
3. Length and weight.
4. Head and chest circumferences.
5. Vital signs:
   a. Axillary temperature.
   b. Respirations (check rate, character, rhythm).
   c. Apical pulse.
6. General physical assessment (**Table 4.14**) and reflexes (**Table 4.15**).
7. Estimate of gestational age (**Table 4.16**).

B. Analysis/nursing diagnosis:

1. *Altered health maintenance* related to separation from maternal support system.
2. *Impaired skin integrity* related to umbilical stump; incontinence of urine and meconium stool; skin penetration by scalp electrode, injections, heel stick, scalpel during cesarean birth; abrasion from obstetric forceps.
3. *Ineffective airway clearance* related to excessive mucus.
4. *Pain* related to environmental stimuli.
5. *Ineffective thermoregulation* related to immature temperature regulation mechanism.

(text continues on page 205)

Table 4.14

Physical Assessment of the Term Neonate

Criterion	Average Values and Normal Variations	Deviations from Normal
Vital Signs		
Heart rate	120–140/min, irregular, especially when crying, and functional murmur	Faint sound—pneumomediastinum; and heart rate <100 beats/min or >180 beats/min
Respiratory rate	30–60/min with short periods of apnea, irregular; vigorous and loud cry	Distress—flaring of nares, retractions, tachypnea, grunting, excessive mucus, <30 respirations/min or >60 respirations/min; cyanosis
Temperature	Stabilizes about 8–10 hours after birth; 36.5–37°C (97.7–98.6°F) axillary	Unreliable indicator of infection due to environmental influences
Blood pressure	60–80/40–50; varies with change in activity level	Hypotension: with RDS Hypertension: coarctation of aorta
Measurements		
Weight	3400 gm (7½ lbs); range: 5 lb 8 oz–8 lb 13 oz	Birth weight <2500 gm: preterm or SGA infant; >4000 gm: LGA infant, evaluate mother for gestational diabetes
Length	50 cm (20 inches); range: 18–22 inches	
Chest circumference	2 cm (¾ inch) less than head circumference	If relationship varies, check for reason
Head circumference	33–35 cm (13–14 inches)	Check for microcephalus and macrocephalus
General Assessment		
Muscle tone	Good tone and generalized flexion; full range of motion; spontaneous movement	Flaccid, and persistent tremor or twitching; movement limited; asymmetrical
Skin color	Mottling, acrocyanosis, and physiological jaundice; petechiae (over presenting part), milia, mongolian spotting, lanugo, and vernix caseosa	• Pallor, cyanosis, or jaundice within 24 hours of birth • Petechiae or ecchymoses elsewhere; all rashes, except erythema toxicum; pigmented nevi; hemangioma; and yellow vernix
Head	Molding of fontanels and suture spaces; one fourth of body length	Cephalohematoma, caput succedaneum, sunken or bulging fontanels, closed sutures; excessively wide sutures

Continued

Table 4.14

Physical Assessment of the Term Neonate—cont'd

Criterion	Average Values and Normal Variations	Deviations from Normal
Hair	Silky, single strands, lies flat; grows toward face and neck	Fine, wooly; unusual swirls, patterns, hairline; coarse
Eyes	Edematous eyelids, conjunctival hemorrhage; grayish-blue to grayish-brown; blink reflex, usually no tears; uncoordinated movements may focus for a few seconds; good placement on face; cornea is bright and shiny; pupillary reflex equal and reactive to light; eyebrows distinct	Epicanthal folds (in non-Asians); discharges; agenesis; opaque lenses; lesions; strabismus; "doll's eyes" beyond 10 days; absence of reflexes
Nose	Appears to have no bridge; should have no discharge; preferential nose breathers; sneezes to clear nose	Discharge and choanal atresia; malformed; flaring of nares beyond first few moments of life
Mouth	*Epstein's pearls* on gum ridges; tongue does not protrude and moves freely, symmetrically; uvula in midline; reflexes present; sucking, rooting, gag, extrusion	*Cleft lip or palate;* teeth, cyanosis, circumoral pallor; asymmetrical lip movement; excessive saliva; thrush; incomplete or absent reflexes
Ears	Well formed, firm; notch of ear should be on straight line with outer canthus	Low placement, clefts; tags; malformed; lack of cartilage
Face	Symmetrical movements and contours	*Facial palsy* (7th cranial nerve); looks "funny"
Neck	Short, freely movable; some head control	Wry neck, webbed neck; restricted movement; masses; distended veins; absence of head control
Chest	Enlarged breasts, "*witch's milk*"; barrel shaped; both sides move synchronously; nipples symmetrical	Flattened, funnel-chested, asynchronous movement; lack of breast tissue; fracture of clavicle(s); supernumerary or widely spaced nipples; bowel sounds
Abdomen	Dome shaped, abdominal respirations, soft; may have small umbilical hernia; umbilical cord well formed, containing three vessels; dry around base; bowel sounds within 2 hours of birth; voiding; passage of meconium	Scaphoid shaped, omphalocele, diastasis recti, and distention; umbilical cord containing two vessels; redness or drainage around base of cord
Genitalia		
Girl	Large labia; may have pseudomenstruation, smegma; vaginal orifice open; increased pigmentation; ecchymosis and edema following breech birth; pink-stained urine (uric acid crystals)	Agenesis and imperforate hymen; ambiguous labia widely separated, fecal discharge per vagina; *epispadias or hypospadias*
Boy	Pendulous scrotum covered with rugae, and testes usually descended; voids with adequate stream; increased pigmentation; edema and ecchymosis following breech birth	*Phimosis, epispadias,* or *hypospadias;* ambiguous; scrotum smooth and testes undescended *Hydrocele:* collection of fluid in the sac surrounding the testes
Extremities	Synchronized movements, freely movable through full range of motion; legs appear bowed, and feet appear flat; attitude of general flexion; arms longer than legs; grasp reflex; palmar and sole creases; normal contour	Fractures, brachial nerve palsy, *clubbed foot,* phocomelia or amelia, unusual number or webbing of digits, and abnormal palmar creases; poor muscle tone; asymmetry; hypertonicity; unusual hip contour and click sign (*hip dysplasia*); hypermobility of joints
Back	Spine straight, easily movable, and flexible; may have small pilonidal dimple at base of spine; may raise head when prone	Fusion of vertebrae: pilonidal dimple with tuft of hair; *spina bifida,* agenesis of part of vertebral bodies; limitation of movement; weak or absent reflexes
Anus	Patent, well placed; "wink" reflex	Imperforate, and absence of "wink" (absence of sphincter muscle); fistula

Table 4.14

Physical Assessment of the Term Neonate—cont'd

Criterion	Average Values and Normal Variations	Deviations from Normal
Stools	Meconium within first 24 hours; transitional—days 2–5; *breastfed:* loose, golden yellow; *bottle-fed:* formed, light yellow (see **Table 4.17**)	Light-colored meconium (dry, hard), or absent with distended abdomen (*cyctic fibrosis* or *Hirschsprung's disease*); diarrhetic
Laboratory Values		
Hemoglobin (cord)	13.6–19.6 gm/dL	Evaluate for anemia and persistent polycythemia
Serum bilirubin	2–6 mg/dL	Hyperbilirubinemia (*term:* 15 mg or more; *preterm:* 10 mg or more)
Blood glucose	40 mg/dL for *term;* >30 mg/dL for *preterm*	Identify hypoglycemia before overt or asymptomatic hypoglycemia—do Dextrostix on all suspected infants (LGA or SGA neonates, or neonates of mothers who are diabetic)
*Neurological Examination**	Specific to gestational age and state of wakefulness	
1. Behavioral patterns		
a. Feeding	• Variations in interest, hunger; usually feeds well within 48 hours	• Lethargic. Poor suck, poor coordination with swallow, choking, cyanosis
b. Social	• Crying is lusty, strong, and soon indicative of hunger, pain, attention seeking. • Responds to cuddling, voice by quietness and increased alertness	• Absent; no focusing on person holding him/her; unconsolable
c. Sleep-wakefulness	• Two periods of reactivity: at birth, and 6–8 hours later. Stabilization, with wakeful periods about every 3–4 hours	• Lethargy, drowsiness • Disorganized pattern
d. Elimination	• Stooling: *see* Stools • Urination First few days: 3–4 qd End of first week: 5–6 qd Later: 6–10 qd, with adequate hydration	*See* Stools Diminished number: dehydration
2. Reflex response	Bilateral, symmetrical response (see **Table 4.15**)	Absent, hyperactive, incomplete, asynchronous
3. Sensory capabilities		
a. Vision	• Limited accommodation, with clearest vision within 7–8 inches. Focuses and follows by 15 minutes of age. Prefers patterns to plain.	Absence of these responses may be due to absence of or diminished acuity or to sensory deprivation
b. Hearing	• By 2 minutes of age, can move in direction of sound: responds to high pitch by "freezing," followed by agitation; to low pitch (crooning) by relaxing	Absence of response: deafness
c. Touch	• Soothed by massaging, warmth, weightlessness (as in water bath)	Unable to be comforted: possible drug dependence
d. Smell	• By fifth day, can distinguish between mother's breasts and those of another woman	Newborns who are cocaine-addicted avoid eye contact
e. Taste	• Can distinguish between sweet and sour	
f. Motor	• Coordinates body movement to parent's voice and body movement	Absence

*Based on Brazelton's method.

MATERNAL/INFANT

Table 4.15

Assessment: Normal Newborn Reflexes*

Reflex	Description	Implications of Deviations from Normal Patterns
Moro (startle)	Symmetrical *abduction* and *extension* of arms with fingers extended in response to sudden movement or loud noise	Asymmetrical reflex may indicate brachial (Erb's) palsy or fractured clavicle
Tonic neck (fencing)	When head turned to one side, arm and leg on *that* side *extend,* and *opposite* arm and leg *flex*	Asymmetry may indicate cerebral lesion, if persistent
Rooting and sucking	With stimulus to cheek, turns *toward* stimulus, opens mouth, sucks	Absence of response may indicate prematurity, neurological problem, or depressed infant (or not hungry)
Palmar grasp	If palm stimulated, fingers *curl;* holds adult finger briefly	Asymmetry may indicate neurological involvement
Plantar grasp	Pressure on sole will elicit *curling* of toes	Absence/asymmetry associated with defects of lower spinal column
Stepping/dancing	If held in upright position with feet in contact with hard surface, alternately raises feet	Asymmetry may indicate neurological problem
Babinski	Stroking the sole in a upward fashion elicits *hyperextension* of toes	Same as for plantar grasp
Crawling	When placed in prone position, attempts to crawl	Absence may indicate prematurity or depressed infant

*Reflexes are good indicators of the neurological system in infants who are well, but not in neonates who are sick. Infants with infections may not show normal reflexes yet have an intact neurological system.

MATERNAL/INFANT

Table 4.16

Estimation of Gestational Age: Common Clinical Parameters

Characteristic	Preterm	Term
Head	Oval—narrow biparietal; large in proportion to body; face looks like "old man"	Square-shaped biparietal prominences; 1/4 body length
Ears: form, cartilage	Soft, flat, shapeless	Pinna firm; erect from head
Hair: texture, distribution	Fine, fuzzy, or wooly; clumped; appears at 20 weeks	Silk; single strands apparent
Sole creases	Starting at ball of foot: 1/3 covered with creases by 36 weeks, 2/3 by 38 weeks	Entire sole heavily creased
Breast nodules	0 mm at 36 weeks; 4 mm at 37 weeks	10 mm or more
Nipples	No areolae	Formed; raised above skin level
Genitalia		
Girl	Clitoris large, labia gaping	Labia larger, meet in midline
Boy	Small scrotum, rugae on inferior surface only, and testes undescended	Scrotum pendulous, covered with rugae; testes usually descended
Skin: texture, opacity	Visible abdominal veins; thin, shiny	Few indistinct larger veins; thick, dry, cracked, peeling
Vernix	Covers body by 31–33 weeks	Small amount in creases or absent at term; post-term: dry, wrinkled
Lanugo	Apparent at 20 weeks; by 33–36 weeks, covers shoulders	Minimal or no lanugo (depends on parental ethnicity)
Muscle tone	Hypotonia; extension of arms and legs	Hypertonia; well flexed
Posture	Froglike	Attitude of general flexion

Table 4.16

Estimation of Gestational Age: Common Clinical Parameters—cont'd

Characteristic	Preterm	Term
Head lag	Head lags; arms have little or no flexion	Head follows trunk; strong arm flexion
Scarf sign	Elbow can extend to opposite axilla	Elbow to midline only; infant resists
Square window	90 degrees	0 degrees
Ankle dorsiflexion	90 degrees	0 degrees
Popliteal angle	180 degrees	<90 degrees
Heel-to-ear maneuver	Touches ear easily	90 degrees
Ventral suspension	Hypotonia; "rag-doll"	Good caudal and cephalic tone
Reflexes		
Moro	Apparent at 28 weeks; good, but no adduction	Complete reflex with adduction; disappears 4 months postterm
Grasp	Fair at 28 weeks; arm is involved at 32 weeks	Strong enough to sustain weight for a few seconds when pulled up; hand, arm, shoulder involved
Cry	24 weeks: weak; 28 weeks: high-pitched; 32 weeks: good	Lusty; can persist for some time
Length	Under 47 cm (18½ inches), usually	50 cm (20 inches); range: 18–22 inches
Weight	Under 2500 gm (5 lb 5 oz)	3400 gm (7½ lb); range: 5 lb 8 oz–8 lb 13 oz

C. Nursing care plan/implementation:

1. Goal: *promote effective gas transport.*
   a. Maintain patent airway—to promote effective gas exchange and respiratory function.
   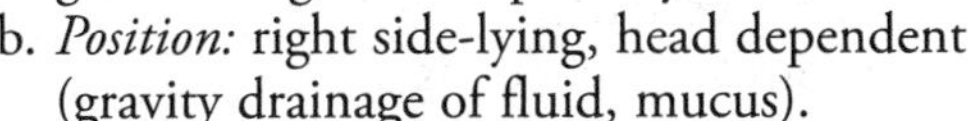
   b. *Position:* right side-lying, head dependent (gravity drainage of fluid, mucus).
   c. Suction prn with bulb syringe for mucus.
2. Goal: *establish/maintain thermal stability.*
   a. *Avoid* chilling—to prevent metabolic acidosis.
   b. Dry, wrap, and apply hat.
   c. Place in heated crib.
   d. Monitor vital signs hourly until stable.
3. Goal: *reduce possibility of blood loss.*
   a. Check cord clamp for security.
   b. Administer vitamin K injection, as ordered, in anterior or lateral thigh muscle—to stimulate blood coagulability.
4. Goal: *prevent infection.*
   a. Administer antibiotic treatment to eyes (if not performed in birth room)—to prevent ophthalmia neonatorum.
   b. Treat cord stump (alcohol), as ordered.
   c. Use standard precautions.
5. Goal: *promote comfort and cleanliness.* Admission bath when temperature stable.
6. Goal: *promote nutrition, hydration, elimination.*
   a. Encourage breastfeeding within 1 hour after birth.
   b. Check blood sugar (Dextrostix or Chem-strip) at 30 minutes, 1, 2, and 4 hours for infants at risk for hypoglycemia (e.g., SGA, LGA, infant of diabetic mother).
   c. First feeding at 1 to 4 hours of age with sterile water (or formula) if permissible and if not breastfeeding.
   d. Note voiding or meconium stool; report if failure to void or defecate within 24 hours.
7. Goal: *promote bonding.*
   a. Encourage parent-infant interaction (holding, touching, eye contact, talking to infant).
   b. Encourage breastfeeding within 1 hour of birth, if applicable.
   c. Encourage parent participation in infant care—to develop confidence and competence in caring for newborn.
      (1) Assist with initial efforts at feeding.
      (2) Discuss and demonstrate positioning and burping techniques.
      (3) Demonstrate/assist with basic care procedures, as necessary:
         (a) Bath.
         (b) Cord care.
         (c) Diapering.
         (d) Aid parents in distinguishing normal vs. abnormal newborn characteristics.

8. Goal: *health teaching*—to provide anticipatory guidance for discharge.
   a. Facilitate sibling bonding.
   b. Describe/discuss normal newborn behavior:
      (1) *Sleeping*—almost continual (wakes only to feed) or 12 to 16 hours daily.
      (2) *Feeding*—from every 2 to 3 hours to longer intervals; establish own pattern; babies who are breastfed feed more often.
      (3) *Weight loss*—5% to 10% in first few days; regained in 7 to 14 days.
      (4) *Stools*—(**Table 4.17**).
      (5) *Cord care*—cord drops off in 7 to 10 days
         (a) Keep clean and dry.
         (b) Alcohol may be applied to stump, or it may be allowed to dry naturally.
         (c) HIV precautions.
      (6) *Circumcision care*
         (a) Keep clean and dry; heals rapidly.
         (b) Watch for bleeding.
         (c) Petroleum jelly, gauze prn, if ordered.
         (d) Do *not* remove yellowish exudate.
      (7) *Physiological jaundice*—occurs 24 to 72 hours after birth.
         (a) Nonpathologic.
         (b) Need for hydration.
      (8) Identify need for newborn screening test after ingestion of milk (done routinely at 24 hours of age and later). Includes screen for congenital hypothyroidism and galactosemia (see **Table 11.2, Chapter 11,** for other newborn screening procedures).
      (9) Describe suggested sensory *stimulation* modalities (mobiles, color, music).
      (10) Discuss *safety* precautions:
         (a) Position on back for sleep.
         (b) Infant seat for travel and home safety.
         (c) Maintaining contact/control over infant to prevent falls, drowning in bath.
         (d) Instruct parents in infant cardiopulmonary resuscitation (CPR).
         (e) *Hepatitis B vaccination*—first dose can be given at 24 to 48 hours of life; second dose at 1 month; third dose at 6 months. If infant born to mother who is infected, hepatitis B vaccine and hepatitis B immune globulin should be administered within 12 hours of birth.
      (11) Describe signs of *common health problems* to be reported promptly:
         (a) Diarrhea, constipation.
         (b) Colic, vomiting.
         (c) Rash, jaundice.
         (d) Differentiation from normal patterns.

D. Evaluation/outcome criteria:

1. Infant demonstrates successful transition to independent life:
   a. Breastfeeds well.
   b. Normal feeding, sleeping, elimination patterns.
   c. No evidence of infection or abnormality.
2. Mother/family evidences bonding.
   a. Eye contact.
   b. Stroking, cuddling.
   c. Crooning, calling baby by name, talking to infant.
3. Mother demonstrates comfort and skill in basic newborn care.
4. Mother verbalizes understanding of subjects discussed:
   a. Safety precautions.
   b. Health maintenance actions.
   c. Signs of normal infant behavior and health.

Table 4.17

Infant Stool Characteristics

Age	Bottle-fed	Breastfed	Implications of Abnormal Patterns
1 day	Meconium	Meconium	Absence may indicate obstruction, atresia
2–5 days (transitional)	Greenish yellow, loose	Greenish yellow, loose, frequent	*Note*—At any time:
>5 days	Yellow to brown, firm, 2–4 daily, foul odor	Bright golden yellow, loose, 6–10 daily	*Diarrhea*—greenish, mucus or blood tinged, or forceful expulsion, may indicate infection *Constipation*—dry, hard stools or infrequent or absent stools may indicate obstruction

Complications During the Neonatal Period: The High-Risk Newborn

I. GENERAL OVERVIEW—Successful newborn adaptation to the demands of independent extrauterine life may be complicated by environmental insults during the *prenatal* period or those arising in the period immediately surrounding birth. The nursing role focuses on minimizing the effect of present and emerging health problems and on facilitating and supporting a successful transition to extrauterine life.

II. GENERAL ASPECTS—common neonatal risk factors:

A. Gestational age profile (see **Tables 4.15** and **4.16**):
   1. Prematurity.
   2. Dysmaturity.
   3. Postmaturity.

B. Congenital disorders.

C. Birth trauma.

D. Infections.

III. DISORDERS AFFECTING PROTECTIVE FUNCTIONS: NEONATAL INFECTIONS

A. Assess for intrauterine infections.

B. Oral thrush (mycotic stomatitis).
   1. **Pathophysiology**—local inflammation of oral mucosa due to fungal infection.
   2. **Etiology:**
      a. Organism—*Candida albicans.*
      b. More common in newborn who is vulnerable (i.e., sick, debilitated; those receiving antibiotic therapy).
   3. Mode of transmission—direct contact with:
      a. Maternal birth canal, hands, and linens.
      b. Contaminated feeding equipment, staff's hands.
   4. **Assessment:**
      a. White patches on oral mucosa, gums, and tongue that bleed when touched.
      b. Occasional difficulty swallowing.
   5. **Analysis/nursing diagnosis:**
      a. *Pain* related to irritation of oral mucous membrane secondary to oral moniliasis.
      b. *Altered nutrition, less than body requirements* related to irritability and poor feeding.
   6. **Nursing care plan/implementation:** Goal: *prevent cross-contamination.*
      a. Aseptic technique; good hand washing.
      b. Give medications as ordered:
         (1) Aqueous gentian violet, 1% to 2%: apply to infected area with swab.
         (2) Nystatin (Mycostatin)—instill into mouth with medicine dropper, or apply to lesions with swab, *after* feedings. *Note:* Before medicating, feed sterile water to rinse out milk.
   7. **Evaluation/outcome criteria:**
      a. Oral mucosa intact, lesions healed, no evidence of infection.
      b. Feeds well; maintains weight or regains weight lost, if any.

C. Neonatal sepsis
   1. **Pathophysiology**—generalized infection; may overwhelm infant's immature immune system.
   2. **Etiology:**
      a. Prolonged rupture of membranes.
      b. Long, difficult labor.
      c. Resuscitation procedures.
      d. Maternal infection (e.g., β-hemolytic streptococcus vaginosis).
      e. Aspiration—amniotic fluid, formula, mucus.
      f. Iatrogenic (nosocomial)—caused by infected health personnel or equipment.
   3. **Assessment:**
      a. Respirations—irregular, periods of apnea.
      b. Irritability or lethargy.
   4. **Analysis/nursing diagnosis:**
      a. *Fatigue* related to increased oxygen needs.
      b. *High risk for infection* related to septic condition.
   5. **Nursing care plan/implementation:**
      a. Cultures (spinal, urine, blood).
      b. Check vitals.
      c. Monitor respirations.
      d. Give medications, as ordered.
   6. **Evaluation/outcome criteria:**
      a. Responds to medical/nursing regimen (all assessment findings within normal limits).
      b. Parent(s) verbalize understanding of diagnosis, treatment; demonstrate appropriate techniques in participating in care (as possible).
      c. Parent(s) demonstrate effective coping with situation; express satisfaction with care.

IV. DISORDERS AFFECTING NUTRITION: INFANT OF THE DIABETIC MOTHER (IDM)

A. Pathophysiology—hyperplasia of pancreatic beta cells → increased insulin production → excessive deposition of glycogen in muscles, subcutaneous fat, and tissue growth. Results in fetal:
   1. *Macrosomia*—LGA infant.
   2. *Enlarged internal organs*—common.
      a. Cardiomegaly.
      b. Hepatomegaly.
      c. Splenomegaly.
   3. Neonatal—inadequate carbohydrate reserve to meet energy needs.

4. Associated with *increased incidence of:*
   a. Congenital anomalies (five times average incidence with pregestational diabetes) includes cardiac, pelvic, and spinal anomalies.
   b. Preterm birth: respiratory distress syndrome (RDS); increased insulin needs prenatally lead to decreased surfactant production.
   c. Fetal dystocia—due to CPD.
   d. Neonatal metabolic problems:
      (1) Hypoglycemia.
      (2) Hypocalcemic tetany.
      (3) Metabolic acidosis.
      (4) Hyperbilirubinemia.

B. Etiology—high circulating maternal glucose levels during fetal growth and development; loss of maternal glucose supply following birth; decreased hepatic gluconeogenesis.

C. Assessment:
1. Characteristics of IDM.
2. Hypoglycemia—Dextrostix or Chem-strip to heel stick at:
   a. 30 minutes × 2.
   b. 1, 2, and 4 hours of age; before meals × 4 or until stable.
   c. Chem-strip: if less than 20 mg/dL, must draw glucose STAT.
   d. Hypoglycemia laboratory values for preterm and term infants: under 45 mg/dL.
   e. Behavioral signs—tremors; twitching, hypotonia, seizures.
3. Gestational age, since macrosomia may mask prematurity.
4. Hypocalcemia—usually within first 24 hours
   a. Irritability.
   b. Coarse tremors, twitching, convulsions.
5. Birth injuries:
   a. Fractures: clavicle, humerus, skull.
   b. Brachial palsy.
   c. Intracranial hemorrhage/signs of increased intracranial pressure.
   d. Cephalohematoma.
6. Respiratory distress:
   a. Nasal flaring.
   b. Expiratory grunt.
   c. Sternal retraction.
   d. Intercostal retractions.
   e. Cyanosis—central.
7. Jaundice.

D. Analysis/nursing diagnosis:
1. *High risk for injury* related to CPD, dystocia.
2. *Altered cardiopulmonary tissue perfusion* related to placental insufficiency, RDS.
3. *Impaired gas exchange* related to RDS.
4. *Altered nutrition, less than body requirements,* related to hypoglycemia, hypocalcemia.
5. *Risk for altered endocrine/metabolic processes* related to hyperbilirubinemia and kernicterus.

E. Nursing care plan/implementation:
1. Hypoglycemia—administer formula or IV glucose, as ordered (may cause rebound effect).
2. Preterm/immature—institute preterm care prn.
3. Hypocalcemia—administer oral or IV calcium gluconate, as ordered.
4. Inform pediatrician **immediately** of signs of:
   a. Jaundice.
   b. Hyperirritability.
   c. Birth injury.
   d. Increased intracranial pressure/hemorrhage

F. Evaluation/outcome criteria:
1. Infant makes successful transition to extrauterine life.
2. Infant responds to medical/nursing regimen. Experiences minimal or no metabolic disturbances (hypoglycemia, hypocalcemia, hyperbilirubinemia).
3. Infant exhibits normal respiratory function and gas exchange.

V. HYPOGLYCEMIA

A. Pathophysiology—low serum-glucose level → altered cellular metabolism → cerebral irritability, cardiopulmonary problems.

B. Etiology:
1. Loss of maternal glucose supply.
2. Normal physiological activities of respiration, thermoregulation, muscular activity exceed carbohydrate reserve.
3. Decreased hepatic ability to convert amino acids into glucose.
4. More common in:
   a. Infants of diabetic mothers.
   b. Preterm, postterm infants.
   c. SGA infants.
   d. Smaller twin.
   e. Infant of mother with preeclampsia.
   f. Birth asphyxia.

C. Assessment:
1. Jitteriness, tremors, convulsions; lethargy and hypotonia.
2. Sweating; unstable temperature.
3. Tachypnea; apneic episodes; cyanosis.
4. High-pitched, shrill cry.
5. Difficulty feeding.

D. Analysis/nursing diagnosis:
1. *Altered tissue perfusion (fetal)* related to placental insufficiency associated with maternal diabetes, preeclampsia, renal or cardiac disorders; erythroblastosis.

2. *Risk for altered endocrine metabolic processes* related to high incidence of morbidity associated with birth asphyxia.
3. *Impaired gas exchange* related to coexisting RDS.
4. *Altered nutrition, less than body requirements,* related to hypoglycemia.
5. *High risk for injury* related to coexisting infection, metabolic acidosis.

E. Nursing care plan/implementation (see **IV. INFANT OF THE DIABETIC MOTHER, p. 208**).

F. Evaluation/outcome criteria (see **IV. INFANT OF THE DIABETIC MOTHER, p. 208**).

VI. DISORDERS AFFECTING PSYCHOSOCIAL-CULTURAL FUNCTIONS: NEONATE WHO IS DRUG-DEPENDENT (HEROIN)

A. General aspects

1. Maternal drug addiction has been associated with:
   a. Prenatal malnutrition and vitamin deficiencies.
   b. Increased risk of antepartal infections.
   c. Higher incidence of antepartal and intrapartum complications.
2. Infant at risk for:
   a. Intrauterine growth retardation (IUGR).
   b. Prematurity.
   c. Fetal distress.
   d. Perinatal death.
   e. Child abuse.
   f. Sudden infant death syndrome (SIDS) (5–10 times higher than normal).
   g. Learning and behavior disorders.
   h. Poor social adjustment.

B. Pathophysiology—withdrawal of accustomed drug levels → physiological deprivation response.

C. Etiology—repeated intrauterine absorption of heroin/cocaine/methadone from maternal bloodstream → fetal drug dependency.

D. Assessment—degree of withdrawal depends on type and duration of addiction and maternal drug levels at birth.

1. Irritability, hyperactivity, hypertonicity, exaggerated reflexes, tremors, high-pitched cry, difficult to comfort:
   a. *"Step" reflex* (dancing)—infant places both feet on surface; assumes rigid stance—does not "step" or dance.
   b. *"Head-righting" reflex*—holds head rigid; fails to demonstrate head lag.
2. Nasal stuffiness and sneezing; respiratory distress, tachypnea, cyanosis, or apnea.
3. Exaggerated acrocyanosis or mottling in the infant who is warm.
4. Sweating.
5. Hunger—sucks on fists; feeding problems—regurgitation, vomiting, poor feeding, diarrhea, and increased mucus production.
6. Convulsions with abnormal eye-rolling and chewing motions.
7. Developmental lags/mental retardation.

E. Analysis/nursing diagnosis:

1. *High risk for injury* related to convulsions secondary to physiological response to withdrawal, CNS hyperirritability.
2. *Impaired gas exchange* related to respiratory distress secondary to inhibition of reflex clearing of fluid by the lungs.
3. *Altered nutrition, less than body requirements,* related to feeding problems secondary to respiratory distress and GI hypermotility.
4. *High risk for impaired skin integrity* related to scratching secondary to withdrawal symptoms.

F. Nursing care plan/implementation:

1. Goal: *prevent/minimize respiratory distress.*
   a. *Position:* side-lying, head dependent—to facilitate mucus drainage.
   b. Suction prn with bulb syringe for excess mucus—to maintain patent airway.
   c. Monitor respirations and apical pulse.
2. Goal: *minimize possibility of convulsions.*
   a. Decrease environmental stimuli—quiet, touch only when necessary, offer pacifier.
   b. Keep warm, swaddle for comfort.
3. Goal: *maintain nutrition/hydration.*
   a. Food/fluids—oral or IV, as ordered.
   b. I&O.
   c. Daily weight.
4. Goal: *assist in diagnosis of drug and drug level.* Collect all urine and meconium during first 24 hours for toxicological studies.
5. Goal: *maintain/promote skin integrity.*
   a. Mitts over hands—to minimize scratching.
   b. Keep clean and dry.
   c. Medicated ointment/powder, as ordered, q2–4h, to excoriated areas.
   d. Expose excoriated areas to air.
6. Goal: *minimize withdrawal symptoms.* Administer medications, as ordered.
   a. Paregoric elixir—to wean from drug.
   b. Phenobarbital—to reduce CNS hyperirritability, hyperbilirubinemia.
   c. Chlorpromazine (Thorazine), diazepam (Valium)—to tranquilize, reduce hyperirritability. *Note:* Valium is **contraindicated** for the neonate who is jaundiced because it predisposes to hyperbilirubinemia.
   d. Methadone.

MATERNAL/INFANT

7. Goal: *emotional support to mother.*
   a. Encourage verbalization of feelings of guilt, anxiety, fear, concerns.
   b. Refer to social service.

G. Evaluation/outcome criteria:
1. Infant responds to medical/nursing regimen.
   a. Maintains adequate respirations.
   b. Feeds well, gains weight.
   c. No evidence of CNS hyperirritability, convulsions; demonstrates normal newborn reflexes.
2. Infant evidences bonding with parent(s). Responsive to mother's voice.

VII. DISORDERS AFFECTING PSYCHOSOCIAL-CULTURAL FUNCTION: FETAL ALCOHOL SYNDROME (FAS)

A. General aspects:
1. Maternal alcohol abuse has been associated with:
   a. Malnutrition, vitamin deficiencies.
   b. Bone marrow suppression.
   c. Liver disease.
   d. Child abuse.
2. Infant at risk for:
   a. Congenital anomalies (FAS).
   b. Mental deficiency; learning disabilities.
   c. IUGR.

B. Pathophysiology—permanent damage to developing embryonic/fetal structures; cardiovascular anomalies (ventricular septal defects).

C. Etiology—high circulating alcohol levels are lethal to the embryo; lower levels cause permanent cell damage.

D. Assessment:
1. Characteristic craniofacial abnormalities:
   a. Short, palpebral fissure.
   b. Epicanthal folds.
   c. Maxillary hypoplasia.
   d. Micrognathia.
   e. Long, thin upper lip.
2. Short stature.
3. Irritable, hyperactive, poor feeding.
4. High-pitched cry, difficult to comfort.

E. Nursing care plan/implementation:
1. Goal: *reduce irritability.*
   a. Reduce environmental stimuli.
   b. Wrap, cuddle.
   c. Administer sedatives, as ordered.
2. Goal: *maintain nutrition/hydration.*
3. Goal: *emotional support to mother.*

F. Evaluation/outcome criteria (see **VI. NEONATE WHO IS DRUG-DEPENDENT [HEROIN], p. 209**):
1. No respiratory distress.
2. Infant feeding properly.
3. Maternal bonding apparent.
4. Social services—home involvement.

VIII. CLASSIFICATION OF INFANTS BY WEIGHT AND GESTATIONAL AGE

A. Terminology
1. *Preterm, or premature*—37 weeks' gestation or less (usually 2500 gm [5 lb] or less).
2. *Term*—38 to 42 weeks' gestation.
3. *Postterm*—over 42 weeks.
4. *Postmature*—gestation greater than 42 weeks.
5. *Appropriate for gestational age (AGA)*—for each week of gestation, there is a normal range of expected weight (between 10th and 90th percentile).
   a. Term infants weighing 2500 gm or more are usually mature in physiological functions.
   b. If respiratory distress occurs, it is usually related to meconium aspiration syndrome.
6. *SGA or dysmature*—weight falls *below* normal range for age (<10th percentile).
   a. Preeclampsia.
   b. Malnutrition.
   c. Smoking.
   d. Placental insufficiency.
   e. Alcohol syndrome.
   f. Rubella.
   g. Syphilis.
   h. Multifetal gestation (twins, etc.).
   i. Genetic.
   j. Cocaine abuse.
7. *LGA*—*above* expected weight for age (>90th percentile). *Note:* If **preterm,** at risk for **RDS.** If **postterm,** at risk for **aspiration** and **sudden intrauterine death.**
   a. **Etiology:**
      (1) Maternal diabetes or prediabetes.
      (2) Maternal weight gain over 35 lb.
      (3) Maternal obesity.
      (4) Genetic.
   b. *Associated problems:*
      (1) Hypoglycemia.
      (2) Hypocalcemia.
      (3) Hyperbilirubinemia.
      (4) Birth injury (e.g., fractures, Erb-Duchenne paralysis).

B. *Estimation of gestational age*—planning appropriate care for the newborn requires accurate assessment to differentiate between preterm and term infants.

PRETERM INFANT—Born at 37 weeks of gestation or less.

A. Pathophysiology—anatomical and physiological immaturity of body systems compromises ability to adapt to extrauterine environment and independent life.
1. *Interference with* **protective** *functions*
   a. *Temperature regulation*—unstable, due to:
      (1) Lack of subcutaneous fat.

MATERNAL/INFANT

(2) Large body surface area in proportion to body weight.
(3) Small muscle mass.
(4) Absent sweat or shiver responses.
(5) Poor capillary response to changes in environmental temperature.

b. *Resistance to infection*—low, due to:
(1) Lack of immune bodies from mother (these cross placenta *late* in pregnancy).
(2) Inability to produce own immune bodies (immature liver).
(3) Poor WBC response to infection.

c. *Immature liver*
(1) Inability to conjugate bilirubin liberated by normal breakdown of RBCs → increased susceptibility to hyperbilirubinemia and kernicterus.
(2) Immature production of clotting factors and immune globulins.
(3) Inadequate glucose stores → increased susceptibility to hypoglycemia.

2. *Interference with* **elimination:** immature *renal* function—unable to concentrate urine → precarious fluid-electrolyte balance.
3. *Interference with* **sensory-perceptual functions:** CNS—immature → weak or absent reflexes and fluctuating primitive control of vital functions.

B. Etiology: often unknown; preterm labor.

1. *Iatrogenic*—EDD miscalculated for repeat cesarean birth (rare).
2. *Placental factors*
   a. Placenta previa.
   b. Abruptio placentae.
   c. Placental insufficiency.
3. *Uterine factors*
   a. Incompetent cervix.
   b. Overdistention (multifetal gestation, polyhydramnios).
   c. Anomalies (e.g., myomas).
4. *Fetal factors*
   a. Malformations.
   b. Infections (rubella, toxoplasmosis, HIV-positive status, AIDS, cytomegalic inclusion disease).
   c. Multifetal gestations (twins, triplets).
5. *Maternal factors*
   a. Severe physical or emotional trauma.
   b. Coexisting disorders (preeclampsia, hypertension, heart disease, diabetes, malnutrition).
   c. Infections (streptococcus, syphilis, bacterial vaginosis, pyelonephritis, pneumonia, influenza, leukemia, UTI).
6. *Miscellaneous factors*
   a. Close frequency of pregnancies.
   b. Advanced maternal age.
   c. Heavy smoking.
   d. High-altitude environment.
   e. Cocaine use.

C. Factors influencing survival:

1. Gestational age.
2. Lung maturity.
3. Anomalies.
4. Size.

D. Causes of mortality (in order of frequency):

1. Abnormal pulmonary ventilation.
2. Infection.
   a. Pneumonia.
   b. Septicemia.
   c. Diarrhea.
   d. Meningitis.
3. Intracranial hemorrhage.
4. Congenital defects.

E. Disorders affecting fluid-gas transport: RDS

1. **Pathophysiology**—insufficient pulmonary surfactant (lecithin) and insufficient number/maturity of alveoli predispose to atelectasis; alveolar ducts and terminal bronchi become lined with fibrous, glossy membrane.
2. **Etiology:**
   a. Primarily associated with prematurity.
   b. Other *predisposing* factors:
   (1) Fetal hypoxia—due to decreased placental perfusion secondary to maternal bleeding (e.g., abruptio placentae) or hypotension.
   (2) Birth asphyxia.
   (3) Postnatal hypothermia, metabolic acidosis, or hypotension.
3. Factors *protecting* neonate from RDS:
   a. Chronic fetal stress—due to maternal hypertension, preeclampsia, or heroin addiction.
   b. PROM.
   c. Maternal steroid ingestion (e.g., betamethasone).
   d. Low-grade chorioamnionitis.
4. **Assessment:**
   a. Usually appears during first or second day after birth.
   b. Signs of *respiratory distress:*
   (1) Nasal flaring.
   (2) Expiratory grunt.
   (3) Sternal retractions.
   (4) Tachypnea (60 breaths/min or more).
   (5) Cyanosis—central.
   (6) Increasing number and length of apneic episodes.
   (7) Increasing exhaustion.
   c. *Respiratory acidosis*—due to hypercapnea and rising CO_2 level.
   d. *Metabolic acidosis*—due to increased lactic acid levels and falling pH.

MATERNAL/INFANT

5. **Analysis/nursing diagnosis:**
   a. *Impaired gas exchange* related to lack of pulmonary surfactant secondary to preterm birth, intrapartum stress and hypoxia, infection, postnatal hypothermia, metabolic acidosis, or hypotension.
   b. *Altered nutrition, less than body requirements,* related to poor feeding secondary to respiratory distress, ↑ caloric demand.
6. **Nursing care plan/implementation:**
   a. Goal: *reduce metabolic acidosis, increase oxygenation, support respiratory efforts.*
      (1) Ensure warmth (isolette at 97.6°F).
      (2) Warmed, humidified O_2 at lowest concentration required to relieve cyanosis, through hood, nasal prongs, or endotracheal tube.
      (3) Monitor *continuous positive airway pressure (CPAP)*—oxygen–air mixture administered under pressure during inhalation *and* exhalation to maintain alveolar patency.
      (4) *Position:* side-lying or supine with neck slightly extended ("sniffing" position); arms at sides.
      (5) Suction prn with bulb syringe—for excessive mucus.
   b. Goal: *modify care for infant with endotracheal tube.*
      (1) Disconnect tubing at adapter.
      (2) Inject 0.5 mL sterile normal saline (may be omitted).
      (3) Insert sterile suction tube, start suction, rotate tube, withdraw.
      (4) Suction up to 5 seconds.
      (5) Ventilate with bag and mask during procedure.
      (6) Reconnect tubing securely to adapter.
      (7) Auscultate for breath sounds and pulse.
   c. Goal: *maintain nutrition/hydration.*
      (1) Administer fluids, electrolytes, calories, vitamins, minerals PO or IV, as ordered.
      (2) I&O.
   d. Goal: *prevent secondary infections.*
      (1) Strict aseptic technique.
      (2) Hand washing.
   e. Goal: *emotional support of infant.*
      (1) Gentle touching.
      (2) Soft voices.
      (3) Eye contact.
      (4) Rocking.
   f. Goal: *emotional support of parents.*
      (1) Keep informed of status and progess.
      (2) Encourage contact with infant—to promote bonding, understanding of treatment.
   g. Goal: *minimize possibility of iatrogenic disorders associated with oxygen therapy* (see **F.** and **G.,** below).
7. **Evaluation/outcome criteria:**
   a. Respiratory distress treated successfully; infant breathes without assistance.
   b. Infant completes successful transition to extrauterine life.

F. Iatrogenic (oxygen toxicity) disorders: retinopathy of prematurity

1. **Pathophysiology**—intraretinal hemorrhage → fibrosis → retinal detachment → loss of vision.
2. **Etiology**—prolonged exposure to high concentrations of oxygen.
3. **Assessment**—only perceptible retinal change is vasoconstriction. *Note:* Arterial blood gas (PaO_2) readings less than 50 or more than 80 mm Hg.
4. **Nursing care plan/implementation:** Goal: *prevent disorder.* Maintain PaO_2 of 50 to 70 mm Hg.
5. **Evaluation/outcome criteria:**
   a. Successful recovery from respiratory distress.
   b. No evidence of retinopathy.

G. Iatrogenic (oxygen toxicity) disorders: bronchopulmonary dysplasia (BPD)

1. **Pathophysiology**—damage to alveolar cells result in focal emphysema.
2. **Etiology**—positive-pressure ventilation (CPAP and positive end-expiratory pressure [PEEP]) and prolonged administration of high concentrations of oxygen.
3. **Assessment**—monitor for signs of:
   a. Tachypnea.
   b. Increased respiratory effort.
   c. Respiratory distress.
4. **Nursing care plan/implementation:** Goal: *prevent disorder.*
   a. Use of *positive*-pressure devices.
   b. Maintain oxygen concentration *below 80%.*
   c. Supportive care.
   d. Wean off ventilator, as possible.
5. **Evaluation/outcome criteria:**
   a. Successful recovery from respiratory distress.
   b. No evidence of disorder.

H. Intraventricular hemorrhage

1. **Pathophysiology**—rupture of thin, fragile capillary walls within ventricles of the brain (more common in preterm).
2. **Etiology:**
   a. Hypoxia.
   b. Respiratory distress.
   c. Birth trauma.
   d. Birth asphyxia.
   e. Hypercapnia.
3. **Assessment:**
   a. Hypotonia.
   b. Lethargy.
   c. Hypothermia.
   d. Bradycardia.
   e. Bulging fontanels.

f. Respiratory distress or apnea.
g. Seizures.
h. Cry: high-pitched whining.

4. **Nursing care plan/implementation:** Goal: *supportive care* to promote healing.
   a. Monitor vital signs.
   b. Maintain thermal stability.
   c. Ensure adequate oxygenation (may be placed on CPAP).
5. **Evaluation/outcome criteria:**
   a. Condition stable, all assessment findings within normal limits.
   b. No evidence of residual damage.

I. Disorders affecting nutrition

1. **Pathophysiology**—underdeveloped feeding abilities, small stomach capacity, immature enzyme system, fat intolerance.
2. **Etiology**—immature body systems associated with preterm birth.
3. **Assessment:**
   a. Weak suck, swallow, gag reflexes—tendency to aspiration.
   b. Signs of malabsorption and fat intolerance (abdominal distention, diarrhea, weight loss, or failure to gain weight).
   c. Signs of vitamin E deficiency (edema, anemia).
4. **Analysis/nursing diagnosis:**
   a. *Altered nutrition, less than body requirements,* related to poor feeding reflexes, reduced stomach capacity, inability to absorb needed nutrients.
   b. *Impaired gas exchange* related to aspiration.
5. **Nursing care plan/implementation:** Goal: *maintain/increase nutrition.*

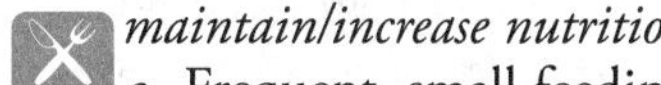

   a. Frequent, small feedings—to *avoid* exceeding stomach capacity, facilitate digestion.
   b. Frequent "burping" during feeding—to *avoid* regurgitation/aspiration.
   c. Supplement vitamin E (alpha-tocopherol) intake, as ordered, in infants who are formula-fed. (*Note:* intake adequate in infants who are breastfed.) *Vitamin E actions:*
      (1) Antioxidant.
      (2) Maintains structure and function of smooth, skeletal, and cardiac muscle.
      (3) Maintains structure and function of vascular tissue, liver, and RBC integrity.
      (4) Coenzyme in tissue respiration.
      (5) Treatment for malnutrition with macrocytic anemia.
   d. Encourage parent/family participation.
6. **Evaluation/outcome criteria:**
   a. Feeds well without regurgitation/aspiration.
   b. Maintains/gains weight.
   c. No evidence of malabsorption, vitamin deficiency.

J. Disorders affecting nutrition/elimination: necrotizing enterocolitis (NEC)

1. **Pathophysiology**—intestinal thrombosis, infarction, autodigestion of mucosal lining, and necrotic lesions; incidence *increased in preterm.*
2. **Etiology**—intestinal ischemia, due to blood shunt to brain and heart in response to:
   a. Fetal distress.
   b. Fetal/neonatal asphyxia.
   c. Neonatal shock.
   d. After birth, may result from:
      (1) Low cardiac output.
      (2) Infusion of hyperosmolar solutions.
   e. Complicated by action of enteric bacteria on damaged intestine.
3. **Assessment**—early identification is **vital.**
   a. Abdominal distention or erythema, or both.
   b. Poor feeding, vomiting.
   c. Blood in stool.
   d. Systemic signs associated with sepsis that may need temporary colostomy or iliostomy:
      (1) Lethargy or irritability.
      (2) Hypothermia.
      (3) Labored respirations or apnea.
      (4) Cardiovascular collapse.
   e. *Medical diagnosis:*
      (1) Increased gastric residual.
      (2) X-ray shows ileus, air in bowel wall.
4. **Analysis/nursing diagnosis:**
   a. *Altered nutrition, less than body requirements,* related to inability to tolerate oral feedings, and gastrointestinal dysfunction secondary to ischemia, thrombosis, or necrosis.
   b. *Constipation* related to paralytic ileus with stasis; diarrhea related to water loss.
   c. *High risk for injury* related to infection, thrombosis, metabolic alterations (acidosis, osmotic diuresis, dehydration, hyperglycemia) due to parenteral nutrition.
   d. *Altered parenting* related to physiological compromise and prolonged hospitalization.
   e. *Impaired skin integrity* when colostomy is necessary.
5. **Nursing care plan/implementation:**
   a. Goal: *supportive care.*
      (1) Rest GI tract: *no oral intake*—to achieve gastric decompression.
      (2) IV fluids, as ordered—to maintain hydration.
   b. Goal: *prevent infection.* Administer antibiotics, as ordered.
   c. Goal: *prevent trauma to skin surrounding stoma.*
6. **Evaluation/outcome criteria:**
   a. Tolerates oral feedings.
   b. Demonstrates weight gain.
   c. Normal stool pattern.

d. Parents are accepting and knowledgeable about care of infant.

POSTTERM INFANT—Over 42 weeks of gestation.

A. General aspects
1. Labor may be hazardous for mother and fetus because:
   a. Large size of infant contributes to cephalopelvic disproportion; obtain estimate of fetal weight (EFW) by ultrasound.
   b. Placental insufficiency → fetal hypoxia; diagnosis by:
      (1) Contraction stress test.
      (2) Nonstress test
      (3) Amniotic fluid index (AFI).
   c. Meconium passage (common physiological response) increases chance of meconium aspiration.

B. Assessment:
1. If postmature skin: dry, wrinkled—due to metabolism of fat and glycogen reserves to meet in utero energy needs.
2. Long limbs, fingernails, and toenails—due to continued growth in utero.
3. Lanugo and vernix—absent.
4. Expression: wide-eyed, alert—probably due to chronic hypoxia (oxygen hunger).
5. Placenta—signs of aging.

C. Analysis/nursing diagnosis: *High risk for injury* related to high incidence of morbidity and mortality due to dystocia or hypoxia.

D. Nursing care plan/implementation:
1. **During labor:**
   a. Goal: *emotional support of mother*—may require cesarean birth due to CPD or fetal distress.
   b. Goal: *continuous electronic monitoring of FHR.* Report *late* decelerations **immediately** (indicate fetal distress).
2. **After birth:**
   a. Goal: *if born vaginally, prompt identification of birth injuries, respiratory distress.* Continual observation.
   b. Goal: *early identification/treatment of emerging signs of complications.*
      (1) *Hypoglycemia*—Dextrostix readings and behavior.
      (2) Administer oral or intravenous glucose, as ordered.

E. Evaluation/outcome criterion: successful transition to extrauterine life (all assessment findings within normal limits).

Congenital Disorders

I. GENERAL OVERVIEW: Genetic abnormalities and environmental insults often lead to congenital disorders of the newborn. Successful transition to independent extrauterine life may pose a major challenge to infants compromised by anatomical or physiological disorders. Knowledge regarding the implications of the neonate's structural or metabolic problems enables the nurse to identify early signs of health problems and to plan, provide, and evaluate appropriate outcome-directed care to safeguard the status of the infant with a congenital disorder.

II. DISORDERS AFFECTING FLUID-GAS TRANSPORT: *congenital heart disease*

A. Pathophysiology—altered hemodynamics, due to persistent fetal circulation or structural abnormalities.
1. *Acyanotic defects*—no mixing of blood in the systemic circulation.
   a. *Patent ductus arteriosus.*
   b. *Atrial septal defect.*
   c. *Ventriclar septal defect.*
   d. *Coarctation of the aorta.*
2. *Cyanotic defects*—unoxygenated blood enters systemic circulation.
   a. *Tetralogy of Fallot.*
   b. *Transposition of the great vessels.*

B. Etiology—unknown. Associated with maternal:
1. Prenatal viral disease (e.g., rubella, coxsackievirus).
2. Malnutrition; alcoholism.
3. Diabetes (poorly controlled).
4. Ingestion of lithium salts.

C. Assessment:
1. *Patent ductus arteriosus* (see **Fig. 5.5, p. 278**).
   a. Characteristic machine murmur, mid to upper left sternal border (cardiomegaly); persists throughout systole and most of diastole; associated with a "thrill."
   b. Widened pulse pressure.
   c. Bounding pulse, tachycardia, "gallop" rhythm.
2. *Atrial septal defect* (see **Fig. 5.3, p. 277**).
   a. Characteristic crescendo-decrescendo systolic ejection murmur.
   b. Fixed S_2 splitting.
   c. Dyspnea, fatigue on normal activity.
   d. *Medical diagnosis*—cardiac catheterization, x-ray.
3. *Ventricular septal defect* (see **Fig. 5.4, p. 278**).
   a. Loud, harsh, pansystolic murmur; heard best at left lower sternal border; radiates throughout precordium. (*Note:* may be absent—due to high pulmonary vascular resistance → equalization of interventricular pressure.)
   b. *Medical diagnosis*—cardiac catheterization, ECG, chest x-ray.
4. *Coarctation of the aorta* (see **p. 279**).
   a. Absent femoral pulse.
   b. Late systolic murmur.

c. Decreased blood pressure in *lower* extremities.
d. *Medical diagnosis:* x-ray.

5. *Tetralogy of Fallot* ("blue" baby) (see **Fig. 5.6, p. 278**).
   a. Acute hypoxic/cyanotic episodes.
   b. Limp, sleepy, exhausted; hypotonic extended position—postepisode.
   c. *Medical diagnosis*—cardiac catheterization.
6. *Transposition of the great arteries* (see **Fig. 5.7, p. 278**).
   a. Cyanotic after crying or feeding.
   b. Progressive tachypnea—attempt to compensate for decreased PaO_2, metabolic acidosis.
   c. Heart sounds vary; consistent with defect.
   d. Signs of CHF.
   e. *Medical diagnosis*—cardiac catheterization, x-ray, ECG.

D. Analysis/nursing diagnosis:

1. *Fluid volume excess* related to persistent fetal circulation, structural abnormalities.
2. *Impaired gas exchange* related to abnormal circulation, secondary to pathology.
3. *Altered nutrition, less than body requirements,* related to exhaustion, dyspnea.

E. Nursing care plan/implementation:

1. Goal: *minimize cardiac workload.*
   a. Minimize crying—snuggle; pacifier—to meet psychological needs.
   b. Keep clean and dry.
2. Goal: *maintain thermal stability*—to reduce body need for oxygen.
3. Goal: *prevent infection.*
   a. Strict aseptic technique; standard precautions.
   b. Hand washing.
4. Goal: *parental emotional support.*
   a. Encourage verbalization of anxiety, fears, concerns.
   b. Keep informed of status.
5. Goal: *health teaching*—explain, discuss:
   a. Diagnostic procedures.
   b. Treatment procedures.
   c. Basic care modalities.
6. Goal: *promote bonding.* Encourage parents to participate in infant care, as possible.
7. Medical-surgical management: surgical intervention/repair of congenital cardiac abnormality.

F. Evaluation/outcome criteria:

1. Experiences no respiratory distress in immediate postnatal period.
2. Completes transfer to high-risk center without incident, if applicable.
3. Surgical intervention successful, where applicable.

III. DISORDERS AFFECTING FLUID-GAS TRANSPORT: *hemolytic disease of the newborn*

A. Rh incompatibility

1. **Pathophysiology** (see **p. 139**).
2. **Etiology** (see **Rh isoimmunization, p. 140**).
3. **Assessment:**
   a. *Prenatal*—maternal Rh titers, amniocentesis.
   b. *Intrapartum*—amniotic fluid color:
      (1) Straw-colored: *mild* disease.
      (2) Golden: *severe* fetal disease.
   c. Direct *Coombs' blood test;* positive test demonstrates Rh antibodies in fetal blood.
4. **Nursing care plan/implementation—exchange transfusion:**
   a. Goal: *health teaching.*
      (1) Explain purpose and process to parents:
         (a) Removes anti-Rh antibodies and fetal cells that are coated with antibodies.
         (b) Reduces bilirubin levels—indicated when 20 mg/dL in term neonate and 15 mg/dL in preterm.
         (c) Corrects anemia—supplies RBCs that will not be destroyed by maternal antibodies.
         (d) Rh-negative type O blood elicits no reaction; maximum exchange is 500 mL; duration of exchange: 45 to 60 minutes.
   b. Goal: *minimize transfusion hazards.*
      (1) Warm blood to room temperature, since cold blood may precipitate cardiac arrest.
      (2) Use only fresh blood—to reduce possibility of hypocalcemia, tetany, convulsions.
      (3) Give calcium gluconate, as ordered, after each 100 mL of transfusion.
   c. Goal: *prepare for transfusion procedure.* Ready necessary equipment—monitor, resuscitation equipment, radiant heater, light.
   d. Goal: *assist with exchange transfusion.*
      (1) Continuous monitoring of vital signs; record baseline, and every 15 minutes during procedure.
      (2) Record: time, amount of blood withdrawn; time and amount injected; medications given.
      (3) Observe for: dyspnea, listlessness, bleeding from transfusion site, cyanosis, cardiovascular irregularity or arrest; coolness of lower extremities.
   e. Goal: *posttransfusion care.*
      (1) **Assessment:**
         (a) Observe for: dyspnea, cyanosis, cardiac arrest or irregularities, jaundice, hypoglycemia; frequent vital signs.
         (b) *Signs of sepsis*—fever, tachycardia, dyspnea, chills, tremors.

(2) **Nursing care plan/implementation:**
(a) Maintain thermal stability—to reduce physiological stress, possibility of metabolic acidosis.
(b) Give oxygen—to relieve cyanosis.
(c) Keep cord moist—to facilitate repeat transfusion, if necessary.
(d) Maintain nutrition/hydration—feed per schedule.

5. **Evaluation/outcome criteria:**
   a. Infant's hemolytic process ceases; bilirubin level drops.
   b. Infant makes successful transition to extrauterine life.
   c. Infant experiences no complications of therapeutic regimen.
   d. Infant shows evidence of bonding.

B. ABO incompatibility

1. **Pathophysiology**—fetal blood carrying antigens A/B enters maternal type O bloodstream → antibody formation → antibodies cross placenta → hemolyze fetal RBCs. *Note:* less severe than Rh reaction.
2. **Etiology:**
   a. Type O mother carries anti-A and anti-B antibodies.
   b. Even first pregnancy is jeopardized if fetal blood enters maternal system.
   c. Reaction possible if fetus is type A, type B, or type AB and mother is type O.
3. **Assessment:**
   a. Jaundice within first 24 hours.
   b. Rising bilirubin levels.
   c. Enlarged liver and spleen.
4. **Nursing care plan/implementation:** Goal: *reduce hazard to newborn.*
   a. Prepare for exchange transfusion with O-negative blood.
   b. Phototherapy may be ordered if bilirubin is 10 mg/dL, and anemia is mild or absent.
   c. Close monitoring of status.
   d. Supportive care.
5. **Evaluation/outcome criteria:**
   a. Infant responds to medical/nursing regimen.
   b. Infant's assessment findings within normal limits.

C. Hyperbilirubinemia

1. **Pathophysiology**—bilirubin, a breakdown product of hemolyzed RBCs, appears at increased levels; exceeds 13 to 15 mg/dL. Bilirubin is safe when bound with albumin and conjugated by user for body excretion; danger is when unconjugated and deposits in CNS.
   a. **WARNING:** There is no "safe" serum bilirubin level; kernicterus is a function of the bilirubin level *and* neonatal age and condition; poor fluid-and-caloric balance subjects the infant (especially the preterm infant) to kernicterus at low serum bilirubin levels.
   b. *Kernicterus*—high bilirubin levels result in deposition of yellow pigment in basal ganglia of brain → irreversible retardation.
2. **Etiology:**
   a. Rh or ABO incompatibility, during first 48 hours.
   b. Resolution of an enclosed hemorrhage (e.g., cephalohematoma).
   c. Infection.
   d. Drug induced—vitamin K injection, maternal ingestion of sulfisoxazole (Gantrisin).
   e. Bile duct blockage.
   f. Albumin-binding capacity is exceeded.
   g. "Breastfeeding jaundice" (e.g., pregnanediol in milk). Breastfeeding is *not* dangerous and not a cause of physiological jaundice.
   h. Dehydration.
   i. Immature liver (interferes with conjugation).
3. **Assessment:**
   a. Jaundice noted after blanching skin to suppress hemoglobin color; noted in sclera or mucosa in dark-skinned neonates; make sure light is adequate; spreads from head down, with increasing severity.
   b. Pallor.
   c. Concentrated, dark urine.
   d. Blood level determination—hemoglobin or indirect bilirubin (unconjugated, unbound bilirubin deposits in CNS).
   e. *Kernicterus*—similar to intracranial hemorrhage.
      (1) Poor feeding or sucking.
      (2) Regurgitation, vomiting.
      (3) High-pitched cry.
      (4) Temperature instability.
      (5) Hypertonicity/hypotonicity.
      (6) Progressive lethargy; diminished Moro reflex.
      (7) Respiratory distress.
      (8) Cerebral palsy, mental retardation.
      (9) Death.
4. **Analysis/nursing diagnosis:**
   a. *Fluid volume (RBC) deficit* related to hemolysis secondary to blood incompatibility.
   b. *High risk for injury* (brain damage) related to kernicterus.
   c. *Altered thought processes* (mental retardation) related to brain damage secondary to kernicterus.
   d. *Knowledge deficit (parental)* related to infant condition.

5. **Nursing care plan/implementation:**
   a. *Medical management:*
      (1) *Prenatal*—amniocentesis.
      (2) *Postnatal*—exchange transfusion, phototherapy.
   b. Goal: *assist bilirubin conjugation through phototherapy.*
      (1) Cover closed eyelids while under light to protect eyes. (If Biliblanket is used, no need to cover eyes.) Remove eye pads when not under light (feeding, cuddling, during parental visits).
      (2) Expose as much skin as possible—to maximize exposure of circulating blood to light. Remove for only brief periods.
      (3) *Change position* q1h—to maximize exposure of circulating blood to light.
      (4) *Note:* any loose green stools as bile is cleared through gut; watch for skin breakdown on buttocks.
      (5) Monitor temperature—to identify hyperthermia. (Not necessary if using Biliblanket.)
      (6) *Push fluids* (to 25% more than average) between feedings—to counteract dehydration. Breast milk has natural laxative effects that help clear bile.
   c. Goal: *health teaching.* Explain, discuss phototherapy, bilirubin levels, implications.
   d. Goal: *emotional support.*
      (1) Encourage verbalization of anxiety, fears, concerns.
      (2) Encourage contact with infant.
      (3) Reassure, as possible.
6. **Evaluation/outcome criteria:**
   a. Infant's hemolytic process ceases; bilirubin level drops.
   b. Infant makes successful transition to extrauterine life.
   c. Infant experiences no complications of therapeutic regimen.
   d. Infant shows evidence of effective bonding.

Emotional Support of the High-Risk Infant

I. GENERAL ASPECTS

A. The high-risk infant has the same *developmental needs* as the healthy term infant:
   1. Social and tactile stimulation.
   2. Comfort and removal of discomfort (hunger, soiling).
   3. Continuous contact with a consistent, parenting person.

B. Treatment for serious physiological compromise may result in:
   1. Isolation.
   2. Sensory deprivation or noxious stimuli.
   3. Emotional stress.

II. ASSESSMENT—signs of neonatal emotional stress:

A. Does not look at person performing care.
B. Does not cry or protest.
C. Poor weight gain; failure to thrive.

III. ANALYSIS/NURSING DIAGNOSIS: *sensory-perceptual alterations related to isolation in isolette, oxygen hood.*

IV. NURSING CARE PLAN/IMPLEMENTATION:

A. Goal: *provide consistent parenting contact.* Assign same nurses whenever possible.
B. Goal: *emotional support.*
   1. Comfort when crying.
   2. Provide positive sensory stimulation. Arrange time to:
      a. Stroke skin.
      b. Hold hand.
      c. Hum, sing, talk.
      d. Hold in en-face position (nurse looking into infant's eyes).
      e. Hold when feeding, if possible.
C. Goal: *encourage parents to participate in care*—to:
   1. Reduce their psychological stress, anxiety, fear.
   2. Promote bonding.
   3. Reduce possibility of later child abuse (higher incidence of child abuse against children who have been high-risk infants).

V. EVALUATION/OUTCOME CRITERIA:

A. Infant demonstrates successful resolution of physiological problems.
B. Parents and infant evidence bonding.
C. Parents express satisfaction with care and result.

General Aspects: Nursing Care of the High-Risk Infant and Family

I. GENERAL OVERVIEW: The birth of a physiologically compromised neonate is psychologically stressful for both infant and family and physiologically stressful for the neonate. Effective, goal-directed nursing care is directed toward:

A. Minimizing physiological and psychological stress.
B. Facilitating/supporting successful coping or adaptation.
C. Encouraging parental attachment/separation/grieving, as appropriate.

II. ASSESSMENT—directed toward determining neonate's present and projected status:

A. Determine neonate's current physical status.

B. Identify specific status and diagnosis-related problems and needs.

C. Describe family psychological status, strengths, and coping mechanisms/skills.

D. Determine medical-surgical/nursing approach to problems—and prognosis.

III. ANALYSIS/NURSING DIAGNOSIS:

A. Parental *anxiety/fear* related to physiological compromise of neonate.

B. *Self-esteem disturbance* related to feelings of guilt or anger.

C. *Ineffective individual coping* related to severe psychological stress.

D. *Knowledge deficit* related to diagnosis, treatment, prognosis of infant.

E. *High risk for altered parenting* related to concern about infant.

IV. NURSING CARE PLAN/IMPLEMENTATION:

A. Goal: *preoperative and postoperative care.*

1. Maintain/improve physiological stability.
   a. Temperature stabilization—keep warm.
   b. Oxygenation:
      (1) Position.
      (2) Administer oxygen, as ordered or necessary.
   c. Nutrition/hydration:
      (1) Administer/monitor IV fluids.
      (2) Oral fluids, as ordered.
      (3) Feed, as status permits.
2. Assist with diagnostic testing.

B. Goal: *emotional support of parents.*

1. Encourage exploring and ventilating feelings.
2. Involve parents in decision-making process.

C. Goal: *health teaching.*

1. Determine knowledge/understanding of problem.
2. Explain/simplify/clarify, as needed, physician's discussions with parents.
3. Describe/explain/discuss neonate's present status and any auxiliary equipment; teach CPR to family.
4. Refer, as needed, to hospital/community resources.

D. Goal: *promote bonding.* Encourage parental participation in care of the neonate.

V. EVALUATION/OUTCOME CRITERIA:

A. Parents verbalize understanding of relevant information; make informed decisions regarding infant care.

B. Parents demonstrate comfort and increasing participation in care of neonate.

C. Infant maintains/increases adequacy of adaptation to extrauterine life.

D. If relevant, parents demonstrate progress in grieving process.

QUESTIONS

Questions

Select the one answer that is best for each question, unless otherwise directed.

1. A client who is 23 years old, gravida 2, para 1 with a twin gestation, is admitted to labor and delivery at 29 weeks' gestation with complaints of lower abdominal pain and decreased fetal movement. Which interventions should a nurse perform? *Select all that apply.*

1. Place the client on electronic fetal monitor.
2. Administer betamethasone IM.
3. Perform nipple stimulation stress test.
4. Limit oral fluid intake.
5. Place client on strict bedrest.

2. A postpartum nurse is caring for a client suspecting of having endometritis. What are the risk factors for developing endometritis? *Select all that apply.*

1. Protracted active phase of labor.
2. Prolonged rupture of membranes.
3. Precipitous delivery.
4. Prolonged latent phase of labor.
5. Internal fetal monitoring.

3. A client who is a 38-year-old gravida 1, para 0 with type 2 non–insulin-dependent diabetes, is 6 weeks pregnant. She asks a clinic nurse how she should manage her diabetes now that she is pregnant. Which would be the most appropriate response by the nurse?

1. "You can control your blood sugar with oral hypoglycemic agents."
2. "You can control your blood sugar with insulin injections."
3. "You can control your blood sugar with dietary changes."
4. "You can control your blood sugar by exercising more."

4. A 26-year-old client, who is a gravida 1, para 1, delivered an 8-pound, 12-ounce female infant over an intact perineum 24 hours ago. Since the client's delivery, an RN has observed that the client does not seem to show a lot of attention to her new infant. The client frequently lets her family take care of changing and holding the newborn. How should the RN interpret the client's behavior?

1. The client seems to doubt her competency as a mother.
2. The client is developing an attachment disorder.
3. The client is showing expected behaviors for the taking-in period.
4. The client is probably suffering from postpartum depression.

5. A physician orders fentanyl 75 mcg IV for a client in early labor. The dose of fentanyl on hand is labeled 100 mcg/2 mL. A nurse should correctly administer ________ mL of fentanyl. *Fill in the blank.*

6. A client who is a 23-year-old primigravida is admitted for induction of labor for macrosomia. Upon assessment, an RN notes the client is having contractions every 2 minutes, lasting 60 seconds in duration. A physician orders misoprostol 25 mcg to be placed in the posterior fornix of the vagina. Which action should be taken by the RN?
   1. Call the physician to clarify the dosage of misoprostol.
   2. Perform a vaginal exam to determine dilation and place the misoprostol as ordered by the physician.
   3. Withhold the dosage and notify the physician of contraction pattern.
   4. Withhold the dosage of misoprostol due to the risks associated with macrosomia.

7. A client who is a 38-year-old multipara had an epidural during her last labor for pain control. She and her husband have chosen to decline any medication during this labor and delivery and ask an RN to help them achieve this goal. To best assist them during the second stage of labor, which action should be taken by the RN?
   1. Perform vigorous perineal massage to decrease pain during delivery.
   2. Encourage patterned breathing to decrease pain during delivery.
   3. Encourage strong pushing between contractions.
   4. Inform the couple about progress toward delivery and all procedures.

8. A client who is a primigravida is admitted in early labor at 38 weeks' gestation. Her physician orders auscultation of fetal heart tones every 30 minutes. The RN knows that the most appropriate time to listen to fetal heart tones is:
   1. For 30 seconds after a contraction.
   2. During a contraction and for 30 seconds after the contraction.
   3. Between the contractions.
   4. During the contractions.

9. A client, who is a gravida 7, para 3, delivers a healthy 6-pound, 4-ounce infant. When an RN performs a postpartum assessment, the client states, "I hope this is our last baby because we can't afford any more children." What is the best response by the nurse?
   1. "You won't have to worry about getting pregnant again until you stop breastfeeding."
   2. "You should discuss this with your physician at your postpartum checkup."
   3. "Perhaps the social worker can help you find a way to budget your finances."
   4. "We can discuss different birth-control methods you can use."

10. A nurse is caring for a client at 35 weeks' gestation who has been admitted to an obstetrics unit with abruptio placentae. Which symptoms are likely to be a result of the placental abruption? *Select all that apply.*
   1. Painless vaginal bleeding.
   2. Tetanic uterine contractions.
   3. Premature rupture of membranes.
   4. Severe abdominal pain.
   5. Rigid, boardlike abdomen.

11. A client delivered a 7-pound, 6-ounce neonate 14 hours ago over a midline episiotomy. Upon assessment, a nurse notes that the client has perineal pain of 7/10 on a numeric scale. Which actions should the nurse take? *Select all that apply.*
   1. Perform perineal hygiene after voiding.
   2. Encourage adequate fluid intake.
   3. Apply an ice pack to her perineum.
   4. Suggest taking a sitz bath several times a day.
   5. Provide topical anesthetics as ordered by the physician.

12. A nurse is providing discharge teaching to a 16-year-old primigravida client. The client is asking questions about her neonate's care. Which methods should be used by the nurse to assist the client in learning to care for her newborn? *Select all that apply.*
   1. Relate stories of the nurse's own personal experiences.
   2. Provide written materials to reinforce teaching.
   3. Demonstrate skills to the client using her own neonate.
   4. Show videotapes to the parent to demonstrate skills.
   5. Tell her to ask her family members for advice about infant care.

13. A client had a vaginal delivery 2 days ago. During the morning assessment, the client complains that excessive perspiration kept her awake all night. She is worried that there is a problem. Which response by a nurse would be the most appropriate?
   1. "You may be experiencing signs of infection."
   2. "Fluids that were retained during pregnancy are normally lost in this manner."
   3. "Maybe you drank too much fluid during the day."
   4. "IV fluids administered during labor sometimes cause sweating."

14. A client is admitted in early labor. The client requests to ambulate to enhance the strength of her contractions. Which event should prompt an RN to return the client to bed and evaluate her condition?
   1. Intense pressure at the peak of contractions.
   2. Warm flushed skin.
   3. Nausea during contractions.
   4. Contractions that are mild and last 60 seconds in duration.

15. A client, 39 weeks' gestation, gravida 2, para 1, is in active labor and reports frequent, painful uterine contractions. Which fetal monitoring pattern would require an *immediate* nursing intervention and why?

Pattern 1

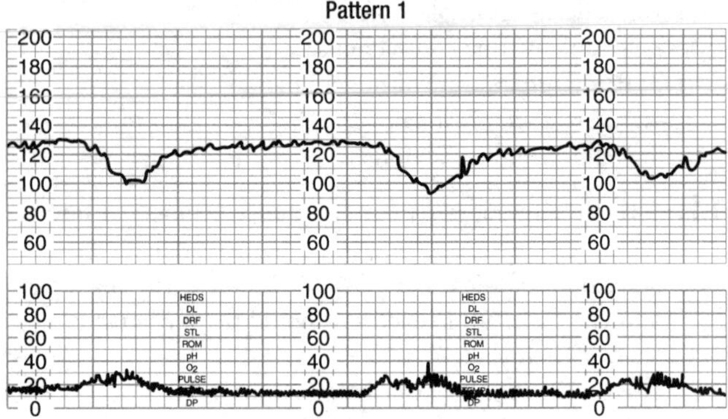

Pattern 2

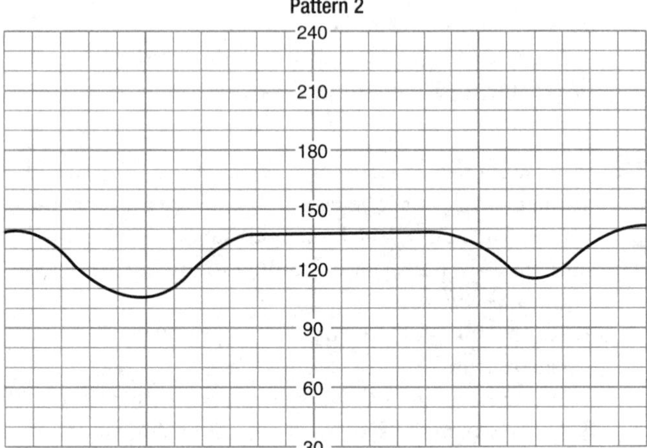

Pattern 3

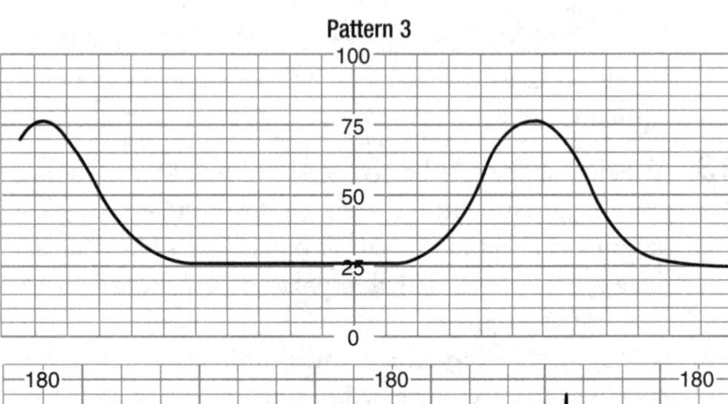

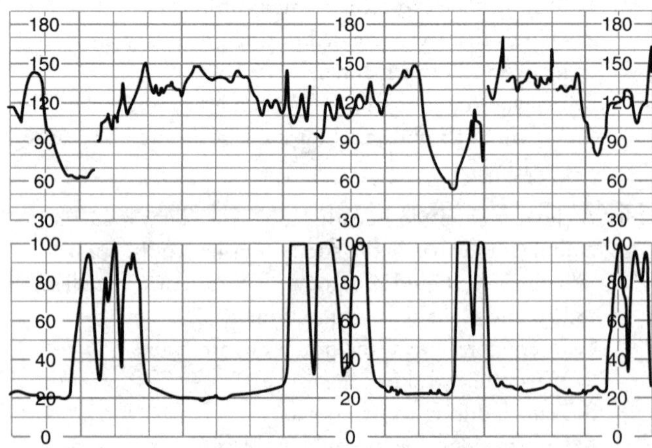

1. Pattern 1 because the tracing shows early decelerations.
2. Pattern 2 because the tracing shows late decelerations.
3. Pattern 3 because the tracing shows variable decelerations.
4. Pattern 3 because the tracing shows late decelerations.

16. A neonate is flaccid at delivery and is not breathing. A pediatrician orders positive-pressure ventilation using a mask attached to wall oxygen. While administering the oxygen, in which position should a nurse place the neonate?

1. On the left side, with the neck slightly flexed.
2. On the back, with the head turned to the left side.
3. On the abdomen, with the head down.
4. On the back, with the neck slightly extended.

17. Which observation of an 8-pound, 4-ounce neonate, if made by an RN, would require an intervention?

1. The neonate's respirations are 36, shallow, and irregular in rate, rhythm, and depth.
2. The neonate's axillary temperature is 96.2°F (35.6°C).
3. Rapid pulsations are visible in the fifth intercostal space, left midclavicular line.
4. There is asynchronous spontaneous movement of the infant's extremities.

18. A client presents to a labor and delivery unit at 38 weeks' gestation. Before applying an external fetal monitor, an RN performs Leopold's maneuver and finds a hard, distinct mass in the upper right quadrant of the client's uterus. Where should the RN anticipate finding the fetal heart tones?

1. Below the umbilicus on the client's left side.
2. Above the umbilicus on the client's left side.
3. Below the umbilicus on the client's right side.
4. Above the umbilicus on the client's right side.

19. A pregnant client expresses concern about her gestational diabetes and asks an RN, "Does this mean I will be diabetic for the rest of my life?" Which is the most appropriate response by the RN?

1. "In most cases, a woman with gestational diabetes will become a diabetic who is insulin-dependent."
2. "If you follow your diabetic diet, you will probably not have anything to worry about."
3. "As long as you don't become pregnant again you will not become a diabetic."
4. "There is a possibility that you may develop type 2 diabetes at some point in the future."

20. A physician orders oxytocin IV at 2 milliunits/minute for the induction of labor. The premixed IV has 15 units of oxytocin in 250 mL of normal saline. A nurse calculates that _______ mL/hr should be administered to the client via an infusion pump. *Fill in the blank.*

21. A client gave birth 40 minutes ago. The placenta has not yet delivered. What is the most appropriate action for an RN to take at this time?

1. Inform the primary health-care provider.
2. Apply traction to the umbilical cord.

3. Prepare the client for surgery.
4. Reassure the client that this is normal.

22. During a routine ultrasound examination, a client, who is 33 weeks pregnant, states that she feels that her heart is pounding. She also reports feeling "hot and sweaty." Which intervention by a nurse is the most appropriate?
   1. Get the client a cool washcloth for her forehead.
   2. Administer nasal oxygen at 12 L/min.
   3. Place the client in Trendelenburg position.
   4. Assist her to a left lateral position.

23. A client who is 32 weeks' gestation presents to a physician's office for a routine prenatal checkup. Leopold's maneuver reveals the fetal position as right occipitoanterior (ROA). At which site would an RN expect to find the fetal heart tone?
   1. Below the umbilicus, on the client's left side.
   2. Below the umbilicus, on the client's right side.
   3. Above the umbilicus, on the client's left side.
   4. Above the umbilicus, on the client's right side.

24. An RN is completing a home visit with a client who delivered a full-term infant 4 days ago. The client states that she is exclusively bottle feeding her infant. Upon assessment, the RN notes white, curdlike patches on the newborn's oral mucous membranes. Which action should the RN take?
   1. Explain that the newborn will need to receive some medication.
   2. Suggest that the newborn's formula be changed.
   3. Remind the caregiver not to let the infant sleep with the bottle.
   4. Determine the baby's blood glucose level.

25. During the examination of a newborn infant, an RN suspects congenital dislocation of the left hip. Which assessment finding would confirm the nurse's suspicion?
   1. Lengthening of the limb on the affected side.
   2. Deformities of the foot and ankle.
   3. Plantar flexion of the foot.
   4. Asymmetry of the gluteal and thigh folds.

26. A nurse is caring for a client who is hospitalized with severe pregnancy-induced hypertension (PIH). What would be an appropriate nursing intervention for this client?
   1. Encourage visitors to spend time with her.
   2. Keep her in the supine position.
   3. Keep her room darkened and limit nursing visits.
   4. Keep her on modified bedrest in a lateral position.

27. The mother of a neonate with a clubfoot feels guilty because she believes she did something during her pregnancy to cause the deformity. A nurse should explain to the mother that the cause of clubfoot is:
   1. Unknown.
   2. Hereditary.
   3. Restricted movement in utero.
   4. An anomaly during embryonic development.

28. A nursing student is preparing to administer an injection of vitamin K, 1 mg IM, to a newborn. The student asks a nurse, "Where should I give the injection?" Which is the most accurate response by the nurse?
   1. Gluteus maximus.
   2. Gluteus minimus.
   3. Vastus lateralis.
   4. Vastus medialis.

29. A client, who is multiparous, delivered a 9-pound, 12-ounce baby girl at 41 3/7 weeks' gestation. After 14 hours of labor, she had an arrest of descent and a cesarean section was performed. While performing an initial newborn assessment, what observations should a nurse expect to find in a neonate of this gestation? *Select all that apply.*
   1. Vernix.
   2. Plethora.
   3. Milia.
   4. Crepitus.
   5. Parchment skin.

30. A client who is at 38 weeks' gestation presents to labor and delivery and states, "I have water leaking down my legs." Which assessment by a nurse is most appropriate in this situation?
   1. Deep tendon reflexes.
   2. Fern test.
   3. Blood pressure check.
   4. Urine test for protein.

31. A nurse performs a sterile vaginal examination on a multiparous client at 37 weeks' gestation. The client is 8 cm dilated, completely effaced, and a +1 station. She tells the nurse, "I can't keep myself from pushing when I have a contraction." Which nursing intervention is most appropriate in this situation?
   1. Encourage her to push through the last 2 cm of dilation.
   2. Assist the client to pant-blow at the peak of contractions.
   3. Readjust the fetal monitor.
   4. Tell the coach that it is not good for the baby if she pushes right now.

32. A client, who is gravida 1, para 0 at 40 weeks' gestation, is in the active phase of labor. The client has had no identified risk factors during her prenatal care. A nurse evaluates the fetal monitor strip at 10:00 hours. The fetal heart rate (FHR) is 130 with moderate variability, and accelerations are present, but no decelerations. At what time should the nurse reevaluate the FHR?
   1. 10:05 a.m.
   2. 10:15 a.m.
   3. 10:30 a.m.
   4. 11:00 a.m.

33. A client, who is gravida 4, para 3 at 39 weeks' gestation, has no identified prenatal risk factors and is in early labor. The client declines electronic fetal monitoring (EFM), stating that she delivered her second baby at home without a monitor and everything went well. What is the most appropriate way for the nurse to handle this situation?

1. Explain that she will need to be on the monitor for about 20 minutes to assess fetal well-being. If the initial tracing is reassuring, the baby may be monitored intermittently.
2. Insist that the fetal monitor be used because there are not enough staff members to adequately monitor her using any other method.
3. Request a change in assignment because of the responsibility if anything were to happen to her baby during labor.
4. Tell her that it is her decision, although continuous EFM is the only effective way to monitor infant well-being during labor.

34. A nurse evaluates a fetal monitor tracing. The nurse should anticipate that an obstetrician will consider performing an amnioinfusion if the electronic fetal monitor tracing reveals:

1. Baseline heart rate = 130, moderate variability present, occasional accelerations and consistent early decelerations.
2. Baseline heart rate = 145, minimal variability present, no accelerations and no decelerations are present.
3. Baseline heart rate = 135, moderate variability present, no accelerations and occasional mild variable decelerations.
4. Baseline heart rate = 120, moderate variability present, and deep variable decelerations with every contraction.

35. A client, who is gravida 1, para 0, presents to labor and delivery because her contractions have become regular, every 5 minutes, and she rates them a 5 on a pain scale of 1 to 10. She talks excitedly with her husband, who is to be her coach. She says that she is pleased that the happy day is finally here, but she is afraid that she will start screaming and she will not be able to handle it when the contractions get stronger. She and her husband have attended childbirth preparation classes. Based on her contractions pattern and her behavior, what are the most likely stage and phase of labor?

1. First stage, active phase.
2. First phase, active stage.
3. First phase, latent stage.
4. First stage, latent phase.

36. Several hours after admission to a birthing center, a client, who is gravida 1, para 0, is dilated 5 cm. The cervix is completely effaced and the fetus is at a +1 station. When a contraction begins, the client kneels on the bed, rests her upper body against her husband, closes her eyes, and sways slowly while humming softly. At the end of the contraction, her husband gently places her on her side and she rests with her eyes closed until the next contraction begins. Which is the most appropriate nursing action for this client?

1. Offer her clear liquids.
2. Offer her an epidural.
3. Offer her pain medication.
4. Encourage her to begin pant-blow breathing.

37. A client, who is gravida 3, para 1, is 8 cm dilated, completely effaced, and a +1 station. She becomes agitated and snaps at her husband and a nurse. She exclaims, "I can't stand this anymore! I want a cesarean section!" What is the most appropriate response by the nurse at this time?

1. "I understand you are in a lot of pain, but you are doing very well and you are almost ready to have this baby."
2. "I will call the doctor and tell him about your request."
3. "Just breathe; you don't need to have a cesarean section."
4. "I understand you want a cesarean section, but you are in the transition phase of labor and your feelings are very common in this stage."

38. A nurse gives a report on a client who is 29 years old, gravida 2, para 1 at 32 weeks' gestation. The fetus is in a vertex presentation and the water bag is intact. A vaginal examination was done 1 hour previously. At that time, the client's cervix was 3 cm dilated and 80% effaced. The station was –2. Continuous EFM is ordered and IV fluids are infusing into the client's left arm. Which is the most important nursing assessment at this time?

1. The frequency and duration of contractions.
2. The patency of the IV infusion.
3. The baseline fetal heart rate.
4. The maternal vital signs.

39. A client delivers a 7-pound, 4-ounce neonate at 38 weeks' gestation. What observations, if found on initial assessment, should a nurse report to a physician? *Select all that apply.*

1. Slight acrocyanosis.
2. Respiratory rate of 20.
3. Consistent heart rate of 145.
4. Pilonidal dimple.
5. Ecchymosis over the occiput.

40. A client, who is gravida 1, para 0, is admitted to labor and delivery for induction of labor at 41 weeks' gestation. Her cervical examination reveals her cervix to be closed and thick and the fetal head is out of the pelvis. Which medications should a nurse anticipate being ordered by a physician? *Select all that apply.*

1. Nifedipine.
2. Cervidil.
3. Prostaglandin gel.
4. Misoprostol.
5. Brethine.

QUESTIONS

41. A 23-year-old client, who is gravida 3, para 2, delivered a baby by vacuum-assisted vaginal delivery 2 days ago. As part of the discharge teaching class, for which conditions should a nurse instruct the client to call a physician? *Select all that apply.*
   1. Pain that is not well controlled by prescription pain medication.
   2. Pain in her calves when walking.
   3. Foul-smelling lochia.
   4. Lochia serosa that is soaking less than a pad every 3 hours.
   5. Soaking more than a pad an hour with lochia.

42. A client, who is a primigravida at 10 weeks' gestation, reports mild uterine cramping and slight vaginal spotting without passage of tissue. When assessed, no cervical dilation is noted. Which is the best action by the nurse?
   1. Anticipate that the woman will be sent home and placed on bedrest.
   2. Prepare the woman for a dilation and curettage.
   3. Notify a grief counselor to assist the woman with the imminent loss of her fetus.
   4. Tell the woman that the doctor will most likely perform a cerclage to help maintain the pregnancy.

43. A client, who is gravida 3, para 2 at 28 weeks' gestation, exhibits glucosuria during her routine prenatal visit. A nurse knows that glucosuria during pregnancy indicates:
   1. An increased glomerular filtration of glucose.
   2. Gestational diabetes.
   3. A need for a 3-hour glucose tolerance test.
   4. A need for small doses of insulin.

44. A client, who is gravida 4, para 1 at 28 weeks' gestation, completes a 1-hour glucose tolerance test. Her 1-hour blood sugar is 150 mg/dL. Which type of follow-up should a nurse recommend to this client?
   1. No follow-up.
   2. A 2000-calorie diet.
   3. A 3-hour glucose tolerance test.
   4. A 2-hour postprandial blood sugar.

45. A client, who is at 32 weeks' gestation, comes to a clinic for a routine prenatal visit. She is having discomfort related to constipation. The nurse should teach the client that the most appropriate measures to alleviate this problem include:
   1. Taking a mild laxative daily.
   2. Adding more protein and fat to the daily diet.
   3. Drinking hot coffee or tea each morning at breakfast.
   4. Drinking 8–10 cups of water and take a daily walk.

46. A client, who is at 26 weeks' gestation, presents for a routine appointment. The client asks a nurse why she is having trouble with constipation during her pregnancy. Which explanation by the nurse would be most accurate?
   1. The intestines are expanded during pregnancy, which causes stool stasis.
   2. The muscle movement of the intestines slows down, which causes dry, hard stools.
   3. The intestines are compressed during pregnancy, which causes stool stasis.
   4. The muscle movement of the intestines speeds up, which causes dry, hard stools.

47. A client, who is gravida 6, para 2, is admitted to labor and delivery in early labor on October 18. A nurse palpates regular uterine contractions every 5 minutes with moderate intensity. A sterile vaginal examination reveals a soft cervix that is 2 cm dilated, 85% effaced, and a –2 station. Which admission information is *most important* in planning this client's nursing care?
   1. The client's LMP was January 2.
   2. The client's blood type is A and Rh+.
   3. The client's hemoglobin is 11 gm/dL.
   4. The client's blood pressure is 100/64 mm Hg.

48. A pregnant client attends a first-trimester class on eating well for pregnancy. Which statement should indicate to a nurse that the client requires additional teaching?
   1. "I should gain around 30 pounds by my due date."
   2. "My strange craving to eat laundry starch is a normal part of pregnancy."
   3. "I need about an extra 300 calories per day during my pregnancy."
   4. "Frozen foods are more nutritious than canned foods."

49. A client, who is 22 years old, gravida 1, para 0, is admitted to an obstetrics unit with contractions every 8 to 10 minutes. A physical assessment reveals that her cervix is 3 cm dilated, 100% effaced, and a 0 station. During the admission process, a nurse asks the couple about their plans for pain relief during labor. The client and her support person state they planned to use prepared childbirth techniques. Based on the information provided, which pain relief method should the nurse expect the couple to use during this phase of labor?
   1. Slow, deep breathing.
   2. Narcotic analgesia.
   3. Local anesthesia.
   4. Rapid, shallow breathing.

50. A client, who is 37 years old, gravida 4, para 3 at 14 weeks' gestation, asks a nurse, "Do you think I'm having a boy? All my other children are girls. If I don't have a boy this time, my husband will really be disappointed in me." Which explanation by the nurse would be most accurate?
   1. "The heartbeat of the baby is fast; that means it's a boy."
   2. "Girls probably run in your family; there's nothing you can do about it."
   3. "The father's sperm determines if the baby is male or female."
   4. "Don't worry; you are carrying this baby low; that means it's a boy."

51. A client at 12 weeks' gestation is at her first prenatal visit. The client is given instructions to get prenatal labs and a multiple marker screen drawn at the laboratory. She asks a nurse about the purpose of the multiple marker screen. The nurse should inform the client that the conditions that may be detected with this test are:
Select all that apply.
1. Gestational diabetes.
2. Edwards' syndrome.
3. Pregnancy-induced hypertension.
4. Trisomy 21.
5. Neural tube defects.

52. A 24-hour-old neonate is icteric with a serum bilirubin level of 14 mg/100 mL. The mother's blood type is O+; the blood type of the baby is B and has a positive direct Coombs' test. The infant is being breastfed. Which measure should a nurse include in the neonate's plan of care?
1. No special measures are necessary; newborns normally get a little jaundiced.
2. Tell the mother to stop breastfeeding and give formula to the baby instead.
3. Place the infant under the bililights and prepare for an exchange transfusion.
4. Encourage the mother to increase the frequency of breastfeeding sessions.

53. A client, who is gravida 2, para 0, has a routine ultrasound at 18 weeks' gestation to confirm her estimated date of delivery; the ultrasound shows the fetus in a breech position. The client asks a nurse "Does this mean I will have to have a C-section?" Which response by the nurse would be most accurate?
1. "If a baby is breech at this gestation, it must always be delivered by cesarean section."
2. "The baby will have more room to turn as your delivery date nears."
3. "You can probably deliver normally; most babies are born breech."
4. "Many babies are breech at this gestation; most turn to head-down by term."

54. A laboring client, who is gravida 1, para 0, has had no change in her cervix for 2 hours and remains 9 to 10 cm dilated. The fetal head has remained at 0 station. A sterile vaginal examination reveals a position of occiput posterior. Which action by the nurse would be most appropriate?
1. Prepare the client for a forceps rotation.
2. Assist the client to a hands-and-knees position.
3. Assist the client to a supine position.
4. Prepare the client for a cesarean delivery.

55. A client with preterm contractions at 34 weeks' gestation is dilated to 3 cm. A physician orders an amniocentesis for fetal lung maturity. Which laboratory test will provide the most information to a nurse about fetal lung maturity?
1. Human chorionic gonadotropin (HCG).
2. Phosphatidylglycerol (PG).
3. α-Fetoprotein (AFP).
4. Partial thromboplastin time (PTT).

56. A client, who is gravida 6, para 4, has a routine ultrasound at 16 weeks' gestation. The ultrasound shows that the client is carrying dizygotic twins. She asks a nurse what the difference is between monozygotic and dizygotic twins. Which explanation by the nurse would be most accurate?
1. "Monozygotic twins come from two different eggs and sperm."
2. "Monozygotic twins come from one egg and two sperm."
3. "Dizygotic twins come from one fertilized egg that splits."
4. "Dizygotic twins come from two different eggs and sperm."

57. A client, who is 18 years old, presents to a prenatal clinic because her menstrual period is 9 days late. She tells a nurse, "I'm sure I'm pregnant because my period is late and my breasts are tender." Which response by the nurse would be most appropriate?
1. "A missed menstrual period and breast tenderness are probable signs of pregnancy."
2. "A missed menstrual period and breast tenderness are presumptive signs of pregnancy."
3. "A missed menstrual period and breast tenderness are positive signs of pregnancy."
4. "A missed menstrual period and breast tenderness are negative signs of pregnancy."

58. A client who is gravida 2, para 1 is seen in an emergency department at 14 weeks' gestation with bright red vaginal bleeding and severe lower abdominal cramping. Which assessment finding is the *most important* observation at this time?
1. Increased temperature.
2. Increased pulse pressure.
3. Increasing heart rate.
4. Increased blood pressure.

59. An anesthetist has just placed an epidural catheter dosed with bupivacaine hydrochloride (Marcaine) in a client in labor who is gravida 2, para 1 at 39 weeks' gestation. For which side effect should a nurse observe this client?
1. Hypotension.
2. Hypertension.
3. Hypoventilation.
4. Hyperventilation.

60. A nurse assesses a client who is 40 years old, gravida 11, para 9 at 14 weeks' gestation, and has a history of thromboembolitic disease. The client is placed on daily heparin therapy. Which laboratory test will be the *most important* for this client?
1. Prothrombin time.
2. Partial thromboplastin time.

3. Bleeding time.
4. D-dimer.

61. A client, who is 36 years old, has been trying to get pregnant for about 5 months. At her physician appointment, she states that she knows she should take folic acid supplements but dislikes taking pills. Which foods that are high in folic acid should a nurse suggest? *Select all that apply.*
1. Salmon.
2. Spinach.
3. Orange juice.
4. Asparagus.
5. Chicken.

62. A client has just completed the second stage of labor and has begun the third stage of labor. Which nursing action has *priority* at this time?
1. Promotion of the bonding process.
2. Administration of an oxytocic medication.
3. Encouraging the client to push.
4. Physical assessment of the neonate.

63. A client, who delivered a full-term infant 45 minutes ago, is carefully examining her newborn during the initial breastfeeding. She asks a nurse, "My baby's head is shaped like a bullet! Will it stay like that?" Which response by the nurse is most accurate?
1. "That is called a caput. It usually lasts for 3 or 4 days."
2. "That is called a hemangioma. It will probably last a few months."
3. "That is called a cephalohematoma. It usually lasts for a few weeks."
4. "That is called molding. It usually lasts for a few days."

64. A client, who is 20 years old, delivered her first baby 2 days ago. She is exclusively breastfeeding and has been discharged home by her physician. A nurse has completed discharge teaching on newborn care. Which statement by the client would indicate a need for further teaching?
1. "I should nurse my baby whenever he acts hungry and for as long as he wants to nurse."
2. "If my baby has at least one wet diaper and one bowel movement a day, he is getting enough to eat."
3. "I should dress my baby in clothing I would be comfortable in, plus a light blanket."
4. "I should clean the cord stump with alcohol every day until it falls off."

65. A client, who is gravida 3, para 2, has a spontaneous vaginal delivery of a 6-pound baby girl over an intact perineum. She has an epidural for relief of labor pain. She is currently in the fourth stage of labor. Which nursing goal would be most appropriate for the client at this time?
1. The client's episiotomy will remain clean, dry, and intact.
2. The client will turn, cough, and deep breathe 10 times an hour.
3. The client will ambulate in the room without assistance.
4. The client will maintain physiological homeostasis.

66. A client, who is 19 years old, gravida 1, para 0, is admitted to labor and delivery with HELLP syndrome at 28 weeks' gestation. A nurse knows that management for her condition should include:
Select all that apply.
1. Administration of corticosteroid.
2. Administration of an IV fluid bolus.
3. Liver function tests.
4. Administration of tocolytics.
5. Bedrest in the left lateral position.

67. A nurse assesses a client who is 15 years old, gravida 1, para 0, and is 11 weeks' gestation. Which prenatal laboratory test would indicate a risk factor for this client?
1. White blood cell count = 12,000.
2. Hematocrit = 32%.
3. Hemoglobin = 9 gm/dL.
4. Random serum glucose = 105 gm/dL.

68. A client, who is gravida 3, para 2 at 37 weeks' gestation, is 5 cm dilated, 80% effaced, and a +1 station. She received epidural anesthesia with bupivacaine hydrochloride (Marcaine) for contraction pain 1 hour ago. Which nursing assessment is *most important* for this client at this time?
1. Assessing the client hourly for respiratory depression.
2. Assessing the client hourly for uterine atony.
3. Assessing the client hourly for bladder distention.
4. Assessing the client hourly for hypertension.

69. A client, who is gravida 1, para 0, arrives in a labor and delivery unit at 38 weeks' gestation with mild irregular contractions. A sterile vaginal examination reveals the following: cervical dilation of 3 cm, 60% effaced, –1 station, and membranes intact. An external fetal monitor is placed and the fetal heart tracing reveals a baseline of 130 bpm, moderate variability, and accelerations to the 150s during contractions. Based on this information, which nursing action would be most appropriate?
1. Turn the client to her left side and administer oxygen.
2. Prepare the client for an immediate operative delivery.
3. Begin an intravenous infusion for hydration.
4. Send the client home and encourage her to ambulate.

70. A client, who delivered 8 weeks ago, is exclusively breastfeeding, and asks for information on birth control methods that do not interfere with breast milk production. Which statement should indicate to a nurse that the client needs further instruction?
1. "Breastfeeding itself is effective at preventing pregnancy."
2. "Using condoms would be a good choice for me."
3. "I can use Depo-Provera and breastfeed without problems."
4. "I can use contraceptive foam for birth control."

71. A nurse assesses a client who delivered an 8-pound, 6-ounce infant 2 hours ago. Which assessment findings are considered "normal" in a client during this time? *Select all that apply.*
   1. Fundus firm, at the umbilicus.
   2. Fundus firm, 2 fingerbreadths below the umbilicus.
   3. Bluish-white fluid expressed from her breasts.
   4. Lochia serosa, moderate amount.
   5. Moderate lochia rubra.

72. A client delivered an 8-pound, 9-ounce neonate at 39 weeks' gestation. Which observations, if found during the initial assessment, are normal findings and do not need to be reported to a physician? *Select all that apply.*
   1. Heart rate of 170 at rest.
   2. Respiratory rate of 46.
   3. Circumoral cyanosis.
   4. Caput succedaneum over the occiput.
   5. Mongolian spots.

73. A client with type 1 insulin-dependent diabetes presents to a prenatal clinic at 17 weeks' gestation for α-fetoprotein testing. She asks a nurse why this test is being performed. Which explanation by the nurse would be most accurate?
   1. "This test is to determine the sex of your baby."
   2. "This test is to determine glycemic control."
   3. "This test is screening for neural tube defects."
   4. "This test is to determine fetal lung maturity."

74. A client entered the fourth stage of labor 30 minutes ago. During an assessment, a nurse notes that there is constant trickling of bright red vaginal blood in the presence of a contracted uterus midline at the umbilicus. Which action by the nurse would be most appropriate in this situation?
   1. Massage the fundus.
   2. Call the physician.
   3. Have the client empty her bladder.
   4. Increase the oxytocin infusion.

75. A client, who is a gravida 3, para 1, presents to labor and delivery at 41 4/7 weeks' gestation for induction of labor. Her cervix is 2 cm dilated, 80% effaced, and a –3 station. A nurse anticipates that, in preparation for labor, a physician will likely order: *Select all that apply.*
   1. Hemabate 250 mcg IM.
   2. Pitocin at 2 milliunits/min IV.
   3. Betamethasone 6 mg IM.
   4. Cytotec 200 mcg PO.
   5. Cervidil 10 mg vaginally.

76. A client, gravida 2, para 0, is admitted to a labor and delivery unit at 35 weeks' gestation. Her blood pressure is 180/110 mm Hg, pulse 88, respirations 18, and temperature 98.6°F. Her urine dipstick shows 3+ proteinuria and a physical assessment reveals 3+ deep tendon reflexes. A physician orders magnesium sulfate to be infused at 2 gm/hr. Which action by a nurse indicates understanding of the possible side effects of magnesium sulfate?
   1. Placing a sign over the bed not to check blood pressure in the right arm.
   2. Placing a padded tongue blade at the bedside.
   3. Inserting a Foley catheter.
   4. Darkening the room.

77. A nurse enters the room of a client who is a 22-year-old primigravida who was 39 weeks' gestation. The infant was delivered using vacuum extraction 3 hours ago. The client is in tears and says "When I first delivered, the baby breastfed for almost an hour, now the baby won't wake up enough to take the nipple!" Which intervention would be most appropriate in this case?
   1. Instruct the client to supplement breastfeeding with formula; the baby isn't waking up because there isn't enough milk.
   2. Instruct the client to wake the baby by changing the baby's diaper.
   3. Instruct the client to let the baby sleep, because babies cluster-feed, and frequently sleep for several hours after the initial breastfeeding.
   4. Instruct the client to submerge the baby into a bath of lukewarm water to wake the baby up so that the baby will breastfeed.

78. A client, who is gravida 3, para 0 at 39 weeks' gestation, is admitted to a labor and delivery unit in active labor. The physician performs an amniotomy. Which assessment finding should a nurse anticipate after the amniotomy?
   1. Fetal heart tones 90 bpm.
   2. A moderate amount of straw-colored fluid.
   3. A small amount of greenish fluid.
   4. A small segment of the umbilical cord.

79. A client, who is gravida 1, para 0, is admitted to labor and delivery with spontaneous rupture of membranes. A vaginal examination reveals clear fluid and the cervix is 2 cm dilated. Based on the information provided, which statement should a nurse expect this client to make?
   1. "We have a name picked out for the baby."
   2. "I need to push when I have a contraction."
   3. "I can't concentrate if anyone is touching me."
   4. "When can I get my epidural?"

80. A client, who is gravida 2, para 0 at 38 weeks' gestation, is having sharp decreases in fetal heart rate from a baseline of 130 bpm to 90 to 110 bpm during the contractions. Which action should a nurse take *first?*
   1. Reposition the monitor.
   2. Turn the client to her left side.
   3. Ask the client to ambulate.
   4. Prepare the client for delivery.

81. A client, who is gravida 1, para 0, is dilated to 6 cm, 100% effaced, and a 0 station for the past 2 hours

without any change in her cervix. A physician orders oxytocin (Pitocin) augmentation. When evaluating the effectiveness of IV oxytocin augmentation, which outcome should a nurse anticipate?

1. A painless delivery.
2. Cervical effacement.
3. Infrequent contractions.
4. Progressive cervical dilation.

82. A client, who is gravida 1, para 0 at 37 weeks' gestation, is admitted to labor and delivery in active labor. A vaginal examination reveals a footling breech presentation. Which action should the nurse take *first?*

1. Anticipate the need for a cesarean section.
2. Apply the fetal heart monitor.
3. Place the client in genupectoral position.
4. Perform an ultrasound exam.

83. A client, who is gravida 2, para 1, is admitted to a birthing center. A nurse is using a Doppler to check fetal heart tones. The nurse finds fetal heart tones of 160 to 170 bpm. A vaginal examination reveals that the cervix is 4 cm dilated, with intact membranes and a –1 station. The nurse decides to apply an external fetal monitor rather than an internal monitor. Which is the best rationale for this decision?

1. The cervix is closed.
2. The membranes are still intact.
3. The fetal heart tones are within normal limits.
4. The contractions are intense enough for insertion of an internal monitor.

84. A client, who is gravida 1, para 0, presents to labor and delivery with contractions every 3 minutes. The client states that she has not felt the baby move for the last 2 hours. What action should the nurse take *first?*

1. Call the physician.
2. Place the client on an external fetal monitor.
3. Start an IV.
4. Obtain maternal vital signs.

85. A client, who is gravida 3, para 2, is 8 cm dilated, 100% effaced, and a 0 station. When evaluating the fetal monitor tracing, a nurse notes baseline heart rate 170 bpm, minimal variability, and consistent late decelerations. What is the most likely explanation of this pattern?

1. The fetus is asleep.
2. The umbilical cord is compressed.
3. There is a head compression.
4. There is uteroplacental insufficiency.

86. A client, who is gravida 4, para 3, is 4 cm dilated, 80% effaced, and a +1 station. Assessment of the fetal monitor tracing reveals baseline 140 bpm, moderate variability, and accelerations and variable decelerations to 100 bpm. Which action should a nurse take *first?*

1. Notify her physician.
2. Give a 500-mL bolus IV.
3. Reposition the client.
4. Readjust the monitor.

87. A gravida 4, para 2 client with gestational diabetes is having nonstress tests twice a week. A nurse evaluates the fetal monitor strip. Which fetal heart rate pattern should the nurse interpret as reassuring?

1. A baseline fetal heart rate of 170–180 bpm.
2. Baseline variability of 25–35 bpm.
3. Variable decelerations to 100 bpm.
4. Acceleration of FHR with fetal movements.

88. A client, who is gravida 3, para 2, receives an epidural for labor pain relief. A nurse knows the client will need to have a Foley catheter placed if the epidural is in place longer than 1 hour. Which is the best rationale for this nursing action?

1. The bladder fills more rapidly because of the medication used for the epidural.
2. Her level of consciousness is such that she is in a trancelike state.
3. The sensation of the bladder filling is diminished or lost.
4. She is embarrassed to ask for the bedpan that frequently.

89. A woman is practicing natural family planning methods. She asks a nurse about the most likely time for her to conceive. The nurse explains that conception is most likely to occur when:

1. Estrogen levels are low.
2. Luteinizing hormone is high.
3. The endometrial lining is thin.
4. The progesterone level is low.

90. A client tells a nurse that she plans to use the rhythm method of birth control. The nurse instructs the client that the success of this method depends on the:

1. Age of the client.
2. Frequency of intercourse.
3. Regularity of the menses.
4. Range of the client's temperature.

91. A 34-year-old client with type 1 diabetes since age 5 asks a nurse for advice regarding methods of birth control. Which method of birth control is the best choice for a client with type 1 diabetes?

1. Intrauterine device.
2. Oral contraceptives.
3. Diaphragm.
4. Contraceptive patch.

92. A client presents to an emergency department at 8 weeks' gestation. A physician suspects that the client has an ectopic (tubal) pregnancy. When performing an initial assessment, which symptom should a nurse recognize as consistent with a diagnosis of ectopic (tubal) pregnancy?

1. Painless vaginal bleeding.
2. Abdominal cramping.
3. Throbbing pain in the upper quadrant.
4. Sudden, stabbing pain in the lower quadrant.

93. A client, who is 10 weeks' gestation, has been having severe nausea for the past 3 weeks. She tells a nurse that she cannot eat anything. She has been diagnosed with hyperemesis gravidarum and is at risk for developing:
1. Respiratory alkalosis without dehydration.
2. Metabolic acidosis with dehydration.
3. Respiratory acidosis without dehydration.
4. Metabolic alkalosis with dehydration.

94. A client presents to a prenatal clinic and tells a physician that she thinks she might be pregnant because she has not has a period for about 5 months. Which is the most definitive sign of pregnancy?
1. Elevated human chorionic gonadotropin.
2. The presence of fetal heart tones.
3. Uterine enlargement.
4. Breast enlargement and tenderness.

95. A client, who is gravida 3, para 2 at 39 weeks' gestation with poorly controlled gestational diabetes, has just given birth via cesarean section. A nurse will expect that the neonate will most likely be:
1. Hypoglycemic, small for gestational age.
2. Hyperglycemic, large for gestational age.
3. Hypoglycemic, large for gestational age.
4. Hyperglycemic, small for gestational age.

96. A client, who is 44 years old, gravida 3, para 2, has just delivered a newborn suspected of having trisomy 21. Which characteristics should a nurse observe in an infant with this condition? *Select all that apply.*
1. Simian creases.
2. Increased muscle tone.
3. Flat appearance of the face.
4. Small tongue.
5. Upward-slanting eye creases.

97. A nursing student is performing an initial newborn assessment. The newborn is observed to have a cephalohematoma. What are the likely causes of this condition? *Select all that apply.*
1. Scheduled cesarean delivery.
2. Prolonged latent phase of labor.
3. Prolonged second stage of labor.
4. Vacuum-assisted vaginal delivery.
5. Breech presentation.

98. A client, who is 24 years old, gravida 4, para 3, has had no prenatal care and does not know when her last menstrual period was. She presents to labor and delivery completely dilated and crowning. She precipitously delivers a 5-pound, 6-ounce infant. The client's urine toxicology screen shows methamphetamines. The client admits that she uses methamphetamine daily. Which observations should a nurse expect in the neonate that would be consistent with methamphetamine exposure in utero? *Select all that apply.*
1. Cleft lip.
2. Irritability.
3. Clubfoot.
4. Hyperbilirubinemia.
5. Gastroschisis.

99. An 18-year-old client chooses oral contraceptives as her method of birth control. Which instruction should be included in a nurse's teaching regarding oral contraceptives?
1. Weight gain should be reported to the physician.
2. An alternate method of birth control is needed when taking antibiotics.
3. If the client misses one or more pills, two pills should be taken per day for 1 week.
4. Nausea or stomach upset should be reported to the physician.

100. A 27-year-old client, who is gravida 3, para 1, presents to a labor and delivery unit at 33 weeks' gestation. She tells a nurse that she woke up this morning in a pool of blood about the size of an orange, but she has no abdominal cramping or pain. The nurse's *first* action should be to:
1. Assess the fetal heart tones.
2. Check for cervical dilation.
3. Check for firmness of the uterus.
4. Obtain maternal vital signs.

ANSWERS

Answers/Rationales/Tips

1. CORRECT ANSWERS: 1, 2. Answer 1 is correct because placing the client on an electronic fetal monitor is an appropriate intervention to evaluate uterine contractions and determine fetal well-being. Evaluate of fetal well-being is very important for this client because of her complaint of decreased fetal movement. Answer 2 is correct because betamethasone is a corticosteroid used to help stimulate fetal lung maturity in infants who are preterm. **Answer 3** is incorrect because performing a nipple stimulation test is inappropriate for a client who is in preterm labor; stimulating nipples may stimulate uterine contractions, which is *contraindicated* in preterm labor. **Answer 4** is incorrect because adequate hydration (*not* limiting oral fluids) is important to decrease uterine contraction in clients who are in preterm labor. **Answer 5** is incorrect because placing the client on strict bedrest increases the chance of developing deep vein thrombosis. *Modified* bedrest is the appropriate management for this client.

■ **TEST-TAKING TIP:** ***Eliminate Answers 3 and 4 because these actions are contraindicated in preterm labor. Since pregnancy increases the chance for developing blood clots,*** **strict** ***bedrest also increases the chance of developing blood clots; therefore, eliminate Answer 5 also.***

Content Area: Maternity, Intrapartum; ***Integrated Process:*** Nursing Process, Implementation; ***Cognitive Level:*** Application; ***Client Need/Subneed:*** Physiological Integrity/Physiological Adaptation/Alterations in Body Systems

2. CORRECT ANSWERS: 1, 2, 5. Answer 1 is correct because a risk factor for developing an infection postpartum is a long active phase of labor. Answer 2 is correct because prolonged

rupture of membranes (longer than 24 hours) is a risk factor for developing postpartum endometritis. **Answer 3** is incorrect because prolonged *labor, not precipitous* delivery, is associated with an increased risk of postpartum endometritis. **Answer 4** is incorrect because a long *active* phase, *not latent* phase, of labor is associated with a higher risk of endometritis. **Answer 5 is correct because internal fetal monitoring can act as a conduit for transmission of bacteria into the uterine cavity during labor and delivery, increasing the risk of developing postpartum endometritis.**

■ **TEST-TAKING TIP:** *Endometritis is an infection (not to be confused with endometriosis, which is* **dysfunctional** *uterine bleeding). Focus on the conditions that increase a chance for infection:* **long** *labor,* **long ago** *rupture of membranes, and an* **internal** *conduit.*

Content Area: Maternity, Postpartum; ***Integrated Process:*** Nursing Process, Analysis; ***Cognitive Level:*** Application; ***Client Need/Subneed:*** Physiological Integrity/Physiological Adaptation/Pathophysiology

3. **CORRECT ANSWER: 2.** **Answer 1** is incorrect because oral hypoglycemic agents cross the placenta and can *cause fetal anomalies* during the first trimester of pregnancy. **Answer 2 is correct because insulin does not cross the placenta and is safe for use in pregnancy.** **Answer 3** is incorrect because *only gestational diabetes* can be treated with diet during pregnancy. **Answer 4** is incorrect because *only gestational diabetes* can be treated with exercise during pregnancy.

■ **TEST-TAKING TIP:** *This client had diabetes* **before** *pregnancy and is asking how to manage her blood sugar. Eliminate the options that are only for controlling* **gestational** *diabetes.*

Content Area: Maternity, Antepartum; ***Integrated Process:*** Teaching and Learning; ***Cognitive Level:*** Application; ***Client Need/Subneed:*** Physiological Integrity/Reduction of Risk Potential/Potential for Complications from Surgical Procedures and Health Alterations

4. **CORRECT ANSWER: 3.** **Answer 1** is incorrect because, according to Rubin, maternal role attachment develops over about a 3- to 10-month period, so it is *too early* to make this determination. **Answer 2** is incorrect because attachment is an ongoing process that occurs *gradually.* **Answer 3 is correct because this client is demonstrating normal behavior for the taking-in period, which, according to Rubin, includes dependence and passivity that may last up to 3 days after delivery.** **Answer 4** is incorrect because a client experiencing postpartum depression *consistently* demonstrates anxiety, confusion, or other signs and symptoms (i.e., feelings of worthlessness or guilt, tearfulness, hopelessness and feeling empty inside, lack of joy in new baby).

■ **TEST-TAKING TIP:** *Consider the time that has passed since delivery and what stage of adaptation the new mother is experiencing. Three of the options focus on* **problems** *(e.g., doubting competency, attachment disorder, depression). Select the one option that is "normal."*

Content Area: Maternity, Postpartum; ***Integrated Process:*** Nursing Process, Analysis; ***Cognitive Level:*** Application; ***Client Need/Subneed:*** Health Promotion and Maintenance/Ante/Intra/Postpartum and Newborn Care

5. **CORRECT ANSWER: 1.5.** **The calculation is completed by dividing 100 mcg/2 mL; there are 50 mcg/1 mL, 25 mcg/0.5 mL. Therefore, 75 mcg is 1.5 mL of fentanyl.**

■ **TEST-TAKING TIP:** *Calculate how many milligrams (mg) are in each milliliter (mL). The calculation is easier when you are dealing with 1 mL.*

Content Area: Maternity, Intrapartum; ***Integrated Process:*** Nursing Process, Analysis; ***Cognitive Level:*** Analysis; ***Client Need/Subneed:*** Physiological Integrity/Pharmacological and Parenteral Therapies/Dosage Calculation

6. **CORRECT ANSWER: 3.** **Answer 1** is incorrect because this is an appropriate dosage of misoprostol for induction of labor; no clarification is needed for this order. **Answer 2** is incorrect because this client is already having very frequent uterine contractions and placing misoprostol is *contraindicated* for this client. **Answer 3 is correct because this client is having very frequent uterine contractions and placing misoprostol is contraindicated for this client. The physician should be notified of the contraction pattern and withholding the misoprostol dose.** **Answer 4** is incorrect because macrosomia is an indication for induction of labor; however, this client is not a candidate for placement of misoprostol due to the frequency of her uterine contractions.

■ **TEST-TAKING TIP:** *Consider that misoprostol cannot be removed once it is given vaginally and the contractions caused by the medication can result in uterine hyperstimulation. Focus on the two options that state: do not give ("withhold").*

Content Area: Maternity, Intrapartum; ***Integrated Process:*** Nursing Process, Implementation; ***Cognitive Level:*** Application; ***Client Need/Subneed:*** Physiological Integrity/Pharmacological and Parenteral Therapies/Adverse Effects/Contraindications/Interactions

7. **CORRECT ANSWER: 4.** **Answer 1** is incorrect because vigorous perineal massage does *not* decrease pain during delivery; gentle perineal massage may be used by some practitioners to decrease perineal tearing. **Answer 2** is incorrect because the second stage of labor is the pushing stage and coaching with patterned breathing is used to decrease pain during the *first stage* of labor. **Answer 3** is incorrect because pushing should be performed *during* the peak of the contractions, not between, to enhance progress toward delivery. **Answer 4 is correct because keeping the couple informed decreases anxiety, increases confidence in their ability to cope with an unmedicated labor and delivery, and helps accomplish their goals.**

■ **TEST-TAKING TIP:** *Remember the stages of labor and that the correct coaching for a woman who is pushing (second stage of labor) is different than during the first stage of labor.*

Content Area: Maternity, Intrapartum; ***Integrated Process:*** Nursing Process, Implementation; ***Cognitive Level:*** Application; ***Client Need/Subneed:*** Health Promotion and Maintenance/Ante/Intra/Postpartum and Newborn Care

8. CORRECT ANSWER: 2. **Answer 1** is incorrect because auscultation should be performed to hear decelerations of the fetal heart rate. Correct procedure includes listening for decelerations *during* a contraction and for 30 seconds *after* the contraction, to make sure that there are no audible decelerations. **Answer 2 is correct because this is the correct procedure for fetal heart tone auscultation.** **Answer 3** is incorrect because this answer doesn't include listening *during* the contraction for decelerations; therefore, it is incomplete. **Answer 4** is incorrect because this answer doesn't include listening *after* the contraction. Late decelerations may not be heard.

■ **TEST-TAKING TIP:** *The reason for obtaining fetal heart tones is to ensure that the fetus is not having any fetal distress. Eliminate the answers that do not provide complete assessment for fetal distress.*

Content Area: Maternity, Intrapartum; *Integrated Process:* Nursing Process, Assessment; *Cognitive Level:* Application; *Client Need/Subneed:* Health Promotion and Maintenance/ Ante/Intra/Postpartum and Newborn Care

9. CORRECT ANSWER: 4. **Answer 1** is incorrect because breastfeeding is *not* a reliable method of birth control. **Answer 2** is incorrect because ovulation may occur *before* the 6-week postpartum checkup, and may lead to an unwanted pregnancy. **Answer 3** is incorrect because, although a referral to a social worker may assist in providing information about available resources, it will *not* prevent an unwanted pregnancy. **Answer 4 is correct because it is appropriate to discuss birth control at the time when the client is asking questions and is receptive to teaching.**

■ **TEST-TAKING TIP:** *The client is asking about birth control. Eliminate the answers where the nurse doesn't focus on birth control or that contain incorrect advice (Answer 1).*

Content Area: Maternity, Postpartum; *Integrated Process:* Communication and Documentation; *Cognitive Level:* Application; *Client Need/Subneed:* Psychosocial Integrity/ Therapeutic Communications

10. CORRECT ANSWERS: 2, 3, 4, 5. **Answer 1** is incorrect because painless vaginal bleeding is a symptom of *placenta previa, not* abruptio placentae. **Answer 2 is correct because a placental abruption causes tetanic uterine contractions in response to the placenta detaching from the uterine wall. Answer 3 is correct because premature rupture of membranes is associated with placental abruption. Answer 4 is correct because severe abdominal pain is a symptom of placental abruption; and uterine contractions, in response to the placenta detaching from the uterine wall, cause severe pain. Answer 5 is correct because a rigid, boardlike abdomen is a symptom of placental abruption; and uterine contractions, in response to the placenta detaching from the uterine wall, cause severe pain. The uterus stays contracted, causing the rigid abdomen.**

■ **TEST-TAKING TIP:** *Note the difference between abruption (pain) and previa (painless). Four options = pain; one option = painless. Both are placenta complications, but are very different in manifestation of symptoms.*

Content Area: Maternity, Antepartum; *Integrated Process:* Nursing Process, Analysis; *Cognitive Level:* Comprehension; *Client Need/Subneed:* Physiological Integrity/Physiological Adaptation/Pathophysiology

11. CORRECT ANSWERS: 2, 3, 4, 5. **Answer 1** is incorrect because, although perineal hygiene can decrease the chance for infection, perineal hygiene after voiding will *not* be helpful in decreasing her perineal pain. Using the peri bottle during urination can decrease the pain caused by urination. **Answer 2 is correct because staying well hydrated by drinking plenty of water can be helpful in decreasing pain caused by constipation. Straining with bowel movements will stretch the episiotomy scar and perineum and can cause pain. Avoid constipation by eating fiber-rich foods such as fresh fruits and vegetables. Answer 3 is correct because applying an ice pack is helpful in decreasing perineal pain by decreasing perineal edema. Answer 4 is correct because taking a sitz bath several times a day can decrease the pain by increasing the circulation to the perineum. Answer 5 is correct because topical anesthetics, as ordered by the physician, can decrease the perineal pain by slowing down the rate at which pain sensors in the skin send pain messages to the brain, and by reducing perineal swelling.**

■ **TEST-TAKING TIP:** *The key concept in this question is the treatment and prevention of perineal pain related to the delivery. Choose the interventions that decrease pain.*

Content Area: Maternity, Postpartum; *Integrated Process:* Nursing Process, Implementation; *Cognitive Level:* Application; *Client Need/Subneed:* Health Promotion and Maintenance/ Ante/Intra/Postpartum and Newborn Care

12. CORRECT ANSWERS: 2, 3, 4. **Answer 1** is incorrect because relating personal experiences is *not* an appropriate method of teaching or reinforcing learning. **Answer 2 is correct because providing written materials is a suitable method for reinforcing teaching. Answer 3 is correct because demonstrating skills to the client using her own neonate is an acceptable method that involves the parent in learning skills using her own infant. Answer 4 is correct because showing videotapes to the parent is a common and appropriate method to demonstrate skills.** **Answer 5** is incorrect because telling her to ask her family members for advice about infant care is *not* an appropriate method of teaching neonatal care. Using standardized materials for instruction, providing feedback about neonatal care and answering the client's questions are appropriate methods. Simply telling the client to ask her family members does not provide instruction for the client.

■ **TEST-TAKING TIP:** *Appropriate teaching methods include visual information such as videotapes and written materials, the kinesthetic method using the infant, and auditory materials such as a recording of discharge instructions.*

Content Area: Maternity, Postpartum; *Integrated Process:* Teaching and Learning; *Cognitive Level:* Analysis; *Client Need/Subneed:* Health Promotion and Maintenance/Principles of Teaching and Learning

13. CORRECT ANSWER: 2. **Answer 1** is incorrect because this response could unnecessarily worry the client. Excessive perspiration may be a sign of infection, but there is no additional information in the stem that would lead to that possibility. **Answer 2 is correct because this explanation is factually true. Fluids are retained during pregnancy and lost in this manner. This is called postpartum diuresis and is commonly experienced about 24 to 48 hours after delivery.** **Answer 3** is incorrect because speculating about the client's intake is not an appropriate response to her concerns. **Answer 4** is incorrect because it assumes that the client had IV fluids administered during labor and does not address her concerns about having "a problem."

■ **TEST-TAKING TIP:** ***Consider why the client is asking the question—she is concerned about developing a problem; eliminate responses that do not address her concern.***

Content Area: Maternity, Postpartum; *Integrated Process:* Communication and Documentation; *Cognitive Level:* Application; *Client Need/Subneed:* Health Promotion and Maintenance/Ante/Intra/Postpartum and Newborn Care

14. CORRECT ANSWER: 1. Answer 1 is correct because intense pressure at the peak of contractions may indicate the client is completely dilated and is close to delivery. A return to bed and a vaginal examination are needed to confirm this possibility. **Answer 2** is incorrect because warm flushed skin *is a common finding* during labor and is not indicative of a need for reevaluation. **Answer 3** is incorrect because nausea during contractions *is a common finding* during labor and is not indicative of a need for reevaluation. **Answer 4** is incorrect because contractions that are mild will probably not result in cervical change; therefore, this finding does not require a reevaluation.

■ **TEST-TAKING TIP:** ***Consider the reason for reevaluating the client. Eliminate responses that are common to all clients in labor, such as skin flushing and nausea, and are not specific to this client's condition.***

Content Area: Maternity, Intrapartum; *Integrated Process:* Nursing Process, Assessment; *Cognitive Level:* Analysis; *Client Need/Subneed:* Physiological Integrity/Reduction of Risk Potential/Potential for Alterations in Body Systems

15. CORRECT ANSWER: 2. **Answer 1** is incorrect because the pattern here is *early* decelerations and is caused by compressions of the fetal head descending through the birth canal. *No* nursing intervention is needed. **Answer 2 is correct because the pattern is *late* decelerations and is caused by uteroplacental insufficiency. The fetal heart rate is tachycardic, baseline heart rate of 180 bpm with decreased baseline variability. The nurse must immediately attempt to correct the pattern by turning the client on her side and giving a fluid bolus and oxygen mask. The physician must also be notified immediately.** **Answer 3** is incorrect because this pattern is *variable* decelerations, caused by compression of the umbilical cord. The fetus demonstrates good oxygen reserve since the baseline variability is normal and the fetal heart rate rapidly returns to baseline after the deceleration. Immediate intervention in this type of pattern is not required, but continued close observation of the pattern is needed. **Answer 4** is incorrect because this pattern is *variable* decelerations, caused by compression of the umbilical cord. The fetus demonstrates good oxygen reserve since the baseline variability is normal and the fetal heart rate rapidly returns to baseline after the deceleration. Immediate intervention in this type of pattern is not required, but continued close observation of the pattern is needed.

■ **TEST-TAKING TIP:** ***To determine the type of deceleration, draw a line from the lowest part of the deceleration down to the uterine contraction to establish the relationship as early, variable, or late between the deceleration and the uterine contraction.***

Content Area: Maternity, Intrapartum; *Integrated Process:* Nursing Process, Analysis; *Cognitive Level:* Analysis; *Client Need/Subneed:* Physiological Integrity/Physiological Adaptation/Medical Emergencies

16. CORRECT ANSWER: 4. **Answer 1** is incorrect because the left side, with the neck slightly flexed, will prevent proper ventilation. **Answer 2** is incorrect because the back, with the head turned to the left side, will prevent proper ventilation. **Answer 3** is incorrect because placing the neonate on the abdomen, with the head down, will prevent ventilation and may cause suffocation. **Answer 4 is correct because placing the neonate on the back, with the neck slightly extended, will open the airway and facilitate ventilation.**

■ **TEST-TAKING TIP:** ***Picture the positions described and eliminate the ones that prevent air exchange.***

Content Area: Child Health, Newborn; *Integrated Process:* Nursing Process, Implementation; *Cognitive Level:* Application; *Client Need/Subneed:* Physiological Integrity/Reduction of Risk Potential/Potential for Complications of Diagnostic Tests/Treatments/Procedures

17. CORRECT ANSWER: 2. **Answer 1** is incorrect because these *are normal* findings in a neonate. **Answer 2 is correct because this subnormal temperature indicates prematurity, infection, low environment temperature, inadequate clothing, and/or dehydration and requires an intervention.** **Answer 3** is incorrect because these *are normal* findings in a neonate. **Answer 4** is incorrect because these *are normal* findings in a neonate.

■ **TEST-TAKING TIP:** ***Identify which answers are within normal ranges for a neonate and eliminate these options.***

Content Area: Child Health, Newborn; *Integrated Process:* Nursing Process, Assessment; *Cognitive Level:* Application; *Client Need/Subneed:* Physiological Integrity/Reduction of Risk Potential/Potential for Alterations in Body Systems

18. CORRECT ANSWER: 4. **Answer 1** is incorrect because, when the fetal head is in the upper right quadrant, the body will be on the right side with the fetal hands and feet on the left side. The heart tones would not be audible on the left side. **Answer 2** is incorrect because the fetus is in a breech position, so the heart tones would be upper quadrant on the right side, not the left side, because the hands and feet are on the left side. **Answer 3** is incorrect because the fetal head is in the upper right quadrant; the body will be on the right side with the heart tones in the upper quadrant above the umbilicus, not below the umbilicus, which would be a vertex position. **Answer 4 is correct because the fetal head is in the upper right quadrant, the body will be on the right side with the heart tones in the upper quadrant above the umbilicus.**

■ TEST-TAKING TIP: *Picture the position of the fetus and the heart on the side where the head is palpable.*

Content Area: Maternity, Intrapartum; *Integrated Process:* Nursing Process, Assessment; *Cognitive Level:* Application; *Client Need/Subneed:* Health Promotion and Maintenance/ Ante/Intra/Postpartum and Newborn Care

19. CORRECT ANSWER: 4. **Answer 1** is incorrect because, in most cases, a woman with gestational diabetes will *not* become a diabetic who is insulin dependent, but rather has a high chance of developing type 2 diabetes in the future. **Answer 2** is incorrect because, even with following a diabetic diet, there is still a high chance of developing type 2 diabetes in the future. **Answer 3** is incorrect because, even if there are no subsequent pregnancies, there is still a high chance of developing type 2 diabetes in the future. **Answer 4 is correct because there is about a 75% chance that a woman with gestational diabetes will develop type 2 diabetes in the future.**

■ TEST-TAKING TIP: *Eliminate the answer that gives false reassurance. Telling a client she has nothing to worry about is not an appropriate response.*

Content Area: Maternity, Antepartum; *Integrated Process:* Communication and Documentation; *Cognitive Level:* Application; *Client Need/Subneed:* Physiological Integrity/ Reduction of Risk Potential/Potential for Alterations in Body Systems

20. CORRECT ANSWER: 2. **The answer is calculated as follows:**

15 units/250 mL or 60 units/1000 mL = 0.06 units/mL (concentration of the drug)
0.06 units/hr (60 minutes = 0.001 units/min)
0.001 units/min × 1000 (for conversion to milliunits) = 1 milliunit/min × 2 = 2 milliunits/min infusion rate

■ TEST-TAKING TIP: *Pay attention to the concentration of the oxytocin and the final calculation. The concentration is 15 units/250 mL, but the conversion must be done to milliunits per minute or the answer will be incorrect.*

Content Area: Maternity, Intrapartum; *Integrated Process:* Nursing Process, Analysis; *Cognitive Level:* Analysis; *Client Need/Subneed:* Physiological Integrity/Pharmacological and Parenteral Therapies/Dosage Calculation

21. CORRECT ANSWER: 3. **Answer 1** is incorrect because the primary health-care provider should still be present until after the delivery of the placenta. **Answer 2** is incorrect because the primary health-care provider may sometimes apply gentle tension to the cord to facilitate delivery of the placenta, but this is not the role of the RN; and traction on the cord will increase the risk of complication, such as uterine inversion. **Answer 3 is correct because the client has not delivered the placenta within 40 minutes; the physician will explore the uterus and may determine that the client has a placenta accreta, which would require surgical intervention.** **Answer 4** is incorrect because the normal time frame for delivery of the placenta is 5 to 30 minutes. Most placentas deliver within 5 minutes, but 40 minutes is longer than the expected time frame for this stage.

■ TEST-TAKING TIP: *Know the stages and phases of labor and the expected time frame for each of these stages.*

Content Area: Maternity, Intrapartum; *Integrated Process:* Nursing Process, Implementation; *Cognitive Level:* Application; *Client Need/Subneed:* Physiological Integrity/Physiological Adaptation/Alterations in Body Systems

22. CORRECT ANSWER: 4. **Answer 1** is incorrect because the client's symptoms are related to vena cava syndrome and are a result of low blood pressure. Assisting her to her side will likely resolve the problem. **Answer 2** is incorrect because nasal oxygen is *not needed* and the flow rate is far *too high* for a nasal cannula. Assisting the mother to a lateral Sims' position will improve her blood pressure and reduce her symptoms. **Answer 3** is incorrect because this position is indicated for a client in shock. This client should be positioned on her *side* to alleviate symptoms. **Answer 4 is correct because changing to a left lateral position helps to alleviate vena cava compression from the gravid uterus, and will reduce her discomfort.**

■ TEST-TAKING TIP: *Think about the underlying reason for this client's symptoms. Focus on the options that relate to positioning, and eliminate the option that is used for shock.*

Content Area: Maternity, Antepartum; *Integrated Process:* Nursing Process, Implementation; *Cognitive Level:* Analysis; *Client Need/Subneed:* Physiological Integrity/Physiological Adaptation/Hemodynamics

23. CORRECT ANSWER: 2. **Answer 1** is incorrect because the fetal heart tones would be heard below the umbilicus on the right side, *not* on the *left* side, which would then be LOA position. **Answer 2 is correct because the fetal head and back are pressing against the right side of the client's abdomen; the fetal heart tones would be heard below the umbilicus on the right side.** **Answer 3** is incorrect because the fetal heart tones would be heard *above* the umbilicus in *breech* presentation. **Answer 4** is incorrect because the fetal heart tones would be heard *above* the umbilicus in *breech* presentation.

■ **TEST-TAKING TIP:** ***Picture the situation described. It may be helpful for you to draw this out so that you can imagine where the heartbeat would be found.***

Content Area: Maternity, Antepartum; ***Integrated Process:*** Nursing Process, Analysis; ***Cognitive Level:*** Application; ***Client Need/Subneed:*** Health Promotion and Maintenance/Ante/Intra/Postpartum and Newborn Care

24. CORRECT ANSWER: 1. Answer 1 is correct because the newborn most likely has thrush (oral candidiasis): white plaque on the oral mucous membranes, gums, or tongue. Treatment usually includes good hand washing and nystatin (Mycostatin). **Answer 2** is incorrect because thrush in newborns is caused by poor hand washing or exposure to *Candida* during vaginal birth. Changing formula is unnecessary and will not cure the thrush. **Answer 3** is incorrect because thrush in newborns is *not* caused by bottle propping. Tooth decay is related to sleeping with a bottle. **Answer 4** is incorrect because thrush in newborns is caused by poor hand washing or exposure to *Candida* during vaginal birth, *not* glucose.

■ **TEST-TAKING TIP:** ***Consider the outcome for each option; will the intervention solve the issue? If not, eliminate the answer.***

Content Area: Child Health, Newborn; ***Integrated Process:*** Nursing Process, Implementation; ***Cognitive Level:*** Analysis; ***Client Need/Subneed:*** Physiological Integrity/Physiological Adaptation/Alterations in Body Systems

25. CORRECT ANSWER: 4. **Answer 1** is incorrect because the femur on the affected side is shortened, *not* lengthened. **Answer 2** is incorrect because deformities of the foot and ankle are *not* symptoms of congenital hip dislocation. **Answer 3** is incorrect because plantar flexion of the foot is seen with clubfoot, and is *not* a symptom of congenital hip dislocation. **Answer 4 is correct because asymmetry of the gluteal and thigh folds is caused by restricted movement on the affected side, which is a symptom of congenital hip dislocation.**

■ **TEST-TAKING TIP:** ***Form a mental image of the deformity and read the options carefully. Note the anatomical proximity between "hip" in the stem and "gluteal and thigh." Eliminate the other three options that refer to the lower extremity: ". . . limb" (Answer 1); ". . . foot and ankle" (Answer 2); ". . . foot" (Answer 3).***

Content Area: Child Health, Newborn; ***Integrated Process:*** Nursing Process, Assessment; ***Cognitive Level:*** Application; ***Client Need/Subneed:*** Physiological Integrity/Reduction of Risk Potential/System Specific Assessments

26. CORRECT ANSWER: 4. **Answer 1** is incorrect because the management of a client with severe pregnancy-induced hypertension (PIH) includes *reducing* stimulation to decrease her chance of developing seizures. **Answer 2** is incorrect because severe PIH can decrease perfusion to the placenta and the supine position can also decrease perfusion, leading to fetal distress. **Answer 3** is incorrect because, although the management of a client with severe PIH includes reducing stimulation to decrease her chance of developing seizures, it should not include "limiting nursing visits." The client requires *frequent* observation by a nurse. **Answer 4 is correct because modified bedrest in a lateral position can decrease the client's blood pressure and increase the placental perfusion.**

■ **TEST-TAKING TIP:** ***Read options carefully. Both parts of the answer must be true to have the answer be the correct option.***

Content Area: Maternity, Antepartum; ***Integrated Process:*** Nursing Process, Implementation; ***Cognitive Level:*** Application; ***Client Need/Subneed:*** Physiological Integrity/Physiological Adaptation/Alterations in Body Systems

27. CORRECT ANSWER: 1. Answer 1 is correct because the cause of clubfoot isn't known, but it is not related to anything a woman did during pregnancy to cause the malformation. **Answer 2** is incorrect because clubfoot isn't hereditary, although it can occur with other congenital spinal malformations. **Answer 3** is incorrect because evidence shows that clubfoot isn't caused by the position of the fetus in the uterus. **Answer 4** is incorrect because the cause of clubfoot is unknown and not due to a problem during embryo development.

■ **TEST-TAKING TIP:** ***The client is concerned about exposure to something during pregnancy that resulted in this condition. Basically, two of the choices are the same, an anomaly during development and a heredity condition; therefore, eliminate these options.***

Content Area: Child Health, Newborn; ***Integrated Process:*** Nursing Process, Implementation; ***Cognitive Level:*** Application; ***Client Need/Subneed:*** Physiological Integrity/Physiological Adaptation/Pathophysiology

28. CORRECT ANSWER: 3. **Answer 1** is incorrect because the gluteus maximus is never an appropriate injection site for a newborn because nerve damage can occur when performing an injection in this site. **Answer 2** is incorrect because the gluteus minimus is never an appropriate injection site for a newborn because nerve damage can occur when performing an injection in this site. **Answer 3 is correct because the vastus lateralis is the proper injection site; it is a large muscle and avoids the nerve tracts.** **Answer 4** is incorrect because the vastus medialis is not an appropriate injection site for a newborn because nerve damage can occur when performing an injection in this site.

■ **TEST-TAKING TIP:** ***Eliminate the gluteal muscles; they are never a correct injection site for an infant. Then picture the infant's thigh and the muscles that make up the thigh to choose the correct injection site.***

Content Area: Child Health, Newborn; ***Integrated Process:*** Nursing Process, Implementation; ***Cognitive Level:*** Application; ***Client Need/Subneed:*** Physiological Integrity/Pharmacological and Parenteral Therapies/Medication Administration

29. CORRECT ANSWERS: 3, 5. Answer 1 is incorrect because vernix is *usually absorbed* in neonates who are past their estimated date of delivery. **Answer 2** is incorrect because plethora is an indication of a *high hematocrit* and is *not* a normal finding in a neonate of any gestation. **Answer 3 is correct because milia are clogged sebaceous glands usually found on the nose and are a normal finding in all gestational ages. Answer 4** is incorrect because crepitus is the crunching, crackling, or popping sounds and sensations that are felt under the skin when palpating the clavicles in a neonate who is suspected of having a *fractured clavicle.* **Answer 5 is correct because parchment skin is a *common* finding in *postdates* neonates. The neonate who is postdates absorbs the vernix, which protects the skin. When the vernix is absorbed, the skin dries out and begins to peel off in large sheets that resemble parchment.**

■ **TEST-TAKING TIP:** ***The question is focusing on evaluation of a neonate who has passed the estimated date of delivery. Think about what a neonate who is "postdates" looks like: dry, peeling, and wrinkled.***

Content Area: Child Health, Newborn; ***Integrated Process:*** Nursing Process, Assessment; ***Cognitive Level:*** Application; ***Client Need/Subneed:*** Health Promotion and Maintenance/ Ante/Intra/Postpartum and Newborn Care

ANSWERS

30. CORRECT ANSWER: 2. Answer 1 is incorrect because deep tendon reflexes are a part of *every* labor assessment and are *not specific* to rupture of membranes. **Answer 2 is correct because the fern test is done to check for ruptured membranes. It is positive if the amniotic sac has broken. Answer 3** is incorrect because a blood pressure check is a part of *every* labor assessment and is *not specific* to rupture of membranes. **Answer 4** is incorrect because a urine test for protein is a part of *every* labor assessment and is *not specific* to rupture of membranes.

■ **TEST-TAKING TIP:** ***When you see "assessment" or "evaluation" in the stem of the question, think about an assessment specific to this case and not applicable in general.***

Content Area: Maternity, Intrapartum; ***Integrated Process:*** Nursing Process, Implementation; ***Cognitive Level:*** Application; ***Client Need/Subneed:*** Physiological Integrity/Reduction of Risk Potential/System Specific Assessments

31. CORRECT ANSWER: 2. Answer 1 is incorrect because pushing before the cervix is completely dilated can result in *cervical tears.* **Answer 2 is correct because assisting the client to pant-blow at the peak of contractions will help her to avoid pushing before her cervix is completely dilated. Answer 3** is incorrect because readjusting the fetal monitor will not help the client avoid pushing and damaging her cervix. **Answer 4** is incorrect because telling the coach that it is not good for the baby if she pushes right now is not directly helping the client avoid pushing and it is unnecessarily trying to scare her into compliance. The baby will not be affected by pushing too early.

■ **TEST-TAKING TIP:** ***The goal of the question is to directly assist the client in coping with increased pressure. Look for the intervention that will provide direct support.***

Content Area: Maternity, Intrapartum; ***Integrated Process:*** Nursing Process, Implementation; ***Cognitive Level:*** Application; ***Client Need/Subneed:*** Health Promotion and Maintenance/ Ante/Intra/Postpartum and Newborn Care

32. CORRECT ANSWER: 3. Answer 1 is incorrect because this client in labor is a low risk with a reassuring fetal heart rate tracing. Five minutes is too frequent for a client who is a low risk. **Answer 2** is incorrect because this client in labor is a low risk with a reassuring fetal heart rate tracing. Fifteen minutes is too frequent for a low-risk client. It is an appropriate interval for a client who is high risk. **Answer 3 is correct because reevaluating the fetal heart rate tracing every 30 minutes is the recommended interval for a client who is low risk. Answer 4** is incorrect because 60 minutes is too long an interval for a client in active labor.

■ **TEST-TAKING TIP:** ***Two key concepts guide the interval of evaluating the fetal heart rate tracing: the risk factors (in this case, none) and the phase of labor (in this case, active labor).***

Content Area: Maternity, Intrapartum; ***Integrated Process:*** Nursing Process, Implementation; ***Cognitive Level:*** Application; ***Client Need/Subneed:*** Health Promotion and Maintenance/ Ante/Intra/Postpartum and Newborn Care

33. CORRECT ANSWER: 1. Answer 1 is correct because studies have shown that intermittent monitoring is a safe and effective method for monitoring fetal well-being for a low-risk pregnancy. This client fits the criteria for intermittent monitoring. In addition, the use of intermittent monitoring may depend on the hospital's policy and procedure. Answer 2 is incorrect because the client has the right to refuse any medical procedure and it is inappropriate to tell clients there are not enough staff members to care for them during labor. **Answer 3** is incorrect because changing assignments does not deal with the underlying problem—the client's desire to avoid electronic fetal monitoring. **Answer 4** is incorrect because, although the nurse is acknowledging the client's decision-making rights, continuous EFM is *not the only effective* way to monitor infant well-being during labor; and the statement could be perceived by the client as manipulating her into accepting the electronic fetal monitoring.

■ **TEST-TAKING TIP:** ***Watch out for the word "only." The choice with that absolute word is usually wrong.***

Content Area: Maternity, Antepartum; ***Integrated Process:*** Communication and Documentation; ***Cognitive Level:*** Application; ***Client Need/Subneed:*** Health Promotion and Maintenance/Ante/Intra/Postpartum and Newborn Care

34. CORRECT ANSWER: 4. Answer 1 is incorrect because this is a *normal* baseline heart rate, with a *benign* pattern of head compressions; no intervention is needed for this pattern. **Answer 2** is incorrect because this pattern may be indicative of hypoxia, maternal drug administration, or fetal sleep. An amnioinfusion will *not* relieve this pattern. **Answer 3** is incorrect because this is a *normal* baseline heart rate, with mild variable decelerations. In the presence of normal baseline variability, an amnioinfusion is not needed to relieve mild variable decelerations. **Answer 4 is correct because this pattern has the potential for prolonged decelerations and fetal distress. An amnioinfusion will help cushion the umbilical cord compression and relieve or decrease the severity of the variable decelerations.**

■ **TEST-TAKING TIP:** *Try drawing the pattern out from the description on a piece of paper. Seeing the pattern may help you focus on the physiology of the pattern and the interventions needed. Focus on the lowest heart rate and the word "deep" variable decelerations.*

Content Area: Maternity, Antepartum; ***Integrated Process:*** Nursing Process, Planning; ***Cognitive Level:*** Application; ***Client Need/Subneed:*** Physiological Integrity/Reduction of Risk Potential/Vital Signs Changes/Abnormalities

35. CORRECT ANSWER: 4. Answer 1 is incorrect because the active phase of the first stage of labor usually is associated with behavior that is self-focused and requires concentration to breathe with the contractions. This client is excited and talkative, suggesting she is in early labor or the latent phase. **Answer 2** is incorrect because there is *no first phase* of labor; it is the first stage of labor. **Answer 3** is incorrect because there is *no first phase* of labor; it is the first stage of labor. **Answer 4 is correct because this client is excited and talkative, suggesting she is in early labor or the latent phase of the first stage of labor.**

■ **TEST-TAKING TIP:** *Remember stages and phases of labor. There are* **four stages** *of labor, with the first stage having* **three phases** *of labor: latent, active and transition.*

Content Area: Maternity, Intrapartum; ***Integrated Process:*** Nursing Process, Analysis; ***Cognitive Level:*** Analysis; ***Client Need/Subneed:*** Health Promotion and Maintenance/ Ante/Intra/Postpartum and Newborn Care

36. CORRECT ANSWER: 1. Answer 1 is correct because the client is coping well with her labor and, with the partner's support, is using prepared childbirth techniques. Offering clear liquids would be an appropriate nursing action during the active phase of labor. Answer 2 is incorrect because offering her an epidural when she is coping well is not an appropriate nursing action. If the client asked for pain relief, then offering an epidural would then be an appropriate option. **Answer 3** is incorrect because offering her pain medication when she is coping well is not an appropriate nursing action. If the client asked for pain relief, then offering pain medication would be an appropriate option. **Answer 4** is incorrect because pant-blow breathing is a technique used during *transition* phase of labor; this client is in the active phase of labor.

■ **TEST-TAKING TIP:** *Two of the alternatives are essentially the same: offering an epidural and offering pain medication; therefore, eliminate both of those choices.*

Content Area: Maternity, Intrapartum; ***Integrated Process:*** Nursing Process, Implementation; ***Cognitive Level:*** Analysis; ***Client Need/Subneed:*** Health Promotion and Maintenance/ Ante/Intra/Postpartum and Newborn Care

37. CORRECT ANSWER: 4. Answer 1 is incorrect because this response *does* validate her feelings, *but* it promises the client something that may not be true; she may have a while before delivery. **Answer 2** is incorrect because calling the doctor and "passing the buck" to him or her does nothing for the client's pain and coping. **Answer 3** is incorrect because this response promises the client something that may not be true (she may need a cesarean section to deliver), and it does nothing to validate her feelings. **Answer 4 is correct because it validates the client's feelings, gives an explanation for her condition, and does not promise anything to the client.**

■ **TEST-TAKING TIP:** *Validating a client's feelings is important to let her know that you hear her and understand her. Eliminate the choices that do not validate the client's feelings.*

Content Area: Maternity, Intrapartum; ***Integrated Process:*** Communication and Documentation; ***Cognitive Level:*** Application; ***Client Need/Subneed:*** Health Promotion and Maintenance/Ante/Intra/Postpartum and Newborn Care

38. CORRECT ANSWER: 1. Answer 1 is correct because this client is at 32 weeks' gestation, multipara, and 3 cm dilated. The contractions are the most important assessment in a client who is in preterm labor. If the contractions are close together, tocolytics will be required to decrease the contractions. If there are rare or no contractions, the nurse can focus on other assessments. Answer 2 is incorrect because the client is preterm and her contractions are the most important assessment for this client. If her contractions are regular or close together, tocolytics will be required to decrease the contractions. The patency of the IV infusion is not the most important assessment in a client with preterm labor. **Answer 3** is incorrect because the client is preterm and her contractions are the most important assessment. The fetal heart rate is an important assessment for all clients in labor, but the most important assessment for this woman who is preterm with a cervix that is dilated and effaced is the frequency and duration of the contractions. If the client is having regular contractions, tocolytics may be required to stop her uterine contractions. **Answer 4** is incorrect because the maternal vital signs are a common part of the assessment for all obstetric clients, but this client is preterm and her contractions are the most important assessment. If the client is having regular contractions, tocolytics may need to be ordered to stop the uterine contractions.

■ **TEST-TAKING TIP:** *Consider the gestational age, and which assessment is the most important to perform at the beginning of the shift for a client who is in preterm labor.*

Content Area: Maternity, Intrapartum; ***Integrated Process:*** Nursing Process, Assessment; ***Cognitive Level:*** Analysis; ***Client Need/Subneed:*** Physiological Integrity/Reduction of Risk Potential/System Specific Assessments

39. CORRECT ANSWERS: 2, 4. **Answer 1** is incorrect because slight acrocyanosis, a bluish color of the extremities, is a benign, *normal* part of neonatal transition and is common during the first 24 to 48 hours after birth. It does not require any intervention, and does not need to be reported to the physician. **Answer 2 is correct because the normal respiratory rate is 30 to 60 breaths/min. A rate of 20 is abnormal after birth and may indicate apnea and respiratory distress, and should be reported to the physician.** **Answer 3** is incorrect because a heart rate of 145 is in the *normal* range of 110 to 160, and does not need to be reported to the physician because it is within the *normal* limits for this infant. **Answer 4 is correct because a pilonidal dimple may be a sign of spina bifida occulta, and requires further evaluation by a physician.** **Answer 5** is incorrect because ecchymosis (bruising) over the back of the fetal head is a *normal* finding related to the pressure of the presenting part on the fetal head resulting in bruising, and doesn't need to be reported to the physician.

■ TEST-TAKING TIP: *Do not be distracted by the word "consistent," which in this case means* **consistently normal.**

Content Area: Child Health, Newborn; *Integrated Process:* Nursing Process, Assessment; *Cognitive Level:* Application; *Client Need/Subneed:* Physiological Integrity/Reduction of Risk Potential/Potential for Alterations in Body Systems

40. CORRECT ANSWERS: 2, 3, 4. **Answer 1** is incorrect because nifedipine is a *calcium channel blocker* that is used to treat *preterm labor, not* to *induce* labor. **Answer 2 is correct because cervidil is a prostaglandin E_2 vaginal insert used to help ripen the cervix for induction of labor. Answer 3 is correct because prostaglandin gel is a ripening agent used to help ripen the cervix for induction of labor. Answer 4 is correct because misoprostol is a prostaglandin E_1 analog used to help ripen the cervix for induction of labor.** **Answer 5** is incorrect because Brethine (terbutaline) is an *asthma* drug, which is a beta-adrenergic that relaxes the smooth muscles of the uterus. It is *not* a drug used to induce labor.

■ TEST-TAKING TIP: *The key information in the stem is that the client has an unripe cervix (closed, thick, and fetal head out of the pelvis). Select drugs that ripen the cervix for induction of labor. Eliminate the calcium channel blocker and the beta-adrenergic drugs.*

Content Area: Maternity, Intrapartum; *Integrated Process:* Nursing Process, Analysis; *Cognitive Level:* Analysis; *Client Need/Subneed:* Physiological Integrity/Pharmacological and Parenteral Therapies/Expected Effects/Outcomes

41. CORRECT ANSWERS: 1, 2, 3, 5. **Answer 1 is correct because pain that is not well controlled by pain medication can be indicative of a postpartum complication, such as *endometritis,* and the physician should be notified. Answer 2 is correct because pain in her calves while walking may be a sign of *thrombophlebitis,* and the physician should be notified. Answer 3 is correct because foul-smelling lochia is a symptom of *endometritis,* and the physician should be notified.** **Answer 4** is incorrect because lochia serosa that is soaking less than a pad every 3 hours is *normal* for a client who is postpartum, and does not need to be reported to the physician. **Answer 5 is correct because soaking more than a pad an hour may be a sign of *retained placental fragments,* and the physician should be notified.**

■ TEST-TAKING TIP: *Reportable conditions are: "pain," "foul-smelling," and "soaking more . . . ."*

Content Area: Maternity, Postpartum; *Integrated Process:* Nursing Process, Implementation; *Cognitive Level:* Analysis; *Client Need/Subneed:* Physiological Integrity/Reduction of Risk Potential/Potential for Alterations in Body Systems

42. CORRECT ANSWER: 1. **Answer 1 is correct because this client is experiencing a *threatened* abortion. At this gestation, there is no medical intervention to prevent miscarriage. Bedrest is the expected management.** **Answer 2** is incorrect because this client is experiencing a *threatened* abortion; a dilation and curettage would be expected for a client who had passed some tissue, had a dilated cervix, and *had an incomplete abortion.* **Answer 3** is incorrect because this client is experiencing a *threatened* abortion; notifying a grief counselor to assist the woman with the imminent *loss* of her fetus is unnecessary. **Answer 4** is incorrect because this client is experiencing a threatened abortion; a cerclage is usually done *after the first trimester* for an *incompetent cervix.*

■ TEST-TAKING TIP: *To remember the different types of abortions, the cervix and the passage of tissue are the key. If the cervix is not dilated and no tissue is passed, it is a threatened abortion. If the cervix is dilated and tissue is passed, then imminent abortion is likely to occur.*

Content Area: Maternity, Antepartum; *Integrated Process:* Nursing Process, Implementation; *Cognitive Level:* Analysis; *Client Need/Subneed:* Physiological Integrity/Reduction of Risk Potential/Potential for Alterations in Body Systems

43. CORRECT ANSWER: 1. **Answer 1 is correct because glucosuria is most often secondary to the pregnancy-related increased glomerular filtration of glucose without an increased tubular reabsorption.** **Answer 2** is incorrect because the finding of glucose in the urine of a woman who is pregnant does *not* mean that she has gestational diabetes. **Answer 3** is incorrect because, although glucosuria is an indication to perform glucose testing, the initial test would be a *1-hour* screening test and *not* the 3-hour test, which is only done *if* the 1-hour glucose tolerance test is *abnormal.* **Answer 4** is incorrect because small doses of insulin would be *unnecessary* in the *absence* of a diagnosis of diabetes.

■ TEST-TAKING TIP: *Glucosuria is a screening test that may indicate the presence of gestational diabetes, but it is not*

diagnostic for gestational diabetes. Eliminate the answers that indicate glucosuria is a diagnosis for gestational diabetes.
Content Area: Maternity, Antepartum; ***Integrated Process:*** Nursing Process, Analysis; ***Cognitive Level:*** Application; ***Client Need/Subneed:*** Health Promotion and Maintenance/ Ante/Intra/Postpartum and Newborn Care

44. CORRECT ANSWER: 3. **Answer 1** is incorrect because, since the screening 1-hour glucose tolerance test was abnormal, the 3-hour glucose tolerance test follow-up *is needed.* **Answer 2** is incorrect because, even though the 1-hour test result was abnormal, a diagnosis of gestational diabetes cannot be made on that value alone; therefore, there is no immediate need for dietary control. **Answer 3 is correct because the abnormal 1-hour test results should be followed up by a 3-hour glucose tolerance test.** **Answer 4** is incorrect because, even though the 1-hour test result was abnormal, a diagnosis of gestational diabetes cannot be made on that value alone; therefore, there is no immediate need for postprandial blood sugar monitoring.
■ TEST-TAKING TIP: *The 1-hour glucose tolerance test is a* **screening** *test for gestational diabetes; the 3-hour glucose tolerance test is the* **diagnostic test** *for gestational diabetes. Eliminate the answers that are interventions for a diagnosis of gestational diabetes.*
Content Area: Maternity, Antepartum; ***Integrated Process:*** Nursing Process, Planning; ***Cognitive Level:*** Application; ***Client Need/Subneed:*** Physiological Integrity/Reduction of Risk Potential/Potential for Alterations in Body Systems

45. CORRECT ANSWER: 4. **Answer 1** is incorrect because laxatives stimulate the intestinal tract, but also can initiate uterine *contractions,* which can be a cause of preterm labor contractions. **Answer 2** is incorrect because high-fat and high-protein foods *contribute* to constipation. **Answer 3** is incorrect because caffeine can cause *tachycardia* in the fetus and its use during pregnancy is discouraged. **Answer 4 is correct because pregnancy slows intestinal motility due to the influence of progesterone. Increasing fluid intake and exercise stimulates peristalsis and can relieve the discomfort of constipation.**
■ TEST-TAKING TIP: *Exclude interventions that involve drugs (laxative, caffeine) to relieve the common complaint of constipation. Suggesting natural measures for common pregnancy complaints are safer in pregnancy.*
Content Area: Maternity, Antepartum; ***Integrated Process:*** Teaching and Learning; ***Cognitive Level:*** Application; ***Client Need/Subneed:*** Physiological Integrity/Basic Care and Comfort/Elimination

46. CORRECT ANSWER: 2. **Answer 1** is incorrect because the intestines do *not* increase in diameter due to pregnancy. **Answer 2 is correct because, during pregnancy, progesterone causes peristalsis to slow the intestines so that more nutrients can be absorbed.** **Answer 3** is incorrect because compression of the intestines during pregnancy does *not contribute* to constipation. **Answer 4** is incorrect because, during pregnancy, there is a decrease, *not* an increase, in intestinal motility.
■ TEST-TAKING TIP: *When there are similar answers, read the answer carefully to determine the differences.*
Content Area: Maternity, Antepartum; ***Integrated Process:*** Nursing Process, Implementation; ***Cognitive Level:*** Application; ***Client Need/Subneed:*** Physiological Integrity/Basic Care and Comfort/Elimination

47. CORRECT ANSWER: 1. **Answer 1 is correct because, when using Naegele's rule, this client's EDD is October 8th. This makes the client 41 weeks and 3 days' gestation on admission. This is the most important factor in planning her nursing care since this is a postdates pregnancy.** **Answer 2** is incorrect because blood type A with Rh+ does *not* present any problems in client care; but, maternal blood type O and/or Rh– blood types can cause severe jaundice in the newborn due to maternal antibodies that destroy fetal RBCs. **Answer 3** is incorrect because hemoglobin of 11 gm/dL is physiological anemia, caused by the increase in plasma volume in pregnancy. It is not a true anemia. **Answer 4** is incorrect because this is a *normal* blood pressure in pregnancy. The maternal blood pressure normally decreases by 5 to 10 mm Hg in both systolic and diastolic pressures. This decrease is due to peripheral vasodilation caused by pregnancy hormones.
■ TEST-TAKING TIP: *Think about which of the answers represents a risk factor for the pregnancy. Does that answer correspond to a risk factor or a normal value for pregnancy? Note that three options focus on "blood." Choose the option that is different.*
Content Area: Maternity, Intrapartum; ***Integrated Process:*** Nursing Process, Assessment; ***Cognitive Level:*** Analysis; ***Client Need/Subneed:*** Health Promotion and Maintenance/ Ante/Intra/Postpartum and Newborn Care

48. CORRECT ANSWER: 2. **Answer 1** is incorrect because the suggested weight gain for pregnancy *is* between 25 and 35 lb. **Answer 2 is correct because strange cravings called pica are not a normal part of pregnancy and may be associated with iron deficiency.** **Answer 3** is incorrect because about 300 calories *is* the additional calories needed in pregnancy. **Answer 4** is incorrect because canned foods lose some nutrients in processing. Foods that are frozen have less processing and may be more nutritious.
■ TEST-TAKING TIP: *Be sure to read the question carefully. By asking which response requires additional teaching, the question is asking for an* **incorrect** *response.*
Content Area: Maternity, Antepartum; ***Integrated Process:*** Nursing Process, Evaluation; ***Cognitive Level:*** Analysis; ***Client Need/Subneed:*** Physiological Integrity/Basic Care and Comfort/Nutrition and Oral Hydration

49. CORRECT ANSWER: 1. Answer 1 is correct because this client is in the latent phase of labor; their plan is to use prepared childbirth techniques. Slow, deep breathing and relaxation techniques are used to relieve contraction pain during this phase. **Answer 2** is incorrect because minimizing the use of narcotics is preferred when prepared childbirth techniques are used. **Answer 3** is incorrect because local anesthesia is used for numbing the perineum *immediately before delivery* of the fetus during the *second stage* of labor. **Answer 4** is incorrect because rapid, shallow breathing can lead to hyperventilation and is *inappropriate for any* phase of labor.

■ **TEST-TAKING TIP:** *Eliminate the two options that focus on drugs, which would be the opposite of the couple's desire to use prepared childbirth techniques.*

Content Area: Maternity, Intrapartum; ***Integrated Process:*** Nursing Process, Planning; ***Cognitive Level:*** Application; ***Client Need/Subneed:*** Health Promotion and Maintenance/ Ante/Intra/Postpartum and Newborn Care

50. CORRECT ANSWER: 3. **Answer 1** is incorrect because the heart rate of the fetus is *unrelated* to the gender of the fetus. The range for the fetal heart rate is 110 to 160 bpm *regardless* of gender. **Answer 2** is incorrect because the mother has two X chromosomes; the father has both X and Y chromosomes, and *his sperm* determines the sex of the fetus. **Answer 3 is correct because meiosis results in the X and Y chromosomes of the male splitting so that each sperm carries either an X or a Y chromosome, thus determining the gender of the fetus.** **Answer 4** is incorrect because how the mother carries the fetus is *unrelated* to the gender. How a fetus is carried is related to maternal uterine and abdominal muscle tone. The gender of the fetus does not determine how high or low it is carried.

■ **TEST-TAKING TIP:** *Eliminate the options that are myths about pregnancy. Choose the option that is scientifically based.*

Content Area: Maternity, Antepartum; ***Integrated Process:*** Teaching and Learning; ***Cognitive Level:*** Application; ***Client Need/Subneed:*** Health Promotion and Maintenance/ Ante/Intra/Postpartum and Newborn Care

51. CORRECT ANSWERS: 2, 4, 5. **Answer 1** is incorrect because gestational diabetes cannot be detected in the multiple marker screen; the correct screening test is a *1-hour glucose tolerance* test. **Answer 2 is correct because Edwards' syndrome (trisomy 18) is one of the conditions that may be detected by the multiple marker screen. It is a severe, usually lethal developmental disorder. It is characterized by cranial, neurological, facial, cardiac, and GI malformations.** **Answer 3** is incorrect because pregnancy-induced hypertension cannot be detected in the multiple marker screen. Serial blood pressure readings, urine protein, and liver and renal function tests are the screening tests for pregnancy-induced hypertension. **Answer 4 is correct because Down syndrome (trisomy 21) is one of the conditions that may be detected by the multiple marker screen. Answer 5 is correct because neural tube defects are conditions that may be detected by the multiple marker screen.**

■ **TEST-TAKING TIP:** *Select the three options that are congenital (Answers 2, 4, and 5). Multiple marker screen is usually performed about* **16 weeks' gestation;** *gestational diabetes and pregnancy-induced hypertension are conditions that are usually found during the* **third trimester** *of pregnancy.*

Content Area: Maternity, Antepartum; ***Integrated Process:*** Nursing Process, Analysis; ***Cognitive Level:*** Application; ***Client Need/Subneed:*** Health Promotion and Maintenance/ Ante/Intra/Postpartum and Newborn Care

52. CORRECT ANSWER: 4. **Answer 1** is incorrect because bilirubin levels in excess of 12 mg/100 mL at 24 hours of age may indicate the presence of a *pathological* process. This client's jaundice is most likely due to an ABO incompatibility. **Answer 2** is incorrect because breastfeeding jaundice occurs around the *third* day of age. Encouraging early and frequent feedings at the breast lowers neonatal bilirubin levels. This client developed high serum bilirubin at 24 hours of age. **Answer 3** is incorrect because bililight therapy *requires an order* from the physician. Exchange transfusions for ABO incompatibilities are *seldom necessary.* **Answer 4 is correct because early and frequent breastfeeding tends to lower serum bilirubin levels and avoids dehydration that increases the serum bilirubin level.**

■ **TEST-TAKING TIP:** *The risk factor for this client is the ABO incompatibility. Eliminate the answer that refers to the level being normal, or the answer that deals with jaundice related to breastfeeding.*

Content Area: Child Health, Newborn; ***Integrated Process:*** Nursing Process, Implementation; ***Cognitive Level:*** Analysis; ***Client Need/Subneed:*** Physiological Integrity/Physiological Adaptation/Alterations in Body Systems

53. CORRECT ANSWER: 4. **Answer 1** is incorrect because the fetus usually turns to vertex by term. If the fetus remains in a breech position, a cesarean delivery is the recommended method of delivery. **Answer 2** is incorrect because the uterus becomes *more crowded, not* less, as pregnancy progresses. **Answer 3** is incorrect because few fetuses (3%–4%) are in a breech position by delivery; a *cesarean delivery* is the recommended method of delivery for a fetus in breech presentation. **Answer 4 is correct because approximately 96% of fetuses in a breech position will turn to a vertex position by term.**

■ **TEST-TAKING TIP:** *The key to this question is the gestational age. At 18 weeks' gestation, many fetuses are breech, and most will turn by full term.*

Content Area: Maternity, Antepartum; ***Integrated Process:*** Communication and Documentation; ***Cognitive Level:*** Application; ***Client Need/Subneed:*** Health Promotion and Maintenance/Ante/Intra/Postpartum and Newborn Care

54. CORRECT ANSWER: 2. **Answer 1** is incorrect because use of forceps when the client is not completely dilated is *not acceptable* practice according to the American College of Obstetricians and Gynecologists. **Answer 2 is correct because maternal position changes such as sitting, kneeling, lateral, or hands and knees can assist fetal head rotation from an occipitoposterior to an occipitoanterior position.** **Answer 3** is incorrect because, in the supine position, the gravid uterus compresses the pelvic blood vessels and compromises uteroplacental blood flow. This position not only has *no effect* on rotation of the fetal head, but *can cause decreased* perfusion to the placenta. **Answer 4** is incorrect because cesarean delivery should be considered only if adequate contractions are documented and there is still *no change* in the cervical dilation.

■ TEST-TAKING TIP: *This question is asking for the intervention to rotate the fetal head from occipitoposterior to occipitoanterior. Which action assists the fetus to rotate?*

Content Area: Maternity, Intrapartum; *Integrated Process:* Nursing Process, Implementation; *Cognitive Level:* Application; *Client Need/Subneed:* Health Promotion and Maintenance/Ante/Intra/Postpartum and Newborn Care

55. CORRECT ANSWER: 2. **Answer 1** is incorrect because human chorionic gonadotropin (HCG) is a hormone produced by the developing placenta that prevents the corpus luteum from deteriorating and secretes estrogen and progesterone, which *maintains the pregnancy* for the first 20 weeks of gestation. It is found in *maternal blood and urine.* **Answer 2 is correct because phosphatidylglycerol (PG) is a major phospholipid of surfactant. The presence of PG in amniotic fluid indicates fetal lung maturity.** **Answer 3** is incorrect because α-fetoprotein (AFP) is a plasma protein that is produced by the fetus. Abnormally high or low levels can indicate *fetal anomalies.* AFP levels are drawn from *maternal blood.* **Answer 4** is incorrect because partial thromboplastin time (PTT) levels are drawn to determine if *anticoagulant* drugs are at a therapeutic level in women with thromboembolic disease.

■ TEST-TAKING TIP: *The key to this question is choosing the proper laboratory test. Eliminate the alternative that is obviously not specific to pregnancy.*

Content Area: Maternity, Intrapartum; *Integrated Process:* Nursing Process, Assessment; *Cognitive Level:* Comprehension; *Client Need/Subneed:* Physiological Integrity/Reduction of Risk Potential/Laboratory Values

56. CORRECT ANSWER: 4. **Answer 1** is incorrect because monozygotic twins (identical) develop from *one* fertilized egg that *splits into identical* halves early in embryonic development. **Answer 2** is incorrect because monozygotic twins (identical) develop from *one* fertilized egg that splits into identical halves early in embryonic development. Once an egg has been penetrated by a *single sperm,* chemical changes take place that prevent multiple sperm fertilization. **Answer 3** is incorrect because dizygotic twins develop from *two different eggs* fertilized by *two different* sperm. **Answer 4 is correct because dizygotic twins develop from two different eggs fertilized by two different sperm.**

■ TEST-TAKING TIP: *When there are two alternatives that seem similar, read the answers very carefully to determine the correct answer. Look at the root prefix:* mono = *one, and* di = *two (2 eggs, 2 sperm).*

Content Area: Maternity, Antepartum; *Integrated Process:* Nursing Process, Implementation; *Cognitive Level:* Application; *Client Need/Subneed:* Health Promotion and Maintenance/Ante/Intra/Postpartum and Newborn Care

57. CORRECT ANSWER: 2. **Answer 1** is incorrect because *probable* signs of pregnancy are: Hegar's sign, ballottement, positive pregnancy test, and Goodell's sign, which are *objective* signs. **Answer 2 is correct because presumptive signs of pregnancy are: amenorrhea, fatigue, breast tenderness and enlargement, morning sickness, and quickening, which are more subjective signs.** **Answer 3** is incorrect because the *only positive* signs of pregnancy are: auscultation of fetal heart tones, visualization of the fetus by ultrasound, and fetal movement felt by the health-care provider. **Answer 4** is incorrect because amenorrhea and breast tenderness are *presumptive* signs of pregnancy, not negative signs.

■ TEST-TAKING TIP: *Missed periods and breast tenderness are associated with pregnancy. Eliminate Answer 4, which states that they are negative signs of pregnancy. There are* three *positive signs of pregnancy that are objective and determined by the health-care provider; thus, Answer 3 can also be eliminated.*

Content Area: Adult Health, Women's Health; *Integrated Process:* Nursing Process, Implementation; *Cognitive Level:* Application; *Client Need/Subneed:* Health Promotion and Maintenance/Ante/Intra/Postpartum and Newborn Care

58. CORRECT ANSWER: 3. **Answer 1** is incorrect because an increased temperature may be a sign of infection; however, this client's major symptom is *bleeding, not infection.* **Answer 2** is incorrect because the client is at a high risk for excess blood loss. The pulse pressure *decreases* with hemorrhage. **Answer 3 is correct because an increased pulse in the presence of visible bleeding indicates excessive blood loss.** **Answer 4** is incorrect because increased blood pressure at this stage of pregnancy would be a sign of a hydatidiform mole or chronic hypertension; *decreased* blood pressure is a sign of *hemorrhage.*

■ TEST-TAKING TIP: *Note that all the answers have "increased" as the first word. Since the client's symptoms are indicative of hemorrhage, the vital sign that increases with hemorrhage is heart rate (pulse).*

Content Area: Maternity, Antepartum; *Integrated Process:* Nursing Process, Analysis; *Cognitive Level:* Analysis; *Client Need/Subneed:* Physiological Integrity/Physiological Adaptation/Alterations in Body Systems

59. CORRECT ANSWER: 1. Answer 1 is correct because, with epidural anesthesia, the sympathetic nerves are also blocked by the medication, resulting in vasodilation and hypotension. **Answer 2** is incorrect because hypertension is *not* a side effect of epidural anesthesia. **Answer 3** is incorrect because hypoventilation does *not* occur when bupivacaine is used as the anesthetic agent. If epidural narcotics are used, hypoventilation can occur. **Answer 4** is incorrect because hyperventilation is *not* a side effect of epidural anesthesia; it is more likely to occur during *painful contractions.* Epidural anesthesia helps to relieve contraction pain.

■ **TEST-TAKING TIP:** *The question has "hypo-" and "hyper-" options for respirations and blood pressure. Think about the physiology behind these options and eliminate the three options that do not fit with epidural analgesia.*

Content Area: Maternity, Intrapartum; *Integrated Process:* Nursing Process, Assessment; *Cognitive Level:* Application; *Client Need/Subneed:* Physiological Integrity/Pharmacological and Parenteral Therapies/Expected Effects/Outcomes

60. CORRECT ANSWER: 2. **Answer 1** is incorrect because prothrombin time is assessed to maintain correct dosages of *warfarin* (*Coumadin*). Coumadin crosses the placental barrier and is *contraindicated* in pregnancy. **Answer 2 is correct because partial thromboplastin time is evaluated to determine the effectiveness of heparin therapy.** **Answer 3** is incorrect because a bleeding time is not routinely performed on women who are pregnant, and it is *unnecessary* for a pregnant woman on *heparin* therapy. **Answer 4** is incorrect because D-dimer tests are ordered, along with other laboratory tests and imaging scans, to help rule out and diagnose conditions that cause hypercoagulability. Since this client already has a history of thromboembolitic disease, the D-dimer is unnecessary.

■ **TEST-TAKING TIP:** *The question is asking which test should be used for monitoring* this *client's* heparin *therapy. Choose the test that reflects monitoring heparin effectiveness.*

Content Area: Maternity, Antepartum; *Integrated Process:* Nursing Process, Assessment; *Cognitive Level:* Analysis; *Client Need/Subneed:* Physiological Integrity/Reduction of Risk Potential/Laboratory Values

61. CORRECT ANSWERS: 2, 3, 4. **Answer 1** is incorrect because salmon is *not* a good source of folic acid. **Answer 2 is correct because spinach is the richest source of folic acid, with about 130 mcg per serving. The recommended folic acid intake is 600 mcg/day during pregnancy. Answer 3 is correct because orange juice is a good source of folic acid, with about 100 mcg per serving. Answer 4 is correct because asparagus is a good source of folic acid, with about 130 mcg per serving.** **Answer 5** is incorrect because chicken is *not* a good source of folic acid.

■ **TEST-TAKING TIP:** *Leafy greens and citrus foods are the highest in folic acid content.*

Content Area: Maternity, Antepartum; *Integrated Process:* Nursing Process, Implementation; *Cognitive Level:* Application; *Client Need/Subneed:* Physiological Integrity/Basic Care and Comfort/Nutrition and Oral Hydration

62. CORRECT ANSWER: 4. **Answer 1** is incorrect because promoting the bonding process as soon as possible after birth is important, but the evaluation of the *newborn's* physical stability is most important at this time. **Answer 2** is incorrect because oxytocin should not be administered *until after the placenta* is delivered, which usually occurs *within 30 minutes* after delivery of the infant. **Answer 3** is incorrect because the third stage of labor is the stage of delivery of the *placenta.* The placenta will *spontaneously separate* from the uterine wall and be expelled by uterine contractions. Maternal pushing is not needed. **Answer 4 is correct because the client has just delivered; the placenta has not delivered yet. The newborn's physical condition and Apgar scoring is a priority at 1 and 5 minutes after delivery.**

■ **TEST-TAKING TIP:** *The key to this question is the wording, "has begun the third stage of labor," the delivery of the placenta. Once the placenta has delivered, the client would be in the fourth stage of labor.*

Content Area: Maternity, Intrapartum; *Integrated Process:* Nursing Process, Analysis; *Cognitive Level:* Analysis; *Client Need/Subneed:* Health Promotion and Maintenance/Ante/Intra/Postpartum and Newborn Care

63. CORRECT ANSWER: 4. **Answer 1** is incorrect because caput succedaneum is an area of generalized edema of the scalp on the presenting part of the fetal skull, usually the occiput. **Answer 2** is incorrect because a hemangioma (also known as "stork bites") are pink areas on the upper eyelids, nose, upper lip, lower occiput, and the nape of the neck that are transient, and usually resolve within a few months. **Answer 3** is incorrect because a cephalohematoma is a collection of blood between the skull bone and the periosteum. It does not cross suture lines and may last up to several months. **Answer 4 is correct because molding is an overlapping of the fetal skull bones at the occiput of the skull. The infant skull has a bullet-shaped appearance that quickly resolves.**

■ **TEST-TAKING TIP:** *Visualize the different conditions described in the options. Eliminate the options that do not fit with the shape of the head. In this question, a tip is to choose the shortest time period (few days, not weeks or months).*

Content Area: Child Health, Newborn; *Integrated Process:* Nursing Process, Implementation; *Cognitive Level:* Application; *Client Need/Subneed:* Health Promotion and Maintenance/Ante/Intra/Postpartum and Newborn Care

64. CORRECT ANSWER: 2. **Answer 1** is incorrect because breast-fed infants *should be* fed on demand. Breast milk is more completely and quickly digested than formula. It is important not to limit infant sucking time at the breast because it is directly related to breast milk production. **Answer 2 is correct because an infant who is exclusively breastfed should have**

at least four to six wet diapers daily. Adequate urinary output is a reliable indicator of adequate intake of breast milk. **Answer 3** is incorrect because the infant *should be* dressed as parents would dress themselves. Overdressing can cause prickly heat rash. Wrapping the infant in a light blanket maintains body temperature and makes the infant feel secure. **Answer 4** is incorrect because the cord stump *should be* cleaned with the solution ordered by the health-care provider daily until it falls off. Some providers may prefer natural drying, without using any alcohol for treating the cord.

■ **TEST-TAKING TIP:** ***This question is asking which answer is not correct. Be careful when reading and answering this type of question so that you do not pick out the first correct response rather than the proper*** **incorrect** ***response.***

Content Area: Child Health, Newborn; ***Integrated Process:*** Nursing Process, Evaluation; ***Cognitive Level:*** Analysis; ***Client Need/Subneed:*** Health Promotion and Maintenance/Ante/Intra/Postpartum and Newborn Care

65. CORRECT ANSWER: 4. Answer 1 is incorrect because the client *doesn't have* an episiotomy. **Answer 2** is incorrect because pulmonary hygiene is important in clients with a *respiratory* condition, or those who have undergone a *cesarean* section. **Answer 3** is incorrect because epidural anesthesia takes approximately an hour to wear off. The client will be *unable* to ambulate during this time. In addition, all clients who are postpartum should be *assisted* with ambulation the first few times out of bed. **Answer 4 is correct because maintaining physiological homeostasis is the most important goal during the fourth stage of labor, the immediate postpartum period. The most common complication of the fourth stage of labor is uterine atony and hemorrhage.**

■ **TEST-TAKING TIP:** ***The question states the client has an intact perineum; therefore, eliminate the obvious answer that discusses an episiotomy (Answer 1). Choose the answer with the most*** **general** ***content (i.e., physiological homeostasis), rather than*** **specific** ***behaviors (i.e., "turn, cough . . ." and ". . . ambulate without assistance").***

Content Area: Maternity, Postpartum; ***Integrated Process:*** Nursing Process, Implementation; ***Cognitive Level:*** Analysis; ***Client Need/Subneed:*** Health Promotion and Maintenance/Ante/Intra/Postpartum and Newborn Care

66. CORRECT ANSWERS: 1, 3, 5. Answer 1 is correct because the client who is 28 weeks' gestation with HELLP syndrome will most likely have to be delivered before reaching full-term gestation. Administration of corticosteroid to help mature the *fetal lungs* would be an appropriate part of management for this client. **Answer 2** is incorrect because an IV fluid bolus is *not* an appropriate management for a client with increased blood pressure in HELLP syndrome. A fluid bolus can lead to fluid *overload* and increase third spacing of fluid, with possible pulmonary edema. **Answer 3 is correct because elevated liver function tests are a part of the HELLP syndrome; following serial liver function tests will be a part of the management of this client's condition. Worsening liver function would be an indicator for early delivery.** **Answer 4** is incorrect because this client is admitted for HELLP, *not* preterm labor. Although she is preterm, tocolytics are not appropriate management for HELLP syndrome. Delivery is the *only* treatment for HELLP syndrome. **Answer 5 is correct because bedrest in the left lateral position would be a part of the management to *decrease blood pressure* in this client.**

■ **TEST-TAKING TIP:** ***The key for this question is HELLP syndrome. The fact that the client is preterm is important for administration of corticosteroids for fetal lung maturity. Do not get distracted by the early gestation for treatment and eliminate the answer that refers to tocolytics (Answer 4).***

Content Area: Maternity, Antepartum; ***Integrated Process:*** Nursing Process, Implementation; ***Cognitive Level:*** Application; ***Client Need/Subneed:*** Physiological Integrity/Physiological Adaptation/Alterations in Body Systems

67. CORRECT ANSWER: 3. Answer 1 is incorrect because white blood cell counts indicate the presence or absence of infection. The *normal* range for WBCs in pregnancy is 9000 to 15,000. There is no evidence of infection. **Answer 2** is incorrect because the *normal* hematocrit in pregnancy ranges from 32% to 45%. **Answer 3 is correct because the normal hemoglobin in pregnancy ranges from 11 to 12 gm/dL. This client is a teenager who is pregnant and is anemic.** **Answer 4** is incorrect because the *normal* serum glucose in pregnancy ranges from 65 to 110 gm/dL.

■ **TEST-TAKING TIP:** ***Knowing common laboratory values will help to eliminate the three options that are normal, and therefore*** **not** ***risk factors (Answers 1, 2, and 4).***

Content Area: Maternity, Antepartum; ***Integrated Process:*** Nursing Process, Assessment; ***Cognitive Level:*** Application; ***Client Need/Subneed:*** Physiological Integrity/Reduction of Risk Potential/Laboratory Values

68. CORRECT ANSWER: 3. Answer 1 is incorrect because Marcaine is an anesthetic agent and does *not* cause respiratory depression. Respiratory depression is associated with *epidural narcotics.* **Answer 2** is incorrect because uterine atony is *not* an effect of epidural anesthesia. **Answer 3 is correct because the client may not sense the urge to void due to decreased sensation to the area. Bladder distention can interfere with descent of the fetus and cause pain.** **Answer 4** is incorrect because maternal *hypotension, not* hypertension, is a side effect of epidural anesthesia.

■ **TEST-TAKING TIP:** ***All the answers involve assessment on an hourly basis; therefore, focus on the differences between the alternatives. Eliminate the three options that are not an effect of epidural anesthesia.***

Content Area: Maternity, Intrapartum; ***Integrated Process:*** Nursing Process, Assessment; ***Cognitive Level:*** Analysis; ***Client Need/Subneed:*** Physiological Integrity/Pharmacological and Parenteral Therapies/Expected Effects/Outcomes

69. CORRECT ANSWER: 4. **Answer 1** is incorrect because turning the client to her left side and administering oxygen is an intervention for *fetal distress* and there is no evidence of fetal distress. **Answer 2** is incorrect because this is a reassuring fetal heart pattern; no immediate nursing actions other than *comfort measures* are necessary. **Answer 3** is incorrect because the client is in *no need* for fluid volume expansion; neither she nor the fetus is in distress. **Answer 4 is correct because this client is in prodromal labor. The fetal heart pattern is reassuring. There is no reason to admit the client to the hospital at this time. Ambulation at home may stimulate labor and descent of the presenting part, and decrease hospitalization time.**

■ **TEST-TAKING TIP:** *The key to this question is the stage and phase of labor. Prodromal labor in a primipara can last several days. The fetal heart tracing is reassuring; therefore, the client can be safely discharged. Note that three of the options are* active *interventions (give O_2, "immediate operative delivery," start IV). Choose the one that is a different option from the others ("send the client home").*

Content Area: Maternity, Intrapartum; *Integrated Process:* Nursing Process, Implementation; *Cognitive Level:* Analysis; *Client Need/Subneed:* Health Promotion and Maintenance/ Ante/Intra/Postpartum and Newborn Care

70. CORRECT ANSWER: 1. **Answer 1 is correct because high prolactin levels with exclusive breastfeeding can delay ovulation for up to 6 months. However, it is a very unpredictable method of birth control.** **Answer 2** is incorrect because condoms are a mechanical barrier method that does *not interfere* with breastfeeding. **Answer 3** is incorrect because Depo-Provera is an injectable form of progestin that prevents pregnancy for 3 months. It *is safe* for use during lactation once the milk supply is established. **Answer 4** is incorrect because contraceptive foam has no hormones to affect lactation, and *is safe* for use during the postpartum period.

■ **TEST-TAKING TIP:** *This question is asking for the incorrect answer. Be careful when reading the stem so that you do not choose the first correct response rather than the incorrect response.*

Content Area: Maternity, Postpartum; *Integrated Process:* Nursing Process, Evaluation; *Cognitive Level:* Analysis; *Client Need/Subneed:* Health Promotion and Maintenance/ Lifestyle Choices

71. CORRECT ANSWERS: 1, 5. **Answer 1 is correct because the fundus is usually at about the level of the umbilicus 2 hours after delivery.** **Answer 2** is incorrect because the fundus is not found 2 fingerbreadths below the umbilicus *until about 48 hours* after delivery. **Answer 3** is incorrect because bluish-white fluid in milk does not come in *until 3 to 4 days* after delivery, *not* 2 hours after delivery. **Answer 4** is incorrect because lochia serosa does not occur until about *5 days after* delivery, lasting about 5 days. **Answer 5 is correct because moderate lochia rubra is a normal finding 2 hours after delivery.**

■ **TEST-TAKING TIP:** *The key to this question is the time frame after delivery. Choose the options that apply to a client 2 hours after delivery.*

Content Area: Maternity, Postpartum; *Integrated Process:* Nursing Process, Evaluation; *Cognitive Level:* Application; *Client Need/Subneed:* Health Promotion and Maintenance/ Ante/Intra/Postpartum and Newborn Care

72. CORRECT ANSWERS: 2, 4, 5. **Answer 1** is incorrect because the normal heart rate at rest is 110 to 160. A rate of 170 is *tachycardia,* which is not normal after birth, and may indicate neonatal sepsis. This needs to be reported to the physician. **Answer 2 is correct because the normal respiratory rate is 30 to 60 breaths/min. This finding does not require any intervention and does not need to be reported to the physician.** **Answer 3** is incorrect because circumoral cyanosis, a bluish color around the mouth, is an *abnormal* finding and requires further assessment, including pulse oximetry. Findings need to be reported to the physician. **Answer 4 is correct because caput succedaneum is edema over the back of the fetal head caused by pressure over the presenting part of the fetal head and it resolves spontaneously. This finding does not require any intervention and does not need to be reported to the physician.** **Answer 5 is correct because mongolian spots are a normal finding in dark-skinned neonates. This finding does not require any intervention and does not need to be reported to the physician.**

■ **TEST-TAKING TIP:** *Note the key word in the stem—* **normal**—*and eliminate the two answers that pertain to abnormal findings.*

Content Area: Child Health, Newborn; *Integrated Process:* Nursing Process, Assessment; *Cognitive Level:* Analysis; *Client Need/Subneed:* Physiological Integrity/Physiological Adaptation/Alterations in Body Systems

73. CORRECT ANSWER: 3. **Answer 1** is incorrect because analysis of amniotic fluid from *amniocentesis* allows determination of fetal gender. **Answer 2** is incorrect because glycemic control is determined by *hemoglobin A_{1c}*, a maternal blood test. **Answer 3 is correct because the α-fetoprotein (AFP) is a maternal blood test that screens for possible neural tube defects (the most common anomaly) in fetuses of a client with diabetes. It can also indicate the presence of Down syndrome.** **Answer 4** is incorrect because the presence of phosphatidylglycerol and the *L/S* ratio determine fetal lung maturity. It is obtained from *amniotic fluid.*

■ **TEST-TAKING TIP:** *The most important fact in this question is that the client with insulin-dependent diabetes has a higher risk for having a fetus with neural tube defects, and the AFP test screens for this possibility.*

Content Area: Maternity, Antepartum; *Integrated Process:* Nursing Process, Implementation; *Cognitive Level:* Application; *Client Need/Subneed:* Physiological Integrity/Reduction of Risk Potential/Diagnostic Tests

74. CORRECT ANSWER: 2. **Answer 1** is incorrect because fundal massage would be an appropriate intervention for uterine atony. Symptoms of *uterine atony would* reveal a constant trickle of bright red blood in the presence of a *boggy uterus.* In this case it is in the presence of a *contracted* uterus. **Answer 2 is correct because a constant trickling of bright red vaginal blood in the presence of a contracted uterus may be an unrepaired laceration of the birth canal. The physician must be notified so that the laceration can be repaired.** **Answer 3** is incorrect because excessive bleeding caused by a full bladder would reveal a uterus that was *above* the umbilicus and *deviated to the right* side. In this case the uterus is *midline at* the umbilicus. **Answer 4** is incorrect because increasing the rate of an infusion of oxytocin would *not correct* the problem of a lacerated birth canal.

■ TEST-TAKING TIP: *When there is a postpartum hemorrhage, the first consideration is uterine atony. Do not immediately assume that all postpartum bleeding is uterine atony. This client had a contracted uterus, so you must consider other reasons for bleeding that may require a medical, not a nursing, intervention.*

Content Area: Maternity, Intrapartum; *Integrated Process:* Nursing Process, Implementation; *Cognitive Level:* Analysis; *Client Need/Subneed:* Physiological Integrity/Reduction of Risk Potential/Potential for Complications of Diagnostic Tests/Treatments/Procedures

75. CORRECT ANSWERS: 2, 5. **Answer 1** is incorrect because Hemabate is used to control *postpartum hemorrhage,* and is *contraindicated* for induction of labor. **Answer 2 is correct because pitocin at 2 milliunits/min IV is an appropriate dose for induction of labor in a client who is past her estimated date of delivery.** **Answer 3** is incorrect because betamethasone is used to *stimulate fetal lung maturity* in preterm gestation, and is *not used* for induction of labor. **Answer 4** is incorrect because Cytotec *is* used for induction of labor, *but* 200 mcg is *too high* a dose for induction of labor and may cause uterine hyperstimulation and uterine rupture. The normal dose of Cytotec for induction is 25 mcg vaginally or 50 mcg orally. **Answer 5 is correct because cervidil 10 mg vaginally is an appropriate method to induce labor.**

■ TEST-TAKING TIP: *Focus on the agents used to induce labor (Answers 2 and 5). Eliminate those medications that are used in postpartum hemorrhage and preterm labor (Answers 1 and 3) but are not used to induce labor.*

Content Area: Maternity, Intrapartum; *Integrated Process:* Nursing Process, Analysis; *Cognitive Level:* Application; *Client Need/Subneed:* Physiological Integrity/Pharmacological and Parenteral Therapies/Expected Effects/Outcomes

76. CORRECT ANSWER: 4. **Answer 1** is incorrect because checking the blood pressure in the right arm has *no association* with the side effects of magnesium sulfate. **Answer 2** is incorrect because this intervention is *contraindicated* in a seizure. It acts to occlude the airway and prevent proper ventilation. **Answer 3** is incorrect because inserting a Foley catheter is *not associated* with any side effects of magnesium sulfate. It may be used to carefully measure output and signs of worsening preeclampsia, but not for side effects of magnesium sulfate. **Answer 4 is correct because magnesium sulfate side effects include headaches and seizures. Darkening the room can help reduce the occurrence of these side effects.**

■ TEST-TAKING TIP: *This question is asking about the* **side effects** *of magnesium sulfate and* **not about treatments** *for preeclampsia. Eliminate the options that do not treat side effects.*

Content Area: Maternity, Intrapartum; *Integrated Process:* Nursing Process, Implementation; *Cognitive Level:* Application; *Client Need/Subneed:* Physiological Integrity/Pharmacological and Parenteral Therapies/Adverse Effects/Contraindications/Interactions

77. CORRECT ANSWER: 3. **Answer 1** is incorrect because this infant's initial alertness and eagerness are followed by an increasingly deeper sleep. This infant is only 3 hours old, and the client should be instructed to wait for the infant to wake up. At about 20 to 24 hours of age, the baby will be awake more often and be more interested in nursing. **Answer 2** is incorrect because this infant is in a *normal sleep state* and does not need to be awakened for a feeding. **Answer 3 is correct because the infant's suckling reflex is greatest from 45 minutes to 2 hours after birth. The baby may nurse several times close together (cluster feedings) and then sleep several hours without nursing.** **Answer 4** is incorrect because this infant is in a *normal sleep state* and does not need to be awakened for a feeding. In addition, the client should be instructed to sponge bathe, *not submerse,* the infant until the cord falls off.

■ TEST-TAKING TIP: *Is this a normal newborn infant behavior? Or, is this a problem? Remember that* **normal** *newborn infants are demand-fed and the normal feeding pattern is cluster feeding 8 to 12 times in a 24-hour period. The infant's initial alertness and eagerness are followed by an increasingly deeper sleep. At about 20 to 24 hours of age, the baby will be awake more often and be more interested in nursing. Eliminate the two options that call for waking the baby who is in a normal sleep state (Answers 2 and 4).*

Content Area: Maternity, Postpartum; *Integrated Process:* Teaching and Learning; *Cognitive Level:* Application; *Client Need/Subneed:* Health Promotion and Maintenance/Ante/Intra/Postpartum and Newborn Care

78. CORRECT ANSWER: 2. Answer 1 is incorrect because fetal heart tones less than 110 bpm is bradycardia and *not* a *normal* finding after amniotomy. **Answer 2 is correct because a moderate amount of straw-colored fluid is a normal color and an amount of amniotic fluid that is expected after the artificial rupture of membranes. Answer 3** is incorrect because a small amount of greenish fluid is meconium staining, *not* a *normal result* after amniotomy. **Answer 4** is incorrect because a small segment of the umbilical cord would be a prolapsed cord, which is an obstetric *emergency.*

■ **TEST-TAKING TIP:** *This question is asking which finding is* **normal** *after rupture of membranes. Think about the normal color and consistency of amniotic fluid.*

Content Area: Maternity, Intrapartum; ***Integrated Process:*** Nursing Process, Planning; ***Cognitive Level:*** Application; ***Client Need/Subneed:*** Physiological Integrity/Reduction of Risk Potential/Diagnostic Tests

79. CORRECT ANSWER: 1. Answer 1 is correct because this client is a primigravida at 2 cm dilated. This is the first stage of labor, and latent phase. Typically, clients in this stage of labor are not in much pain, and are excited and talkative about what is happening. Answer 2 is incorrect because the urge to push during a contraction occurs during the *transition* phase of labor, *not* the latent phase. **Answer 3** is incorrect because inability to concentrate during a contraction happens during the *active* phase of labor, *not* the latent phase of labor. **Answer 4** is incorrect because clients usually ask for an epidural when they are in pain during the *active* or transition phase of labor. The epidural is generally given when the client is in active labor, *not* latent phase.

■ **TEST-TAKING TIP:** *The best answer is based on identifying the stage and phase of labor based on her cervical dilation, and the typical response of a woman in the latent phase of labor.*

Content Area: Maternity, Intrapartum; ***Integrated Process:*** Nursing Process, Analysis; ***Cognitive Level:*** Analysis; ***Client Need/Subneed:*** Health Promotion and Maintenance/ Ante/Intra/Postpartum and Newborn Care

80. CORRECT ANSWER: 2. Answer 1 is incorrect because this action will do *nothing* to resolve the *decelerations* of the fetal heart tones. This would be an appropriate action if there was an inconsistent or broken tracing. **Answer 2 is correct because the first action the nurse should take is to turn the client to her left side, which may help resolve the variable decelerations. Answer 3** is incorrect because asking the client to ambulate may make the variable decelerations *worse,* especially if the reason for the decelerations is cord compression. **Answer 4** is incorrect because preparing the client for delivery is not the first action the nurse should take, since it will not resolve the decelerations.

■ **TEST-TAKING TIP:** *Envision the type of decelerations that occur during a contraction and think about the actions that would resolve the pattern of decelerations.*

Content Area: Maternity, Intrapartum; ***Integrated Process:*** Nursing Process, Implementation; ***Cognitive Level:*** Analysis; ***Client Need/Subneed:*** Health Promotion and Maintenance/ Ante/Intra/Postpartum and Newborn Care

81. CORRECT ANSWER: 4. Answer 1 is incorrect because oxytocin makes the contractions *more painful.* Painless delivery would not be a measure of the effectiveness of IV oxytocin. **Answer 2** is incorrect because this client was *already 100%* effaced before the oxytocin augmentation was started. **Answer 3** is incorrect because infrequent contractions would mean the oxytocin was not effective. IV oxytocin *increases* the frequency of the contractions. **Answer 4 is correct because this client has uterine dystocia, and the effectiveness of the oxytocin infusion is measured by a change in the dilation of the cervix.**

■ **TEST-TAKING TIP:** *Restate this question to ask, how would the nurse know if oxytocin augmentation is working?*

Content Area: Maternity, Intrapartum; ***Integrated Process:*** Nursing Process, Evaluation; ***Cognitive Level:*** Analysis; ***Client Need/Subneed:*** Physiological Integrity/Pharmacological and Parenteral Therapies/Expected Effects/Outcomes

82. CORRECT ANSWER: 1. Answer 1 is correct because the client will need a cesarean section as quickly as possible to avoid a vaginal delivery and possible head entrapment. Answer 2 is incorrect because applying the fetal heart monitor is important, but does not facilitate preparation for the cesarean section. **Answer 3** is incorrect because placing the client in genupectoral position is appropriate for a *prolapsed cord, not* for footling breech presentation. **Answer 4** is incorrect because the vaginal examination has already revealed a footling breech; getting an ultrasound is not a priority at this time.

■ **TEST-TAKING TIP:** *Eliminate the interventions that* delay *getting the client ready for a cesarean section.*

Content Area: Maternity, Intrapartum; ***Integrated Process:*** Nursing Process, Implementation; ***Cognitive Level:*** Analysis; ***Client Need/Subneed:*** Physiological Integrity/Reduction of Risk Potential/Potential for Complications from Surgical Procedures and Health Alterations

83. CORRECT ANSWER: 2. Answer 1 is incorrect because the cervix is 4 cm *dilated, not* closed. **Answer 2 is correct because the nurse cannot artificially rupture the amniotic membranes in order to apply an internal fetal monitor. The only choice for continuous fetal monitoring is an external fetal monitor. Answer 3** is incorrect because the fetal heart tones show *tachycardia,* which is an indicator that continuous fetal monitoring is needed to ensure fetal well-being. **Answer 4** is incorrect because, when the contractions are intense enough, there is *no need* for insertion of an internal monitor. The purpose of an internal uterine monitor is to ensure the strength of the contractions.

■ TEST-TAKING TIP: *Think about the purpose of fetal monitoring and the difference between external and internal monitoring. The membranes must be ruptured to place an internal monitor. This client has intact membranes, so only an external monitor can be used on this client.*
Content Area: Maternity, Intrapartum; *Integrated Process:* Nursing Process, Implementation; *Cognitive Level:* Analysis; *Client Need/Subneed:* Health Promotion and Maintenance/ Ante/Intra/Postpartum and Newborn Care

84. CORRECT ANSWER: 2. **Answer 1** is incorrect because an assessment should be completed *before* calling the physician. **Answer 2 is correct because decreased fetal movement may be a sign of hypoxia in the fetus or a fetal demise. Placing the client on a fetal monitor will assist the nurse to evaluate the fetal well-being.** **Answer 3** is incorrect because starting an IV *will not* demonstrate fetal well-being, or do anything about evaluating the decreased fetal movement. **Answer 4** is incorrect because maternal vital signs are not as crucial at this time. Evaluating the fetus is most important when a client presents with decreased fetal movement.
■ TEST-TAKING TIP: *The key word is* fetal. *Focus on what is the most important evaluation of fetal status. Calling the physician is always required, but an assessment needs to be completed so the physician can understand the condition.*
Content Area: Maternity, Intrapartum; *Integrated Process:* Nursing Process, Implementation; *Cognitive Level:* Analysis; *Client Need/Subneed:* Health Promotion and Maintenance/ Ante/Intra/Postpartum and Newborn Care

85. CORRECT ANSWER: 4. **Answer 1** is incorrect because fetal sleep can manifest as minimal variability—but this fetus also has tachycardia and late decelerations, which are *not* associated with fetal sleep. **Answer 2** is incorrect because umbilical cord compression is manifested by *variable* decelerations, *not late* decelerations or tachycardia. **Answer 3** is incorrect because head compressions are *early* decelerations that mirror the contractions, *not late* decelerations or tachycardia. **Answer 4 is correct because late decelerations are indicative of uteroplacental insufficiency, and tachycardia can be a sign of hypoxia as well.**
■ TEST-TAKING TIP: *Picture the fetal heart tracing and the physiology behind each of the patterns. Evaluate a fetal heart rate tracing the same way every time: baseline, variability, accelerations, and finally, decelerations.*
Content Area: Maternity, Intrapartum; *Integrated Process:* Nursing Process, Analysis; *Cognitive Level:* Analysis; *Client Need/Subneed:* Physiological Integrity/Reduction of Risk Potential/Potential for Complications from Surgical Procedures and Health Alterations

86. CORRECT ANSWER: 3. **Answer 1** is incorrect because the nurse should try to resolve the variable decelerations *before* notifying the physician. **Answer 2** is incorrect because, although giving a 500-mL bolus IV is part of the intervention to resolve variable decelerations, repositioning the client is the *first* action the nurse should take. **Answer 3 is correct because repositioning the client will help to alleviate the variable decelerations. This should be the first action of the nurse.** **Answer 4** is incorrect because readjusting the monitor does *nothing* to resolve the variable decelerations.
■ TEST-TAKING TIP: *Assess the fetal monitor strip in the same way each time: What is the baseline and is it normal? What is the variability and is it normal? Are there accelerations? Are there decelerations and what types of decelerations are present? What interventions are appropriate for each type of deceleration?*
Content Area: Maternity, Intrapartum; *Integrated Process:* Nursing Process, Implementation; *Cognitive Level:* Analysis; *Client Need/Subneed:* Physiological Integrity/Reduction of Risk Potential/Potential for Complications from Surgical Procedures and Health Alterations

87. CORRECT ANSWER: 4. **Answer 1** is incorrect because a baseline fetal heart rate of 170 to 180 bpm is *tachycardia* and is *nonreassuring*. **Answer 2** is incorrect because baseline variability of 25 to 35 bpm is *marked* variability, and *not* a characteristic of a *reassuring* fetal heart rate pattern. **Answer 3** is incorrect because variable decelerations to 100 bpm are a result of *cord compression* and are *not* a characteristic of a *reassuring* fetal heart rate pattern. **Answer 4 is correct because accelerations are correlated with fetal movement and adequate oxygen reserves in the fetus.**
■ TEST-TAKING TIP: *Remember the characteristics of normal fetal heart rate patterns in the same way every time: baseline heart rate 110 to 160 bpm, baseline variability 6 to 25 bpm, accelerations and no decelerations.*
Content Area: Maternity, Antepartum; *Integrated Process:* Nursing Process, Evaluation; *Cognitive Level:* Application; *Client Need/Subneed:* Health Promotion and Maintenance/ Ante/Intra/Postpartum and Newborn Care

88. CORRECT ANSWER: 3. **Answer 1** is incorrect because the bladder fills more rapidly because of the fluid *bolus* given before the epidural, *not the medication* used for the epidural. **Answer 2** is incorrect because the epidural does *not* affect the level of consciousness. **Answer 3 is correct because the sensation of the bladder filling is diminished or lost when the client has an epidural.** **Answer 4** is incorrect because there is no information in the stem that would indicate that she is embarrassed to ask for the bedpan that frequently. Even if that were the case, the *bladder sensation* is diminished when the client has an epidural.
■ TEST-TAKING TIP: *Restate this question as "What are the side effects of epidural anesthetics for a client in labor?"*
Content Area: Maternity, Intrapartum; *Integrated Process:* Nursing Process, Analysis; *Cognitive Level:* Application; *Client Need/Subneed:* Physiological Integrity/Basic Care and Comfort/Elimination

89. CORRECT ANSWER: 2. Answer 1 is incorrect because, during the ovulatory phase, the developing follicles produce estrogen, which is critical for the buildup of the uterine lining. To conceive, the estrogen levels need to be *elevated.* **Answer 2 is correct because the luteinizing hormone surge is responsible for triggering ovulation, or the release of the egg from the ovary, and conception. Answer 3** is incorrect because, during the ovulatory phase, the developing follicles produce estrogen, which is critical for the buildup of the uterine lining. The lining must be *thick* to nourish the fertilized egg. **Answer 4** is incorrect because progesterone is the reproductive hormone that is actually produced by the corpus luteum (a part of the ovary from which the mature egg bursts during ovulation). The levels need to be *elevated* for conception to occur.

■ **TEST-TAKING TIP:** ***Review the hormones responsible for fertility and the role of each in conception. Eliminate the obvious response that does not refer to hormone production because the endometrial lining must be conductive to a pregnancy for conception to occur.***

Content Area: Adult Health, Family Planning; ***Integrated Process:*** Teaching and Learning; ***Cognitive Level:*** Application; ***Client Need/Subneed:*** Health Promotion and Maintenance/Self-Care

90. CORRECT ANSWER: 3. Answer 1 is incorrect because the age of the client has *nothing* to do with the success of the method. **Answer 2** is incorrect because the *timing* of intercourse, *not* the *frequency* of intercourse, is the important factor. **Answer 3 is correct because the effectiveness of the rhythm method depends on how consistent her cycle is and how accurately the couple tracks when she could be ovulating. Answer 4** is incorrect because, although the range of the client's temperature can be important, the regularity of the menstrual cycle and commitment to timing the intercourse is more critical.

■ **TEST-TAKING TIP:** ***Remember that the rhythm method is based on predicting ovulation, and having a regular menstrual cycle is the most important factor.***

Content Area: Adult Health, Family Planning; ***Integrated Process:*** Teaching and Learning; ***Cognitive Level:*** Application; ***Client Need/Subneed:*** Health Promotion and Maintenance/Lifestyle Choices

91. CORRECT ANSWER: 3. Answer 1 is incorrect because intrauterine devices have a higher rate of infection. A client with diabetes should be protected from the risk of developing a pelvic infection due to the intrauterine device. **Answer 2** is incorrect because oral hormonal contraceptive methods can affect the carbohydrate metabolism and insulin utilization in clients with type 1 diabetes. **Answer 3 is correct because barrier methods (e.g., diaphragm) are the best choice for a client with diabetes since they do not have the undesirable side effects that the other methods have. Answer 4** is incorrect because a contraceptive patch is a hormonal contraceptive method that can affect the carbohydrate metabolism and insulin utilization in clients with type 1 diabetes.

■ **TEST-TAKING TIP:** ***Oral contraceptives and contraceptive patches utilize the same hormones; eliminate both choices because they both are basically the same choice.***

Content Area: Adult Health, Family Planning; ***Integrated Process:*** Teaching and Learning; ***Cognitive Level:*** Application; ***Client Need/Subneed:*** Health Promotion and Maintenance/Lifestyle Choices

92. CORRECT ANSWER: 4. Answer 1 is incorrect because painless vaginal bleeding is a symptom of *placenta previa.* Ectopic pregnancy is a painful condition. **Answer 2** is incorrect because abdominal cramping is related to *threatened or imminent abortion.* Ectopic pregnancy is characterized by sharp pain. **Answer 3** is incorrect because throbbing pain in the upper quadrant is not a characteristic of ectopic pregnancy. The fallopian tubes are in the *lower* quadrant. **Answer 4 is correct because sudden, stabbing pain in the lower quadrant is a symptom of ectopic pregnancy. The pain is related to the stretching of the fallopian tube in the lower abdominal quadrant.**

■ **TEST-TAKING TIP:** ***Eliminate Answer 3, which states the pain is in the upper quadrant; fallopian tubes are in the lower quadrant.***

Content Area: Maternity, Antepartum; ***Integrated Process:*** Nursing Process, Assessment; ***Cognitive Level:*** Application; ***Client Need/Subneed:*** Physiological Integrity/Physiological Adaptation/Medical Emergencies

93. CORRECT ANSWER: 2. Answer 1 is incorrect because hyperemesis leads to metabolic acidosis, *not* respiratory alkalosis. Hyperemesis also *includes dehydration.* **Answer 2 is correct because hyperemesis leads to metabolic acidosis and dehydration. Answer 3** is incorrect because hyperemesis leads to *metabolic* acidosis, *not* respiratory acidosis. Hyperemesis also *includes dehydration.* **Answer 4** is incorrect because, if the client has *prolonged vomiting,* it can lead to metabolic alkalosis. This client has *only* nausea and dehydration for a 3-day period.

■ **TEST-TAKING TIP:** ***Hyperemesis results in metabolic acidosis. Eliminate the options with respiratory acidosis and alkalosis.***

Content Area: Maternity, Antepartum; ***Integrated Process:*** Nursing Process, Analysis; ***Cognitive Level:*** Analysis; ***Client Need/Subneed:*** Physiological Integrity/Physiological Adaptation/Fluid and Electrolyte Imbalances

94. CORRECT ANSWER: 2. Answer 1 is incorrect because elevated human chorionic gonadotropin can been seen in a *hydatidiform mole.* **Answer 2 is correct because the presence of fetal heart tones is a positive sign of pregnancy. Answer 3** is incorrect because uterine enlargement can be a result of a *tumor,* a *hydatidiform mole,* or *myomata.* **Answer 4** is incorrect because breast enlargement and tenderness can be caused by hormonal fluctuations of the *normal menstrual* cycle.

■ **TEST-TAKING TIP:** ***Remember that the positive signs of pregnancy are limited to: fetal heart tones, fetal outline on ultrasound or x-ray, and fetal movement felt by an examiner.***

Content Area: Maternity, Antepartum; *Integrated Process:* Nursing Process, Assessment; *Cognitive Level:* Comprehension; *Client Need/Subneed:* Physiological Integrity/Reduction of Risk Potential/System Specific Assessments

95. CORRECT ANSWER: 3. **Answer 1** is incorrect because, with poorly controlled gestational diabetes, the neonate will likely be hypoglycemic, but *large* for gestational age, *not* small for gestational age. **Answer 2** is incorrect because, with poorly controlled gestational diabetes, the neonate will likely be hypoglycemic, *not hyperglycemic.* Answer 3 is correct because, with poorly controlled gestational diabetes, the neonate will likely be hypoglycemic and large for gestational age. **Answer 4** is incorrect because, with poorly controlled gestational diabetes, the neonate will likely be *hypoglycemic, not* hyperglycemic.

■ TEST-TAKING TIP: *Focus on pairs of responses: hypo- versus hyper- and small versus large. In poorly controlled gestational diabetes, the fetus produces excess insulin, which acts as a growth hormone in the fetus; the neonate is likely to be large for gestational age.*

Content Area: Child Health, Newborn; *Integrated Process:* Nursing Process, Analysis; *Cognitive Level:* Analysis; *Client Need/Subneed:* Physiological Integrity/Physiological Adaptation/Alterations in Body Systems

96. CORRECT ANSWERS: 1, 3, 5. Answer 1 is correct because simian creases are a typical finding in a newborn with trisomy 21. **Answer 2** is incorrect because *decreased, not* increased, muscle tone is typical of newborns with trisomy 21. Answer 3 is correct because flat appearance of the face is typical of newborns with trisomy 21. **Answer 4** is incorrect because *large* tongue, *not* small tongue, is typical of newborns with trisomy 21. Answer 5 is correct because upward-slanting eye creases are typical of newborns with trisomy 21.

■ TEST-TAKING TIP: *Read the answers carefully; in two of the options, the typical characteristics of trisomy 21 are the opposite of the characteristics listed here. If not carefully read, the wrong choice can be made.*

Content Area: Child Health, Newborn; *Integrated Process:* Nursing Process, Assessment; *Cognitive Level:* Application; *Client Need/Subneed:* Physiological Integrity/Physiological Adaptation/Pathophysiology

97. CORRECT ANSWERS: 3, 4. **Answer 1** is incorrect because cephalohematoma is an area of bleeding underneath one of the cranial bones usually caused by a difficult birth. A scheduled cesarean delivery does *not* result in trauma to the fetal head with a result of cephalohematoma. **Answer 2** is incorrect because prolonged latent phase does not necessarily mean a difficult birth. A prolonged latent phase is fairly common in clients who are primigravida. This is the phase of labor when the cervix is less than 4 cm dilated. Answer 3 is correct because prolonged second stage of labor is a long pushing stage that may result in a cephalohematoma, caused by the fetal head being in the birth canal for a prolonged period. Answer 4 is correct because vacuum-assisted vaginal delivery may result in a cephalohematoma caused by the application of a vacuum extractor. **Answer 5** is incorrect because breech presentation does *not* result in fetal head trauma; therefore, cephalohematoma does not form on the fetal head.

■ TEST-TAKING TIP: *Remember that cephalohematoma is the collection of blood and is a result of trauma to the fetal head. When there is no trauma, such as with cesarean section or breech presentation, you can eliminate those options.*

Content Area: Child Health, Newborn; *Integrated Process:* Nursing Process, Analysis; *Cognitive Level:* Application; *Client Need/Subneed:* Health Promotion and Maintenance/Ante/Intra/Postpartum and Newborn Care

98. CORRECT ANSWERS: 1, 2, 3, 5. Answer 1 is correct because the developing fetus appears to be vulnerable to DNA damage from methamphetamine exposure because it hasn't yet developed the enzymes that protect it against free radicals. Methamphetamines can cause neural tube defects such as cleft lip and palate. Answer 2 is correct because, when a neonate is withdrawing from methamphetamine, there is an increased incidence of irritability, inability to be consoled, and difficulty sleeping. Answer 3 is correct because methamphetamine exposure can cause skeletal malformations such as clubfoot. **Answer 4** is incorrect because hyperbilirubinemia is *not* associated with exposure to methamphetamines. Answer 5 is correct because gastroschisis—when all of the intestines are outside of the body—is a common birth defect in methamphetamine-exposed infants.

■ TEST-TAKING TIP: *Methamphetamines are manufactured with a variety of toxic chemicals that can cause DNA damage in the developing fetus. Many defects can be attributed to methamphetamine exposure in utero.*

Content Area: Child Health, Newborn; *Integrated Process:* Nursing Process, Assessment; *Cognitive Level:* Application; *Client Need/Subneed:* Physiological Integrity/Pharmacological and Parenteral Therapies/Adverse Effects/Contraindications/Interactions

99. CORRECT ANSWER: 2. **Answer 1** is incorrect because weight gain is a *common side* effect of oral contraceptives that does not need to be reported to the physician. Answer 2 is correct because an alternate method of birth control is needed when taking antibiotics due to the decreased effectiveness of oral contraceptives when taking antibiotics. **Answer 3** is incorrect because, if the client misses one or more pills, two pills should be taken on the day that the client remembers; and two pills the *next day* if two pills are missed, *not* two pills for a week. **Answer 4** is incorrect because nausea and stomach upset are common side effects of oral contraceptives that do not need to be reported to the physician.

■ TEST-TAKING TIP: *Eliminate the common side effects of oral contraceptives that do not need to be reported to the physician.*

Content Area: Adult Health, Family Planning; *Integrated Process:* Teaching and Learning; *Cognitive Level:* Application; *Client Need/Subneed:* Physiological Integrity/Pharmacological and Parenteral Therapies/Expected Effects/Outcomes

100. CORRECT ANSWER: 1. Answer 1 is correct because the client likely has a placenta previa. Assessing the fetal heart tones for signs of fetal distress is the most important action. **Answer 2** is incorrect because the client likely has a placenta previa, and a cervical examination is *contraindicated.* **Answer 3** is incorrect because the client likely has a placenta previa. The uterus is firm with minimal relaxing with a placental abruption. **Answer 4** is incorrect because, although the client likely has a placenta previa and obtaining maternal vital signs is important, assessing the *fetal heart tones* for signs of fetal distress is the *most* important action.

■ **TEST-TAKING TIP:** ***Know the difference between placenta previa and placental abruption. A previa has painless bleeding and an abruption has pain with or without bleeding.***
Content Area: Maternity, Intrapartum; ***Integrated Process:*** Nursing Process, Implementation; ***Cognitive Level:*** Analysis; ***Client Need/Subneed:*** Physiological Integrity/Physiological Adaptation/Alterations in Body Systems

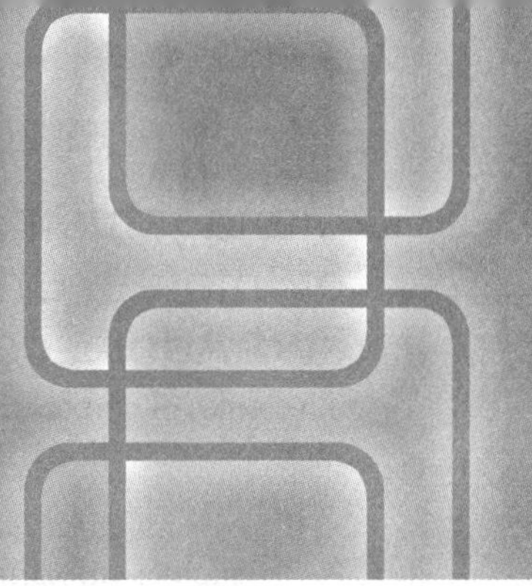

CHAPTER 5

Health Promotion and Maintenance

Nursing Care of the Pediatric Client

Kathleen E. Snider • Denise Wall Parilo

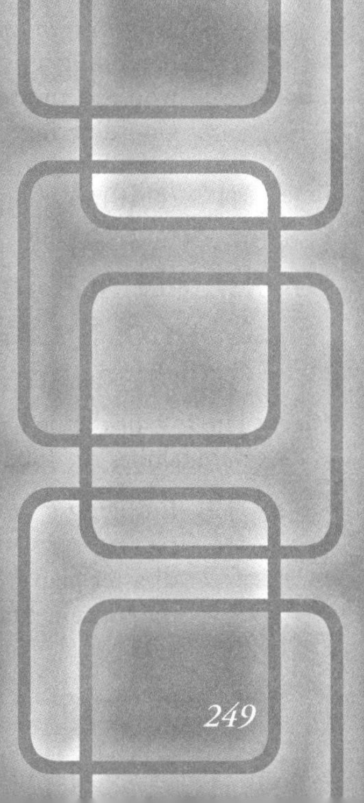

Management of Care of Infants, Children, and Adolescents

The role of the pediatric nurse in *management of care* includes the following:

1. Serving as an *advocate* for the child and family, such as informing the child and family of all treatments and procedures.
2. Coordinating clinical *case management* to provide access to high-quality clinical resources appropriate to the level of care needed, such as referring a child to an acute rehabilitation facility following spinal cord injury.
3. Coordinating *continuity of care* across the health-care delivery continuum, such as discussing the needs of the child and family with the home-care nurse before the child's discharge in a spica cast.
4. *Delegating* care to and *supervising* care among various members of the health-care delivery team, such as assigning a float nurse to care for selected clients on the pediatrics unit.
5. Completing *incident/irregular occurrence/variance reports* as needed, including filing, monitoring, and analyzing reports of drug reactions to a new medication.
6. Working toward *continuous quality improvement,* such as studying incident reports of accidents on the pediatrics unit to determine what changes in practice are needed to increase client safety.
7. Suggesting *organ donation* to selected families when appropriate—for example, asking the family whose 16-year-old child has been declared brain dead about the possibility of organ donation.
8. Collaborating with other members of the health-care team *in consultation and referrals,* such as requesting a psychiatric consultation for a child who is depressed.
9. Coordinating *resource management,* such as reminding the unlicensed assistive personnel (UAP) to stamp all equipment charge forms used for each child.

Safety and Infection Control for Infants, Children, and Adolescents

The role of the pediatric nurse in *safety and infection control* includes the following:

1. Engaging in *disaster planning* activities—for example, the nurse reads and thoroughly reviews the disaster plan for the health-care facility in which the nurse is practicing.
2. Engaging in activities designed to *prevent errors,* such as identifying pediatric clients only by their name bands or by a reliable adult who knows the child.
3. *Handling hazardous and infectious materials* appropriately—for example, always disposing of contaminated waste in a clearly marked biohazard container.
4. Using *medical and surgical asepsis,* such as using sterile gloves and technique when changing a surgical incision dressing.

Prevention and Early Detection of Disease in Infants, Children, and Adolescents

The role of the pediatric nurse in the *prevention and early detection of disease* includes the following:

1. Engaging in *disease prevention* activities (e.g., washing hands thoroughly before and after providing client care).
2. Participating in *health promotion programs,* such as teaching a class on accident prevention to parents of infants and young children.
3. Conducting *health screening* as needed, such as performing the Denver II developmental assessment on age-appropriate clients (1 month to 6 years) in the pediatric clinic as part of routine screening.
4. Teaching families about and administering *immunizations* as ordered—signs/symptoms of reactions, providing parents with an immunization record card after administering immunization(s).
5. Discussing *lifestyle choices* with older children and adolescents, as appropriate (e.g., discussing risks associated with body piercing and tattooing).

Coping and Adaptation in Infants, Children, and Adolescents

The role of the pediatric nurse in *coping and adaptation* includes the following:

1. Understanding and respecting *religious and spiritual influences on children's health* (e.g., allowing families to engage in dying and death rituals according to their spiritual beliefs) (see **Table 5.1**).
2. Helping clients engage in problem-solving related to *situational role changes,* such as discussing transportation and child care issues with the parents of a child who is newly diagnosed with leukemia.

Table 5.1

Stages of Spiritual Development in Childhood

Stage	Characteristics
Infancy (Stage 0: *undifferentiated*)	• No concept of right/wrong • No convictions to guide behavior • Beginnings of a faith are established with the development of basic trust through relationships with the primary caregiver
Toddler/Preschooler (Stage 1: *intuitive-projective*)	**Toddlers:** • Imitate the religious gestures and behaviors of others without comprehending the meaning or significance of the activities **Preschoolers:** • Assimilate some of the values and beliefs of their parents • Parents' attitudes toward moral codes and religious beliefs convey to child what they consider good and bad • Follow parental beliefs as part of daily lives rather than through an understanding of their basic concepts
School-age (Stage 2: *mythical-literal*)	• Spiritual development parallels cognitive development • Closely related to child's experiences and social interactions • Develop strong interest in religion • Accept existence of a deity • Petitions to an omnipotent being are important and expected to be answered • Good behavior is rewarded/bad behavior is punished • Conscience is bothered when they disobey • Have reverence for many thoughts and matters • Able to articulate own faith • May even question validity of faith
Preadolescent (Stage 3: *synthetic-convention*)	• Become increasingly aware of spiritual disappointments • Recognize that prayers are not always answered (at least on their own terms) • Begin to reason, to question some of the established parental religious standards • May drop or modify some religious practices
Adolescent (Stage 4: *individuating-reflexive*)	• Become more skeptical • Begin to compare parent's religious standards with the standards of others • Attempt to determine which to adopt and incorporate into their own set of values • Begin to compare religious standards with the scientific viewpoint • Time of "searching" rather than "reaching" • Uncertain about many religious ideas but will not achieve profound insights until late adolescence or early adulthood

PEDIATRICS

GROWTH AND DEVELOPMENT

I. INFANT (28 DAYS TO 1 YEAR)

A. Erikson's theory of personality development

1. *Central task:* basic trust vs. mistrust; central person: primary caregiver/maternal person.
2. *Behavioral indicators*
   a. Crying is only means of communicating needs.
   b. Quieting usually means needs are met.
   c. Fear of strangers at 6 to 8 months.
3. **Parental guidance/teaching**
   a. Must meet infant's needs consistently—cannot "spoil" infant by holding, comforting.
   b. Neonatal *reflexes* fade between 4 and 6 months, replaced with increase in purposeful behavior (e.g., babbling, reaching).
   c. *Fear of strangers* is normal—indicates attachment between infant and primary caregiver.
   d. Child may repeat over and over newly learned behaviors (e.g., sitting or standing).
   e. *Weaning* can begin around the time child begins walking.
   f. Review *Preventive Care Timeline* and *Recommended Health Screenings* **(Tables 5.2 and 5.3)** with parents of infants.
4. For additional information about behavioral concerns for each age group, see **Tables 5.4** and **5.5.**

B. Physical growth (by 1 year)

1. *Height* (length): 50% increase by first birthday.
2. *Weight*
   a. Doubles by 4 to 7 months, triples by 1 year.
   b. Gains 5 to 7 oz/wk in first 6 months of life.
   c. Gains 3 to 5 oz/wk in second 6 months of life.
3. *Vital signs:* see **Table 5.6.**

(text continues on page 255)

Table 5.2

Child Preventive Care Timeline

Clinical Preventive Services for Normal-Risk Children

IMMUNIZATION

Month/ Years of Age	B	1m	2m	4m	6m	12m	15m	18m	2y	3y	4y	6y	7-10y	11-12y	13-18y
Hepatitis B (HepB)	1		2				3								
Rotavirus (RV)			1	2	3										
Polio (IPV)*			1	2			3				4				
Haemophilus influenzae type B (HIB)*			1	2	3		4								
Pneumococcal Disease (PCV)			1	2	3		4						High-Risk Groups		
Diphtheria, Tetanus, Pertussis (DTaP, Tdap)			1	2	3		4				5			Tdap	
Measles, Mumps, Rubella (MMR)							1				2				
Chickenpox (VZV)							1				2				
Hepatitis A (Hep A)							2 Doses						High-Risk Groups		
Influenza										Yearly					
Meningococcal (MCV)											High-Risk Groups			Once	
Human Papillomavirus (HPV)†														3 Doses	

SCREENING

Years of Age	B	1y	2y	3y	4y	5y	6y	7y	8y	9y	10y	11y	12y	13y	14-18y
Newborn Screening: PKU, Sickle cell hemoglobinopathies, Hypothyroidism															
Hearing															
Head Circumference		Periodically													
Height and Weight									Periodically						
Lead															
Vision Screening															
Blood Pressure										Periodically					
Dental Health										Periodically					
Alcohol Use														Adolescents	
Chlamydia														Adolescents	

COUNSELING

Years of Age	B	1y	2y	3y	4y	5y	6y	7y	8y	9y	10y	11y	12y	13y	14-18y
Development, nutrition, physical activity, safety, unintentional injuries and poisonings, violent behaviors and firearms, STIs and HIV, family planning, tobacco use, drug use									As appropriate for age						

[shaded] Recommended by most U.S. authorities. [outlined box] Recommended by CDC for high-risk groups.

This is an **example** of a typical schedule that indicates the recommended ages for routine administration of currently licensed childhood vaccines for children through age 18 years. Any dose not administered at the recommended age should be administered at any subsequent visit when indicated and feasible. Keep current on vaccine recommendations by going to the **Centers for Disease Control and Prevention Web site: www.cdc.gov/vaccines.**

*Schedules may vary according to vaccine type.

†The human papillomavirus vaccine may also be given in three doses to males between the ages of 9 and 19 years to prevent genital warts. On October 25, 2011, CDC recommended that boys get HPV also.

Modified from *Child Health Guide: Put Prevention into Practice.* U.S. Department of Health and Human Services, Agency for Healthcare Research and Quality, updated January 2003. Modified from *Recommended Immunization Schedule for Persons Aged 0 Through 6 Years* and from *Recommended Immunization Schedule for Persons Aged 7 Through 10 Years,* U.S. Department of Health and Human Services, Centers for Disease Control and Prevention, 2011.

Table 5.3

Recommended Health Screenings for Infants, Children, and Adolescents: Specific Conditions

Area of Concern	Screening Method	Recommendations
Neonatal metabolic and genetic screening: Hypothyroidism Sickle cell anemia PKU	Blood tests: Serum T_3/T_4 levels ↓ Sickledex ↓ Phenylalanine levels ↓	All are done in immediate neonatal period, within first few days of life. Testing for PKU must be done after infant has ingested formula or breast milk for 48–72 hours.
Lead poisoning (see **Table 5.2**)	Blood lead level (BLL)	Centers for Disease Control and Prevention (CDC) recommends universal or targeted screening for all children. • At a minimum, all children should have BLL drawn between 1–2 years, or earlier if needed. • BLL should also be done on any child between 3–6 years who has never been tested. • Those children at high risk (e.g., live in older home with lead in paint and plumbing, have sibling or friend with lead poisoning) should be screened earlier and more frequently.
Hyperlipidemia	Serum cholesterol levels	• Routinely at 2–4 years, 6 years, 10 years, 11–14 years, 15–17 years, and 18–21 years. • May be done earlier or more frequently with risk factors such as diabetes, hypertension, parent with high cholesterol level.
Cystic fibrosis	Genetic studies, sweat test	• Screen children who have sibling or other family members with CF. • Screen family members of child with CF.
Tuberculosis	Mantoux or PPD	First test done at age 12–15 months; repeated prn based on risk and exposure.
Latex allergies	Health history	During each routine visit, but especially important preoperatively or before procedures or children with ongoing urinary catheterizations (e.g., in myelomeningocele).

PEDIATRICS

Table 5.4

Pediatric Behavioral Concerns: Nursing Implications and Parental Guidance

Behavioral Concern	Nursing Implications/Parental Guidance
Teething	Begins around age 4 months—infant may seem unusually fussy and irritable but should *not* run a fever. Provide relief with teething rings, acetaminophen, topical preparations.
Thumb sucking	Need to "suck" varies: may be due to hunger, frustration, loneliness. Do *not* stop *infant* from doing this—usually stops by preschool years. If behavior persists, evaluate need for attention, peer play.
Temper tantrums	Normal in the *toddler*—occurs in response to frustration. *Avoid* abrupt end to play or making excessive demands. Offer only allowable choices. Once a decision is verbalized, *avoid* sudden changes of mind. Provide diversion to achieve cooperation. If it occurs, best means to handle is to *ignore* the outburst.
Toilet training	Assess child for readiness: awareness of body functions, form of mutual communication, physical control over sphincters. Use child-size seat. *No* distractions (food, toys, books). Offer praise for success *or* efforts (never shame accidents).
Discipline	*Not* for infant. Can begin with *toddler,* within limits. Be consistent and clear. *Avoid* excessively strict measures.
Sibling rivalry	Fairly common, normal. Allow older child to "help." Give each child "special" time, with individual attention.

Continued

Table 5.4

Pediatric Behavioral Concerns: Nursing Implications and Parental Guidance—cont'd

Behavioral Concern	Nursing Implications/Parental Guidance
Masturbation	Normal, common in *preschooler.* Set firm limits. *Avoid* overreacting.
Lying	• *In preschooler:* not deliberate; child is often unable to differentiate between "real" and "lie," and by saying something often feels it makes a thing real. • *In older child:* may indicate problems and need for professional attention if persists. Serve as role model—no "white lies."
Cursing	*Avoid* overreacting. Defuse use of "the word" by simply stating "not here, not now." Distract, change subject, substitute activity. Serve as role model by own language.
"Accidents" (enuresis)	*Occasional*—common and normal through preschool. *If frequent*—need complete physical examination to rule out pathology. "Training": after dinner—*avoid* fluids; before bed—toilet (perhaps awaken once during night). *Never* put back into diapers or attempt to shame.
Smoking/drinking	May begin in *older school-age* child or adolescent. Serve as role model with own habits.

Table 5.5

Pediatric Sleep and Rest Norms: Nursing Implications and Parental Guidance

Pediatric Sleep and Rest Norms	Nursing Implications/Parental Guidance
INFANT: 16–20 hr/day	
3 months: nocturnal pattern	No set schedule can be predetermined.
6 months: 1–2 naps, with 12 hr at night	If waking at night after age 3 mo, investigate hunger as a probable cause.
12 months: 1 nap, with 12 hr at night	Monitor behavior to determine sleep needs: Alert, active? Growing, developing? Routine fairly well established.
TODDLER: 12–14 hr/night	
"Dawdles" at bedtime.	Set firm, realistic limits.
Dependency on security object.	Place favorite blanket or toy in crib/bed.
May ask to sleep with bottle.	**Avoid** "bottle mouth syndrome" (caries).
May rebel against going to sleep.	Establish bedtime "ritual."
PRESCHOOL: 10–12 hr/night	
Gives up afternoon nap.	May regress in behavior when tired; provide "quiet time" in place of nap.
Difficulty falling asleep/nighttime waking.	**Avoid** overstimulation in evening.
Fear of dark.	Leave night-light on, door open.
Enuresis.	Occasional accidents are normal.
May begin to have nightmares.	Comfort child but leave in own bed.
SCHOOL-AGE: 8–12 hr/night	
Nightmares common.	Comfort child but leave in own bed.
Awakens early in morning.	Important that child play/relax after school.
May not be aware he or she is tired.	Remind about bedtime.
Likes to stay up late.	"Privilege" of later bedtime can be "awarded" as child gets older.
Slumber parties.	Permit, as good opportunity to socialize.
ADOLESCENT: 10–14 hr/night	
Need for sleep increases greatly.	Needs vary greatly among individuals.
May complain of excessive fatigue.	Related to rapid growth rate and overall increased activity.

Table 5.6

Normal Vital Signs: Measurements and Variations with Age

Age (yr)	Heart Rate (beats/min)	Respiratory Rate (breaths/min)	Blood Pressure (mm Hg)
Newborn	120–160	30–40	70/55
1	100–140	25–35	90/55
2	80–120	20–30	90/56
5	70–100	18–24	95/56
10	60–90	18–22	102/62
14	55–90	16–20	110/65
18	55–90	16–18	116/68

Adapted from Hockenberry, M, & Wilson, D: *Wong's Nursing Care of Infants and Children,* ed 8. Mosby, St. Louis, 2007.

4. *Cardiac system*
   a. Heart begins to function effectively.
   b. Decreased heart rate, increased blood pressure from neonatal values.
5. *Pulmonary system*
   a. Predisposed to upper respiratory infections due to anatomical differences (e.g., eustachian tube is shorter and straighter in infant).
   b. Decreased respiratory rate from neonatal values.
6. *Gastrointestinal system*
   a. Swallowing improves.
   b. Stomach enlarges to hold greater volume.
   c. Digests more complex foods as enzymes increase (by 4–6 months).
7. *Genitourinary system*
   a. Immature; waste products poorly eliminated.
   b. Easily prone to fluid and electrolyte imbalances.
8. *Immune system*
   a. Functional by 2 months.
   b. Produces IgG and IgM antibodies.
9. *Neurological system*
   a. Fontanels:
      (1) Anterior—open or patent through first 12–18 months.
      (2) Posterior—closed by 2 months.
   b. Head circumference increases as brain grows rapidly.
   c. Neurological reflexes (e.g., Landau, parachute) appear; neonatal reflexes (e.g., Moro, rooting) disappear.
10. *Sensory*
    a. Hearing improves from "quieting" to a sound, to locating a sound easily and turning toward it.
    b. Vision improves from 8 to 18 inches, to searching for hidden objects and following moving objects.
11. *Teething*
    a. Generally begins around 6 months.
    b. First two teeth: lower central incisors.
    c. By 1 year: six to eight teeth.

C. Denver II Developmental Assessment: See **Table 5.7.**

1. *Birth to 3 months*
   a. Personal-social: smiles responsively, then spontaneously.
   b. Fine motor-adaptive:
      (1) Follows 180 degrees, past midline.
      (2) Grasps rattle.
      (3) Holds hands together.
   c. Language: laughs/squeals; vocalizes without crying.
   d. Gross motor: while on stomach, lifts head 45 to 90 degrees, able to hold head steady and erect; rolls over, from stomach to back.
2. *4 to 6 months*
   a. Personal-social: works for toy; feeds self (bottle).
   b. Fine motor-adaptive: palmar grasp, reaches for objects.
   c. Language: turns toward voice, imitates speech.
   d. Gross motor: some weight-bearing on legs; no head lag when pulled to sitting; sits with support.
3. *7 to 9 months*
   a. Personal-social
      (1) Indicates wants.
      (2) Plays pat-a-cake, waves bye-bye.
   b. Fine motor-adaptive: takes two cubes in hands and bangs them together; passes cube hand to hand; crude pincer grasp.
   c. Language: "dada," "mama," nonspecific, jabbers.
   d. Gross motor: creeps on hands and knees; gets self up to sitting; pulls self to standing; stands holding on.

Table 5.7

Facts About the DENVER II Developmental Assessment

Parents' Questions	Nurse's Best Response
"Will this be used as a measure of my child's IQ?"	"No, it is a screening test for your child's development."
"What ages can be tested?"	"Infants through preschoolers, *or* from 1 month to 6 years."
"What will they test?"	"There are four areas: personal-social, fine motor-adaptive, language, gross motor."
"Can I stay with my child?"	"Yes, in fact it is preferred you be there."
"If my child fails, does it mean he is retarded?"	"No, this is not a diagnostic tool but rather a screening test."
"If he fails, what do we do?"	"Repeat the test in a week or two to rule out temporary factors."
"Why didn't my child accomplish everything?"	"He is not expected to."
"Why did my child score so poorly?"	"Perhaps it's a bad day for the child, he isn't feeling up to par, etc."

4. *10 to 12 months*
   a. Personal-social
      (1) Plays ball.
      (2) Imitates activities.
      (3) Drinks from cup.
   b. Fine motor-adaptive: neat pincer grasp.
   c. Language: "dada," "mama," specific.
   d. Gross motor: stands alone well; walks holding on; stoops and recovers.

D. Nursing interventions/parental guidance, teaching:

1. *Play*
   a. First year—generally solitary.
   b. Visual stimulation
      (1) Best color: red.
      (2) *Toys:* mirrors, brightly colored pictures.
   c. Auditory stimulation
      (1) Talk and sing to infant.
      (2) *Toys:* musical mobiles, rattles, bells.
   d. Tactile stimulation
      (1) Hold, pat, touch, cuddle, swaddle/keep warm; rub body with lotion.
      (2) *Toys:* various textures; nesting and stacking; plastic milk bottle with blocks to dump in, out.
   e. Kinetic stimulation
      (1) Cradle, stroller, carriage, infant seat, car rides, furniture strategically placed for walking.
      (2) *Toys:* cradle gym, push-pull.
2. *Safety*
   a. Refer to **Tables 3.7, 3.8,** and **3.9** for additional information on safety and infection control.
   b. *Note:* Most common accident during first 12 months is the aspiration of foreign objects.
      (1) Keep small objects out of reach.
      (2) Use one-piece pacifier only.
      (3) *No* nuts, raisins, hot dogs, popcorn.
      (4) *No* toys with small, removable parts.
      (5) *No* balloons or plastic bags.
   c. *Falls*
      (1) Raise crib rails.
      (2) *Never* place child on high surface unsupervised.
      (3) Use restraining straps in seats, high chairs, etc.
   d. *Poisoning*
      (1) Check that paint on toys/furniture is *lead-free.*
      (2) Treat all medications as drugs, never as "candy."
      (3) Store all poisonous substances in locked cabinet, closet.
      (4) Have telephone number of Poison Control Center on hand.
      (5) Instruct in use of syrup of ipecac, if indicated. The use of syrup of ipecac is controversial in children (see **p. 312**).
   e. *Burns*
      (1) Use microwave oven to heat refrigerated formula only; heat only 4 oz or more for about 30 seconds. Test formula on top of your hand, not inside wrist.
      (2) Check temperature of bath water; *never* leave infant alone in bath.
      (3) Special care with cigarettes, hot liquids.
      (4) Do *not* leave infant in sun.
      (5) Cover all electrical sockets.
      (6) Keep electrical wires out of sight/reach.
      (7) *Avoid* tablecloths with overhang.
      (8) Put guards around heating devices.
   f. *Motor vehicles*
      (1) Use only federally approved car seat for all car rides; safest position is rear-facing in middle of back seat (from *birth to 20 pounds,* and as close to *1 year* of age as possible).

PEDIATRICS

(2) *Never* leave stroller behind parked car.
(3) Do *not* allow infant to crawl near parked cars or in driveway.

II. TODDLER (1–3 YEARS)

A. Erikson's theory of personality development

1. *Central task:* autonomy vs. shame and doubt; central person(s): parent(s)
2. *Behavioral indicators*
   a. Does not separate easily from parents.
   b. Negativistic.
   c. Prefers rituals and routine activities.
   d. Active physical explorer of environment.
   e. Begins attempts at self-assertion.
   f. Easily frustrated by limits.
   g. Temper tantrums.
   h. May have favorite "security object."
   i. Uses "mine" for everything—does not understand concept of sharing.
3. **Parental guidance/teaching**
   a. *Avoid* periods of prolonged separation if possible.
   b. *Avoid* constantly saying "no" to toddler.
   c. *Avoid* "yes/no" questions.
   d. Stress that child may use "no" even when he or she means "yes."
   e. Establish and maintain rituals (e.g., toilet training, going to sleep).
   f. Offer opportunities for play, *with* supervision.
   g. Allow child to feed self.
   h. Offer only allowable choices.
   i. Best method to handle temper tantrums: ignore them.
   j. Keep security object with child, if so desired.
   k. Do not force toddler to "share."
   l. Review *Preventive Care Timeline* and *Recommended Health Screenings* (see **Tables 5.2** and **5.3**) with parents of toddlers.
4. Additional information about behavioral concerns for each age group may be found in **Tables 5.4** and **5.5.**

B. Physical growth (by 3 years)

1. *Height*
   a. Slow, steady growth at 2 to 4 inches/yr, mainly in *legs* rather than trunk.
   b. Adult height is roughly *twice* child's height at 2 years of age.
2. *Weight*
   a. Slow, steady growth at 4 to 6 lb/yr.
   b. Birth weight *quadruples* by 2.5 years of age.
3. *Vital signs:* refer to **Table 5.6.**
4. *Cardiac system*
   a. Heart begins to function more efficiently.
   b. Decreased heart rate, slight increase in blood pressure from infant values.
5. *Pulmonary system*
   a. Mainly abdominal breathing.
   b. Lumina of bronchial vessels ↑ in size → decrease in lower respiratory system infections.
   c. Decreased respiratory rate from infant values.
6. *Gastrointestinal system*
   a. Increased capacity → three-meals-a-day feeding schedule.
   b. Gastric juices increase in acidity → decrease in GI infections.
   c. Possible voluntary control of anal sphincter.
7. *Genitourinary system*
   a. Bladder capacity increases; to determine bladder capacity in ounces, add 2 to the child's age (e.g., 2-year-old has a bladder capacity of 4 oz or 120 mL).
   b. Ability to "hold" urine increases.
   c. Possible voluntary control of urethral sphincter.
8. *Immune system*
   a. Possible immunity from intrauterine life/maternal transfer disappears.
   b. Gradual increase in IgA, IgD, and IgE antibodies.
9. *Neurological system*
   a. Anterior fontanel closed by 12–18 months.
   b. Brain increases to 90% of adult size.
   c. Progressive increase in intelligence.
   d. Myelinization of spinal cord is complete.
10. *Sensory*
    a. Hearing evidences basic auditory skills.
    b. Vision shows evidence of convergence and accommodation; full binocular vision developed; visual acuity: 20/40.
11. *Teething*
    a. Introduce toothbrushing as a "ritual."
    b. By 30 months: all 20 primary teeth present.
    c. First dental checkup should be between 12 and 18 months.
12. *Musculoskeletal system*
    a. Lordosis: abdomen protrudes.
    b. Walks like a duck: wide-based gait, side-to-side.

C. Denver II Developmental Assessment (see **Table 5.7**)

1. *12 to 18 months*
   a. Personal-social
      (1) Imitates housework.
      (2) Uses spoon, spilling little.
      (3) Removes own clothes.
      (4) Drinks from cup.
      (5) Feeds doll.
   b. Fine motor-adaptive
      (1) Scribbles spontaneously.
      (2) Builds tower with two to four cubes.

c. Language
(1) Three to six words other than "mama," "dada."
(2) Points to at least one named body part.
d. Gross motor
(1) Kicks ball forward.
(2) Walks up steps.
2. *19 to 24 months*
a. Personal-social
(1) Puts on clothing.
(2) Washes and dries hands.
(3) Brushes teeth with help.
b. Fine motor-adaptive
(1) Builds tower with four to six cubes.
(2) Imitates vertical line.
c. Language
(1) Combines two or three words.
(2) Speech partially understandable.
(3) Names picture.
d. Gross motor
(1) Throws ball overhand.
(2) Jumps in place.
3. *2 to 3 years*
a. Personal-social
(1) Puts on T-shirt.
(2) Can name a friend.
b. Fine motor-adaptive
(1) Thumb wiggles.
(2) Builds tower of eight cubes.
c. Language
(1) Knows two verbs and two adjectives.
(2) Names one color.
d. Gross motor
(1) Balances on one foot briefly.
(2) Pedals tricycle.

D. Nursing interventions/parental guidance:
1. *Play:* toddler years—generally parallel.
2. *Toys*—stimulate multiple senses simultaneously:
a. Push-pull.
b. Riding toys (e.g., straddle horse or car).
c. Small, low slide or gym.
d. Balls, in various sizes.
e. Blocks—multiple shapes, sizes, colors.
f. Dolls, trucks, dress-up clothes.
g. Drums, horns, cymbals, xylophones, toy piano.
h. Pounding board and hammer, clay.
i. Finger paints, chalk and board, thick crayons.
j. Wooden puzzles with large pieces.
k. Toy record player with kiddie records.
l. Talking toys: dolls, read-along books, phones.
m. Sand, water, soap bubbles.
n. Picture books, photo albums.
o. Nursery rhymes, songs, music.
3. *Safety*
a. Refer to **Tables 3.7, 3.8, and 3.9** for additional information on safety and infection control.
b. Accidents are the leading cause of death among toddlers.
c. *Motor vehicles:* most accidental deaths in children under age 3 are related to motor vehicles.
(1) Use only federally approved car seat for all car rides, through age 8 or 60 lb.
(2) Follow manufacturer directions carefully.
(3) Make car seat part of routine for toddler.
d. *Drowning*
(1) Always supervise child near water: bathtub, pool, hot tub, lake, ocean.
(2) Keep bathroom locked to prevent drowning in toilet.
e. *Burns*
(1) Turn pot handles *in* when cooking.
(2) Do *not* allow child to play with electrical appliances.
(3) Decrease water temperature in house to avoid scald burns.
f. *Poisonings:* most common in 2-year-olds.
(1) Consider every nonfood substance a hazard and place out of child's sight/reach.
(2) Keep all medications, cleaning materials, etc., in clearly marked containers in locked cabinets.
(3) Instruct in use of syrup of ipecac, if indicated by Poison Control Center (see **p. 312**).
g. *Falls*
(1) Provide barriers on open windows.
(2) *Avoid* gates on stairs—child can strangle on gate.
(3) Move from crib to bed.
h. *Choking: avoid* food on which child might choke:
(1) Fish with bones.
(2) Fruit with seeds, pits, or "skin."
(3) Nuts, raisins.
(4) Hot dogs.
(5) Chewing gum.
(6) Hard candy.
(7) "Coin-cut" foods.

III. PRESCHOOLER (3–5 YEARS)

A. Erikson's theory of personality development
1. *Central task:* initiative vs. guilt; central person(s): basic family unit.
2. *Behavioral indicators*
a. Attempts to perform activities of daily living (ADLs) independently.
b. Attempts to make things for self/others.
c. Tries to "help."

PEDIATRICS

d. Talks constantly: verbal exploration of the world ("Why?").
e. Extremely active, highly creative imagination: fantasy and magical thinking.
f. May demonstrate fears: "monsters," dark rooms, etc.
g. Able to tolerate short periods of separation.

3. **Parental guidance/teaching**
   a. Encourage child to dress self by providing simple clothing.
   b. Remind to go to bathroom (tends to "forget").
   c. Assign small, simple tasks or errands.
   d. Answer questions patiently, simply; do *not* offer child more information than what the child is asking for.
   e. Normal to have "imaginary playmates."
   f. Offer realistic support and reassurance with regard to fears.
   g. Expose to a variety of experiences: zoo, train ride, shopping, sleigh riding, etc.
   h. Enroll in preschool/nursery school program; kindergarten at 5 years.
   i. Review *Preventive Care Timeline* and *Recommended Health Screenings* (see **Tables 5.2** and **5.3**) with parents of preschoolers.
4. Additional information about behavioral concerns for each age group may be found in **Tables 5.4 and 5.5.**

B. Physical growth (by 5 years)

1. *Height and weight*
   a. Continued slow, steady growth.
   b. Generally grows more in *height* than weight.
   c. Posture: appears taller and thinner; "lordosis" of toddler gradually *disappears.*
2. *Vital signs:* see **Table 5.6.**
3. *Cardiac system*
   a. Increased heart size (4 times larger than at birth); heart function is comparable to a healthy adult (by 5 years).
   b. Heart assumes vertical position in thoracic cavity.
   c. May hear "splitting" of heart sounds, as well as innocent murmurs on auscultation.
   d. Decreased heart rate, steady blood pressure from toddler values.
4. *Pulmonary system*
   a. Increase in amount of lung tissue.
   b. Adult-like lung sounds heard on auscultation.
   c. Decreased respiratory rate from toddler values.
5. *Gastrointestinal system*
   a. Continued increase in size.
   b. Position is straighter and more upright than adult stomach → more rapid emptying (defecation, vomiting).
   c. Lining still sensitive to roughage and spices.
   d. Elimination controlled.
6. *Genitourinary system*
   a. Bladder remains palpable above symphysis pubis.
   b. Needs to void frequently, or "accidents" may occur despite sphincter control.
   c. Low-grade urinary tract infections common.
7. *Immune system*
   a. Growth of lymphoid tissue (especially tonsils).
   b. Illnesses (especially respiratory) tend to be more localized.
   c. Continued increase in IgA and IgG.
8. *Neurological system*
   a. "Handedness" (right or left) is established.
9. *Sensory*
   a. Vision—far-sightedness is improving; visual acuity: 20/30.
   b. Vision and hearing screening should be conducted before kindergarten, and annually thereafter.
10. *Teeth*
    a. All 20 primary or deciduous teeth ("baby teeth") should be present.
    b. Annual dental checkups; continue daily brushing.

C. Denver II Developmental Assessment/ developmental norms: see **Table 5.7.**

1. *3 years*
   a. Personal-social
      (1) Dresses without help.
      (2) Plays board/card games.
   b. Fine motor-adaptive
      (1) Picks longer of two lines.
      (2) Copies circle, intersecting lines.
      (3) Draws person, three parts.
   c. Language
      (1) Comprehends "cold," "tired," "hungry."
      (2) Comprehends prepositions: "over," "under."
      (3) Names four colors.
   d. Gross motor
      (1) Pedals tricycle; hops, skips on alternating feet.
      (2) Broad jumps, jumps in place.
      (3) Balances on one foot.
2. *4 years*
   a. Personal-social
      (1) Brushes own teeth, combs own hair.
      (2) Dresses without supervision.
      (3) Knows own age and birthday.
      (4) Ties own shoes.
   b. Fine motor-adaptive
      (1) Draws person with six body parts.
      (2) Copies square.
   c. Language
      (1) Knows opposite analogies (two of three).
      (2) Defines seven words.

d. Gross motor
(1) Balances on each foot for 5 seconds.
(2) Can walk heel-to-toe.

3. *5 years*
a. Personal-social
(1) Interested in money.
(2) Knows days of week, seasons.
b. Fine motor-adaptive
(1) Prints name.
c. Language
(1) Counts to 10.
(2) Verbalizes number sequences (e.g., telephone number).
d. Gross motor
(1) Attempts to ride bike.
(2) Rollerskates, jumps rope, bounces ball.
(3) Backward heel-toe walk.

D. Nursing interventions/parental guidance:

1. *Play:* preschool years—associative and cooperative.
a. Likes to play house, "work," school, firehouse.
b. "Arts and crafts": color, draw, paint dot-to-dot, color by number, cut and paste, simple sewing kits.
c. Ball, rollerskate, jump rope, jacks.
d. Swimming.
e. Puzzles, blocks (e.g., Lego blocks).
f. Tricycle, then bicycle (with/without training wheels).
g. Simple card games and board games.
h. Costumes and dress-up: "make-believe."

2. *Safety:* Emphasis shifts from protective supervision to teaching simple safety rules. Preschoolers are "the great imitators" of parents, who now serve as role models.
a. Refer to **Tables 3.7, 3.8, and 3.9** for additional information on safety and infection control.
b. Teach child car/*street* safety rules.
c. Convertible safety seats should be used until child weighs at least 40 lb.
d. Teach child not to go with strangers or accept gifts or candy from strangers.
e. Teach child danger of *fire,* matches, flame: "drop and roll."
f. Teach child rules of *water* safety; provide swimming lessons.
g. Provide adult supervision, frequent checks on activity/location. Despite safety teaching, preschooler is still a child and may be unreliable.

IV. SCHOOL AGE (6–12 YEARS)

A. Erikson's theory of personality development

1. *Central task:* industry vs. inferiority; central person(s): school, neighborhood friend(s).

2. *Behavioral indicators*
a. Moving toward complete independence in ADLs.
b. May be very competitive—wants to achieve in school, at play.
c. Likes to be alone occasionally, may seem shy.
d. Prefers friends and peers to siblings.

3. **Parental guidance/teaching**
a. Be accepting of the child as he or she *is.*
b. Offer consistent support and guidance.
c. *Avoid* authoritative or excessive demands on child.
d. Respect need for privacy.
e. Assign household tasks, errands, chores.
f. Review *Preventive Care Timeline* and *Recommended Health Screenings* (see **Tables 5.2** and **5.3**) with parents of school-age children.

4. Additional information about behavioral concerns for each age group may be found in **Tables 5.4** and **5.5.**

B. Physical growth (by 12 years)

1. *Height and weight*
a. Almost *double* in weight from 6 to 12 years.
b. Period of slow, steady growth.
c. 1 to 2 inches/yr.
d. 3 to 6 lb/yr.
e. Girls and boys differ in size at end of school-age years.

2. *Vital signs:* refer to **Table 5.6.**

3. *Cardiac system*
a. Increased size of left ventricle (to meet demands for increased blood to growing structures).
b. Decreased heart rate, increased blood pressure from preschool values.

4. *Pulmonary system*
a. Front sinuses develop (by 7 years).
b. Lymphatic tissue completes growth (by 9 years).
c. Remains well oxygenated on exertion.
d. Continued decrease in respiratory rate from preschool values; using intercostal muscles more effectively for breathing.

5. *Gastrointestinal system*
a. Higher metabolic rate requires adequate food and fluids to ensure nutrition and hydration.
b. Food retained in stomach for longer periods of time.

6. *Genitourinary system*
a. Bladder capacity increase continues.
b. Kidneys mature.
c. Less likely to have fluid and electrolyte (F/E) imbalance as increased conservation of water occurs.

7. *Immune system*
   a. Growth of lymphoid tissue increases, then plateaus, then decreases.
   b. Continued improvement noted with body's increased ability to localize infections.
8. *Neurological system*
   a. Central nervous system matures.
   b. Myelinization continues → increase in both fine motor-adaptive and gross motor skills.
9. *Sensory*
   a. Vision: 20/20 vision well established between 9 and 11 years.
   b. Should be screened for vision/hearing annually, usually in school.
10. *Teeth*
   a. Begins to lose primary teeth around sixth birthday.
   b. Eruption of permanent teeth, including molars; 28 permanent teeth (by 12 years).
   c. Dental screening annually, daily brushing.
11. *Pubescence* (preliminary physical changes of adolescence)
   a. Average age of onset: girls at 10, boys at 12.
   b. Beginning of growth spurt.
   c. Some sexual changes may start to occur.

C. Developmental norms

1. *6 to 8 years*
   a. Dramatic, exuberant, boundless energy.
   b. Alternating periods: quiet, private behavior.
   c. Conscientious, punctual.
   d. Wants to care for own needs but needs reminders, supervision.
   e. Oriented to time and space.
   f. Learns to read, tell time, follow map.
   g. Interested in money—asks for "allowance."
   h. Eagerly anticipates upcoming events, trips.
   i. Can bicycle, swim, play ball.
2. *9 to 11 years*
   a. Worries over tasks; takes things seriously, yet also developing sense of humor—likes to tell jokes.
   b. Keeps room, clothes, toys relatively tidy.
   c. Enjoys physical activity, has great stamina.
   d. Very enthusiastic at work and play; has lots of energy—may fidget, drum fingers, tap foot.
   e. Wants to work to earn money: mow lawn, baby-sit, deliver papers.
   f. Loves secrets (secret clubs).
   g. Very well behaved outside own home (or with company).
   h. Uses tools, equipment; follows directions, recipes.
   i. By 12th birthday: paradoxical stormy behavior, onset of adolescent conflicts.

D. Nursing interventions/parental guidance:

1. *Play*
   a. Wants to win, likes competitive games.
   b. Prefers to play with same-sex children.
   c. Enjoys group, team play.
   d. Loves to do magic tricks and other "show-off" activities (e.g., puppet shows, plays, singing).
   e. Likes to collect things: cards, compact discs.
   f. Does simple scientific experiments, computer games.
   g. Has hobbies: needlework, woodwork, models.
   h. Enjoys pop music, musical instruments, videos, posters.
2. *Safety* (see **Table 3.7**)
   a. As passenger: use specially designed car restraints until age 8 or 60 lbs, then safety belts. Teach child not to distract driver.
   b. As pedestrian: teach bike, street safety.
   c. Teach how to swim, rules of water safety.
   d. Sports: teach safety rules.
   e. Adult supervision still necessary; serve as role model for safe activities.
   f. Teach about "stranger danger" and online safety.
   g. Suggest Red Cross courses on first aid, water safety, babysitting, etc.
   h. Refer to **Tables 3.7, 3.8, and 3.9** for additional information on safety and infection control.

V. ADOLESCENT (12–18 YEARS)

A. Erikson's theory of personality development

1. *Central task:* identity vs. role confusion; central person(s): peer group.
2. *Behavioral indicators*
   a. Changes in body image related to sexual development.
   b. Awkward and uncoordinated in the beginning.
   c. Much interest in opposite sex: girls become romantic.
   d. Wants to be exactly like peers.
   e. Becomes hostile toward parents, adults, family.
   f. Concerned with vocation, life after high school.
3. **Parental guidance/teaching**
   a. Offer firm but realistic limits on behavior.
   b. Continue to offer guidance, support.
   c. Allow child to earn own money, control own finances.
   d. Assist adolescent to develop positive self-image.
   e. Review *Preventive Care Timeline* and *Recommended Health Screenings* (see **Tables 5.2** and **5.3**) with parents of adolescents.
4. Additional information about behavioral concerns for each age group may be found in **Tables 5.4** and **5.5.**

PEDIATRICS

B. Physical growth (by 18 years)

1. *Height and weight*
   a. Adolescent growth spurt lasts 24 to 36 months.
   b. Growth in height commonly *ceases* at 16 to 17 years in girls, 18 to 20 years in boys.
   c. Boys gain more weight than girls, are generally taller and heavier.
2. *Vital signs* approximately those of the adult (see **Table 5.6**).
3. *Cardiac system*
   a. Increased heart size and strength to near-adult values.
   b. Decreased heart rate, increased blood pressure from school-age values.
4. *Pulmonary system*
   a. Lungs increase in size to near-adult levels, but not as rapidly as other body systems (may explain lack of energy).
   b. System is "mature" by 12 years.
   c. Continued decreased respiratory rate from school-age values.
5. *Gastrointestinal system*
   a. Continued need for increased calories.
6. *Genitourinary system*
   a. Fully developed; bladder can hold 700 mL.
7. *Immune system*
   a. Fully developed; infections become increasingly rare in an adolescent who is healthy.
   b. Lymphoid tissue matures and regresses.
8. *Neurological system*
   a. Fully developed.
9. *Sensory*
   a. Fully developed.
10. *Teeth:* 32 permanent teeth by 18 to 21 years.
11. *Sexual changes*
    a. *Girls*
       (1) Changes in nipple and areola; development of breast buds.
       (2) Growth of pubic hair.
       (3) Change in vaginal secretions.
       (4) Menstruation—average onset between 12 and 13 years of age; range 8 to 15 years.
       (5) Growth of axillary hair.
       (6) Ovulation.
    b. *Boys*
       (1) Enlargement of genitalia.
       (2) Growth of pubic, axillary, facial, and body hair.
       (3) Lowering of voice.
       (4) Production of sperm; nocturnal emission ("wet dreams").

C. Developmental norms

1. *Motor development*
   a. *Early (12–15 years)*—awkward, uncoordinated, poor posture, decrease in energy and stamina.
   b. *Later (15–18 years)*—increased coordination and better posture; more energy and stamina.
2. *Cognitive*
   a. Academic ability and interest vary greatly.
   b. "Think about thinking"—period of introspection.
3. *Emotional*
   a. Same-sex best friend, leading to strong friendship bonds.
   b. Highly romantic period for boys and girls.
   c. May be moody, unpredictable, inconsistent.
4. *Social*
   a. Periods of highs and lows, sociability and loneliness.
   b. Turmoil with parents—related to changing roles, desire for increased independence.
   c. Peer group is important socializing agent—conformity increases sense of belonging.
   d. Friendships: same-sex best friend advancing to heterosexual "relationships."

D. Nursing interventions/parental guidance:

1. *Play*
   a. School-related group activities and sports.
   b. Develops talents, skills, and abilities.
   c. Television—watches soap operas, romantic movies, sports.
   d. Develops interest in art, writing, poetry, musical instrument.
   e. Girls: increased interest in makeup and clothes.
   f. Boys: increased interest in mechanical and electronic devices.
2. *Safety* (see **Table 3.7**)
   a. Motor vehicles (cars and motorcycles)—as *passenger* or as *driver.*
   b. Encourage driver education; serve as positive role model.
   c. Teach rules of safety for water sports.
   d. Teach about "stranger danger" and online safety.
   e. Wants to earn money but still needs guidance: advocate safe job, reasonable hours.

DEVELOPMENTAL DISABILITIES

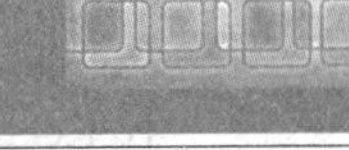

I. DOWN SYNDROME

A. *Introduction:* Down syndrome (trisomy 21) is a chromosomal abnormality involving an extra chromosome #21 and resulting in 47 chromosomes instead of the normal 46 chromosomes. As a consequence, the child usually has varying degrees of mental retardation, characteristic facial and physical features, and other congenital anomalies. Down syndrome is the most common chromosomal disorder, occurring in approximately 1 of 800 to 1000 live births. Perinatal risk factors include advanced maternal age, especially with the first pregnancy (although average maternal age is now 25-28 years for an infant with Down's); paternal age is thought to be a related factor. Multiple causality is suspected.

B. Assessment:

1. *Physical characteristics*
   a. Brachycephalic (small, round *head*) with oblique palpebral fissures (almond-shaped *eyes*) and *Brushfield* spots (speckling of *iris*)—depressed *nasal* bridge ("saddle nose") and small, low-set *ears.*
   b. Mouth
      (1) Small oral cavity with protruding tongue causes difficulty sucking and swallowing.
      (2) Delayed eruption/misalignment of teeth.
   c. Hands
      (1) Clinodactyly—incurved little finger.
      (2) Simian crease—transverse palmar crease.
   d. Muscles: hypotonic ("floppy baby") with hyperextensible joints.
   e. Skin: dry, cracked.
2. Genetic studies reveal an extra chromosome #21 ("trisomy 21").
3. *Intellectual characteristics*
   a. Mental retardation—varies from severely retarded to low-average intelligence.
   b. Most fall within "trainable" range, or IQ of 36 to 51 ("moderate mental retardation").
4. *Congenital anomalies/diseases*
   a. 40% to 45% have congenital heart defects: mortality highest in clients with Down syndrome and cyanotic heart disease.
   b. GI: tracheoesophageal fistula (TEF), Hirschsprung's disease.
   c. Thyroid dysfunction, especially hypothyroidism.
   d. Visual defects: cataracts, strabismus.
   e. Hearing loss.
   f. Increased incidence of leukemia.
5. *Growth and development*
   a. Slow growth, especially in height.
   b. Delay in developmental milestones.
6. *Sexual development*
   a. Delayed or incomplete.
   b. Women—small number have had offspring (majority have had abnormality).
   c. Men—infertile.
7. *Aging*
   a. Premature aging, with shortened life expectancy.
   b. Death—generally related to respiratory complications: repeated infections, pneumonia, lung disease.

C. Analysis/nursing diagnosis:

1. *Risk for aspiration* related to hypotonia.
2. *Altered nutrition, less than body requirements,* related to hypotonia or congenital anomalies.
3. *Altered growth and development* related to Down syndrome.
4. *Self-care deficit* related to Down syndrome.
5. *Altered family processes* related to birth of an infant with a congenital defect.
6. *Knowledge deficit* related to Down syndrome.

D. Nursing care plan/implementation:

1. Goal: *prevent physical complications.*
   a. Respiratory
      (1) Use bulb syringe to clear nose, mouth.
      (2) Vaporizer.
      (3) Frequent position changes.
      (4) *Avoid* contact with people with upper respiratory infections.
   b. Aspiration
      (1) Small, more frequent feedings.
      (2) Burp well during/after infant feedings.
      (3) Allow sufficient time to eat.
      (4) *Position after meals:* head of bed elevated, right side—or on stomach, with head to side.
   c. Observe for signs and symptoms of: heart disease, constipation/GI obstruction, leukemia, thyroid dysfunction.
2. Goal: *meet nutritional needs.*
   a. Suction (before meals) to clear airway.
   b. Adapt feeding techniques to meet special needs of infant/child (e.g., use long, straight-handled spoon).
   c. Monitor height and weight.
   d. As child grows, monitor caloric intake (tends toward obesity with advancing age).
   e. Offer foods *high in bulk* to prevent constipation related to hypotonia.
3. Goal: *promote optimal growth and development.*
   a. Encourage parents to enroll infant/toddler in early stimulation program and to follow through with suggested exercises at home.
   b. Preschool/school-age: special education classes.
   c. Screen frequently, using Denver II to monitor development.
   d. Help parents focus on "normal" or positive aspects of infant/child.
   e. Help parents work toward realistic goals with their child.
4. Goal: *health teaching.*
   a. Explain that tongue-thrust behavior is normal and that child should be re-fed.
   b. Before adolescence—counsel parents and child about delay in sexual development, decreased libido, marriage and family relations.
   c. In severe cases, assist parents to deal with issue of placement/institutionalization.

E. Evaluation/outcome criteria:

1. Physical complications are prevented.
2. Adequate nutrition is maintained.
3. Child attains optimal level of growth and development.

II. ATTENTION DEFICIT–HYPERACTIVITY DISORDER (ADHD); BEHAVIORAL DISORDER (DSM-IV)

A. *Introduction:* As defined by the American Psychiatric Association (APA), this diagnostic term includes a persistent pattern of inattention or hyperactivity-impulsivity. The exact cause and pathophysiology remain unknown. The major symptoms include a greatly shortened attention span and difficulty in integrating and synthesizing information. This disorder is three times more common in boys than girls, with onset before age 7; the diagnosis is based on the child's history rather than on any specific diagnostic test.

B. Assessment:

1. The behaviors exhibited by children with ADHD are not unusual behaviors seen in children. The behavior of children with ADHD *differs* from the behavior of non-ADHD children in both *quality* and *appropriateness:*
   a. Motor activity is excessive.
   b. Developmentally "younger" than chronological age.
2. Inattention
   a. Does not pay attention to detail.
   b. Does not listen when spoken to.
   c. Does not do what he or she is told to do.
3. Hyperactivity
   a. Fidgets and squirms excessively.
   b. Cannot sit quietly.
   c. Has difficulty playing quietly.
   d. Seems to be constantly in motion, moving or talking; always "on."
4. Impulsiveness
   a. Blurts out answers before question is completed.
   b. Has difficulty awaiting turn. Interrupts others.

C. Analysis/nursing diagnosis:

1. *Altered thought processes* related to inattention and impulsiveness.
2. *Impaired physical mobility* related to hyperactivity.
3. *Risk for injury* related to impulsivity.
4. *Self-esteem disturbance* related to hyperactivity and impulsivity.
5. *Knowledge deficit* related to behavioral modification program, medications, and follow-up care.

D. Nursing care plan/implementation:

1. Goal: *teach family and child about ADHD.*
   a. Provide complete explanation about disorder, probable course, treatment, and prognosis.
   b. Answer questions directly, simply.
   c. Encourage family to verbalize; offer support.
2. Goal: *provide therapeutic environment* using principles of behavior modification and/or psychotherapy.
   a. Reduce extraneous or distracting stimuli.
   b. Reduce stress by decreasing environmental expectations (home, school).
   c. Provide firm, consistent limits.
   d. Special education programs.
   e. Special attention to safety needs.
3. Goal: *reduce symptoms by means of prescribed medication.*
   a. Medications: *Ritalin* and *Cylert*—both are CNS stimulants but have a paradoxical calming effect on the child's behavior. *Tofranil* and *Norpramin*—both are tricyclic antidepressants that ↑ action of norepinephrine and serotonin in nerve cells, but also can have paradoxical calming effect on child's behavior. Must monitor for development of tics and arrhythmias.
   b. *Health teaching* (child *and* parents).
      (1) Need to take medication regularly, as ordered. *Avoid* taking medication late in the day because it may cause insomnia; monitor neurological and cardiac status. Assess for ↓ appetite → ↓ weight; *avoid* caffeine.
      (2) Need for long-term administration, with probable decreased need as child nears adolescence.
4. Goal: *provide safe outlet for excess energy.*
   a. Alternate planned periods of outdoor play with schoolwork or quiet indoor play.
   b. Channel energies toward safe, large-muscle activities: running track, swimming, bicycling, hiking.

E. Evaluation/outcome criteria:

1. Family and child verbalize understanding of "attention deficit disorders."
2. Therapeutic environment enhances socially acceptable behavior.
3. Medication taken regularly, with behavioral improvements noted.
4. Excess energy directed appropriately.

PSYCHOSOCIAL-CULTURAL FUNCTIONS

Refer to **Table 5.8** for information on the nursing care of hospitalized infants and children as it relates to key developmental differences.

PEDIATRICS

Table 5.8

Nursing Care of Hospitalized Infants and Children: Key Developmental Differences

Age	Assessment: Reaction to Hospitalization	Nursing Care Plan/Implementation: Key Nursing Behaviors
Infant	Difficult to assess needs, pain Wants primary caretaker	Close observation, must look at behavioral cues Rooming-in
Toddler	Separation anxiety Frustration, loss of autonomy Regression Fears intrusive procedures	Rooming-in Punching bag, pounding board, clay Behavior modification Axillary temperatures
Preschooler	• Fearful • Fantasy about illness/hospitalization (may feel punished, abandoned) • Peak of body mutilation fear • Behavior problems: aggressive, manipulative • Regression	Therapeutic play with puppets, dolls Therapeutic play with puppets, dolls Care with dressings, casts, IMs; invasive procedures Clear, consistent limits Behavior modification
School Age	Cooperative Quiet, may withdraw May complain of being bored	• Use diagrams, models to teach • Indirect interview: tell story, draw picture • Involve in competitive game with peer; encourage peers to call, send get well cards, and visit
Adolescent	Fears loss of control Competitive—afraid of "failing" Difficulty with body image Does not want to be separated from peers Rebellious behavior	Provide privacy; allow to make some decisions Provide tutor prn; get books and homework Provide own clothes; give realistic feedback Telephone in room; liberal visiting; teen lounge Set clear rules; form teen support group

NEUROLOGICAL SYSTEM

I. BACTERIAL MENINGITIS

A. Assessment:

1. Abrupt onset: initial sign may be a seizure, following an episode of upper respiratory infection (URI)/acute otitis media.
2. Chills and fever.
3. Vomiting; may complain of headache, neck pain (older children).
4. Photophobia.
5. Alterations in level of consciousness: delirium, stupor, increased intracranial pressure.
6. Nuchal rigidity (older children).
7. Opisthotonos position: head is drawn backward into overextension; bulging fontanel (most significant finding in infants).
8. Hyperactive reflexes related to CNS irritability.

B. Analysis/nursing diagnosis:

1. *Risk for infection* related to communicability of meningitis.
2. *Risk for injury* related to CNS irritability and seizures.
3. *Pain* related to nuchal rigidity, opisthotonos position, increased muscle tension.
4. *Sensory/perceptual alterations* related to seizures and changes in level of consciousness.
5. *Altered nutrition, less than body requirements,* related to fever and poor oral intake.
6. *Knowledge deficit* regarding diagnostic procedures, condition, treatment, prognosis.

C. Nursing care plan/implementation:

1. Goal: *prevent spread of infection.*
   a. Institute standard precautions.
   b. Enforce strict hand washing.
   c. Institute and maintain *respiratory isolation* for minimum of 24 hours after starting IV antibiotics, at which time child is no longer considered to be communicable and can be removed from isolation.
   d. Supervise all visitors in isolation techniques.
   e. Identify family members and others at high risk: do cultures (*Haemophilus influenzae, Escherichia coli,* etc.); possibly begin prophylactic antibiotics (e.g., rifampin). Lumbar puncture (LP) is the definitive diagnostic test.
   f. Treat with IV antibiotics (as ordered) as soon as possible after admission (after cultures are obtained); continue 10 to 14 days (until cerebrospinal fluid [CSF] culture is negative and child appears clinically improved).
   g. Anticipate large-dose IV medications only—administer *slowly* in *dilute* form to prevent phlebitis.
   h. Restrain as needed to maintain IV.

PEDIATRICS

2. Goal: *promote safety and prevent injury/seizures.*
   a. Maintain seizure precautions. Give anticonvulsants, as ordered (e.g., phenytoin).
   b. Place child near nurses' station for maximum observation; provide private room for isolation.
   c. Minimize stimuli: quiet, calm environment.
   d. Restrict visitors to immediate family.
   e. *Position:* Head of bed (HOB) slightly elevated to decrease intracranial pressure. (If opisthotonos: side-lying, for comfort and safety.)
3. Goal: *maintain adequate nutrition.*

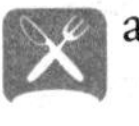

   a. NPO or *clear liquids* initially; supplement with IVs, because child may be unable to coordinate sucking and swallowing.
   b. Offer diet for age, as tolerated—child may experience anorexia (due to disease) or vomiting (due to increased intracranial pressure).
   c. Monitor I&O, daily weights.

D. Evaluation/outcome criteria:
1. No spread of infection noted; immunize all children against *H. influenzae* type B
2. Safety maintained.
3. Adequate nutrition and fluid intake maintained.
4. Child recovers without permanent neurological damage (e.g., seizure disorders, hydrocephalus).

II. REYE SYNDROME

A. *Introduction:* Reye syndrome, first described as a disease entity in the mid-1960s, is a multisystem disorder primarily affecting children between 6 and 12 years of age. Although **not** truly a "communicable disease," studies have confirmed a relationship between aspirin administration during a viral illness (e.g., chickenpox, flu) and the onset of Reye syndrome. The exact cause remains unknown. Reye syndrome is characterized by acute metabolic encephalopathy and fatty degeneration of the visceral organs, particularly the liver. Earlier diagnosis, more sophisticated monitoring equipment, and more aggressive treatment have greatly improved the survival rate of children with Reye syndrome. Recovery is generally rapid in those children who do survive, though they may suffer certain deficits.

B. Assessment:
1. Onset typically follows a viral illness, just as child appears to be recovering.
2. *Early signs and symptoms:*
   a. Rapidly progressing behavioral changes: irritability, agitation, combativeness, hostility, confusion, apathy, lethargy.
   b. Vomiting, which becomes progressively worse.
3. Rapidly progressive neurological deterioration:
   a. Cerebral edema and increased intracranial pressure.
   b. Alteration in level of consciousness from lethargy through coma, decerebrate posturing, and respiratory arrest.
4. Liver biopsy reveals liver dysfunction, necrosis, and failure:
   a. *Elevated* serum alanine aminotransferase (ALT) (serum glutamic-pyruvic transaminase [SGPT]), aspartate aminotransferase (AST) (serum glutamic-oxaloacetic transaminase [SGOT]), lactate dehydrogenase (LDH), serum ammonia levels.
   b. Severe hypoglycemia.
   c. *Increased* prothrombin time, coagulation defects, and bleeding.

C. Analysis/nursing diagnosis:
1. *Altered cerebral tissue perfusion* related to cerebral edema and increased intracranial pressure.
2. *Altered hepatic tissue perfusion* related to fatty degeneration of the liver.
3. *Risk for injury* related to coagulation defects and bleeding.
4. *Knowledge deficit* related to diagnosis, course of disease, treatment, and prognosis.

D. Nursing care plan/implementation:
1. Goal: *reduce intracranial pressure.*
   a. Child is admitted to pediatric intensive care unit (PICU) for intensive nursing care, continuous observation, and monitoring.
   b. Monitor neurological status and vital signs continuously.
   c. Assist with/prepare for numerous invasive procedures, including endotracheal (ET) tube/mechanical ventilation and intracranial pressure (ICP) monitor.
   d. Monitor closely for the development of seizures; institute seizure precautions.
   e. *Position:* elevate HOB 30 to 45 degrees.
   f. Administer medications as ordered:
      (1) Osmotic diuretics (e.g., mannitol) to decrease ICP.
      (2) Diuretics (e.g., *Lasix*) to decrease CSF production.
      (3) Anticonvulsants (e.g., *Dilantin*, phenobarbital).
      (4) Vitamin K, fresh frozen plasma, or platelet transfusions for overt or covert bleeding.
2. Goal: *restore and maintain fluid and electrolyte balance, including perfusion of liver.*
   a. Administer IV fluids per physician's order—usually 10% glucose (or higher).
   b. Strict I&O.

PEDIATRICS

c. Prepare for/assist with Foley catheter placement, central venous pressure (CVP) monitor, ICP monitor, nasogastric (NG) tube, etc.
d. Monitor serum electrolyte laboratory values.

3. Goal: *prevent injury and possible bleeding.*
   a. Observe child for petechiae, unusual bruising, oozing from body orifices or tubes, frank hemorrhage.
   b. Check all urine and stool for occult blood.
   c. Monitor laboratory values, including prothrombin time (PT), partial thromboplastin time (PTT), platelets.
   d. Administer blood products per physician's order.
4. Goal: *provide parents with thorough understanding of Reye syndrome.*
   a. Primary nurse assigned to provide care and follow through with teaching.
   b. Encourage parents' presence, even in PICU—explain all equipment and procedures in simple, direct terms.
   c. Provide factual, honest, and complete information regarding disease, diagnosis, and prognosis.

E. Evaluation/outcome criteria:

1. Intracranial pressure is reduced and normal neurological functioning is restored.
2. Fluid and electrolyte balance is restored.
3. No clinical evidence of bleeding is found.
4. Parents express understanding of Reye syndrome.

III. HYDROCEPHALUS

A. *Introduction:* Hydrocephalus, known to the layperson as "water on the brain," is actually a syndrome resulting from disturbances in the dynamics of CSF. The accumulation of this fluid causes enlargement and dilation of the ventricles of the brain and increased ICP. If untreated, severe brain damage will result; treatment is a surgical shunting procedure that allows CSF to drain from the ventricles of the brain to another, less harmful area within the body: most commonly the peritoneal cavity, less often the jugular vein or right atrium of the heart. Hydrocephalus can develop as the result of a *congenital malformation* (e.g., Arnold-Chiari malformation); can be *associated with other congenital defects* (e.g., spina bifida); or can be acquired secondary to infection (e.g., meningitis), trauma, or neoplasm.

B. Assessment:

1. *Head:* increased circumference—earliest sign of hydrocephalus in the infant (more than 1 inch/mo).
2. *Fontanels:* tense and bulging without head enlargement.
3. *Veins:* dilated scalp veins.
4. **"Setting sun"** sign: sclera visible above pupil; pupils are sluggish, with unequal response to light.
5. *Cry:* shrill, high pitched.
6. Developmental milestones: delayed.
7. *Reflexes:* persistence of neonatal reflexes; hyperactive reflexes.
8. Feeds poorly.
9. *Signs of increased ICP:*
   a. Vomiting.
   b. Irritability.
   c. Seizures.
   d. *Decreased* pulse.
   e. *Decreased* respirations.
   f. *Increased* blood pressure.
   g. Widened pulse pressure.
10. History may reveal other CNS defects (e.g., spina bifida), infection (e.g., meningitis), trauma, or neoplasm.

C. Analysis/nursing diagnosis:

1. *Altered cerebral tissue perfusion* related to increased intracranial pressure.
2. *Impaired skin integrity* related to enlarged head size and lack of motor coordination.
3. *Altered nutrition, less than body requirements,* related to anorexia and vomiting.
4. *Anxiety* related to diagnosis and uncertain outcome.
5. *Knowledge deficit* regarding care of the child with a shunt and follow-up care.

D. Nursing care plan/implementation:

1. Goal: *monitor neurological status.*
   a. Measure head circumference daily, and note any abnormal increase.
   b. Perform neurological checks at least every 4 hours to monitor for signs of increased ICP.
   c. Report signs of increased ICP **STAT** to physician.
   d. Assist with diagnostic procedures/treatments: *ventricular tap, computed tomography* (CT) scan, etc.
2. Goal: *health teaching to reduce parental anxiety.*
   a. Do preoperative teaching regarding the shunt procedure: stress need to remove excessive CSF to relieve pressure on brain; done as soon as possible after diagnosis is established.
   b. Stress early diagnosis and prompt shunting procedure to minimize the risk of long-term neurological complications.
   c. Offer realistic information regarding prognosis:
      (1) Surgically treated, with continued follow-up care: 80% survival rate.

(2) Of these survivors, 50% are completely normal and 50% have some degree of neurological disability (such as inattentiveness or hyperactivity).

3. Goal: *provide postoperative shunt care.*

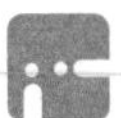

a. *Position:*

(1) Flat in bed for 24 hours to prevent subdural hematoma.

(2) Gradually increase the angle of elevation of HOB, as ordered by surgeon.

(3) On the *nonoperative side,* to prevent mechanical pressure and obstruction to shunt.

b. Monitor head circumference daily to note any abnormal increase that might indicate malfunctioning shunt.

c. Monitor vital signs; monitor for signs of increased ICP.

d. Monitor for possible complications:

(1) Infection.

(2) Malfunction of shunt: increased ICP.

4. Goal: *provide discharge teaching to parents regarding home care of the child with a shunt.*

a. Stress need for long-term follow-up care.

b. Discuss feeding techniques, care of skin (especially scalp), need for stimulation.

c. Prepare parents for shunt revisions to be done periodically as child grows.

d. Teach parents signs and symptoms of shunt malfunctioning (i.e., of increased ICP or infection) and to report these promptly to physician.

e. Encourage parents to enroll infant in "early infant stimulation" program to maximize developmental potential.

f. Stress need to monitor development at frequent intervals, make referrals prn.

E. Evaluation/outcome criteria:

1. Neurological functioning is maintained or improved.
2. Adequate nutrition is maintained.
3. No impairment of skin integrity occurs.
4. Parents' anxiety is relieved; they verbalize understanding of how to care for child after discharge.

IV. FEBRILE SEIZURES

A. *Introduction:* Febrile seizures are *transient* neurological disorders of childhood, affecting perhaps as many as 3% of all children. Although the exact cause of febrile seizures remains uncertain, they seem to be a relatively transient problem that occurs exclusively in the presence of high, spiked fevers. Children in the infant and toddler stages (6 months to 3 years) appear to be most susceptible to febrile seizures, and they are twice as common in boys as in girls. There also appears to be an increased susceptibility within families, suggesting a possible genetic predisposition. *Note:* Epilepsy is discussed in **Chapter 6.**

B. Assessment:

1. History usually reveals presence of URI or gastroenteritis.
2. Occurs with a sudden rise in fever: often spiked and quite high (102°F or higher) vs. prolonged temperature elevation.

C. Analysis/nursing diagnosis:

1. *Risk for injury* related to seizures.
2. *Knowledge deficit* related to prevention of future seizures, care of child having a seizure, and possible long-term effects.

D. Nursing care plan/implementation:

1. Goal: *reduce fever/prevent further elevation of fever.*

a. Administer antipyretics, as ordered: acetaminophen only (*not* aspirin).

b. Use cool, loose, cotton clothes to decrease heat retention.

c. *Avoid* shivering, which increases metabolic rate and temperature.

d. Encourage child to drink *cool fluids.*

e. Monitor temperature hourly.

f. Minimize stimulation, frustration for child.

2. Goal: *teach parents about care of child who experiences febrile seizure.*

a. Discuss how to prevent seizures from recurring: best method is to prevent temperature from rising over 102°F (see **Goal 1**).

b. Discuss how to handle seizures if they do recur: prevent injury, maintain airway, etc.

c. Answer questions simply and honestly:

(1) 25% of children with one febrile seizure will experience a recurrence.

(2) 75% of recurrences occur within 1 year.

(3) Reassure parents of the benign nature of febrile seizures; 95% to 98% of children with febrile seizures do not develop epilepsy or neurological damage.

E. Evaluation/outcome criteria:

1. Fever is kept below 102°F; additional seizures are prevented.
2. Parents verbalize their understanding of how to care for child at home.

RESPIRATORY SYSTEM

I. ACUTE OTITIS MEDIA

A. *Introduction:* Acute bacterial ear infection *(acute otitis media)* is common in young children, primarily because their eustachian tube is shorter and

PEDIATRICS

straighter than the adult's; this allows for ready drainage of infected mucus from URIs directly into the middle ear. In *some* cases, acute otitis media precedes the onset of *bacterial meningitis,* an extremely serious and potentially fatal disease. Bacterial meningitis is a ***medical emergency,*** requiring early detection and prompt, aggressive therapy to prevent permanent neurological damage or death. Serous otitis (chronic) may result in hearing impairment or loss but is not likely to result in meningitis (Refer to Myringotomy, **Table 5.22**).

B. Assessment:
1. Fever.
2. Pain in affected ear. An infant who is prelingual may not complain of pain but may tug at ear, cry, shake head, refuse to lie down.
3. Malaise, irritability, anorexia (possibly vomiting).
4. May have symptoms and signs of URI: rhinorrhea, coryza, cough.
5. Diminished response to sound.

C. Analysis/nursing diagnosis:
1. *Pain* related to pressure of pus/purulent material on eardrum.
2. *Risk for injury/infection* related to complication of meningitis.

D. Nursing care plan/implementation:
1. Goal: *eradicate infection and prevent further complications (meningitis).* Administer antibiotics as ordered.
2. Goal: *relieve pain and promote comfort.*
   a. Administer decongestants as ordered.
   b. Offer analgesics/antipyretics to provide symptomatic relief and to decrease fever.
3. Goal: *health teaching.*
   a. Teach parents that the child needs to finish all medication, even though child will seem clinically better within 24 to 48 hours.
   b. Review appropriate measures to control fever: antipyretics, cool sponges.

E. Evaluation/outcome criteria:
1. Infection is eradicated, no complications.
2. Child appears to be comfortable.

II. PEDIATRIC RESPIRATORY INFECTIONS

A. Assessment: general assessment of infant/child with respiratory distress. *Note:* Additional information about specific respiratory infections may be found in **Table 5.9.**
1. Restlessness—*earliest* sign of hypoxia.
2. Difficulty sucking/eating—parents may state the infant or child has "poor appetite."
3. Expiratory grunt, nasal flaring, retractions.
4. Changes in vital signs: fever, tachycardia, tachypnea.
5. Cough: productive/nonproductive.
6. Wheeze: expiratory/inspiratory.
7. Hoarseness or aphonic crying.
8. Dyspnea or prostration.
9. Dehydration—related to increase in insensible fluid loss and poor PO intake.
10. Color change (pallor, cyanosis)—*later* sign of respiratory distress.

B. Analysis/nursing diagnosis:
1. *Ineffective airway clearance* related to infection or obstruction.
2. *Fluid volume deficit* related to excessive losses through normal routes, discomfort and inability to swallow.
3. *Anxiety* related to hypoxia.
4. *Risk for injury* related to spread of infection.
5. *Knowledge deficit* related to disease process, infection control, home care, and follow-up.

C. Nursing care plan/implementation:
1. Goal: *relieve respiratory distress by reducing swelling and edema and liquefying secretions.*
   a. Environment: age- and disease-appropriate oxygen delivery system (see **Table 5.10**).
   b. Administer oxygen as ordered.
   c. *Position:* semi-Fowler's or in infant seat to promote maximum expansion of the lungs; small blanket or diaper roll under neck to keep airway patent; change position at least q2h to prevent pooling of secretions.
   d. Suction/postural drainage and percussion prn.
   e. Tape diapers loosely and use only loose-fitting clothing to *avoid* pressure on abdominal organs, which could impinge on diaphragm and impede respirations.
   f. Administer medications: antibiotics, bronchodilators, steroids.
   g. Monitor temperature q4h/prn; reduce fever with acetaminophen, cool sponges, hypothermia blanket.
2. Goal: *observe for potential respiratory failure related to exhaustion or complete airway obstruction.*
   a. Place in room near nurses' station for maximum observation.
   b. Monitor vital signs: q1h during acute phase, then q4h.
   c. Place emergency equipment near bedside prn: endotracheal tube, tracheostomy set.
   d. Monitor closely for signs of impending respiratory failure: increased rapid, shallow respirations, progressive hoarseness/aphonia, deepening cyanosis.
   e. Report adverse changes in condition STAT to physician.
3. Goal: *maintain normal fluid balance.*
   a. May be NPO initially to prevent aspiration.
   b. IVs until severe distress subsides and child is able to suck and swallow.

PEDIATRICS

Table 5.9

Pediatric Respiratory Infections

Name	Definition	Age Group	Etiology	Assessment: Definitive Clinical Signs and Symptoms	Plan: Specifics of Treatment	Prognosis
Upper Airway Infections						
Croup (acute spasmodic laryngitis)	Paroxysmal attacks (spasms of larynx)	3 months–3 years	Viral (possible allergy or psychogenic)	• Most common onset at night • Inspiratory stridor • "Croupy" barking cough • Dyspnea • Anxiety	• Teach parents—turn on hot water in bathroom and close door (steam); warm temperature will not relieve the congestion • Common to treat at home	Excellent (but likely to recur)
Epiglottitis	Extremely acute, severe, and rapid, progressive swelling (due to infection) of epiglottis and surrounding tissue	1–8 years	Bacterial (*H. influenzae* type b)	• Abrupt onset—rapid progression; **medical emergency** • Dyspnea • Dysphagia • Sit up/chin thrust/mouth open • Thick muffled voice • Cherry red, swollen epiglottis	• Do *not* visualize epiglottis unless airway support is immediately available • Will need endotracheal tube or tracheostomy for 24–48 hr to maintain patent airway IV ampicillin for 10–14 days to treat bacterial infection IV corticosteroids (e.g., Solu-Cortef) to reduce inflammation	Very good if detected and treated early Prevent via Hib immunization
Laryngotracheobronchitis (LTB)	Acute infection of lower respiratory tract: larynx, trachea, and bronchi	3 months–8 years	Viral (possible secondary bacterial infection)	• Inspiratory stridor • High fever • Signs and symptoms of severe respiratory distress • Hoarseness, progressing to aphonia and respiratory arrest without treatment	Hospitalization: • Tracheostomy set at bedside • Racemic epinephrine/steroids • Antibiotics if cultures are positive	Good
Lower Airway Infection						
Bronchiolitis/respiratory syncytial virus (RSV)	Acute viral infection of lower respiratory tract (small, low bronchioles), with resultant trapping of air	Infants 2–12 months (peak at 2–5 months)	Respiratory syncytial virus 80% of cases	• Hyperinflation of alveoli • Scattered areas of atelectasis • Acute, severe respiratory distress for first 48–72 hours, followed by rapid recovery	Supportive care during acute phase: • Hospitalization • High humidity • Oxygen • IV fluids • Clear liquids • Ribavirin (not given everywhere) • RespiGam or Synagis may be given as prophylaxis	Excellent (less than 1% mortality rate)

Table 5.10

Comparison of Common Oxygen Delivery Systems

System	Advantages	Disadvantages
Cannula	• Provides low-moderate oxygen concentration (22%–40%) • Child can talk/eat without altering FIO_2 • Possibility of more complete observation of child because nose/mouth remain unobstructed • Relatively comfortable and inexpensive	• Difficulty in controlling O_2 concentrations if child breathes through mouth • Must have patent nasal passages • Possibility of causing abdominal distention/discomfort/vomiting • Can cause drying/bleeding of nasal mucosa
Hood	• Achievement of high O_2 concentrations; FIO_2 up to 1.00 • Quick recovery time of FIO_2 • Free access to infant's chest for assessment	• Moist environment may lead to skin irritation and prevent quick assessment of color or respiratory effort • Need to remove infant for feeding and weighing
Mask	• Various sizes available • Delivers higher, more precise FIO_2 concentrations than cannula • Comfortable for older children who are quiet and do not struggle	• Accumulation of moisture on face leading to skin irritation • Possibility of aspiration of vomitus • Eating disrupts O_2 delivery • Not well tolerated by most children due to fear of suffocation
Tent	• Achievement of lower O_2 concentrations (FIO_2 of 0.3–0.5) • Child receives increased inspired O_2 concentrations even while eating • Child can move around in bed and play while receiving O_2 and humidity	• Necessity for tight fit around bed to prevent leakage of O_2 and maintain specific O_2 concentrations • Child is difficult to see/assess • Cool/wet tent environment will decrease body temperature, increasing O_2 requirements • Inspired O_2 levels will fall whenever tent is entered for caregiving purposes

c. Monitor hydration status: I&O, urine specific gravity, weight.

d. When resuming PO fluids—start with sips of clear liquids, advance slowly as tolerated: Pedialyte, clear broth, gelatin, popsicles, fruit juices, ginger ale.

e. **Avoid** milk/milk products, which may cause increased mucus production.

4. Goal: *provide calm, secure environment.*
   a. During acute distress: remain with child/family (do **not** leave unattended).
   b. Keep crying to a minimum to prevent severe hypoxia and to reduce the body's demand for oxygen.
   c. *Avoid* painful/intrusive procedures if possible.
   d. Organize nursing care to provide planned periods of uninterrupted rest.
   e. Allow parents to room-in, and encourage their participation in care of their child to keep the child relatively calm and reduce anxiety.
   f. Allow child to keep favorite toy or security object.
5. Goal: *provide parents with teaching, as necessary.*
   a. *Short term:* discuss equipment, treatments, procedures; offer frequent progress reports, answer parents' questions.
   b. *Long term:* how to handle recurrences, how to check temperature at home, medications for fever, when to call physician about respiratory problem.

D. Evaluation/outcome criteria:

1. No further evidence of respiratory distress.
2. Resumption of normal respiratory pattern.
3. Normal fluid balance maintained/restored.
4. Parents verbalize their concerns and express confidence in their ability to care for their child after discharge.

III. LONG-TERM RESPIRATORY DYSFUNCTION: ASTHMA

A. *Introduction:* Asthma is generally considered a chronic, lower airway disorder characterized by heightened airway reactivity with bronchospasm and obstruction. The exact cause of asthma is unknown; however, it is believed to include an allergic reaction to one or more allergens, or "triggers," that either precipitate or aggravate asthmatic exacerbation. The child usually exhibits other symptoms of allergy, such as infantile eczema or hay fever; in addition, 75% of children with asthma have a positive family history for asthma. The onset is usually before age 5 and the disorder remains with the child throughout life, although some children experience dramatic

PEDIATRICS

improvement in their asthma with the onset of puberty. Most children do *not* require continuous medication. Early relief of symptoms with a combination of drugs can reverse bronchospasm.

B. Assessment:

1. Expiratory wheeze.
2. General signs and symptoms of respiratory distress, including: anxiety, cough, shortness of breath, crackles, cyanosis due to obstruction within the respiratory tract, use of accessory muscles of respirations.
3. Cough: hacking, paroxysmal, nonproductive; especially at night.
4. *Position* of comfort for breathing: sitting straight up, leaning forward, which is the position for optimal lung expansion.
5. Peak expiratory flow rate (PEFR) is in the *yellow* zone (50%–80% of personal best) or in the *red* zone (<50% of personal best).

C. Analysis/nursing diagnosis:

1. *Ineffective airway clearance* related to bronchospasm.
2. *Anxiety* related to breathlessness.
3. *Knowledge deficit,* actual or risk for potential, related to disease process, treatment, and prevention of future asthmatic attacks.
4. *Activity intolerance* related to dyspnea and bronchospasm.

D. Nursing care plan/implementation:
Treatment is aimed toward *improvement of ventilation, correction of dehydration and acidosis,* and *management of concurrent infection.*

1. Goal: *provide patent airway and effective breathing patterns.*
   a. Initiate oxygen therapy (by tent, face mask, or cannula), as ordered, to relieve hypoxia, with high humidity (to liquefy secretions).
   b. Administer bronchodilators, as ordered, to relieve the obstruction: epinephrine (1:1000), nebulized albuterol, *Atrovent.* Inhalers may be used with metered-dose inhalers (MDIs) to ensure proper delivery of the medication.
   c. Administer corticosteroids as ordered (PO or IV) to reduce inflammation, relieve edema (prednisone, *Decadron*) and decrease bronchial hyperreactivity.
   d. Administer antibiotics as ordered; infection is commonly either a trigger or complication of asthma.
   e. *Note:* methylxanthines (theophylline, aminophylline) are third-line agents that are rarely used to treat asthma.
2. Goal: *relieve anxiety.*
   a. Provide relief from hypoxia (refer to **Goal 1**), which is the chief source of anxiety.
   b. Remain with child, offer support.
   c. Administer sedation as ordered.
   d. Encourage parents to remain with child.
3. Goal: *teach principles of prophylaxis.*

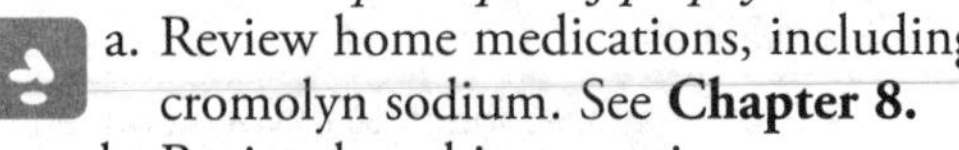

   a. Review home medications, including cromolyn sodium. See **Chapter 8.**
   b. Review breathing exercises.
   c. Discuss precipitating factors ("triggers") and offer suggestions on how to avoid them.
   d. Teach how to use peak expiratory flowmeter to monitor respiratory status and determine need for treatment.
   e. Introduce need for child to assume control over own care.

E. Evaluation/outcome criteria:

1. Adequate oxygenation provided, as evidenced by pink color of nailbeds and mucous membranes and ease in respiratory effort.
2. Anxiety is relieved.
3. Child verbalizes confidence in, and demonstrates mastery of, skills needed to care for own asthma.

IV. CYSTIC FIBROSIS

A. *Introduction:* Cystic fibrosis is a generalized dysfunction of the exocrine glands that produces multisystem involvement. The disorder is inherited as an autosomal recessive defect. The mutated gene responsible for CF is located on the long arm of chromosome 7 (*CFTR*). The basic problem is one of *thick, sticky, tenacious mucous secretions that obstruct* the ducts of the exocrine glands, thus affecting their ability to function. Cystic fibrosis is found in all races and socioeconomic groups, although there is a significantly lower incidence in Asians and African Americans. It is a chronic disease with no known cure and guarded prognosis; median age at death in the United States is 31 years. Those born in the late 1990s can be expected to survive into their 40s with new therapies.

B. Assessment:

1. Newborn: *meconium ileus.*
2. Frequent, recurrent *pulmonary infections:* bronchitis, bronchopneumonia, pneumonia, and ultimately chronic obstructive pulmonary disease (COPD) due to mechanical obstruction of respiratory tract caused by thick, tenacious mucous gland secretions.
3. *Malabsorption syndrome:* failure to gain weight, distended abdomen, thin arms and legs, lack of subcutaneous fat due to disturbed absorption of nutrients that results from the inability of pancreatic enzymes to reach intestinal tract.
4. *Steatorrhea:* bulky, foul-smelling, frothy, fatty stools in increased amounts and frequency (predisposed to rectal prolapse).
5. Parents may note that child *"tastes salty"* when kissed, due to excessive loss of sodium and chloride in sweat.

6. *Sweat test* reveals high sodium and chloride levels in child's sweat, unique to children with cystic fibrosis.
7. Sexual development:
   a. *Boys/Men:* sterile (due to aspermia).
   b. *Girls/Women:* difficulty conceiving and bearing children (due to increased viscosity of cervical mucus, which acts as a plug in the cervical os and mechanically blocks the entry of sperm).

C. Analysis/nursing diagnosis:
1. *Ineffective breathing patterns* related to thick, viscid secretions.
2. *Altered nutrition, less than body requirements,* related to diarrhea and poor intestinal absorption of nutrients.
3. *Decreased cardiac output* related to COPD and decreased compliance of lungs.
4. *Activity intolerance* related to respiratory compromise.
5. *Self-esteem disturbance* related to body image changes.
6. *Knowledge deficit* related to disease process, treatments, medications, genetics.
7. *Risk for noncompliance* related to complicated and prolonged treatment regimen.

D. Nursing care plan/implementation:
1. Goal: *assist child to expectorate sputum.*
   a. Perform postural drainage and percussion as prescribed: first thing in morning, between meals, before bedtime, *not* after meals to prevent aspiration.
   b. Administer nebulizer treatments, expectorants, mucolytics, bronchodilators. *Avoid* or limit use of medications that suppress cough mechanism.
   c. Provide for exercises that promote position changes and keep sputum moving up and out.
   d. Encourage *high fluid intake* to keep secretions liquefied.
   e. Suction, administer oxygen prn.
2. Goal: *prevent infection.*
   a. Standard precautions to prevent infection.
   b. Evaluate carefully, check continually for potential infection (especially respiratory); report to physician promptly.
   c. Limit contact with staff or visitors (especially children) with infection.
   d. Administer antibiotics as ordered, to *treat* respiratory infections and *prevent* overwhelming sepsis.
   e. May be placed on *prophylactic* antibiotic therapy *between* episodes of infection.
   f. Teach importance of prevention of infection at home: adequate nutrition, frequent medical checkups, stay away from known sources of infection.
3. Goal: *maintain adequate nutrition.*

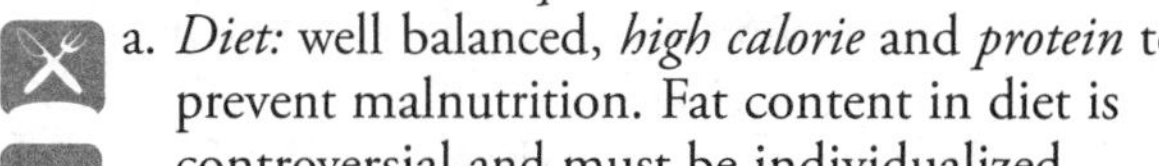

   a. *Diet:* well balanced, *high calorie* and *protein* to prevent malnutrition. Fat content in diet is controversial and must be individualized.
   b. Administer *pancreatic enzyme* (Pancrease, Ultrase) immediately before *every* meal and *every* snack to enhance the absorption of vital nutrients, especially fats.
   c. If child is unable to swallow capsules, take capsule apart and sprinkle on food at beginning of meal or mix with chilled applesauce.
   d. Administer water-miscible preparations of *fat-soluble vitamins* (A, D, E, K), multivitamins, and iron.
   e. Encourage *extra salt* intake to compensate for excessive sodium losses in sweat (unless congestive heart failure [CHF] is present); especially important in hot weather, after physical exertion, febrile periods.
   f. Encourage *extra fluid* intake (e.g., *Gatorade*) to *prevent* dehydration/electrolyte imbalance, ↑ thickening of mucous secretions.
   g. Daily I&O and weights to monitor nutritional and hydration status.
   h. Encourage child to assume gradually increasing responsibility for choosing own foods within dietary restrictions.
4. Goal: *teach child and family about cystic fibrosis.*
   a. Discuss diagnostic procedures: sweat test, stool specimens.
   b. Review multiple medications: use, effects, side/toxic effects.
   c. Stress need to care for pulmonary system (major cause of mortality/morbidity).
   d. Teach various treatments: postural drainage, nebulizers, oxygen therapy, breathing exercise.
   e. Encourage child to assume as much responsibility for own care as possible: medications, treatments, diet.
   f. Promote development of healthy attitude toward disease/prognosis (no known cure). Heart/lung transplantation may be considered as an option.
   g. Refer to appropriate community agencies for assistance with home care.
   h. Assist with genetic counseling.
   i. Discuss sexual concerns with adolescent.
5. Goal: *promote compliance with treatment regimen.*
   a. Encourage child to verbalize anger or frustration at being "different"/body image alterations.

b. Suggest alternatives to chest physical therapy (CPT) (e.g., yoga/standing on head).
c. Offer "rewards" for compliance: going swimming with friends or other types of peer activities.

E. Evaluation/outcome criteria:

1. Child can clear own airway, expectorate sputum.
2. Child is maintained in infection-free state.
3. Adequate nutrition is maintained.
4. Child and family verbalize understanding of the disease.
5. Child complies with rigors of treatment.

V. APNEA-RELATED DISORDERS

A. Apnea of infancy

1. *Introduction:* Apnea of infancy is the unexplained cessation of breathing for 20 seconds or longer in an apparently healthy, full-term infant who is more than 37 weeks of gestation. It is usually diagnosed by the second month of life and is generally thought to resolve during the first 12 to 15 months of life. The exact cause is unknown. The association between apnea of infancy and sudden infant death syndrome (SIDS) is still controversial. However, infants experiencing significant apnea without a known cause are thought to be at increased risk for SIDS and must be treated accordingly. The diagnosis of apnea of infancy (AOI) is made when no identifiable cause for the apparent life-threatening event (ALTE) is found.
2. **Assessment:**
   a. Unexplained cessation of breathing (apnea) for 20 seconds or longer.
   b. Bradycardia.
   c. Color change: cyanosis or pallor.
   d. Limp, hypotonic.
   e. Diagnostic tests, including cardiopneumogram, pneumocardiogram, and polysomnography.
3. **Analysis/nursing diagnosis:**
   a. *Ineffective breathing patterns* related to apnea.
   b. *Anxiety, fear* related to apnea and threat of infant's death.
   c. *Knowledge deficit* regarding home care of infant on an apnea monitor and infant cardiopulmonary resuscitation (CPR).
4. **Nursing care plan/intervention:**
   a. Goal: *maintain effective breathing pattern.*
      (1) Apnea monitor on infant at all times, including at home.
      (2) Place in room near nurses' station for maximum observation with a nurse or parent present at all times.
      (3) Suction, oxygen, and resuscitation equipment readily available if needed.
      (4) Observe for apnea or bradycardia; note duration and associated symptoms—color change, change in muscle tone.
      (5) If apnea occurs, use gentle stimulation to start infant breathing again. If ineffective, begin CPR **(Figs. 5.1** and **5.2).**
      (6) If suctioning is needed, do it gently for the shortest time and least number of times possible to maintain patent airway. *Note:* Repeated, vigorous suctioning is associated with prolonged periods of apnea.
      (7) Medications: respiratory stimulant drugs (such as theophylline or caffeine) may be given until 2 to 3 months have passed without an episode of apnea.
      (8) *Positions:* side-lying or supine; *never* prone, to prevent SIDS.
      (9) Feedings: smaller and more frequent; *avoid* overfeeding, which can lead to reflux and apnea.
   b. Goal: *teach parents how to care for their infant at home* **(Table 5.11).**
      (1) Thoroughly explain discharge plans to parents; encourage questions and discussion.
      (2) Begin teaching use of apnea monitor and infant CPR techniques several days before discharge; allow parents to handle the monitor and become thoroughly familiar with its use.
      (3) Provide parents with emergency response numbers and community health nurse referral.
      (4) Stress need for at least *1 year of ongoing care* with constant use of monitor, or 2 to 3 months without an episode requiring intervention.
      (5) Discuss need for support and refer to local self-help/support group.
      (6) Encourage parents to take time for themselves if a reliable caregiver is available who is trained in use of monitor and infant CPR.
5. **Evaluation/outcome criteria:**
   a. Effective breathing pattern is established.
   b. Parents verbalize their concerns and express confidence in their ability to care for their infant at home.

B. Sudden infant death syndrome (SIDS)

1. *Introduction:* SIDS is the *sudden, unexpected* death of an apparently healthy infant under 1 year of age, which remains *unexplained* after a complete postmortem examination. Various

PEDIATRICS

	Objectives	ACTIONS		
		Adult	Child (1 year to puberty)	Infant (up to 1 year)
A. RECOGNITION	1. Determine unresponsiveness.	Tap victim or gently shake shoulder. Say, "Are you okay?" Speak loudly.		
	2. Determine breathlessness.	Check for absent breathing or abnormal breathing (such as agonal gasps).	Check for absent breathing or only agonal gasps.	
	3. Determine pulselessness.	Feel for carotid pulse (no more than 10 seconds).		Feel for brachial pulse (no more than 10 seconds).
	4. Recognize emergency and get help.	Activate EMS. Get Automated External Defibrillator (AED), if available. Deploy AED as soon as available but do not delay CPR.		
B. CPR	5. Start CPR.	Use CAB sequence: Compression, Airway, Breathing.		
C. COMPRESSION	6. Begin chest compressions: Landmark check.	Imagine a line drawn between the nipples of the chest.		
	7. Position hands.	Place hand(s) at center of breastbone between nipples.		*Single rescuer:* Place 2 fingers just between nipple line. *Two-person rescuer:* use 2 thumb-encircling hands technique.
	8. Push hard.	Depress at least 2 inches.	Depress at least 1/3 depth of chest, about 2 inches.	Depress at least 1/3 depth of chest, about 1.5 inches.
	9. Push fast.	Perform compressions at a rate of at least 100 per minute.		
	10. Allow chest recoil.	Allow chest to recoil completely between compressions.		
	11. Minimize interruptions.	Limit interruptions to 10 seconds or less while performing compressions. Two-person rescuers should rotate every 2 minutes.		
		Perform compressions only if not CPR proficient and continue to step 15. If proficient, continue to steps 12-15.		
D. AIRWAY	12. Open airway.	Perform head tilt–chin lift (or jaw thrust, if trauma suspected).		
E. BREATHING	13. Provide ventilations until advanced airway established.	Give 2 breaths for every 30 compressions (1 or 2 rescuers).	Give 2 breaths for every 30 compressions for single rescuer; give 2 breaths for every 15 compressions for 2 rescuers.	
	14. Provide ventilations with advanced airway in place.	Provide 1 breath every 6-8 seconds during uninterrupted CPR; one second per breath. Observe for chest rise.		
F. DEFIBRILLATION	15. Defibrillate.	Apply and deploy AED as soon as available. Minimize interruptions in compressions before and continue compressions immediately after shock delivered.		

Figure 5.1 CPR recommendations for the healthcare provider. If victim is breathing or resumes effective breathing, place in recovery position; (1) move head, shoulders, and torso simultaneously; (2) turn onto side; (3) leg not in contact with ground may be bent and knee moved forward to stabilize victim; (4) victim should not be moved in any way if trauma is suspected and should not be placed in recovery position if rescue breathing or CPR is required. (Modified from CPR Overview: 2010 American Heart Association guidelines for cardiopulmonary resuscitation and emergency cardiovascular care. Circulation, 122[18 Suppl 3], 2010. Adapted from Hockenberry, M, & Wilson, D: *Wong's Nursing Care of Infants and Children,* ed 8. Mosby, St. Louis, 2007.)

theories have been suggested, none proved; research is ongoing. It has been suggested that prone sleeping position, cigarette smoke, and excessive swaddling may be associated with SIDS. It is the third leading cause of death between 1 month and 1 year, affecting almost 2500 infants annually.

2. **Assessment:**
   a. Sudden, unexplained death in otherwise "normal" infant; occurs exclusively during sleep.

Signs of life-threatening obstruction: truly choking child ***cannot speak***, becomes ***cyanotic***, and ***collapses***.				
	Objectives	**ACTIONS**		
		Adult	**Child (1 year to puberty)**	**Infant (up to 1 year)**
CONSCIOUS VICTIM	1. Determine airway obstruction.	Ask, "Are you choking?" Determine if victim can cough or speak.		Observe breathing difficulty, ineffective cough, no strong cry.
	2. Act to relieve obstruction.	Perform up to 5 subdiaphragmatic abdominal thrusts.		Give 5 back blows. Give 5 chest thrusts.
	3. Be persistent.	Repeat Step 2 until obstruction is relieved or victim becomes unconscious.		
VICTIM WHO BECOMES UNCONSCIOUS	4. Position the victim and get help.	Turn on back as a unit, supporting head and neck, face up, arms by sides. Call out, "Help!" Activate EMS. If second rescuer available, have person activate EMS.		
	5. Start CPR.	Use CAB sequence: Compression, Airway, Breathing. Perform a series of 30 chest compressions first. Do **not** perform pulse check.		
	6. Open airway.	Perform head tilt–chin lift (do **not** tilt too far for infants).		
	7. Look for foreign object.	If you see foreign body, remove it. Do **not** perform a blind finger sweep.		
	8. Give rescue breaths.	Attempt to give 2 rescue breaths.		
	9. Continue CPR.	Continue with chest compressions and attempted ventilations until obstruction is relieved. After 2 minutes of CPR, activate EMS if this has not already been done.		

Figure 5.2 Foreign body airway obstruction management. (Modified from CPR Overview: 2010 American Heart Association guidelines for cardiopulmonary resuscitation and emergency cardiovascular care. Circulation, 122[18 Suppl 3], 2010. Adapted from Hockenberry, M, & Wilson, D: *Wong's Nursing Care of Infants and Children,* ed 8. Mosby, St. Louis, 2007.)

Table 5.11

Guidelines for Home Care of Infant on Apnea Monitor

1. Show the parents how to connect the monitor leads.
2. Remind parents to remove the leads unless they are connected to the infant.
3. Stress that the infant must be on the monitor whenever respirations are not being directly observed and that a trained person must be present in the home at all times in case the alarm sounds.
4. Teach parents **not** to adjust the monitor to eliminate false alarms.
5. Explain that the infant will need direct observation whenever loud noises could obscure the monitor alarm (e.g., dishwasher, vacuum).
6. Teach parents what to look for when alarm sounds (i.e., loose monitor leads vs. apnea).
7. Teach parents how to assess the infant for an episode of apnea (i.e., lack of respirations, duration, color, muscle tone).
8. Teach the parents to first use gentle physical stimulation if the infant experiences an apnea spell (e.g., touching the face or stroking the soles of the feet).
9. Demonstrate infant CPR to be used if tactile stimulation is not effective in reestablishing respirations.
10. Encourage parents to keep emergency numbers posted near the telephone.
11. Explain that monitor will not interfere with normal growth and development. Encourage the parents to promote normal growth and development as much as possible.

Also refer to **Table 3.9,** Safety Considerations, **p. 94.**

b. Note overall appearance of infant (differentiate from child abuse).
c. Obtain history from parents—note affect or how parents are dealing with grief.

3. **Analysis/nursing diagnosis:**
   a. *Dysfunctional grieving* related to loss of infant.
   b. *Knowledge deficit* related to SIDS.
4. **Nursing care plan/implementation:**
   a. *Immediate goal:* support parents who are grieving.
      (1) Stress that nothing could have been done to prevent the death.
      (2) Allow parents to express grief emotions; provide privacy.

(3) Offer parents opportunity to see, hold infant.
(4) Explain purpose of autopsy (physician to obtain consent).
(5) Contact spiritual advisor: priest, rabbi, minister.
(6) Assist parents to plan what to tell siblings.

b. *Ongoing goal:* provide factual information regarding SIDS.
(1) Offer information that is known about SIDS in simple, direct terms **(Table 5.12).**
(2) Answer questions honestly.
(3) Give parents printed literature on SIDS.
(4) Refer to local/national SIDS foundation group.

c. *Long-term goal:* assist family to resolve grief.
(1) Track progress of other siblings.
(2) Refer to local perinatal bereavement group.
(3) Consider subsequent pregnancy to be at risk for:
(a) Attachment/bonding.
(b) SIDS recurrence.

5. **Evaluation/outcome criteria:**
a. Parents are able to express their grief and receive adequate support.
b. Parents raise questions about SIDS and can understand answers.
c. Family's grief is resolved; in time, normal family dynamics resume.

CARDIOVASCULAR SYSTEM

I. CONGENITAL HEART DISEASE (CHD)

A. *Introduction:* There are more than 35 documented types of congenital heart defects, which occur in 5 to 8 per 1000 live births. For the purpose of this review, only five *major* defects are given. These are presented in **Figures 5.3** through **5.7.** *Note:* The

(text continues on page 279)

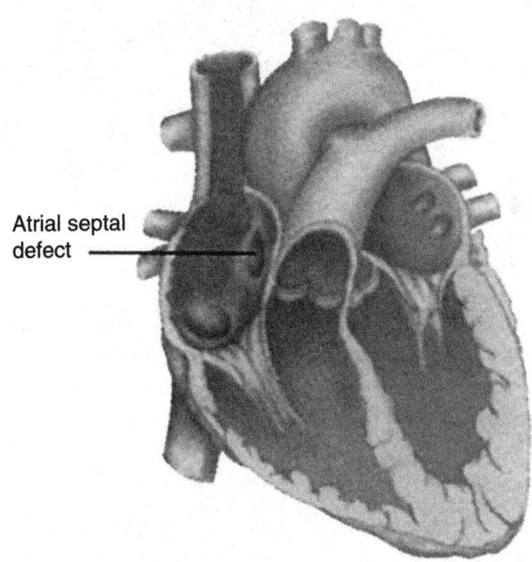

Figure 5.3 Atrial septal defect. An opening between the two atria, allowing oxygenated blood and unoxygenated blood to mix. Left-to-right shunting of blood occurs due to the higher pressure on the left side of the heart. (From Ashwill, JW & James, SR: *Nursing Care of Children: Principles and Practice.* WB Saunders, Philadelphia, 2007.)

PEDIATRICS

Table 5.12

SIDS: What to Tell Families

Concern	Facts
Cause	Unknown (possibly related to delayed maturation of cardiorespiratory system)
Incidence	Almost 2500 cases annually; leading cause of death between ages 1 month and 1 year
When	Occurs during *sleep* (nap, night)
Age	Peak at 2–4 months; 95% of cases occur by age *6 months*
Sex	More common in boys
Race	More common in African Americans, Native Americans, and Hispanics
Season	More common in *winter*, peaks in January
Siblings	May have greater incidence
Perinatal	More common in preterm infants, in *multiple* births, in infants with *low Apgar scores*, and with maternal smoking
Socioeconomic	More common in lower socioeconomic classes
Feeding habits	More common in infants who are bottle-fed, less common in infants who are breastfed.
Means of prevention	*Supine* (on back) sleeping position (mnemonic: "back to sleep"); *avoid* soft bedding and overheating during sleep; *avoid* cigarette smoking in house.

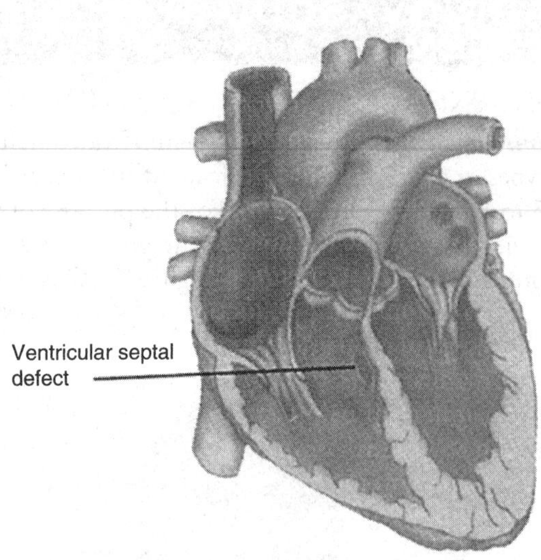

Figure 5.4 Ventricular septal defect. An opening between the two ventricles, allowing oxygenated and unoxygenated blood to mix. Shunting of blood occurs due to the higher pressure on the left side of the heart. Ventricular septal defects are classified as membranous or muscular according to location in the septum. (From Ashwill, JW & James, SR: *Nursing Care of Children: Principles and Practice.* WB Saunders, Philadelphia, 2007.)

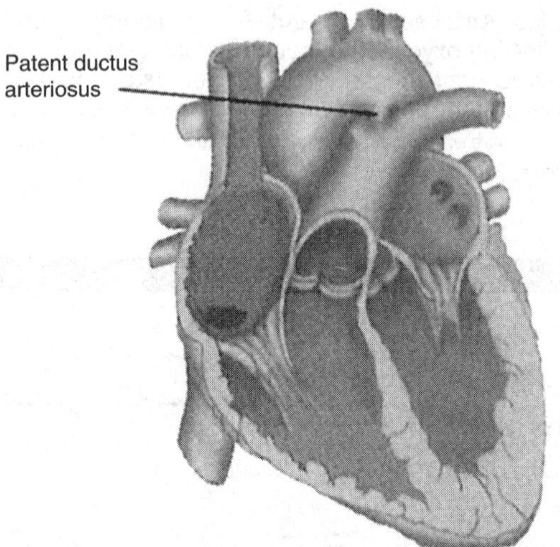

Figure 5.5 Patent ductus arteriosus. An artery that connects the aorta and the pulmonary artery during fetal life. It generally closes spontaneously within a few hours to several days after birth. Allows abnormal blood flow from the high-pressure aorta to the low-pressure pulmonary artery, resulting in a left-to-right shunt. (From Ashwill, JW & James, SR: *Nursing Care of Children: Principles and Practice.* WB Saunders, Philadelphia, 2007.)

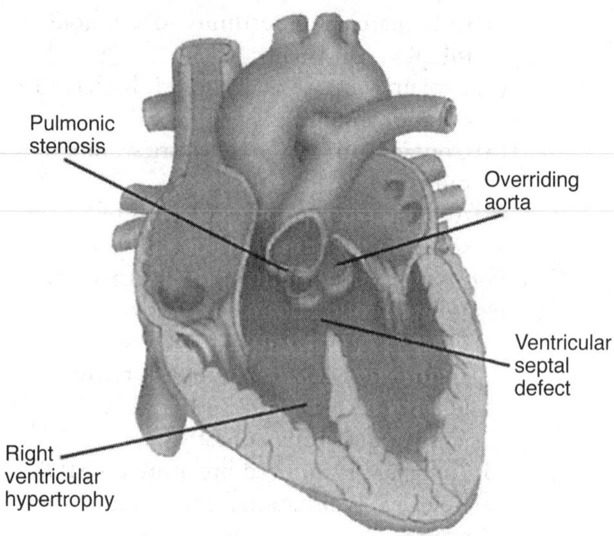

Figure 5.6 Tetralogy of Fallot. Four cardiac anomalies make up tetralogy of Fallot: a ventricular septal defect, pulmonary stenosis, an overriding aorta, and right ventricular hypertrophy. There are other associated defects in certain cases. Pulmonary stenosis results in reduction of pulmonary blood flow; the ventricular septal defect allows mixing of oxygenated and unoxygenated blood. (From Ashwill, JW & James, SR: *Nursing Care of Children: Principles and Practice.* WB Saunders, Philadelphia, 2007.)

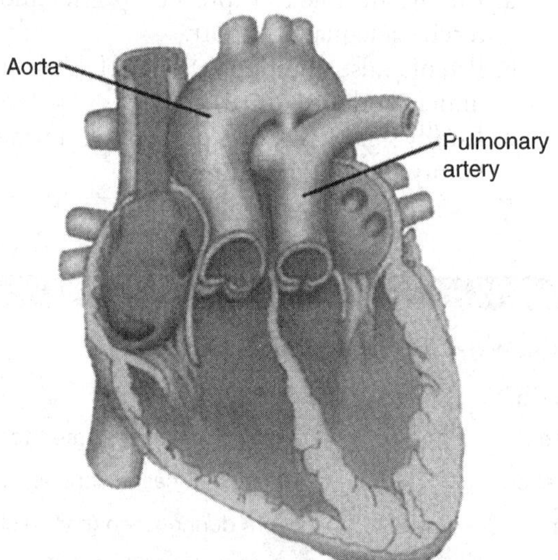

Figure 5.7 Transposition of the great arteries. The aorta and the pulmonary artery are reversed; that is, the aorta rises from the right instead of the left ventricle, and the pulmonary artery arises from the left instead of the right ventricle. Systemic venous blood (unoxygenated blood) returns to the right side of the heart to pass through the aorta back to the body without being oxygenated because of bypassing the lungs. The pulmonary venous blood (oxygenated blood) enters the left side of the heart, returning to the lungs via the pulmonary artery. The systemic (unoxygenated) and pulmonary (oxygenated) circulations are totally separate. There must be some opening (i.e., patent ductus arteriosus or septal defect) to allow blood to mix. (From Ashwill, JW & James, SR: *Nursing Care of Children: Principles and Practice.* WB Saunders, Philadelphia, 2007.)

content has been synthesized for ease in review and recall; for additional study aids, the student may wish to refer to **Tables 5.13** and **5.14. Chapter 6** also contains information on congestive heart failure, and **Chapter 8** covers the most commonly used drugs, including digoxin and furosemide (*Lasix*).

B. Assessment:

1. Exact cause unknown, but related factors include:
   a. Familial history of CHD, especially in siblings, parents.
   b. Presence of other genetic defects in infant (e.g., Down syndrome, trisomy 13 or 18).
   c. History of maternal prenatal infection with rubella, cytomegalovirus, etc.
   d. High-risk maternal factors:
      (1) Age: under 18 years, over 40 years.
      (2) Weight: under 100 lb, over 200 lb.
      (3) Maternal type 1 (insulin-dependent) diabetes.
   e. Maternal history of drinking during pregnancy, with resultant "fetal alcohol syndrome."
   f. Extracardiac defects, including tracheoesophageal fistula, renal agenesis, and diaphragmatic hernia.

Table 5.13

Comparison of Acyanotic and Cyanotic Heart Disease

Feature	Acyanotic	Cyanotic
Shunting of blood	L → R	R → L
Cyanosis	*Not usual* (unless congestive heart failure)	*Always;* "blue babies"
Surgery	Usually done in one stage—technically simple	Usually done in several stages—technically complex
Prognosis	Very good/excellent	Guarded
Major types	1. Atrial septal defect (ASD) 2. Ventricular septal defect (VSD) 3. Patent ductus arteriosus (PDA) 4. Coarctation of the aorta (COA)	1. Tetralogy of Fallot (ToF) 2. Transposition of the great vessels (TGV)

Table 5.14

Overview of the Most Common Types of Congenital Heart Disease

Type of Defect	Medical Treatment	Surgical Treatment	Prognosis
Acyanotic			
Atrial septal defect (ASD)	Clinical trials using device closure during cardiac catheterization	Open chest/open heart surgery with closure through patch (recommended age: preschooler).	Excellent, with survival rate greater than 99%
Ventricular septal defect (VSD)	Clinical trials using device closure during cardiac catheterization	*Palliative treatment:* pulmonary banding; *definitive repair:* same as for **ASD**	Excellent, with 95% or greater survival rate
Patent ductus arteriosus (PDA)	In newborns, attempt pharmacological closure with indomethacin (prostaglandin inhibitor)	Open chest: surgical division or ligation of the patent ductus	Excellent, with survival rate greater than 99%
Coarctation of the aorta (COA)	Infants or children with CHF: digoxin and diuretics	Open chest: resection of coarcted portion of aorta with end-to-end anastomosis within first 2 years of life Nonsurgical: balloon angioplasty	Fair—less than 5% mortality rate
Cyanotic			
Tetralogy of Fallot (ToF)	None—supportive prn	Often done in *stages* with definitive repair accomplished within first year of life	Fair—less than 5% mortality rate
Transposition of the great vessels (TGV)	None—supportive prn	Arterial switch procedure during first weeks of life	Guarded—5%–10% mortality rate

2. Most frequent parental complaint: *difficulty feeding.*
   a. Infant must be awakened to feed.
   b. Has weak suck.
   c. May turn blue when eating, especially with cyanotic defects.
   d. Infant takes overly long time to feed.
   e. Falls asleep during feeding, without finishing.
3. Nursing observations
   a. *Most frequent symptom*—tachycardia, as body attempts to compensate for lack of oxygen (hypoxia): heart rate over 160 beats/min.
   b. Tachypnea, corresponding to heart rate: respirations over 60 breaths/min.
   c. Cyanosis due to hypoxia:
      (1) *Not* with acyanotic defects (unless CHF is present).
      (2) *Always* with cyanotic defects ("blue infants").
   d. Failure to grow at a normal rate: slow weight gain, height and weight below the norm due to difficulty feeding and hypoxia.
   e. Developmental delays related to weakened physical condition.
   f. Frequent respiratory infections associated with increased pulmonary blood flow or aspiration.
   g. Dyspnea on exertion due to hypoxia, shunting of blood.
   h. Murmurs may or may not be present (e.g., patent ductus arteriosus [PDA] machinery murmur).
   i. Changes in blood pressure (e.g., coarctation—*increased* blood pressure in arms; *decreased* blood pressure in legs).
   j. Possible congestive heart failure—refer to **Chapter 6.** *Note:* Infants may *not* demonstrate distended neck veins and may have difficult-to-detect generalized edema if not yet walking—check for facial, scrotal edema.
   k. Cyanotic heart defects:
      (1) **"Tet spells"**—choking spells with paroxysmal dyspnea: severe hypoxia, deepening cyanosis; relieved by placing infant in knee-chest position, which alters cardiopulmonary dynamics, thus increasing the flow of blood to the lungs.
      (2) Clubbing of fingers and toes—due to chronic hypoxia.
      (3) Polycythemia (increased red blood cells [RBCs]) with possible thrombi/emboli formation.

C. Analysis/nursing diagnosis:

1. *Ineffective breathing pattern* related to tachypnea and respiratory infection.
2. *Activity intolerance* related to tachycardia and hypoxia.
3. *Altered nutrition, less than body requirements,* related to difficulty in feeding.
4. *Risk for infection* related to poor nutritional status.
5. *Knowledge deficit* related to diagnostic procedures, condition, surgical/medical treatments, prognosis.

D. Nursing care plan/implementation:

1. Goal: *promote adequate oxygenation.*
   a. Administer oxygen per physician's order/prn.
   b. Use loose-fitting clothing; tape diapers loosely to *avoid* pressure on abdominal organs, which could impinge on diaphragm and impede respiration.
   c. *Position:* neck slightly hyperextended to keep airway patent; place in knee-chest position to relieve "tet spell" (choking spell).
   d. Suction prn to clear the airway.
   e. Administer *digoxin,* per physician's order, to slow and strengthen heart's pumping action (refer to **Chapter 8** and to **Table 5.6** for pediatric pulse rate norms).
   f. Monitor pulse oximetry, as ordered.
2. Goal: *reduce workload of heart to conserve energy.*
   a. *Position:* infant seat, semi-Fowler's to promote maximum expansion of the lungs.
   b. Provide pacifier to promote psychological rest.
   c. Organize nursing care to provide periods of uninterrupted rest.
   d. Adjust physical activity according to child's condition, capabilities to conserve energy.
   e. Provide diversion, as tolerated, to meet developmental needs yet conserve energy.
   f. *Avoid* extremes of temperature to avoid the stress of hypothermia/hyperthermia, which will increase the body's demand for oxygen.
   g. Administer diuretics (*Lasix*), per physician's order, to eliminate excess fluids, which increase the heart's workload. *Note:* Refer to **Chapter 8.**
3. Goal: *provide for adequate nutrition.*
   a. May need standard infant formula with ↑ caloric density to minimize fluid retention and meet nutritional needs.
   b. Discourage foods with high or added sodium to minimize fluid retention.
   c. I&O, daily/weekly weights, and monitor for rate of growth.
   d. Limit PO feedings to 20 minutes to *avoid* overtiring infant. Supplement PO feeding with gavage feeding (prn with physician's order) to meet fluid and caloric needs.
   e. Encourage foods *high in potassium* (prevent hypokalemia) and *high in iron* (prevent anemia). *Note:* Refer to **Chapter 9.**

4. Goal: *prevent infection.*
   a. Standard precautions to prevent infection.
   b. Use good hand-washing technique.
   c. Limit contact with staff/visitors (especially children) with infections.
   d. Monitor for early symptoms and signs of infection; report STAT.
5. Goal: *meet teaching needs of client, family.*
   a. Explain diagnostic procedures: blood tests, x-rays, urine, ECG, echocardiogram, cardiac catheterization.
   b. Explain condition/treatment/prognosis (see **Table 5.14**).
   c. Review nutrition and medications.
   d. Discuss how to adjust realistically to life with congenital heart disease, activity restrictions, etc.

E. Evaluation/outcome criteria:

1. Child's level of oxygenation is maintained, as evidenced by pink color in nailbeds and mucous membranes (for both light- and dark-skinned children) and ease in respiratory effort.
2. Energy is conserved, thus reducing the heart's workload as evidenced by vital signs within normal limits.
3. The child's fluid and caloric requirements are met, allowing for physical growth to occur at normal or near-normal rate.
4. The family (and child, when old enough) verbalize their understanding of the type of CHD, its treatment, and prognosis.
5. The family and child demonstrate adequate coping mechanisms to deal with CHD.

II. RHEUMATIC FEVER

A. *Introduction:* Rheumatic fever is an acute, systemic, inflammatory disease affecting multiple organs and systems: heart, joints, CNS, collagenous tissue, etc. Thought to be autoimmune in nature, it most commonly follows a streptococcus infection (**Fig. 5.8**) and occurs primarily in school-age children. In addition, it tends to recur, and the risk of permanent heart damage increases with each subsequent attack of rheumatic fever.

B. Assessment:

1. *Major manifestations* (modified Jones criteria)
   a. *Carditis:* tachycardia, cardiomegaly, murmur, congestive heart failure (CHF).
   b. *Migratory polyarthritis:* swollen, hot, red, and excruciatingly painful large joints; migratory and reversible.
   c. *Sydenham's chorea* (St. Vitus' dance): sudden, aimless, irregular movements of the extremities; involuntary facial grimaces, speech disturbances, emotional lability, muscle weakness; completely reversible.

PEDIATRICS

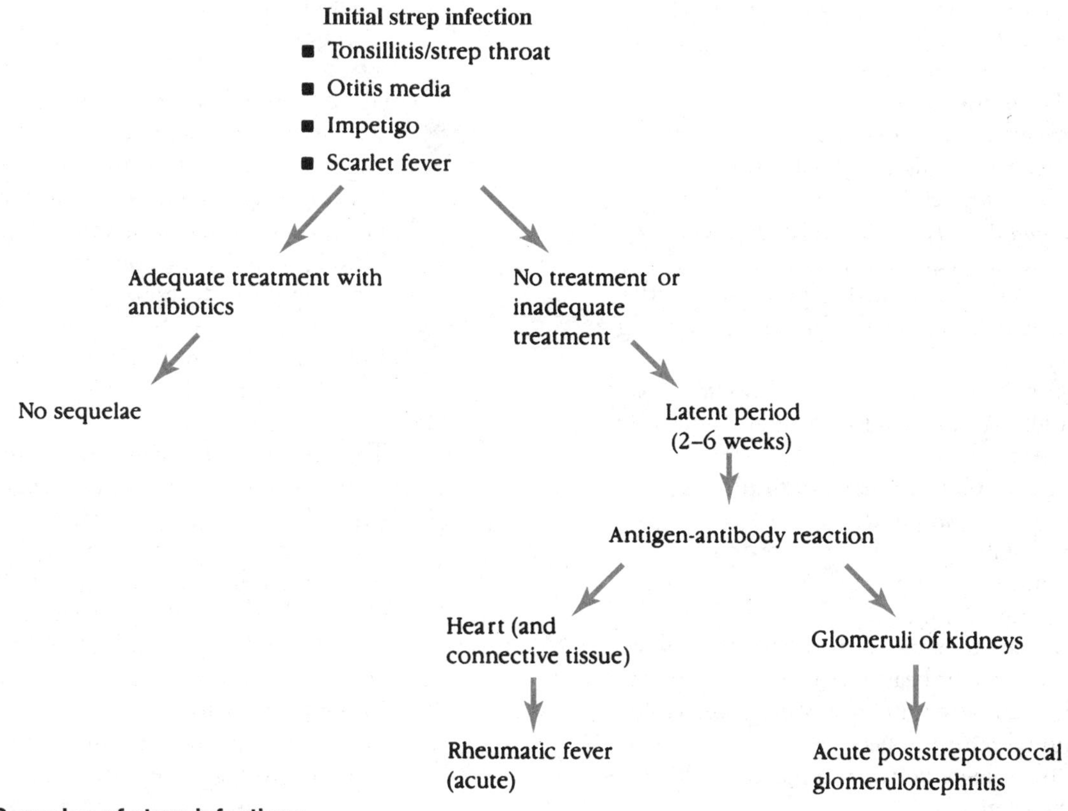

Figure 5.8 **Sequelae of strep infections.**

d. *Erythema marginatum:* reddish pink rash most commonly found on the trunk; nonpruritic, macular, clear center, wavy but clearly marked border; transient.
e. *Subcutaneous nodules:* small, round, freely movable, and painless swellings usually found over the extensor surfaces of the hands/feet or bony prominences; resolve without any permanent damage.

2. *Minor manifestations*
   a. Clinical
      (1) Previous history of rheumatic fever.
      (2) Arthralgia.
      (3) Fever—normal in morning, rises in midafternoon, normal at night.
   b. Laboratory
      (1) *Increased* erythrocyte sedimentation rate (ESR).
      (2) *Positive* C-reactive protein.
      (3) Leukocytosis.
      (4) Anemia.
      (5) *Prolonged* P-R/Q-T intervals on ECG.
3. Supportive evidence
   a. Recent history of streptococcus infection:
      (1) Strep throat/tonsillitis.
      (2) Otitis media.
      (3) Impetigo.
      (4) Scarlet fever.
   b. Positive throat culture for streptococcus.
   c. *Increased* antistreptolysin-O (ASO) titer: indicates presence of streptococcus antibodies; begins to rise in 7 days, reaches maximum level in 4 to 6 weeks.

C. Analysis/nursing diagnosis:

1. *Decreased cardiac output* related to carditis.
2. *Pain* related to migratory polyarthritis.
3. *Risk for injury* related to chorea.
4. *Diversional activity deficit* related to lengthy hospitalization and recuperation.
5. *Knowledge deficit* related to preventing cardiac damage, relieving discomfort, and preventing injury.
6. *Ineffective management of therapeutic regimen* with long-term antibiotic therapy and follow-up care.

D. Nursing care plan/implementation:

1. Goal: *prevent cardiac damage.*
   a. Hospitalization, with strict bedrest.
   b. Monitor apical pulse for changes in rate, rhythm, murmurs.
   c. Evaluate tolerance of increased activity by apical rate: if heart rate increases by more than 20 beats/min over resting rate, child should return to bed.
   d. Offer *low-sodium diet* to prevent fluid retention.
   e. Administer oxygen, digoxin/*Lasix* as ordered (if CHF develops). *Note:* Refer to **Chapter 6** for additional information on CHF.
2. Goal: *relieve discomfort.*
   a. Use bed cradle to keep linens from resting on painful joints.
   b. Administer aspirin as ordered to relieve pain.
   c. Move child carefully, minimally—support joints.
   d. Do *not* massage; do *not* perform range-of-motion (ROM) exercises; do *not* apply splints; do *not* apply heat/cold. All these treatments will cause increased pain and are *not needed,* because *no* permanent deformities will result from this type of arthritis.
3. Goal: *promote safety and prevent injury related to chorea.*
   a. Use side rails: elevated, padded.
   b. Restrain in bed if necessary.
   c. *No* oral temperatures—child may bite thermometer.
   d. Spoon-feed—no forks or knives, to prevent injury to oral cavity.
   e. Assist with all aspects of ADLs until child can care for own needs.
4. Goal: *provide diversion as tolerated.*
   a. Encourage quiet diversional activities: hobbies, reading, puzzles.
   b. Get homework, books; provide tutor as condition permits.
   c. Encourage contact with peers: telephone calls, letters, cards.
5. Goal: *encourage child and family to comply with long-term antibiotic therapy.*
   a. Begin antibiotics immediately, to eradicate any lingering streptococcus infection.
   b. Duration of prophylaxis varies (5 years → lifelong) and depends on cardiac involvement.
   c. Stress need to adhere to prescribed prophylaxis schedule.
   d. Enlist child's cooperation with therapy (e.g., "hero" badge).
6. Goal: *health teaching.*
   a. To encourage compliance with prolonged bedrest—stress that ultimate prognosis depends on amount of cardiac damage.
   b. Teach necessity for long-term prophylactic therapy, for example, during dental work, childbirth, surgery (to prevent subacute bacterial endocarditis [SBE]). Instruct adolescents to *avoid* body piercing and tattooing for same rationale.
   c. Teach rationale: permanent cardiac damage (mitral valve) is more likely to occur with subsequent attacks of rheumatic fever.

E. Evaluation/outcome criteria:

1. No permanent cardiac damage occurs.
2. Child is free from discomfort or is able to tolerate discomfort.
3. Injuries are avoided.
4. Child's need for diversional activity is met.
5. Child/family comply with long-term antibiotic therapy/prophylactic therapy.

III. KAWASAKI DISEASE (MUCOCUTANEOUS LYMPH NODE SYNDROME)

A. *Introduction:* Kawasaki disease (mucocutaneous lymph node syndrome) is an acute, febrile, multisystem disorder believed to be autoimmune in nature. Affecting primarily the *skin* and *mucous membranes of the respiratory tract, lymph nodes,* and *heart,* Kawasaki disease has a low fatality rate (<2%), although vasculitis and cardiac involvement (coronary artery changes) may result in major complications in as many as 20% to 25% of children with this disease. The disease is not believed to be communicable, and the exact cause remains unknown; *geographic* (living near fresh water) and *seasonal* (late winter, early spring) outbreaks do occur. Kawasaki disease occurs in *both* boys and girls between 1 and 14 years of age; 80% of cases occur in children *under age 5 years.* It is more common among children of Japanese or Korean descent, although children from any ethnic background may be affected. It may be preceded by URI or exposure to a freshly cleaned carpet. A complete and apparently *spontaneous* recovery occurs within 3 to 4 weeks in the majority of cases. Treatment, which is primarily symptomatic, does not appear to either enhance recovery or prevent complications, although recent research indicates that life-threatening complications and long-term disability may be avoided or minimized with early treatment (i.e., gamma globulin) to reduce cardiovascular damage.

B. Assessment:

1. Abrupt onset with high fever (102° to 106°F) lasting more than 5 days that does *not* remit with the administration of antibiotics and antipyretics.
2. Conjunctivitis—bilateral, nonpurulent.
3. Oropharyngeal manifestations:
   a. Dry, red, cracked lips.
   b. Oropharyngeal reddening and a "strawberry" tongue.
4. Peeling (desquamation) of the palms of the hands and the soles of the feet; begins at the fingertips and the tips of the toes; as peeling progresses, hands and feet become very red, sore, and swollen.
5. Cervical lymphadenopathy.
6. Generalized erythematous rash on trunk and extremities, without vesicles or crusts.
7. Irritability, anorexia.
8. Arthralgia and arthritis.
9. Panvasculitis of coronary arteries: formation of aneurysms and thrombi; CHF, myocarditis, pericardial effusion, arrhythmias, mitral insufficiency, myocardial infarction (MI).
10. Three phases: *acute* (onset of fever) → *subacute* (resolution of fever and all outward clinical signs) → *convalescent* (without clinical signs but laboratory values remain abnormal).
11. Laboratory tests:
    a. *Elevated:* ESR.
    b. *Elevated:* white blood cell (WBC) count.
    c. *Elevated:* platelet count.

C. Analysis/nursing diagnosis:

1. *Hyperthermia* related to high, unremitting fever.
2. *Altered oral mucous membrane and impaired swallowing* related to oropharyngeal manifestations.
3. *Impaired skin integrity* related to desquamation.
4. *Fluid volume deficit* related to high fever and poor oral intake.
5. *Altered tissue perfusion* (cardiovascular, potential/actual) related to vasculitis or thrombi.
6. *Knowledge deficit* related to disease course, treatment, prognosis.

D. Nursing care plan/implementation:

1. Goal: *reduce fever.*
   a. Monitor temperature every 2 hours or prn.
   b. Administer **aspirin** (*not* acetaminophen [Tylenol]) per physician's order. (*Note:* aspirin is the drug of choice to reduce fever; also has anti-inflammatory effect and antiplatelet effect. Dose is 100 mg/kg/day in divided doses q6h. Monitor for signs of salicylate toxicity.)
   c. Tepid sponge baths or hypothermia blanket per physician's order.
   d. Offer frequent cool fluids.
   e. Apply cool, loose-fitting clothes; use cotton bed linens only (no heavy blankets).
   f. Seizure precautions.
2. Goal: *provide comfort measures to oral cavity to ease the discomfort of swallowing.*
   a. Good oral hygiene with soft sponge and diluted hydrogen peroxide.
   b. Apply petroleum jelly to lips.
   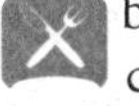
   c. *Bland* foods in small amounts at frequent intervals.
   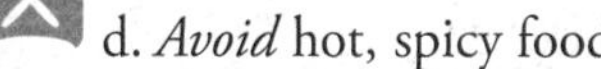
   d. *Avoid* hot, spicy foods.
   e. Offer favorite foods from home or preferred foods from hospital selection.

3. Goal: *prevent infections and promote healing of skin.*
   a. Monitor skin for desquamation, edema, rash.
   b. Keep skin clean, dry, well lubricated.
   c. *Avoid* soap to prevent drying.
   d. Gentle handling of skin to minimize discomfort.
   e. Provide sheepskin to lie on.
   f. Prevent scratching and itching—apply cotton mittens if necessary.
   g. Bedrest; *elevate* edematous extremities.
4. Goal: *prevent dehydration and restore normal fluid balance.*
   a. Strict I&O.
   b. Monitor urine specific gravity q8h for increase (dehydration) or decrease (hydration).
   c. Monitor vital signs for fevers, tachycardia, arrhythmia.
   d. Monitor skin turgor, mucous membranes, anterior fontanel for dehydration.
   e. Force fluids.
   f. IV fluids per physician's order.
5. Goal: *prevent cardiovascular complications.*
   a. ECG monitor—report arrhythmias or tachycardia.
   b. Administer aspirin (see **Goal 1**) and high-dose IV gamma globulin.
   c. Monitor for signs and symptoms of CHF: tachycardia, tachypnea, dyspnea, crackles, orthopnea, distended neck veins, dependent edema.
   d. Monitor circulatory status of extremities—check for possible development of thrombi.
   e. Stress need for long-term follow-up, including ECGs and echocardiograms, possible cardiac catheterization (if coronary artery abnormalities exist at 1 year after disease).

E. Evaluation/outcome criteria:
1. Fever returns to normal.
2. Oral cavity heals, and child is able to swallow.
3. Skin heals, and no infection occurs.
4. Normal fluid balance is restored.
5. Normal cardiovascular functioning is reestablished, and no complications occur.
6. Parents/child verbalize their understanding of Kawasaki disease.

GASTROINTESTINAL SYSTEM

Structural Defects

I. CLEFT LIP AND CLEFT PALATE

A. *Introduction:* Cleft lip and cleft palate are congenital facial malformations resulting from faulty embryonic development; there appear to be multiple factors involved in the exact etiology: mutant genes, chromosomal abnormalities, teratogenic agents, etc. The infant may be born with cleft lip alone, cleft palate alone, or with both cleft lip and cleft palate. Cleft lip and palate may occur unilaterally or bilaterally. **Table 5.15** compares these conditions.

PEDIATRICS

Table 5.15

Comparison of Cleft Lip and Cleft Palate

Dimension	Cleft Lip Only	Cleft Palate Only	Both Cleft Lip and Cleft Palate
Incidence	1/7800 More common among boys	1/2000 More common among girls	Most common facial malformation More common among boys More common among Caucasians than African Americans
Surgical repair	"Cheiloplasty" Often done in a single stage Timing: age 6–12 weeks	Palatoplasty Often done in staged repairs Timing: age 12–18 months (controversial; usually done prior to development of faulty speech habits)	Lip always repaired before palate to enhance parent-infant attachment, bonding
Position postoperatively	*Never* on abdomen	*Always* on abdomen	
Feeding postoperatively	*No* sucking Use Breck feeder or Asepto syringe	*No* sucking • Use wide-bowl spoon or plastic cup	
Nursing care postoperatively	Elbow restraints Lessen crying	Elbow restraints Lessen crying	OK to show parents pictures of "before" and "after" repair

Table 5.15

Comparison of Cleft Lip and Cleft Palate—cont'd

Dimension	Cleft Lip Only	Cleft Palate Only	Both Cleft Lip and Cleft Palate
Long-term concerns	Bonding, attachment Social adjustment—potential threat to self-image	Defective speech—refer to speech therapist Abnormal dentition—refer to orthodontist Hearing loss—refer to pediatric eye, ear, nose, throat specialist/physician	

B. Assessment:

1. *Cleft lip*—obvious facial defect, readily detectable at time of birth.
2. *Cleft palate*—must feel inside infant's mouth to check for presence of palatal defect and to note extent of defect: soft palate only or soft palate *and* hard palate.
3. *Both*—major problems with feeding: difficult to feed, noisy sucking, swallows excessive amounts of air, prone to aspiration.
4. Parent-infant attachment (bonding) may be adversely affected due to "loss of perfect infant," multiple hospitalizations; note amount and quality of parent-infant interaction.

C. Analysis/nursing diagnosis:

1. *Altered nutrition, less than body requirements,* related to physical defect.
2. *Impaired physical mobility* (postoperative) related to postoperative care requirements.
3. *Altered parenting* related to birth of child with obvious facial defect.
4. *Knowledge deficit,* actual or risk for, potential, related to treatment and follow-up.

D. Nursing care plan/implementation:

1. Goal: *maintain adequate nutrition.*
   a. *Preoperative:* first encourage parents to watch nurse feed infant, then teach parents proper feeding techniques:
      (1) Use *Breck* feeder or Asepto syringe.
      (2) Deposit formula on back of tongue to facilitate swallowing and to prevent aspiration.
      (3) Rinse mouth with sterile water after feedings, to prevent infection.
      (4) Feed slowly, with child in sitting position, to prevent aspiration.
      (5) Burp frequently, because infant will swallow air along with formula due to the defect.
      (6) Monitor weight.
   b. *Postoperative*
      (1) Begin with *clear liquids* when child has fully recovered from anesthesia (see **Table 5.15**).
      (2) Monitor weight gain carefully, to ensure adequate rate of growth.
      (3) **No** sucking for either cleft lip or palate repair until incision is healed.
      (4) Avoid stretching or pulling at incision site; metal "Logan bow" may be used as external brace for cleft lip repair.
2. Goal: *promote parent-infant attachment.*
   a. Show no discomfort handling infant; convey acceptance.
   b. Stay with parents the first time they see/hold infant.
   c. Offer positive comments about infant.
   d. Give positive reinforcement to parents' initial attempts at parenting.
   e. Encourage parents to assume increasing independence in care of their infant.
   f. Allow rooming-in on subsequent hospitalizations.
3. Goal: *teach parents particulars of feeding and need for long-term follow-up care.*
   a. Teach parents regarding long-term concerns (see **Table 5.15**).
   b. Make necessary *referrals* before discharge:
      (1) Specialists: speech, dentition, hearing.
      (2) Home health nurse.
      (3) Social service.
      (4) Disabled children's services for financial assistance.
      (5) Local craniofacial malformations support group.
   c. Refer parents to genetic counseling services because of mixed genetic/environmental etiology.
   d. Encourage parents to promote self-esteem in infant/child as child grows and develops.

E. Evaluation/outcome criteria:

1. Adequate nutrition is provided, and infant grows at "normal" rate for age.
2. Parent-infant attachment is formed.
3. Parents verbalize confidence in their ability to care for infant.

PEDIATRICS

II. TRACHEOESOPHAGEAL FISTULA

A. *Introduction:* Tracheoesophageal fistula (TEF) is a congenital anomaly resulting from faulty embryonic development; although there are numerous "types" of TEF, the major problem is an anatomical defect that results in an abnormal connection between the trachea (respiratory tract) and the esophagus (GI system) (**Fig. 5.9**). No exact cause has been identified; however, infants born with TEF are often premature, with a maternal history of polyhydramnios. Diagnosis should be made immediately, within hours after birth, and preferably before feeding (to avoid aspiration pneumonia). Associated anomalies include: CHD, anorectal malformations, and genitourinary anomalies.

B. Assessment:

1. Perinatal history: maternal polyhydramnios, premature birth.
2. *Most important system* affected is *respiratory:*
   a. Shortly after birth, infant has excessive amounts of mucus.
   b. Mucus bubbles or froths out of nose and mouth as infant literally "exhales" mucus.
   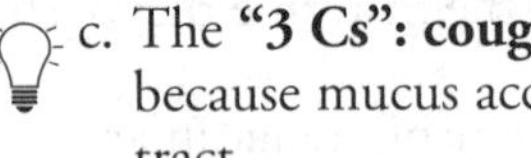
   c. The **"3 Cs": coughing, choking, cyanosis**—because mucus accumulates in respiratory tract.
   d. "Pinks up" with suctioning, only to experience repeated respiratory distress within a short time as mucus builds up again.
   e. Aspiration pneumonia occurs early.
   f. Respiratory arrest may occur.
3. *Second* system affected is GI:
   a. Abdominal distention because excessive air enters stomach with each breath infant takes.
   b. Inability to aspirate stomach contents when attempting to pass NG tube.
   c. If all these signs are not correctly interpreted and feeding is attempted, infant takes two to three mouthfuls, coughs and gags, and forcefully "exhales" formula through nostrils.

C. Analysis/nursing diagnosis:

1. *Ineffective breathing pattern/ineffective airway clearance* related to excess mucus.
2. *Altered nutrition, less than body requirements,* related to inability to take fluids by mouth.
3. *Anxiety* related to surgery, condition, preterm delivery, and uncertain prognosis.
4. *Knowledge deficit* regarding discharge care of infant related to gastrostomy tube, feeding.

D. Nursing care plan/implementation:

1. Goal: *prepare neonate for surgery.*
   a. Stress to parents that surgery is *only* possible treatment.
   b. Allow parents to see neonate before surgery to promote bonding and attachment.
   c. Maintain NPO—provide IV fluids, monitor I&O, gastrostomy tube.
   d. *Position:* elevate HOB 20 to 30 degrees to prevent aspiration.
   e. Administer warmed, humidified oxygen, as ordered, to relieve hypoxia and to prevent cold stress.

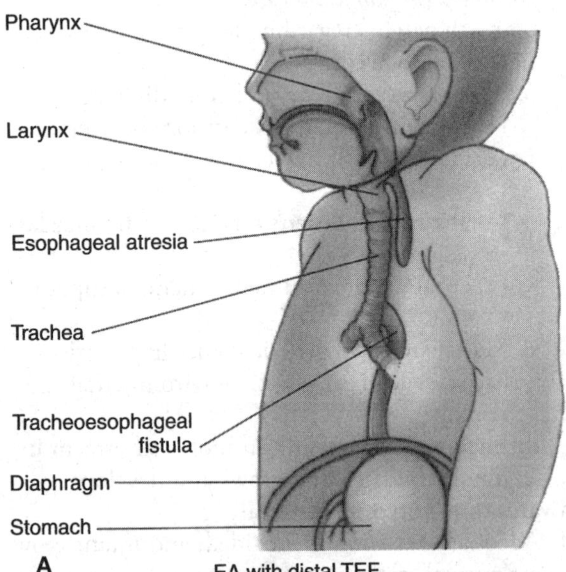

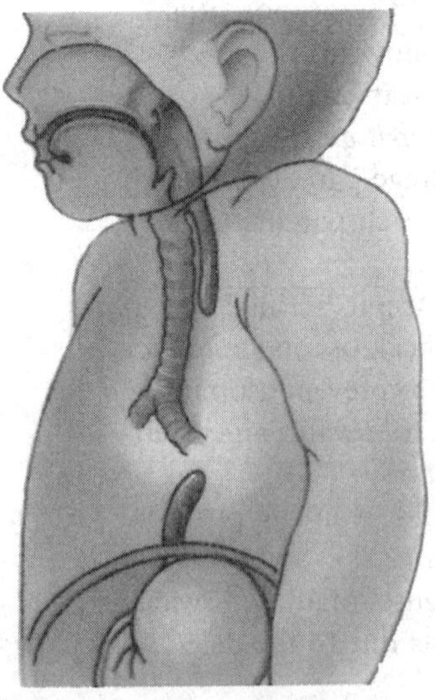

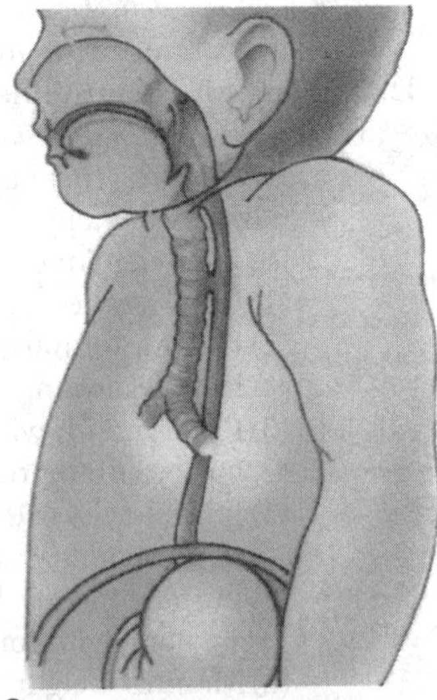

Figure 5.9 Esophageal malformations. *EA* = esophageal atresia; *TEF* = tracheoesophageal fistula. *(A)* The esophagus ends in a blind pouch with a fistula between the distal esophagus and trachea. *(B)* Esophageal atresia without fistula. *(C)* Tracheoesophageal fistula without esophageal atresia. (From Bowden, VR, Dickey, SB, & Greenberg, CS: *Children and Their Families: The Continuum of Care.* WB Saunders, Philadelphia, 1999, p 105.)

2. Goal (**postoperative**): *maintain patent airway.*
   a. *Position:* elevate HOB 20 to 30 degrees.
   b. Care of chest tubes (open-chest procedure).
   c. Care of endotracheal tube/ventilator (neonate frequently requires ventilatory assistance for 24 to 48 hours postoperatively).
   d. Monitor for symptoms and signs of pneumonia (most common postoperative complication):
      (1) Aspiration.
      (2) Hypostatic, secondary to anesthesia.
   e. Monitor for symptoms and signs of respiratory distress syndrome (preterm infant).
   f. Use special precautions when suctioning: "suction with marked catheter" to avoid exerting undue pressure on newly sutured trachea.
   g. Administer prophylactic/therapeutic antibiotics, as ordered.
   h. Administer warmed, humidified oxygen, as ordered; monitor arterial blood gases (ABGs).
3. Goal: *maintain adequate nutrition.*
   a. 48 to 72 hours postoperatively: IV fluids only.
   b. Maintain NPO for 10 to 14 days, until esophagus is fully healed (offer pacifier).
   c. When condition is stable: begin gastrostomy tube (G-tube) feedings, as ordered.
      (1) Start with small amounts of clear liquids.
      (2) Gradually increase to full-strength formula.
      (3) *Postoperative:* leave G-tube open and elevated slightly above level of stomach to prevent aspiration if infant vomits.
      (4) Offer pacifier ad lib.
   d. Between *10th and 14th postoperative day:* begin oral feedings.
      (1) Start with clear liquids again.
      (2) Note ability to suck and swallow.
      (3) Offer small amounts at frequent intervals.
      (4) May need to supplement postop feeding with G-tube feeding prn.
   e. Monitor weight, I&O.
4. Goal: *prepare parents to successfully care for the infant after discharge.*
   a. Teach parents that infant will probably be discharged with G-tube in place; teach care of G-tube at home.
   b. Teach parents symptoms and signs of most common long-term problems (i.e., *esophageal reflux, stricture formation*).
      (1) Refusal to eat solids or swallow liquids.
      (2) Dysphagia.
      (3) Increased coughing or choking.
   c. Stress need for long-term follow-up care.
   d. Offer realistic encouragement, because prognosis is generally good.

E. Evaluation/outcome criteria:
1. Neonate survives immediate surgical repair without untoward difficulties.
2. Patent airway is maintained; adequate oxygenation is provided.
3. Adequate nutrition is maintained; infant begins to gain weight and grow.
4. Parents verbalize confidence in ability to care for infant on discharge.

Obstructive Disorders

I. HYPERTROPHIC PYLORIC STENOSIS

A. *Introduction:* Hypertrophic pyloric stenosis (HPS) causes obstruction of the upper GI tract, but the infant frequently does not have symptoms until 2 to 4 weeks of age. HPS results in thickening, or hypertrophy, of the pyloric sphincter located at the distal end of the stomach; this causes a mechanical intestinal obstruction that becomes increasingly evident as the infant begins to consume larger amounts of formula during the early weeks of life. Pyloric stenosis is five times more common in *boys* than girls and is most often found in full-term Caucasian infants. The exact etiology remains unknown; however, there does seem to be a genetic predisposition.

B. Assessment:
1. Classic symptom is *vomiting:*
   a. Begins as nonprojectile at age 2 to 4 weeks.
   b. Advances to projectile at age 4 to 6 weeks.
   c. Vomitus is non–bile stained (stomach contents only).
   d. Most often occurs shortly after a feeding.
   e. Major problem is the mechanical obstruction of the flow of stomach contents to the small intestine due to the anatomical defect of stenosis of the pyloric sphincter.
   f. *No* apparent nausea or pain, as evidenced by the fact that infant eagerly accepts a second feeding after episode of vomiting.
   g. Metabolic alkalosis develops due to loss of hydrochloric acid.
2. Inspection of abdomen reveals:
   a. Palpable olive-shaped *mass* in right upper quadrant.
   b. Visible peristaltic *waves,* moving from left to right across upper abdomen.
3. *Weight:* fails to gain or loses.
4. *Stools:* constipated, diminished in number and size—due to loss of fluids with vomiting.
5. Signs of *dehydration* may become evident **(Table 5.16).**
6. Upper GI series and ultrasonography reveal:
   a. Delayed gastric emptying.
   b. Elongated and narrowed pyloric canal.

Table 5.16

Signs and Symptoms of Dehydration in Infants and Young Children

- *Weight loss* (most important to assess):
  - *Mild dehydration:* <5% weight loss
  - *Moderate dehydration:* 5%–9% weight loss
  - *Severe dehydration:* 10%–15% weight loss
- *Skin:* gray, cold to touch, poor skin turgor (check skin across abdomen)
- *Mucous membranes:* dry oral buccal mucosa; salivation absent
- *Eyes:* sunken eyeballs; absence of tears when crying
- *Anterior fontanel* (in infant): sunken
- *Shock: increased* pulse, *increased* respirations, *decreased* blood pressure
- *Urine:* oliguria, *increased* specific gravity, ammonia odor
- *Alterations in level of consciousness:* irritability, lethargy, stupor, coma, possible seizures
- *Metabolic acidosis* (with diarrhea)
- *Metabolic alkalosis* (with vomiting)

C. Analysis/nursing diagnosis:

1. *Fluid volume deficit* related to vomiting.
2. *Altered nutrition, less than body requirements,* related to vomiting.
3. *Risk for injury/infection* related to altered nutritional state.
4. *Impaired skin integrity* related to dehydration and altered nutritional state.
5. *Knowledge deficit* related to cause of disease, treatment and surgery, prognosis, and follow-up care.

D. Nursing care plan/implementation:

1. Goal (**preoperative**): *restore fluid and electrolyte balance.*

   a. Generally NPO, with IVs preoperatively to provide fluids and electrolytes.
   b. Observe and record I&O, including vomiting and stool.
   c. Weight: check every 8 hours or daily.
   d. Monitor laboratory data.
2. Goal (**postoperative**): *provide adequate nutrition.*

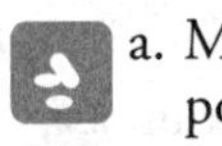

   a. Maintain NPO with IVs for 4 to 6 hours postoperatively, as ordered (*can* offer pacifier).
   b. Follow specific feeding regimen ordered by doctor—generally start with clear fluids in small amounts hourly, increasing slowly as tolerated. Full feeding schedule reinstated within 48 hours. Offer pacifier between feedings.
   c. **Fed only by RN for 24 to 48 hours,** because vomiting tends to continue in immediate postoperative period.
   d. Burp well—before, during, and after feeding.

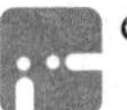

   e. *Position* after feeding: high Fowler's turned to right side; minimal handling after feeding to prevent vomiting.
3. Goal (**preoperative and postoperative**): *institute preventive measures to avoid infection or skin breakdown.*
   a. Use good hand-washing technique.
   b. Administer good skin care, especially in diaper area (urine is highly concentrated); give special care to any reddened areas.
   c. Give mouth care when NPO or after vomiting.
   d. Tuck diaper down below suture line to prevent contamination with urine (postoperatively).
   e. Note condition of suture line—report any redness or discharge immediately.
   f. Screen staff and visitors for any sign of infection.
4. Goal: *do discharge teaching to prepare parents to care for infant at home.*
   a. Teach parents that defect is anatomical and unrelated to their parenting behavior/skill.
   b. Demonstrate feeding techniques, and remind parents that vomiting may still occur.
   c. Stress that repair is complete; this condition will *never* recur.
   d. Instruct parents in care of the suture line: no baths for 10 days, tuck diaper down, report any signs of infection promptly.
   e. Offer follow-up referrals as indicated.

E. Evaluation/outcome criteria:

1. Infant survives surgical repair without untoward difficulties (including infection/skin breakdown).
2. Adequate nutrition is maintained, and infant begins to grow and gain weight.
3. Parents verbalize confidence in their ability to care for their infant on discharge.

II. HIRSCHSPRUNG'S DISEASE (congenital aganglionic megacolon)

A. *Introduction:* Hirschsprung's disease is a congenital anomaly of the lower GI tract, but the diagnosis often is not established until the infant is 6 to 12 months old. The major problem is a functional obstruction of the colon caused by the congenital anatomical defect of lack of nerve cells in the walls of the colon, resulting in the *absence* of peristalsis. Hirschsprung's disease is four times more common in *boys* than girls and is frequently noted in children with *Down* syndrome.

B. Assessment:

1. In the newborn, failure to pass meconium (in addition to other signs and symptoms of intestinal obstruction).
2. *Obstinate constipation*—history of inability to pass stool without stool softeners, laxatives, or

PEDIATRICS

enemas; persists despite all attempts to treat medically.
3. *Stools* are infrequent and tend to be thin and ribbonlike.
4. *Vomiting:* bile stained, flecked with bits of stool (breath has fecal odor), due to GI obstruction and eventual backing up of stools.
5. Abdominal distention can be severe enough to impinge on respirations, due to GI obstruction and retention of stools.
6. Anorexia, nausea, irritability due to severe constipation.
7. Malabsorption results in *anemia, hypoproteinemia,* and loss of subcutaneous fat.
8. Visible peristalsis and palpable fecal masses may also be detected.

C. Analysis/nursing diagnosis:
1. *Constipation* related to impaired bowel functioning.
2. *Altered nutrition, less than body requirements,* related to poor absorption of nutrients.
3. *Risk for injury/infection* related to malnutrition.
4. *Pain* related to surgery and treatments.
5. *Knowledge deficit* regarding care of the child with a colostomy and follow-up care.

D. Nursing care plan/implementation:
1. Goal (**preoperative**): *promote optimum nutritional status, fluid and electrolyte balance.*
   a. Monitor for signs and symptoms of progressive intestinal obstruction: measure abdominal girth daily.
   b. Administer IV fluids, as ordered—may include total parenteral nutrition (TPN) or intravenous lipids.
   c. Daily weights, I&O, urine specific gravity.
   d. Monitor for possible dehydration.
   e. *Diet: low* residue.
2. Goal (**preoperative**): *assist in preparing bowel for surgery.*
   a. Teach parents what will be done and why—enlist their cooperation as much as possible.
   b. Insert NG tube, connect to low suction to achieve and maintain gastric decompression.
   c. *Position:* semi-Fowler's.
   d. Bowel is cleansed with a series of isotonic saline (0.9%) enemas.
   e. Administer oral antibiotics and colonic irrigations to decrease bacteria.
   f. Take axillary temperatures *only.*
   g. If child can understand, prepare for probable colostomy using pictures, dolls (usual age at surgery is 10 to 16 months).
3. Postoperative goals: same as for adult having major abdominal surgery or a colostomy (see **Chapter 6**).
4. Goal (**postoperative**): *discharge teaching to prepare parents to care at home for infant with a colostomy.*
   a. Home care of colostomy of infant is essentially same as for adult (see **Chapter 6**).
   b. Teach parents to keep written records of stools: number, frequency, consistency.
   c. Teach parents to tape diaper below colostomy to prevent irritation.
   d. Because colostomy is usually temporary, discuss:
      (1) Second-stage repair (closure and pull-through) done when the child weighs approximately 20 lb.
      (2) Possible difficulties in toilet training.
   e. Stress need for long-term follow-up care.
   f. Make referral to home care if indicated.

E. Evaluation/outcome criteria:
1. Infant is prepared for surgery and tolerates procedure well.
2. Postoperative recovery is uneventful.
3. Parents verbalize confidence in ability to care at home for infant with a colostomy and verbalize their understanding that second surgery will be needed to close the colostomy.

III. INTUSSUSCEPTION

A. *Introduction:* Intussusception is the apparently spontaneous telescoping of one portion of the intestine into another, resulting in a mechanical obstruction of the lower GI tract. There is no known cause, and intussusception is three times more common in *boys* than girls; the child with intussusception is usually between 3 and 36 months of age.

B. Assessment:
1. Typically presents with sudden onset in child who is healthy, thriving.
2. *Pain:* paroxysmal, colicky, abdominal, with intervals when the child appears normal and comfortable.
3. *Stools:* "currant-jelly," bloody, mixed with mucus.
4. *Vomiting* due to intestinal obstruction.
5. *Abdomen:* distended, tender, with palpable, sausage-shaped mass in right upper quadrant (RUQ).
6. *Late signs:* fever, shock, signs of peritonitis as the compressed bowel wall becomes necrotic and perforates.

C. Analysis/nursing diagnosis:
1. *Fluid volume deficit* related to diarrhea and vomiting.
2. *Pain* related to bowel-wall ischemia, necrosis, and death.
3. *Risk for injury/infection* related to bowel-wall perforation and peritonitis.
4. *Knowledge deficit* regarding the disease, medical or surgical treatment, and prognosis.

PEDIATRICS

D. Nursing care plan/implementation:

1. Goal: *assist with attempts at medical treatment.*
   a. Explain to parents that a barium enema will be given to the child in an attempt to reduce the telescoping through hydrostatic pressure (succeeds in 75% of cases).
   b. Stress that if this treatment is not successful, or if perforation of the bowel wall has already occurred, surgery will be necessary.
   c. If medical treatment is apparently successful, monitor child for 24 to 36 hours for recurrence before discharge.
2. *Preoperative and postoperative goals:* same as for adult with major abdominal surgery (see **Chapter 6**).
3. Goal: *discharge teaching to prepare parents for care of the child at home.*
   a. Stress that recurrence is rare (10%) and most often occurs within the first 24 to 36 hours after reduction.
   b. Other teaching: same as for adult going home after bowel surgery (see **Chapter 6**).

E. Evaluation/outcome criteria:

1. Infant tolerates medical-surgical treatment and completely recovers.
2. Parents verbalize confidence in ability to care for infant after discharge.

PEDIATRICS

Disorders of Motility

I. ACUTE GASTROENTERITIS (AGE)

A. *Introduction:* In infants and young children, gastroenteritis is a common acute illness that can rapidly progress to dehydration, hypovolemic shock, and severe electrolyte disturbances.

B. Assessment:

1. Diarrhea: often watery, green, explosive, contains mucus and blood.
2. Abdominal cramping and pain, often accompanied by bouts of diarrhea.
3. Dehydration: see **Table 5.16.**
4. Irritability, restlessness, alterations in level of consciousness.
5. Electrolyte disturbances: see Chapter 6.

C. Analysis/nursing diagnosis:

1. *Fluid volume deficit* related to vomiting and diarrhea.
2. *Altered nutrition, less than body requirements,* related to AGE and its treatment (i.e., dietary restrictions).
3. *Pain* related to abdominal cramping, diarrhea.
4. *Impaired skin integrity* related to diarrhea.
5. *Altered tissue perfusion* related to dehydration and hypovolemia.
6. *Knowledge deficit* regarding diagnosis, dietary restrictions, treatment.

D. Nursing care plan/implementation:

1. Goal: *prevent spread of infection.*
   a. Standard precautions to prevent infection.
   b. Enforce strict hand washing.
   c. Institute and maintain *enteric precautions*—follow policies regarding linens, excretions, specimens ("double-bag, special tag").
   d. Tape diapers snugly; keep hands out of mouth.
   e. Obtain stool culture to identify causative organism; then administer antibiotics as ordered.
   f. Identify family members and others at high risk, obtain cultures.
2. Goal: *restore fluid and electrolyte balance.*
   a. Administer IV fluids and electrolytes as ordered.
   b. Monitor for appropriate response to therapy: decreased specific gravity, good skin turgor, normal vital signs.
   c. Monitor weight, I&O, specific gravity.
   d. Oral feedings—oral rehydration therapy (ORT) with Pedialyte or comparable solution; resume normal diet as quickly as possible.
   e. Ongoing assessment of stools: note **A**mount, **C**olor, **C**onsistency, **T**iming (**ACCT**).
3. Goal: *maintain or restore skin integrity.*
   a. Frequent diaper changes.
   b. Keep perineal area clean and dry.
   c. Apply protective ointments (e.g., petroleum jelly, A and D emollient ointment).
   d. If feasible, expose reddened buttocks to air (but *not* with explosive diarrhea).
4. Goal: *provide discharge teaching to parents.*
   a. Careful review of diet to be followed at home.
   b. Review principles of food preparation and storage to prevent infection.
   c. Instruct in disposal of stools at home.
   d. Emphasize importance of good hygiene.

E. Evaluation/outcome criteria:

1. No spread of infection noted.
2. Fluid and electrolyte balance normal.
3. No skin breakdown noted.
4. Parents verbalize understanding of home care.

GENITOURINARY SYSTEM

Genitourinary Tract Disorder

I. HYPOSPADIAS

A. *Introduction:* Hypospadias is a congenital anatomical defect of the male genitourinary tract, readily detected at birth through simple visual examination. In hypospadias, the urethral opening is located on the ventral surface of the penile shaft; this makes voiding in the standing position virtually impossible, which creates potential for serious psychological problems. Ideally, staged surgical repair should be completed *by 6 to 18 months of age,* before body image is developed or castration fears are evident.

B. Assessment:

1. Urethral opening is located on ventral surface of penis.
2. May be accompanied by "chordee"—ventral curvature of the penis due to a fibrous band of tissue.
3. Rare: ambiguous genitalia, resulting in need for chromosomal studies to determine sex of neonate.

C. Analysis/nursing diagnosis:

1. *Altered urinary elimination* related to congenital anatomical defect of penis.
2. *Pain* related to surgery and treatments.
3. *Self-esteem disturbance* related to anatomical defect in penis and resulting disturbance in ability to void standing up.
4. *Knowledge deficit* related to condition, surgeries, outcome.

D. Nursing care plan/implementation:

1. Goal: *promote normal urinary function.*
   a. Teach family that surgery is done in several stages, beginning in the early months of life and finishing by age 18 months.
   b. Provide age-appropriate information to child regarding condition, surgery.
   c. *Preoperative* teaching with child: simulate anticipated postoperative urinary drainage apparatus and dressings on dolls; allow child to handle and play with them *now,* but stress need *not* to touch postoperatively.
   d. *Postoperatively:* Monitor urinary drainage apparatus; note hourly urine output, color, appearance (should be clear yellow, *no* blood).
2. Goal: *promote self-esteem.*
   a. Do *not* scold child if he exposes penis, dressings, catheters, etc.
   b. Reassure parents that preoccupation with penis is normal and will pass.
   c. Encourage calm, matter-of-fact acceptance of, and *avoid* strict discipline for this behavior, which could affect the child negatively.

E. Evaluation/outcome criteria:

1. Child is able to void in normal male pattern.
2. Child does not experience disturbances in self-concept and has normal self-esteem.

Kidney Tumor

I. WILMS' TUMOR (NEPHROBLASTOMA)

A. *Introduction:* Wilms' tumor, a malignant tumor of the kidney, is the most common form of renal cancer in children. Peak incidence occurs at 3 years of age, with a slightly higher incidence in *boys* than girls. Ninety percent of the cases occur unilaterally; the treatment of choice is nephrectomy (and adrenalectomy) followed by chemotherapy and radiation.

B. Assessment:

1. Most common sign: abdominal mass (firm, nontender).
2. Most often first found by parent changing diaper; felt as a mass over the kidney area.
3. Intravenous pyelogram (IVP), abdominal ultrasound, and CT confirm the diagnosis.
4. Metastasis occurs most frequently to the lungs: pain in chest, cough, dyspnea.

C. Analysis/nursing diagnosis: *altered urinary elimination* (other diagnoses depend on stage of tumor and presence of metastasis—similar to adult with cancer).

D. Nursing care plan/implementation:

1. Goal: *promote normal urinary function.*
   a. Inform family that surgery is scheduled as soon as possible after confirmed diagnosis (within 24–48 hours).
   b. Explain to family that the preferred surgical approach is nephrectomy (and adrenalectomy).
   c. *Preoperative:* do ***not palpate abdomen*** because the tumor is highly friable, and palpation increases the risk of metastasis.
   d. *Postoperative nursing care:* similar to care of adult with nephrectomy (see **Chapter 6**).
   e. *Postoperative care also includes long-term radiation therapy and chemotherapy* (actinomycin D, vincristine, Adriamycin; see **Chapters 6** and **8**).
2. Goal: *discharge teaching to prepare parents to care for child at home.*
   a. Teach parents need for long-term follow-up care with specialists: oncologist, urologist.
   b. Answer questions regarding prognosis, offering realistic hope.
      (1) Children with localized tumor: 90% survival rate.
      (2) Children with metastasis: 50% survival rate.

E. Evaluation/outcome criteria:

1. Child is able to maintain normal urinary elimination.
2. Parents verbalize their understanding of home care for the child.

PEDIATRICS

Glomerular Diseases

I. NEPHROSIS

Nephrosis (idiopathic nephrotic syndrome) is a chronic renal disease having no known cause, variable pathology, and no known cure. It is thought that several different pathophysiological processes adversely affect the glomerular membranes of the kidneys, resulting in increased permeability to protein. This "leakage" of protein into the urine results in massive *proteinuria,* severe *hypoproteinemia,* and total body edema. A chronic disease, nephrosis often has its onset during the preschool years but is characterized by periods of exacerbation and remission throughout the childhood years.

The nursing care plan for the child with nephrosis is very similar to that for the adult with compromised renal functioning. Refer to **Chapters 8 and 9** for additional information about dietary restrictions and medications; refer to **Table 5.17** for a chart comparing nephrosis and nephritis.

II. ACUTE POSTSTREPTOCOCCAL GLOMERULONEPHRITIS

A. *Introduction:* Acute poststreptococcal glomerulonephritis (APSGN) is a bilateral inflammation of the glomeruli of the kidneys and is the most common noninfectious renal disease of childhood. It occurs most frequently in early school-age

Table 5.17

Comparison of Nephrosis and Acute Poststreptococcal Glomerulonephritis

Factor	Nephrosis (Nephrotic Syndrome)	Acute Poststreptococcal Glomerulonephritis (APSGN)
Illness type	Chronic	Acute
Illness course	Characterized by periods of exacerbations and remissions during many years	Predictable, self-limiting, typically lasting 4–10 days (acute edematous phase)
Cause	Unknown	Group A β-hemolytic streptococci
Age at onset	2–4 years	Early school-age children; peaks at 6–7 years
Sex	More common among boys	More common among boys
Major signs and symptoms:		
General	Syndrome with variable pathology: massive proteinuria, hypoalbuminemia, severe edema, hyperlipidemia	Hematuria, hypertension
Blood pressure	Normal or decreased	Elevated
Edema	Generalized and severe	Periorbital and peripheral
Proteinuria	Massive	Moderate
Serum protein level	*Decreased* (6.1–7.9 g/dL)	Slightly decreased
Serum lipid level	*Elevated*	Normal
Potassium level	Normal (3.5–5 mEq/L)	*Increased*
Treatment	Symptomatic—no known cure; prednisone, cyclophosphamide, furosemide	Penicillin (EES), hydralazine, furosemide (sources are divided regarding use of prophylactic antimicrobials)
Diet	*Decrease* sodium, *increase* protein (unless azotemia develops)	*Decrease* sodium, *decrease* potassium, *decrease* protein (if azotemia develops)
Fluid restrictions	Seldom necessary	Necessary if output is significantly reduced
Specific nursing care	Treat at home if possible; good skin care; prevent infection	Treat in hospital during acute phase; monitor vital signs, especially blood pressure; on discharge, stress need to restrict strenuous activity until microscopic hematuria is gone
Prognosis	Fair; subject to long-term steroid treatment and social isolation related to frequent hospitalizations/confinement during relapses; 20% suffer chronic renal failure	Good; stress that recurrence is *rare* because specific immunity is conferred

children, with a peak age of onset of 6 to 7 years; it is twice as common in boys as in girls. Like rheumatic fever, acute glomerulonephritis is thought to be the result of an antigen-antibody reaction to a streptococcus infection (see **Fig. 5.8**); however, unlike rheumatic fever, it does *not* tend to recur, because specific immunity is conferred following the first episode of APSGN. (Further information about APSGN is found in **Table 5.17.)**

B. Assessment:

1. Typical concerns from family about urine: change in color/appearance of urine (thick, reddish brown; decreased amounts).
2. *Acute edematous phase*—usually lasts 4 to 10 days.
   a. Laboratory examination of urine:
      (1) Severe **hematuria.**
      (2) Mild proteinuria.
      (3) *Increased* specific gravity.
   b. **Hypertension**
      (1) Headache.
      (2) Potential hypertensive encephalopathy leading to seizures, increased intracranial pressure.
   c. Mild-moderate edema: chiefly periorbital; increased weight due to fluid retention.
   d. General:
      (1) Abdominal pain.
      (2) Malaise.
      (3) Anorexia.
      (4) Vomiting.
      (5) Pallor.
      (6) Irritability.
      (7) Lethargy.
      (8) Fever.
3. *Diuresis phase:*
   a. Copious diuresis.
   b. Decreased body weight.
   c. Marked clinical improvement.
   d. Decrease in gross hematuria, but microscopic hematuria may persist for weeks/months.

C. Analysis/nursing diagnosis:

1. *Fluid volume excess* related to decreased urine output.
2. *Pain* related to fluid retention.
3. *Altered nutrition, less than body requirements,* related to anorexia and vomiting.
4. *Impaired skin integrity* related to immobility.
5. *Activity intolerance* related to fatigue.
6. *Knowledge deficit* related to disease process, treatment, and follow-up care.

D. Nursing care plan/implementation:

1. Goal: *monitor fluid balance, observing carefully for complications.*
   a. Check and record blood pressure at least every 4 hours to monitor hypertension.
   b. Monitor daily weights.
   c. Urine: strict I&O; specific gravity and dipstick for blood every void.
   d. Note edema: extent, location, progression.
   e. Adhere to fluid restrictions if ordered.
   f. Monitor for possible development of hypertensive encephalopathy (seizures, increased intracranial pressure); report any changes STAT to physician.
   g. Administer medications as ordered:
      (1) *Antibiotics*—eradicate any lingering streptococcus infection; controversial.
      (2) *Antihypertensives* (e.g., Apresoline).
      (3) Rarely use diuretics—limited value.
      (4) If CHF develops—may use digoxin.
      (5) Refer to **Chapter 8** for additional information on medications.
2. Goal: *provide adequate nutrition.*

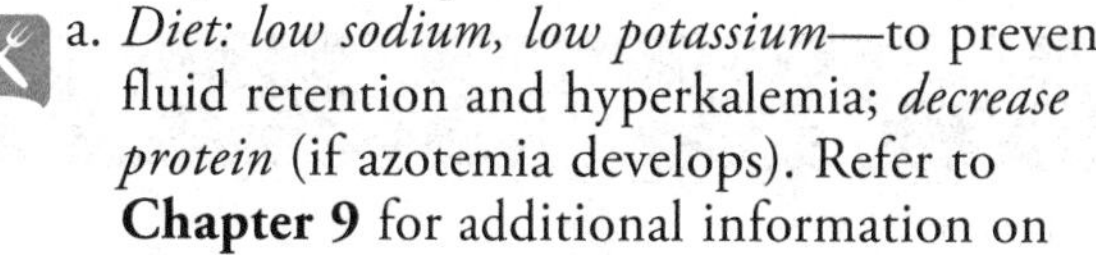

   a. *Diet: low sodium, low potassium*—to prevent fluid retention and hyperkalemia; *decrease protein* (if azotemia develops). Refer to **Chapter 9** for additional information on diets.
   b. Stimulate appetite: offer small portions, attractively prepared; meals with family or other children; offer preferred foods, if possible; encourage parents to bring in special foods (e.g., culturally related preferences).
3. Goal: *provide reasonable measure of comfort.*
   a. Encourage parental visiting.
   b. Provide for positional changes, give good skin care.
   c. Provide appropriate diversion, as tolerated.
4. Goal: *prevent further infection.*
   a. Use good hand washing technique.
   b. Screen staff, other clients, visitors (especially children) to limit contact with people who are infectious.
   c. Administer antibiotics if ordered (usually only for children with positive cultures).
   d. Keep warm and dry, stress good hygiene.
   e. Note possible sites of infection: increased skin breakdown secondary to edema.
5. Goal: *teach child and family about APSGN/discharge planning.*
   a. Teach how to check urine at home: dipstick for protein and blood. (*Note:* occult hematuria may persist for months.)
   b. Teach activity restriction: **no** strenuous activity until hematuria is completely resolved.
   c. Teach family how to prepare low-sodium, low-potassium diet.
   d. Arrange for follow-up care: physician, home health nurse.
   e. *Stress:* subsequent recurrences are *rare* because specific immunity is conferred.

E. Evaluation/outcome criteria:
1. No permanent renal damage occurs.
2. Normal fluid balance is maintained/restored.
3. Adequate nutrition is maintained.
4. No secondary infections occur.
5. Child/family verbalize their understanding of the disease, its treatment, and its prognosis.

ENDOCRINE SYSTEM

I. DIABETES MELLITUS TYPE 1

Diabetes mellitus type 1 was formerly called insulin-dependent diabetes mellitus (IDDM) and juvenile-onset diabetes. Diabetes mellitus is fully covered in **Chapter 6.** Only the differences between adults and children are covered in **Table 5.18.**

HEMATOLOGICAL SYSTEM

I. LEUKEMIA

A. *Introduction:* Known as "cancer of the blood," leukemia is the most common form of childhood cancer, with an incidence of 4/100,000. Acute leukemia is basically a malignant proliferation of white blood cell (WBC) precursors triggered by an unknown cause and affecting all blood-forming organs and systems throughout the body. The onset is typically insidious, and the disease is most common in preschoolers (age 2–6 years).

B. Assessment:
1. Major problem—leukopenia: *decreased* WBCs/*increased* blasts (overproduction of immature, poorly functioning WBCs).
2. Bone marrow dysfunction results in:
   a. *Neutropenia:* multiple prolonged infections.
   b. *Anemia:* pallor, weakness, irritability, shortness of breath.
   c. *Thrombocytopenia:* bleeding tendencies (petechiae, epistaxis, bruising).
3. Infiltration of reticuloendothelial system (RES): hepatosplenomegaly, abdominal pain, lymphadenopathy.
4. Leukemic invasion of CNS: increased intracranial pressure/leukemic meningitis.
5. Leukemic invasion of bone: pain, pathological fractures, hemarthrosis.

C. Analysis/nursing diagnosis:
1. *Risk for infection* related to neutropenia.
2. *Risk for injury* related to thrombocytopenia.
3. *Altered nutrition, less than body requirements,* related to loss of appetite, vomiting, mouth ulcers.
4. *Pain* related to disease process and treatments (e.g., hemarthrosis, bone pain, bone marrow aspiration).

PEDIATRICS

Table 5.18

Differences Between Type 1 and Type 2 Diabetes Mellitus

Variable	Type 1 (Insulin-Dependent) Diabetes Mellitus	Type 2 (Non–Insulin-Dependent) Diabetes Mellitus
Endogenous (naturally occurring) insulin	*Absolute* deficiency of insulin; pancreas produces no insulin	*Relative* insufficiency of insulin
Dependence on exogenous insulin	Total dependence on insulin injections for remainder of life	Varies; disease may be controlled by combination of: diet, exercise, oral hypoglycemics, and insulin injections
Typical onset	Abrupt	Insidious
Age at onset	Anytime during childhood years; usually before age 20	Most common between age 40 and 60 years, but ↑ incidence in children with obesity, lack of exercise, diet high in "junk" food
Weight at onset	Normal or sudden, unexplained loss of weight	Overweight or obese
Gender	Slightly more common in boys than girls	More common in women than men
Ethnicity	More common in Caucasians	More common in Hispanics and Native Americans
Ketoacidosis	Relatively common	Relatively rare
Ease of control/stability	Unstable, difficult to achieve steady blood sugar level	Stable, easier to achieve steady blood sugar level
Presenting symptoms	Polyuria, polyphagia, polydipsia (**"three Ps"**)	More commonly related to long-term complications (e.g., changes in vision or kidney function)
Complications	Occur more frequently and at relatively younger age because of younger age at onset of disease; rate 80% or greater	Occur less frequently, and often not seen until later adult years; rate is variable

5. *Activity intolerance* related to infection and anemia.
6. *Self-esteem disturbance* related to disease process and treatments (e.g., loss of hair with chemotherapy, moon face with prednisone).
7. *Anticipatory grieving* related to life-threatening illness.
8. *Knowledge deficit* related to diagnosis, treatment, prognosis.

D. Nursing care plan/implementation:

1. Goal: *maintain infection-free state.*
   a. Standard precautions to prevent infection.
   b. Use good hand washing technique.
   c. Ongoing evaluation of sites for potential infection (e.g., gums).
   d. Provide meticulous oral hygiene.
   e. Keep record of vital signs, especially temperature.
   f. Provide good skin care.
   g. Screen staff and visitors (especially children)—restrict anyone with infection.
   h. *Protective isolation/reverse isolation* to minimize exposure to potentially life-threatening infection.
   i. Discharge planning: return to school, but isolate from chickenpox or known communicable diseases.
2. Goal: *prevent injury.*
   a. *Avoid* IMs/IVs if possible, due to bruising and bleeding tendencies.
   b. Do *not* give aspirin or medications containing aspirin, which will interfere with platelet formation, thus increasing the risk of bleeding.
   c. Use soft toothbrush to *avoid* trauma to gums, which may cause bleeding and infection.
   d. *Avoid* "per rectum" suppositories, due to probable rectal ulcers.
   e. Supervise play/activity carefully to promote safety and prevent excessive bruising or bleeding.
3. Goal: *promote adequate nutrition.*
   a. *Diet:* high *calorie*, high *protein,* high *iron.*
   b. Encourage *extra fluids* to prevent constipation or dehydration.
   c. I&O, daily weights, to monitor fluid and nutritional status.
   d. Allow child to be involved with food selection/preparation; allow child almost any food he or she tolerates, to encourage better dietary intake.
   e. Thoroughly wash/peel fresh fruits and vegetables if child is neutropenic (or *avoid* eating these foods).
   f. Serve frequent, small snacks to increase fluid and caloric consumption.
   g. Offer dietary supplements to increase caloric intake.
   h. Encourage local anesthetics such as dextromethorphan throat lozenges (*Chloraseptic*) before meals to allow child to eat without pain from oral mucous membrane ulcers.
4. Goal: *relieve pain.*
   a. Offer supportive alternatives: extra company, back rub. Offer complementary therapies: meditation, visualization (if age appropriate).
   b. Administer medications regularly, before pain becomes excessive.
   c. Use beanbag chair for positional changes.
   d. *Avoid* excessive stimulation (noise, light), which may heighten perception of pain.
5. Goal: *promote self-esteem.*
   a. Stress what child can still do to keep the child as independent as possible.
   b. Encourage performance of ADLs as much as possible to foster a sense of independence.
   c. Provide diversion/activity as tolerated.
   d. Give lots of positive reinforcement to enhance a sense of accomplishment.
   e. Provide realistic feedback on child's appearance; offer suggestions, such as a wig or cap to cover alopecia secondary to chemotherapy.
   f. Encourage early return to peers/school to avoid social isolation.
6. Goal: *prevent complications related to leukemia/prolonged immobility/treatments.*
   a. Inspect skin for breakdown, especially over bony prominences, due to poor nutritional intake and limited mobility due to bone pain.
   b. Anticipate need for and administer (per physician's order) multiple transfusions of platelets, packed red blood cells (RBCs), etc.
   c. Check for hemorrhagic cystitis; *push fluids* (especially with *Cytoxan*).
   d. Check for constipation or peripheral neuropathy (especially with *vincristine*). Refer to **Chapter 8** for specific information on chemotherapy.
7. Goal: *assist child and parents to cope with life-threatening illness.*
   a. Teach rationale for repeated hospitalizations, multiple invasive tests/treatments, long-term follow-up care.
   b. Encourage compliance with all aspects of therapy, to increase chances of survival.
   c. Support family members and their coping mechanisms.
   d. Offer factual information regarding ultimate prognosis ("80% cure" for acute lymphocytic leukemia [ALL]).
   e. If death appears imminent, assist family to cope with dying and death.

E. Evaluation/outcome criteria:
1. Child is maintained in infection-free state.
2. Injuries are prevented or kept to a minimum.
3. Adequate nutrition is maintained.
4. Child is free from pain or can live with minimum level of pain.
5. Child's self-esteem is maintained; child is treated as living (not dying).
6. Complications are prevented or kept to a minimum.
7. Child and family use positive coping mechanisms to deal with illness.

II. SICKLE CELL ANEMIA

A. *Introduction:* Sickle cell anemia is a congenital hemolytic anemia resulting from a defective hemoglobin (Hgb) molecule (hemoglobin S). It is most common in African Americans (8% have sickle cell trait) and in people of Mediterranean, Hispanic, and Middle Eastern descent. The diagnosis is usually made during the toddler or preschool years, during the first crisis episode following an infection. There is also the need to differentiate between *sickle cell trait* (Sickledex test) and *sickle cell anemia* (hemoglobin electrophoresis). Sickle cell anemia has no known cure.

B. Assessment:
1. Increased susceptibility to infection (cause: unknown; most common cause of death in children under 5 years).
2. Inherited as autosomal recessive disorder **(Fig. 5.10).**
3. Precipitated by conditions of low oxygen tension, dehydration, vascular obstruction, increased blood viscosity, infection.
4. Signs of anemia:
   a. Pallor (in dark-skinned children, do not rely on pallor alone—check hemoglobin [Hgb] and hematocrit [Hct]).
   b. Jaundice, due to excessive hemolysis.
   c. Irritability, lethargy, anorexia, malaise.
5. **Vaso-occlusive crisis:** severe pain (variable sites, e.g., chest, back, abdomen), fever, swelling of hands and feet, joint pain and swelling, all related to hypoxia, ischemia, and necrosis at the cellular level. Most common; usually non–life threatening.

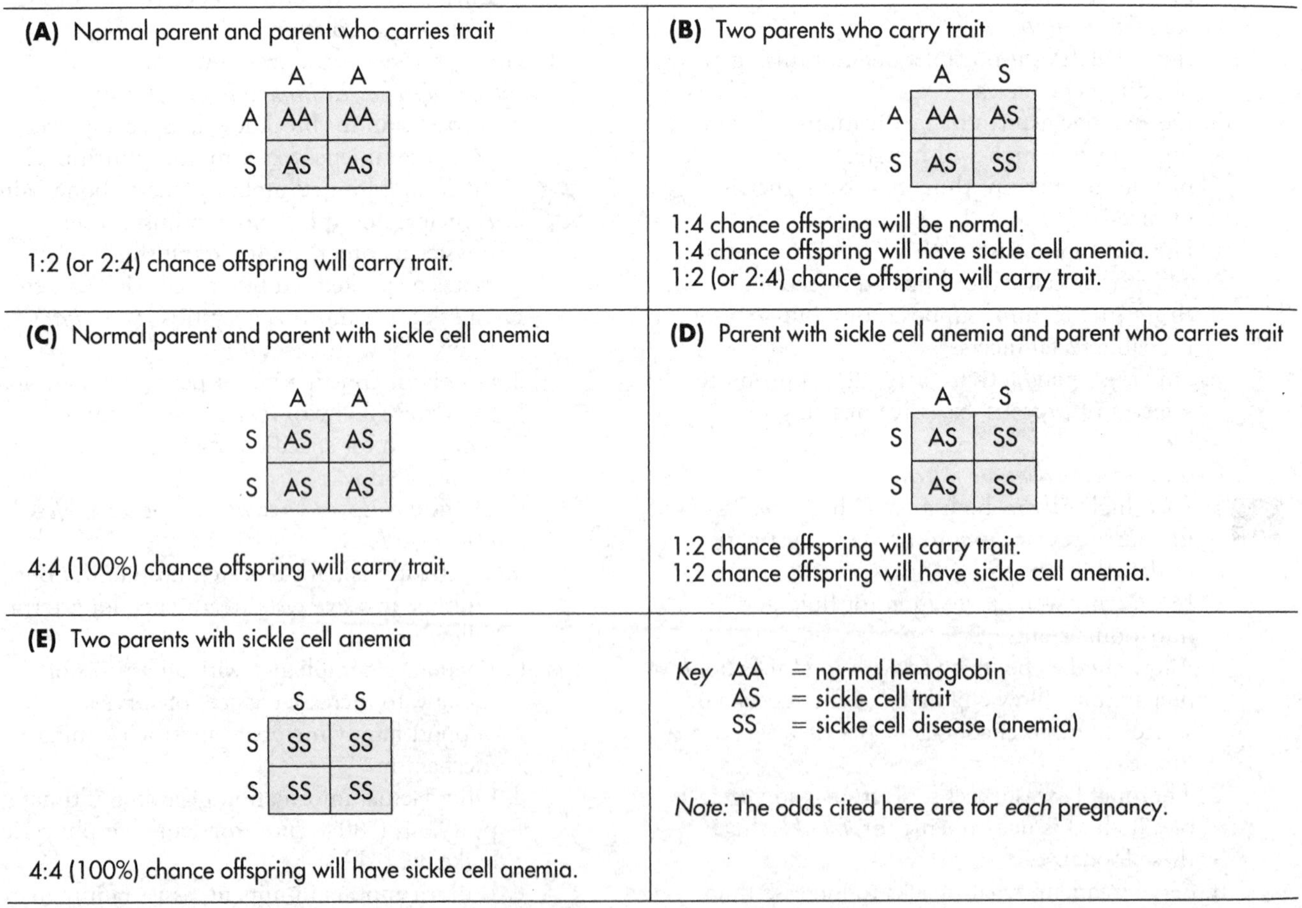

(A) Normal parent and parent who carries trait

	A	A
A	AA	AA
S	AS	AS

1:2 (or 2:4) chance offspring will carry trait.

(B) Two parents who carry trait

	A	S
A	AA	AS
S	AS	SS

1:4 chance offspring will be normal.
1:4 chance offspring will have sickle cell anemia.
1:2 (or 2:4) chance offspring will carry trait.

(C) Normal parent and parent with sickle cell anemia

	A	A
S	AS	AS
S	AS	AS

4:4 (100%) chance offspring will carry trait.

(D) Parent with sickle cell anemia and parent who carries trait

	A	S
S	AS	SS
S	AS	SS

1:2 chance offspring will carry trait.
1:2 chance offspring will have sickle cell anemia.

(E) Two parents with sickle cell anemia

	S	S
S	SS	SS
S	SS	SS

4:4 (100%) chance offspring will have sickle cell anemia.

Key
AA = normal hemoglobin
AS = sickle cell trait
SS = sickle cell disease (anemia)

Note: The odds cited here are for *each* pregnancy.

Figure 5.10 Genetic transmission of sickle cell anemia.

PEDIATRICS

6. **Splenic sequestration crisis:** blood is sequestered (pooled) in spleen; precipitous drop in hemoglobin levels and blood pressure, increased pulse rate, shock, and ultimately death from profound anemia and cardiovascular collapse.

C. Analysis/nursing diagnosis:
1. *Altered tissue perfusion* related to anemia and occlusion of vessels.
2. *Pain* related to vaso-occlusion.
3. *Impaired physical mobility* related to pain, immobility.
4. *Knowledge deficit* related to disease process and treatment (e.g., prevention of sickling or infection; genetic counseling).

D. Nursing care plan/implementation:
1. Goal: *prevent sickling.*
   a. *Avoid* conditions of low oxygen tension (hypoxia), which causes RBCs to assume a sickled shape.
   b. Provide continuous *extra fluids* to prevent dehydration, which causes sluggish circulation. State specific amounts to be consumed rather than "encourage fluids." *Avoid* temperature extremes.
   c. *Avoid* activities that may result in overheating, to prevent dehydration; suggest appropriate clothes; limit time in sun.
   d. If dehydrated due to acute illness, supplement with IV fluids and additional oral fluids to reestablish fluid balance.
2. Goal: *maintain infection-free state.*
   a. *Standard precautions* to prevent infection.
   b. Use good hand washing technique.
   c. Evaluate carefully, check continually for potential infection sites, which may either lead to death due to sepsis or precipitate sickle cell crisis.
   d. Teach importance of prevention of sickle cell crisis: adequate fluids and nutrition; frequent medical checkups; keep away from known sources of infection.
   e. Stress need to report early signs of infection (**chest crisis**) promptly to physician.
   f. Need to balance prevention of infection with child's need for a "normal" life.
   g. Administer yearly influenza vaccine.
3. Goal: *provide supportive therapy during crisis.*
   a. Provide bedrest/hospitalization during crisis to decrease the body's demand for oxygen.
   b. Relieve pain due to infarction of tissues by administering pain medications as ordered; handle gently and use proper positioning techniques.
   c. Apply heat *(never cold)* to affected painful areas to increase blood flow (vasodilation) and oxygen supply.
   d. Administer oxygen, as ordered, to relieve hypoxia and prevent further sickling.
   e. Administer blood transfusions, as ordered, to correct severe anemia. *Complication:* If hypertransfusion programs are implemented, child may develop "iron overload." *Desferal* chelates the iron so that it can be excreted through the urine or bile to help reduce this complication.
   f. Standard medications: hydroxyurea, folic acid.
   g. Monitor fluid and electrolyte balance: I&O, weight, electrolytes.
   h. Perform ADLs for child if unable to care for own needs; encourage self-care as soon as possible to promote independence. *Avoid* stress and fatigue.
4. Goal: *teach child and family about sickle cell anemia.*
   a. Provide factual information based on child's developmental level.
   b. When asked, offer information regarding prognosis (no known cure).
   c. Encourage child to live as normally as possible.
   d. Genetic screening and counseling (see **Fig. 5.10**).

E. Evaluation/outcome criteria:
1. Sickling is prevented or kept to a minimum.
2. Child is maintained in infection-free state.
3. Child/family verbalize that they can cope adequately with crisis.
4. Child/family verbalize their understanding about disease, its management, and its prognosis.

III. HEMOPHILIA

A. *Introduction:* Hemophilia is a bleeding disorder inherited as a sex-linked (X-linked) recessive trait; that is, it occurs only in men but is transmitted by women carriers who are symptom free **(Fig. 5.11)**. Hemophilia results in a deficiency of one or more clotting factors; it is necessary to determine which clotting factor is deficient and to what extent. Classic hemophilia (hemophilia A), a lack of clotting factor VIII, accounts for 75% of all cases of hemophilia.

B. Assessment:
1. Major problem is bleeding.
   a. In *newborn* boy: abnormal bleeding from umbilical cord, prolonged bleeding from circumcision site.
   b. In *toddler* boy: excessive bruising, possible intracranial bleeding, prolonged bleeding from cuts or lacerations.
   c. *General:* hemarthrosis, petechiae, epistaxis, frank hemorrhage anywhere in body, anemia.

(A) "Normal" male and female with trait

	X	Y
X*	X*X	X*Y
X	XX	XY

1:4 chance will be female with trait.
1:4 chance will be male with hemophilia.
1:2 (or 2:4) chance will be "normal" female/male.

(B) Male with hemophilia and "normal" female

	X*	Y
X	XX*	XY
X	XX*	XY

1:2 (or 2:4) chance will be female with trait.
1:2 (or 2:4) chance will be "normal" male.

(C) Male with hemophilia and female with trait

	X*	Y
X*	X*X*	X*Y
X	X*X	XY

1:2 (or 2:4) chance will be female with trait.
1:4 chance will be "normal" male.
1:4 chance will be male with hemophilia.

Key
XY = normal male
X*Y = male with hemophilia
XX = normal female
X*X = female carrying hemophilia trait
X*X* = female with possible relative lack of clotting factor–*not* a true hemophiliac (von Willebrand's disease).

Note: The odds cited here are for *each* pregnancy.

Figure 5.11 **Genetic transmission of hemophilia.**

2. Need to determine which clotting factor is deficient/missing and extent of deficiency:
   a. *Mild:* child has 5% to 50% of normal amount of clotting factor.
   b. *Moderate:* child has 1% to 5% of normal amount of clotting factor.
   c. *Severe:* child has less than 1% of normal amount of clotting factor.
3. Definitive test: PTT

C. Analysis/nursing diagnosis:
1. *Risk for injury* related to bleeding tendencies.
2. *Pain* related to hemarthrosis.
3. *Impaired physical mobility* related to bleeding and pain.
4. *Knowledge deficit* related to home care and follow-up.

D. Nursing care plan/implementation:
1. Goal: *prevent injury and possible bleeding.*
   a. Provide an environment that is as safe as possible (e.g., toys with no sharp edges, child's safety scissors).
   b. Use soft toothbrush to prevent trauma to gums. Wear safety equipment in PE; no contact sports.
   c. When old enough to shave, use only electric razor (no straight-edge razors).
   d. *Avoid* IMs/IVs—but when absolutely necessary, treat as arterial puncture; that is, apply direct pressure to the site for at least 5 min after withdrawing needle.
   e. Do **not** use aspirin or medication containing aspirin (prolongs bleeding/clotting time). Caution with NSAIDs (inhibit platelet function).
2. Goal: *control bleeding episodes when they occur.*
   a. Local measures: *RICE* (**R**est, **I**ce, **C**ompression, **E**levation); keep immobilized during acute bleeding episodes only. For epistaxis: child should sit up and lean slightly forward.
   b. Systemic measures: administer clotting *antihemophilic factor* (factor VIII or DDAVP) via IV infusion. *Note:* These are blood products, so a transfusion reaction is possible.
   c. *Note:* cryoprecipitate (a blood product) is no longer used due to risk of transmission of hepatitis and HIV.
3. Goal: *prevent long-term disability related to joint degeneration.*
   a. Keep *immobilized* during period of acute bleeding and for 24 to 48 hours afterward to allow blood to clot and to prevent dislodging the clot.
   b. Administer prescribed pain medications *before* physical therapy sessions.
   c. Begin prescribed exercise program, starting with passive range of motion (ROM) and gradually advancing to active ROM, then full exercise program, as tolerated, to maintain maximum joint function. Monitor weight to prevent ↑ strain on joints (especially knees).
   d. **Avoid:** prolonged immobility, braces, splints—which can lead to permanent deformities and loss of mobility.
4. Goal: *promote independence in management of own care.*
   a. Encourage child to assume responsibility for choosing safe activities.

b. Encourage child to attend regular school as much as possible; provide support through school nurse.
c. Advise child to wear Medic Alert bracelet.
d. Caution parents to *avoid* overprotecting child.
e. Offer child chance to self-limit activities within appropriate limits (parents can offer guidance).
f. Assist child to cope with life-threatening disorder with no known cure.

5. Goal: *health teaching.*
a. Between 9 and 12 years of age: child can be taught to self-administer clotting factor IV (before this, family can perform).
b. As child enters adolescence: begin to discuss issues such as realistic vocations, insurance coverage, genetic transmission (see **Fig. 5.11**).

E. Evaluation/outcome criteria:
1. Serious injuries are prevented; bleeding is kept to a minimum.
2. Episodes of bleeding are controlled by prompt, effective intervention.
3. There are no long-term disabilities.
4. Child is able to manage own care independently, with minimum supervision.

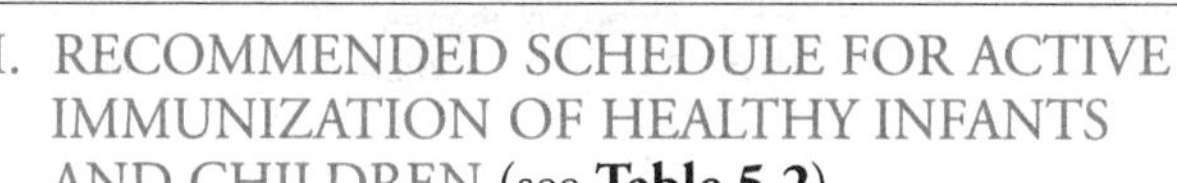

IMMUNOLOGICAL SYSTEM

I. RECOMMENDED SCHEDULE FOR ACTIVE IMMUNIZATION OF HEALTHY INFANTS AND CHILDREN (see **Table 5.2**).

II. ASSESSMENT: common side effects of immunizations (occur 24 to 48 hours after immunization except as noted):
A. Soreness, redness, tenderness, or lump at injection site.
B. Fever: brief, mild to moderate.
C. Crankiness and fussiness; anorexia; drowsiness.
D. Measles—coryza and rash 7 to 10 days after immunization.
E. Rubella—arthralgia and arthritis-like symptoms 2 weeks after immunization.

III. NURSING INTERVENTIONS/HOME CARE for infant or child who has been immunized:
A. Explain to parents the reason for each immunization and common side effects.
B. Suggest acetaminophen for fever or discomfort.
C. Extra affection and closeness—cuddling, soothing, rocking.
D. Teach parents to notify physician of untoward, serious, or prolonged side effects.

IV. CONTRAINDICATIONS/PRECAUTIONS TO IMMUNIZATIONS
A. Child who has a severe febrile illness (e.g., URI, gastroenteritis, or any fever).
B. Child with alteration in skin integrity: rash, eczema.
C. Child with alteration in immune system; steroids; chemotherapy, radiation therapy; human immunodeficiency virus (HIV)/acquired immunodeficiency syndrome (AIDS) (no live virus vaccine).
D. Child with a known allergic reaction to previous immunization or substance in the immunization.
E. Recent recipient of blood/blood products.

V. CHILDHOOD COMMUNICABLE DISEASES (**Table 5.19**). Basic principles of care:
A. Standard precautions to prevent communicability/infection.
B. Fever control with acetaminophen.
C. Extra fluids for hydration.
D. General home care procedures: comfort measures/supportive care.

Streptococcus Infections/Sequelae

Introduction: Group A β-hemolytic streptococcus is a common infectious organism that causes illness in children and is highly contagious. In themselves, the diseases caused by streptococcus do not seem very serious (e.g., strep throat, otitis media, impetigo, or scarlet fever). The most common treatment for strep is a full course of antibiotic therapy: 10 days of penicillin (or, if allergic, erythromycin). With adequate therapy, generally no sequelae are seen. If the strep is *not* treated, or is only partially treated, the sequelae include serious systemic diseases, with potentially long-term effects. If the effect is manifested primarily in the *heart (carditis),* it is *acute rheumatic fever.* If the effect is manifested primarily in the *kidneys,* it is *acute glomerulonephritis* (see **Fig. 5.10**).

INTEGUMENTARY SYSTEM

I. INFANTILE ECZEMA (ATOPIC DERMATITIS)
A. *Introduction:* Eczema is an allergic skin reaction, most commonly to foods (e.g., cow's milk, eggs). It is most common in *infants* and young children (under 2 years). Infantile eczema generally undergoes permanent, spontaneous remission by age 3 years; however, approximately 50% of children who have had infantile eczema develop asthma during the preschool or school-age years.

(text continues on page 306)

PEDIATRICS

Table 5.19

Communicable Diseases of Childhood

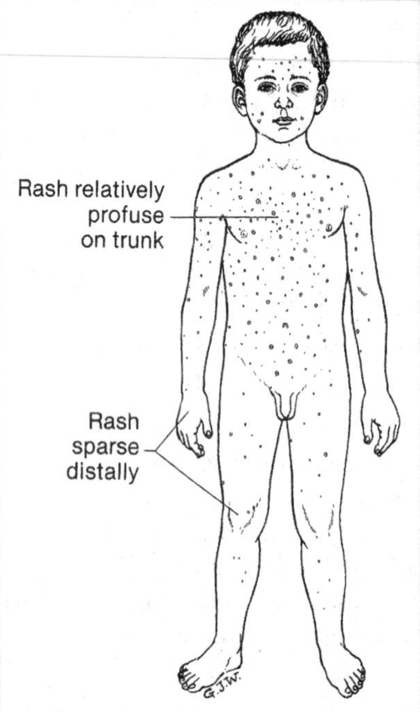

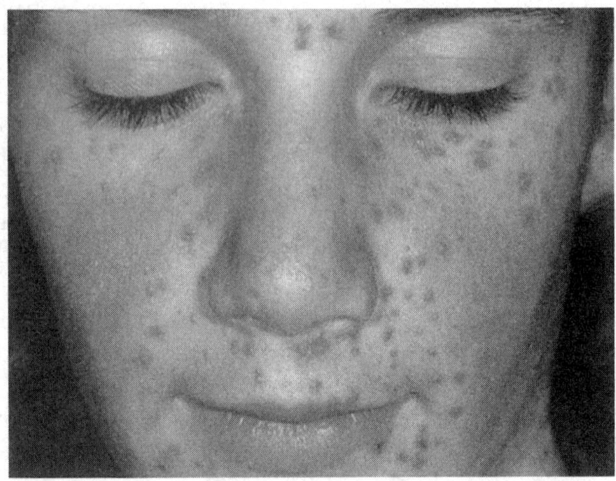

Chickenpox (varicella). (From Habif, TP: *Clinical Dermatology: A Color Guide to Diagnosis and Therapy,* ed 3. St. Louis, Mosby, 1996.)

Disease

Chickenpox (Varicella)
Agent: Varicella-zoster virus (VZV)

Source: Primary secretions of respiratory tract of person who is infected and to a lesser degree skin lesions (scabs not infectious)

Transmission: Direct contact, droplet (airborne) spread, and contaminated objects

Incubation period: 2–3 weeks, usually 13–17 days

Period of communicability: Probably 1 day before eruption of lesions (prodromal period) to 6 days after first crop of vesicles when crusts have formed

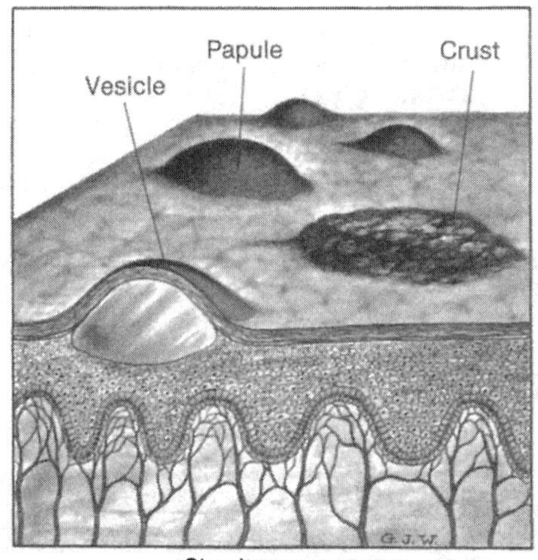

Simultaneous stages of lesions in chickenpox

Table 5.19

Communicable Diseases of Childhood—cont'd

Clinical Manifestations	Therapeutic Management/Complications	Nursing Considerations
Prodromal stage: Slight fever, malaise, and anorexia for first 24 hours; rash highly pruritic; begins as macule, rapidly progresses to papule and then vesicle (surrounded by erythematous base, becomes umbilicated and cloudy, breaks easily and forms crusts); all three stages (papule, vesicle, crust) present in varying degrees at one time. *Distribution:* Centripetal, spreading to face and proximal extremities but sparse on distal limbs and less on areas not exposed to heat (i.e., from clothing or sun) *Constitutional signs and symptoms:* Elevated temperature from lymphadenopathy, irritability from pruritus	 *Specific:* Antiviral agent acyclovir (Zovirax), varicella-zoster immune globulin (VZIG) after exposure in children who are high risk. 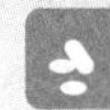 *Supportive:* Diphenhydramine hydrochloride or antihistamines to relieve itching; skin care to prevent secondary bacterial infection *Complications:* • Secondary bacterial infections (abscesses, cellulitis, pneumonia, sepsis) • Encephalitis • Varicella pneumonia • Hemorrhagic varicella (tiny hemorrhages in vesicles and numerous petechiae in skin) • Chronic or transient thrombocytopenia	Maintain strict isolation in hospital. Isolate child in home until vesicles have dried (usually 1 week after onset of disease), and isolate children who are high risk from children who are infected. Administer skin care: give bath and change clothes and linens daily; administer topical calamine lotion; keep child's fingernails short and clean; apply mittens if child scratches. Keep child cool (may decrease number of lesions). Lessen pruritus; keep child occupied. Remove loose crusts that rub and irritate skin. Teach child to apply pressure to pruritic area rather than scratch it. If older child, reason with child regarding danger of scar formation from scratching.  *Avoid* use of aspirin; use of acetaminophen controversial.

Continued

Table 5.19

Communicable Diseases of Childhood—cont'd

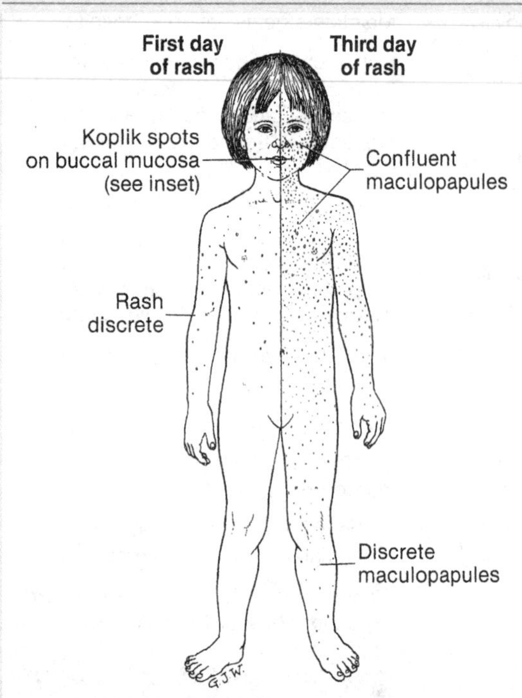

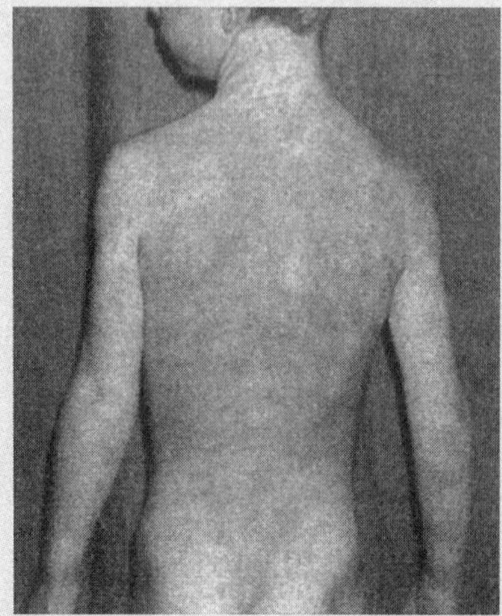

Measles (rubeola). (From Seidel, HM and others: *Mosby's Guide to Physical Examination,* ed 3. St. Louis, Mosby, 1995.)

Disease

Measles (Rubeola)
Agent: Virus

Source: Respiratory tract secretions, blood, and urine of person who is infected

Transmission: Usually by direct contact with droplets of person who is infected

Incubation period: 10–20 days

Period of communicability: From 4 days before to 5 days after rash appears but mainly during prodromal (catarrhal) stage

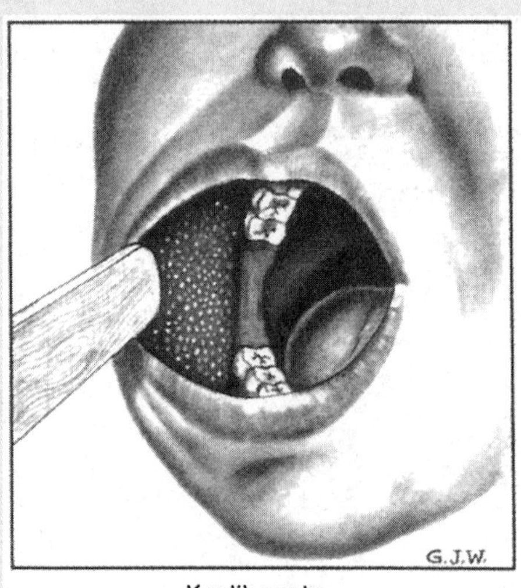

Koplik spots

Mumps
Agent: Paramyxovirus

Source: Saliva of people who are infected

Transmission: Direct contact with or droplet spread from a person who is infected

Incubation period: 14–21 days

Period of communicability: Most communicable immediately *before* and *after* swelling begins

PEDIATRICS

Table 5.19

Communicable Diseases of Childhood—cont'd

Clinical Manifestations	Therapeutic Management/Complications	Nursing Considerations
Prodromal (catarrhal) stage: Fever and malaise, followed in 24 hours by coryza, cough, conjunctivitis, *Koplik's spots* (small, irregular red spots with a minute, bluish-white center first seen on buccal mucosa opposite molars 2 days before rash); symptoms gradually increase in severity until second day after rash appears, when they begin to subside *Rash:* Appears 3–4 days after onset of prodromal stage; begins as erythematous maculopapular eruption on face and gradually spreads downward; more severe in earlier sites (appears confluent) and less intense in later sites (appears discrete); after 3–4 days assumes brownish appearance, and fine desquamation occurs over areas of extensive involvement *Constitutional signs and symptoms:* Anorexia, malaise, generalized lymphadenopathy	 Vitamin A supplementation *Supportive:* Bedrest during febrile period Antipyretics Antibiotics to prevent secondary bacterial infection in high-risk children *Complications:* Otitis media Pneumonia Bronchiolitis Obstructive laryngitis and laryngotracheitis Encephalitis	Isolation until fifth day of rash; if hospitalized, institute respiratory precautions. Maintain bedrest during prodromal stage; provide quiet activity. *Fever:* Instruct parents to administer antipyretics; *avoid* chilling; if child is prone to seizures, institute appropriate precautions (fever spikes to 104°F [40°C] between fourth and fifth days). *Eye care:* Dim lights if photophobia present; clean eyelids with warm saline solution to remove secretions or crusts; keep child from rubbing eyes; examine cornea for signs of ulceration.  *Coryza/cough:* Use cool mist vaporizer; protect skin around nares with layer of petrolatum; encourage fluids and soft, bland foods. *Skin care:* Keep skin clean; use tepid baths as necessary.
Prodromal stage: Fever, headache, malaise, and anorexia for 24 hours, followed by "earache" that is aggravated by chewing *Parotitis:* By third day, parotid gland(s) (either unilateral or bilateral) enlarge(s) and reach(es) maximum size in 1–3 days; accompanied by pain and tenderness *Other manifestations:* Submaxillary and sublingual infection, orchitis, and meningoencephalitis	 *Symptomatic and supportive:* Analgesics for pain and antipyretics for fever Intravenous fluid may be necessary for child who refuses to drink or vomits because of meningoencephalitis *Complications:* Sensorineural deafness Postinfectious encephalitis Myocarditis Arthritis Hepatitis Epididymo-orchitis Sterility (extremely rare in adult men)	Isolation during period of communicability; institute respiratory precautions during hospitalization. Maintain bedrest during prodromal phase until swelling subsides. 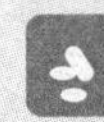 Give analgesics for pain; if child is unwilling to chew medication, use elixir form. 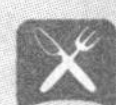 Encourage fluids and soft, bland foods; *avoid* foods that require chewing. Apply hot or cold compresses to neck, whichever is more comforting. To relieve orchitis, provide warmth and local support with tight-fitting underpants (stretch bathing suit works well).

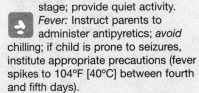

Continued

Table 5.19

Communicable Diseases of Childhood—cont'd

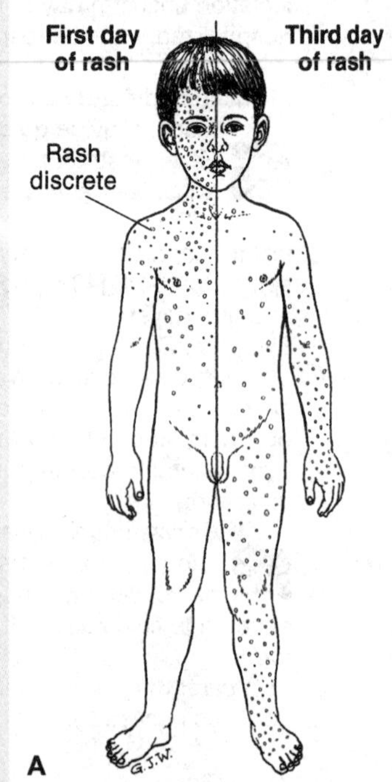

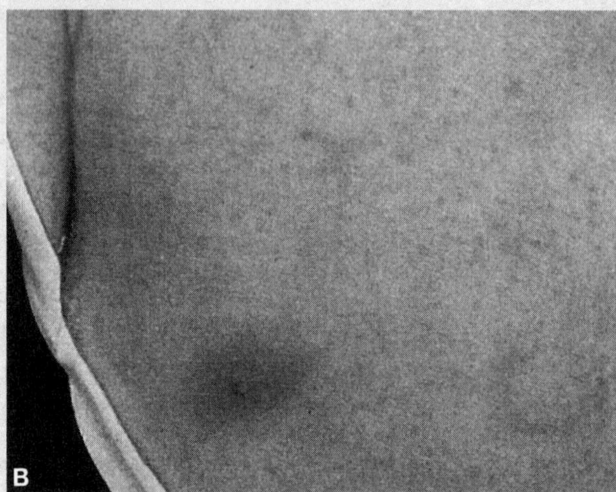

Rubella (German Measles). (A) Progression of rash. **(B)** Appearance of rash. (From Habif, TP: *Clinical Dermatology: A Color Guide to Diagnosis and Therapy,* ed 3. St. Louis, Mosby, 1996.)

Disease

Rubella (German Measles)

Agent: Rubella virus

Source: Primarily nasopharyngeal secretions of persons with apparent or inapparent infection; virus also present in blood, stool, and urine

Transmission: Direct contact and spread via person who is infected; indirectly via articles freshly contaminated with nasopharyngeal secretions, feces, or urine

Incubation period: 14–21 days

Period of communicability: 7 days *before* to approximately 5 days *after* appearance of rash

Scarlet Fever

Agent: Group A β-hemolytic streptococci

Source: Usually from nasopharyngeal secretions of person who is infected and carriers

Transmission: Direct contact with person who is infected, or droplet spread indirectly by contact with contaminated articles, ingestion of contaminated milk or other food

Incubation period: 2–4 days, with range of 1–7 days

Period of communicability: During incubation period and clinical illness, approximately 10 days; during first 2 weeks of carrier phase, although may persist for months

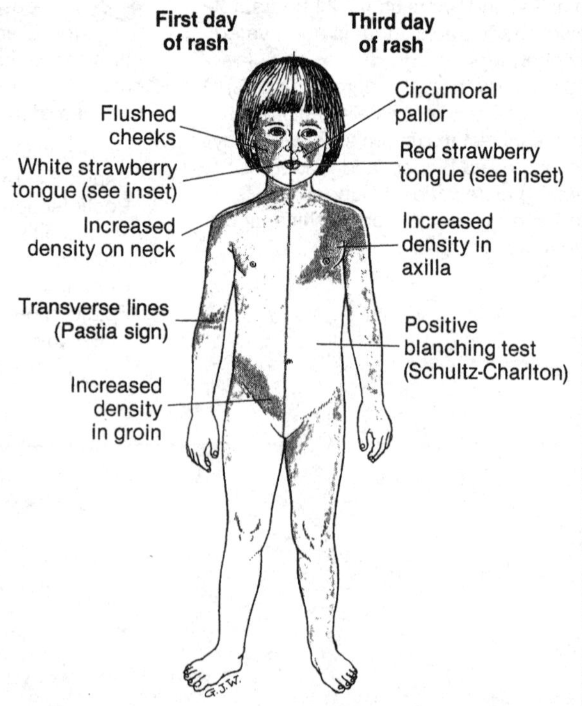

Scarlet Fever.

PEDIATRICS

Table 5.19

Communicable Diseases of Childhood—cont'd

Clinical Manifestations	Therapeutic Management/Complications	Nursing Considerations
Prodromal stage: Absent in children, present in adults and adolescents; consists of: low-grade fever, headache, malaise, anorexia, mild conjunctivitis, coryza, sore throat, cough, and lymphadenopathy; lasts for 1–5 days, subsides 1 day after appearance of rash *Rash:* First appears on face and rapidly spreads downward to neck, arms, trunk, and legs; by end of *first* day, body is covered with a discrete, pinkish red maculopapular exanthema; disappears in same order as it began and is usually gone by *third* day *Constitutional signs and symptoms:* Occasionally low-grade fever, headache, malaise, and lymphadenopathy	 No treatment necessary other than antipyretics for low-grade fever and analgesics for discomfort *Complications:* Rare (arthritis, encephalitis, or purpura); most benign of all childhood communicable diseases; greatest danger is teratogenic effect on fetus	Reassure parents of benign nature of illness in child who is affected. Use comfort measures as necessary. Isolate child from women who are pregnant.
Prodromal stage: Abrupt high fever, pulse increased out of proportion to fever, vomiting, headache, chills, malaise, abdominal pain *Enanthema:* Tonsils enlarged, edematous, reddened, and covered with patches of exudate; in severe cases appearance resembles membrane seen in diphtheria; pharynx is edematous and beefy red; during *first 1–2 days* tongue is coated and papillae become red and swollen (*white strawberry tongue*); by *fourth or fifth day* white coat sloughs off, leaving prominent papillae (*red strawberry tongue*); palate is covered with erythematous punctate lesions *Exanthema:* Rash appears within *12 hours* after prodromal stage; red pinhead-sized punctate lesions rapidly become generalized but are absent on face, which becomes flushed with striking circumoral pallor; rash is more intense in folds of joints; by *end of first week* desquamation begins (fine, sandpaper-like on torso; sheetlike sloughing on palms and soles), which may be complete by 3 weeks or longer	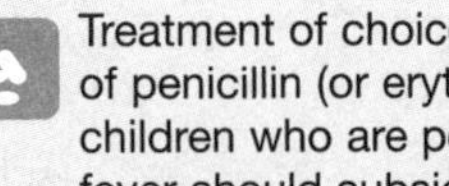 Treatment of choice is a full course of penicillin (or erythromycin for children who are penicillin-sensitive); fever should subside 24 hr after beginning therapy 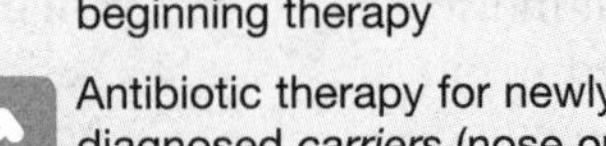 Antibiotic therapy for newly diagnosed *carriers* (nose or throat cultures positive for streptococci) 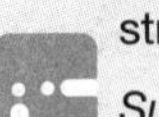 *Supportive measures:* Bedrest during febrile phase, analgesics for sore throat *Complications:* Otitis media Peritonsillar abscess Sinusitis Glomerulonephritis Carditis, polyarthritis (uncommon)	Institute *respiratory precautions* until 24 hours after initiation of treatment.  Ensure compliance with oral antibiotic therapy (intramuscular benzathine penicillin G [Bicillin] may be given if parents' reliability in giving oral drugs is questionable). Maintain bedrest during febrile phase; provide quiet activity during convalescent period.  Relieve discomfort of sore throat with analgesics, gargles, lozenges, antiseptic throat sprays (*Chloraseptic*), and inhalation of cool mist.  Encourage fluids during febrile phase; *avoid* irritating liquids (citrus juices) or rough foods; when child is able to eat, begin with soft diet. Advise parents to consult practitioner if fever persists after beginning therapy. Discuss procedures for preventing spread of infection.

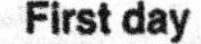

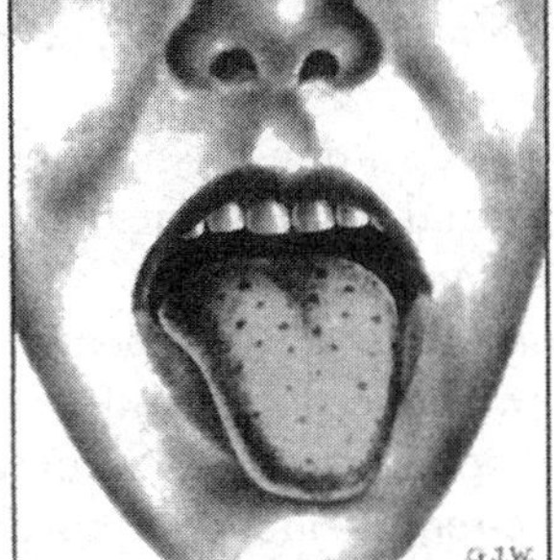

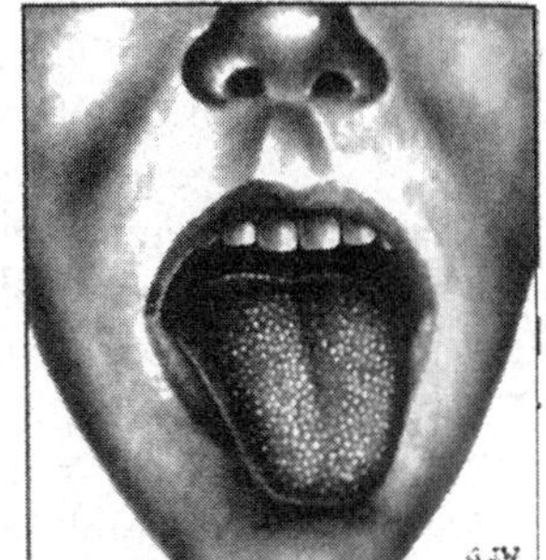

Strawberry tongue. (From Wong, D: *Whaley and Wong's Nursing Care of Infants and Children*, ed 7. Mosby, St. Louis, 2003.)

PEDIATRICS

B. Assessment:

1. Erythematous lesions, beginning on cheeks and spreading to rest of face and scalp.
2. May spread to rest of body, especially in flexor surfaces (e.g., antecubital space).
3. Lesions may ooze or crust over.
4. Severe pruritus, which may lead to secondary infection.
5. Lymphadenopathy near site of rash.
6. Unaffected skin tends to be dry and rough.
7. Systemic manifestations are rare—but child may be irritable, cranky.

C. Analysis/nursing diagnosis:

1. *Impaired tissue integrity* related to lesions.
2. *Pain* related to pruritus.
3. *Risk for (secondary) infection* related to breaks in the skin (first line of defense) and itching.
4. *Knowledge deficit* related to care of child with eczema, prognosis, how to prevent exacerbations.

D. Nursing care plan/implementation:

1. Goal: *promote healing of lesions.*
   a. *Wet method:* frequent tepid baths (up to four times a day) followed by immediate application of a lubricant while the skin is still moist; **no soap** or use very mild, nonperfumed soap (e.g., Dove, Neutrogena); most useful method if child lives in a *dry* climate.
   b. *Dry method:* infrequent baths; cleanse skin with nonlipid, hydrophilic agent (e.g., Cetaphil); most useful method if child lives in a *humid* climate.
   c. Can add cornstarch to bath water to relieve itching and promote healing; keep skin well hydrated by applying emollients containing petrolatum or lanolin, which are occlusive and prevent evaporation of moisture.
   d. Apply wet soaks with Burow's solution (aluminum acetate solution; topical astringent and antiseptic); wet soaks should not be used for more than 3 days at a time
   e. Protect child from possible sources of infection; *standard precautions* to prevent infection.
   f. **Absolutely no** immunizations during acute exacerbations of eczema because of the possibility of an overwhelming dermatitis, allergic reaction, shock, or even death.
   g. Apply topical creams/ointments as prescribed: A and D emollient ointment, hydrocortisone cream to promote healing.
2. Goal: *provide relief from itching/keep child from scratching.*
   a. Administer systemic oral antihistamines as ordered (e.g., *Benadryl* or *Atarax*) to break itch-scratch cycle. Most useful at bedtime when itching tends to increase.
   b. Keep nails trimmed short—may need mittens (preferable not to use elbow restraints, because the antecubital space is a common site for eczema).
   c. Use clothes and bed linens that are nonirritating, that is, pure cotton (**no** wool or blends).
   d. Institute *elimination/hypoallergenic diet:*
      (1) *No* milk or milk products.
      (2) Change to lactose-free formula (e.g., Isomil).
      (3) *Avoid:* eggs, wheat, nuts, beans, chocolate.
   e. *No* stuffed animals or hairy dolls.
3. Goal: *provide discharge planning/teaching for parents and child.*
   a. Include all above information.
   b. Include information on course of disease: characterized by exacerbations and remissions throughout early years.
   c. Include information on prognosis: 50% to 60% will go into spontaneous (and permanent) remission during preschool years; 40% to 50% will develop asthma/hay fever during school-age years.

E. Evaluation/outcome criteria:

1. Lesions heal well, without secondary infection.
2. Adequate relief from itching is achieved.
3. Parents verbalize understanding of eczema, prognosis, and how to prevent exacerbations.

II. INFESTATIONS

A. Lice (pediculosis)

1. *Introduction:* In children, the most common form of lice is *pediculosis capitis*, or head lice. This parasite feeds on the scalp, and its saliva causes severe itching. Head lice are frequently associated with the sharing of combs and brushes, hats, and clothing; thus, they are more common in girls, especially those with long hair. Lice are also associated with overcrowded conditions and poor hair hygiene.
2. **Assessment:**
   a. Severe itching of scalp.
   b. Visible eggs/nits on shafts of hair.
3. **Analysis/nursing diagnosis:**
   a. *Impaired skin integrity* related to infestation of scalp with lice.
   b. *Risk for impaired skin integrity* related to severe pruritus of scalp.
   c. *Knowledge deficit* related to transmission and prevention of disease and treatment regimen.
4. **Nursing care plan/implementation:**
   a. Goal: *eradicate lice infestation.* Apply permethrin (*Nix*) as drug of choice for infants and children—rub shampoo in for 4 to 5 minutes, then comb with fine-tooth comb to remove dead lice and nits (eggs).

b. Goal: *prevent spread of lice.*
(1) Wear gloves and cap to protect self.
(2) Inspect other family members; treat prn with pediculocide.
(3) Wash all clothes and linens to kill any lice that may have fallen off the child's hair.
(4) Encourage short hair, if acceptable.
(5) Teach preventive measures: do *not* share comb, brushes, hats.

5. **Evaluation/outcome criteria:** lice are eradicated and do not spread.

B. **Pinworms** (enterobiasis)

1. *Introduction:* In children, the most common helminthic infestation is pinworms. Infestation usually occurs when the child places fingers (and the pinworm eggs) into the mouth. Breaking the *anus-to-mouth* contamination cycle can best be accomplished by good hygiene, especially hand washing before eating and after toileting. If one family member has pinworms, it is highly likely that other family members are also infested; therefore, treat the entire family to eradicate the parasite. Pinworms are easily eradicated with antiparasitic medications.
2. **Assessment:**
a. Intense perianal itching.
b. Visible pinworms in the stool.
c. Vague abdominal discomfort.
d. Anorexia and weight loss.
3. **Analysis/nursing diagnosis:**
a. *Risk for infection/injury* related to the anus-to-mouth contamination cycle of pinworm infestation, severe rectal itching.
b. *Knowledge deficit* related to transmission and prevention of disease and treatment regimen.
4. **Nursing care plan/implementation:**
a. Goal: *eradicate pinworm infestation.* Treat all family members simultaneously with an antiparasitic agent (e.g., *Vermox, Povan*).
b. Goal: *prevent spread of pinworms.*
(1) Launder all underwear, bed linens, and towels in hot soapy water to kill eggs.
(2) Teach family members the importance of good hygiene, especially hand washing before eating (or preparing food) and after toileting. Stress to children to keep their fingers out of their mouths.
5. **Evaluation/outcome criteria:** Pinworms are eradicated and do not spread; reinfestation does not occur.

MUSCULOSKELETAL AND NEUROMUSCULAR SYSTEMS

Orthopedic conditions in infants and children are many and varied, but treatment is based on basic principles of nursing care. **Table 5.20** and **Figs. 5.12** and **5.13** offer a quick review of the major pediatric orthopedic conditions.

PEDIATRICS

Table 5.20

Common Pediatric Orthopedic Conditions

Condition	Definition	Age at Onset/Sex Difference	Treatment	Nursing Considerations
Congenital Musculoskeletal Disorders				
Clubfoot	Downward, inward rotation of one or both feet: talipes equinovarus (95%)	Newborn (congenital); twice as common in *boys*	Series of casts changed weekly followed by *Denis Browne splint* and then corrective shoes (severe cases—surgery)	• Care of child in cast/brace. • Stress need for follow-up. • Encourage compliance.
Developmental dysplasia of the hip (see Fig. 5.12)	Abnormal development of hip joint (most frequently unilateral)	Newborn (congenital); more common in *girls*	*Newborn—Pavlik harness; older infant or toddler*—possible surgery, spica cast	• Early identification. • Care of child in traction/cast: check circulation; turn q2h while cast is wet. • Encourage compliance. • Check for other anomalies (e.g., spina bifida).

Continued

Table 5.20

Common Pediatric Orthopedic Conditions—cont'd

Condition	Definition	Age at Onset/Sex Difference	Treatment	Nursing Considerations
Congenital Musculoskeletal Disorders				
Legg-Calvé-Perthes disease	Aseptic necrosis of the head of the femur (cause unknown)	*Peak:* 4–8 years; *range:* 3–12 years; 5 times more common in *boys;* 10 times more common in Caucasians than non-Caucasians	Conservative therapy lasts 2–4 years, usually begins with bedrest and traction, followed by non–weight-bearing devices such as brace, cast	• Early identification. • Care of child in traction/cast: check for frayed pulley ropes. • Provide diversion. • Assist child and family to cope with child's prolonged immobility.
Scoliosis (see Fig. 5.13)	Lateral curvature of the spine (cause unknown)	Adolescence; more common in *girls*	Braces specific to type of curvature; halo-pelvic traction; *Harrington rod;* Luque, Cotrel-Dubousset, or Dwyer/Zielke instrumentation	• Care of child in traction/cast/brace. • Teach that brace is worn 16–23 hr/day, 7 days/wk for 6 months–2 years. • Encourage compliance. • Promote positive self-image.
Acquired Defect				
Osteomyelitis	Most frequently occurring bone infection among children	5–14 years; twice as common in *boys*	Blood cultures to diagnose causative organisms—select appropriate antibiotic; bedrest, immobilization with splint or cast	• Care of child in splint/cast. • Provide diversion. • Pain medications/antibiotics per physician order.
Joint Disorder				
Juvenile idiopathic arthritis (JIA) (formerly known as juvenile rheumatoid arthritis)	Chronic systemic inflammatory disease (cause unknown)	*Peak:* 1–3 years and 8–10 years; more common in *girls*	Prevent joint deformity by exercise, splints, medications (NSAIDs, SAARDs, corticosteroids, biological agents [Etanercept], cytotoxic agents); relieve symptoms (as per adult with arthritis)	• Care of child in brace/splint. • Provide diversion. • Encourage compliance.
Bone Tumor				
Osteosarcoma	Most frequently occurring bone cancer among children	Adolescence (10–25 years); more common in *boys* and men	Limb salvage procedure; amputation → prosthesis; chemotherapy	• Prepare child for loss of limb • Help cope with prosthesis, life-threatening illness • Assist with grieving process

PEDIATRICS

I. CEREBRAL PALSY

A. *Introduction: Cerebral palsy (CP)* is the most common permanent physical disability of childhood. It is a neuromuscular disorder of the pyramidal motor system resulting in debilitating impaired voluntary muscle control. The damage appears to be fixed and nonprogressive, and the cause is unknown. However, although a variety of factors have been implicated in the etiology of CP, it is now known that CP results more commonly from prenatal brain abnormalities.

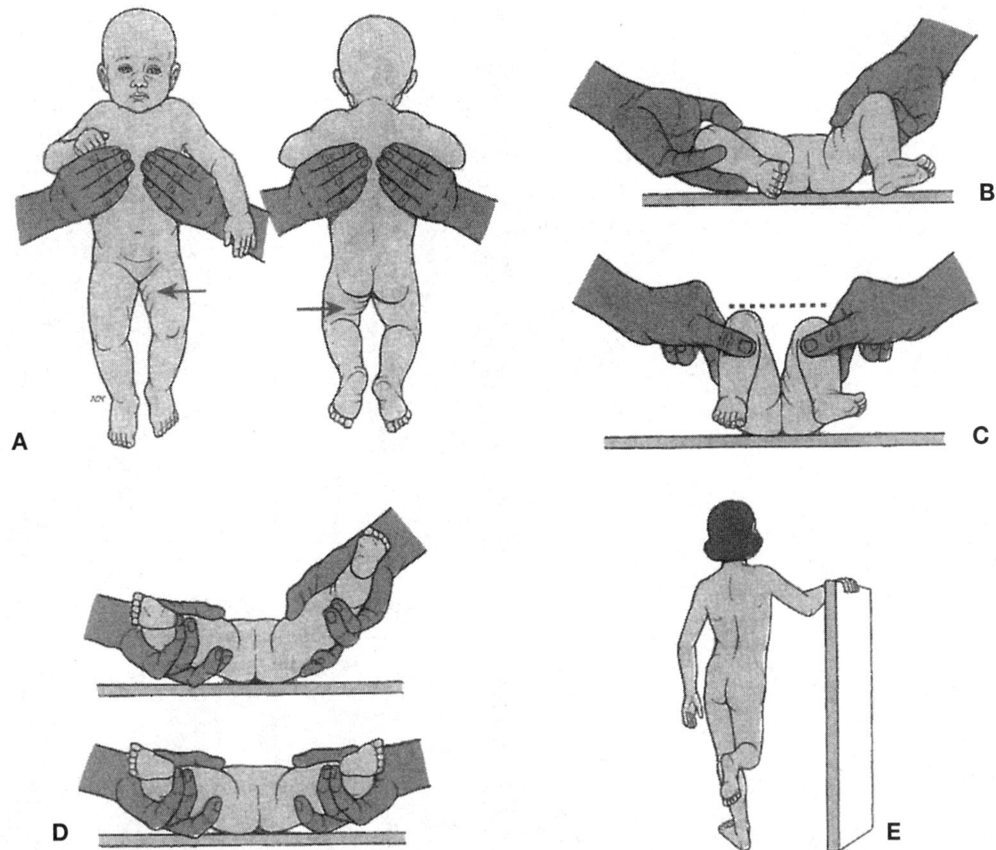

Figure 5.12 **Signs of developmental dysplasia of the hip.** *(A)* Asymmetry of gluteal and thigh folds. *(B)* Limited hip abduction as seen in flexion. *(C)* Apparent shortening of the femur, as indicated by the level of the knees in flexion. *(D)* Ortolani click (if infant is under 4 weeks of age). *(E)* Positive Trendelenburg sign or gait (if child is weight bearing). (From Hockenberry, M, & Wilson, D: *Wong's Nursing Care of Infants and Children*, ed 8. Mosby, St. Louis, 2007.)

B. Assessment:

1. Most common type of cerebral palsy—*spastic.*
   a. Delayed developmental milestones.
   b. Tongue thrust with difficulty swallowing and sucking. Poor weight gain. Aspiration may occur.
   c. Increased muscle tone: "scissoring" (legs crossed, toes pointed).
   d. Persistent neonatal reflexes.
   e. Associated problems:
      (1) Mental retardation in 30% of children with cerebral palsy (70% are normal).
      (2) Sensory impairment: vision, hearing.
      (3) Orthopedic conditions: congenital dysplasia of hip, clubfoot.
      (4) Dental problems: malocclusion.
      (5) Seizures.

C. Analysis/nursing diagnosis:

1. *Ineffective airway clearance* related to hyperactive gag reflex and possible aspiration.
2. *Altered nutrition, less than body requirements,* related to difficulty sucking and swallowing.
3. *Fluid volume deficit* related to difficulty sucking and swallowing.
4. *Impaired verbal communication* related to difficulty with speech.
5. *Sensory/perceptual alterations* related to potential vision and hearing defects.
6. *Risk for injury* related to difficulty controlling voluntary muscles.
7. *Self-esteem disturbance* related to disability.
8. *Note:* Because the level of disabilities with CP can vary, the nurse must select those diagnoses that apply, and clearly specify the individual child's limitations in any diagnostic statements.

D. Nursing care plan/implementation:

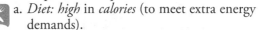

1. Goal: *maintain patent airway.*
   a. Have suction and oxygen readily available.
   b. Use feeding and positioning techniques to maintain patent airway.
   c. Institute prompt, aggressive therapy for URIs, to prevent the possible development of pneumonia.
2. Goal: *promote adequate nutrition.*
    a. *Diet: high* in *calories* (to meet extra energy demands).

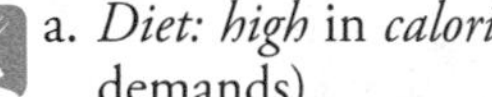

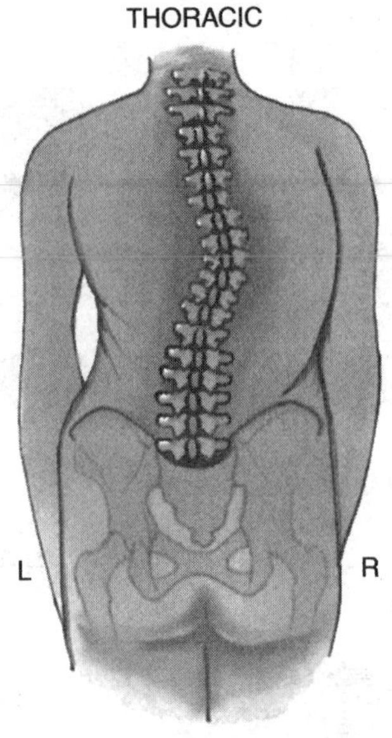
THORACIC
L
R
90% occur on the right side above T-11

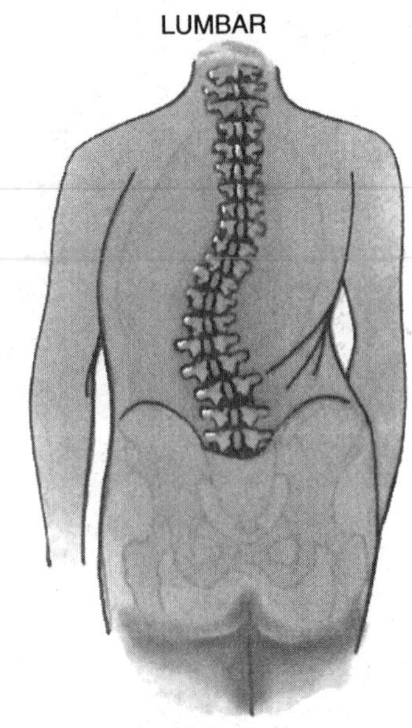
LUMBAR
70% occur on the left side at L-1 or lower

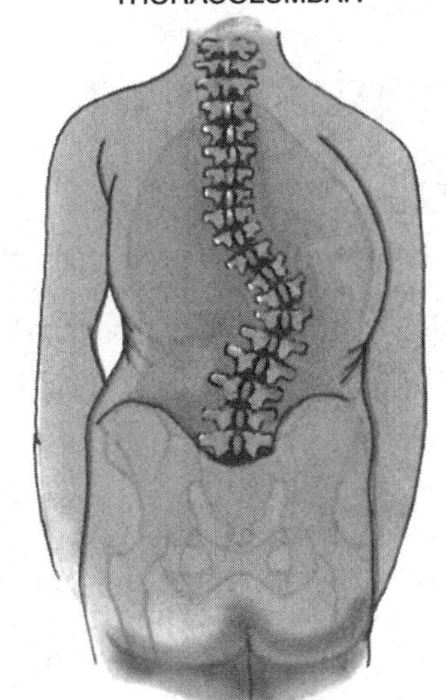
THORACOLUMBAR
80% occur on the right side at T-11 – T-12

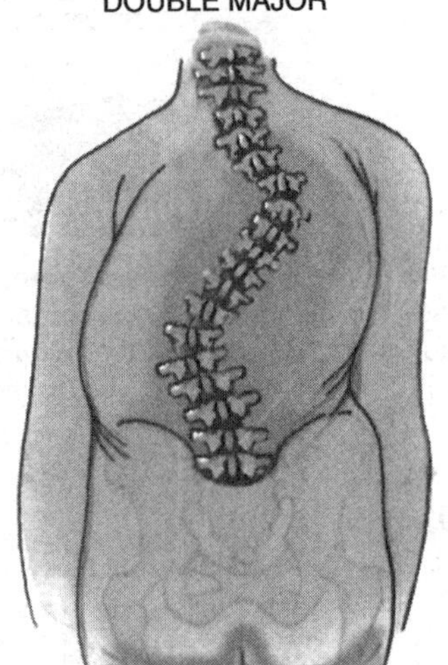
DOUBLE MAJOR
Usually involves right-sided and left-sided lumbar curves
Curve location is determined by the level of the apical vertebra

Figure 5.13 The four major curve patterns in idiopathic scoliosis. (From Bowden, VR, Dickey, SB, & Greenberg, CS: *Children and Their Families: The Continuum of Care.* WB Saunders, Philadelphia, 1999.)

   b. Ensure balanced diet of basic foods that can be easily chewed. Refer to dentist for early dental care.
   c. Provide feeding utensils that promote independence.
   d. Feed in upright position.
   e. Relaxed mealtimes, decreased emphasis on manners, cleanliness.
   f. Monitor I&O, weight gain.
3. Goal: *facilitate verbal communication.*
   a. Refer to speech therapist.
   b. Speak slowly, clearly to child.
   c. Use pictures or actual objects to reinforce speech.
4. Goal: *prevent injury.* Refer to information on safety throughout growth and development sections, **pp. 256–257, 258, 260, 261, Table 3.9, p. 94, and Table 3.10, pp. 94–95.**
   a. Use individually designed chairs with restraints for positioning and safety.
   b. Provide protective helmet to prevent head trauma.
   c. Implement seizure precautions.
5. Goal: *provide early detection of and correction for vision and hearing defects.*
   a. Arrange for screening tests.
   b. Assist family with obtaining corrective devices: eyeglasses, hearing aids.

6. Goal: *promote locomotion.*
   a. Encourage "infant stimulation" program to assist infant in reaching developmental milestones.
   b. *Refer to physical therapy* for exercise program.
   c. Incorporate play into exercise routine.
   d. Use devices that promote locomotion: parallel bars, crutches, and braces.
   e. Surgical approach may be needed to relieve contractures.
   f. Medications: focus on ↓ excessive motion and tension; antianxiety agents, skeletal muscle relaxants, Botox injections, baclofen pump (IT).
7. Goal: *encourage independence in ADLs.*
   a. Adapt clothing, feeding utensils, etc., to facilitate self-help.
   b. Encourage child to perform ADLs as much as possible; offer positive reinforcement.
   c. Assist parents to have realistic expectations for their child; *avoid* excessively high expectations that might increase frustration.
8. Goal: *promote self-esteem.*
   a. Praise child for each accomplishment or for sincere effort.
   b. Help child dress and groom self daily in an attractive "normal" manner for developmental level and age.
   c. Encourage child to form friendships with children with similar problems.
   d. Enroll child in special education classes to meet the child's educational needs.
   e. Encourage parents to expose child to wide variety of experiences.

E. Evaluation/outcome criteria:
1. Patent airway and adequate oxygenation maintained.
2. Adequate nutrition maintained, and child begins to grow and gain weight.
3. Child has an acceptable means of verbal communication.
4. Safety is maintained.
5. Vision and hearing within normal limits using corrective devices prn.
6. Child is as mobile as possible, given disabilities.
7. Child is performing ADLs, within capabilities.
8. Child has positive self-image/self-esteem.

II. SPINA BIFIDA (MYELODYSPLASIA)

A. *Introduction:* Three different types of spina bifida:
1. *Spina bifida occulta*—a "hidden" bony defect without herniation of the meninges or cord; not visible externally, no symptoms are present, and no treatment is needed.
2. Spina bifida cystica—visible defect of the spine with external saclike protrusion.
   a. *Meningocele* (**Table 5.21**).
   b. *Myelomeningocele*—see **Table 5.21.** Most serious type of spina bifida cystica and also most common.
   The remainder of this section deals with *myelomeningocele* exclusively.

B. Assessment:
1. Congenital defect.
2. Readily detected by visual inspection in delivery room: round, bulging sac filled with fluid, usually in lumbosacral area.

PEDIATRICS

Table 5.21

Comparison of Two Major Types of Spina Bifida

Dimension	Meningocele	Myelomeningocele
Contents of sac	Meninges and cerebrospinal fluid	Meninges, cerebrospinal fluid, spinal cord
Transillumination	Present	Absent
Percentage of total cases	25%	75%
Motor function	Present	Absent
Sensory function	Present	Absent
Urinary/fecal incontinence	Absent	Present
Associated orthopedic anomalies	Rare	Developmental dysplasia of the hip, *clubfoot*
Other anomalies	Rare	*Hydrocephalus* (90%–95%)
Treatment	Surgery	Surgery
Major *short-term* complication	Infection (meningitis)	Infection (meningitis)
Major *long-term* complication	None	Chronic urinary tract infection leading to renal disease/failure
Prognosis	Excellent	Guarded

3. *Sensation and movement:* complete lack below the level of the lesion.
4. *Urinary:* retention, with overflow incontinence.
5. *Fecal:* constipation, fecal impaction, oozing of liquid stool around impaction.
6. 80% to 85% develop signs and symptoms of hydrocephalus.
7. May have associated orthopedic anomalies: clubfoot, developmental hip dysplasia.

C. Analysis/nursing diagnosis:

1. *Risk for injury/infection* related to rupture of the sac.
2. *Altered urinary elimination* related to urinary retention and overflow incontinence.
3. *Impaired skin integrity* related to immobility.
4. *Constipation* related to fecal incontinence and impaired innervation.

D. Nursing care plan/implementation:

1. Goal: *prevent rupture of the sac and possible infection (preoperative).*
   a. *Position: no* pressure on sac; *prone,* to prevent contamination with urine or stool.
   b. *No* clothing or diapers, to *avoid* pressure on sac.
   c. Place in heated isolette to maintain body temperature. *Avoid* radiant heat, which can dry and crack the sac.
   d. Keep sac covered with sterile, moist, nonadherent dressing (sterile normal saline) to prevent drying, cracking, and leakage of CSF; change every 2 to 4 hours; document appearance of sac with each dressing change to note signs and symptoms of infection, leaks, abrasions, or irritation.
   e. Enforce *strict aseptic technique* to prevent infection (leading cause of morbidity/mortality in neonatal period).
   f. *Avoid* repeated latex exposure (e.g., gloves, catheters) to decrease risk of latex allergy.
2. Goal: *prevent infection in postoperative period.*
   a. *Position:* prone, side-lying, or partial side-lying.
   b. Use myelomeningocele apron (specific type of dressing) to prevent urine or stool from contaminating suture line.
   c. Administer antibiotics as ordered.
   d. Use *strict aseptic techniques* in dressing changes; standard precautions to prevent infection.
3. Goal: *prevent urinary retention and UTI.*
   a. Monitor I&O, offer extra fluids to flush kidneys.
   b. Keep urethral meatus clean of stool to prevent ascending bacterial infection.
   c. Monitor urinary output for retention.
   d. Administer antibiotics/urinary tract antiseptics as ordered.
4. Goal: *prevent complications of prolonged immobility or associated orthopedic anomalies.*
   a. *Position:* hips abducted.
   b. Use positional devices, rotating pressure mattress/flotation mattress.
   c. *Refer to physical therapy* for ROM exercises.
   d. Make necessary referrals for care of possible clubfoot/developmental hip dysplasia.
5. Goal: *monitor for possible development of hydrocephalus.* Occurs in 90% to 95% of infants born with myelomeningocele.

E. Evaluation/outcome criteria:

1. Integrity of sac is maintained until surgery is done.
2. No infection occurs.
3. Adequate patterns of urinary and bowel elimination are achieved with necessary support.
4. Complications of immobility, orthopedic anomalies are prevented or treated promptly.

ACCIDENTS: INGESTIONS AND POISONINGS

I. GENERAL PRINCIPLES OF TREATMENT FOR INGESTIONS AND POISONINGS

A. *Prevention:* refer to section on toddler safety, **p. 258.**

B. How to induce vomiting:

1. Drug of choice—*syrup of ipecac* (available over the counter; does not require a physician's order). If families with young children keep this medication on hand it should be administered **only** if directed by Poison Control Center. *Note:* Safety of ipecac has been questioned due to esophageal tears (when misused) and anorexia nervosa/bulimia (when abused).
2. Dose:
   a. 30 mL for adolescents over 12 years; repeat dosage once if vomiting has not occurred within 20 minutes.
   b. 15 mL for children 1 to 12 years; repeat dosage once if vomiting has not occurred within 20 minutes. *Note:* Do *not* administer to infants *less than 1 year of age* without physician's order.
   c. 10 mL for infants 6 to 12 months; do *not* repeat dosage.
3. Follow dose of ipecac with 4 to 8 oz of tap water or as much water as child will drink. In young children, give water first because child may refuse to drink anything else after tasting the ipecac.
4. The child *must* vomit the syrup of ipecac to avoid its being absorbed and causing

potentially fatal cardiotoxicity (cardiac arrhythmias, atrial fibrillation, severe heart block). If child does not vomit within 20 minutes of second dose, summon paramedics; gastric lavage may be indicated upon arrival in emergency department. Do **not** manually stimulate gagging because gagging may ↑ vagal response → significant bradycardia.

C. When **not** to induce vomiting:
1. Child is stuporous or comatose.
2. Poison ingested is a corrosive substance or petroleum distillate.
3. Child is having seizures.
4. Child is in severe shock.
5. Child has lost the gag reflex.

II. SALICYLATE POISONING

A. Assessment:
1. Determine how much aspirin was ingested, when, which type.
2. Evaluate salicylate levels: normal, 0; therapeutic range = 15 to 30 mg/dL; *toxic,* >30 mg/dL.
3. *Early* identification of *mild toxicity:*
   a. Tinnitus (ringing in the ears).
   b. Changes in vision, dizziness.
   c. Sweating.
   d. Nausea, vomiting, abdominal pain.
4. *Immediate* recognition of salicylate *poisoning:*
   a. Hyperventilation (*earliest* sign).
   b. Fever—may be extremely high (105° to 106°F).
   c. Respiratory alkalosis or metabolic acidosis.
   d. *Late* signs: bleeding tendencies, severe electrolyte disturbances, liver or kidney failure.

B. Analysis/nursing diagnosis:
1. *Ineffective breathing patterns* related to hyperventilation/respiratory alkalosis.
2. *Fluid volume deficit* (dehydration) related to increased insensible loss of fluids through hyperventilation, increased loss of fluids through vomiting, and increased need for fluids due to hyperpyrexia (fever).
3. *Risk for injury* related to bleeding.
4. *Anxiety* related to parental/child feelings of guilt, uncertainty as to outcome, invasive nature of treatments.
5. *Knowledge deficit* regarding accident prevention.

C. Nursing care plan/implementation:
1. Goal: *promote excretion of salicylates.*
   a. If possible, induce vomiting using syrup of ipecac (save, bring to emergency department).
   b. Assist with gastric lavage, if appropriate.
   c. Administer activated charcoal as early as possible.
   d. Administer IV fluids, as ordered.
   e. Assist with hemodialysis, as ordered, to promote excretion of salicylates and fluids.
2. Goal: *restore fluid and electrolyte balance.*
   a. Monitor I&O, urinalysis, specific gravity.
   b. Prepare sodium bicarbonate, administer as ordered to correct metabolic acidosis.
   c. Monitor IV fluids and electrolytes.
   d. NPO initially (NG tube).
3. Goal: *reduce temperature.*
   a. **No** aspirin or acetaminophen, which might further complicate bleeding tendencies or lead to liver or kidney damage.
   b. Supportive measures: cool soaks, ice packs to armpits/groin, hypothermia blanket.
4. Goal: *prevent bleeding and possible hemorrhage.*
   a. Monitor urine and stools for occult blood.
   b. Insert NG tube to detect gastric bleeding.
   c. Observe for petechiae, bruising; monitor laboratory values for Hct and Hgb.
   d. Administer vitamin K as ordered to correct bleeding tendencies.
5. Goal: *health education to prevent another accidental poisoning.*
   a. Teach principles of poison prevention.
   b. Stress need to avoid accidental overdose with over-the-counter medications or dosage mix-ups.
   c. Allow child/parents to verbalize guilt, but *avoid* blaming or scapegoating.

D. Evaluation/outcome criteria:
1. Aspirin is successfully removed from child's body without permanent damage.
2. Fluid and electrolyte balance is restored and maintained.
3. Child is afebrile.
4. Bleeding is controlled, no hemorrhage occurs.
5. No further episodes of poisoning occur.

III. ACETAMINOPHEN POISONING

A. Assessment:
1. Determine how much acetaminophen was ingested, when, and which type.
2. Evaluate acetaminophen levels: normal = 0; therapeutic range = 15 to 30 mcg/mL; toxic = 150 mcg/mL 4 hours after ingestion.
3. *Initial period* (2–4 hours after ingestion): malaise, nausea, vomiting, anorexia, diaphoresis, pallor.
4. *Latent period* (1–3 days after ingestion): clinical improvement with asymptomatic rise in liver enzymes.
5. *Hepatic involvement* (may last 7 days or may be permanent): pain in RUQ, jaundice, confusion, hepatic encephalopathy, clotting abnormalities.
6. Gradual recuperation.

PEDIATRICS

B. Analysis/nursing diagnosis:
1. *Altered tissue perfusion* (liver) related to hepatic necrosis.
2. *Fluid volume deficit* related to increased loss of fluids secondary to vomiting and diaphoresis.
3. *Risk for injury* related to bleeding and clotting disorders.
4. *Anxiety* related to parental/child feelings of guilt, uncertainty as to outcome, and invasive nature of treatments.
5. *Knowledge deficit* regarding accident prevention.

C. Nursing care plan/implementation:
1. Goal: *promote excretion of acetaminophen.*
   a. If possible, induce vomiting; save, bring to emergency department.
   b. Assist with gastric lavage, if appropriate.
   c. Administer activated charcoal.
   d. Assist with obtaining acetaminophen level 4 hours after ingestion.
2. Goal: *prevent permanent liver damage.*
   a. Treatment must begin as soon as possible; therapy begun later than 10 hours after ingestion has no value.
   b. Administer the antidote (acetylcysteine [*Mucomyst*]) per physician's order. Usually administered in cola or through NG tube because of offensive odor. Given as one loading dose and 17 maintenance doses.
   c. Monitor hepatic functioning—assist with obtaining specimens and check results frequently; be aware that liver enzymes will rise and peak within 3 days and then should rapidly return to normal.
3. Goal: *restore fluid and electrolyte balance.*
   a. Monitor vital signs and perform neurological checks every 2 to 4 hours and prn.
   b. Monitor I&O; urine analysis, including specific gravity; and weight.
   c. Monitor IV fluids as ordered.
4. Goal: *prevent bleeding.*
   a. Assist in monitoring child's PT; notify physician of significant changes.
   b. Monitor urine and stool for occult blood.
   c. Observe for and report any petechiae or unusual bruising.
5. Goal: *health education to prevent another accidental poisoning.* (See **Goal 5, Nursing care plan/implementation,** Salicylate poisoning.)

D. Evaluation/outcome criteria:
1. Acetaminophen is successfully removed from child's body.
2. Normal liver function is reestablished.
3. Fluid and electrolyte balance is restored and maintained.
4. No further episodes of poisoning occur.

PEDIATRICS

IV. LEAD POISONING (PLUMBISM)

A. *Introduction:* Lead poisoning is a heavy-metal poisoning that occurs from ingestion or inhalation of lead. In children, this is most common in the *toddler* age group (1–3 years) and is usually a *chronic* type of poisoning that occurs as the result of repeated ingestions of lead. Older plumbing is one source of lead. Children who engage in the practice of *pica,* the ingestion of nonnutritive substances, often ingest lead in flecks of lead-based paint from plumbing, walls, furniture, or toys. In addition, research demonstrates that the parent-child relationship is a significant variable in lead poisoning; typically, there is a lack of adequate parental supervision that enables the child to engage in pica repeatedly over a fairly long time, until symptoms of lead poisoning become evident. (**Fig. 5.14** shows the pathophysiological effects of lead poisoning.)

B. Assessment:
1. Investigate history of pica.
2. Evaluate parent-child relationship.
3. *Chronic lead poisoning:* vague, crampy abdominal pain; constipation; anorexia and vomiting; listlessness.
4. Neurological, renal, hematological effects: see **Fig. 5.14.**
5. "Blood lead line"—bluish-black line seen in gums.
6. X-rays: lead lines in long bones and flecks of lead in GI tract.
7. *Elevated* serum blood lead levels: ≥ 20 mcg/dL requires clinical management; ≥ 45 mcg/dL requires parenteral chelating therapy.

C. Analysis/nursing diagnosis:
1. *Altered thought processes* related to neurotoxicity.
2. *Activity intolerance* (and *risk for infection*) related to anemia.
3. *Altered urinary elimination* related to excretion of lead by kidneys.
4. *Pain* related to lead poisoning and its treatment.
5. *Knowledge deficit* related to etiology of lead poisoning.

D. Nursing care plan/implementation:
1. Goal: *promote excretion of lead.*
   a. Administer chelating agents (EDTA [IM or IV], BAL [IM only]) as ordered. Chelation therapy typically continues over several days, with multiple treatments daily.
   b. Monitor kidney function carefully: the treatment itself is potentially nephrotoxic. Maintain adequate oral intake of fluids.
   c. Institute seizure precautions.
2. Goal: *prevent reingestion of lead.*
   a. Determine primary source of poisoning.
   b. Eliminate source from child's environment before discharge.

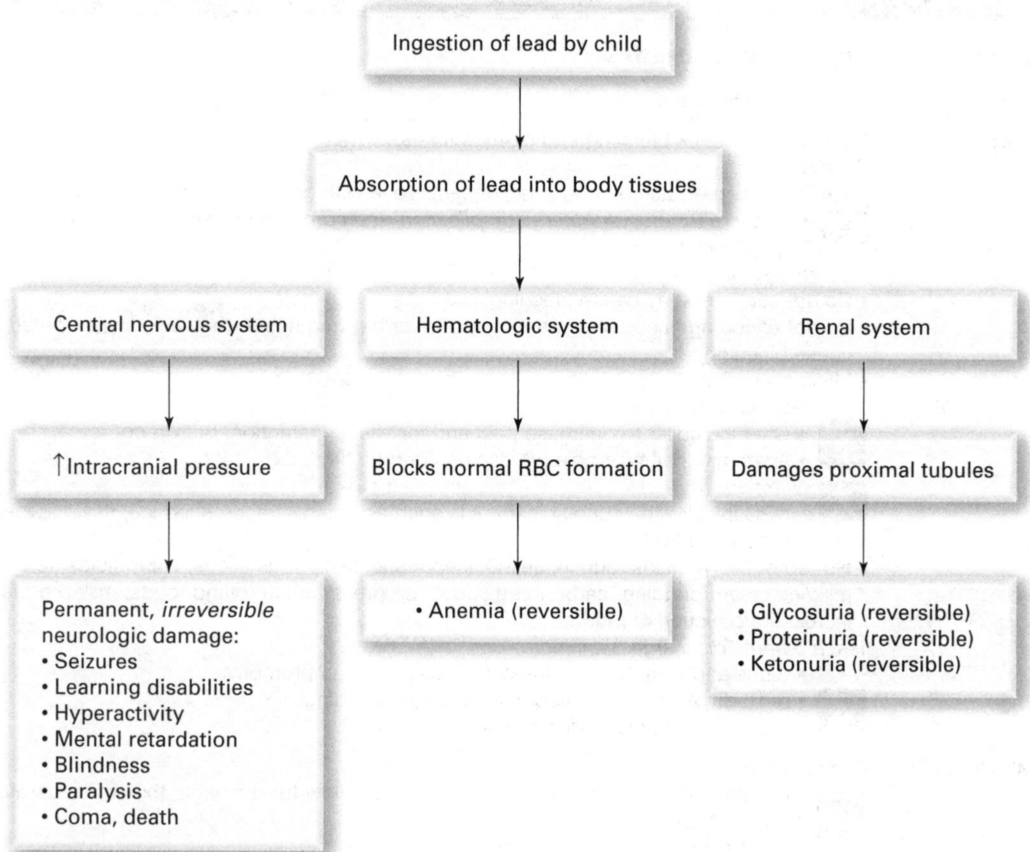

Figure 5.14 Pathophysiological effects of lead poisoning.

c. Follow up with home care referral.
   (1) Screen other siblings prn.
   (2) Monitor blood lead level of all children in the home.

3. Goal: *assist child to cope with multiple painful injections when treated with IM chelation therapy.*
   a. Prepare child for treatment regimen.
   b. Stress that this is *not* a punishment.
   c. Rotate sites as much as possible.
   d. May use a local anesthetic (e.g., procaine, injected simultaneously with chelating agent to decrease pain of injections).
   e. Apply warm soaks to injection sites: may help lessen pain.
   f. Encourage child to self-limit gross muscle activity (which increases pain).
   g. Offer child safe outlets for anger, fear, frustration—punching bag, pounding board, clay.
   h. Offer opportunity for medical play with empty syringes, etc.
4. Goal: *health teaching.*
   a. Stress (to child and parents) that removing the lead is the only way to prevent permanent, irreversible neurological damage (irreversible damage may have *already* occurred).
   b. Teach that the chelating agent binds with the lead and promotes its excretion through the kidneys.

E. Evaluation/outcome criteria:
1. Lead is successfully removed from child's body without permanent damage.
2. No further episodes of lead poisoning.
3. Child copes successfully with the disease and its treatment.

PEDIATRIC SURGERIES: NURSING CONSIDERATIONS

I. In general, basic care principles for children are the same as for adults having surgery.

II. EXCEPTIONS:

A. Children should be prepared according to their developmental level and learning ability.

B. Children cannot sign own surgical consent form; to be done by parent or legal guardian.

C. Parents should be actively involved in the child's care.

III. See **Table 5.22,** which reviews specific nursing care for the most common pediatric surgical procedures.

Table 5.22

Pediatric Surgeries: Nursing Considerations

Surgical Procedure	Specific Nursing Care
TONSILLECTOMY	*Preoperative:* check bleeding and clotting times. *Postoperative:* • *Position*—place on abdomen or semiprone with head turned to side to prevent aspiration. • *Observe for most frequent complication—hemorrhage* (frequent swallowing, emesis of bright red blood, shock). *Prevent bleeding:* • Do *not* suction—may cause bleeding. • Do *not* encourage coughing, clearing throat, or blowing nose—may aggravate operative site and cause bleeding. • Minimize crying. *Decrease pain:* • Offer ice collar to decrease pain and for vasoconstriction, but do *not* force. • Acetaminophen for pain (*no* aspirin, ibuprofen). 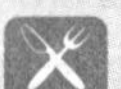 *Nutrition:* • NPO initially, then cool, clear fluids such as cool water, crushed ice, flavored icepops, dilute (noncitrus) fruit juice. • **No** red or brown fluids (punch, Jell-O, icepops, colas), citrus juices, warm fluids (tea, broth), toast, milk/ice cream/pudding, carbonated sodas; progress to soft, bland foods; milk products can increase production of mucus. *Teach parents/discharge planning:* • Signs and symptoms of infection; call physician promptly. • 5–10 days postoperatively, expect slight bleeding. • Continue soft, bland diet as tolerated.
MYRINGOTOMY ("tubes")	*Postoperative:* 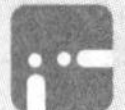 • *Position*—place with operated ear down, to allow for drainage. Expect moderate amount of purulent drainage initially. • Keep external ear canal clean and dry. *Teach parents/discharge planning:* • Need to keep water out of ear—use special ear plugs when bathing or swimming. • "Tubes" will remain in place 3–7 months and then fall out spontaneously (with healing of eardrum).
APPENDECTOMY	(Observe same principles of preoperative and postoperative care as for adult GI surgery.) 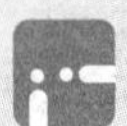 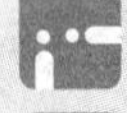 • NPO until bowel sounds return (24–48 hours). • If appendix ruptured preoperatively or intraoperatively, *position* in semi-Fowler's and implement wound precautions; administer antibiotics as ordered. 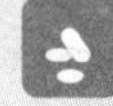 • Monitor for signs and symptoms of peritonitis. • Typical course: speedy recovery, with discharge in about 2–3 days and excellent prognosis.
HERNIORRHAPHY (umbilical/inguinal)	*Umbilical:* increased incidence in infants who are of African descent. *Inguinal:* increased incidence in boys. *Preoperative:* monitor for possible complications of strangulation. Routine postoperative GI surgery care. Prognosis—excellent, with discharge 24–48 hours postoperatively.

SELECTED PEDIATRIC EMERGENCIES

For a quick review, use this index to locate content on 19 pediatric emergencies that are covered in this book.

PEDIATRICS

Questions

Select the one answer that is best for each question, unless otherwise directed.

1. A nurse is caring for a child diagnosed with syndrome of inappropriate antidiuretic hormone (SIADH). Which laboratory test would the nurse be *least* likely to obtain?
1. Urine specific gravity.
2. Blood glucose.
3. Serum sodium.
4. Urine osmolality.

2. A physician prescribes digoxin (Lanoxin) for a toddler with congestive heart failure (CHF). Before administering the medication, it is *most important* for the nurse to:
1. First obtain an apical heart rate.
2. Determine the serum potassium.
3. Review the child's admission electrocardiogram (ECG).
4. Mix the medication with a pleasant-tasting food.

3. A nurse prepares to administer spironolactone (Aldactone) to an infant with congenital heart disease. The nurse understands that the main purpose of this medication is to:
1. Preserve the patent ductus arteriosus.
2. Cause vasodilation of the blood vessels.
3. Prevent the secretion of potassium.
4. Block aldosterone, which leads to diuresis.

4. Which symptom(s), if present in a child, should a nurse recognize as being characteristic of Kawasaki disease? *Select all that apply.*
1. Strawberry tongue.
2. High fever.
3. Irritability.
4. Cough.
5. Desquamation of the extremities.
6. Elevated ESR.

5. Which orders should a nurse question for a 5-month-old infant with hypoplastic left heart syndrome who is hospitalized awaiting the second stage of surgical repair? *Select all that apply.*
1. Call physician for oxygen saturations below 85%.
2. Daily weights.
3. Hold digoxin (Lanoxin) for heart rate less than 80 beats per minute.
4. Strict I&O.
5. Enfamil formula ad lib.

6. A nurse would be most correct in withholding digoxin (Lanoxin) prescribed to an infant if the heart rate falls below which parameter?
1. Below 100 beats per minute.
2. Below 120 beats per minute.
3. Below 140 beats per minute.
4. Below 160 beats per minute.

7. A hospitalized child is experiencing sickle cell vaso-occlusive crisis. The child is currently receiving an intravenous (IV) fluid bolus, pain medication every 4 hours, and warm compresses to the extremities per physician orders. During the midday assessment, the child reports no pain. Which action should a nurse take?
1. Continue to apply warm compresses per physician order.
2. Hold the next dosage of pain medication.
3. Hold the next round of warm compresses.
4. Contact the physician for a change in orders.

8. What should be the expected weight of an infant at 12 months of age whose birth weight was 3600 grams?
1. 5600 grams.
2. 7200 grams.
3. 11 kilograms.
4. 15 kilograms.

9. An infant in a newborn nursery is identified as having phenylketonuria (PKU). What is the *best* initial source of nutrients for an infant with this diagnosis?
1. Maternal breast milk.
2. Pregestimil.
3. Lofenalac.
4. Isomil.

10. In assessing the reflexes of a 15-month-old child, which finding would indicate that the child is experiencing normal development?
1. Positive Babinski reflex.
2. Asymmetric tonic neck reflex.
3. Positive patellar reflex.
4. Presence of doll's eye reflex.

11. A child with type 1 diabetes is receiving insulin based on carbohydrate intake. The child's insulin-to-carbohydrate ratio is 15:1. Of the items listed on the child's lunch menu shown below, the child ate 2 slices of bread, a slice of cheese, a glass of milk, a cup of soup, and half of a banana. How many units of insulin should the nurse administer based on the client's carbohydrate count? Round to the nearest whole number.

Food Item:	Carbohydrates:
Banana	22 g
Glass of low-fat milk	10 g
Bread slice	15 g
Cheese slice	Free
Cup of soup	10 g

1. 2 units.
2. 3 units.
3. 4 units.
4. 5 units.

12. A nurse is caring for a child with acute glomerulonephritis. Which nursing assessment should be the nurse's *first priority* when caring for this child?
 1. Obtaining a daily weight.
 2. Palpating extremities frequently for edema.
 3. Assessing urine for hematuria.
 4. Obtaining the child's blood pressure every shift.

13. In developing a plan of care for a hospitalized preschooler, a nurse recognizes that it is most essential to consider:
 1. That the child may believe the hospitalization is a punishment.
 2. Ways to provide visitation from peers.
 3. How to incorporate play activities with other children.
 4. Ways to promote privacy and independence.

14. A nurse assesses a child who is 12 hours status post–tonsillectomy and adenoidectomy. The child reports feeling nauseated and shows the nurse a moderate amount of red-tinged vomitus in the emesis basin. Which action should the nurse take *first?*
 1. Administer an antiemetic as ordered.
 2. Offer the child ice chips as tolerated.
 3. Report the findings to the physician.
 4. Apply bilateral pressure to the child's neck.

15. The parents of a 2-year-old child ask a nurse how to best assist the child to accomplish developmental tasks at this age. What is the best response by the nurse?
 1. "Make sure that the child's siblings insist that the child share toys at playtime."
 2. "Since the child understands the word 'no,' use this word frequently to establish house rules."
 3. "Ask grandparents and other child care providers to follow your home schedule as much as possible."
 4. "Attend to the child quickly during temper tantrums by hugging and offering reassurance."

16. An infant is hospitalized following a febrile seizure. When a nurse teaches the infant's family about the prevention of future seizures, what would be the nurse's best recommendation?
 1. Place the child in a tepid bath during the next febrile illness.
 2. Administer antipyretics around the clock the next time the child has a fever.
 3. Contact the physician for antibiotics if the child becomes feverish again.
 4. Take the child's temperature frequently during the next illness.

17. A toddler with Kawasaki disease is being evaluated by a primary care clinic nurse 1 week following discharge. The nurse understands that it is *a priority* to instruct the parents to contact the clinic immediately if the child:
 1. Throws frequent temper tantrums.
 2. Is exposed to someone with chickenpox.
 3. Experiences night terrors.
 4. Develops a low-grade fever.

18. A child arrives in an emergency department with a chief complaint of asthma exacerbation. Which assessment information is most important for the nurse to obtain *first?*
 1. Whether the child has been taking asthma medications as prescribed.
 2. When the child began having symptoms.
 3. Whether the child is able to speak in full sentences.
 4. The child's ABG levels.

19. A child is seen in an emergency department following the ingestion of lighter fluid. Which nursing action is of the *highest priority* at this time?
 1. Induce vomiting.
 2. Determine the amount of poison ingested.
 3. Assess the respiratory system.
 4. Administer Mucomyst as ordered.

20. A nurse prepares to administer a chelating agent to a child with lead poisoning. Which laboratory tests should be obtained *prior* to the administration of this agent?
 1. BUN and creatinine.
 2. PT, PTT.
 3. Urine specific gravity.
 4. CBC.

21. A nurse is caring for a child with meningococcemia who is on a ventilator. This morning, the nurse finds the child's mother sitting at the bedside, crying. The mother tells the nurse, "I thought it was the flu. This is my fault because I should have come to the hospital earlier." What is the best action by the nurse in response to the mother's statements?
 1. Tell the mother not to worry since many parents and even physicians frequently mistake meningitis symptoms for other infectious conditions.
 2. Make a referral to social services.
 3. Call the child's father and explain that the mother needs emotional support from him.
 4. Remind the mother that she did seek proper treatment as soon as she became concerned, and review the special care the child is receiving now.

22. An infant is admitted for probable pyloric stenosis. A physician orders IV fluids and makes the infant NPO pending a surgical consult. The infant is crying vigorously and the parents express frustration that they cannot feed their baby even though the surgery is not yet definite. Which is the best action for the nurse to take now?
 1. Explain to the parents that feeding an infant with pyloric stenosis can lead to electrolyte imbalances from possible vomiting.
 2. Offer the parents a pacifier for the infant.
 3. Place a call to the surgeon to find out how long it will be before the consult.
 4. Feed the infant a small amount of Pedialyte since the surgical repair for this condition will most likely not occur until the following day.

QUESTIONS

23. A 1-day-old infant, born at 39 weeks' gestation, weighs 4 pounds, 7 ounces at birth. A pediatrician diagnoses the neonate with intrauterine growth restriction (IGR). An RN observes the newborn to be irritable, difficult to console, restless, fist-sucking, and demonstrating a high-pitched, shrill cry. Based on these assessment data, the RN should:

1. Increase stimulation of the baby by handling the infant as much as possible.
2. Schedule routine feeding times every 3 to 4 hours.
3. Encourage stimulation by rubbing the infant's back and head.
4. Tightly swaddle the infant in a flexed position.

24. A nurse performs a scoliosis screening at a local school. Which assessment finding by the nurse would *least* likely result in a scoliosis referral?

1. Unilateral rib hump noted when the child is bent forward.
2. Asymmetrical hip height noted when the child is standing erect.
3. Uneven wear noted on the bottom of the child's pant legs.
4. Rounded shoulders noted when the child is standing erect.

25. Which conditions in children and/or adolescents should a nurse identify as being associated with metabolic alkalosis? *Select all that apply.*

1. Pyloric stenosis.
2. Diabetes.
3. Renal failure.
4. Bulimia nervosa.
5. Aspirin ingestion.

26. A child is admitted for treatment of lead poisoning. A nurse recognizes that the *priority* nursing diagnosis for this child is:

1. *Alteration in comfort related to abdominal pain.*
2. *Alteration in nutrition related to pica.*
3. *Pain related to chelation therapy.*
4. *Alteration in neurologic functioning.*

27. A newborn arrives in a neonatal intensive care unit with a myelomeningocele. A physician writes orders to keep the infant in the prone position. A nurse should know that the most important rationale behind this order is to:

1. Prevent infection.
2. Promote circulation in the lower extremities.
3. Prevent trauma to the meningeal sac.
4. Promote comfort.

28. A child, hospitalized with nephrotic syndrome, has been receiving corticosteroids for a week. What should the nurse recognize as *early* evidence that the child is responding well to treatment?

1. Decreased general edema.
2. Increased urinary output.
3. Improved general appetite.
4. Hemoglobin and hematocrit within normal limits.

29. A nurse is performing discharge teaching with the parents of a preschooler diagnosed with cystic fibrosis. What part of the teaching plan will best assist the parents to prevent future pulmonary infections in this child?

1. Teaching the parents proper administration of pancreatic enzymes.
2. Emphasizing the need for regular and consistent chest physiotherapy.
3. Stressing the need to seek prompt medical attention for increased work of breathing.
4. Instructing the parents to monitor the child's daily fluid intake for adequacy.

30. The mother of a child asks a clinic nurse how to safety-proof the home. What should the nurse recognize as the most effective means to prevent accidental poisoning?

1. Keep the Poison Control Center phone number near the phone.
2. Store poisons in the garage rather than in the home.
3. Scan the home from the child's eye level and remove accessible toxins.
4. Tell children where toxic substances are kept and instruct them not to go there.

31. A nurse visits the home of a toddler. With what aspect of the home environment would the nurse be most concerned?

1. Power cords plugged into capped electrical outlets.
2. Presence of a television in the child's bedroom.
3. A swimming pool located in the backyard.
4. Cooking pot handle turned toward the front of the stove.

32. An infant is admitted to a pediatric unit with labored breathing and moderate amounts of thick nasal secretions. What nursing intervention is most likely to improve the infant's oxygenation?

1. Frequent suctioning of the nares with a nasal olive.
2. Providing supplemental oxygen via nasal cannula.
3. Strict monitoring of oxygen saturation levels.
4. Placing the child in an infant seat.

33. A client is attending a newborn discharge class and asks a nurse about the bump on the infant's head. Upon assessment, the neonate has a large, diffuse swelling on the left occiput that crosses the sagittal suture line. The nurse should explain to the mother that:
Select all that apply.

1. This is a collection of blood under the skull bone of the infant.
2. It is edematous swelling that overlies the periosteum.
3. It leads to hyperbilirubinemia in the infant.
4. It will require no treatment to resolve.
5. It is caused by pressure on the fetal head before delivery.

34. A child with status post–Harrington rod placement for the correction of scoliosis is being cared for on the pediatric unit. The child suddenly experiences facial sweating and complains of a headache. A nurse notes also a slower heart rate on the monitor. What action should the nurse take *first?*
1. Call the surgeon immediately.
2. Assess patency of the urinary catheter.
3. Administer pain medication as ordered.
4. Complete a neurological assessment.

35. What assessment findings should a nurse expect in a child with acute post-streptococcal glomerulonephritis? *Select all that apply.*
1. Severe hematuria.
2. Pallor.
3. Decreased urine specific gravity.
4. Weight gain.
5. Headache.
6. Massive proteinuria.

36. In doing a child's admission assessment, which signs and symptoms should a nurse recognize as most likely related to rheumatic fever?
1. Vomiting and diarrhea.
2. Arthralgia and muscle weakness.
3. Conjunctivitis and red, cracked lips.
4. Bradycardia and hypotension.

37. When preparing an intramuscular injection for a 1-week-old infant, which needle would be the most appropriate for the nurse to select?
1. 18 G, ⅞ inch.
2. 21 G, 1 inch.
3. 25 G, ⅝ inch.
4. 25 G, 1½ inch.

38. A young child diagnosed with iron-deficiency anemia is prescribed a liquid iron supplement. A nurse provides the parents with instructions on administration and should be certain to advise them that:
1. The medication should be given along with the child's morning cereal breakfast.
2. The child may experience some pale-colored stools.
3. The child should be permitted to sip the medication from a medicine cup.
4. The medication can be mixed with a small amount of fruit juice.

39. A child is receiving chemotherapy for the treatment of osteosarcoma. Which morning laboratory result must a nurse report *immediately* to the physician?
1. Absolute neutrophil count of 1200.
2. Platelet count of 150,000.
3. Urine dipstick positive for heme.
4. WBC count of 4500.

40. A nurse prepares to administer digoxin to an infant. Where is the most appropriate location for the nurse to assess the infant's heart rate?

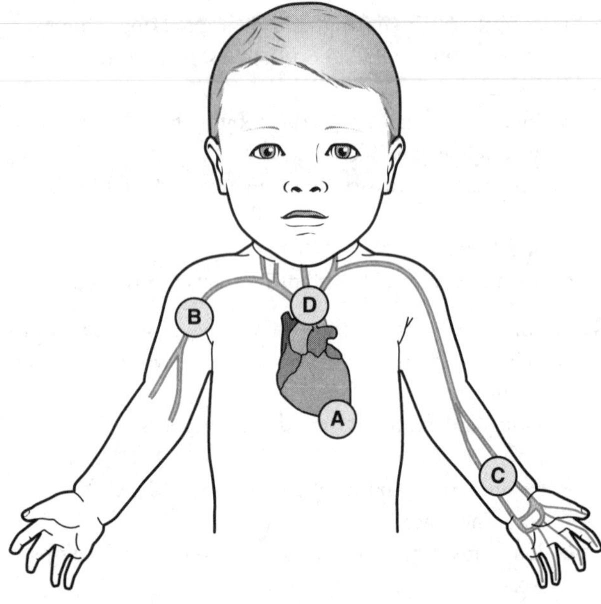

1. A.
2. B.
3. C.
4. D.

41. Which statement made by the mother of a child with cystic fibrosis should indicate to a nurse that the mother is in need of further teaching regarding the administration of pancreatic enzymes?
1. "I'll crush the capsules and mix with my child's food."
2. "The capsule can be broken and its contents sprinkled onto food."
3. "I may need to give more enzymes with larger meals."
4. "I will administer the enzymes 30 minutes after the meal."

42. A nurse is working with a nursing student in the care of a young child status post-appendectomy. The student checks the current order of IV gentamicin and discovers the ordered dose is above the safe dose range based on the child's weight. What should be the nurse's *first* action?
1. Check the child's recent lab work.
2. Contact the physician.
3. Order a hearing test.
4. Obtain an order for BUN and creatinine.

43. A child with type 1 diabetes is being prepared for discharge from a hospital. What should a nurse include as part of the teaching regarding diabetes care?
1. Expect hypoglycemic episodes to always occur after meals.
2. Insulin dosage may need to be decreased during sports activities.

3. The child should not self-administer injections until the teen years.
4. Insulin should never be administered during febrile illnesses.

44. An LVN/LPN from an orthopedic unit is floated to a child health unit. In creating assignments, which child should the charge nurse *avoid* assigning to the LVN/LPN?
1. A 10-year-old in traction for a fractured femur.
2. An 8-year-old child with Legg-Calvé-Perthes disease.
3. A 4-year-old with osteogenesis imperfecta.
4. A teenager receiving chemotherapy for osteosarcoma.

45. A nurse performs a head-to-toe assessment on a newborn. Which finding should be of *greatest* concern to the nurse?
1. Capillary refill time of 2 seconds.
2. Transient mottling of the skin.
3. Irregular respirations.
4. Negative Babinski reflex.

46. The parent of a young child phones an advice nurse to report that the child is ill. The child has a reddish pinpoint rash most concentrated in the axilla and groin areas, a high fever, flushed cheeks, and abdominal pain. The parent also reports that the child's tongue is dark red with white spots. A nurse should recognize these symptoms as indicative of which infection?
1. Mumps.
2. Measles.
3. Scarlet fever.
4. Varicella.

47. Where should the nurse place the stethoscope on an infant to best auscultate bronchial breath sounds?

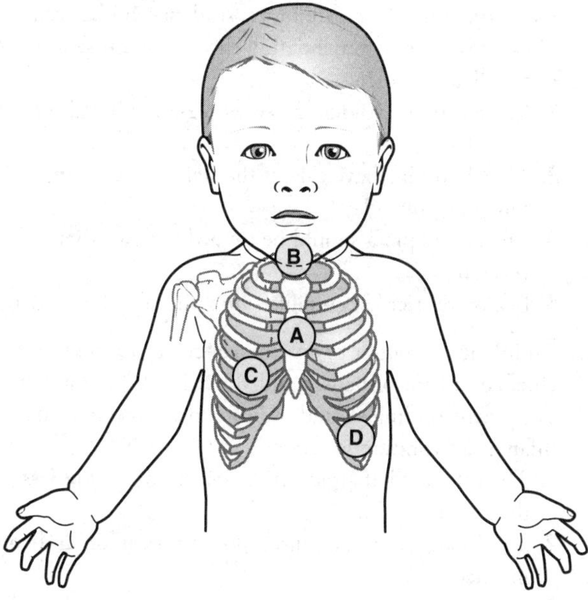

1. A.
2. B.
3. C.
4. D.

48. A nurse is planning to teach a child safety class to a group of new parents. When preparing a lesson regarding car seats, what should the nurse recommend?
1. Children should be seated in the rear of the car until 6 years of age.
2. Infants should face forward in an infant seat until 20 pounds.
3. Children should face the rear of the car until as close to 1 year of age as possible.
4. Make sure to use the automobile air bags as these enhance the safety of car seats.

49. Which would be an *abnormal* finding when doing a well-child checkup on a 1-week-old infant?
1. An audible "clunk" during the Ortolani test.
2. Symmetrical gluteal folds when the infant is held upright.
3. Negative Barlow test.
4. Symmetrical knee height when the infant is supine.

50. A physician orders penicillin 200,000 units/kg/day IV q6h for a child weighing 16 kg. The penicillin on hand comes prepared in a concentration of 250,000 units/mL. In order to administer the correct dose, a nurse calculates that _______ mL of penicillin should be administered to the child. *Fill in the blank.*

51. Which nursing intervention should a nurse perform on a young child suspected of having a diagnosis of acute epiglottitis whose oxygen saturation measures 93% on room air?
1. Allow the child to sit in a position of comfort.
2. Provide small amounts of liquid orally via a syringe.
3. Inspect the child's nares to assess degree of swelling.
4. Apply 100% oxygen via mask.

52. A nurse teaches a child with spina bifida how to perform urinary self-catheterization. Which steps should the nurse include in the teaching? *Place each correct step in sequential order.*

_______ 1. Wash hands.
_______ 2. Open latex catheter package.
_______ 3. Lubricate tip of catheter.
_______ 4. Wash catheter with soap and water.
_______ 5. Cleanse perineum with Betadine swabs.

53. A child recovering from abdominal surgery removes the nasogastric tube accidentally. A nurse replaces the nasogastric tube and places it to low wall suction. Two hours later, the nurse discovers that there is no drainage from the tube. What should be the nurse's *first* action?
1. Ask the child to change position.
2. Place an urgent call to the surgeon.
3. Flush the tube with 10 mL of sterile water.
4. Check the suction mechanism and settings.

54. A charge nurse is seated in front of a bank of cardiac monitors on a pediatric unit. There are four children receiving cardiac monitoring. Which finding should the charge nurse communicate *at once* to the child's nurse?
1. A heart rate of 50 in a 15-year-old adolescent who is sleeping.
2. A heart rate of 190 in a 1-month-old infant who is crying.
3. A heart rate of 160 in a 2-year-old child who is walking in the hallway.
4. A heart rate of 75 in a 5-year-old child who is watching television.

55. A school-age child visits a school nurse and states that a family member has been behaving inappropriately by touching the child near the groin area. What should be the school nurse's *priority* action?
1. Make a report to the proper child protective authorities as mandated by law.
2. Contact the child's parents to share what the child has reported.
3. Question the child to determine all of the details of the inappropriate touching.
4. Provide the child with a safe and calm environment in which to continue the discussion.

56. Which child would be the best roommate for a 9-year-old child with myelodysplasia who is hospitalized for a foot infection?
1. A 13-year-old with juvenile idiopathic arthritis.
2. A 10-year-old with a fractured femur.
3. An 8-year-old status post-appendectomy.
4. A 6-year-old with bacterial meningitis.

57. A 7-year-old child is hospitalized for a tonsillectomy. What are *priority* nursing actions when caring for this child after surgery? *Select all that apply.*
1. Advancing diet as tolerated.
2. Encouraging coughing to clear the throat.
3. Monitoring PT and PTT.
4. Administering pain medication around the clock.
5. Suctioning mouth and throat frequently.

58. A nurse is caring for a child newly diagnosed with congenital heart disease. The nurse should monitor the child with the understanding that the *earliest* sign of heart failure is:
1. Audible lung crackles.
2. Increased heart rate.
3. Weight gain.
4. Generalized edema.

59. When teaching a class on home safety to new parents, on which type of exposure should a nurse focus as the *primary* cause of lead poisoning in children?
1. Ingesting paint dust or chips from an old home.
2. Having a parent who works near lead products.
3. Riding in a car that uses leaded gasoline.
4. Chewing on pencils with lead tips.

60. A school nurse is preparing to teach a group of teenagers how to prevent meningitis. What aspect of meningitis prevention should the nurse be certain to include in the presentation?
1. Getting a meningitis vaccine is the only way to guarantee prevention.
2. Refraining from sharing food and drinks is a good way to prevent meningitis infection.
3. Avoiding team sports is one way to stop the spread of meningitis infection.
4. Meningitis prevention methods should be employed whenever children are in crowds.

61. When providing anticipatory guidance to the parents of a child with hemophilia, a nurse should stress that:
1. Active range-of-motion exercise should be used to treat sore joints.
2. Aspirin should be given for minor bumps and bruises.
3. Warm compresses should be applied to wounds to promote circulation.
4. A soft toothbrush should be used to promote oral health.

62. When providing client teaching to the caregivers of a young child with sickle cell disease, a nurse should stress that:
1. The child's diet should include whole grains and leafy green vegetables.
2. Immunizations should be delayed until the child enters school.
3. There is a 50% chance that the child's future offspring will have sickle cell anemia.
4. The parents should request IV Demerol if the child is hospitalized with pain crisis.

63. A school nurse advises the dietary staff that a special lunch tray must be created for a student who has celiac disease. What recommendation should the nurse provide to the dietary staff?
1. Make sure the student has a whole-grain bread roll each day.
2. The child may have cake if the staff is celebrating someone's birthday.
3. The child's pizza should be topped with a variety of vegetables.
4. Beans and rice are suitable side dishes for this student.

64. An infant is brought to an emergency department with a chief complaint of nausea and vomiting. Which nursing assessment finding should indicate to a nurse that the infant's dehydration is severe?
1. The infant is lethargic with a urinary output of less than 1 mL/kg/hr.
2. The infant has weak pulses, poor skin turgor, and cool, mottled skin.
3. The infant has warm skin, increased pulse, and capillary refill of 2 seconds.
4. The infant is irritable, with dry mucous membranes and increased respirations.

QUESTIONS

65. Where is the best location for a nurse to auscultate a murmur created by pulmonic stenosis?

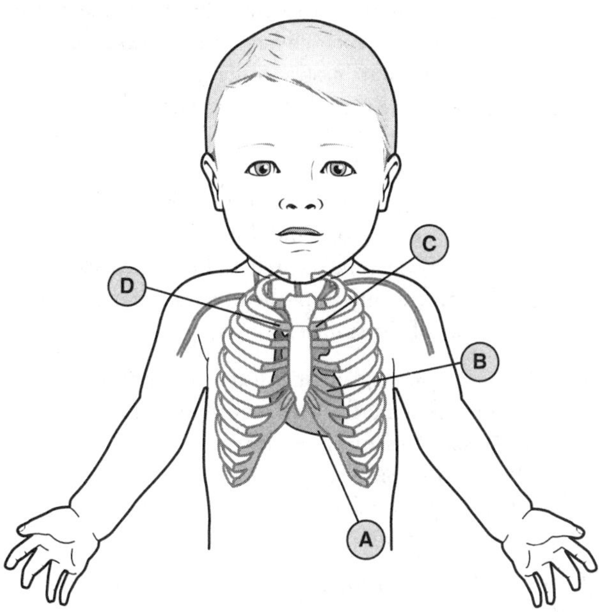

1. A.
2. B.
3. C.
4. D.

66. When visiting the home of a school-age child who is dying, what would be the best action by a hospice nurse?
1. Speak softly (whisper) when speaking in the child's presence.
2. Provide as little interaction with the child as possible.
3. Avoid correcting the child who is in denial about dying.
4. Rely on the parents for pain assessment.

67. A nurse is preparing to administer an unpleasant-tasting liquid medication to a toddler. What is the best method for administering this medication?
1. Mix the medication with a cup of ice cream to mask the taste.
2. Ask the child to choose between two types of fluids as a chaser.
3. Request the parents hold the child firmly so the nurse can place the medication into the mouth.
4. Offer the child a toy out of the toy box as a reward if the child agrees to take the medication.

68. A nursing student prepares to administer eyedrops to a young child. What action by the nursing student should cause a registered nurse to intervene?
1. The student positions the child supine with head extended.
2. After administration, the student asks the child to close eyes and move them around.
3. The student schedules medication administration to occur just before lunchtime.
4. Prior to administration, the student pulls the lower lid down, forming a sac.

69. A nurse admits a teenager in sickle cell crisis to a pediatric unit. The child has an elevated heart rate but normal blood pressure, respiratory rate, and temperature. The child has an oxygen saturation of 98% on room air and rates pain in the extremities at an 8 on a 1-to-10 numeric pain rating scale. Which actions should the nurse perform at this time? Prioritize the nurse's actions by placing each correct intervention in *priority order.*

_________ 1. Administer oxygen.
_________ 2. Obtain the child's weight.
_________ 3. Administer IV fluids as ordered.
_________ 4. Monitor I&O.
_________ 5. Obtain an order for pain medication via PCA.
_________ 6. Apply cool, moist compresses to extremities.

70. A school nurse is creating an informational brochure for parents regarding the treatment of head lice. What form of treatment should the nurse caution *against?*
1. Applying repeated doses of permethrin for as long as it takes until the infestation clears.
2. Washing all clothing and linens in hot water followed by drying them in a hot dryer.
3. Wearing gloves when washing the child's hair or inspecting for nits.
4. Removing nits daily from the child's hair with a fine-tooth comb.

71. The parents of a newborn infant ask a nurse how to prevent future ear infections. What is the best advice the nurse should provide these parents?
1. Avoid crowds during the winter months.
2. Allow the baby to bottle-feed in the supine position.
3. Make sure the baby receives the DTaP vaccine as scheduled.
4. Continue breastfeeding as close to the baby's first birthday as possible.

72. A nurse enters the room of a child following the placement of a ventriculoperitoneal shunt. The child is sitting up in bed, crying, and has vomited a small amount on the bed linens. What are the *priority* nursing actions? *Select all that apply.*
1. Complete a neurological assessment.
2. Place the child in the supine position.
3. Administer the antiemetic as ordered.
4. Complete a pain assessment.
5. Increase the child's IV rate.

73. A charge nurse is creating nursing assignments for a pediatric unit when one of the oncoming nurses calls to say, "Sorry, I'll be a few minutes late since I have a child home ill with the chickenpox." What type of assignment would be most acceptable for the nurse who will be late?
1. Any assignment is fine as long as the nurse wears a mask.
2. The nurse needs an assignment that does not include children with neutropenia.
3. The nurse should not be given an assignment and should be called off.
4. Any care assignment is acceptable, without restrictions.

74. A nurse assesses the respiratory status of an infant. Which finding should be of *most* concern to the nurse?
1. Tachypnea.
2. Scattered rhonchi.
3. Expiratory grunt.
4. Abdominal breathing.

75. While suctioning a child with a tracheostomy tube in place, a nurse discovers that the suction catheter will not advance inside the tracheostomy tube and the child is becoming pale and anxious, with noticeable suprasternal retractions. What should be the nurse's *priority* action?
1. Change the tracheostomy tube at once.
2. Instill normal saline into the tracheostomy tube and attempt suctioning again.
3. Obtain a pulse oximetry reading.
4. Auscultate lung sounds.

76. While preparing for an admission, a nurse hears the alarm sound on the cardiac monitor of a child in the next bed. The nurse views the screen and sees what appears to be ventricular fibrillation. What is the best *initial* action by the nurse?
1. Call out for help.
2. Assess the child.
3. Begin chest compressions.
4. Press the "Code Blue" button.

77. Which response to hospitalization is a nurse *most* likely to observe in a 4-year-old child?
1. Fearfulness of loud noises and sudden movements.
2. Frequent crying outbursts and agitation.
3. Urinary frequency and fear of mutilation.
4. Boredom or loneliness.

78. A 13-year-old client diagnosed with beta-thalassemia is hospitalized for blood transfusion. What are the *priority* nursing diagnoses related to this child's care? *Select all that apply.*
1. *Risk for infection.*
2. *Impaired elimination.*
3. *Risk for injury.*
4. *Disturbed body image.*
5. *Chronic pain.*
6. *Activity intolerance.*

79. A 3-year-old child is hospitalized with multiple fractures as a result of a car accident. What is the best way for a nurse to assess this child's pain level?
1. Ask the child to rate pain using a numeric pain rating scale.
2. Rely on vital sign measurements as a way to verify pain ratings.
3. Employ the FACES pain scale with every nursing assessment.
4. Try to have the child describe the pain's intensity and quality.

80. A nurse prepares to insert a nasogastric tube in a 10-month-old child. Which actions should the nurse take to complete this procedure? Prioritize the nurse's actions by placing each correct step in *sequential order.*
________ **1.** Aspirate gastric contents.
________ **2.** Have the child begin a bottle feeding.
________ **3.** Place child supine with head and neck elevated.
________ **4.** Inject 10 mL of air into the tube while auscultating the stomach.
________ **5.** Tape tube securely to infant's cheek.
________ **6.** Measure from the infant's earlobe to the area of the stomach.

81. What is the *priority* nursing diagnosis for an infant receiving treatment for hyperbilirubinemia?
1. *Imbalanced body temperature.*
2. *Alteration in elimination.*
3. *Deficient fluid volume.*
4. *Interrupted family processes.*

82. Which assessment findings would cause a nurse to withhold scheduled immunizations in a child? *Select all that apply.*
1. Current cold symptoms (e.g., runny nose, cough).
2. History of recent blood transfusion.
3. Currently taking corticosteroids.
4. Mild diarrhea without symptoms of dehydration.
5. Family history of penicillin allergy.
6. Positive for HIV.

83. A nurse and nursing student are caring for a child who sustained a head injury as a result of a fall from a play structure. The nurse knows the nursing student is prepared to care for the child when the student states:
1. "I will be sure to let you know if the child's pupils become fixed and dilated."
2. "I will keep the child straight in the supine position."
3. "I will look for any changes in the child's respirations, pulse, or blood pressure."
4. "I will notify the physician if the child becomes sleepy."

84. A child diagnosed with hypopituitarism is to begin receiving daily injections. At what time should a nurse instruct the child's parents to administer the injection each day?
1. Before breakfast.
2. At bedtime.
3. With lunch.
4. Any time the child prefers.

85. An infant is hospitalized for congenital adrenal hyperplasia (CAH). Which medication should a nurse anticipate to be part of the child's treatment plan?
1. Insulin.
2. Cortisone.
3. Growth hormone.
4. Thyroid hormone.

86. A child hospitalized with hydrocephalus is being treated with an externalized ventricular drain (EVD). A nurse begins the afternoon assessment and discovers that the drain is positioned several inches below the child's ear level. What should be the nurse's *priority* action?
1. Raise the drain to the child's ear level.
2. Leave the drain as is and monitor the CSF drainage hourly.
3. Quickly elevate the head of the bed.
4. Clamp the drain and complete a neurological assessment.

87. A nurse is planning to teach a group of 10-year-old children about drug and alcohol prevention. Which characteristics of this age group are important for the nurse to consider when developing the teaching plan? *Select all that apply.*
1. These children are achievement-oriented.
2. They expect good behavior to be rewarded.
3. Their problem-solving approach tends to be concrete and systematic.
4. The central persons in their lives tend to be friends.
5. These children are nearing puberty.

88. A nurse visits the home of a young child to administer the Denver II developmental assessment. The child is unable to perform several required items, and the parent expresses concern regarding the child's performance. What is the best way for the nurse to respond to the parent's concerns?
1. Reassure the parent that the Denver II is not a measure of the child's IQ.
2. Offer the parent some skill-building activities and explain that the child will be reassessed in 2 weeks.
3. Advise the parent that the child's primary physician will be notified and will make any necessary referrals.
4. Tell the parent that it is not unusual for children to fail the Denver II.

89. A nurse is caring for a child with tetralogy of Fallot. Which assessment findings should the nurse expect? *Select all that apply.*
1. Ventricular septal defect (VSD).
2. Atrial septal defect (ASD).
3. Overriding aorta.
4. Pulmonic stenosis.
5. Right ventricular hypertrophy.
6. Patent ductus arteriosus (PDA).
7. Left-to-right shunting of blood.
8. Aortic stenosis

90. The parents of a child recently discharged with acute spasmodic laryngitis contact a nurse to report that the child continues to have croupy coughing spells at nighttime but is otherwise fine. What should the nurse recommend?
1. Contact the child's physician for another round of antibiotics.
2. Treat the spasms by sitting in the bathroom while a hot shower runs.
3. Bring the child back to the emergency department as soon as possible.
4. Elevate the child's head at bedtime using pillows.

91. A 12-month-old child with infantile eczema is seen at the clinic for several open lesions on the arms and legs. What should a nurse caution the child's parents against?
1. Initiating a diet free of milk products.
2. The use of topical hydrocortisone cream.
3. Adding cornstarch to bath water.
4. Immunization during eczema exacerbations.

92. A nurse is working with a nursing student in caring for an infant who has just returned from the surgical recovery area following a cleft lip repair. Which action by the nursing student should cause the nurse to intervene?
1. Placement of elbow restraints on the infant.
2. Offering the parents a regular bottle with which to feed the infant.
3. Positioning the infant in the semi-Fowler's position.
4. Advising the parents of a plan to administer pain medication around the clock.

93. A school-age child visits a school nurse with complaints of dizziness and shaking. The nurse confirms that the child has a history of type 1 diabetes mellitus when the child becomes diaphoretic and begins to faint. What should be the nurse's *first* action?
1. Administer an injection of glucagon.
2. Activate EMS.
3. Squeeze glucose gel into the cheek.
4. Test the child's blood sugar.

94. A nurse should suspect Hirschsprung's disease in a child who has which type of stooling pattern?
1. Pale gray stools.
2. Currant-jelly stools.
3. Loose, yellow stools.
4. Thin, ribbon-like stools.

95. A nurse attempts to give a newborn infant the first bottle feeding. While sucking, the infant becomes cyanotic and coughs, and formula is seen coming out of the infant's nose. What should be the nurse's *first* action?
1. Auscultate the lungs.
2. Suction the child's airway.
3. Obtain an order for an x-ray.
4. Contact the physician.

96. A nurse is caring for a newborn infant diagnosed with hypospadias. The parents ask when the surgical repair will be complete. The nurse knows that the most likely time for completion of the surgical repair will be:
1. Within the first month of life.
2. Not until the child reaches puberty.
3. Nearer the child's first birthday.
4. Before the child begins school.

97. A clinic nurse has a follow-up appointment with an adolescent with juvenile idiopathic arthritis (JIA). What topic should be the nurse's *top priority?*
1. Sleep patterns.
2. Participation in daily exercise.
3. Information regarding JIA support groups.
4. Avoidance of alcohol use.

98. An RN and LVN/LPN are working as a team on a pediatric unit. Which task should the RN perform rather than delegating to the LVN/LPN?
1. Obtain a 12-lead ECG on a 10-year-old.
2. Change the dressing and examine the decubitus ulcer of a preschooler.
3. Administer a gavage feeding to an infant with failure to thrive.
4. Check the blood sugar of a teen in DKA.

99. A clinic nurse prepares to perform a physical assessment on a preschool child. What are the appropriate actions for the nurse to take when preparing for and performing the examination? *Prioritize* the nurse's actions by placing each correct step in sequential order.

_______ **1.** Allow child to keep underpants on.
_______ **2.** Allow child to undress in private.
_______ **3.** Ask child's preference for parental involvement.
_______ **4.** Inspect ears, eyes, and mouth.
_______ **5.** Proceed in head-to-toe direction.
_______ **6.** Gain cooperation with bright objects as a distraction.

100. A child is admitted with acute exacerbation of asthma. A physician orders 100% oxygen via mask. Which physician order should be a nurse's *next* priority?
1. Continuous inhaled albuterol.
2. IV Solu-Medrol 2 mg/kg loading dose.
3. IV fluids at maintenance rate.
4. Chest x-ray.

ANSWERS

Answers/Rationales/Tips

1. CORRECT ANSWER: 2. Answer 1 is incorrect because this is a measure of urine concentration, which provides the practitioner information regarding the child's degree of fluid retention from excessive ADH production. **Answer 2 is correct because obtaining a blood glucose level is not expected for a child diagnosed with SIADH since the priority measures involve blood and urine osmolality. Blood glucose is a likely laboratory test in a child with diabetes insipidus. Answer 3** is incorrect because a child with SIADH should be monitored closely for hyponatremia due to abnormal fluid retention. **Answer 4** is incorrect because this is a measure of urine concentration, which provides the practitioner information regarding the child's degree of fluid retention from excessive ADH production.

■ **TEST-TAKING TIP:** *Note how three of the answer options are useful in assessing fluid shifts while one is not. The stem of the question calls for the "least likely" laboratory test. Select the answer that does not belong to the group.*
Content Area: Child Health, Endocrine; ***Integrated Process:*** Nursing Process, Analysis; ***Cognitive Level:*** Analysis; ***Client Need/Subneed:*** Physiological Integrity/Reduction of Risk Potential/Laboratory Values

2. CORRECT ANSWER: 1. Answer 1 is correct because the apical heart rate must always be obtained by the nurse prior to the administration of digoxin (Lanoxin) to a child. Unless otherwise prescribed, the medication is typically withheld for a heart rate below 90 to 110 bpm in young children. Answer 2 is incorrect because, although the potassium level may be affected by the combined administration of digoxin (Lanoxin) with diuretics, the most important nursing action is to determine whether the apical heart rate meets the parameter for safe digoxin (Lanoxin) administration. **Answer 3** is incorrect because the heart rate and *not* the ECG waveform should be assessed prior to digoxin (Lanoxin) administration. **Answer 4** is incorrect since mixing the medication with a food or fluid is generally unnecessary due to the medication's sweet taste. Additionally, mixing with foods/fluids poses the risk that the child will refuse the mixture and the nurse may be unable to determine how much medication the child ingested.

■ **TEST-TAKING TIP:** *Since the main action of the drug is to slow the heart rate, the nurse should monitor the heart rate for signs of toxicity. The best answer is based upon the key safety parameter for this medication.*
Content Area: Child Health, Cardiovascular; ***Integrated Process:*** Nursing Process, Implementation; ***Cognitive Level:*** Application; ***Client Need/Subneed:*** Physiological Integrity/Pharmacological and Parenteral Therapies/Medication Administration

3. CORRECT ANSWER: 4. Answer 1 is incorrect since spironolactone (Aldactone) does *not affect* the ductus arteriosus. **Answer 2** is incorrect since spironolactone (Aldactone) does *not cause* vasodilation. **Answer 3** is incorrect because, although spironolactone (Aldactone) is a potassium-sparing diuretic, the main purpose of the medication is to *remove excess* fluid through diuresis. **Answer 4 is correct because spironolactone (Aldactone) is a diuretic that blocks aldosterone. Use of this medication is common among children with congenital heart disease for the prevention and treatment of congestive heart failure.**

■ **TEST-TAKING TIP:** *When unsure about medications and their actions, it is sometimes helpful to examine the root of the medication name. Spironolactone (Aldactone) begins with "A-L-D" as does the hormone aldosterone. The mechanism of action of spironolactone (Aldactone) is to inhibit aldosterone, thereby preventing water and sodium retention.*
Content Area: Child Health, Cardiovascular; ***Integrated Process:*** Nursing Process, Analysis; ***Cognitive Level:*** Application; ***Client Need/Subneed:*** Physiological Integrity/Pharmacological and Parenteral Therapies/Expected Effects/Outcomes

4. CORRECT ANSWERS: 1, 2, 3, 5, 6. Answer 1 is correct because strawberry tongue is a symptom of Kawasaki disease (mucocutaneous lymph node syndrome), occurring as the skin of the tongue sloughs off, leaving a bright red tongue with white spots. Answer 2 is correct because a symptom of Kawasaki disease is high fever lasting more than 5 days. Answer 3 is correct because irritability is a symptom of Kawasaki disease. **Answer 4** is incorrect since a cough is not a symptom of Kawasaki disease. Answer 5 is correct because the child with Kawasaki disease may experience peeling of the hands (on palms and fingertips) and feet (on soles and tips of toes) following the initial inflammatory rash on these areas. Answer 6 is correct because an elevated erythrocyte sedimentation rate (ESR) is a symptom of Kawasaki disease. Elevated ESR is indicative of an inflammatory process, which would include Kawasaki disease.
■ TEST-TAKING TIP: *When given the option to select more than one answer, review each option carefully since each may be correct. Do not assume that only a few in the list must be correct.*
Content Area: Child Health, Infectious Disease; *Integrated Process:* Nursing Process, Assessment; *Cognitive Level:* Analysis; *Client Need/Subneed:* Physiological Integrity/Physiological Adaptation/Pathophysiology

5. CORRECT ANSWERS: 1, 3, 5. Answer 1 is correct because the nurse should question an order that requires the nurse to call the physician for an oxygen saturation that *is* appropriate for an infant waiting surgical repair for a severe cyanotic heart defect. **Answer 2** is incorrect because this *is* an appropriate order; the infant with a heart defect *should* be weighed daily to assist in monitoring fluid status. Answer 3 is correct because this parameter is too low. The heart rate should be at least 100 when administering digoxin (Lanoxin) to an infant. **Answer 4** is incorrect because this *is* an appropriate order; the infant with a heart defect *should* have strict monitoring of intake and output (I&O). Answer 5 is correct because an infant with a congenital heart defect frequently requires formula with extra calories per ounce. Regular Enfamil formula would *not* provide sufficient calories.
■ TEST-TAKING TIP: *Read the stem carefully. The question asks for the identification of orders that should* not *be implemented.*
Content Area: Child Health, Cardiovascular; *Integrated Process:* Nursing Process, Analysis; *Cognitive Level:* Analysis; *Client Need/Subneed:* Physiological Integrity/Reduction of Risk Potential/Potential for Alterations in Body Systems

6. CORRECT ANSWER: 1. Answer 1 is correct because digoxin (Lanoxin) should be withheld if the heart rate of the infant falls below 90 to 110 beats per minute (bpm). If digoxin (Lanoxin) is given when the infant's heart rate is 100, the resulting cardiac output may not be adequate. **Answer 2** is incorrect because the nurse would cautiously administer digoxin to an infant with an apical heart rate below 120 bpm if the infant's heart rate was at least 90 bpm. **Answer 3** is incorrect because the nurse would administer the medication to an infant with an apical heart rate below 140 bpm if the infant's heart rate was at least 90 bpm. **Answer 4** is incorrect because the nurse would administer the medication to an infant with an apical heart rate below 160 bpm if the infant's heart rate was at least 90 bpm.
■ TEST-TAKING TIP: *Recall that the minimum apical heart rate for an infant to receive digoxin (Lanoxin) is 90 to 110 bpm. The nurse would administer the medication if the infant's apical heart rate was 120, 140, or 160 bpm.*
Content Area: Child Health, Cardiovascular; *Integrated Process:* Nursing Process, Assessment; *Cognitive Level:* Application; *Client Need/Subneed:* Physiological Integrity/Pharmacological and Parenteral Therapies/Medication Administration

7. CORRECT ANSWER: 1. Answer 1 is the correct response since the child is currently receiving a fluid bolus, which may be providing temporary improvement of pain symptoms. Ongoing application of warm compresses will continue to promote circulation in the extremities, thereby preventing pain. Once the fluid bolus is completed, the nurse should reassess the child's pain and circulation. **Answer 2** is incorrect because around-the-clock dosing of pain medication is the best way to prevent pain in a child with a chronic painful condition such as sickle cell crisis. **Answer 3** is incorrect because cessation of the warm compresses may lead to decreased circulation in the extremities, resulting in a recurrence of the pain. **Answer 4** is incorrect because both warm compresses and pain medication should be continued to prevent recurrence of pain. A change in orders is not necessary at this time, and the nurse should reassess the child following the IV fluid bolus.
■ TEST-TAKING TIP: *Whenever a client is in the middle of receiving a prescribed treatment, such as a fluid bolus, the nurse should continue supportive measures until the treatment is complete and the nurse is able to reassess. Choose the one option that is different–"continue."*
Content Area: Child Health, Cardiovascular; *Integrated Process:* Nursing Process, Implementation; *Cognitive Level:* Analysis; *Client Need/Subneed:* Physiological Integrity/Physiological Adaptation/Alterations in Body Systems

8. CORRECT ANSWER: 3. **Answer 1** is incorrect because 5600 gm would be *too little* weight gain. **Answer 2** is incorrect because the infant's birth weight should double by 4 to 7 months of age. Answer 3 is correct because an infant is expected to triple its birth weight in the first year of life; therefore, 11 kilograms (11,000 grams) is the best answer of the options given. **Answer 4** is incorrect because 15 kg would be too much weight gain compared to what is expected.
■ TEST-TAKING TIP: *Note that the answer options may only approximate the answer that is calculated. Choose the answer that most closely approximates your calculation.*
Content Area: Child Health, Growth and Development; *Integrated Process:* Nursing Process, Analysis; *Cognitive Level:* Analysis; *Client Need/Subneed:* Health Promotion and Maintenance/Developmental Stages and Transitions

9. CORRECT ANSWER: 1. **Answer 1 is correct because the child with PKU is missing the enzyme needed to digest the amino acid phenylalanine. Maternal breast milk has many beneficial properties and it contains low levels of phenylalanine. Therefore, breast milk should be given until laboratory findings demonstrate the child is not tolerating the breast milk.** **Answer 2** is incorrect because Pregestimil is an example of a formula containing *excessive* amounts of phenylalanine and is *contraindicated* for an infant with PKU. **Answer 3** is incorrect. Although Lofenalac is a formula specially made for infants with PKU and contains very low amounts of phenylalanine, maternal breast milk is the *best* initial source of nutrients. **Answer 4** is incorrect because Isomil is an example of a formula containing *excessive* amounts of phenylalanine and is *contraindicated* for an infant with PKU.

■ TEST-TAKING TIP: *Note that the stem of the question asks for the best "initial" source of nutrients. Breastfeeding should be started first, and then special formulas may be considered if necessary.*

Content Area: Child Health, Gastrointestinal; *Integrated Process:* Nursing Process, Analysis; *Cognitive Level:* Application; *Client Need/Subneed:* Physiological Integrity/Basic Care and Comfort/Nutrition and Oral Hydration

10. CORRECT ANSWER: 3. **Answer 1** is incorrect because the Babinski reflex is a normal *newborn* reflex. This reflex should *disappear* well before the child reaches 15 months of age, and its persistence should be considered abnormal. **Answer 2** is incorrect because the tonic neck reflex is a normal *newborn* reflex. This reflex should *disappear* well before the child reaches 15 months of age, and its persistence should be considered abnormal. **Answer 3 is correct because a positive patellar reflex is part of a normal assessment. The reflex is obtained when the practitioner strikes the patellar tendon, causing the leg to kick.** **Answer 4** is incorrect because the doll's eye reflex is a normal *newborn* reflex. This reflex should *disappear* well before the child reaches 15 months of age, and its persistence should be considered abnormal.

■ TEST-TAKING TIP: *Make sure to note when the stem of a question asks you to identify the* normal *finding or the* abnormal *finding. In this question, three options would be* abnormal *since they are* newborn *reflexes. Recall that a 15-month-old should have the same reflexes as an adult, including a positive patellar reflex.*

Content Area: Child Health, Neurological; *Integrated Process:* Nursing Process, Assessment; *Cognitive Level:* Application; *Client Need/Subneed:* Health Promotion and Maintenance/Developmental Stages and Transitions

11. CORRECT ANSWER: 3. **To solve this calculation, first add up the total amount of carbohydrates consumed by using the menu as a reference. The total carbohydrates consumed are 61. Next, divide the 61 total carbohydrates by 15 to arrive at 4.06. Rounded to the nearest whole number, the correct response equals 4 units of insulin.** **Answer 1** is incorrect because 2 units is an insufficient amount of insulin. **Answer 2** is incorrect because 3 units is an insufficient amount of insulin. **Answer 3 is correct because 4 units of insulin would be required to metabolize 61 carbohydrates based on an insulin-to-carbohydrate ratio of 15:1.** **Answer 4** is incorrect because 5 units is an excessive amount of insulin.

■ TEST-TAKING TIP: *When utilizing carbohydrate counts, be sure to account for partial ingestion of foods as well as extra servings of food items.*

Content Area: Child Health, Endocrine; *Integrated Process:* Nursing Process, Analysis; *Cognitive Level:* Analysis; *Client Need/Subneed:* Physiological Integrity/Pharmacological and Parenteral Therapies/Medication Administration

12. CORRECT ANSWER: 1. **Answer 1 is correct because of primary concern in the child with glomerulonephritis is the monitoring of fluid balance. The nurse should obtain a weight for this child at the same time and on the same scale daily to monitor for changes.** **Answer 2** is incorrect because edema is expected in a child with glomerulonephritis and is part of the diagnostic assessment. Although the nurse should assess edema regularly, increased frequency of this assessment is not needed and is not the highest priority of care. **Answer 3** is incorrect because gross hematuria is expected in a child with glomerulonephritis and is part of the diagnostic assessment. The presence of blood in the child's urine may last for some months; therefore, this is not the highest priority. **Answer 4** is incorrect because a major complication of glomerulonephritis is hypertensive encephalopathy. The nurse should obtain blood pressure at least every 4 hours; once per shift is insufficient monitoring.

■ TEST-TAKING TIP: *Since glomerulonephritis involves improper kidney functioning, focus on responses dealing with fluid status. The best answer calls for monitoring complications of fluid imbalance with appropriate frequency.*

Content Area: Child Health, Genitourinary; *Integrated Process:* Nursing Process, Assessment; *Cognitive Level:* Application; *Client Need/Subneed:* Physiological Integrity/Reduction of Risk Potential/System Specific Assessments

13. CORRECT ANSWER: 1. **Answer 1 is correct because preschoolers may perceive hospitalization as a punishment. The nurse should create a plan of care that reassures the child and helps the child understand the reasons for hospitalization.** **Answer 2** is incorrect because providing peer visitation is a high priority for *adolescents.* Preschoolers are most concerned with having parents present during hospitalization. **Answer 3** is incorrect because, although preschoolers should be provided play opportunities, group play is most essential for the *school-age child* who craves interaction with children of the same age. **Answer 4** is incorrect because privacy and independence are most important to *adolescents.*

■ TEST-TAKING TIP: *Recall that preschoolers are magical thinkers and may create their own explanations for events. Only one option reflects this developmental theory, making it the best answer.*

Content Area: Child Health, Hospitalization; *Integrated Process:* Nursing Process, Analysis; *Cognitive Level:* Analysis;

ANSWERS

Client Need/Subneed: Health Promotion and Maintenance/Developmental Stages and Transitions

14. CORRECT ANSWER: 3. Answer 1 is incorrect because administering an antiemetic fails to recognize the seriousness of the child's symptoms, thereby placing the child in danger. **Answer 2** is incorrect because offering ice chips may induce further vomiting and is contraindicated in the client who is nauseated. **Answer 3 is correct because the appearance of moderate red-tinged vomitus could indicate hemorrhage in the surgical area. The physician should be notified immediately of this potentially harmful complication. Answer 4** is incorrect because the application of pressure to the child's neck is contraindicated and would not resolve potential incisional bleeding and might block the carotid arteries, thereby causing harm to the child.

■ **TEST-TAKING TIP:** ***When the stem of a question appears to indicate active bleeding in a client, it is likely to be a medical emergency. The proper initial response is to stop the bleeding if possible. In this case, the bleeding is in the airway so only the physician is capable of stopping the bleeding.***

Content Area: Child Health, Respiratory; **Integrated Process:** Nursing Process, Implementation; **Cognitive Level:** Application; **Client Need/Subneed:** Physiological Integrity/Reduction of Risk Potential/Potential for Complications from Surgical Procedures and Health Alterations

15. CORRECT ANSWER: 3. Answer 1 is incorrect because toddlers have not mastered the concept of sharing, so insisting that the child share toys will likely result in frustration. **Answer 2** is incorrect because children at this age are increasingly negative. Their negativity is reinforced when parents use the word "no" frequently; avoidance of the word is suggested whenever possible **Answer 3 is correct because toddlers prefer predictable schedules and routines. The child will feel more comfortable if the home schedule is implemented when away from the parents. Answer 4** is incorrect because temper tantrums will extinguish more rapidly if the child is ignored rather than given positive reinforcement.

■ **TEST-TAKING TIP:** ***Toddlers are in the stage of autonomy and have a need to control their environment; therefore, choose the option that assists in this goal.***

Content Area: Child Health, Growth and Development; **Integrated Process:** Nursing Process, Implementation; **Cognitive Level:** Application; **Client Need/Subneed:** Health Promotion and Maintenance/Developmental Stages and Transitions

16. CORRECT ANSWER: 2. Answer 1 is incorrect because tepid baths are contraindicated in the treatment of fevers as they cause shivering, which leads to a further elevation in temperature. **Answer 2 is correct because febrile seizures are thought to occur when a child who is ill has a sudden high fever. To prevent this situation, the parents should be instructed to administer an antipyretic around the clock during the next febrile illness. Answer 3** is incorrect because antibiotics are not indicated for every childhood illness and antipyretic administration is the best way to prevent a spike in body temperature. **Answer 4** is incorrect because, although the parents should monitor the child's temperature, the administration of an antipyretic is the best prevention measure for febrile seizures.

■ **TEST-TAKING TIP:** ***The question asks how to* prevent *febrile seizures. The responses that assess temperature (Answer 4) and treat infection (Answer 3) should therefore be eliminated. Of the remaining two options, one is contraindicated and cannot be the correct response.***

Content Area: Child Health, Neurological; **Integrated Process:** Nursing Process, Implementation; **Cognitive Level:** Application; **Client Need/Subneed:** Physiological Integrity/Reduction of Risk Potential/Potential for Complications from Surgical Procedures and Health Alterations

17. CORRECT ANSWER: 2. Answer 1 is incorrect because temper tantrums are normal in this age group, and children with Kawasaki disease may experience the symptom of irritability for some time after treatment. **Answer 2 is correct because children with Kawasaki disease are placed on aspirin therapy, so exposure to chickenpox puts the child at risk for Reye syndrome. Answer 3** is incorrect because night terrors can occur in toddlers and are a normal part of development. **Answer 4** is incorrect because a low-grade fever can be related to minor infections, unlike the high, unremitting fever present in Kawasaki disease.

■ **TEST-TAKING TIP:** ***The word "*****immediately*****" in the stem of the question implies urgency, so you should look for a concern that must be addressed urgently. The behavioral issues listed would not require such attention (even if they were abnormal for the age group) and can be readily eliminated.***

Content Area: Child Health, Infectious Disease; **Integrated Process:** Nursing Process, Implementation; **Cognitive Level:** Application; **Client Need/Subneed:** Physiological Integrity/Reduction of Risk Potential/Potential for Complications from Surgical Procedures and Health Alterations

18. CORRECT ANSWER: 3. Answer 1 is incorrect because knowing whether the child has been taking medications is not part of the initial physical assessment. **Answer 2** is incorrect because knowing when the child began having symptoms is not part of the initial physical assessment. **Answer 3 is correct because the nurse should first assess the child's airway to determine the severity of respiratory symptoms. One way to assess shortness of breath is to determine whether the child speaks in full sentences, short phrases, or barely at all. Answer 4** is incorrect because the nurse should first assess the airway. ABGs (arterial blood gases) may be obtained later if ordered by the practitioner.

■ **TEST-TAKING TIP:** ***The question asks what the nurse should do* first. *Remember the nursing process–first* assess *the ABCs (airway, breathing, circulation). The other three responses contain information that could be obtained subsequent to the initial physical assessment.***

Content Area: Child Health, Respiratory; **Integrated Process:** Nursing Process, Implementation; **Cognitive Level:** Application; **Client Need/Subneed:** Physiological Integrity/Reduction of Risk Potential/System Specific Assessments

19. CORRECT ANSWER: 3. Answer 1 is incorrect because inducing vomiting is *contraindicated* for the ingestion of a hydrocarbon. **Answer 2** is incorrect because, although it is helpful to know the approximate amount of poison ingested, the highest priority upon admission is to assess the child for symptoms of *aspiration*. **Answer 3 is correct because, when a child ingests a hydrocarbon such as lighter fluid, there is an immediate danger of aspiration. Therefore, the nurse's first priority is to assess the lungs. Answer 4** is incorrect because Mucomyst (*N*-acetylcysteine) is the treatment for an overdose of *acetaminophen* and is *not* indicated in the treatment of hydrocarbon ingestion.

■ **TEST-TAKING TIP:** ***Any time a child ingests a poison, the nurse should first assess for aspiration.***

Content Area: Child Health, Poisoning; ***Integrated Process:*** Nursing Process, Implementation; ***Cognitive Level:*** Application; ***Client Need/Subneed:*** Physiological Integrity/Reduction of Risk Potential/Potential for Alterations in Body Systems

20. CORRECT ANSWER: 1. Answer 1 is correct because the chelating agent binds with lead and is excreted by the kidneys; therefore, normal kidney function should be established beforehand; blood urea nitrogen (BUN) and creatinine provide the best evidence of function. Answer 2 is incorrect because these laboratory tests would provide evidence of liver and *not* kidney function. **Answer 3** is incorrect because urine specific gravity is *not* a specific test of kidney function. **Answer 4** is incorrect because a complete blood count (CBC) is *not* a specific test of kidney function.

■ **TEST-TAKING TIP:** ***First consider the organ system best represented by the laboratory tests. If kidney function is of primary importance, the best response is the test that best demonstrates normal functioning.***

Content Area: Child Health, Poisoning; ***Integrated Process:*** Nursing Process, Analysis; ***Cognitive Level:*** Analysis; ***Client Need/Subneed:*** Physiological Integrity/Reduction of Risk Potential/Laboratory Values

21. CORRECT ANSWER: 4. Answer 1 is incorrect because, although meningitis symptoms are sometimes mistaken for other conditions, this action does little to refocus the mother's attention away from her guilt. **Answer 2** is incorrect because it is appropriate for a parent to express guilty feelings in this situation, and a referral to social services is not necessary based solely on the mother's statements. **Answer 3** is incorrect because contacting the father would violate the trusting relationship that the mother has built with the nurse. **Answer 4 is correct because the mother's statement expresses guilt feelings about the child's condition. A nurse needs to validate that the mother did seek treatment appropriately, and assist the mother to focus on what is happening now to help her child recover.**

■ **TEST-TAKING TIP:** ***An essential component of the nurse-client relationship is trust. The best response incorporates both validation of the mother's efforts to help her child and reassurance that the child is receiving appropriate care.***

Content Area: Child Health, Infectious Disease; ***Integrated Process:*** Communication and Documentation; ***Cognitive Level:*** Application; ***Client Need/Subneed:*** Psychosocial Integrity/Therapeutic Communications

22. CORRECT ANSWER: 1. Answer 1 is correct because the best action for the nurse is to help the parents understand that the NPO status is to avoid vomiting. This message should be delivered while expressing empathy for the situation. Answer 2 is incorrect because simply offering a pacifier does not address the parents' concern about feeding the infant. **Answer 3** is incorrect because knowing how long it will be until the surgeon arrives does not address the parents' concern about feeding the infant, and may actually increase their frustration if the surgeon is not able to arrive until many hours later. **Answer 4** is incorrect because this will likely result in more vomiting, which can lead to electrolyte imbalances. This action also directly violates a written order.

■ **TEST-TAKING TIP:** ***Helping families understand the treatment plan is always important in child health and is best done in combination with an empathetic and problem-solving approach.***

Content Area: Child Health, Gastrointestinal; ***Integrated Process:*** Nursing Process, Implementation; ***Cognitive Level:*** Analysis; ***Client Need/Subneed:*** Psychosocial Integrity/Therapeutic Communications

23. CORRECT ANSWER: 4. Answer 1 is incorrect because this infant needs comfort and security with *decreased* stimulation. Increasing stimulation will not meet this infant's needs. **Answer 2** is incorrect because this infant will benefit from small, frequent feedings on *demand* rather than a schedule that may increase stimulation by arousing the infant to eat on a defined schedule. **Answer 3** is incorrect because this infant needs comfort and security with *decreased* stimulation. Increasing stimulation by rubbing will increase the infant's irritability. **Answer 4 is correct because tightly swaddling the baby promotes the infant's comfort and security and decreases the stimulation that may contribute to the infant's irritability.**

■ **TEST-TAKING TIP:** ***The focus is on decreasing the irritability in the infant. Choose the interventions that will decrease stimulation and enhance security for the infant.***

Content Area: Child Health, Newborn; ***Integrated Process:*** Nursing Process, Implementation; ***Cognitive Level:*** Application; ***Client Need/Subneed:*** Health Promotion and Maintenance/Ante/Intra/Postpartum and Newborn Care

24. CORRECT ANSWER: 4. Answer 1 is incorrect because a unilateral rib hump *is* indicative of scoliosis. **Answer 2** is incorrect because asymmetrical hip height *is* indicative of scoliosis. **Answer 3** is incorrect because uneven pant lengths *may be* indicative of scoliosis. **Answer 4 is correct because the nurse is least likely to refer a child for scoliosis follow-up based on an assessment finding of rounded shoulders. This finding may simply reflect the child's**

ANSWERS

poor posture or in severe cases may indicate the condition of *kyphosis*, not scoliosis.

■ TEST-TAKING TIP: *Screening for scoliosis does involve assessing for differences between the right and left side of the child's body when standing erect (**Answer 2**) and when bent forward (**Answer 1**) at 90 degrees. The stem asks for "least likely" as the best response.*

Content Area: Child Health, Musculoskeletal; *Integrated Process:* Nursing Process, Assessment; *Cognitive Level:* Analysis; *Client Need/Subneed:* Health Promotion and Maintenance/Health Screening

25. CORRECT ANSWERS: 1, 4. **Answer 1 is correct because children with pyloric stenosis experience loss of stomach acid from excessive vomiting.** **Answer 2** is incorrect because a complication of diabetes is diabetic *ketoacidosis,* not metabolic alkalosis. **Answer 3** is incorrect because this condition results in metabolic *acidosis* due to build-up of uric acid. **Answer 4 is correct because children with bulimia nervosa vomit frequently, resulting in a loss of stomach acid.** **Answer 5** is incorrect because aspirin (acetylsalicylic acid) ingestion results in metabolic *acidosis* due to the large intake of acid.

■ TEST-TAKING TIP: *Recall that metabolic alkalosis is caused by excess loss of acid or excess intake of base.*

Content Area: Child Health, Acid-Base; *Integrated Process:* Nursing Process, Analysis; *Cognitive Level:* Analysis; *Client Need/Subneed:* Physiological Integrity/Physiological Adaptation/Fluid and Electrolyte Imbalances

26. CORRECT ANSWER: 4. **Answer 1** is incorrect because, although the child may experience discomfort, the effects of lead on the central nervous system have a higher priority. **Answer 2** is incorrect because, although the child may exhibit the symptom of pica, nutritional effects of lead poisoning are of a lesser priority than neurologic effects. **Answer 3** is incorrect because, although the child may experience pain with injections of the chelating agent, the effects of lead on the central nervous system have a higher priority. **Answer 4 is correct because the priority nursing diagnosis for this child is *alteration in neurologic functioning due to the effects of lead on the central nervous system.***

■ TEST-TAKING TIP: *The question asks for the highest priority nursing diagnosis. Only one diagnosis leads to death, so it ranks as the top priority.*

Content Area: Child Health, Poisoning; *Integrated Process:* Nursing Process, Assessment; *Cognitive Level:* Application; *Client Need/Subneed:* Safe and Effective Care Environment/Management of Care/Establishing Priorities

27. CORRECT ANSWER: 3. **Answer 1** is incorrect because, although prevention of infection is a top priority, trauma to the sac could permanently affect the function of the lower extremities while infection may be treated with antibiotics. **Answer 2** is incorrect because the rationale for placing the infant in the prone position is *not* to promote increased *circulation.* **Answer 3 is correct because the most important rationale for the prone position is to prevent damage to the meningeal sac, which could result in damage to the nerves and infection.** **Answer 4** is incorrect because, although a newborn may prefer the prone position, the rationale for this intervention is *not* to promote *comfort.*

■ TEST-TAKING TIP: *Two of the main priorities of care for an infant with myelomeningocele are to prevent infection and prevent damage to the meningeal sac. To identify the most important, think about which complication is more apt to cause irreversible damage.*

Content Area: Child Health, Neurological; *Integrated Process:* Nursing Process, Planning; *Cognitive Level:* Analysis; *Client Need/Subneed:* Physiological Integrity/Reduction of Risk Potential/Potential for Complications from Surgical Procedures and Health Alterations

28. CORRECT ANSWER: 2. **Answer 1** is incorrect because, although decreasing edema is a sign of improvement, this is *not* the earliest sign. **Answer 2 is correct because the earliest sign that a child with nephrotic syndrome is improving is an increase in urine output.** **Answer 3** is incorrect because a child's appetite should improve as the nephrotic syndrome resolves, but children's appetites can vary for a number of reasons. This sign would not necessarily signify that the child is or is not getting better. **Answer 4** is incorrect because resolution of anemia would be a *later* sign of improvement.

■ TEST-TAKING TIP: *Note the word* "earliest" *in the stem of the question. To arrive at the best answer, order the possible correct responses from early to late signs of improvement.*

Content Area: Child Health, Genitourinary; *Integrated Process:* Nursing Process, Evaluation; *Cognitive Level:* Analysis; *Client Need/Subneed:* Physiological Integrity/Pharmacological and Parenteral Therapies/Expected Effects/Outcomes

29. CORRECT ANSWER: 2. **Answer 1** is incorrect because, although proper nutrition does help prevent infection, regular and consistent pulmonary toilet has a greater preventive effect. **Answer 2 is correct because chest physiotherapy (CPT) is essential to help loosen sticky respiratory secretions and facilitate sputum removal in the child with cystic fibrosis. Failure to implement this treatment would create a ready environment for pulmonary infection.** **Answer 3** is incorrect because increased work of breathing would most likely occur after an infection has already begun. **Answer 4** is incorrect because, although proper hydration helps loosen respiratory secretions, regular and consistent pulmonary toilet has a greater preventive effect.

■ TEST-TAKING TIP: *Recall that, in a child with cystic fibrosis, the respiratory tract is filled with thick, tenacious secretions. The best answer focuses on the loosening and removal of the secretions through CPT.*

Content Area: Child Health, Respiratory; *Integrated Process:* Nursing Process, Implementation; *Cognitive Level:* Analysis; *Client Need/Subneed:* Physiological Integrity/Reduction of Risk Potential/System Specific Assessments

30. CORRECT ANSWER: 3. **Answer 1** is incorrect because, although this is the proper place to post the Poison Control Center phone number, having the number does *not prevent* ingestion from taking place. **Answer 2** is incorrect because children may come into contact with poisonous substances in the garage just as easily as they do in the home. **Answer 3 is correct because the parents should bend down and view the home from the child's eye level to better examine potential access to poisonous substances. This includes checking all storage areas inside and outside the home that are easily accessible and those that may be reached by children when climbing.** **Answer 4** is incorrect because simply instructing children to stay away from poisonous substances will *not ensure* they follow these instructions and might in fact increase the curiosity of children.

■ TEST-TAKING TIP: ***The best way to prevent ingestions is to keep harmful substances out of the reach of children. Choose the option that has the greatest likelihood of accomplishing this goal.***

Content Area: Child Health, Poisoning; *Integrated Process:* Nursing Process, Implementation; *Cognitive Level:* Application; *Client Need/Subneed:* Safe and Effective Care Environment/ Safety and Infection Control/Home Safety

31. CORRECT ANSWER: 4. **Answer 1** is incorrect because capped electrical outlets are less accessible to children and provide some degree of electrocution prevention. **Answer 2** is incorrect because the presence of a television in the child's bedroom is not a safety hazard. **Answer 3** is incorrect because, although having a swimming pool introduces the risk of drowning, the risk of burn injury from the pot handle is a more immediate danger. **Answer 4 is correct because toddlers like to reach for objects. Having pot handles turned toward the front of the stove creates the potential for the child to pull the pot and its contents onto the child, causing a severe burn injury. The parents should be instructed to turn handles toward the back of the stove and consider placing a safety guard at the front of the stove.**

■ TEST-TAKING TIP: ***Look for the option in closest proximity to the child, then consider the potential severity of the injury. The pot handle is readily accessible to the child and can lead to severe burns.***

Content Area: Child Health, Growth and Development; *Integrated Process:* Nursing Process, Assessment; *Cognitive Level:* Analysis; *Client Need/Subneed:* Safe and Effective Care Environment/Safety and Infection Control/Home Safety

32. CORRECT ANSWER: 1. **Answer 1 is correct because infants are obligatory nose breathers. A nurse should attempt to keep nasal passages open through frequent suctioning with a nasal olive.** **Answer 2** is incorrect because, although supplemental oxygen may be necessary, its delivery via nasal cannula will be *ineffective* in an infant whose nares are blocked with thick secretions. **Answer 3** is incorrect because monitoring oxygen saturations does nothing to improve oxygenation. Rather, the nurse must intervene by suctioning in order to improve saturation levels. **Answer 4** is incorrect because placing the child in an infant seat does promote lung expansion through upright positioning, but the effect will be *minimal* if the child's nares are blocked with thick secretions.

■ TEST-TAKING TIP: ***Pay attention to both the child's symptoms and physical development in order to select the correct response. The symptom of thick nasal secretions must be addressed in terms of the infant's unique respiratory pattern of nose breathing. Only one response focuses on clearing the airway in order for the other interventions to be more successful.***

Content Area: Child Health, Respiratory; *Integrated Process:* Nursing Process, Implementation; *Cognitive Level:* Application; *Client Need/Subneed:* Physiological Integrity/Reduction of Risk Potential/Potential for Alterations in Body Systems

33. CORRECT ANSWERS: 2, 4, 5. **Answer 1** is incorrect because this neonate has caput succedaneum, a collection of *fluid* and *not blood.* Cephalohematoma is a collection of blood under the skull bones and does not cross the suture lines. **Answer 2 is correct because caput succedaneum is an edematous swelling that overlies the periosteum.** **Answer 3** is incorrect because caput succedaneum is a collection of fluid, *not* blood; therefore, there is *no* increased chance of hyperbilirubinemia that is associated with cephalohematoma. **Answer 4 is correct because the only management is observation. No treatment is needed for caput succedaneum.** **Answer 5 is correct because caput succedaneum is the result of pressure on the fetal head before delivery.**

■ TEST-TAKING TIP: ***Remember that caput succedaneum*** **crosses** ***the suture lines and cephalohematoma does not. Answer 1 relates to Answer 3; therefore, you can eliminate both, as they both relate to collection of blood in*** **cephalohematoma.** ***This infant has*** **caput succedaneum.**

Content Area: Child Health, Newborn; *Integrated Process:* Nursing Process, Implementation; *Cognitive Level:* Application; *Client Need/Subneed:* Health Promotion and Maintenance/ Ante/Intra/Postpartum and Newborn Care

34. CORRECT ANSWER: 2. **Answer 1** is incorrect because the nurse should *first assess* the likely causes of the symptoms before calling the surgeon. **Answer 2 is correct because the child is experiencing symptoms of autonomic dysreflexia, an excessive stimulation of the sympathetic nervous system that is a potential complication of spinal cord surgery. Since bladder distention can lead to this problem, the nurse should first assess the urinary catheter for obstruction or malfunction.** **Answer 3** is incorrect because the headache is a symptom of the high blood pressure caused by the autonomic dysreflexia, and administering pain medication will *not resolve* the headache. **Answer 4** is incorrect because, although a neurological assessment is an important priority of care, the nurse should *first* investigate the potential *cause of* the symptoms.

■ TEST-TAKING TIP: ***When deciding between the option to phone the physician or perform additional assessments, think about what the nurse might find with the assessment that has the potential to resolve the problem or provide the physician with additional, necessary information. In this case, the nurse should suspect bladder distention, investigate urinary catheter functioning, and fix any malfunction as a way to resolve the problem without first contacting the physician.***

ANSWERS

Content Area: Child Health, Musculoskeletal; ***Integrated Process:*** Nursing Process, Implementation; ***Cognitive Level:*** Application; ***Client Need/Subneed:*** Physiological Integrity/Reduction of Risk Potential/Potential for Complications from Surgical Procedures and Health Alterations

35. CORRECT ANSWERS: 1, 2, 4, 5. Answer 1 is correct because the child with acute glomerulonephritis has large amounts of red blood cells in the urine due to ruptured glomerular capillaries. Answer 2 is correct because pallor is a symptom of acute glomerulonephritis as a result of anemia. **Answer 3** is incorrect because urine specific gravity *increases* with the fluid *retention* of acute glomerulonephritis. Answer 4 is correct because the child with acute glomerulonephritis gains weight due to fluid retention. Answer 5 is correct because the child with acute glomerulonephritis may have a headache as a result of hypertension caused by hypervolemia. **Answer 6** is incorrect because proteinuria is mild, *not* massive for the child with acute glomerulonephritis. Massive proteinuria is a symptom of *nephrotic* syndrome.

■ TEST-TAKING TIP: *Look for answers that go together. Hematuria (Answer 1) results in pallor (Answer 2); weight gain (Answer 4) from fluid retention goes with headache from hypertension (Answer 5).*

Content Area: Child Health, Genitourinary; ***Integrated Process:*** Nursing Process, Assessment; ***Cognitive Level:*** Analysis; ***Client Need/Subneed:*** Physiological Integrity/Physiological Adaptation/Alterations in Body Systems

36. CORRECT ANSWER: 2. **Answer 1** is incorrect because vomiting and diarrhea are not part of the diagnostic criteria for rheumatic fever and are symptoms common to many other illnesses. Answer 2 is correct because symptoms of rheumatic fever include muscle weakness and arthralgia. **Answer 3** is incorrect because together these are symptoms of Kawasaki disease, *not* rheumatic fever. **Answer 4** is incorrect because children with rheumatic fever are likely to experience *tachycardia.* In addition, hypotension is *not* part of the diagnostic criteria for rheumatic fever.

■ TEST-TAKING TIP: *The question contains the word "rheumatic," which is related to joints. Only one answer option contains a symptom associated with joints (arthralgia), which should help you narrow your choice.*

Content Area: Child Health, Infectious Disease; ***Integrated Process:*** Nursing Process, Assessment; ***Cognitive Level:*** Application; ***Client Need/Subneed:*** Physiological Integrity/Physiological Adaptation/Pathophysiology

37. CORRECT ANSWER: 3. **Answer 1** is incorrect since an 18-gauge (G) needle would be too large a diameter for a newborn infant. **Answer 2** is incorrect since a 21-gauge, 1-inch needle would be too large for a newborn infant. Answer 3 is correct because the most appropriate needle to select for use in administering IM injection to a 1-week-old infant would be a 25 gauge, 5/8 inch long. **Answer 4** is incorrect since a 1 1/2-inch needle would be far too long for a newborn infant and also for most children.

■ TEST-TAKING TIP: *Recall that the gauge of the needle gets* **larger** *as the number gets* **smaller** *(i.e., an 18 G is larger than a 25 G). The best answer contains both the smallest gauge and the shortest length.*

Content Area: Child Health, Medication Administration; ***Integrated Process:*** Nursing Process, Implementation; ***Cognitive Level:*** Application; ***Client Need/Subneed:*** Physiological Integrity/Pharmacological and Parenteral Therapies/Medication Administration

38. CORRECT ANSWER: 4. **Answer 1** is incorrect because the iron supplement is best absorbed *between* meals. Additionally, a bowl of cereal is likely to contain milk, which would impair the absorption of iron. **Answer 2** is incorrect because iron supplementation is more likely to cause *dark*-colored stools. **Answer 3** is incorrect because the medication is best administered at the *back* of the mouth to avoid staining the child's teeth. Answer 4 is correct since iron is best absorbed in the presence of vitamin C. The liquid iron supplement may be mixed with fruit juices such as orange juice to make the medication more palatable while also increasing the absorption.

■ TEST-TAKING TIP: *Remember that a frequent recommendation is to administer iron supplements with orange juice. Fruit juices contain vitamin C, or ascorbic acid, which makes Answer 4 the best answer.*

Content Area: Child Health, Medication Administration; ***Integrated Process:*** Teaching and Learning; ***Cognitive Level:*** Application; ***Client Need/Subneed:*** Physiological Integrity/Pharmacological and Parenteral Therapies/Medication Administration

39. CORRECT ANSWER: 3. **Answer 1** is incorrect because an absolute neutrophil count (ANC) of 1200 is just below the normal range of 1500 or greater. This slightly low value is not unexpected for a child with cancer who is receiving chemotherapy. An ANC of less than 500 should be reported since this would meet the criteria for neutropenia. **Answer 2** is incorrect because this is within the range of normal (150,000 to 400,000) for the platelet count. If the platelet count fell below 100,000, the physician should be notified. Answer 3 is correct because a positive urine dipstick for the presence of red blood cells could indicate hemorrhagic cystitis, a complication of chemotherapy agents, including cyclophosphamide and ifosfamide. This finding should be communicated immediately to the physician. **Answer 4** is incorrect because a white blood cell (WBC) count of 4500 is just below the range of normal (5000 to 10,000), which is expected for a child receiving chemotherapy.

■ TEST-TAKING TIP: *When given laboratory values, consider both the range of normal values as well as expected values for given medical conditions. Pay attention to those values that are abnormal for the child even with the stated diagnosis and treatment.*

Content Area: Child Health, Oncology; ***Integrated Process:*** Nursing Process, Evaluation; ***Cognitive Level:*** Analysis; ***Client Need/Subneed:*** Physiological Integrity/Reduction of Risk Potential/Laboratory Values

40. CORRECT ANSWER: 1. Answer 1 is correct because, prior to digoxin administration, all children should have their apical pulse assessed by auscultation at the apex of the heart. The heartbeats are best heard at the apex of the heart, making this the best location for assessing the heart rate. **Answer 2** is incorrect because this location is best for assessing the *brachial pulse.* This is not the best location for assessing heart rate because the brachial artery may be difficult to palpate, leading to inaccurate assessment. **Answer 3** is incorrect because this location is best for assessing the *radial pulse.* This is not the best location for assessing heart rate because the radial artery may be difficult to palpate, leading to inaccurate assessment. **Answer 4** is incorrect because heart beats are best heard at the *apex* of the heart, *not* the base of the heart, making the apex the best location for auscultation and assessment of heart rate.

■ **TEST-TAKING TIP:** *The correct response does not vary with the child's age. A nurse must assess the apical heart rate, not simply the pulse rate, prior to digoxin administration.*

Content Area: Child Health, Cardiovascular; ***Integrated Process:*** Nursing Process, Assessment; ***Cognitive Level:*** Application; ***Client Need/Subneed:*** Physiological Integrity/Pharmacological and Parenteral Therapies/Medication Administration

41. CORRECT ANSWER: 1. Answer 1 is correct because this statement by the mother indicates more teaching is needed, since crushing the capsule would destroy the enteric coating on the enzyme beads, leading to their destruction in the acid environment of the stomach. **Answer 2** is incorrect because this statement demonstrates *appropriate* knowledge. **Answer 3** is incorrect because this statement demonstrates *appropriate* knowledge. **Answer 4** is incorrect because this statement demonstrates *appropriate* knowledge. Pancreatic enzymes must be administered within 30 minutes of the ingestion of food.

■ **TEST-TAKING TIP:** *Make sure to look for an* incorrect *statement when the stem says "further teaching is needed."*

Content Area: Child Health, Respiratory; ***Integrated Process:*** Nursing Process, Evaluation; ***Cognitive Level:*** Analysis; ***Client Need/Subneed:*** Physiological Integrity/Pharmacological and Parenteral Therapies/Medication Administration

42. CORRECT ANSWER: 1. Answer 1 is correct because the nurse should first check the child's recent laboratory work to see if a gentamicin level has been done. The physician may have increased the dose of IV gentamicin above the safe dose range if the child's gentamicin level fell below that which is effective. The safe dose range is the starting point for this medication, but the dose is then increased or decreased to achieve therapeutic blood levels. **Answer 2** is incorrect because the nurse should *first* discover if the dose was changed to achieve a therapeutic blood level. **Answer 3** is incorrect because, although gentamicin may be ototoxic, the nurse should *first* discover if the dose was changed to achieve a therapeutic blood level. **Answer 4** is incorrect because, although gentamicin may be nephrotoxic, the nurse should *first* discover if the dose was changed to achieve a therapeutic blood level.

■ **TEST-TAKING TIP:** *Note that two of the options (Answers 3 and 4) require consultation with the physician, so they are subsumed under the "contact the physician" response. Then, to decide between the first two answers, consider that the nurse should review the* assessment *data first to determine whether a call to the physician is even necessary.*

Content Area: Child Health, Medication Administration; ***Integrated Process:*** Nursing Process, Implementation; ***Cognitive Level:*** Application; ***Client Need/Subneed:*** Physiological Integrity/Pharmacological and Parenteral Therapies/Medication Administration

43. CORRECT ANSWER: 2. **Answer 1** is incorrect because hypoglycemia is more likely to occur just *prior to* meals. **Answer 2 is correct since the body becomes more sensitive to insulin with physical activity, and it may be necessary to reduce the child's insulin dosage with sports participation.** **Answer 3** is incorrect because self-administration of insulin depends on developmental readiness rather than age. Children as young as early school age may be capable of giving injections with caregiver supervision. **Answer 4** is incorrect because insulin is not contraindicated during febrile illnesses. The dosage of insulin may increase, decrease, or stay the same depending on the child's needs.

■ **TEST-TAKING TIP:** *Be wary of answer options that contain extreme terms such as "never" or "always."*

Content Area: Child Health, Endocrine; ***Integrated Process:*** Teaching and Learning; ***Cognitive Level:*** Application; ***Client Need/Subneed:*** Physiological Integrity/Physiological Adaptation/Illness Management

44. CORRECT ANSWER: 4. **Answer 1** is incorrect because the LVN/LPN should *have* experience caring for clients in traction for bone fractures. **Answer 2** is incorrect because the LVN/LPN *has* experience caring for clients with alterations in bone health. Legg-Calvé-Perthes disease involves necrosis of the femoral head. **Answer 3** is incorrect because the LVN/LPN floated from the orthopedic unit *may have* experience caring for clients with osteogenesis imperfecta since this is a chronic condition. **Answer 4 is correct because the child with osteosarcoma is receiving chemotherapy, which requires continuous monitoring for complications. This child would not be an appropriate client for the LVN/LPN due to the need for frequent assessment by a registered nurse.**

■ **TEST-TAKING TIP:** *Note the key word "avoid" and look for the incorrect answer as the best choice. When determining the proper assignment for this LPN/LVN, consider the scope of practice. In this case, only the child receiving chemotherapy would require too much expertise and too high a level of assessment.*

ANSWERS

Content Area: Child Health, Musculoskeletal; *Integrated Process:* Nursing Process, Analysis; *Cognitive Level:* Analysis; *Client Need/Subneed:* Safe and Effective Care Environment/ Management of Care/Delegation

45. CORRECT ANSWER: 4. **Answer 1** is incorrect because a capillary refill time of 2 seconds is a normal finding. Extended refill time would be a concern. **Answer 2** is incorrect because transient mottling of the skin is likely caused by a decrease in environmental temperature or as a result of stress. *Sustained* mottling of the skin would be cause for concern. **Answer 3** is incorrect because irregular, periodic breaths are normal findings in an infant. Apneic spells or respirations that never sustain any pattern would be a concern. **Answer 4 is correct because the newborn should have a positive Babinski, or plantar, reflex. This reflex occurs when the toes extend in response to the stroking of the sole of the foot. A negative finding should occur in *older* infants and adults and is noted when the toes demonstrate a flexor response.**

■ TEST-TAKING TIP: *The key word in the stem of the question is "newborn." Look for the assessment finding that is abnormal for a newborn.*

Content Area: Child Health, Newborn; *Integrated Process:* Nursing Process, Assessment; *Cognitive Level:* Analysis; *Client Need/Subneed:* Health Promotion and Maintenance/Health Screening

46. CORRECT ANSWER: 3. **Answer 1** is incorrect because, although children with mumps have a fever, the other symptoms are not present. **Answer 2** is incorrect because children with measles have a fever and rash, but the rash spreads from the face to the rest of the body, becoming more prominent in the upper body. The other symptoms are not present. **Answer 3 is correct because these symptoms are classic for scarlet fever. The child develops a high fever, abdominal pain, flushed cheeks, and strawberry tongue, as well as a generalized pinpoint red rash that is more concentrated in the axillae and groin.** **Answer 4** is incorrect because varicella begins with a macular rash, progressing to papular and then vesicular lesions. The child also has a fever but the other symptoms are not present.

■ TEST-TAKING TIP: *Recall that two pediatric infections have the symptom of a strawberry-like tongue: Kawasaki disease and scarlet fever.*

Content Area: Child Health, Infectious Disease; *Integrated Process:* Nursing Process, Assessment; *Cognitive Level:* Application; *Client Need/Subneed:* Physiological Integrity/ Physiological Adaptation/Pathophysiology

47. CORRECT ANSWER: 2. **Answer 1** is incorrect because placing the stethoscope over the sternum will produce *bronchovesicular* breath sounds. **Answer 2 is correct because the nurse is best able to auscultate bronchial breath sounds in an infant by placing the stethoscope over the trachea above the suprasternal notch.** **Answer 3** is incorrect because placing the stethoscope beneath the scapula will produce *bronchovesicular* breath sounds. **Answer 4** is incorrect because placing the stethoscope at the base of the lungs will produce *vesicular* breath sounds.

■ TEST-TAKING TIP: *The word "bronchial" is derived from the word "bronchus." The best place to auscultate breath sounds is over the main bronchus, which is located directly underneath the sternum.*

Content Area: Child Health, Respiratory; *Integrated Process:* Nursing Process, Assessment; *Cognitive Level:* Application; *Client Need/Subneed:* Health Promotion and Maintenance/ Techniques of Physical Assessment

48. CORRECT ANSWER: 3. **Answer 1** is incorrect because children should ride in the back seat until they are *12 years* of age or older. **Answer 2** is incorrect because infants should be *rear* facing rather than forward facing. **Answer 3 is correct because infants should face the rear of the vehicle until they weigh 20 pounds, from birth to as close to the first birthday as possible.** **Answer 4** is incorrect because air bags should be turned off where children are sitting, as air bag deployment could strike a child in the face, causing serious injury.

■ TEST-TAKING TIP: *When deciding whether a child should face the front or the rear of the car, recall that an infant's neck muscles are weak. The safest place for the infant is facing the rear since this would prevent the child's head from flexing forward in a head-on collision.*

Content Area: Child Health, Safety; *Integrated Process:* Nursing Process, Implementation; *Cognitive Level:* Application; *Client Need/Subneed:* Health Promotion and Maintenance/ Health Promotion Programs

49. CORRECT ANSWER: 1. **Answer 1 is correct because an audible, low-pitched, "clunk" during the Ortolani test is caused by the sound of the femur head exiting or entering the acetabulum, indicating hip dislocation.** **Answer 2** is incorrect because symmetrical gluteal and thigh folds are negative signs of hip dislocation. *Asymmetry* would indicate dislocation of the hip. **Answer 3** is incorrect because a *positive* Barlow test would indicate hip dislocation. **Answer 4** is incorrect because *asymmetry* of the knees while the infant is in the supine position would indicate hip dislocation.

■ TEST-TAKING TIP: *Note the key words "abnormal findings." Recall that, when investigating hip dislocation, symmetrical findings are normal, which eliminates Answers 2 and 4. Next, recall that* positive *Ortolani and Barlow tests are pathologic for developmental dysplasia of the hip, which makes Answer 1 the only correct response.*

Content Area: Child Health, Musculoskeletal; *Integrated Process:* Nursing Process, Assessment; *Cognitive Level:* Analysis; *Client Need/Subneed:* Physiological Integrity/ Reduction of Risk Potential/System Specific Assessments

50. **CORRECT ANSWER: 3.2.** To solve this problem, first multiply the ordered 200,000 units per kilogram by the child's weight of 16 kg to get a total of 3,200,000 units per day. Next, divide the total daily units of 3,200,000 by 4 (since the drug is administered every 6 hours) to get a single dose of 800,000 units. Finally, take the single dose of 800,000 units and divide by the 250,000 units per mL to get a total of 3.2 mL.

■ **TEST-TAKING TIP:** ***Approach pharmacology math questions in a stepwise fashion, paying attention to the number of doses given in a 24-hour* day *rather than the* hours *between doses (in this example, divide by 4 doses per day, not by 6 hours between doses).***

Content Area: Child Health, Medication Administration; ***Integrated Process:*** Nursing Process, Implementation; ***Cognitive Level:*** Application; ***Client Need/Subneed:*** Physiological Integrity/Pharmacological and Parenteral Therapies/Dosage Calculation

51. **CORRECT ANSWER: 1.** **Answer 1 is correct because the child with acute epiglottitis is likely to be restless and agitated due to the progressive airway obstruction. The child should be allowed to maintain a position of comfort (e.g., sitting upright) to avoid further agitation and impaired oxygenation.** **Answer 2** is incorrect because placing any item in the child's mouth is contraindicated with a diagnosis of acute epiglottitis because this may lead to complete airway obstruction. **Answer 3** is incorrect because the inspection of the child's nares is likely to agitate the child, and is also unnecessary since the primary area of swelling is in the epiglottis and not the nares. **Answer 4** is incorrect because the child *is* maintaining oxygenation at this time and the application of a mask on a young child is likely to create anxiety, which will decrease oxygenation.

■ **TEST-TAKING TIP:** ***Children with epiglottitis are at risk for complete airway obstruction. Note that all but one of the answer options requires a nursing intervention near the child's nose or mouth, which may cause distress. Select the option that will not agitate the child further.***

Content Area: Child Health, Respiratory; ***Integrated Process:*** Nursing Process, Implementation; ***Cognitive Level:*** Application; ***Client Need/Subneed:*** Physiological Integrity/Reduction of Risk Potential/Potential for Alterations in Body Systems

52. **CORRECT ANSWERS: 1, 3, 4.** **Answer 1 is correct as the first step because the child should wash hands prior to the procedure to prevent infection.** **Answer 2** is incorrect because children with spina bifida are at increased risk for *latex allergy* and should *not* utilize latex catheters. **Answer 3 is correct as the second step because lubricating jelly should be applied.** **Answer 4 is correct because, after insertion and removal of the catheter, the third (and last) step is to cleanse the catheter for storage.** **Answer 5** is incorrect because the child should cleanse the perineum with soap and water, *not* Betadine.

■ **TEST-TAKING TIP:** ***Since self-catheterization is done at home, remember that the procedure is clean, not sterile.* Start and end with washing *(Answers 1 and 4). The child may reuse catheters as long as they are properly cleaned and stored.***

Content Area: Child Health, Neurological; ***Integrated Process:*** Nursing Process, Implementation; ***Cognitive Level:*** Application; ***Client Need/Subneed:*** Physiological Integrity/Basic Care and Comfort/Elimination

53. **CORRECT ANSWER: 4.** **Answer 1** is incorrect because the nurse should *first assess* the suction. Although changing position may help move the tip of the tube from a potential blockage in the stomach, it is more effective to aspirate and irrigate the tube in this situation. **Answer 2** is incorrect because the nurse should *first assess* the situation and attempt to resolve the issue before consulting the surgeon. **Answer 3** is incorrect because the nurse should *first assess* the suction. If the suction is working properly, the nurse should check placement before instilling anything into the tube. **Answer 4 is correct because the most likely cause of poor drainage is ineffective suction. The suction tubing may have become dislodged or the settings may have been altered. A nurse should inspect this first, then continue to problem-solve if needed.**

■ **TEST-TAKING TIP:** ***Look for nursing actions that are the least invasive. Checking the suction settings can be done quickly and easily without disturbing the child.***

Content Area: Child Health, Gastrointestinal; ***Integrated Process:*** Nursing Process, Evaluation; ***Cognitive Level:*** Application; ***Client Need/Subneed:*** Physiological Integrity/Reduction of Risk Potential/Potential for Complications of Diagnostic Tests/Treatments/Procedures

54. **CORRECT ANSWER: 3.** **Answer 1** is incorrect because teenagers have heart rates that generally range from 55 to 90. However, children who are athletic may have even lower heart rates, especially at rest. **Answer 2** is incorrect because, although an infant's heart rate ranges from 120 to 160, the rate can near 200 with vigorous crying. If the infant were at rest, a rate of 190 would be suspicious. **Answer 3 is correct because the normal heart rate in a 2-year-old child is from 80 to 120 beats per minute. Even though the child is active, this heart rate is quite high and should be investigated further.** **Answer 4** is incorrect because this is within the range of normal (70 to 100) for a 5-year-old child.

■ **TEST-TAKING TIP:** ***Pay particular attention to the child's activity level when evaluating heart rates. An elevated heart rate during normal or restful activity is more of a concern than a decreased heart rate at rest or an elevated heart rate during vigorous activity.***

Content Area: Child Health, Cardiovascular; ***Integrated Process:*** Nursing Process, Assessment; ***Cognitive Level:*** Analysis; ***Client Need/Subneed:*** Physiological Integrity/Physiological Adaptation/Alterations in Body Systems

55. **CORRECT ANSWER: 1.** **Answer 1 is correct because the nurse's priority is to fulfill the legal duties of a mandated reporter by contacting the agency responsible for taking reports of suspected child abuse.** **Answer 2** is incorrect because the nurse should not discuss the allegations with the child's family members as this may interfere with an investigation. **Answer 3** is incorrect because further questioning by the nurse may harm the investigation. Questioning victims of suspected child abuse should be left to professionals skilled in this procedure. **Answer 4** is incorrect because, although the nurse should provide a safe environment for the child, the nurse should not continue the discussion without the presence of the proper authorities.

■ TEST-TAKING TIP: ***Look to eliminate answers that contain only partially correct responses. Answer 4 is only half right and therefore can be eliminated. Of the remaining options, only Answer 1 contains an action that the nurse must always do when suspecting child abuse.***

Content Area: Child Health, Abuse; ***Integrated Process:*** Nursing Process, Implementation; ***Cognitive Level:*** Application; ***Client Need/Subneed:*** Safe and Effective Care Environment/ Management of Care/Legal Rights and Responsibilities

56. CORRECT ANSWER: 2. **Answer 1** is incorrect because, although this child is likely to have mobility problems, pairing a teenager with a 9-year-old may be problematic as they may not share similar interests. **Answer 2 is correct because this child is close in age and development and is likely to be immobilized in the injured leg due to a cast and/or traction. Since the child with myelodysplasia is likely to have impaired mobility in the infected foot or even complete paralysis of both lower extremities, these children share similar limitations and the nursing staff can encourage them to play video games or participate in suitable activities.** **Answer 3** is incorrect because, although the child is in the same age range, the physical needs are not alike. The child status post-appendectomy may be NPO and have a nasogastric tube for a few days but will then be prodded to ambulate and increase activity. Neither of these situations matches well with the child with myelodysplasia. **Answer 4** is incorrect because a child with bacterial meningitis is contagious until after 24 hours of antibiotic therapy. Also, a 6-year-old child is not the best playmate for a 9-year-old child.

■ TEST-TAKING TIP: ***To select the best roommate for a pediatric client, first eliminate the children who do not share* developmental needs. *Next, eliminate those who are potentially* infectious *to the child in question. Finally, match the child with a roommate who has* similar care *needs.***

Content Area: Child Health, Hospitalization; ***Integrated Process:*** Nursing Process, Planning; ***Cognitive Level:*** Analysis; ***Client Need/Subneed:*** Safe and Effective Care Environment/ Management of Care/Concepts of Management

57. CORRECT ANSWERS: 1, 3, 4. **Answer 1 is correct because, following tonsillectomy, the child may begin oral intake after surgery, beginning with ice chips and progressing as tolerated to avoid vomiting, which could injure the surgical site.** **Answer 2** is incorrect because coughing should be discouraged as this puts stress on the tonsillectomy site and causes bleeding. **Answer 3 is correct because increased bleeding times put the child at risk for hemorrhage at the tonsillectomy site, which could compromise the airway. Answer 4 is correct because the nurse should expect that the child will have pain from the tonsillectomy. Pain control is best achieved with around-the-clock dosing. Without adequate pain control, the child may cry, putting stress on the surgical site.** **Answer 5** is incorrect because frequent oral suctioning puts stress on the tonsillectomy site and causes bleeding.

■ TEST-TAKING TIP: ***Consider that the surgical area for tonsillectomy is in the child's throat. Potential hemorrhage in this area could lead to serious respiratory compromise; therefore, priority nursing actions should be to monitor and protect the* airway.**

Content Area: Child Health, Respiratory; ***Integrated Process:*** Nursing Process, Planning; ***Cognitive Level:*** Analysis; ***Client Need/Subneed:*** Physiological Integrity/Reduction of Risk Potential/Potential for Complications from Surgical Procedures and Health Alterations

58. CORRECT ANSWER: 2. **Answer 1** is incorrect because lung crackles indicate fluid in the lungs, which occurs after the increase in heart rate is no longer effective in compensating for poor cardiac functioning. **Answer 2 is correct because the body tries to compensate for a failing heart by first increasing the heart rate as a way to increase circulating blood volume.** **Answer 3** is incorrect because weight gain occurs more *slowly* over time as the kidneys attempt to retain fluid in response to the poor cardiac output. **Answer 4** is incorrect because generalized edema occurs more *slowly* over time as the kidneys attempt to retain fluid in response to the poor cardiac output.

■ TEST-TAKING TIP: ***Note how three of the answers are similar in that they describe fluid retained in the wrong area. Only one answer is an effort to prevent fluid retention, and is therefore the* earliest *sign of failure.***

Content Area: Child Health, Cardiovascular; ***Integrated Process:*** Nursing Process, Assessment; ***Cognitive Level:*** Application; ***Client Need/Subneed:*** Physiological Integrity/Physiological Adaptation/Alterations in Body Systems

59. CORRECT ANSWER: 1. **Answer 1 is correct because the primary means of lead exposure in children results from ingestion. The presence of lead-based paint should be suspected in homes built prior to the late 1970s when these paints were discontinued. Children can ingest paint chips or dust by chewing on contaminated surfaces such as windowsills, and they can become exposed by playing in contaminated soil.** **Answer 2** is incorrect because this is a means of exposure, but not the most *common* means. **Answer 3** is incorrect because leaded gasoline is not permitted for on-road vehicles. **Answer 4** is incorrect since pencil lead does not contain lead, but graphite, and is not a source of lead poisoning in children.

■ TEST-TAKING TIP: ***To determine the most likely source of exposure, consider that an ingested poison is absorbed most easily. Two answers describe ingestion, but one answer can be generalized to a greater population of children (*many *children live in old homes, while only* some *would chew on pencils). Even if lead is possibly contained in pencils, not enough children would be exposed to make that the primary route of exposure.***

Content Area: Child Health, Poisoning; ***Integrated Process:*** Nursing Process, Analysis; ***Cognitive Level:*** Analysis; ***Client Need/Subneed:*** Safe and Effective Care Environment/Safety and Infection Control/Home Safety

60. CORRECT ANSWER: 2. **Answer 1** is incorrect because the meningitis vaccine is only effective against some strains, and the vaccine is not a guarantee that the child will never become infected. **Answer 2 is correct because meningitis is primarily spread through contact with droplets that arise from the nasopharynx of a person who is infected. Teenagers should be taught to not share food, drinks, or any other item that touches the nose or mouth of another person.** **Answer 3** is incorrect because children should not avoid group activities for fear of infection. Team sports should not be avoided, but participants must have their own water bottles. **Answer 4** is incorrect because prevention methods should be employed whether children are in crowds or in small groups. It is never recommended that children share items touching the nose or mouth of other children.

■ TEST-TAKING TIP: ***The primary focus of infection prevention is to encourage behavior change. However, prevention methods should not expect individuals to make extreme and unrealistic behavioral changes. Teenagers especially are not going to avoid group activities (team sports, crowds) since peer groups are important. The easiest behavior to change is to avoid sharing drinks and food.***

Content Area: Child Health, Infectious Disease; ***Integrated Process:*** Nursing Process, Planning; ***Cognitive Level:*** Application; ***Client Need/Subneed:*** Safe and Effective Care Environment/Safety and Infection Control/Standard/Transmission-based/Other Precautions

61. CORRECT ANSWER: 4. **Answer 1** is incorrect because joint pain is often related to hemarthrosis, which should first be treated with immobilization and then later with *passive,* not *active,* range of motion. **Answer 2** is incorrect because aspirin is *contraindicated* for the child with hemophilia as it increases the risk of bleeding. **Answer 3** is incorrect because *ice* should be applied to injuries to promote *vasoconstriction.* Warm compresses are not recommended because these lead to *vasodilation* and potential bleeding. **Answer 4 is correct because a soft toothbrush will prevent trauma to the child's gums (i.e., bleeding) while keeping the teeth clean.**

■ TEST-TAKING TIP: ***Since the key concern in hemophilia is bleeding, look for the answer that is least likely to cause harm by increasing bleeding tendencies. Only Answer 4 prevents trauma.***

Content Area: Child Health, Hematological; ***Integrated Process:*** Nursing Process, Implementation; ***Cognitive Level:*** Application; ***Client Need/Subneed:*** Physiological Integrity/Reduction of Risk Potential/Potential for Complications from Surgical Procedures and Health Alterations

62. CORRECT ANSWER: 1. **Answer 1 is correct because these foods are high in fiber and folic acid. Fiber prevents constipation, a potential side effect of pain medication, and folic acid is needed for healthy red blood cell production.** **Answer 2** is incorrect because children with sickle cell anemia are at high risk for infection and *should be* properly immunized. **Answer 3** is incorrect because the odds of the child's offspring having sickle cell anemia cannot be determined without knowing the genetic status of the person with whom the client conceives a child. **Answer 4** is incorrect because the use of Demerol in children with sickle cell anemia is *contraindicated* since it carries an increased risk of seizure activity.

■ TEST-TAKING TIP: ***When a question has only one correct response (instead of several* good *responses and one* best *response), look for the response that seems* reasonable. *A diet with healthy foods is reasonable and correct for this child.***

Content Area: Child Health, Hematological; ***Integrated Process:*** Nursing Process, Planning; ***Cognitive Level:*** Application; ***Client Need/Subneed:*** Physiological Integrity/Reduction of Risk Potential/Potential for Complications from Surgical Procedures and Health Alterations

63. CORRECT ANSWER: 4. **Answer 1** is incorrect because whole grains contain gluten. **Answer 2** is incorrect because cake is made with wheat flour, which contains gluten. **Answer 3** is incorrect because pizza dough is made with wheat flour, which contains gluten. **Answer 4 is correct because beans and rice are acceptable foods for a child with celiac disease, who requires a gluten-free diet.**

■ TEST-TAKING TIP: ***Recall that any food item made with wheat flour is unacceptable for a child with celiac disease. Choose the foods that do not contain flour.***

Content Area: Child Health, Gastrointestinal; ***Integrated Process:*** Nursing Process, Implementation; ***Cognitive Level:*** Application; ***Client Need/Subneed:*** Physiological Integrity/Basic Care and Comfort/Nutrition and Oral Hydration

64. CORRECT ANSWER: 2. **Answer 1** is incorrect because, although the infant with severe dehydration may have decreased or absent urinary output, lethargy and decreased urine output alone may also be indicative of moderate dehydration. **Answer 2 is correct because these symptoms describe a child with significantly diminished circulation as a result of dehydration. An infant with severe dehydration has weak to absent pulses, poor skin turgor, and cool, discolored skin.** **Answer 3** is incorrect because these are symptoms of an infant with mild to moderate dehydration. **Answer 4** is incorrect because these are symptoms of an infant with moderate dehydration. The infant with severe dehydration may be lethargic, may have parched mucous membranes, and may experience an abnormally irregular respiratory pattern.

■ TEST-TAKING TIP: ***The stem of the question asks you to identify the most* severe *symptoms. It is helpful to rank the answer options from best to worst in order to identify the most severe description.***

Content Area: Child Health, Gastrointestinal; ***Integrated Process:*** Nursing Process, Analysis; ***Cognitive Level:*** Analysis; ***Client Need/Subneed:*** Physiological Integrity/Physiological Adaptation/Alterations in Body Systems

65. CORRECT ANSWER: 3. **Answer 1** is incorrect because the apical area is a better location to listen for *mitral valve* clicks. **Answer 2** is incorrect because the lower left sternal border is a better location to listen for the murmur of a *ventricular septal defect.* **Answer 3 is correct because the pulmonic area, located at the upper left sternal border, is directly over the pulmonary artery, making the murmur best heard at this location.** **Answer 4** is incorrect because the

ANSWERS

upper right sternal border is a better location to hear *aortic valve clicks.*

■ TEST-TAKING TIP: ***Since the defect involves the pulmonary artery, visualize the heart's anatomy as it sits in the chest and place the stethoscope closest to the pulmonary artery.***

Content Area: Child Health, Cardiovascular; ***Integrated Process:*** Nursing Process, Assessment; ***Cognitive Level:*** Analysis; ***Client Need/Subneed:*** Physiological Integrity/Reduction of Risk Potential/System Specific Assessments

66. CORRECT ANSWER: 3. Answer 1 is incorrect because the nurse should speak in a normal tone of voice rather than a whisper. Children may interpret whispers as an indication that death should not be talked about. **Answer 2** is incorrect because the nurse should always interact with the child, even if the child is comatose or not verbally responsive, because children may be able to hear the nurse even if they do not respond. **Answer 3 is correct because many children use denial as a defense mechanism in the face of their own death. A nurse should *not* take away the child's defenses; rather, the nurse should be honest when answering the child's questions while allowing the child to accept death when ready. Answer 4** is incorrect because a school-age child should be able to report pain to the nurse. The parents may assist in the pain assessment since they know their child best; deferring to the parents denies the child a voice in the given treatment.

■ TEST-TAKING TIP: ***Look for the answer that supports a trusting nurse-client relationship. Answers 1, 2, and 4 describe interventions that prevent interaction with the child. Answer 3 allows the child to express feelings, building trust between the nurse and child.***

Content Area: Child Health, End-of-Life Care; ***Integrated Process:*** Nursing Process, Planning; ***Cognitive Level:*** Application; ***Client Need/Subneed:*** Psychosocial Integrity/End of Life Care

67. CORRECT ANSWER: 2. Answer 1 is incorrect because mixing medications with food may not improve the taste. Also, once the medication is mixed with food, there is typically more volume for the child to swallow since the child must take all the food to get all the medication. **Answer 2 is correct because the child should be given a choice of fluid chaser to wash the unpleasant taste out of the mouth following ingestion of the medication. The child is not given a choice of whether or not to take the medication. Answer 3** is incorrect because it is best for the nurse to elicit the cooperation of the child rather than forcing the medication into the mouth. **Answer 4** is incorrect because offering the child a toy does not guarantee that the child will agree to take the medication. Additionally, if the nurse gives a toy this time, the child will expect a similar reward with each dose of this medication.

■ TEST-TAKING TIP: ***Toddlers need to be provided with real, not false, choices. A nurse should calmly tell the child that the medication must be swallowed, then work with the child to find the least offensive way to accomplish this task.***

Content Area: Child Health, Medication Administration; ***Integrated Process:*** Nursing Process, Implementation; ***Cognitive Level:*** Comprehension; ***Client Need/Subneed:*** Physiological Integrity/Pharmacological and Parenteral Therapies/Medication Administration

68. CORRECT ANSWER: 3. Answer 1 is incorrect because this *is* proper positioning for the child receiving an optic medication. **Answer 2** is incorrect because the child *should be* instructed to close the eyelids while moving the eyes around so as to better distribute the medication. **Answer 3 is correct because eyedrops should be administered when they are least likely to interfere with an activity that requires effective vision. A nurse should intervene and advise the student that the child should eat lunch first. Answer 4** is incorrect because this *is* proper technique for the administration of eyedrops.

■ TEST-TAKING TIP: ***Look for the action that is* not *okay and therefore needs an intervention.***

Content Area: Child Health, Medication Administration; ***Integrated Process:*** Nursing Process, Evaluation; ***Cognitive Level:*** Application; ***Client Need/Subneed:*** Physiological Integrity/Pharmacological and Parenteral Therapies/Medication Administration

69. CORRECT ANSWERS: 2, 3, 5, 4. Answer 1 is incorrect because the child's respiratory assessment did *not* reveal a need for supplemental oxygen at this time. Routine use of oxygen is *not* recommended for a child with sickle cell disease because it will *not* reverse sickling or treat pain. **Answer 2 is correct because the nurse must *first* obtain an accurate weight before determining safe dosages of ordered medications and IV fluids. Additionally, the child's weight will be used to determine whether I&O are meeting appropriate targets. Answer 3 is correct because IV fluid administration is a *priority* treatment for the child in sickle cell crisis. After the child's weight is obtained, the nurse may safely administer the ordered IV fluids, being sure to calculate that the amount and rate is appropriate. Answer 4 is correct because the nurse should monitor intake and output for adequacy since hydration status is an important part of this child's assessment. I&O monitoring should take place *after* the child has been weighed and is *started* on IV fluids and medications. Answer 5 is correct because the child needs effective pain management, yet this is a lower priority than fluid administration. A teenager with a chronic painful condition is an excellent candidate for PCA (patient-controlled analgesia). Answer 6** is incorrect because *warm* compresses, not *cool* compresses, should be used to facilitate circulation in affected extremities.

■ TEST-TAKING TIP: ***When placing options in sequential order, consider whether assessments should be done before or after interventions. In child health, IV fluids and medications are based upon the child's weight; therefore, the weight should be assessed before these treatments can be safely administered.***

Content Area: Child Health, Hematology; ***Integrated Process:*** Nursing Process, Analysis; ***Cognitive Level:*** Analysis; ***Client Need/Subneed:*** Physiological Integrity/Reduction of Risk Potential/Potential for Alterations in Body Systems

70. CORRECT ANSWER: 1. Answer 1 is correct because, although permethrin is an over-the-counter medication for the treatment of pediculosis (head lice), repeated doses may become toxic over time; parents should be cautioned against such treatments. A nurse should stress that nonpharmacologic treatments such as nit removal may be more effective and pose less risk to the child. **Answer 2** is incorrect because this *is* the recommended method for killing nits or lice contained in linen and clothing. **Answer 3** is incorrect because this *is* recommended as a way to prevent nits or lice from being transferred to the parents during treatment of pediculosis. **Answer 4** is incorrect because this *is* recommended treatment for children with pediculosis. This treatment should be continued until no nits remain.

■ TEST-TAKING TIP: *Note the words in the stem "caution against," and choose the option that is different from the others (e.g., pharmacologic treatments, which pose a greater risk to the child than nonpharmacologic treatments).*

Content Area: Child Health, Infectious Disease; ***Integrated Process:*** Nursing Process, Planning; ***Cognitive Level:*** Application; ***Client Need/Subneed:*** Safe and Effective Care Environment/Safety and Infection Control/Standard/Transmission-based/Other Precautions

71. CORRECT ANSWER: 4. **Answer 1** is incorrect because, although avoiding crowds during winter months may decrease the incidence of respiratory infections in general, this is not the best way to prevent otitis media. **Answer 2** is incorrect because feeding the infant in a supine rather than upright position *increases* the risk of otitis media since the bottle's contents may leak into the pharyngeal cavity, creating a medium for bacterial growth. **Answer 3** is incorrect because *pneumococcal* vaccine, not the DTaP (diphtheria, tetanus, and acellular pertussis) may prevent otitis media. The pneumococcal vaccine inoculates against infection by *Streptococcus pneumoniae,* one of the common causes of ear infection in children. Answer 4 is correct because infants who are exclusively breastfed have a decreased incidence of otitis media (ear infections) compared to those who are formula-fed.

■ TEST-TAKING TIP: *Select the response that is* most specific *for prevention of otitis media, not respiratory infections in general.*

Content Area: Child Health, Infectious Disease; ***Integrated Process:*** Nursing Process, Implementation; ***Cognitive Level:*** Application; ***Client Need/Subneed:*** Safe and Effective Care Environment/Safety and Infection Control/Standard/Transmission-based/Other Precautions

72. CORRECT ANSWERS: 1, 3, 4. Answer 1 is correct because the nurse should assess the child thoroughly to determine whether the child's neurological status has changed since the last assessment. **Answer 2** is incorrect because this child should be placed with the head of bed *elevated* to prevent increase of ICP. Answer 3 is correct because nausea and vomiting are common following neurosurgery. The antiemetic should be administered because vomiting needs to be prevented since it increases intracranial pressure (ICP). Answer 4 is correct because determining the child's pain level should be part of the physical assessment. It is expected that the child may have pain from this surgery. **Answer 5** is incorrect because increasing the child's IV rate could lead to increased ICP and should not be done without an order.

■ TEST-TAKING TIP: *The priority of care for children recovering from neurosurgery is monitoring and preventing increased ICP. Select the actions that will not increase ICP.*

Content Area: Child Health, Neurological; ***Integrated Process:*** Nursing Process, Implementation; ***Cognitive Level:*** Analysis; ***Client Need/Subneed:*** Physiological Integrity/Reduction of Risk Potential/Potential for Alterations in Body Systems

73. CORRECT ANSWER: 3. **Answer 1** is incorrect since wearing a mask will not guarantee that the nurse, if infected, will not transmit the virus to hospitalized children. **Answer 2** is incorrect since all pediatric clients could be at risk if the oncoming nurse is not immune to varicella. The charge nurse cannot assume that the nurse is immune. Answer 3 is correct because the nurse has been exposed to someone with varicella (chickenpox). The charge nurse must first determine the nurse's varicella immune status before permitting the nurse to provide care. **Answer 4** is incorrect since all pediatric clients could be at risk if the oncoming nurse is not immune to varicella. The charge nurse cannot assume that the nurse is immune.

■ TEST-TAKING TIP: *Choose the one answer that states "not be given an assignment." Varicella is easily transmitted among close contacts such as family members. Even though most adults have immunity to chickenpox, this can only be verified with a varicella titer.*

Content Area: Child Health, Infectious Disease; ***Integrated Process:*** Nursing Process, Implementation; ***Cognitive Level:*** Analysis; ***Client Need/Subneed:*** Safe and Effective Care Environment/Safety and Infection Control/Standard/Transmission-based/Other Precautions

74. CORRECT ANSWER: 3. **Answer 1** is incorrect because, although tachypnea does occur with respiratory distress, tachypnea *also* occurs during well states. **Answer 2** is incorrect because, although scattered rhonchi are indicative of respiratory infection, the child may have rhonchi and *not* experience respiratory distress. Answer 3 is correct because grunting respirations indicate that the infant is attempting to increase positive airway pressure to prevent airway collapse. **Answer 4** is incorrect because infants are abdominal breathers. This is an *expected* finding.

■ TEST-TAKING TIP: *Consider that grunting noises are usually heard when an individual exerts extra effort at something. Grunting during respiration is an indication that the child is working hard to breathe.*

Content Area: Child Health, Respiratory; ***Integrated Process:*** Nursing Process, Assessment; ***Cognitive Level:*** Analysis; ***Client***

Need/Subneed: Physiological Integrity/Reduction of Risk Potential/System Specific Assessments

75. CORRECT ANSWER: 1. Answer 1 is correct because the child is displaying symptoms of respiratory distress due to tracheostomy occlusion since the nurse is unable to pass the catheter through the tracheostomy tube. This is an emergency requiring the nurse to promptly change the tracheostomy tube. **Answer 2** is incorrect because this action puts the child at risk by *delaying* insertion of a new tracheostomy tube. **Answer 3** is incorrect because this action puts the child at risk by *delaying* insertion of a new tracheostomy tube. **Answer 4** is incorrect because this action puts the child at risk by *delaying* insertion of a new tracheostomy tube.

■ **TEST-TAKING TIP:** *If there is enough evidence in the stem of a question that a client is experiencing a* respiratory emergency, *the best answer is to provide necessary action to resolve the emergency rather than taking time to gather additional assessment data.*

Content Area: Child Health, Respiratory; ***Integrated Process:*** Nursing Process, Implementation; ***Cognitive Level:*** Analysis; ***Client Need/Subneed:*** Physiological Integrity/Physiological Adaptation/Medical Emergencies

76. CORRECT ANSWER: 2. **Answer 1** is incorrect because the nurse is taking action before first assessing the child. **Answer 2 is correct because the nurse should *first assess* the child's physical condition before assuming that the monitor is accurate. The monitor could be displaying an artifact as a result of the child's activity.** **Answer 3** is incorrect because the nurse is taking action before first assessing the child. **Answer 4** is incorrect because the nurse is taking action before first assessing the child.

■ **TEST-TAKING TIP:** *In this question the priority is assessment* before *action.*

Content Area: Child Health, Cardiovascular; ***Integrated Process:*** Nursing Process, Implementation; ***Cognitive Level:*** Application; ***Client Need/Subneed:*** Physiological Integrity/Reduction of Risk Potential/Potential for Alterations in Body Systems

77. CORRECT ANSWER: 3. **Answer 1** is incorrect since these behaviors would be expected in an *infant,* not a preschooler. **Answer 2** is incorrect since these behaviors would be expected in a *toddler,* not a preschooler. **Answer 3 is correct since preschoolers have great concerns over body mutilation and may demonstrate somatic symptoms as a response to the stress of hospitalization.** **Answer 4** is incorrect since these behaviors would be expected in a *school-age* child or adolescent, not a preschooler.

■ **TEST-TAKING TIP:** *Focus on the* age *of the child. Preschoolers are vulnerable to threats of* bodily *harm. Look for the best answer that describes this fear.*

Content Area: Child Health, Hospitalization; ***Integrated Process:*** Nursing Process, Assessment; ***Cognitive Level:*** Application; ***Client Need/Subneed:*** Health Promotion and Maintenance/Developmental Stages and Transitions

78. CORRECT ANSWERS: 1, 3, 4, 6. Answer 1 is correct because children with beta-thalassemia are at increased risk for infection due to the impaired oxygen-carrying capacity of their blood. **Answer 2** is incorrect because elimination is *not* a problem with beta-thalassemia. **Answer 3 is correct because these children are at risk for injury from an increased destruction of red blood cells. As red blood cells die, iron is released with deposits in the liver and spleen, enlarging these organs and impairing their function while also causing vomiting from abdominal pressure. Answer 4 is correct because these children may experience bone deformities, growth retardation, and delayed maturation of the sexual organs. These symptoms (e.g., broad forehead, short stature, immature appearance) may be troubling for an adolescent, whose main concern is to fit in with the peer group.** **Answer 5** is incorrect because these children do *not* experience chronic pain. **Answer 6 is correct because chronic hypoxia results from the production of abnormal red blood cells. If the body does not have sufficient red blood cell production, oxygen is not supplied to the tissues adequately, leading to activity intolerance and fatigue.**

■ **TEST-TAKING TIP:** *Risk for infection (Answer 1) and injury (Answer 3) and circulation (Answer 6) are high priorities on Maslow's hierarchy of needs–followed by self-esteem related to body image (Answer 4).*

Content Area: Child Health, Hematology; ***Integrated Process:*** Nursing Process, Analysis; ***Cognitive Level:*** Analysis; ***Client Need/Subneed:*** Physiological Integrity/Physiological Adaptation/Hemodynamics

79. CORRECT ANSWER: 3. **Answer 1** is incorrect because the child is too young to provide a numeric pain rating. **Answer 2** is incorrect because vital signs are transient and should not be used to verify pain ratings. A nurse should assume that a child with multiple fractures is telling the truth about pain. **Answer 3 is correct because the FACES pain rating scale can be used with children as young as 3 years of age, and pain should be investigated with every nursing assessment.** **Answer 4** is incorrect because young children have minimal language skills and do not understand the difference between descriptive qualities such as dull and sharp.

■ **TEST-TAKING TIP:** *Recall that the FACES pain scale uses drawings of smiling and frowning faces to elicit children's pain ratings. Simple assessment tools are best suited for young children, while more descriptive and finite tools are better suited for children in later stages of cognitive development.*

Content Area: Child Health, Pain; ***Integrated Process:*** Nursing Process, Assessment; ***Cognitive Level:*** Comprehension; ***Client Need/Subneed:*** Health Promotion and Maintenance/Developmental Stages and Transitions

80. CORRECT ANSWERS: 3, 1, 5. Answer 1 is correct because, once the tube is inserted, placement must be verified by both auscultation and aspiration of gastric contents. **Answer 2** is incorrect since feeding the infant prior to, during, or immediately after the procedure may cause vomiting and would contradict the gavage feeding order. **Answer 3 is correct because the child should first be placed on the back with the chest elevated prior to NG tube placement, to prevent aspiration if the child gags during the procedure.** **Answer 4** is incorrect because 10 mL of air is *too much.* No more than 5 mL should be used in young children because the extra air can cause discomfort and lead to abdominal distention. **Answer 5 is correct because taping the tube to the cheek after it has been inserted prevents the child from being able to get fingers around the tube and pull it out.** **Answer 6** is incorrect because the tube should be measured *first* from the *tip of the nose,* extended to the earlobe, and then extended to the area past the xiphoid process. This measurement technique provides the best estimation of the length of tube necessary for stomach placement.

■ TEST-TAKING TIP: ***Note that the nursing tasks related to NG tube insertion are similar for adults and children–the differences pertain to tube sizes and volume of air/fluid.***

Content Area: Child Health, Gastrointestinal; ***Integrated Process:*** Nursing Process, Implementation; ***Cognitive Level:*** Application; ***Client Need/Subneed:*** Physiological Integrity/Basic Care and Comfort/Nutrition and Oral Hydration

81. CORRECT ANSWER: 3. **Answer 1** is incorrect because, although elevated body temperature is a concern during phototherapy treatment, the main complication of elevated temperature is dehydration, making fluid volume deficiency the highest priority. **Answer 2** is incorrect because a change in stooling patterns is expected as the body eliminates the bilirubin and is not of concern. **Answer 3 is correct because an infant with hyperbilirubinemia will have increased fluid needs due to increased insensible fluid losses from phototherapy treatment and increased fluid losses resulting from loose stools as the bilirubin is eliminated through the bowels. Failure to monitor and treat potential fluid volume imbalances can quickly put the infant at risk for dehydration.** **Answer 4** is incorrect because a diagnosis of interrupted family processes is not the highest priority for maintaining physiological integrity.

■ TEST-TAKING TIP: ***Consider which nursing diagnosis is the most life-threatening to identify the nurse's top priority. Infants are particularly susceptible to fluid imbalances and can become seriously compromised because of health conditions and treatments that affect fluid status.***

Content Area: Child Health, Hematological; ***Integrated Process:*** Nursing Process, Analysis; ***Cognitive Level:*** Analysis; ***Client Need/Subneed:*** Physiological Integrity/Reduction of Risk Potential/Potential for Alterations in Body Systems

82. CORRECT ANSWERS: 2, 3, 6. **Answer 1** is incorrect because the common cold is not a contraindication for receiving immunizations; it does not cause a decreased response to vaccines. Young children have many mild cold viruses each year; avoiding immunizations during these times may cause a child to miss many immunizations. **Answer 2 is correct because antibodies present in the transfused blood can inhibit the immune response to the immunization. Answer 3 is correct because corticosteroids can suppress the immune response, limiting the effectiveness of immunization.** **Answer 4** is incorrect because *mild* diarrheal illness is not a contraindication to immunization. However, moderate to *severe* diarrhea is a contraindication since the child's immune response may not be sufficient if immunizations are administered. **Answer 5** is incorrect because *penicillin* allergy is not a contraindication to immunization. Allergy to *streptomycin* is a contraindication for IPV (inactivated polio vaccine), and allergy to *neomycin* is a contraindication for MMR (measles, mumps, and rubella), IPV, and varicella. **Answer 6 is correct because a child with HIV should not receive immunizations that contain live viruses (e.g., varicella), as these may lead to infection.**

■ TEST-TAKING TIP: ***Mild to moderate illness is not a contraindication for immunization. The child must be significantly immunocompromised or at risk for diminished immune response for the nurse to withhold immunization.***

Content Area: Child Health, Infectious Disease; ***Integrated Process:*** Nursing Process, Analysis; ***Cognitive Level:*** Analysis; ***Client Need/Subneed:*** Health Promotion and Maintenance/Immunizations

83. CORRECT ANSWER: 3. **Answer 1** is incorrect since the student should recognize and alert the nurse to *more subtle ocular* changes, such as sluggishness or unequal reactions, prior to the time that the pupils become fixed and dilated and the child is in a potentially irreversible state. **Answer 2** is incorrect because the child should be straight, but with the head of bed slightly *elevated.* **Answer 3 is correct because this statement is evidence that the student understands that alterations in any of these vital signs could be an indication of worsening condition and should be promptly noted.** **Answer 4** is incorrect because sleeping is a *normal* behavior for children, especially if they have been examined frequently throughout the day. The student should assess the child frequently, waking the child as necessary *without assuming* that a sleeping child warrants a call to the practitioner.

■ TEST-TAKING TIP: ***Think: vital signs! Nurses should monitor clients with head injury for changes in vital signs because these may indicate problems with neurological functioning.***

Content Area: Child Health, Neurological; ***Integrated Process:*** Nursing Process, Evaluation; ***Cognitive Level:*** Analysis; ***Client Need/Subneed:*** Physiological Integrity/Reduction of Risk Potential/System Specific Assessments

84. CORRECT ANSWER: 2. **Answer 1** is incorrect because this is not the optimal time for growth hormone injections. **Answer 2 is correct because the child will be receiving growth hormone injections and these should be timed to simulate the body's normal growth hormone peak that occurs within the first 2 hours of sleep.** **Answer 3** is incorrect because this is not the optimal time for growth hormone injections. **Answer 4** is incorrect because allowing the child to choose the injection time may not meet the goal of bedtime injections and may result in varying times each day.

■ TEST-TAKING TIP: *Eliminate the two answers that relate to eating times and eliminate "anytime." The administration of hormone replacement therapy should always attempt to mimic the body's normal secretory patterns (2 hours of sleep).*

Content Area: Child Health, Endocrine; *Integrated Process:* Nursing Process, Implementation; *Cognitive Level:* Application; *Client Need/Subneed:* Physiological Integrity/Pharmacological and Parenteral Therapies/Medication Administration

85. CORRECT ANSWER: 2. **Answer 1** is incorrect because insulin is *not* part of the treatment plan for a child with CAH. **Answer 2 is correct since the child with congenital adrenal hyperplasia (CAH) is given cortisone to stop the increased production of adrenocorticotropic hormone (ACTH), thereby inhibiting adrenocorticoid secretion and virilization of girls/early genital development in boys.** **Answer 3** is incorrect because growth hormone is used to treat hypopituitarism, *not* CAH. **Answer 4** is incorrect because thyroid hormone is used to treat *hypothyroidism.*

■ TEST-TAKING TIP: *The adrenal glands synthesize corticosteroids. Only one answer option is a corticosteroid–cortisone.*

Content Area: Child Health, Endocrine; *Integrated Process:* Nursing Process, Planning; *Cognitive Level:* Application; *Client Need/Subneed:* Physiological Integrity/Pharmacological and Parenteral Therapies/Expected Effects/Outcomes

86. CORRECT ANSWER: 4. **Answer 1** is incorrect because simply raising the EVD to the proper level does not assess if the child is currently experiencing symptoms from improper EVD positioning. **Answer 2** is incorrect because the EVD should not remain "as is" at a level below the ventricles. **Answer 3** is incorrect because elevating the head of the bed will exacerbate the cerebrospinal fluid (CSF) drainage, since the EVD will become even lower than the level of the ventricles. **Answer 4 is correct because the external ventricular drain (EVD) should be at the level of the ventricles, or at the child's ear level. When the EVD is too low, CSF can drain quickly and lead to neurologic complications. A nurse should prevent the CSF from draining any further and assess the child.**

■ TEST-TAKING TIP: *Since tubes and drains work by pressure, the lower the drain, the less pressure required to induce drainage.*

Content Area: Child Health, Neurological; *Integrated Process:* Nursing Process, Implementation; *Cognitive Level:* Application; *Client Need/Subneed:* Physiological Integrity/Reduction of Risk Potential/Potential for Alterations in Body Systems

87. CORRECT ANSWERS: 1, 2, 3, 4, 5. **Answer 1 is correct because this is a developmental characteristic of the school-age child. The teaching plan should include activities that allow the children to succeed, such as games with a drug-free focus. Answer 2 is correct because this is a developmental characteristic of the school-age child. The teaching plan should provide for rewards (e.g., giving children pencils with fun slogans in exchange for signing a no-drug pledge form). Answer 3 is correct because this is a developmental characteristic of the school-age child. The teaching plan should include basic steps for avoiding substance abuse, such as ways to refuse substances when offered by peers. Answer 4 is correct because this is a developmental characteristic of the school-age child. The teaching plan should remind children that the majority of their peers do not abuse illicit substances. Answer 5 is correct because this is a developmental characteristic of the school-age child. The teaching plan should include discussions regarding physical and emotional consequences of substance abuse in boys and girls.**

■ TEST-TAKING TIP: Every *answer in a "select all that apply" question may be correct. Select all of the answers if they are all applicable.*

Content Area: Child Health, Growth and Development; *Integrated Process:* Nursing Process, Planning; *Cognitive Level:* Application; *Client Need/Subneed:* Health Promotion and Maintenance/Developmental Stages and Transitions

88. CORRECT ANSWER: 2. **Answer 1** is incorrect because, although the Denver II is not an IQ test, it does provide information regarding the child's developmental level in the areas of language, personal-social, fine motor-adaptive, and gross motor. **Answer 2 is correct because a "suspect" Denver II should be repeated in 1 to 2 weeks to rule out factors such as fatigue or illness that may influence the child's performance. The parent is also provided some skill-building activities to enjoy with the child to encourage development.** **Answer 3** is incorrect because the nurse should not refer the child to the physician until a second Denver II is suspect. In addition, the nurse is able to make necessary referrals to developmental specialists without first notifying the physician. **Answer 4** is incorrect because this is not accurate and provides false hope in the event the child does have developmental delay.

■ TEST-TAKING TIP: *When parents express concern regarding their child's health or development, the nurse should discuss the next step in plan of care, while also providing the parents with tools* they *can use now.*

Content Area: Child Health, Growth and Development; *Integrated Process:* Nursing Process, Implementation; *Cognitive Level:* Application; *Client Need/Subneed:* Health Promotion and Maintenance/Developmental Stages and Transitions

89. CORRECT ANSWERS: 1, 3, 4, 5, 7. Answer 1 is correct because a VSD is one of the components of tetralogy of Fallot. **Answer 2** is incorrect because an ASD is *not* a component of tetralogy of Fallot. Answer 3 is correct because an overriding aorta is one of the components of tetralogy of Fallot. Answer 4 is correct because pulmonic stenosis is one of the components of tetralogy of Fallot. Answer 5 is correct because right ventricular hypertrophy is one of the components of tetralogy of Fallot. **Answer 6** is incorrect because a PDA is *not* a component of tetralogy of Fallot. Answer 7 is correct because the blood flows from left to right in a child with tetralogy of Fallot through the VSD. **Answer 8** is incorrect because aortic stenosis is *not* a component of tetralogy of Fallot.

■ TEST-TAKING TIP: *The "tetra" in "tetralogy" signifies the number 4. Recall that there are* four defects *in the heart of a child with tetralogy of Fallot: VSD, pulmonic stenosis, an overriding aorta, and right ventricular hypertrophy.*

Content Area: Child Health, Cardiovascular; *Integrated Process:* Nursing Process, Assessment; *Cognitive Level:* Application; *Client Need/Subneed:* Physiological Integrity/Physiological Adaptation/Alterations in Body Systems

90. CORRECT ANSWER: 2. **Answer 1** is incorrect since croup is caused by a virus and is *not* treatable with antibiotics. Answer 2 is correct because the humidity of the shower will create an environment that is soothing to the child's airway. Cool-mist humidifiers are also recommended for the child's room to relieve the symptoms of spasmodic croup. Any of the croup syndromes may be treated with humidified air. In the case of acute spasmodic laryngitis, both warm mist and cool mist are acceptable interventions since the problem is airway spasm rather than severe inflammation. **Answer 3** is incorrect because paroxysmal attacks may last for some time; the child is best treated with supportive care *at home,* and the presence of attacks is not an indication for further hospitalization. **Answer 4** is incorrect because this intervention is *not* likely to prevent laryngeal spasms and may cause the child to be more anxious, which could induce an attack.

■ TEST-TAKING TIP: *Note that the word "spasmodic" in the stem of the question is also in the correct answer ("spasms").*

Content Area: Child Health, Respiratory; *Integrated Process:* Nursing Process, Implementation; *Cognitive Level:* Application; *Client Need/Subneed:* Physiological Integrity/Reduction of Risk Potential/Potential for Alterations in Body Systems

91. CORRECT ANSWER: 4. **Answer 1** is incorrect because a hypoallergenic diet *may* alleviate the severity of eczema symptoms. **Answer 2** is incorrect because hydrocortisone creams *are* recommended in the treatment of eczema. **Answer 3** is incorrect because adding cornstarch to bathwater *may relieve* itching and promote the healing of the lesions. Answer 4 is correct because the child should *not* receive immunizations during an acute exacerbation of eczema (atopic dermatitis), as this may lead to complications such as allergic reaction. The child with atopic dermatitis is experiencing an inflammatory response. Care should be directed at relieving inflammation and avoiding exposure to substances thought to trigger an immune response.

■ TEST-TAKING TIP: *Note that the question calls for what* not *to do.*

Content Area: Child Health, Integumentary; *Integrated Process:* Nursing Process, Implementation; *Cognitive Level:* Application; *Client Need/Subneed:* Physiological Integrity/Reduction of Risk Potential/Potential for Alterations in Body Systems

92. CORRECT ANSWER: 2. **Answer 1** is incorrect because restraints *are* indicated in the care of a child who has had a cleft lip repair, to prevent the child from poking or pulling at the suture line. Answer 2 is correct because the infant should not be fed using a regular bottle. Postoperative feedings for the child with a cleft lip should be administered through special feeders to minimize trauma to the suture line. Since a cleft lip repair involves only the child's upper lip, the nurse should perform interventions that reduce the risk of damage or infection at the operative location. **Answer 3** is incorrect because this *is* the correct position for a child following cleft lip repair, to promote drainage of mucus and decrease risk of aspiration. **Answer 4** is incorrect because the child *should* be given pain medication on a schedule, to minimize pain-induced crying episodes that can put undue tension on the suture line.

■ TEST-TAKING TIP: *The question calls for an answer about what is* not *okay.*

Content Area: Child Health, Gastrointestinal; *Integrated Process:* Nursing Process, Implementation; *Cognitive Level:* Application; *Client Need/Subneed:* Safe and Effective Care Environment/Management of Care/Supervision

93. CORRECT ANSWER: 1. Answer 1 is correct because the child is demonstrating symptoms of severe hypoglycemia and the nurse must administer an emergency dose of glucagon to prevent the child from going into shock. **Answer 2** is incorrect because the nurse should *first* administer the emergency dose of glucagon, *then* contact emergency medical services (EMS). **Answer 3** is incorrect because the child is becoming unresponsive, and placing anything into the mouth would be contraindicated due to the risk of aspiration. **Answer 4** is incorrect because the child has sufficient symptoms of hypoglycemia that need *immediate* treatment.

■ TEST-TAKING TIP: *The key piece of information in the stem of the question is that the child is beginning to lose*

consciousness. A nurse must act quickly in this situation and assume that it is due to low blood sugar, because waiting to differentiate between hyper- and hypoglycemia could be life-threatening.
Content Area: Child Health, Endocrine; *Integrated Process:* Nursing Process, Implementation; *Cognitive Level:* Application; *Client Need/Subneed:* Physiological Integrity/ Physiological Adaptation/Alterations in Body Systems

94. CORRECT ANSWER: 4. **Answer 1** is incorrect because pale gray stools are associated with conditions related to insufficient bile output (e.g., cirrhosis). **Answer 2** is incorrect because currant-jelly stools are associated with a diagnosis of *intussusception.* **Answer 3** is incorrect because loose, yellow stools are *normal* for a breastfed newborn. **Answer 4 is correct because the child with Hirschsprung's disease will have infrequent stools that appear thin and ribbon-like.**
■ TEST-TAKING TIP: *Since Hirschsprung's disease results in obstruction of the lower GI tract, the expected stooling pattern will reflect stools that have become compressed by the obstruction.*
Content Area: Child Health, Gastrointestinal; *Integrated Process:* Nursing Process, Assessment; *Cognitive Level:* Comprehension; *Client Need/Subneed:* Physiological Integrity/Basic Care and Comfort/Elimination

95. CORRECT ANSWER: 2. **Answer 1** is incorrect because, although the nurse should assess the child's lungs for possible aspiration, the first action is to clear the airway. **Answer 2 is correct because the nurse's first action should be to clear the child's airway of formula. Since this is the infant's first feeding, the nurse should suspect a tracheoesophageal fistula (TEF) and should not attempt to feed the child again.** **Answer 3** is incorrect because an x-ray may be obtained *after* the child's airway is stabilized. **Answer 4** is incorrect because the nurse should first stabilize the airway and assess the child before contacting the physician.
■ TEST-TAKING TIP: *It is helpful to remember the 3 C's of TEF: coughing, choking, and cyanosis. A nurse's top priority should be the airway of an infant with these symptoms.*
Content Area: Child Health, Respiratory; *Integrated Process:* Nursing Process, Implementation; *Cognitive Level:* Application; *Client Need/Subneed:* Physiological Integrity/ Reduction of Risk Potential/Potential for Alterations in Body Systems

96. CORRECT ANSWER: 3. **Answer 1** is incorrect because this is *too early* for completion of the surgical repair. Delaying surgery for several months to a year allows time to treat the infant with male hormones to increase the amount of penile tissue prior to surgery. Additionally, surgery on newborns carries an increased risk of complications and should be avoided unless medically necessary. **Answer 2** is incorrect because the surgical repair is completed *much earlier.* **Answer 3 is correct because the surgical repair of hypospadias generally begins within the first few months of life and continues in stages, finishing between 6 and 18 months of age, before the child begins toilet training.** **Answer 4** is incorrect because the surgical repair is completed *much earlier.*
■ TEST-TAKING TIP: *Since toilet training and the development of body image begins in toddlerhood, hypospadias repair is best completed prior to this state of development.*
Content Area: Child Health, Genitourinary; *Integrated Process:* Nursing Process, Implementation; *Cognitive Level:* Comprehension; *Client Need/Subneed:* Physiological Integrity/Reduction of Risk Potential/Potential for Alterations in Body Systems

97. CORRECT ANSWER: 4. **Answer 1** is incorrect because, although children with JIA frequently have sleep disturbances, this is not the top priority. **Answer 2** is incorrect because, although children with JIA should participate in regular exercise, this is not the top priority. **Answer 3** is incorrect because the child should be informed of support groups, but this is not the top priority. **Answer 4 is correct because adolescents with JIA are frequently prescribed medications that are taxing to the liver, including NSAIDs, such as naproxen sodium, and SAARDs (slower-acting antirheumatic drugs), such as methotrexate. Alcohol abuse could cause serious complications when taking these medications. A nurse's top priority takes into consideration that the adolescent is facing increasing peer pressure to drink alcohol, which could lead to hepatotoxicity.**
■ TEST-TAKING TIP: *The best answer is what* not *to do (i.e., what to avoid).*
Content Area: Child Health, Musculoskeletal; *Integrated Process:* Nursing Process, Implementation; *Cognitive Level:* Analysis; *Client Need/Subneed:* Physiological Integrity/ Reduction of Risk Potential/Potential for Alterations in Body Systems

98. CORRECT ANSWER: 2. **Answer 1** is incorrect because the RN *could* delegate this task to the LVN/LPN. **Answer 2 is correct because the RN should change the wound dressing and assess the condition of the decubitus.** **Answer 3** is incorrect because the RN *could* delegate this task to the LVN/LPN. **Answer 4** is incorrect because the RN *could* delegate this task to the LVN/LPN.
■ TEST-TAKING TIP: *When the task involves* **assessment** *and* **analysis** *of assessment findings, the RN should not delegate it to the LVN/LPN.*
Content Area: Child Health, Hospitalization; *Integrated Process:* Nursing Process, Implementation; *Cognitive Level:* Application; *Client Need/Subneed:* Safe and Effective Care Environment/Management of Care/Delegation

99. CORRECT ANSWERS: 3, 1, 5, 4. **Answer 1 is correct because the preschool child may feel more comfortable keeping underpants on during the assessment because a common fear of preschoolers is genital mutilation.** **Answer 2** is incorrect since it would be *unsafe* to leave a preschool child alone in an examination room to undress. This intervention would be appropriate for an *adolescent.* **Answer 3 is correct because the nurse should first ask the child if the parents should participate in the procedure. The child should be given options for parent participation, such as whether parents should be present, if the child would like help undressing, and if the child would prefer to sit on the parent's lap or sit alone on the examination table. Answer 4 is correct because, although the nurse proceeds in a head-to-toe direction, inspecting eyes, ears, and mouth is invasive and is best performed at the *end* of the assessment in order to not disrupt the rest of the examination. Answer 5 is correct because the nurse should proceed in a head-to-toe direction while keeping the most invasive assessments for the end.** **Answer 6** is incorrect because this technique is appropriate for *infants,* not preschoolers.

■ **TEST-TAKING TIP:** ***Because preschool children's central task is initiative vs. guilt, they benefit from interventions that offer independence in decision making.***

Content Area: Child Health, Growth and Development; ***Integrated Process:*** Nursing Process, Implementation; ***Cognitive Level:*** Application; ***Client Need/Subneed:*** Health Promotion and Maintenance/Developmental Stages and Transitions

100. CORRECT ANSWER: 1. **Answer 1 is correct because the nurse's priority is to alleviate airway inflammation, and administration of a beta agonist such as albuterol is recommended.** **Answer 2** is incorrect because the loading dose of Solu-Medrol (methylprednisolone) should be administered *after* starting albuterol treatments. **Answer 3** is incorrect because IV fluids can be given *after* starting albuterol treatments. **Answer 4** is incorrect because a chest x-ray can be obtained *after* starting albuterol treatments.

■ **TEST-TAKING TIP:** ***Airway is the first priority, especially in children with asthma. Begin treatments that have quick effects on oxygen exchange, then administer long-acting medications and gather assessment data.***

Content Area: Child Health, Respiratory; ***Integrated Process:*** Nursing Process, Implementation; ***Cognitive Level:*** Analysis; ***Client Need/Subneed:*** Physiological Integrity/Reduction of Risk Potential/Potential for Alterations in Body Systems

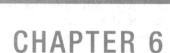

CHAPTER 6

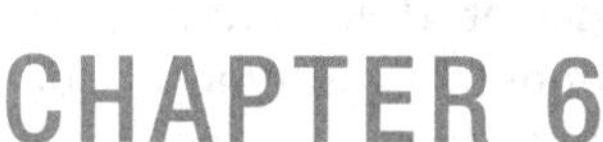

Physiological Integrity

Nursing Care of the Adult Client

Robyn Marchal Nelson

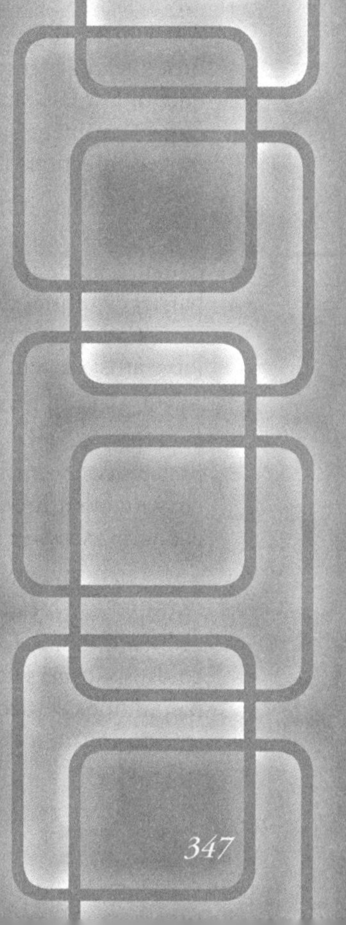

ASSESSMENT OF THE ADULT CLIENT

Assessment is the process of gathering a comprehensive database about the client's present, past, and potential health problems, as well as a description of the client as a whole in his or her environment. It includes a comprehensive nursing history, a physical examination, and laboratory/x-ray data, and it concludes with the formulation of nursing diagnoses.

The Health Insurance Portability and Accountability Act of 1996 (HIPAA) strengthened the privacy protections for consumers. Communications are confidential, and the client needs to give permission for other family members to remain in the room—particularly when asking sensitive questions on pregnancies, abortions, drug use, or multiple sex partners (see **Chapter 3, pp. 81–82**).

Subjective Data

Nursing History

The nursing history obtains data for planning and implementing nursing actions.

I. GENERAL HEALTH INFORMATION: reason for admission; duration of present illness; previous hospitalization; history of illnesses; diagnostic procedures before admission; allergies—type and severity of reactions; medications taken at home—over-the-counter (OTC) and prescription medications, and alternative/complementary therapies.

II. INFORMATION RELATIVE TO GROWTH AND DEVELOPMENT: age; menarche—age at onset; heavy menses; dysmenorrhea; vaginal discharge; date of last Pap smear; pregnancies; abortions; miscarriages; last menstrual period; history of sexually transmitted infections (STIs).

III. INFORMATION RELATIVE TO PSYCHOSOCIAL FUNCTIONS: feelings (anger, denial, fear, anxiety, guilt, lifestyle changes); language barriers; cultural needs; family support; spiritual needs; religious preference; history of trauma/rape; job status; current stressors.

IV. INFORMATION RELATIVE TO NUTRITION: appetite—normal, changes; dietary habits; food preferences or intolerances; difficulty swallowing or chewing; dentures; use of caffeine/alcohol; weight changes; excessive thirst, hunger, sweating.

V. INFORMATION RELATIVE TO FLUID AND GAS TRANSPORT: difficulty breathing; shortness of breath; home O_2 use; history of cough/smoking; colds; sputum; swelling of extremities; chest pain; palpitations; varicosities; excessive bruising; blood transfusions; excessive bleeding.

VI. INFORMATION RELATIVE TO PROTECTIVE FUNCTIONS: skin problems—rash, itch; current treatment; unusual hair loss.

VII. INFORMATION RELATIVE TO COMFORT, REST, ACTIVITY, MOBILITY: usual activity (activities of daily living [ADLs]); present ability and restrictions; rest and sleep pattern; weakness; joint or muscle stiffness, pain, or swelling; occupation; interests.

VIII. INFORMATION RELATIVE TO ELIMINATION: bowel habits; changes—constipation, diarrhea; ostomy; emesis; nausea; voiding—retention, frequency, dysuria, incontinence.

IX. INFORMATION RELATIVE TO SENSORY/PERCEPTUAL FUNCTIONS: pain—verbal report, acute/chronic, treatment, quality, location, precipitating factors, duration; limitations in vision (glasses), hearing, touch, smell; orientation to person, place, time; confusion; headaches; fainting; dizziness; convulsions.

Objective Data

I. GENERAL —provides information on the client as a whole.

A. *Race, sex, apparent age* in relation to stated age.

B. *Nutritional status*—well hydrated and developed or obesity, cachexia—include weight.

C. *Apparent health status*—general good health or mild, moderate, severe debilitation.

D. *Posture and motor activity*—erect, symmetrical, balanced gait and muscle development, or ataxic, circumducted, scissor, or spastic gait; slumped or bent-over posture; scoliosis, lordosis, kyphosis; mild, moderate, or hyperactive motor responses.

E. *Behavior*—alert; oriented to person, time, place; hears and comprehends instructions, or tense, anxious, angry; uses abusive language; slightly or largely unresponsive; delusions, hallucinations.

F. *Odors*—noncontributory, or acetone, alcohol, fetid breath, incontinent of urine or feces.

II. PHYSICAL ASSESSMENT—requires knowledge of normal findings, organization, and keen senses (i.e., visual, auditory, touch, smell). For abnormal findings, refer to the *Assessment* section of each health problem discussed.

A. *Components*

1. *Inspection*—uses observations to detect deviations from normal.
2. *Auscultation*—used to perceive and interpret sounds arising from various organs, particularly heart, lungs, and bowel.
3. *Palpation*—used to assess for discomfort, temperature, pulsations, size, consistency, and texture.

4. *Percussion*—technique used to elicit vibrations produced by underlying organ structures; used less frequently in nursing practice.
   a. Flat—normal percussion; note over muscle or bone.
   b. Dull—normal percussion; note over organs such as liver.
   c. Resonance—normal percussion; note over lungs.
   d. Tympany—normal percussion; note over stomach or bowel.

B. *Approach*—head to toe
1. *General appearance*—well or poorly developed or nourished. Color (black, white, jaundiced, pale). In distress (acutely or chronically)?
2. *Vital signs*—blood pressure (which arm or both, orthostatic change); pulse (regular or irregular, orthostatic change); respirations (labored or unlabored, wheeze); temperature (axillary, rectal, temporal [forehead], tympanic membrane, or oral); weight; height **(Table 6.1).**
3. *Skin, hair, and nails*—pigmentation, scars, lesions, bruises, turgor. Describe or draw rashes.
   a. Skin color:
      (1) Red—fever, allergic reaction, carbon monoxide (CO) poisoning, burn.
      (2) White (pallor)—excessive blood loss, fright.
      (3) Blue (cyanosis)—hypoxemia, peripheral vasoconstriction, shock.
      (4) Mottled—cardiovascular embarrassment, shock.
   b. Skin temperature:
      (1) Hot, dry—excessive body heat (heatstroke).
      (2) Hot, wet—reaction to increased internal or external temperature.
      (3) Cool, dry—exposure to cold.
      (4) Cool, clammy—shock.
4. *Head*—scalp, skull (configuration), scars, tenderness, bruits.
5. *Neck*—suppleness. Trachea, larynx, thyroid, blood vessels (jugular veins, carotid arteries).
6. *Nodes*—any cervical, supraclavicular, axillary, epitrochlear, inguinal lymphadenopathy? If so, size of nodes (in centimeters), consistency (firm, rubbery, tender), mobile or fixed.
7. *Eyes:*
   a. **External eye.** Conjunctivae, sclerae, lids, cornea, pupils (including reflexes), visual fields, extraocular motions.
   b. **Fundus.** Disk, blood vessels, pigmentation.
8. *Ears*—shape of pinnae, external canal, discharge, tympanic membrane, acuity, air conduction versus bone conduction *(Rinne test)*, lateralization *(Weber test)*.
9. *Nose*—nares (symmetry), septum, mucosa, polyps, discharge, flaring.
10. *Mouth and throat*—lips, teeth (loose, dental hygiene, odor), tongue (size, papillation, position), buccal mucosa, palate, tonsils, oropharynx.
11. *Chest*
   a. **Inspection.** Contour, symmetry, expansion, retractions.
   b. **Palpation.** Expansion, rib tenderness, tactile fremitus.
   c. **Percussion.** Diaphragmatic excursion, dullness.
   d. **Auscultation.** Crackles, rubs, wheezes, egophony, pectoriloquy.
      (1) Use diaphragm or bell. Normal sounds over alveoli—*vesicular.* Large airway or abnormal sounds—*bronchial or bronchovesicular.* Adventitious sounds—*crackles or wheezes.*
      (2) *Crackles*—discontinuous noises heard on auscultation; caused by popping open of air spaces; usually associated with increased fluid in the lungs; formerly called *rales* and *rhonchi.*

ADULT

Table 6.1

Factors Affecting Vital Signs

Factor	Infection (Fever)	↓H&H (Hypovolemia)	↓BS (Insulin Shock)	↑BS/DKA (Hyperglycemia)	Narcotic (CNS Depression)	Anxiety (Fear)	Pain (Acute)	Acute MI	↑K+ (Hyperkalemia)	↓K+ (Hypokalemia)	Exercise
T	↑	↓	↓	↑	↓	Normal	Normal	Normal	Normal	Normal	↑
HR	↑	↑	Normal/↑	↑	↓	↑	↑	↓	↓	↑	↑
RR	↑	↑	Normal	↑	↓	↑	↑	↑	Shallow	Shallow	↑
BP	Normal	↓	Normal/↑	↓	↓	↑	↑	↓	Normal/↑	↓	↑

From Myers, Ehren: *RNotes.* FA Davis, Philadelphia, 2009.

(3) *Wheezes*—high-pitched, whistling sounds made by air flowing through narrowed airways.
(4) *Stridor*—harsh, high-pitched, heard during inspiration and expiration; life threatening.

12. *Breasts*—symmetry, retraction, lesions, nipples (inverted, everted), masses, tenderness, discharge.
13. *Heart:*
    a. **Inspection.** Point of maximal impulse (PMI), chest contour.
    b. **Palpation.** Point of maximal impulse (PMI), thrills, lifts, thrusts.
    c. **Auscultation.** Heart sounds, gallops, murmurs, rubs. Use diaphragm for high-pitched sounds of normal heart sounds (S_1 and S_2) and bell for abnormal sounds (S_3 and S_4).
14. *Abdomen:*
    a. **Inspection.** Scars (draw these), contour, masses, vein pattern.
    b. **Auscultation.** Bowel sounds, rubs, bruits. Use diaphragm. Auscultate *after* inspection and *before* palpation and percussion. Listen to each quadrant for at least 1 minute. If bowel sounds are present, they will be heard in lower right quadrant (area of ileocecal valve). *Hypoactivity*—every minute; *normal*—every 15 to 20 seconds; *hyperactivity*—about every 3 seconds.
    c. **Percussion**—organomegaly, hepatic dullness.
    d. **Palpation**—tenderness, masses, rigidity, liver, spleen, kidneys.
    e. **Hernia**—femoral, inguinal, ventral, umbilical.
15. *Genitalia:*
    a. **Male.** Penile lesions, discharge, scrotum, testes. Circumcised?
    b. **Female.** Labia, discharge, odor, Bartholin's and Skene's glands, vagina, cervix. Bimanual examination of internal genitalia.
16. *Rectum*—perianal lesions, sphincter tone, tenderness, masses, prostate, stool color, occult blood.
17. *Extremities*—pulses (symmetry, bruits, perfusion). Joints (mobility, deformity). Cyanosis, edema. Varicosities. Muscle mass. Grips equal.
18. *Back*—contour of spine, tenderness. Sacral edema.
19. *Neurological:*
    a. **Mental status.** Alertness, memory, judgment, mood.
    b. **Cranial nerves** (I–XII) **(Fig. 6.1).**
    c. **Cerebellum.** Gait, finger-nose, heel-shin, tremors.
    d. **Motor.** Muscle mass, strength; deep tendon reflexes. Pathological or primitive reflexes.
    e. **Sensory.** Touch, pain, vibration. Heat and cold as indicated.

III. ROUTINE LABORATORY STUDIES—see **Appendix A** for normal ranges.

A. *Hematology:*
1. Complete blood count—detects presence of anemia, infection, allergy, and leukemia.
2. Prothrombin time—increase may indicate liver disease or cancer.
3. Serology (Venereal Disease Research Laboratories [VDRL])—determines presence of syphilis; false-positive result may indicate collagen dysfunction.

B. *Urinalysis:*
1. Specific gravity—measures ability of kidney to concentrate urine. Fixed specific gravity indicates renal tubular dysfunction.
2. Protein—indicates glomerular dysfunction.
3. Albumin, white blood cells (WBCs), and pus—indicate renal infection.
4. Sugar and acetone—presence indicates metabolic disorder.

C. *Chest x-ray*—detects tuberculosis or other pulmonary dysfunctions, as well as changes in size or configuration of heart.

D. *Electrocardiogram (ECG or EKG)*—detects rhythm and conduction disturbances, presence of myocardial ischemia or necrosis, and ventricular hypertrophy.

E. *Blood chemistries*—detect deviation in electrolyte balance, presence of tissue damage, and adequacy of glomerular filtration.

IV. PREVENTIVE CARE

A. Checkup visits recommended every 1 to 3 years until age 65 and then yearly thereafter. **Table 6.2** lists suggested timelines.

B. Individuals with *special risk factors* may need more frequent and additional types of preventive care.
1. *Diabetes*—eye, foot examinations; urine, blood sugar tests.
2. *Drug abuse*—AIDS, tuberculosis (TB) tests; hepatitis immunization.
3. *Alcoholism*—influenza, pneumococcal immunizations; TB test.
4. *Overweight*—blood sugar test, triglycerides, blood pressure.
5. *Homeless, recent refugee or immigrant*—TB test.
6. *High-risk sexual behavior*—AIDS, syphilis, gonorrhea, chlamydia (every year for women who are sexually active), hepatitis tests.
7. *Pregnancy*—rubella blood test (prior to first pregnancy).
8. *Cancer*—colonoscopy, mammography, x-ray.

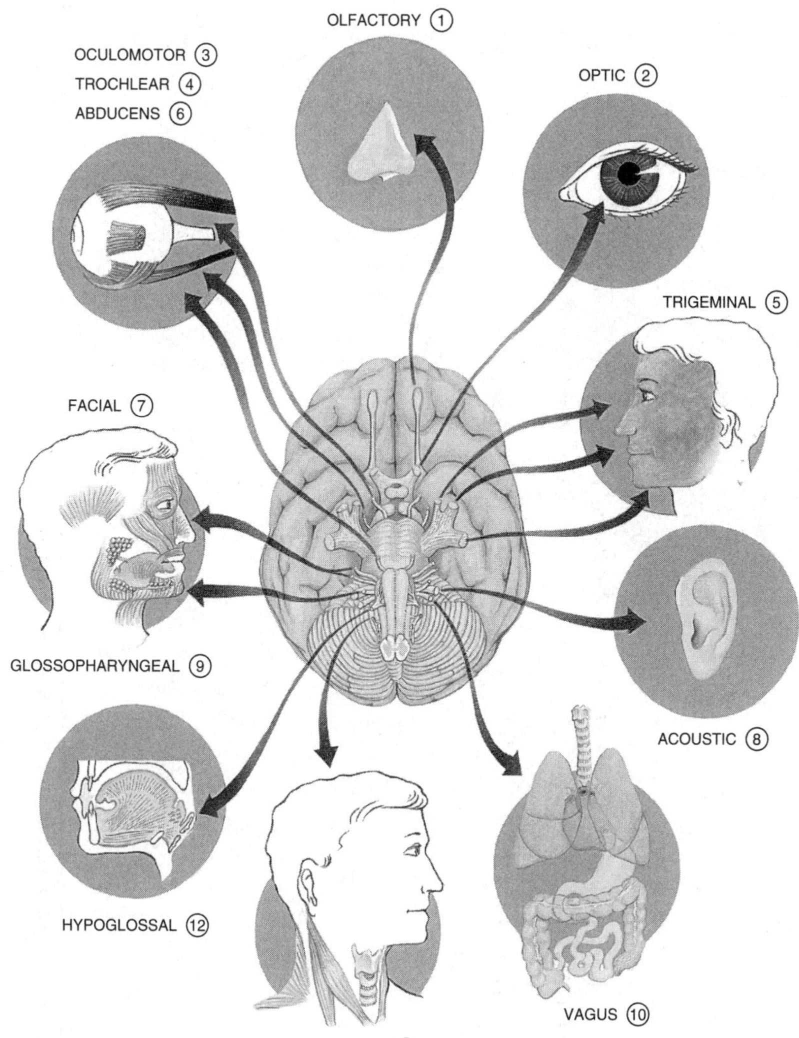

Figure 6.1 **Cranial nerves and their distributions.** (From Venes, D [ed]: *Taber's Cyclopedic Medical Dictionary,* ed 21. FA Davis, Philadelphia, 2009.)

C. *Adult immunizations*—prevention of disease and reduction in the severity of disease **(Table 6.3).**

Assessment is followed by *analysis* of data and formulation of a *nursing diagnosis.* Possible nursing diagnoses are given in the following sections.

GROWTH AND DEVELOPMENT

Young Adulthood (20 to 30 Years of Age)

I. STAGE OF DEVELOPMENT—PSYCHOSOCIAL STAGE: intimacy versus isolation.

II. PHYSICAL DEVELOPMENT (see also **Chapter 7**)

A. *At the height* of bodily vigor.

B. *Maximum* level of strength, muscular development, height, and cardiac and respiratory capacity; also, period of peak sexual capacity for men.

III. COGNITIVE DEVELOPMENT

A. Close to *peak* of intelligence, memory, and abstract thought.

B. Maximum ability to solve problems and learn new skills.

IV. SOCIALIZATION

A. Has a vision of the future and imagines various possibilities for self.

B. Defines and tests out what can be accomplished.

C. Seeks out a mentor to emulate as a guiding, though transitional, figure; the mentor is usually a mixture of parent, teacher, and friend who serves as a role model to support and facilitate the developing vision of self.

D. Grows from a beginning to a fuller understanding of own authority and autonomy.

E. Transfers an interest into an occupation or profession; crucial work choice may be made after one has knowledge, judgment, and self-understanding,

(text continues on page 355)

ADULT

Table 6.2

Preventive Care Timelines

	Years of Age												
	18	25	30	35	40	45	50	55	60	65	70	75	<
Tests													
Blood Pressure							Every 2 Years						
Height & Weight							Periodically						
Cholesterol					Men			Every 2–3 Years (Men & Women)					
Hearing												Periodically	
Mammography				Baseline					Yearly (Women)				
Pap Smear (Cervical Cancer)					Every 1–3 Years (Women)								
Sigmoidoscopy/Colonoscopy										Every 3–5 Years			
and/or										and/or			
Stool Occult Blood (FOBT)										Yearly			
Blood									At Least Every 3–4 Years				
Examinations													
Dental, Oral Health							Yearly						
Vision/Glaucoma							Every 2–4 Years				Every 1–2 Years		
Breast (by Doctor)			Every 1–3 Years (Women)						Every Year (Women)				
Exam for Cancer: thyroid, mouth, skin, ovaries, testicles (monthly between ages 19–40), lymph nodes, rectum (40+), prostate (men 50+)			Every 3 Years						Yearly				
Bone Density (Osteoporosis)								Every 2 Years				Yearly	
Health Guidance													
• Smoking, Alcohol & Drugs • Sexual Behavior, AIDS • Eating Disorders, Nutrition, Physical Activity, Weight Management • Violence & Guns, Injuries • Family Planning • Occupational Health • Folate (Women 12–45), Aspirin (Men 40+)							Periodically						

Upper age limits should be individualized for each person
- Recommended by most major authorities
- Recommended by some major authorities

Source: Office of Disease Prevention and Health Promotion, in cooperation with the agencies of the Public Health Service, U.S. Department of Health and Human Services.

Table 6.3

2011 Recommended Adult Immunization Schedule

Recommended adult immunization schedule, by vaccine and age group — United States, 2011

VACCINE ▼ / AGE GROUP ►	19–26 years	27–49 years	50–59 years	60–64 years	≥65 years
Influenza[1,*]	1 dose annually				
Tetanus, diphtheria, pertussis (Td/Tdap)[2,*]	Substitute 1-time dose of Tdap for Td booster; then boost with Td every 10 years				Td booster every 10 years
Varicella[3,*]	2 doses				
Human papillomavirus (HPV)[4,*]	3 doses (females)				
Zoster[5]				1 dose	
Measles, mumps, rubella (MMR)[6,*]	1 or 2 doses		1 dose		
Pneumococcal (polysaccharide)[7,8]	1 or 2 doses				1 dose
Meningococcal[9,*]	1 or more doses				
Hepatitis A[10,*]	2 doses				
Hepatitis B[11,*]	3 doses				

* Covered by the Vaccine Injury Compensation Program

(light shading) For all persons in this category who meet the age requirements and who lack evidence of immunity (e.g., lack documentation of vaccination or have no evidence of previous infection)

(dark shading) Recommended if some other risk factor is present (e.g., based on medical, occupational, lifestyle, or other indications)

(no shading) No recommendation

Vaccines that might be indicated for adults, based on medical and other indications — United States, 2011

VACCINE ▼ / INDICATION ►	Pregnancy	Immunocompromising conditions (excluding human immunodeficiency virus [HIV])[3,5,6,13]	HIV infection[3,6,12,13] CD4+ T lymphocyte count: <200 cells/µL	HIV infection CD4+ T lymphocyte count: ≥200 cells/µL	Diabetes, heart disease, chronic lung disease, chronic alcoholism	Asplenia[12] (including elective splenectomy) and persistent complement component deficiencies	Chronic liver disease	Kidney failure, end-stage renal disease, receipt of hemodialysis	Health-care personnel
Influenza[1,*]	1 dose TIV annually								1 dose TIV or LAIV annually
Tetanus, diphtheria, pertussis (Td/Tdap)[2,*]	Td	Substitute 1-time dose of Tdap for Td booster; then boost with Td every 10 years							
Varicella[3,*]	Contraindicated			2 doses					
Human papillomavirus (HPV)[4,*]		3 doses through age 26 years							
Zoster[5]	Contraindicated				1 dose				
Measles, mumps, rubella[6,*]	Contraindicated			1 or 2 doses					
Pneumococcal (polysaccharide)[7,8]		1 or 2 doses							
Meningococcal[9,*]	1 or more doses								
Hepatitis A[10,*]	2 doses								
Hepatitis B[11,*]					3 doses				

* Covered by the Vaccine Injury Compensation Program

(light shading) For all persons in this category who meet the age requirements and who lack evidence of immunity (e.g., lack documentation of vaccination or have no evidence of previous infection)

(dark shading) Recommended if some other risk factor is present (e.g., on the basis of medical, occupational, lifestyle, or other indications)

(no shading) No recommendation

NOTE: The above recommendations must be read along with the following footnotes.

1. Influenza vaccination

Annual vaccination against influenza is recommended for all persons aged 6 months and older, including all adults. Healthy, nonpregnant adults aged less than 50 years without high-risk medical conditions can receive either intranasally administered live, attenuated influenza vaccine (FluMist), or inactivated vaccine. Other persons should receive the inactivated vaccine. Adults aged 65 years and older can receive the standard influenza vaccine or the high-dose (Fluzone) influenza vaccine. Additional information about influenza vaccination is available at http://www.cdc.gov/vaccines/vpd-vac/flu/default.htm.

2. Tetanus, diphtheria, and acellular pertussis (Td/Tdap) vaccination

Administer a one-time dose of Tdap to adults aged less than 65 years who have not received Tdap previously or for whom vaccine status is unknown to replace one of the 10-year Td boosters, and as soon as feasible to all 1) postpartum women, 2) close contacts of infants younger than age 12 months (e.g., grandparents and child-care providers), and 3) health-care personnel with direct patient contact. Adults aged 65 years and older who have not previously received Tdap and who have close contact with an infant aged less than 12 months also should be vaccinated. Other adults aged 65 years and older may receive Tdap. Tdap can be administered regardless of interval since the most recent tetanus or diphtheria-containing vaccine.

Adults with uncertain or incomplete history of completing a 3-dose primary vaccination series with Td-containing vaccines should begin or complete a primary vaccination series. For unvaccinated adults, administer the first 2 doses at least 4 weeks apart and the third dose 6–12 months after the second. If incompletely vaccinated (i.e., less than 3 doses), administer remaining doses. Substitute a one-time dose of Tdap for one of the doses of Td, either in the primary series or for the routine booster, whichever comes first.

If a woman is pregnant and received the most recent Td vaccination 10 or more years previously, administer Td during the second or third trimester. If the woman received the most recent Td vaccination less than 10 years previously, administer Tdap during the immediate postpartum period. At the clinician's discretion, Td may be deferred during pregnancy and Tdap substituted in the immediate postpartum period, or Tdap may be administered instead of Td to a pregnant woman after an informed discussion with the woman.

The ACIP statement for recommendations for administering Td as prophylaxis in wound management is available at http://www.cdc.gov/vaccines/pubs/acip-list.htm.

Continued

ADULT

Table 6.3

2011 Recommended Adult Immunization Schedule—cont'd

3. Varicella vaccination

All adults without evidence of immunity to varicella should receive 2 doses of single-antigen varicella vaccine if not previously vaccinated or a second dose if they have received only 1 dose, unless they have a medical contraindication. Special consideration should be given to those who 1) have close contact with persons at high risk for severe disease (e.g., health-care personnel and family contacts of persons with immunocompromising conditions) or 2) are at high risk for exposure or transmission (e.g., teachers; child-care employees; residents and staff members of institutional settings, including correctional institutions; college students; military personnel; adolescents and adults living in households with children; nonpregnant women of childbearing age; and international travelers).

Evidence of immunity to varicella in adults includes any of the following: 1) documentation of 2 doses of varicella vaccine at least 4 weeks apart; 2) U.S.-born before 1980 (although for health-care personnel and pregnant women, birth before 1980 should not be considered evidence of immunity); 3) history of varicella based on diagnosis or verification of varicella by a health-care provider (for a patient reporting a history of or having an atypical case, a mild case, or both, health-care providers should seek either an epidemiologic link with a typical varicella case or to a laboratory-confirmed case or evidence of laboratory confirmation, if it was performed at the time of acute disease); 4) history of herpes zoster based on diagnosis or verification of herpes zoster by a health-care provider; or 5) laboratory evidence of immunity or laboratory confirmation of disease.

Pregnant women should be assessed for evidence of varicella immunity. Women who do not have evidence of immunity should receive the first dose of varicella vaccine upon completion or termination of pregnancy and before discharge from the health-care facility. The second dose should be administered 4–8 weeks after the first dose.

4. Human papillomavirus (HPV) vaccination

HPV vaccination with either quadrivalent (HPV4) vaccine or bivalent vaccine (HPV2) is recommended for females at age 11 or 12 years and catch-up vaccination for females aged 13 through 26 years.

Ideally, vaccine should be administered before potential exposure to HPV through sexual activity; however, females who are sexually active should still be vaccinated consistent with age-based recommendations. Sexually active females who have not been infected with any of the four HPV vaccine types (types 6, 11, 16, and 18, all of which HPV4 prevents) or any of the two HPV vaccine types (types 16 and 18, both of which HPV2 prevents) receive the full benefit of the vaccination. Vaccination is less beneficial for females who have already been infected with one or more of the HPV vaccine types. HPV4 or HPV2 can be administered to persons with a history of genital warts, abnormal Papanicolaou test, or positive HPV DNA test, because these conditions are not evidence of previous infection with all vaccine HPV types.

HPV4 may be administered to males aged 9 through 26 years to reduce their likelihood of genital warts. HPV4 would be most effective when administered before exposure to HPV through sexual contact.

A complete series for either HPV4 or HPV2 consists of 3 doses. The second dose should be administered 1–2 months after the first dose; the third dose should be administered 6 months after the first dose.

Although HPV vaccination is not specifically recommended for persons with the medical indications described in Figure 2, "Vaccines that might be indicated for adults based on medical and other indications," it may be administered to these persons because the HPV vaccine is not a live-virus vaccine. However, the immune response and vaccine efficacy might be less for persons with the medical indications described in Figure 2 than in persons who do not have the medical indications described or who are immunocompetent.

5. Herpes zoster vaccination

A single dose of zoster vaccine is recommended for adults aged 60 years and older regardless of whether they report a previous episode of herpes zoster. Persons with chronic medical conditions may be vaccinated unless their condition constitutes a contraindication.

6. Measles, mumps, rubella (MMR) vaccination

Adults born before 1957 generally are considered immune to measles and mumps. All adults born in 1957 or later should have documentation of 1 or more doses of MMR vaccine unless they have a medical contraindication to the vaccine, laboratory evidence of immunity to each of the three diseases, or documentation of provider-diagnosed measles or mumps disease. For rubella, documentation of provider-diagnosed disease is not considered acceptable evidence of immunity.

Measles component: A second dose of MMR vaccine, administered a minimum of 28 days after the first dose, is recommended for adults who 1) have been recently exposed to measles or are in an outbreak setting; 2) are students in postsecondary educational institutions; 3) work in a health-care facility; or 4) plan to travel internationally. Persons who received inactivated (killed) measles vaccine or measles vaccine of unknown type during 1963–1967 should be revaccinated with 2 doses of MMR vaccine.

Mumps component: A second dose of MMR vaccine, administered a minimum of 28 days after the first dose, is recommended for adults who 1) live in a community experiencing a mumps outbreak and are in an affected age group; 2) are students in postsecondary educational institutions; 3) work in a health-care facility; or 4) plan to travel internationally. Persons vaccinated before 1979 with either killed mumps vaccine or mumps vaccine of unknown type who are at high risk for mumps infection (e.g. persons who are working in a health-care facility) should be revaccinated with 2 doses of MMR vaccine.

Rubella component: For women of childbearing age, regardless of birth year, rubella immunity should be determined. If there is no evidence of immunity, women who are not pregnant should be vaccinated. Pregnant women who do not have evidence of immunity should receive MMR vaccine upon completion or termination of pregnancy and before discharge from the health-care facility.

Health-care personnel born before 1957: For unvaccinated health-care personnel born before 1957 who lack laboratory evidence of measles, mumps, and/or rubella immunity or laboratory confirmation of disease, health-care facilities should 1) consider routinely vaccinating personnel with 2 doses of MMR vaccine at the appropriate interval (for measles and mumps) and 1 dose of MMR vaccine (for rubella), and 2) recommend 2 doses of MMR vaccine at the appropriate interval during an outbreak of measles or mumps, and 1 dose during an outbreak of rubella. Complete information about evidence of immunity is available at http://www.cdc.gov/vaccines/recs/provisional/default.htm.

7. Pneumococcal polysaccharide (PPSV) vaccination

Vaccinate all persons with the following indications:

Medical: Chronic lung disease (including asthma); chronic cardiovascular diseases; diabetes mellitus; chronic liver diseases; cirrhosis; chronic alcoholism; functional or anatomic asplenia (e.g., sickle cell disease or splenectomy [if elective splenectomy is planned, vaccinate at least 2 weeks before surgery]); immunocompromising conditions (including chronic renal failure or nephrotic syndrome); and cochlear implants and cerebrospinal fluid leaks. Vaccinate as close to HIV diagnosis as possible.

Other: Residents of nursing homes or long-term care facilities and persons who smoke cigarettes. Routine use of PPSV is not recommended for American Indians/Alaska Natives or persons aged less than 65 years unless they have underlying medical conditions that are PPSV indications. However, public health authorities may consider recommending PPSV for American Indians/Alaska Natives and persons aged 50 through 64 years who are living in areas where the risk for invasive pneumococcal disease is increased.

8. Revaccination with PPSV

One-time revaccination after 5 years is recommended for persons aged 19 through 64 years with chronic renal failure or nephrotic syndrome; functional or anatomic asplenia (e.g., sickle cell disease or splenectomy); and for persons with immunocompromising conditions. For persons aged 65 years and older, one-time revaccination is recommended if they were vaccinated 5 or more years previously and were aged less than 65 years at the time of primary vaccination.

9. Meningococcal vaccination

Meningococcal vaccine should be administered to persons with the following indications:

Medical: A 2-dose series of meningococcal conjugate vaccine is recommended for adults with anatomic or functional asplenia, or persistent complement component deficiencies. Adults with HIV infection who are vaccinated should also receive a routine 2-dose series. The 2 doses should be administered at 0 and 2 months.

Other: A single dose of meningococcal vaccine is recommended for unvaccinated first-year college students living in dormitories; microbiologists routinely exposed to isolates of *Neisseria meningitidis*; military recruits; and persons who travel to or live in countries in which meningococcal disease is hyperendemic or epidemic (e.g., the "meningitis belt" of sub-Saharan Africa during the dry season [December through June]), particularly if their contact with local populations will be prolonged. Vaccination is required by the government of Saudi Arabia for all travelers to Mecca during the annual Hajj.

Meningococcal conjugate vaccine, quadrivalent (MCV4) is preferred for adults with any of the preceding indications who are aged 55 years and younger; meningococcal polysaccharide vaccine (MPSV4) is preferred for adults aged 56 years and older. Revaccination with MCV4 every 5 years is recommended for adults previously vaccinated with MCV4 or MPSV4 who remain at increased risk for infection (e.g., adults with anatomic or functional asplenia, or persistent complement component deficiencies).

10. Hepatitis A vaccination

Vaccinate persons with any of the following indications and any person seeking protection from hepatitis A virus (HAV) infection:

Behavioral: Men who have sex with men and persons who use injection drugs.

Occupational: Persons working with HAV-infected primates or with HAV in a research laboratory setting.

Medical: Persons with chronic liver disease and persons who receive clotting factor concentrates.

Other: Persons traveling to or working in countries that have high or intermediate endemicity of hepatitis A (a list of countries is available at http://wwwn.cdc.gov/travel/ contentdiseases.aspx).

Unvaccinated persons who anticipate close personal contact (e.g., household or regular babysitting) with an international adoptee during the first 60 days after arrival in the United States from a country with high or intermediate endemicity should be vaccinated. The first dose of the 2-dose hepatitis A vaccine series should be administered as soon as adoption is planned, ideally 2 or more weeks before the arrival of the adoptee.

Single-antigen vaccine formulations should be administered in a 2-dose schedule at either 0 and 6–12 months (Havrix), or 0 and 6–18 months (Vaqta). If the combined hepatitis A and hepatitis B vaccine (Twinrix) is used, administer 3 doses at 0, 1, and 6 months; alternatively, a 4-dose schedule may be used, administered on days 0, 7, and 21–30, followed by a booster dose at month 12.

11. Hepatitis B vaccination

Vaccinate persons with any of the following indications and any person seeking protection from hepatitis B virus (HBV) infection:

Behavioral: Sexually active persons who are not in a long-term, mutually monogamous relationship (e.g., persons with more than one sex partner during the previous 6 months); persons seeking evaluation or treatment for a sexually transmitted disease (STD); current or recent injection-drug users; and men who have sex with men.

Occupational: Health-care personnel and public-safety workers who are exposed to blood or other potentially infectious body fluids.

Medical: Persons with end-stage renal disease, including patients receiving hemodialysis; persons with HIV infection; and persons with chronic liver disease.

Other: Household contacts and sex partners of persons with chronic HBV infection; clients and staff members of institutions for persons with developmental disabilities; and international travelers to countries with high or intermediate prevalence of chronic HBV infection (a list of countries is available at http://wwwn.cdc.gov/travel/contentdiseases.aspx).

Hepatitis B vaccination is recommended for all adults in the following settings: STD treatment facilities; HIV testing and treatment facilities; facilities providing drug-abuse treatment and prevention services; health-care settings targeting services to injection-drug users or men who have sex with men; correctional facilities; end-stage renal disease programs and facilities for chronic hemodialysis patients; and institutions and nonresidential day-care facilities for persons with developmental disabilities.

Administer missing doses to complete a 3-dose series of hepatitis B vaccine to those persons not vaccinated or not completely vaccinated. The second dose should be administered 1 month after the first dose; the third dose should be given at least 2 months after the second dose (and at least 4 months after the first dose). If the combined hepatitis A and hepatitis B vaccine (Twinrix) is used, administer 3 doses at 0, 1, and 6 months; alternatively, a 4-dose Twinrix schedule, administered on days 0, 7, and 21 to 30, followed by a booster dose at month 12 may be used.

Adult patients receiving hemodialysis or with other immunocompromising conditions should receive 1 dose of 40 μg/mL (Recombivax HB) administered on a 3-dose schedule or 2 doses of 20 μg/mL (Engerix-B) administered simultaneously on a 4-dose schedule at 0, 1, 2, and 6 months.

12. Selected conditions for which Haemophilus influenzae type b (Hib) vaccine may be used

1 dose of Hib vaccine should be considered for persons who have sickle cell disease, leukemia, or HIV infection, or who have had a splenectomy, if they have not previously received Hib vaccine.

13. Immunocompromising conditions

Inactivated vaccines generally are acceptable (e.g., pneumococcal, meningococcal, influenza [inactivated influenza vaccine]) and live vaccines generally are avoided in persons with immune deficiencies or immunocompromising conditions. Information on specific conditions is available at http://www.cdc.gov/vaccines/pubs/acip-list.htm.

These schedules indicate the recommended age groups and medical indications for which administration of currently licensed vaccines is commonly indicated for adults ages 19 years and older, as of January 1, 2011. For all vaccines being recommended on the adult immunization schedule: a vaccine series does not need to be restarted, regardless of the time that has elapsed between doses. Licensed combination vaccines may be used whenever any components of the combination are indicated and when the vaccine's other components are not contraindicated. For detailed recommendations on all vaccines, including those used primarily for travelers or that are issued during the year, consult the manufacturers' package inserts and the complete statements from the Advisory Committee on Immunization Practices (http:// www.cdc.gov/vaccines/pubs/acip-list.htm).

Report all clinically significant postvaccination reactions to the Vaccine Adverse Event Reporting System (VAERS). Reporting forms and instructions on filing a VAERS report are available at http://www.vaers.hhs.gov or by telephone, 800-822-7967.

Information on how to file a Vaccine Injury Compensation Program claim is available at http://www.hrsa.gov/vaccinecompensation or by telephone, 800-338-2382. Information about filing a claim for vaccine injury is available through the U.S. Court of Federal Claims, 717 Madison Place, N.W., Washington, D.C. 20005; telephone, 202-357-6400.

Additional information about the vaccines in this schedule, extent of available data, and contraindications for vaccination also is available at http://www.cdc.gov/vaccines or from the CDC-INFO Contact Center at 800-CDC-INFO (800-232-4636) in English and Spanish, 24 hours a day, 7 days a week.

Use of trade names and commercial sources is for identification only and does not imply endorsement by the U.S. Department of Health and Human Services.

U.S. Department of Health and Human Services • Centers for Disease Control and Prevention

From http://www.cdc.gov/vaccines/recs/schedules/downloads/adult/2009/adult-schedule-6x4-5-pss.pdf

usually at the end of young adulthood; when the choice is deferred beyond these years, valuable time is lost.

F. Experiments with and chooses a lifestyle.

G. Forms mature peer relationships with the opposite sex.

H. Overcomes guilt and anxiety about the opposite sex and learns to understand the masculine and feminine aspects of self, as well as the adult concept of roles.

I. Learns to take the opposite sex seriously and may choose someone for a long-term relationship.

J. Accepts the responsibilities and pleasures of parenthood.

Adulthood (31 to 45 Years of Age)

I. STAGE OF DEVELOPMENT—PSYCHOSOCIAL STAGE: generativity versus self-absorption.

II. PHYSICAL DEVELOPMENT

A. Gradual decline in biological functioning, although in the late 30s the individual is still near peak.

B. Period of peak sexual capacity for women occurs during the mid-30s.

C. Distinct sense of bodily decline occurs around 40 years of age.

D. *Circulatory* system begins to slow somewhat after 40 years of age.

III. COGNITIVE DEVELOPMENT

A. Takes longer to memorize.

B. Still at peak in abstract thinking and problem-solving.

C. Generates new levels of awareness.

D. Gives more meaning to complex tasks.

IV. SOCIALIZATION

A. Achieves a realistic self-identity.

B. Perceptions are based on reality.

C. Acts on decisions and assumes responsibility for actions.

D. Accepts limitations while developing assets.

E. Delays immediate gratification in favor of future satisfaction.

F. Evaluates mistakes, determines reasons and causes, and learns new behavior.

G. Struggles to establish a place in society.

1. Begins to settle down.
2. Pursues long-range plans and goals.
3. Has a stronger need to be responsible.
4. Invests self as fully as possible in social structure, including work, family, and community.

H. Seeks advancement by improving and using skills, becoming more creative, and pursuing ambitions.

Middle Life (46 to 64 Years of Age)

I. STAGE OF DEVELOPMENT—PSYCHOSOCIAL STAGE: continuation of generativity versus self-absorption.

II. PHYSICAL DEVELOPMENT

A. Failing *eyesight,* especially for close vision, may be one of the first symptoms of aging.

B. Hearing loss is very gradual, especially for low sounds; hearing for *high-pitched* sounds is impaired more readily.

C. There is a gradual loss of *taste* buds in the 50s and gradual loss of sense of *smell* in the 60s, causing the individual to have a diminished sense of taste.

D. *Muscle strength* declines because of decreased levels of estrogen and testosterone; it takes more time to accomplish the same physical task.

E. *Lung* capacity is impaired, which adds to decreased endurance.

F. The *skin* begins to wrinkle, and hair begins graying.

G. *Postural changes* take place because of loss of calcium and reduced activity.

III. COGNITIVE DEVELOPMENT

A. *Memory* begins to decline slowly around age 50 years.

B. It takes longer to *learn* new tasks, and old tasks take longer to perform.

C. *Practical judgment* is increased due to experiential background.

D. May tend to withdraw from mental activity or overcompensate by trying the impossible.

IV. SOCIALIZATION

A. The middle years can be very rewarding if previous stages have been fulfilled.

B. The years of responsibility for raising children are over.

C. Husbands and wives usually find a closer bond.

D. There is less financial strain for those with steady employment.

E. Individuals are usually at the height of their careers; the majority of leaders in their field are in this age group.

F. Self-realization is achieved.

1. There is more inner direction.
2. There is no longer a need to please everyone.
3. Individual is less likely to compare self with others.
4. Individual approves of self without being dependent on standards of others.
5. There is less fear of failure in life because past failures have been met and dealt with.

Early Late Years (65 to 79 Years of Age)

I. STAGE OF DEVELOPMENT—PSYCHOSOCIAL STAGE: ego integrity and acceptance versus despair and disgust.

II. PHYSICAL DEVELOPMENT (see also **Chapter** 7)

A. Continues to decrease in vigor and capacity.
B. Has more frequent aches and pains.
C. Likely to have at least one major illness.

III. COGNITIVE DEVELOPMENT

A. Mental acuity continues to slow down.
B. Judgment and problem-solving remain intact, but the processes may take longer.
C. May have problems in remembering *names and dates.*

IV. SOCIALIZATION

A. Individual is faced with the reality of the experience of physical decline.
B. Physical and mental changes intensify the feelings of aging and mortality.
C. Increasing frequency of death and serious illness among friends, relatives, and associates further reinforces the concept of mortality.
D. Constant reception of medical warnings to follow certain precautions or run serious risks adds to general feeling of decline.
E. Individual is less interested in obtaining the rewards of society and is more interested in using own inner resources.
F. Individuals feel that they have earned the right to do what is important for self-satisfaction.
G. Retirement allows time for expression of own creative energies.
H. Overcomes the splitting of youth and age; gets along well with adolescents.
I. Learns to deal with the reality that only old age remains.
J. Provides moral support to grandchildren; more tolerant of grandchildren than was of own children.
K. Tends to release major authority of family to children while holding self in the role of consultant.

ADULT

Later Years (80 Years of Age and Older)

I. STAGE OF DEVELOPMENT—PSYCHOSOCIAL STAGE: continuation of ego integrity and acceptance versus despair and disgust.

II. PHYSICAL DEVELOPMENT (see also **Chapter** 7)

A. Additional sensory problems occur, including diminished sensation to *touch and pain.*
B. Increase in loss of muscle tone occurs, including *sphincter* (urinary and anal) control.
C. Individual is insecure and unsure about orientation to *space* and sense of *balance,* which may result in falls and injury.

III. COGNITIVE DEVELOPMENT

A. Has better memory for the *past* than the present.
B. *Repetition* of memories occurs.
C. Individual may use *confabulation* to fill in memory gaps.
D. Forgetfulness may lead to serious *safety* problems, and individual may require constant supervision.
E. Increased arteriosclerosis may lead to mental illness (dementia and other cognitive disorders).

IV. SOCIALIZATION

A. Few significant relationships are maintained; deaths of friends, family, and associates cause isolation.
B. Individual may be preoccupied with immediate bodily needs and personal comforts; the *gastrointestinal tract* frequently becomes the major focus.
C. Individuals see that they can provide others with an example of wisdom and courage.
D. Individuals come to terms with themselves.
E. Individuals are concerned with own mortality.
F. Individuals come to terms with the process of dying and prepare for own death.

FLUID AND ELECTROLYTE IMBALANCES

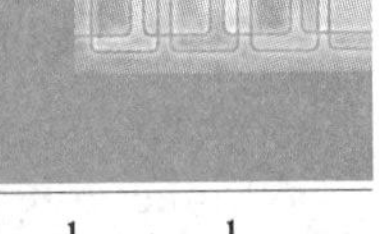

Imbalances in fluid and electrolytes may be due to changes in the total quantity of either substance (deficit or excess), protein deficiencies, or extracellular fluid volume shifts. Clients who are older and very young are particularly susceptible.

I. FLUID VOLUME DEFICIT (dehydration): mechanism that influences fluid balance and sodium levels; decreased quantities of fluid and electrolytes may be caused by *deficient intake* (poor dietary habits, anorexia, and nausea), *excessive output* (vomiting, nasogastric suction, and prolonged diarrhea), or *failure of regulatory mechanism* that influences fluid balance and sodium levels.

A. Pathophysiology: water moves out of the cells to replace a significant water loss; cells eventually become unable to compensate for the lost fluid, and cellular dehydration begins, leading to circulatory collapse.
B. Risk factors:
1. No fluids available.
2. Available fluids not drinkable.
3. Inability to take fluids independently.

4. No response to thirst; does not recognize the need for fluids.
5. Inability to communicate need; does not speak same language.
6. Aphasia.
7. Weakness, comatose.
8. Inability to swallow.
9. Psychological alterations.
10. Overuse of diuretics.
11. Increased vomiting.
12. Fever.
13. Wounds, burns.
14. Blood loss.
15. Endocrine abnormalities (e.g., diabetes insipidus).
16. Diarrhea.

C. Assessment:

1. *Subjective data:*
   a. Thirst.
   b. Behavioral changes: apprehension, apathy, lethargy, confusion, restlessness.
   c. Dizziness.
   d. Numbness and tingling of hands and feet.
   e. Anorexia and nausea.
   f. Abdominal cramps.
2. *Objective data:*
   a. Sudden weight loss of 5%.
   b. *Vital signs:*
      (1) *Decreased* BP; postural changes.
      (2) *Increased* temperature.
      (3) Irregular, weak, rapid pulse.
      (4) *Increased* rate and depth of respirations.
   c. Skin: cool and pale in absence of infection; decreased turgor.
   d. Urine: oliguria to anuria, high specific gravity.
   e. Eyes: soft, sunken.
   f. Tongue: furrows.
   g. Laboratory data:
      (1) Blood—*increased* hematocrit and blood urea nitrogen (BUN).
      (2) Urine—*decreased* 17-ketosteroids; *increased* specific gravity, dark-colored urine.

D. Analysis/nursing diagnosis:

1. *Fluid volume deficit* related to inadequate fluid intake.

E. Nursing care plan/implementation:

1. Goal: *restore fluid and electrolyte balance—increase* fluid intake to hydrate client.
   a. IVs and blood products as ordered; small, frequent drinks by mouth.
   b. Daily weights (same time of day) to monitor progress of fluid replacement.
   c. I&O, hourly outputs (when in acute state).
   d. *Avoid* hypertonic solutions (may cause fluid shift when compensatory mechanisms begin to function).
2. Goal: *promote comfort.*
   a. Frequent skin care (lack of hydration causes dry skin, which may increase risk for skin breakdown).
   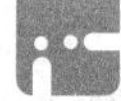
   b. *Position:* change every hour to relieve pressure.
   c. Medications as ordered: *antiemetics, antidiarrheal.*
3. Goal: *prevent physical injury.*
   a. Frequent mouth care (mucous membrane dries due to dehydration; therefore, client is at risk for breaks in mucous membrane, halitosis).
   b. Monitor IV flow rate—observe for circulatory overload, pulmonary edema related to potential fluid shift when compensatory mechanisms begin or client is unable to tolerate rate of fluid replacement.
   c. Monitor vitals, including level of consciousness (*decreasing* BP and level of consciousness indicate continuation of fluid loss).
   d. Prepare for surgery if hemorrhage present (internal bleeding can only be relieved by surgical intervention).

F. Evaluation/outcome criteria:

1. Mentally alert.
2. Moist, intact mucous membranes.
3. Urinary output approximately equal to intake.
4. No further weight loss.
5. Gradual weight gain.

II. FLUID VOLUME EXCESS

(fluid overload): most common cause is an increase in sodium; excessive quantities of fluid and electrolytes may be due to *increased ingestion,* tube feedings, intravenous infusions, multiple tap-water enemas, or a *failure of regulatory systems,* resulting in inability to excrete excesses.

A. Pathophysiology: hypo-osmolar water excess in extracellular compartment leads to intracellular water excess because the concentration of solutes in the intracellular fluid is greater than that in the extracellular fluid. Water moves to equalize concentration, causing swelling of the cells. The most common cause is an increase in sodium.

B. Risk factors:

1. Excessive intake of electrolyte-free fluids.
2. Increased secretion of antidiuretic hormone (ADH) in response to stress, drugs, anesthetics **(Table 6.4).**
3. Decreased or inadequate output of urine.
4. Psychogenic polydipsia.
5. Certain medical conditions: tuberculosis; encephalitis; meningitis; endocrine disturbances; tumors of lung, pancreas, duodenum; heart failure.
6. Inadequate kidney function or kidney failure.

Table 6.4

Diabetes Insipidus (DI) Versus Syndrome of Inappropriate Antidiuretic Hormone (SIADH)

	DI (Fluid Deficit)	SIADH (Fluid Excess)
Pathophysiology:	• Deficiency of ADH → inability to conserve H_2O • Large volumes of hypotonic fluid excreted	• Excessive ADH secreted → water retention, hyponatremia, and hypo-osmolality
Risk factors:	• Head injury • Brain infection • Posterior pituitary tumors • Drugs that inhibit vasopressin (e.g., glucocorticoids, phenytoin, lithium)	• Vasopressin overuse (Rx of DI) or stimulation (chemotherapy) • Small cell carcinoma • Adrenal insufficiency • Myxedema • Anterior pituitary insufficiency
Assessment:	• Polyuria (up to 18 L/day) • Urine specific gravity ↓ • Signs of fluid volume deficit: dry, cool skin; polydipsia; ↓ weight Laboratory: serum Na^+ ↑ initially, then ↓; serum osmolality ↑ initially, then ↓	• Signs of ↓ Na^+—fatigue, headache, ↓ DTR, nausea, anorexia, ↓ mental status • Signs of fluid volume excess: weight gain without edema; tachycardia; tachypnea; crackles
Nursing care plan/implementation:	• Fluids: IV; I/O • Medications: ADH replacement; Pitressin • Education: prepare for hypophysectomy	• Fluids: hypertonic IV (↑ Na^+); I/O • Medications: diuretics; demeclocycline (tetracycline) • Daily weight

C. Assessment:

1. *Subjective data:*
   a. Behavioral changes: irritability, apathy, confusion, disorientation.
   b. Headache.
   c. Anorexia, nausea, cramping.
   d. Fatigue.
   e. Dyspnea.
2. *Objective data:*
   a. Vital signs: *elevated* blood pressure.
   b. Skin: warm, moist; edema—eyelids, facial, dependent, pitting.
   c. Sudden weight gain of 5 lb.
   d. Pink, frothy sputum; productive.
   e. Constant, irritating cough.
   f. Crackles in lungs.
   g. Pulse: bounding.
   h. Engorgement of neck veins in sitting position.
   i. Urine: polyuria, nocturia, pale color.
   j. Laboratory data:
      (1) Blood—*decreasing* hematocrit, BUN.
      (2) Urine—*decreasing* specific gravity.

D. Analysis/nursing diagnosis:

1. *Fluid volume excess* related to excessive fluid intake or decreased fluid output.

E. Nursing care plan/implementation:

1. Goal: *maintain oxygen to all cells.*
   a. *Position:* semi-Fowler's or Fowler's to facilitate improved gas exchange.
   b. Vital signs: prn, minimum q4h.
   c. Fluid restriction.
2. Goal: *promote excretion of excess fluid.*
   a. Medications as ordered: *diuretics.*
   b. Monitor electrolytes, especially Mg^{++}, K^+.
   c. If in kidney failure: may need dialysis; explain procedure.
   d. Assist client during paracentesis, thoracentesis, phlebotomy.
      (1) Monitor vital signs to detect shock.
      (2) Prevent injury by monitoring sterile technique.
      (3) Prevent falling by stabilizing appropriate position during procedure.
      (4) Support client psychologically.
3. Goal: *obtain/maintain fluid balance.*
   a. Daily weights; 1 kg = 1,000 mL fluid.
   b. Measure: all edematous parts, abdominal girth, I&O.
   c. *Limit:* fluids by mouth, IVs, sodium.
   d. Strict monitoring of IV fluids.
4. Goal: *prevent tissue injury.*
   a. Skin and mouth care as needed.
   b. Evaluate feet for edema and discoloration when client is out of bed.
   c. Observe suture line on surgical clients (potential for evisceration due to excess fluid retention).
   d. IV route preferred for parenteral medications; *Z track* if medications are to be given IM

(otherwise injected liquid will escape through injection site).

5. Goal: *health teaching.*

a. Improve nutritional status with *low-sodium* diet.
b. Identify cause that put client at risk for imbalance, methods to avoid this situation in the future.
c. Desired and side effects of diuretics and other prescribed medications.
d. Monitor urinary output, ankle edema; report to health-care manager when fluid retention is noticed.
e. Limit fluid intake when kidney/cardiac function impaired.

F. Evaluation/outcome criteria:

1. Fluid balance obtained.
2. No respiratory, cardiac complications.
3. Vital signs within normal limits.
4. Urinary output improved, no evidence of edema.

III. COMMON ELECTROLYTE IMBALANCES:

Electrolytes are taken into the body in foods and fluids; normally lost through sweat and urine. May also be lost through hemorrhage, vomiting, and diarrhea. Electrolytes have major influences on: body water regulation and osmolality, acid-base regulation, enzyme reactions, and neuromuscular activity. Clinically important electrolytes are:

A. Sodium (Na^+): normal 135 to 145 mEq/L. Most prevalent cation in extracellular fluid. Controls osmotic pressure; essential for neuromuscular functioning and intracellular chemical reactions. Aids in maintenance of acid-base balance. Necessary for glucose to be transported into cells.

1. *Hyponatremia*—sodium deficit, resulting from either a sodium loss or water excess. Serum sodium level below 135 mEq/L; symptoms usually do not occur until below 120 mEq/L unless rapid drop.
2. *Hypernatremia*—excess sodium in the blood, resulting from either high sodium intake, water loss, or low water intake. Serum sodium level above 145 mEq/L.

B. Potassium (K^+): normal 3.5 to 5.0 mEq/L. Direct effect on excitability of nerves and muscles. Contributes to intracellular osmotic pressure and influences acid-base balance. Major cation of the cell. Required for storage of nitrogen as muscle protein.

1. *Hypokalemia*—potassium deficit related to dehydration, starvation, vomiting, diarrhea, diuretics. Serum potassium level below 3.5 mEq/L; symptoms may not occur until below 2.5 mEq/L.
2. *Hyperkalemia*—potassium excess related to severe tissue damage, renal disease, excess administration of oral or IV potassium. Serum potassium level above 5 mEq/L; symptoms usually occur when above 6.5 mEq/L.

C. Calcium (Ca^{++}): normal 4.5 to 5.5 mEq/L. Essential to muscle metabolism, cardiac function, and bone health. Controlled by parathyroid hormone; reciprocal relationship between calcium and phosphorus.

1. *Hypocalcemia*—loss of calcium related to inadequate intake, vitamin D deficiency, hypoparathyroidism, damage to the parathyroid gland, decreased absorption in the GI tract, excess loss through kidneys. Serum calcium level below 4.5 mEq/L.
2. *Hypercalcemia*—calcium excess related to hyperparathyroidism, immobility, bone tumors, renal failure, excess intake of Ca^{++} or vitamin D. Serum calcium level above 5.5 mEq/L.

D. Magnesium (Mg^{++}): normal 1.5 to 2.5 mEq/L. Essential to cellular metabolism of carbohydrates and proteins.

1. *Hypomagnesemia*—magnesium deficit related to impaired absorption from GI tract, excessive loss through kidneys, and prolonged periods of poor nutritional intake. Hypomagnesemia leads to neuromuscular irritability. Serum magnesium level below 1.5 mEq/L.
2. *Hypermagnesemia*—magnesium excess related to renal insufficiency, overdose during replacement therapy, severe dehydration, repeated enemas with Mg^{++} sulfate (epsom salts). Serum magnesium level above 2.5 mEq/L.

E. Table 6.5 provides assessment, analysis/nursing diagnosis, nursing care plan/implementation, and evaluation/outcome criteria of the various electrolyte imbalances.

IV. ACID-BASE BALANCE:

Concentration of hydrogen ions in extracellular fluid is determined by the ratio of bicarbonate to carbonic acid. The normal ratio is 20:1. Even when arterial blood gases are abnormal, if the ratio remains at 20:1, no imbalance will occur. **Table 6.6** shows blood gas variations with acid-base imbalances.

A. Causes of blood gas abnormalities: see **Table 6.7.**

B. Types of acid-base imbalance:

1. *Acidosis:* hydrogen ion concentration *increases* and pH *decreases.*
2. *Alkalosis:* hydrogen ion concentration *decreases* and pH *increases.*
3. *Metabolic imbalances:* bicarbonate is the problem. In primary conditions, the level of bicarbonate is directly *proportional* to pH.
   a. *Metabolic acidosis:* excessive acid is produced or added to the body, bicarbonate is lost, or

(text continues on page 363)

ADULT

ADULT

Table 6.5

Electrolyte Imbalances

Disorder and Related Condition	Assessment: Subjective Data	Assessment: Objective Data	Analysis/Nursing Diagnosis	Nursing Care Plan/Implementation	Evaluation/Outcome Criteria
Hyponatremia • Addison's disease • Starvation • GI suction • Thiazide diuretics • Excess water intake, enemas • Fever • Fluid shifts • Ascites • Burns • Small bowel obstruction • Profuse perspiration	• Apathy, apprehension, mental confusion, delirium • Fatigue • Vertigo, headache • Anorexia, nausea • Abdominal and muscle cramps	• *Pulse:* rapid and weak • *BP:* postural hypotension • Shock, coma • *GI:* weight loss, diarrhea, loss through NG tubes • Muscle weakness	• *Diarrhea* • *Fluid volume excess* • *Altered nutrition, less than body requirements* • *Sensory/perceptual alteration (kinesthetic)*	• *Obtain normal sodium level:* identify cause of deficit, *increase sodium intake* PO (salty foods), IVs—hypertonic solutions • *Prevent further sodium loss:* irrigate NG tubes with saline; hourly I&O to monitor kidney output • *Prevent injury* related to shock, dizziness, decreased sensorium; dangle before ambulation • Skin care	Na^+ 135–145 mEq/L • No complications of shock present • Return of muscle strength • Alert, oriented • Limits intake of plain water
Hypernatremia • High sodium intake • Low water intake • Diarrhea • High fever with rapid respirations • Impaired renal functions • Acute tracheobronchitis	• Lethargy • Restlessness, agitation • Confusion	• *BP and temperature:* elevated • *Neuromuscular:* diminished reflexes • *Skin:* flushed; firm turgor • *GI:* mucous membrane dry, sticky • *GU:* decreased output	• *Fluid volume deficit* • *Fluid volume excess* • *Altered nutrition, less than body requirements* • *Sensory/perceptual alteration (kinesthetic)*	• *Obtain normal sodium level: decrease sodium* intake • I&O to recognize signs and symptoms of complications (e.g., heart failure, pulmonary edema)	Na^+ 135–145 mEq/L • No complaint of thirst • Alert, oriented • Relaxed in appearance • Identifies high-sodium foods to avoid K^+ 3.5–5.0 mEq/L
Hypokalemia *Decreased intake:* • Poor potassium food intake • Excessive dieting • Nausea • Alcoholism • IV fluids without added potassium *Increased loss:* • GI suctioning, vomiting, diarrhea • Ulcerative colitis • Drainage: ostomy, fistulas • Medications: potassium-losing diuretics, digoxin, cathartics • Increased aldosterone production • Renal disorders	• Apathy, lethargy, fatigue, weakness • Irritability, mental confusion • Anorexia, nausea • Leg cramps	• *Muscles:* weakness, paralysis, paresthesia, hyporeflexia. • *Respirations:* shallow to respiratory arrest • *Cardiac:* decreased BP; elevated, weak, irregular pulse; arrhythmias • *ECG:* low, flat T waves; prolonged ST segment; elevated U wave; potential arrest • *GI:* vomiting, flatulence, constipation; decreased motility → distention → paralytic ileus • *GU:* urine not concentrated; polyuria, nocturia; kidney damage • *Speech:* slow	• *Decreased cardiac output* • *Fatigue* • *Altered cardiopulmonary tissue perfusion* • *Ineffective breathing patterns* • *Constipation* • *Bathing/hygiene self-care deficit* • *Impaired home maintenance management* • *Sensory/perceptual alteration (gustatory)*	• *Replace lost potassium: increase potassium* in diet (see **Chapter 9**); liquid PO potassium medications—dilute in juice to aid taste; give potassium only if kidneys functioning • *Prevent injury to tissues:* prevent infiltration, pain, tissue damage • *Prevent potassium loss:* Irrigate NG tubes with saline, not water	• Identifies cause of imbalance • Lists foods to include in diet • Lists signs and symptoms of imbalance • Return of muscle strength • No cardiac arrhythmias

Hyperkalemia • Burns • Crushing injuries • Kidney disease • Excessive infusion or ingestion of K^+ • Adrenal insufficiency • Mercurial poisoning	• Irritability • Weakness, muscle cramps • Nausea, intestinal cramps	• *Muscles:* paresthesia, flaccid muscle paralysis (later) • *Cardiac;* irregular pulse; arrhythmias; bradycardia → asystole • *ECG:* high T waves; depressed ST segment; widened QRS complex; diminished or absent P waves; ventricular fibrillation • *GI:* explosive diarrhea; hyperactive bowel sounds • *Kidney:* scanty to no urine	• *Decreased cardiac output* • *Altered urinary elimination* • *Activity intolerance* • *Ineffective breathing patterns* • *Diarrhea* • *Impaired home maintenance management*	• *Decrease amount of potassium in body;* identify and treat cause of imbalance; give *foods low in K^+; avoid* drugs or IV fluids containing K^+ • If kidney failure present, may need to prepare for dialysis	K^+ 3.5–5.0 mEq/L No complications (e.g., arrhythmias, acidosis, respiratory failure)
Hypocalcemia • Acute pancreatitis • Diarrhea • Peritonitis • Damage to parathyroid during thyroidectomy • Hypothyroidism • Burns • Pregnancy and lactation • Low vitamin D intake • Multiple blood transfusions • Renal disorders • Massive infection	• Fatigue • Tingling/numbness; fingers and circumoral • Abdominal cramps • Palpitations • Dyspnea	• *Muscle spasms:* tonic muscles, carpopedal, laryngeal • *Neuromuscular:* grimacing, hyperirritable facial nerves • Tetany → convulsions • *Orthopedic:* osteoporosis → fractures • *Cardiac:* arrhythmias → arrest • *GI:* diarrhea	• *Pain* • *Diarrhea* • *Altered nutrition, less than body requirements* • *Risk for injury* • *Sensory/perceptual alteration (gustatory)*	• *Prevent tetany* (**medical emergency**): calcium gluconate IV, 2.5–5.0 mL 10% solution; repeated q10 min to maximum dose of 30 mL • *Prevent tissue injury* due to hypoxia and sloughing; administer slowly; *avoid* infiltration • *Prevent injury related to medication administration. Caution:* drug interaction with carbonate, phosphate, digitalis; *avoid* hypercalcemia • *In less acute condition:* increase calcium intake—calcium gluconate or lactate	Ca^{++} 4.5–5.5 mEq/L • No signs of tetany • Absent *Trousseau*'s and *Chvostek*'s signs • Lists foods high in vitamin D and calcium
Hypercalcemia • Parathyroid glands: overactive, tumor • Increased immobility • Decreased renal function • Bone cancer • Increased vitamin D and calcium intake • *Milk-alkali syndrome*—self-administration of antacids; increased milk in diet to relieve GI symptoms	• *Pain:* flank, deep bone, shin splints • Muscle weakness, fatigue • Anorexia, nausea • Headache • Thirst → polyuria	• *Muscles:* relaxed • *GU:* kidney stones • *GI:* increased milk intake, constipation, dehydration • *Neurological:* stupor → coma	• *Decreased cardiac output* • *Constipation* • *Activity intolerance* • *Altered urinary elimination* • *Pain*	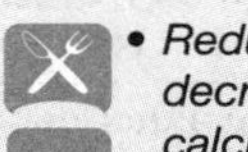 • *Reduce calcium intake: decrease* foods high in *calcium;* identify cause of imbalance; give steroids, diuretics as ordered; isotonic saline IV • *Prevent injury:* prevent pathological fractures (e.g., advanced cancer); prevent renal calculi by *increasing fluid intake*	Ca^{++} 4.5–5.5 mEq/L • No pain reported • No fractures/calculi seen on x-ray examination

Continued

ADULT

Table 6.5

Electrolyte Imbalances—cont'd

Disorder and Related Condition	Assessment: *Subjective Data*	Assessment: *Objective Data*	Analysis/Nursing Diagnosis	Nursing Care Plan/Implementation	Evaluation/Outcome Criteria
Hypomagnesemia • Impaired GI absorption • Prolonged malnutrition or starvation • Alcoholism • Excess loss of magnesium through kidneys, related to increased aldosterone production • Prolonged diarrhea • Draining GI fistulas	Agitation Depression Confusion Paresthesia	• *Muscles:* irritable, tremors, spasticity, tetany → convulsions • *Cardiac:* arrhythmias, tachycardia	• *Risk for injury related to seizure activity* • *Decreased cardiac output*	Provide safety: prevent injury to client who is disoriented; administer magnesium salts PO or IV *Health teaching:* prevention; diet—*high-magnesium* foods: fruits, green vegetables, whole-grain cereals, milk, meats, nuts	Mg^{++} 1.5–2.5 mEq/L
Hypermagnesemia • Renal failure • Diabetic ketoacidosis • Severe dehydration • Antacid therapy	Drowsiness, lethargy	• *Neuromuscular:* loss of deep tendon reflexes • *Respiratory:* depression • *Cardiac:* arrest, hypotension	• *Ineffective breathing pattern* • *Decreased cardiac output* • *Fluid volume deficit* • *Fluid volume excess* • *Altered cardiopulmonary tissue perfusion*	*Obtain normal magnesium level:* IV calcium, fluids; possible dialysis	Mg^{++} 1.5–2.5 mEq/L • No complications (e.g., respiratory depression, arrhythmias) • Identifies magnesium-based antacids (e.g., Gelusil) • Deep tendon reflexes 2+

Table 6.6

Blood Gas Variations with Acid-Base Imbalances

Blood Gas Feature	Normal Value	Value with: Respiratory Acidosis	Respiratory Alkalosis	Metabolic Acidosis	Metabolic Alkalosis
HCO_3 (bicarbonate)	22–26 mm Hg	Normal or ↑	Normal or ↓	↓	↑
Pco_2	35–45 mm Hg	↑	↓	Normal or ↓	Normal or ↑
(Carbonic acid*)	(1.05–1.35)	↑	↓	Normal or ↓	Normal or ↑
pH (hydrogen ion concentration)	7.35–7.45	↓	↑	↓	↑

↑ = increased; ↓= decreased.
*To obtain carbonic acid level, multiply Pco_2 value by 0.03.

Table 6.7

Blood Gas Abnormalities: Causes

Decreased Po_2	*Collapsed alveoli* (atelectasis) 1. Airway obstruction a. By the tongue b. By a foreign body 2. Failure to take deep breaths a. Pain (rib fracture, pleurisy) b. Paralysis of respiratory muscles (spinal cord injury, polio) c. Depression of the respiratory center (head injury, drug overdose) 3. Collapse of the whole lung (pneumothorax) *Fluid in the alveoli* 1. Pulmonary edema 2. Pneumonia 3. Near-drowning 4. Chest trauma *Other gases in the alveoli* 1. Smoke inhalation 2. Inhalation of toxic chemicals 3. Carbon monoxide poisoning *Respiratory arrest*
Elevated Pco_2	*Decreased CO_2 elimination* (hypoventilation) 1. Decreased tidal volume a. Pain (rib fractures, pleurisy) b. Weakness (myasthenia gravis) c. Paralysis (spinal cord injury, polio) 2. Decreased respiratory rate a. Head injury b. Depressant drugs c. Stroke *Increased CO_2 production* 1. Fever 2. Muscular exertion 3. Anaerobic metabolism

acid is retained due to poorly functioning kidneys. *Deficit* of bicarbonate.

b. *Metabolic alkalosis:* excessive acid is lost or bicarbonate or alkali is retained. *Excess* of bicarbonate.

c. As compensatory mechanism, Pco_2 will be *low in metabolic acidosis,* as the body attempts to eliminate excess carbonic acid and elevate pH. Pco_2 will become *elevated in metabolic alkalosis.*

4. *Respiratory imbalances: carbonic acid* is the problem. In primary conditions, Pco_2 is inversely proportional to the pH.
   a. *Respiratory acidosis:* pulmonary ventilation decreases, causing an elevation in the level of carbon dioxide or carbonic acid. *Excess* of Pco_2.
   b. *Respiratory alkalosis:* pulmonary ventilation increases, causing a decrease in the level of carbon dioxide or carbonic acid. *Deficit* of Pco_2.
   c. As a compensatory mechanism, the level of bicarbonate will *increase in respiratory acidosis* and *decrease in respiratory alkalosis.*

C. Assessment: see **Table 6.8.**

D. Analysis/nursing diagnosis:

1. *Impaired gas exchange* related to hyperventilation.
2. *Ineffective breathing pattern* related to decreased thoracic movements.
3. *Ineffective airway clearance* related to retained secretions.
4. *Risk for injury* related to poorly functioning kidneys.
5. *Altered renal tissue perfusion* related to dehydration.
6. *Altered urinary elimination* related to renal failure.

Table 6.8

Acid-Base Imbalances

Disorder and Related Conditions	Assessment: Subjective Data	Assessment: Objective Data	Nursing Care Plan/Implementation	Evaluation/Outcome Criteria
Respiratory Acidosis				
• Acute bronchitis • Emphysema • Respiratory obstruction • Atelectasis • Damage to respiratory center • Pneumonia • Asthmatic attack • Drug overdose	• Headache • Irritability • Disorientation • Weakness • Dyspnea on exertion • Nausea	• Hypoventilation: ↓ rate or rapid and shallow Cyanosis Tachycardia Diaphoresis Dehydration Coma (CO_2 narcosis) • Hyperventilation to *compensate* if no pulmonary pathology present HCO_3, normal $Paco_2$, elevated pH <7.35	• *Assist with normal breathing:* encourage coughing; suction airway; postural drainage; pursed-lip breathing; raise HOB • *Protect from injury:* oxygen as needed; encourage fluids; *avoid* sedation; medications as ordered—*antibiotics, bronchial dilators* • *Health teaching:* identify cause, prevent future episodes; increase awareness regarding risk factors and early signs of impending imbalance; encourage compliance	• Normal acid-base balance obtained • Respiratory rate: 16–20 • No signs of pulmonary infection (e.g., sputum colorless, breath sounds clear) • Demonstrates breathing exercises (e.g., diaphragmatic breathing)
Metabolic Acidosis				
• Diabetic ketoacidosis • Hyperthyroidism • Severe infections • Lactic acidosis in shock • Renal failure → uremia • Prolonged starvation diet; low-protein diet • Diarrhea, dehydration • Hepatitis • Burns	• Headache • Restlessness • Apathy, weakness • Disorientation • Thirst • Nausea, abdominal pain	• *Kussmaul's* respirations: deep, rapid air hunger • ↑ Temperature • Vomiting, diarrhea • Dehydration • Stupor → convulsions → coma HCO_3 below normal $Paco_2$ normal K^+ >5 pH <7.35	• *Restore normal metabolism:* correct underlying problem; sodium bicarbonate PO/IV; sodium lactate; fluid replacement, Ringer's solution; *diet:* high calorie • *Prevent complications: regular* insulin for ketoacidosis; hourly outputs; prepare for dialysis if in kidney failure • *Health teaching:* identify signs and symptoms of primary illness, prevent complications, cardiac arrest; diet instructions	• Normal acid-base balance obtained • No rebound respiratory alkalosis following therapy • No tetany following return of normal pH • Alert, oriented • No signs of K^+ excess
Respiratory Alkalosis				
• Hyperventilation—CO_2 loss • Hypoxia, high altitudes • Fever • Metabolic acidosis • Increased ICP, encephalitis • Salicylate poisoning • After intensive exercise	• Circumoral paresthesia • Weakness • Apprehension	• Increased respirations • Increased neuromuscular irritability; hypereflexia, muscle twitching, tetany, positive *Chvostek's* sign • Convulsions • Unconsciousness • Hypokalemia HCO_3 normal $Paco_2$ decreased pH >7.45	• *Increase carbon dioxide level:* rebreathing into a paper bag; adjusting respirator for CO_2 retention and oxygen inspired; correct hypoxia • *Prevent injury:* safety measures for those who are unconscious; hypothermia for elevated temperature • *Health teaching:* recognize stressful events; counseling if problem is hysteria	• Normal acid-base balance obtained • Recognizes psychological and environmental factors causing condition • Respiratory rate returns to normal limits • No cardiac arrhythmias • Alert, oriented

ADULT

Table 6.8

Acid-Base Imbalances—cont'd

Disorder and Related Conditions	Assessment: Subjective Data	Assessment: Objective Data	Nursing Care Plan/Implementation	Evaluation/Outcome Criteria
Metabolic Alkalosis • Potassium deficiencies • Vomiting • GI suctioning • Intestinal fistulas • Inadequate electrolyte replacement • Increased use of antacids • Diuretic therapy, steroids • Increased ingestion/ injection of bicarbonates	Lethargy Irritability Disorientation Nausea	• *Respirations:* shallow; apnea, decreased thoracic movement; cyanosis • *Pulse:* irregular → cardiac arrest • *Muscles:* twitching → tetany, convulsions • *GI:* vomiting, diarrhea, paralytic ileus HCO_3 elevated above 26 $Paco_2$ normal, K^+ <3.5 pH >7.45	• *Obtain, maintain acid-base balance:* irrigate NG tubes with saline; monitor I&O; IV saline, potassium added; isotonic solutions PO; monitor vital signs • *Prevent physical injury:* monitor for potassium loss, side effects of medications • *Health teaching:* increase sodium when loss expected; instructions regarding self-administration of medications (e.g., baking soda)	• Normal acid-base balance obtained • No signs of potassium deficit • Respiratory rate: 16–20 • No arrhythmias—pulse regular • Lists food sources high in potassium

7. *Fluid volume excess* related to altered kidney function.
8. *Fluid volume deficit* related to diarrhea or dehydration.
9. *Knowledge deficit* (learning need) related to self-administration of antacid medications.

E. Nursing care plan/implementation: see **Table 6.8.**

F. Evaluation/outcome criteria: see **Table 6.8.**

THE PERIOPERATIVE EXPERIENCE

I. PREOPERATIVE PREPARATION

A. Assessment:

1. *Subjective data:*
   a. Understanding of proposed surgery—site, type, extent of hospitalization.
   b. Previous experiences with hospitalization.
   c. Age-related factors.
   d. Allergies—iodine, latex, adhesive tape, cleansing solutions, medications.
   e. Medication/substance use—prescribed, OTC, smoking, alcohol, recreational drugs.
   f. Cultural and religious background.
   g. Concerns or feelings about surgery:
      (1) Exaggerated ideas of surgical risk (e.g., fear of colostomy when none is being considered).
      (2) Nature of anesthesia (e.g., fears of going to sleep and not waking up, saying or revealing things of a personal nature).
      (3) Degree of pain (e.g., may be incapacitating).
      (4) Misunderstandings regarding prognosis.
   h. Identification of significant others as a source of client support or care responsibilities postdischarge.
2. *Objective data:*
   a. Speech patterns indicating anxiety—repetition, changing topics, avoiding talking about feelings.
   b. Interactions with others—withdrawn or involved.
   c. Physical signs of anxiety (i.e., increased pulse, respirations; clammy palms, restlessness).
   d. Baseline physiological status: vital signs; breath sounds; peripheral circulation; weight; hydration status (hematocrit, skin turgor, urine output); degree of mobility; muscle strength.

B. Analysis/nursing diagnosis:

1. *Anxiety* related to proposed surgery.
2. *Knowledge deficit* (learning need) related to incomplete teaching or lack of understanding.
3. *Fear* related to threat of death or disfigurement.
4. *Risk for injury* related to surgical complications.
5. *Ineffective individual coping* related to anticipatory stress.

C. Nursing care plan/implementation:

1. Goal: *reduce preoperative and intraoperative anxiety and prevent postoperative complications.*
   a. *Preoperative teaching:*
      (1) Provide information about hospital nursing routines and preoperative procedures to reduce fear of unknown.
      (2) Explain purpose of diagnostic procedures to enhance ability to cooperate and tolerate procedure.
      (3) Inform about what will occur and what will be expected in the postoperative period:
         (a) Will return to room, postanesthesia care unit, or intensive care unit (ICU).
         (b) Special equipment—monitors, tubes, suction equipment.
         (c) Pain control methods.
   b. *Management of latex allergy if present.* Three forms: *immediate reaction* (most serious, life threatening)—flushing, diaphoresis, pruritus, nausea, vomiting, cramping, hypotension, dyspnea; *delayed response* (most common, discomfort)—localized symptoms 18 to 24 hours after contact; and *contact dermatitis.* Exposure to latex through skin, mucous membranes, inhalation, internal tissue, and intravascular; sources include: gloves, anesthesia masks, tourniquets, ECG electrodes, adhesive tape, warming blankets, elastic bandages, tubes/catheters, irrigation syringes. **Nursing goal:** provide latex-free environment.
2. Goal: *instruct in exercises to reduce complications.*
   a. *Diaphragmatic breathing*—refers to flattening of diaphragm during inspiration, which results in enlargement of upper abdomen; during expiration the abdominal muscles are contracted, along with the diaphragm.
      (1) The client should be in a *flat, semi-Fowler's,* or *side position,* with knees flexed and hands on the midabdomen.
      (2) Have the client take a deep breath through nose and mouth, letting the abdomen rise. Hold breath 3 to 5 seconds.
      (3) Have client exhale through nose and mouth, squeezing out all air by contracting the abdominal muscles.
      (4) Repeat 10 to 15 times, with a short rest after each 5 to prevent hyperventilation.
      (5) Inform client that this exercise will be repeated 5 to 10 times every hour postoperatively.
   b. *Coughing*—helps clear chest of secretions and, although uncomfortable, will not harm incision site.
      (1) Have client lean forward slightly from a sitting position, and place client's hands over incisional site; this acts as a splint during coughing.
      (2) Have client inhale and exhale slowly several times.
      (3) Have client inhale deeply, hold breath 3 seconds, and cough sharply three times while exhaling—client's mouth should be slightly open.
      (4) Tell client to inhale again and to cough deeply once or twice. If unable to cough deeply, client should "huff" cough to stimulate cough.
   c. *Turning and leg exercises*—help prevent circulatory stasis, which may lead to thrombus formation, and postoperative flatus or "gas pains," as well as respiratory problems.
      (1) Tell client to turn on one side with uppermost leg flexed; use side rails to facilitate the movement.
      (2) In a supine position, have client do five repetitions every hour of: ankle pumps, quadriceps-setting exercises, gluteal tightenings, and straight-leg raises.
      (3) Apply intermittent pulsatile compression device or sequential compression device to promote venous return.
3. Goal: *reduce the number of bacteria on the skin to eliminate incision contamination.* **Skin preparation:**
   a. Prepare area of skin wider and longer than proposed incision in case a larger incision is necessary.
   b. Gently scrub with an *antimicrobial* agent.
      (1) Note possibility of allergy to iodine.
      (2) Hexachlorophene should be left on the skin for 5 to 10 minutes.
      (3) If benzalkonium Cl (Zephiran) solution is ordered, do *not* soap skin before use; soap reduces effectiveness of benzalkonium by causing it to precipitate.
   c. Hair should remain *unless* it interferes with surgical procedure.
      (1) Note any nicks, cuts, or irritations, potential infection sites.
      (2) Depilatory creams or clipping of hair is preferred to shaving with a razor; nick may result in cancellation of surgery.
      (3) Skin prep may be done in surgery.

4. Goal: *reduce the risk of vomiting and aspiration during anesthesia; prevent contamination of abdominal operative sites by fecal material.*
   Gastrointestinal tract preparation:
   a. *No* food or fluid at least 6 to 8 hours before surgery.
   b. Remove food and water from bedside.
   c. Place NPO signs on bed or door.
   d. Inform kitchen and oncoming nursing staff that client is NPO for surgery.
   e. Give IV infusions up to time of surgery if dehydrated or malnourished.
   f. Enemas: two or three may be given the evening before surgery with intestinal, colon, or pelvic surgeries; 3 days of cleansing with large intestine procedures.
   g. Possible *antibiotic* therapy to reduce colonic flora with large bowel surgery.
   h. Gastric or intestinal intubation may be inserted the evening before major abdominal surgery.
      (1) Types of tubes:
         (a) *Levin:* single lumen; sufficient to remove fluids and gas from stomach; suction may damage mucosa.
         (b) *Salem sump:* large lumen; prevents tissue-wall adherence.
         (c) *Miller-Abbott:* long single or double lumen; required to remove the contents of jejunum or ileum.
      (2) Pressures: *low* setting with Levin and intestinal tubes; *high* setting with Salem sump; excessive pressures will result in injury to mucosal lining of intestine or stomach.
5. Goal: *promote rest and facilitate reduction of apprehension.*
   a. Medications as ordered: on evening before surgery may give *barbiturate*—pentobarbital (Nembutal), secobarbital (Seconal).
   b. Quiet environment: eliminate noises, distractions.
   c. *Position:* reduce muscle tension.
   d. Back rub.
6. Goal: *protect from injury; ensure final preparation for surgery.* Day of surgery:
   a. Operative permit signed and on chart; physician responsible for obtaining informed consent. Possible blood products consent.
   b. Shower or bathe.
      (1) Dress: hospital pajamas.
      (2) Remove: hairpins (cover hair); nail polish, to facilitate observation of peripheral circulation; jewelry (or tape wedding bands securely); pierced earrings; contact lenses; dentures (store and give mouth care); give valuable personal items to family; chart disposition of items.
   c. Proper identification—check band for secureness and legibility; surgical site (limb) may be marked to prevent error.
   d. Vital signs—baseline data.
   e. Void, to prevent distention and possible injury to bladder.
   f. Give preoperative medication to ensure smooth induction and maintenance of anesthesia—*antianxiety* (e.g., midazolam, diazepam, lorazepam); *narcotics* (e.g., meperidine, morphine, fentanyl); *anticholinergics* (e.g., atropine, glycopyrrolate).
      (1) Administered 45 to 75 minutes before anesthetic induction.
      (2) Side rails up (client will begin to feel drowsy and light-headed).
      (3) Expect complaint of dry mouth if anticholinergics given.
      (4) Observe for side effects—narcotics may cause nausea and vomiting, hypotension, arrhythmias, and/or respiratory depression.
      (5) Quiet environment until transported to operating room (OR).
      (6) Anticipate antibiotics to start "on call" to OR.
   g. Note completeness of chart:
      (1) Surgical checklist completed.
      (2) Vital signs recorded.
      (3) Routine laboratory reports present.
      (4) Preoperative medications given.
      (5) Significant client observations.
   h. Assist client's family in finding proper waiting room.
      (1) Inform family members that the surgeon will contact them after the procedure is over.
      (2) Explain length of time client is expected to be in recovery room.
      (3) Prepare family for any special equipment or devices that may be needed to care for client postoperatively (e.g., oxygen, monitoring equipment, ventilator, blood transfusions).

II. INTRAOPERATIVE PREPARATION—anesthesia: blocks transmission of nerve impulses, suppresses reflexes, promotes muscle relaxation, and in some instances achieves reversible unconsciousness.

A. Intravenous conscious sedation—produces sedation and amnesia in ambulatory procedures, short surgical or diagnostic procedures. Allays fear and anxiety, elevates pain threshold, maintains consciousness and protective reflexes, and returns client quickly to normal activities. Commonly used agents are *benzodiazepines* (midazolam [Versed], diazepam) and *narcotics* (fentanyl [Sublimaze], meperidine, morphine).

B. Regional anesthesia—purpose is to block pain reception and transmission in a specified area. Commonly used drugs are lidocaine HCl, tetracaine HCl, cocaine HCl, and procaine HCl. Types of regional anesthetics:

1. *Topical*—applied to mucous membranes or skin; drug anesthetizes the nerves immediately *below* the area. May be used for bronchoscopic or laryngoscopic examinations. *Side effects:* rare anaphylaxis.
2. *Local infiltration*—used for minor procedures; anesthetic drug is injected directly into the area to be incised, manipulated, or sutured. *Side effects:* rare anaphylaxis.
3. *Peripheral nerve block*—regional anesthesia is achieved by injecting drug into or around a nerve after it passes from vertebral column; procedure is named for nerve involved, such as brachial plexus block. Requires a high degree of anatomical knowledge. *Side effects:* may be absorbed into bloodstream. Observe for: signs of excitability, twitching, changes in vital signs, or respiratory difficulties.
4. *Field block*—a group of nerves is injected with anesthetic as the nerves branch from a major or main nerve trunk. May be used for dental procedures, plastic surgery. *Side effects:* rare.
5. *Epidural anesthesia*—anesthetizing drug is injected into the epidural space of vertebral canal; produces a bandlike anesthesia around body. Frequently used in obstetrics. Rare complications. Slower onset than spinal anesthesia; not dependent on client position for level of anesthesia; no postoperative headaches.
6. *Spinal anesthesia*—anesthetizing drug is injected into the subarachnoid space and mixes with spinal fluid; drug acts on the nerves as they emerge from the spinal cord, thereby inhibiting conduction in the autonomic, sensory, and motor systems.
   a. *Advantages:* rapid onset; produces excellent muscle relaxation.
   b. Utilization: surgery on lower limbs, inguinal region, perineum, and lower abdomen.
   c. *Disadvantages:*
      (1) Loss of sensation below point of injection for 2 to 8 hours—watch for signs of *bladder distention;* prevent injuries by maintaining alignment, keeping bedclothes straightened.
      (2) Client awake during surgical procedure—*avoid* light or upsetting conversations.
      (3) Leakage of spinal fluid from puncture site—keep flat in bed for 24 to 48 hours to prevent headache. Keep well hydrated to aid in spinal fluid replacement.
      (4) Depression of vasomotor responses—frequent checks of vital signs.
7. *Intravenous regional anesthesia*—used in an extremity whose circulation has been interrupted by a tourniquet; the anesthetic is injected into vein, and blockage is presumed to be achieved from extravascular leakage of anesthetic near a major nerve trunk. Precautions as for peripheral nerve block.

C. General anesthesia—a reversible state in which the client loses consciousness due to the inhibition of neuronal impulses in the brain by a variety of chemical agents; may be given intravenously, by inhalation, or rectally.

1. *Side effects:*
   a. Respiratory depression.
   b. Nausea, vomiting.
   c. Excitement.
   d. Restlessness.
   e. Laryngospasm.
   f. Hypotension.
2. **Nursing care plan/implementation**—Goal: *prevent hazardous drug interactions.*
   a. *Notify anesthesiologist* if client is taking any of the following drugs:
      (1) *Antidepressants,* such as Prozac—long half-life; monitor renal and liver function.
      (2) *Antihypertensives,* such as reserpine, hydralazine, and methyldopa—*potentiate* the hypotensive effects of anesthetic agents.
      (3) *Anticoagulants,* such as heparin, warfarin (Coumadin)—increase bleeding times, which may result in excessive *blood loss* or hemorrhage.
      (4) *Aspirin and NSAIDs*—decrease platelet aggregation and may result in increased *bleeding.*
      (5) *Steroids,* such as cortisone—anti-inflammatory effect may *delay* wound healing.
   b. *Stages of inhalation anesthesia and nursing goals:*
      (1) Stage I—extends from beginning of induction to loss of consciousness. **Nursing goal:** *reduce external stimuli,* because all movement and noises are exaggerated for the client and can be highly distressing.
      (2) Stage II—extends from loss of consciousness to relaxation; stage of delirium and

excitement. **Nursing goal:** *prevent injury* by assisting anesthesiologist to restrain client if necessary; maintain a quiet, nonstimulating environment.

(3) Stage III—extends from loss of lid reflex to cessation of voluntary respirations. **Nursing goal:** *reduce risk of untoward effects* by preparing the operative site, assisting with procedures, and observing for signs of complications.

(4) Stage IV—indicates overdose and consists of respiratory arrest and vasomotor collapse due to medullary paralysis. **Nursing goal:** *promote restoration of ventilation and vasomotor tone* by assisting with cardiac arrest procedures and by administering *cardiac stimulants* or *narcotic antagonists* as ordered.

D. Intravenous agents—rapid and pleasant induction of anesthesia. Three categories: *barbiturates* (thiopental), *narcotics,* and *neuromuscular blocking agents* (succinylcholine, curare, pancuronium). Ketamine also used—may produce *emergence delirium.* IV drugs require liver metabolism and renal excretion.

E. Hypothermia—a specialized procedure in which the client's body temperature is lowered to 28° to 30°C (82° to 86°F).

1. Reduces tissue metabolism and oxygen requirements.
2. Used in heart surgery, brain surgery, and surgery on major blood vessels.
3. **Nursing care plan/implementation:**
   a. Goal: *prevent complications.*
      (1) Monitor vital signs for shock.
      (2) Note level of consciousness.
      (3) Record intake and output accurately.
      (4) Maintain good body alignment; reposition to prevent edema, pressure, or discoloration of skin.
      (5) Maintain patent IV.
   b. Goal: *promote comfort.*
      (1) Apply blankets to rewarm and prevent shivering.
      (2) Mouth care.
   c. Goal: *observe for indications of* ***malignant hyperthermia***—common during induction; may occur 24 to 72 hours postoperatively. Genetic defect of muscle metabolism; early sign is unexplained ventricular dysrhythmia, tachypnea, cyanosis, skin mottling; elevated temperature is not reliable indicator.
      (1) Administer 100% O_2.
      (2) Cool with ice packs or cooling blankets.
      (3) Give dantrolene (muscle relaxant) per order.

F. Evaluation/outcome criteria: complete reversal of anesthetic effects (e.g., spontaneous respirations, pupils react to light). No indication of intraoperative complications—cardiac arrest, laryngospasm, aspiration, hypotension, malignant hyperthermia.

III. POSTOPERATIVE EXPERIENCE

A. Assessment:

1. *Subjective data:*
   a. Pain: location, onset, intensity.
   b. Nausea.
2. *Objective data:*
   a. Operative summary:
      (1) Type of operation performed.
      (2) Pathological findings if known.
      (3) Anesthesia and medications received.
      (4) Problems during surgery that will affect recovery (e.g., arrhythmias, bleeding [estimated blood loss]).
      (5) Fluids received: type, amount.
      (6) Need for drainage or suction apparatus.
   b. Observations:
      (1) Patency of airway.
      (2) Vital signs.
      (3) Skin color and dryness.
      (4) Level of consciousness.
      (5) Status of reflexes.
      (6) Dressings.
      (7) Type and rate of IV infusion and blood transfusion.
      (8) Tubes/drains: urinary, chest, Penrose, Hemovac; note color and amount of drainage.

B. Analysis/nursing diagnosis:

1. *Ineffective breathing pattern* related to general anesthesia.
2. *Ineffective airway clearance* related to absent or weak cough.
3. *Risk for aspiration* related to vomiting.
4. *Pain* related to surgical incision.
5. *Altered tissue perfusion* related to shock.
6. *Risk for fluid volume deficit* related to blood loss.
7. *Risk for injury* related to disorientation.
8. *Risk for infection* related to disruption of skin integrity.
9. *Urinary retention* related to anesthetic effects.
10. *Constipation* related to decreased peristalsis.

C. Nursing care plan/implementation—*immediate postanesthesia nursing care:* refers to time following surgery that is usually spent in the recovery room (1 to 2 hours).

1. Goal: *promote a safe, quiet, nonstressful environment.*
   a. Side rails up at all times.
   b. Nurse in constant attendance.
2. Goal: *promote lung expansion and gas exchange.*

3. Goal: *Prevent aspiration and atelectasis.*

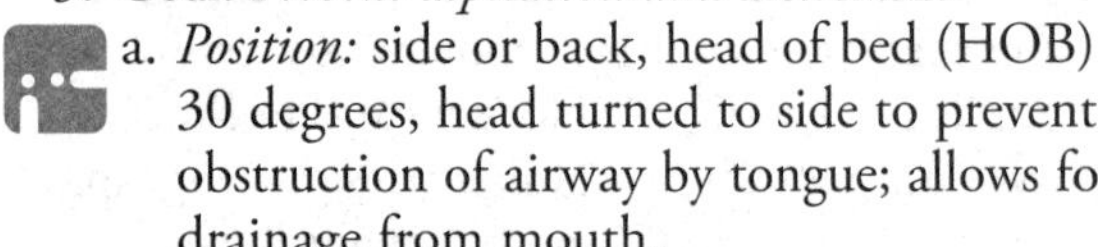

   a. *Position:* side or back, head of bed (HOB) 30 degrees, head turned to side to prevent obstruction of airway by tongue; allows for drainage from mouth.
   b. Airway: leave the oropharyngeal or nasopharyngeal airway in place until client awakens and begins to eject; gagging and vomiting may occur if not removed before pharyngeal reflex returns.
   c. After removal of airway: turn on side in a *lateral position;* support upper arm with pillow.
   d. Suction: remove excessive secretions from mouth and pharynx.
   e. Encourage coughing and deep breathing: aids in upward movement of secretions.
   f. Give humidified oxygen as necessary: reduces respiratory irritation and keeps bronchotracheal secretions soft and moist.
   g. Mechanical ventilation: respirators if needed (see Ventilators in **Chapter 11, p. 836**).
4. Goal: *promote and maintain cardiovascular function.*
   a. Vital signs, as ordered: usually q5–15 min until stable; continuous pulse oximetry.
      (1) Compare with preoperative vital signs.
      (2) **Immediately report:** systolic blood pressure that *drops 20* mm Hg or more, a pressure *below 80* mm Hg, or a pressure that continually drops 5 to 10 mm Hg over several readings; pulse rates *under 60 or over 110* beats/min, or irregularities; respirations *over 30*/min; becoming shallow, quiet, slow; use of neck and diaphragm muscles (symptoms of *respiratory depression*); stridorous breath sounds.
   b. Observe for other alterations in circulatory function—pallor; thready pulse; cold, moist skin; decreased urine output, restlessness.
      (1) **Immediately** report to physician.
      (2) Initiate oxygen therapy.
      (3) Place client in shock position unless contraindicated—feet elevated, legs straight, head *slightly* elevated to increase venous return.
   c. Intravenous infusions: time, rate, orders for added medications.
   d. Monitor *blood transfusions* if ordered: observe for signs of *reaction* (chills, elevated temperature, urticaria, laryngeal edema, and wheezing). **Table 6.9** illustrates the nursing care plan/implementation.
   e. If reaction occurs, **immediately stop** transfusion and notify physician. Send **STAT** urine to laboratory.
5. Goal: *promote psychological equilibrium.*
   a. Reassure on awakening—orient frequently.
   b. Explain procedures even though client does not appear alert.
   c. Answer client's questions briefly and accurately.
   d. Maintain quiet, restful environment.
   e. *Comfort measures:*
      (1) Good body alignment.
      (2) Support dependent extremities to *avoid* pressure areas and possible nerve damage.
      (3) Check for constriction: dressings, clothing, bedding.
      (4) Check IV sites frequently for patency and signs of infiltration (swelling, blanching, cool to touch).
6. Goal: *maintain proper function of tubes and apparatus* (see **Table 11.5, pp. 839–842**).

D. Nursing care plan/implementation—*general postoperative nursing care:* refers to period of time from

(text continues on page 374)

ADULT

Table 6.9

Postoperative Complications

Condition and Etiology	Assessment: Signs and Symptoms	Nursing Care Plan/Implementation
Respiratory Complications—Most Common Are Atelectasis, Pneumonias (Lobar, Bronchial, and Hypostatic), and Pleuritis; Other Complications Are Hemothorax and Pneumothorax		
Atelectasis—undetected preoperative upper respiratory infections, aspiration of vomitus: irritation of the tracheobronchial tree with increased secretions of mucus due to intubation and inhalation anesthesia, a history of heavy smoking, or chronic obstructive pulmonary disease; severe postoperative pain, or high abdominal or thoracic surgery, which inhibits deep breathing; and debilitation or old age, which lowers the client's resistance	*Dyspnea;* ↑ temperature; absent or diminished breath sounds over affected area, asymmetrical chest expansion, ↑ respirations and pulse rate; tracheal shift to affected side when severe; anxiety and restlessness	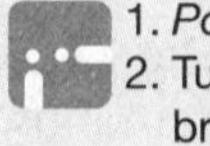 1. *Position:* unaffected side 2. Turn, cough, and deep breathe; encourage use of inspirometer hourly while awake 3. *Postural drainage* 4. Nebulization 5. *Force* fluids if not contraindicated

Table 6.9

Postoperative Complications—cont'd

Condition and Etiology	Assessment: Signs and Symptoms	Nursing Care Plan/Implementation
Pneumonia—see *Atelectasis* for etiology	Rapid, shallow, painful respirations; crackles; diminished or absent breath sounds; asymmetrical lung expansion; chills and fever, productive cough, rust-colored sputum; and circumoral and nailbed cyanosis	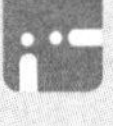 1. *Position of comfort*—semi-Fowler's to high Fowler's 2. *Force* fluids to 3,000 mL/day 3. Provide humidification of air and oxygen therapy 4. Oropharyngeal suction prn 5. Assist during coughing 6. Administer *antibiotics* and *analgesics* as ordered 7. *Diet:* high calorie, as tolerated 8. Cautious disposal of secretions; proper oral hygiene 9. Respiratory treatments as ordered
Pleuritis—see *Atelectasis* for etiology	Knifelike chest pain on inspiration; intercostal tenderness; splinting of chest by client; rapid, shallow respirations; pleural friction rub; ↑ temperature; malaise	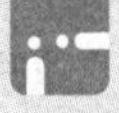 1. *Position: affected* side to splint the chest 2. Manually splint client's chest during cough  3. Administer *analgesics* as ordered
Hemothorax—chest surgery, gunshot or knife wounds, and multiple fractures of chest wall	Chest pain; increased respiratory rate; dyspnea, decreased or absent breath sounds; decreased blood pressure; tachycardia, and *mediastinal shift* may occur (heart, trachea and esophagus, great vessels are pushed toward unaffected side)	1. Observe vital signs closely for signs of shock and respiratory distress 2. Assist with *thoracentesis* (needle aspiration of fluid) 3. Assist with insertion of chest tube to *closed-chest drainage* (see care of water-seal drainage system, **Table 11.5 and Fig.11.2, pp. 840, 843**)
Pneumothorax, closed or tension—thoracentesis (needle nicks the lung), rupture of alveoli or bronchi due to accidental injury, and chronic obstructive lung disease	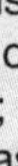 Marked dyspnea, sudden sharp chest pain, subcutaneous emphysema (air in chest wall tissue); cyanosis; tracheal shift to unaffected side; hyperresonance on percussion, decreased or absent breath sounds; increased respiratory rate, tachycardia; asymmetrical chest expansion, feeling of pressure within chest; *mediastinal shift*—severe dyspnea and cyanosis, deviation of larynx and trachea toward unaffected side, deviation either medially or laterally of apex of heart, decreased blood pressure; distended neck veins; increased pulse and respirations	1. Remain with client—keep as calm and quiet as possible; **STAT** chest x-ray 2. *Position:* high Fowler's (sitting) 3. Notify physician through another nurse, and have thoracentesis equipment brought to bedside 4. Administer oxygen as necessary 5. Take vital signs to evaluate respiratory and cardiac function 6. Assist with *thoracentesis* 7. Assist with chest tube insertion and maintenance of *closed-chest drainage*
Circulatory Complications—Shock, Thrombophlebitis, Pulmonary Embolism, and Disseminated Intravascular Coagulation (DIC)		
Shock—hemorrhage, sepsis, decreased cardiac contractility (myocardial infarction, cardiac failure, tamponade), drug sensitivities, transfusion reactions, pulmonary embolism, and emotional reaction to pain or deep fear	Dizziness; fainting; restlessness; anxiety; ↓ LOC *BP:* ↓ or falling *Pulse:* weak, thready *Respirations:* ↑, shallow *Skin:* pale, cool, clammy, cyanotic, ↓ temperature; Oliguria CVP <5 cm H_2O; Thirst	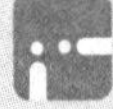 1. *Position:* foot of bed *raised* 20 degrees, knees *straight,* trunk horizontal, head slightly *elevated; avoid* Trendelenburg's position 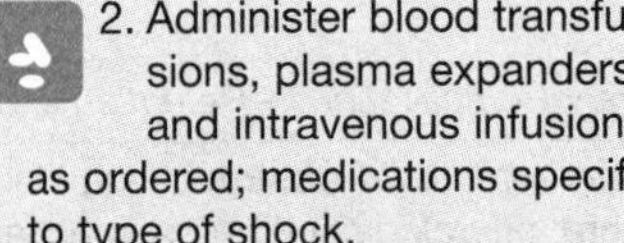 2. Administer blood transfusions, plasma expanders, and intravenous infusions as ordered; medications specific to type of shock. 3. Check: vital signs, CVP, temperature 4. Insert urinary catheter to monitor hourly urine output 5. Administer oxygen as ordered

Continued

Table 6.9

Postoperative Complications—cont'd

Condition and Etiology	Assessment: Signs and Symptoms	Nursing Care Plan/Implementation
Deep vein thrombosis (thrombophlebitis)—injury to vein wall by tight leg straps or leg holders during gynecological surgery; hemoconcentration due to dehydration or fluid loss; stasis of blood in extremities due to postoperative circulatory depression; prolonged immobility; placement of catheters (peripherally inserted central catheter [PICC] line, femoral line) that impede venous flow	Calf pain or cramping in affected extremity, redness and swelling (the left leg is affected more frequently than the right); slight fever, chills; *Homans'* sign and tenderness over the anteromedial surface of thigh; decreased pulse in affected extremity due to swelling and venous congestion	1. Maintain complete bedrest, *avoiding positions* that restrict venous return 2. Apply elastic stockings to prevent swelling and pooling of venous blood 3. Apply warm, moist soaks to area as ordered 4. Administer *anticoagulants* as ordered 5. Use bed cradle over affected limb 6. Provide active and passive ROM exercises in unaffected limb
Pulmonary embolism—obstruction of a pulmonary artery by a foreign body in bloodstream, usually a blood clot that has been dislodged from its original site	*Sudden*, severe stabbing chest pain; *severe* dyspnea; cyanosis; *rapid* pulse; anxiety and apprehension; pupillary dilation; *profuse* diaphoresis; *loss of* consciousness	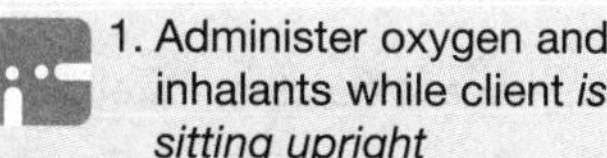 1. Administer oxygen and inhalants while client *is sitting upright* 2. Maintain bedrest and frequent reassurance 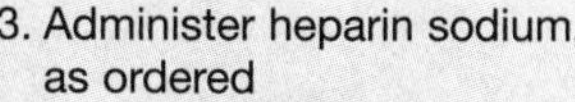 3. Administer heparin sodium, as ordered 4. Administer *analgesics*, such as morphine SO_4, to reduce pain and apprehension
Disseminated Intravascular Coagulation (DIC) (see **p. 429**).		
Wound Complications—Infection, Dehiscence, and Evisceration		
Wound infection—obesity or undernutrition, particularly protein and vitamin deficiencies; *decreased* antibody production in aged; *decreased* phagocytosis in newborn; metabolic disorder, such as diabetes mellitus, Cushing's syndrome, malignancies, and shock; breakdown in aseptic technique	Redness, tenderness, and heat in area of incision; wound drainage; ↑ temperature; ↑ pulse rate.	1. Assist in cleansing and irrigation of wound and insertion of a drain 2. Give *antibiotics* as ordered; observe responses
Wound dehiscence and evisceration—obesity and undernutrition, particularly protein and vitamin C deficiencies; immunosuppression; metabolic disorders, cancer; liver disease; common site is midline abdominal incision, frequently about 7 days postoperatively; precipitating factors include: abdominal distention, vomiting, coughing, hiccups, and uncontrolled motor activity	Slow parting of wound edges with a gush of pinkish serous drainage; or rapid parting with coils of intestines escaping onto the abdominal wall; the latter accompanied by pain and often by vomiting. Client reports "giving" sensation.	1. *Position:* bedrest, low Fowler's or horizontal position 2. Notify physician **STAT** 3. Cover exposed coils of intestines with sterile towels or dressing and keep moist with sterile normal saline 4. Monitor vital signs frequently 5. Remain with client; reassure that physician is coming 6. Prepare for physician's arrival; set up IV, suction equipment, and nasogastric tube; obtain sterile gown, mask, gloves, towels, and warmed normal saline. 7. Notify surgery that client will be returning to operating room
Urinary Complications—Retention and Infections		
Urinary retention—obstruction in bladder or urethra; neurological disease; mechanical trauma as in childbirth or gynecological surgery; psychological conditioning that inhibits voiding in bed; prolonged bedrest; pain with lower abdominal surgery; epidural narcotics	Inability to void within 8 hours postsurgery, despite adequate fluid replacement; palpable bladder, frequent voiding of small amounts of urine or dribbling; suprapubic pain	1. Assist client to stand, or use bedside commode if not contraindicated 2. Provide privacy 3. Reduce tension, provide support 4. Use warm bedpan

Table 6.9

Postoperative Complications—cont'd

Condition and Etiology	Assessment: Signs and Symptoms	Nursing Care Plan/Implementation
		5. Run tap water 6. Place client's feet in warm water 7. Pour warm water over perineum 8. Catheterize if conservative measures fail
Urinary tract infections—urinary retention, bladder distention, repeated or prolonged catheterization	*Urinary:* burning and frequency *Pain:* low back or flank Pyuria, hematuria; ↑ temperature, chills; anorexia; positive urine culture	1. *Push fluids* to 3,000 mL daily, unless contraindicated 2. *Avoid* stimulants such as caffeine 3. Give *antibiotics,* sulfonamides, or acidifying agents as ordered 4. Give perianal care after each bowel movement
Gastrointestinal Complications—Gastric Distention, Paralytic Ileus, and Intestinal Obstruction		
Gastric distention—depressed gastric motility due to sympathoadrenal stress response; idiosyncrasy to drugs: emotions, pain, shock; fluid and electrolyte imbalances	Feeling of fullness, hiccups, overflow vomiting of dark, foul-smelling liquid; severe retention leads to decreased blood pressure (due to pressure on vagus nerve) and other symptoms of shock syndrome	1. Report signs to physician **immediately** 2. Insert or assist in insertion of NG tube; attach to intermittent suction 3. Irrigate NG tube with *saline* (water will deplete electrolytes and result in metabolic alkalosis) 4. Administer IV infusions with electrolytes as ordered
Paralytic ileus—see *Gastric distention*	Greatly decreased or absent bowel sounds, failure of either gas or feces to be passed by rectum; nausea and vomiting; abdominal tenderness and distention; fever; dehydration	1. Notify physician 2. Insert or assist with insertion of *NG tube*; attach to low, intermittent suction 3. Insert rectal tube 4. Administer IV infusion with electrolytes as ordered 5. Irrigate nasogastric tube with saline 6. Assist with insertion of *Miller-Abbott* tube if indicated 7. Administer medications to increase peristalsis as ordered
Intestinal obstruction—due to poorly functioning anastomosis, hernia, adhesions, fecal impaction	Severe, colicky abdominal pains, mild to severe abdominal distention, nausea and vomiting, anorexia and malaise; fever; lack of bowel movement; electrolyte imbalance; high-pitched tinkling bowel sounds	1. Assist with insertion of nasoenteric tube and attach to intermittent suction 2. Maintain IV infusions with electrolytes 3. Encourage nasal breathing to *avoid* air swallowing 4. Check abdomen for distention and bowel sounds every 2 hours 5. Encourage verbalization 6. Plan rest periods for client 7. Administer oral hygiene frequently
Transfusion Reactions—Allergic, Febrile, and Hemolytic		
Allergic and febrile reactions—unidentified antigen or antigens in donor blood or transfusion equipment; previous reaction to transfusions; small thrombi; bacteria; lysed red blood cells	Fever to 103°F, may have *sudden* onset; chills; itching; erythema; urticaria; nausea, vomiting; dyspnea and wheezing, occasionally	1. **Stop** transfusion and notify physician 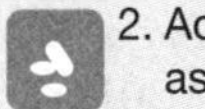 2. Administer *antihistamines,* as ordered 3. Send **STAT** urine to laboratory for analysis

Continued

ADULT

Table 6.9

Postoperative Complications—cont'd

Condition and Etiology	Assessment: Signs and Symptoms	Nursing Care Plan/Implementation
		4. Institute *cooling* measures if indicated 5. Maintain *strict* input and output records 6. Send remaining blood to laboratory for analysis, and order recipient blood sample for *analysis*
Hemolytic reaction—infusion of incompatible blood (less common, more serious)	*Early:* chills and fever; throbbing headache, feeling of burning in face; hypotension; tachycardia; chest, back, or flank pain; nausea, vomiting; feeling of doom; *later:* spontaneous and diffuse bleeding; icterus; oliguria; anuria; hemoglobinuria	1. **Stop infusion immediately;** take vital signs and notify physician 2. Send client blood sample and unused blood to laboratory for analysis 3. Send **STAT** urine to laboratory 4. Save *all* urine for observation of discoloration 5. Administer parenteral infusions to combat shock, as ordered 6. Administer medications as ordered—*diuretics, sodium bicarbonate, hydrocortisone*, and *vasopressors*
Emotional Complications		
Emotional disturbances—grief associated with loss of body part or loss of body image; previous emotional problems; decreased sensory and perceptual input; sensory overload; fear and pain; decreased resistance to stress as a result of age, exhaustion, or debilitation	Restlessness, insomnia, depression, hallucinations, delusions, agitation, suicidal thoughts	1. Report symptoms to physician 2. Encourage verbalization of feelings; give realistic assurance 3. Orient to time and place as necessary 4. Provide safety measures, such as side rails 5. Keep room lit, to reduce incidence of visual hallucinations 6. Administer *tranquilizers* as ordered. 7. Use restraints as a *last* resort

ADULT

admission to the general nursing unit until anticipated recovery and discharge from the hospital (see **Table 6.9** for a review of postoperative complications).

1. Goal: *promote lung expansion, gaseous exchange, and elimination of bronchotracheal secretions.*
   a. Turn, cough, and deep breathe q2h.
   b. Use incentive spirometer as ordered to enable client to observe depth of ventilation.
   c. Administer nebulization as ordered to help mobilize secretions.
   d. Encourage hydration to thin mucous secretions.
   e. Assist in ambulation as soon as allowed.
2. Goal: *provide relief of pain.*
   a. Assess type, location, intensity, and duration; possible causative factors, such as poor body alignment or restrictive bandages.
   b. Observe and evaluate reaction to discomfort. Use scale: 1 to 10 numerical or pictorial.
   c. Use *comfort measures,* such as back rubs and proper ventilation, staying with client and encouraging verbalization.
   d. Reduce incidence of pain: change position frequently; *support dependent* extremities with pillows, sandbags, and footboards; keep bedding dry and straight.
   e. Give *analgesics* or *tranquilizers* as ordered; assure client that they will help.
   f. Observe for desired and untoward effects of medication.
3. Goal: *promote adequate nutrition and fluid and electrolyte balance.*
   a. Parenteral fluids, as ordered.
   b. Monitor blood pressure, I&O to assess adequate, deficient, or excessive extracellular fluid volume.

c. *Diet: liquid* when nausea and vomiting stop and bowel sounds are established; progress as ordered.

4. Goal: *assist client with elimination.*
   a. Encourage voiding within 8 to 10 hours after surgery.
      (1) Allow client to stand or use commode, if not contraindicated.
      (2) Run tap water or soak feet in warm water to promote micturition.
      (3) Catheterization if bladder is distended and conservative treatments have failed.
   b. Maintain accurate I&O records.
   c. Expect bowel function to return in 2 to 3 days.
5. Goal: *facilitate wound healing and prevent infection.*
   a. Incision care: *avoid* pressure to enhance venous drainage and prevent edema.
   b. *Elevate* injured extremities to reduce swelling and promote venous return.
   c. Support or splint incision when coughing.
   d. Check dressings q2h for drainage.
   e. Change dressings on draining wounds prn; *aseptic technique;* protective ointments to reduce skin irritation may be ordered.
   f. Carefully observe wound suction (e.g., *Jackson Pratt*), if applied, for kinking or twisting of the tubes.
6. Goal: *promote comfort and rest.*
   a. Recognize factors that may cause restlessness—fear, anxiety, pain, oxygen lack, wet dressings.
   b. *Comfort measures: analgesics* or *barbiturates;* apply oxygen as indicated; change positions; encourage deep breathing; massage back to reduce restlessness.
   c. Allow rest periods between care—group activities.
   d. Give *antiemetic* for relief of nausea and vomiting, as ordered.
   e. Vigorous oral hygiene (brushing) to prevent "surgical mumps" or parotitis from preoperative atropine or general anesthesia.
7. Goal: *encourage early movement and ambulation to prevent complications of immobilization.*
   a. Turn or reposition q2h.
   b. Range of motion (ROM): passive and active exercises.
   c. Encourage leg exercises.
   d. Use preventive treatments—antiembolic stockings, graduated compression stockings, or external pneumatic compression sleeves:
      (1) With compression stockings, highest pressure (100%) at ankles, lowest pressure (40%) at midthigh.
      (2) Compression sleeves, three chambers sequentially inflated-deflated to stimulate venous return.
   e. Assist with standing or use of commode if allowed.
   f. Encourage resumption of personal care as soon as possible.
   g. Assist with ambulation in room as soon as allowed. *Avoid* prolonged chair sitting because it enhances venous pooling and may predispose to thrombophlebitis. *Elevate* legs when chair sitting.

E. Evaluation/outcome criteria:

1. Incision heals without infection.
2. No complications (e.g., atelectasis, pneumonia, thrombophlebitis).
3. Normal bowel and bladder functions resume.
4. Carries out activities of daily living, self-care.
5. Accepts possible limitations: dietary, activity, body image (e.g., no depression, complies with treatment regimen).

PAIN MANAGEMENT

I. PAIN—the "fifth vital sign" in the care of clients; a complex subjective sensation; unpleasant sensory and emotional experience associated with real or potential tissue damage. *Pain* is considered to be whatever the person experiencing it says it is, existing whenever he or she says it does.

A. Classifications:

1. *Acute pain:* lasts typically less than 1 month; characterized by: tachycardia, tachypnea, increased BP, diaphoresis, dilated pupils. Responsive to analgesics.
2. *Chronic pain:* persists or is recurring for longer than 3 months; often characterized by: lassitude, sleep disturbance, decreased appetite, weight loss, diminished libido, constipation, depression. Rarely responsive to analgesics.
3. *Somatogenic* (organic/physiological):
   a. *Nociceptive:* somatic or visceral pain—sensations, normal pain transmission, such as aching or pressure (e.g., cancer pain, chronic joint and bone pain).
   b. *Neuropathic:* aberrant processes in peripheral and/or central nervous system; part of a defined neurological problem; sensations such as sharp, burning, shooting pain (e.g., nerve compression, polyneuropathy, central pain of stroke, phantom pain after amputation).
4. *Psychogenic* (without organic pathology sufficient to explain pain).

B. Components of pain experience—pain related to:

1. *Stimuli*—sources: chemical, ischemic, mechanical trauma, extremes of heat/cold.
2. *Perception*—viewed with fear by children, can be altered by level of consciousness, interpreted and

influenced by previous and current experience, is more severe when alone at night or immobilized.

3. *Response*—variations in physiological, cultural, and learned responses; anxiety is created; pain seen as justified punishment; pain used as means for attention-getting.

C. **Assessment:**

1. *Subjective data* **(Table 6.10):**
   a. *Site*—medial, lateral, proximal, distal.
   b. *Strength:*
      (1) Certain tissues are more sensitive.
      (2) Change in intensity.
      (3) Based on expectations.
      (4) Affected by distraction or concentration, state of consciousness.
      (5) Described as: slight, medium, severe, excruciating.
   c. *Quality*—aching, burning, crushing, dull, piercing, shifting, throbbing, tingling.
   d. *Antecedent factors*—physical exertion, eating, extreme temperatures, physical and emotional stressors (e.g., fear).
   e. *Previous experience*—influences reaction to pain.
   f. *Behavioral clues*—demanding, worried, irritable, restless, difficult to distract, sleepless.
2. *Objective data:*
   a. *Verbal clues*—moaning, groaning, crying.
   b. *Nonverbal clues*—clenching teeth, grimacing; splinting of body parts, body position, knees drawn up, involuntary reflex movements; tossing/turning, rhythmic rubbing movements; voice pitch and speed; eyes shut.
   c. *Physical clues*—breathing irregularities, abdominal distention; skin color changes, skin temperature changes; excessive salivation, perspiration.
   d. *Time/duration*—onset, duration, recurrence, interval, last occurrence.

D. **Analysis/nursing diagnosis:**

1. *Pain,* acute or chronic, related to specific client condition.
2. *Activity intolerance* related to discomfort.
3. *Sleep pattern disturbance* related to pain.
4. *Fatigue* related to state of discomfort or emotional stress.
5. *Ineffective individual coping* related to chronic pain.

E. **Nursing care plan/implementation:**

1. Goal: *provide relief of pain.*
   a. Assess level of pain; ask client to rate on scale of 0 to 10 (0 = no pain; 10 = worst pain) or smiling/sad faces. Use age-, condition-, and language-appropriate scale **(Table 6.11).**
   b. Determine cause and try nursing *comfort* measures *before* giving drugs:
      (1) *Environmental factors:* noise, light, odors, motion.
      (2) *Physiological needs:* elimination, hunger, thirst, fatigue, circulatory impairment, muscle tension, ventilation, pressure on nerves.
      (3) *Emotional:* fear of unknown, helplessness, loneliness (especially at night).
   c. *Relieve:* anger, anxiety, boredom, loneliness.
   d. Report **sudden, severe, new** pain; pain **not** relieved by medications or comfort measures; pain associated with **casts** or **traction.**
   e. *Remove pain stimulus:*
      (1) Administer pain medication—*nonopioids:* NSAIDs—ketorolac (Toradol); *opioids:* first-line analgesics include morphine, hydromorphone, fentanyl, oxycodone, hydrocodone (see **Table 8.13**); *adjuvants:* local anesthetics, sedatives, muscle relaxants; give at appropriate time intervals; do *not* withhold due to overestimated danger of addiction.

ADULT

Table 6.10

Required Pain Assessment on Admission for Clients Who are Hospitalized

Ask the client: "Do you have pain now?" "Have you had pain in the recent past?"
If "yes" to either question, the following data are obtained:

- Pain intensity (use a scale appropriate for the client population)
- Location (ask client to mark on diagram or point to the site)
- Quality, patterns of radiation, character (use client's own words)
- Onset, duration, variations, and patterns
- Alleviating and aggravating factors
- Present pain management regimen and effectiveness
- Pain management history (medication history, barriers to reporting pain and using analgesics, manner of expressing pain)
- Effects of pain (impact on daily life, function, sleep, appetite, relationships with others, emotions, concentration)
- Client's pain goal (pain intensity and goals related to function, activities, quality of life)
- Physical examination/observation of site(s) of pain

Source: Joint Commission on Accreditation of Healthcare Organizations, Oakbrook Terrace, IL, 1999. (www.jcaho.org)

Table 6.11

Format for Assessing Pain

FIRST, Assess the Pain:	
***F**requency*	Is it intermittent or constant?
***I**ntensity*	What is the quality of the pain? Sharp or dull? Throbbing? Squeezing?
***R**adiation*	Does the pain move to other parts of the body?
***S**everity*	On a scale of 1 to 10, how bad is the pain?
***T**iming*	When did the pain begin? How long does it last? Does anything make it worse or take the pain away? What precedes the pain?

(2) *Avoid* cold (to reduce immediate tissue reaction to trauma).
(3) Apply heat (to relieve ischemia).
(4) Change activity (e.g., restrict activity in cardiac pain).
(5) Change, loosen dressing.
(6) Comfort (e.g., smooth wrinkled sheets, change wet dressing).
(7) Give food (e.g., for ulcer).
(8) Decrease stimulation (e.g., ↓ bright lights, noise, temperature).

f. *Reduce pain receptor reaction.*
(1) Ointment (use as coating).
(2) Local anesthetics.
(3) Padding (of bony prominences).

g. Assist with medical-surgical interventions to *block pain impulse transmission:*
(1) Injection of local anesthetic into nerve (e.g., dental).
(2) Cordotomy—sever anterolateral spinal cord nerve tracts.
(3) Electrical stimulation—transcutaneous (skin surface), percutaneous (peripheral nerve).
(4) Peripheral nerve implant—electrode to major sensory nerve.
(5) Dorsal column stimulator—electrode to dorsal column.

h. *Minimize barriers to effective pain management:*
(1) Achieve "balanced analgesia"; around-the-clock administration of NSAIDs or acetaminophen if possible, continuous infusion, patient-controlled analgesia (PCA); combination therapy (opioids, nonopioids, adjuvants).
(2) Accept client and family report of pain.
(3) Discuss fear of addiction with client family (incidence <1% when opioids taken for pain relief).
(4) Discuss fear of respiratory depression with staff; preventable; related to sedation.

i. *Document response to pain relief measures.*

2. Goal: *use **nonpharmacological methods to reduce pain.***
   a. *Distraction,* such as TV (cerebral cortical activity blocks impulses from thalamus).
   b. *Aromatherapy*—assists in relaxation.
   c. *Hypnosis*—assess appropriateness for use for psychogenic pain and for anesthesia; client needs to be open to suggestion.
   d. *Acupuncture*—assess emotional readiness and belief in it.
3. Goal: *alter interpretation and response to pain.*
   a. Administer *narcotics*—result: no longer sees pain as disturbing.
   b. Administer *hypnotics*—result: changes perception and decreases reaction.
   c. Help client obtain interpersonal satisfaction from ways other than attention received when in pain.
4. Goal: *promote client control of pain and analgesia: patient-controlled analgesia (PCA),* an analgesia administration system designed to maintain optimal serum analgesia levels; safely delivers intermittent bolus doses of a narcotic analgesic; preset to maximum hourly dose.
   a. *Advantages:* decreased client anxiety; improved pulmonary function; fewer side effects.
   b. *Limitations:* requires an indwelling intravenous line; analgesia targets central pain, may not relieve peripheral discomfort; cost of PCA unit.
5. Goal: *health teaching.*
   a. Explain causes of pain and how to describe pain.
   b. Explain that it is acceptable to admit existence of pain.
   c. Relaxation exercises.
   d. Biofeedback methods of pain perception and control.
   e. Proper medication administration (PCA, continuous around-the-clock dosing), when necessary, for self-care.

F. Evaluation/outcome criteria:
1. Verbalizes comfort; awareness of pain decreased.
2. Knows source of pain; how to reduce stimulus and perception.

3. Uses alternative measures for pain relief.
4. Able to cope with pain (e.g., remains active, relaxed appearance; verbal and nonverbal clues of pain absent).

NEUROLOGICAL SYSTEM

I. TRAUMATIC INJURIES TO THE BRAIN

A. Primary trauma:

1. *Concussion*—transient disorder due to injury in which there is brief loss of consciousness due to paralysis of neuronal function; recovery is usually total.
2. *Contusion*—structural alteration of brain tissue characterized by extravasation of blood cells (bruising); injury may occur on side of impact or on opposite side (when cranial contents shift forcibly within the skull with impact).
3. *Laceration*—tearing of brain tissue or blood vessels due to a sharp bone fragment or object or tearing force.
4. *Fracture*—linear (may result in epidural bleed); comminuted or depressed (may tear dura and result in cerebrospinal fluid [CSF] leak); basilar (most serious). Basilar skull fracture may result in meningitis or brain abscess; bleeding from nose or ears; CSF present in drainage; bruising over mastoid process *(Battle sign)* and periorbital ecchymosis (raccoon eyes).

B. Secondary trauma (response to primary trauma):

1. *Hematomas:*
   a. *Subdural*—blood from ruptured or torn vein collects between arachnoid and dura; may be acute, subacute, or chronic.
   b. *Extradural* (epidural)—blood clot located between dura mater and inner surface of skull; most often from tearing of middle meningeal artery; **emergency** condition.
2. *Increased intracranial pressure* (see **II. INCREASED INTRACRANIAL PRESSURE, pp. 379–380**).

C. Mechanisms of injury:

1. Deformation (blow to the head).
2. Acceleration-deceleration (coup-contracoup)—forward and rebounding motion.
3. Rotation (tension, stretching, shearing force).

D. Pathophysiology of impaired CNS functioning:

1. Depressed neuronal activity in reticular activating system → depressed *consciousness* **(Table 6.12).**
2. Depressed neuronal functioning in lower brainstem and spinal cord → depression of reflex activity → decreased eye movements, unequal pupils → decreased response to light stimuli → widely dilated and fixed *pupils.*
3. Depression of respiratory center → altered respiratory pattern → decreased rate → *respiratory arrest.*

E. Risk factors: accidents—automobile, industrial and home, motorcycle, military.

F. Assessment:

1. *Subjective data:*
   a. Headache.
   b. Dizziness, loss of balance.
   c. Double vision.
   d. Nausea.
2. *Objective data:*
   a. Laceration or abrasion around face or head; profuse bleeding from scalp (highly vascular, poor vasoconstrictive abilities).
   b. Drainage from ears or nose (serosanguineous).
   c. Projectile vomiting, hematemesis.
   d. Vital signs indicating increased intracranial pressure (see **II. INCREASED INTRACRANIAL PRESSURE, pp. 379–380**).
   e. Neurological examination:
      (1) *Altered level of consciousness;* a numerical assessment, such as the Glasgow Coma Scale **(Table 6.13),** may be used. The lower the score, the poorer the prognosis, generally.

ADULT

Table 6.12

Levels of Consciousness

Stage	Characteristics
Alertness	Aware of time and place
Automatism	Aware of time and place but demonstrates abnormality of mood (euphoria to irritability)
Confusion	Inability to think and speak in coherent manner; responds to verbal requests but is unaware of time and place
Delirium	Restlessness and violent activity; may not comply with verbal instructions
Stupor	Quiet and uncommunicative; may appear conscious—sits or lies with glazed look; unable to respond to verbal instructions; bladder and rectal incontinence may occur
Semicoma	Unresponsive to verbal instructions but responds to vigorous or painful stimuli
Coma	Unresponsive to vigorous or painful stimuli

Table 6.13

Glasgow Coma Scale

Best eye-opening response	Purposeful and spontaneous: To voice To pain No response Untestable
Best verbal response	Oriented Disoriented Inappropriate words Incomprehensible sounds No response Untestable
Best motor response	Obeys commands Localizes pain Withdraws to pain Flexion to pain Extension to pain No response Untestable

(2) *Pupils*—equal, round, react to light; *or* unequal, dilated, unresponsive to light.
(3) *Extremities*—paresis or paralysis.
(4) *Reflexes*—hypotonia or hypertonia; *Babinski* present (flaring of great toe when sole is stroked).

G. Analysis/nursing diagnosis:

1. *Altered thought processes* related to brain trauma.
2. *Sensory/perceptual alteration* related to depressed neuronal activity.
3. *Risk for injury* related to impaired CNS functioning.
4. *Risk for aspiration* related to respiratory depression.
5. *Self-care deficit* related to altered level of consciousness.
6. *Ineffective breathing pattern* related to CNS trauma.

H. Nursing care plan/implementation:

1. Goal: *sustain vital functions and minimize or prevent complications.*
   a. Patent airway: endotracheal tube or tracheostomy may be ordered.
   b. Oxygen: as ordered (hypoxia increases cerebral edema).
   c. *Position: semiprone* or *prone* (coma position) with head level to prevent aspiration ***(keep off back);*** turn side to side to prevent stasis in lungs.
   d. Vital signs as ordered.
   e. *Neurological check:* pupils, level of consciousness, muscle strength; report changes.
   f. Seizure precautions: padded side rails.

   g. Medications as ordered:
      (1) *Steroids* (dexamethasone [Decadron]).
      (2) *Anticonvulsants* (phenytoin [Dilantin], phenobarbital).
      (3) *Analgesics* **(morphine contraindicated).**
   h. Cooling measures or hypothermia to reduce elevated temperature.
   i. Assist with *diagnostic tests:*
      (1) Lumbar puncture (**contraindicated** with increased intracranial pressure).
      (2) Electroencephalogram (EEG).
   j. *Diet:* NPO for 24 hours, progressing to clear liquids if awake.
   k. Fluids: IVs; nasogastric *tube feedings;* I&O.
   l. Monitor blood chemistries: sodium imbalance common with head injuries.
2. Goal: *provide emotional support and use comfort measures.*
   a. *Comfort:* skin care, oral hygiene; sheepskins; wrinkle-free linen.
   b. Eyes: lubricate q4h with artificial tears if periocular edema present.
   c. ROM—passive, active; physical therapy as tolerated.
   d. *Avoid* restraints.
   e. Encourage verbalization of concerns about changes in body image, limitations.
   f. Encourage family communication.

I. Evaluation/outcome criteria:

1. Alert, oriented—no residual effects (e.g., cognitive processes intact).
2. No signs of increased intracranial pressure (e.g., decreased respirations, increased systolic pressure with widening pulse pressure, bradycardia).
3. No paralysis—regains motor/sensory function.
4. Resumes self-care activities.

II. INCREASED INTRACRANIAL PRESSURE (ICP):

intracranial hypertension associated with altered states of consciousness.

A. Pathophysiology: increases in intracranial blood volume, cerebrospinal fluid, or brain tissue mass → increased intracranial pressure → impaired neural impulse transmission → cellular anoxia, atrophy.

B. Risk factors:

1. Congenital anomalies (hydrocephalus).
2. Space-occupying lesions (abscesses or tumors).
3. Trauma (hematomas or skull fractures).
4. Circulatory problems (aneurysms, emboli).
5. Inflammation (meningitis, encephalitis).

C. Assessment:

1. *Subjective data:*
   a. Headache (early, but nonspecific symptom).
   b. Nausea.
   c. Visual disturbance (diplopia).

ADULT

2. *Objective data:*
   a. Changes in level of consciousness (*early* sign).
   b. Pupillary changes—unequal **(emergency—notify physician, indicates herniation),** dilated, and unresponsive to light (*late* sign).
   c. *Vital signs*—changes are variable.
      (1) *Blood pressure*—gradual or rapid elevation, widened pulse pressure.
      (2) *Pulse*—bradycardia, tachycardia; significant sign is *slowing of pulse as blood pressure rises.*
      (3) *Respirations*—pattern changes (*Cheyne-Stokes,* apneusis, *Biot's*), deep and sonorous; hiccups.
      (4) *Temperature*—moderate elevation.
   d. Projectile vomiting (more common in children).
   e. *Diagnostic test:* head computed tomography (CT)—structural changes.

D. Analysis/nursing diagnosis:
1. *Altered cerebral tissue perfusion* related to increased intracranial pressure.
2. *Altered thought processes* related to cerebral anoxia.
3. *Ineffective breathing pattern* related to compression of respiratory center.
4. *Risk for aspiration* related to unconsciousness.
5. *Self-care deficit* related to altered level of consciousness.
6. *Impaired physical mobility* related to abnormal motor responses.

E. Nursing care plan/implementation: Goal: *promote adequate oxygenation and limit further impairment.*
1. *Vital signs:* report changes **immediately.**
2. Patent airway; keep alkalotic, to prevent increased intracranial pressure from elevated CO_2; hyperventilate if necessary.
3. Give medications as ordered:
   a. *Hyperosmolar diuretics* (mannitol, urea) to reduce brain swelling.
   b. *Steroids* (dexamethasone [Decadron]) for anti-inflammatory action.
   c. *Antacids* or histamine$_2$ (H_2) antagonist to prevent stress ulcer.
4. *Position:* head of bed *elevated* 30 degrees.
5. Fluids: *restrict;* strict I&O.
6. Cooling measures to reduce temperature, because fever increases ICP.
7. Prepare for surgical intervention (see **III. CRANIOTOMY,** following).

F. Evaluation/outcome criteria:
1. No irreversible brain damage—regains consciousness.
2. Resumes self-care activities.

III. CRANIOTOMY: excision of a part of the skull (burr hole to several centimeters) for exploratory purpose and biopsy; to remove neoplasms, evacuate hematomas or excess fluid, control hemorrhage, repair skull fractures, remove scar tissue, repair or excise aneurysms, and drain abscesses; produces minimal neurological deficit.

A. Analysis/nursing diagnosis:
1. *Altered cerebral tissue perfusion* related to edema.
2. *Altered thought processes* related to disorientation.
3. *Self-care deficit* related to continued neurological impairment.
4. Also see nursing diagnosis for **I. TRAUMATIC INJURIES TO THE BRAIN, p. 378; II. D. INCREASED INTRACRANIAL PRESSURE, p. 379;** and **THE PERIOPERATIVE EXPERIENCE, p. 365.**

B. Nursing care plan/implementation:
1. *Preoperative:*
   a. Goal: *obtain baseline measures.*
      (1) Vital signs.
      (2) Level of consciousness.
      (3) Mental, emotional status.
      (4) Pupillary reactions.
      (5) Motor strength and functioning.
   b. Goal: *provide psychological support:* listen; give accurate, brief explanations.
   c. Goal: *prepare for surgery.*
      (1) Cut hair; shave scalp (usually done in surgery); save hair if client/family desire.
      (2) Cover scalp with clean towel.
      (3) Insert indwelling Foley catheter as ordered.
2. *Postoperative:*
   a. Goal: *prevent complications and limit further impairment.*
      (1) *Vital signs (indications of complications):*
         (a) **Decreased blood pressure**—*shock.*
         (b) **Widened pulse pressure**—*increased ICP.*
         (c) **Respiratory failure**—*compression* of medullary *respiratory* centers.
         (d) **Hyperthermia**—disturbance of heat-regulating mechanism; *infection.*
      (2) Neurological:
         (a) Pupils—ipsilateral dilation *(increased ICP),* visual disturbances.
         (b) Altered level of consciousness.
         (c) Altered cognitive or emotional status—disorientation common.
         (d) Motor function and strength—hypertonia, hypotonia, seizures.
      (3) Blood gases, to monitor adequacy of ventilation.
      (4) Dressings: check frequently; *aseptic* technique; reinforce as necessary.
      (5) Observe for:
         (a) CSF leakage (glucose-positive drainage from nose, mouth, ears)—***report immediately.***

ADULT

(b) Periorbital edema—apply light ice compresses as necessary—remove crusts from eyelids; instill lubricant eyedrops.
(6) Check integrity of seventh cranial nerve (facial)—incomplete closure of eyelids.
(7) *Position:*
(a) *Supratentorial surgery* (cerebrum)—*semi-Fowler's* (30-degree elevation); may *not* lie on operative side.
(b) *Infratentorial* (brainstem, cerebellum)—*flat* in bed (prone); may turn to either side but *not* onto back.
(8) Fluids and food: NPO initially; tube feeding until alert and intact gag, swallow, and cough reflexes present. Aspiration risk.
(9) Medications as ordered:
(a) *Osmotic diuretics* (mannitol).
(b) *Corticosteroids* (dexamethasone [Decadron]).
(c) *Mild analgesics* (do *not* mask neurological or respiratory depression).
(d) *Stool softeners* to prevent constipation and straining.
(10) Orient frequently to person, time, place—to reduce restlessness, confusion.
(11) Side rails up for safety.
(12) *Avoid* restraints (may increase agitation and ICP).
(13) Ice bags to head to reduce headache.
(14) Activity: assist with ambulation.

b. Goal: *provide optimal supportive care.*
(1) Cover scalp once dressings are removed (scarves, wigs).
(2) Deal realistically with neurological deficits—facilitate acceptance, adjustment, independence.

c. Goal: *health teaching.*
(1) Prepare for physical, occupational, or speech therapy, as needed.
(2) Activities of daily living.

C. Evaluation/outcome criteria:
1. Regains consciousness—is alert, oriented.
2. Resumes self-care activities within limits of neurological deficits.

IV. EPILEPSY: seizure disorder characterized by sudden transient aberration of brain function; associated with motor, sensory, autonomic, or psychic disturbances.

A. Seizure: involuntary muscular contraction and disturbances of consciousness from abnormal electrical activity.

B. Risk factors:
1. Brain injury.
2. Infection (meningitis, encephalitis).
3. Water and electrolyte disturbances.
4. Hypoglycemia.
5. Tumors.
6. Vascular disorders (hypoxia or hypocapnia).

C. Generalized seizures:
1. *Tonic-clonic* (grand mal) seizures:
a. **Pathophysiology:** increased excitability of a neuron → possible activation of adjacent neurons → synchronous discharge of impulses → vigorous involuntary sustained muscle spasms (*tonic* contractions). Onset of neuronal fatigue → intermittent muscle spasms (*clonic* contractions) → cessation of muscle spasms → fatigue.
b. **Assessment:**
(1) *Subjective data*—aura: flash of light; peculiar smell, sound; feelings of fear; euphoria.
(2) *Objective data:*
(a) *Convulsive stage*—tonic and clonic muscle spasms, loss of consciousness, breath-holding, frothing at mouth, biting of tongue, urinary or fecal incontinence; lasts 2 to 5 minutes.
(b) *Postconvulsion*—headache, fatigue (postictal sleep), malaise, vomiting, sore muscles, choking on secretions, aspiration.

2. *Absence* (petit mal) seizures:
a. **Pathophysiology:** unknown etiology, momentary loss of consciousness (10 to 20 seconds); usually no recollection of seizure; resumes previously performed action.
b. **Assessment**—*objective data:*
(1) Fixation of gaze; blank facial expression.
(2) Flickering of eyelids.
(3) Jerking of facial muscle or arm.

3. *Minor motor* seizures:
a. *Myoclonic*—involuntary "lightning-like" jerking contraction of major muscles; may throw person to the floor; no loss of consciousness.
b. *Atonic*—brief, total loss of muscle tone; person falls to the floor; loss of consciousness (common in children).

D. Partial (focal) seizures:
1. *Partial motor:* arises from region in motor cortex (posterior frontal lobe); most commonly begins in upper extremities, spreading to face and lower extremity *(jacksonian march);* noting progression is important in identifying area of cortex involved.
2. *Partial sensory:* sensory symptoms occur with partial seizure activity; varies with region in brain; transient.
3. *Partial complex* (psychomotor): arises out of anterior temporal lobe; frequently begins with

an aura; characteristic feature is automatism (e.g., lip smacking, chewing, patting body, picking at clothes); lasts from 2 to 3 minutes to 15 minutes; do *not* restrain.

E. Analysis/nursing diagnosis:
1. *Risk for injury* related to convulsive disorder.
2. *Anxiety* related to sudden loss of consciousness.
3. *Self-esteem disturbance* related to chronic illness.
4. *Impaired social interaction* related to self-consciousness.

F. Nursing care plan/implementation (generalized seizures):
1. Goal: *prevent injury during seizure.*
   a. Do *not* force jaw open during convulsion.
   b. Do *not* restrict limbs—protect from injury; place something soft under head (towel, jacket, hands).
   c. Loosen constrictive clothing.
   d. Note: time, level of consciousness, type and duration of seizure.
2. Goal: *postseizure care:*
   a. *Turn on side* to drain saliva and facilitate breathing.
   b. Suction as necessary.
   c. Orient to time and place.
   d. Oral hygiene if tongue or cheek injured.
   e. Check vital signs, pupils, level of consciousness.
   f. Notify physician; medication may need adjusting.
3. Goal: *prevent or reduce recurrences of seizure activity.*
   a. Encourage client to identify precipitating factors.
   b. Moderation in diet and exercise.
   c. Medications as ordered: phenytoin (Dilantin); phenobarbital; carbamazepine (Tegretol); primidone (Mysoline); valproate (Depacon).
4. Goal: *health teaching.*
   a. Medications:
      (1) Actions, side effects (apathy, ataxia, hyperplasia of gums).
      (2) Complications with sudden withdrawal (*status epilepticus*—continuous seizure activity; give diazepam per order, O_2).
   b. Attitude toward life and treatment; adhere to medication program.
   c. Clarify misconceptions, fears—especially about insanity, bad genes.
   d. Maintain activities, interests—expect *no* driving until seizure free for period of time specified by state Department of Motor Vehicles.
   e. *Avoid:* stress; lack of sleep; emotional upset; alcohol.
   f. Relaxation techniques; stress management techniques.
   g. Use Medic Alert band or tag.
   h. Refer to appropriate community resources.

ADULT

G. Evaluation outcome criteria:
1. Avoids precipitating stimuli—achieves seizure control.
2. Complies with medication regimen.
3. Retains independence.

V. TRANSIENT ISCHEMIC ATTACKS (TIAs): temporary, complete, or relatively complete cessation of cerebral blood flow to a localized area of brain, producing symptoms (2 to 30 minutes) ranging from weakness ("drop attacks") and numbness to monocular blindness; an important precursor to stroke. Surgical intervention includes *carotid endarterectomy;* most common postoperative cranial nerve damage causes vocal cord paralysis or difficulty managing saliva and tongue deviation (cranial nerves VII, X, XI, XII); usually temporary; stroke may also occur.

VI. STROKE (cerebrovascular accident [CVA], brain attack): neurologic changes caused by interruption of blood supply to a part of the brain. **Ischemic stroke**—commonly due to thrombosis or embolism; thrombotic strokes more common. **Hemorrhagic stroke**—rupture of cerebral vessel, causing bleeding into the brain tissue; most common after age 50.

A. Pathophysiology: reduced or interrupted blood flow → interruption of nerve impulses down corticospinal tract → decreased or absent voluntary movement on one side of the body (fine movements are more affected than coarse movements); later, autonomous reflex activity → spasticity and rigidity of muscles.

B. Risk factors:
1. Hypertension (modifiable risk factor).
2. Prior ischemic episodes (TIAs).
3. Cardiovascular disease; atrial fibrillation.
4. Oral contraceptives.
5. Emotional stress.
6. Family history.
7. Advancing age.
8. Diabetes mellitus.

C. Assessment:
1. *Subjective data:*
   a. Weakness: sudden or gradual loss of movement of extremities on one side.
   b. Difficulty forming words.
   c. Difficulty swallowing (dysphagia).
   d. Nausea, vomiting.
   e. History of TIAs.
2. *Objective data:*
   a. *Vital signs:*
      (1) *BP—elevated* with thrombosis, normal with embolism. *Widened* pulse pressure with large ischemic strokes or hemorrhage.
      (2) *Temperature—elevated.*
      (3) *Pulse*—normal, slow.

(4) *Respirations*—tachypnea, altered pattern; deep; sonorous.
(5) CT scan of head—negative if no hemorrhage, indicates ischemic stroke.

b. Neurological (vary by type and location of stroke):
(1) Altered level of consciousness; progression to coma with hemorrhage.
(2) Pupils—unequal; vision—homonymous hemianopia.
(3) Ptosis of eyelid, drooping mouth.
(4) Paresis or paralysis (hemiplegia).
(5) Loss of sensation and reflexes.
(6) Incontinence of urine or feces.
(7) Aphasia (see **pp. 383–384**).

D. Analysis/nursing diagnosis:

1. *Impaired physical mobility* related to hemiplegia.
2. *Impaired swallowing* related to paralysis.
3. *Impaired verbal communication* related to aphasia.
4. *Risk for aspiration* related to unconsciousness.
5. *Sensory/perceptual alterations* related to altered cerebral blood flow, visual field blindness.
6. *Altered thought processes* related to cerebral edema.
7. *Self-care deficit* related to paresis or paralysis.
8. *Body image disturbance* related to hemiplegia.
9. *Total incontinence* related to interruption of normal nerve transmission.
10. *Impaired social interaction* related to aphasia or neurological deficit.
11. *Risk for impaired skin integrity* related to immobility.
12. *Unilateral neglect* related to cerebral damage.

E. Nursing care plan/implementation

1. Goal: *reduce cerebral anoxia.*
a. Patent airway:
(1) Oxygen therapy as ordered; suctioning to prevent aspiration.
(2) Turn, cough, deep breathe q2h due to high incidence of aspiration pneumonia.
b. Activity: bedrest, progressing to out of bed as tolerated.
c. *Position:*
(1) Maximize ventilation.
(2) Support with pillows when on side; use hand rolls and arm slings as ordered.

2. Goal: *promote cerebrovascular function and maintain cerebral perfusion.*
a. Vital signs; neurological checks.
b. Medications as ordered:
(1) **Ischemic stroke**—*thrombolytic agents* (recombinant tissue plasminogen activator [r-tPA]) within 3 hours of onset of stroke; *antihypertensives* only if BP >185 mm Hg systolic or 105 mm Hg diastolic; *mannitol* to decrease ICP; heparin **only** if risk for cardiogenic emboli; *antiplatelet agents* (aspirin, ticlopidine, clopidogrel) to decrease risk for thrombus formation.
(2) **Hemorrhagic stroke**—*antihypertensives* for systolic pressure >160 mm Hg; **never** treat with r-tPA; *mannitol* to decrease ICP.
c. *Fluids:* IVs to prevent hemoconcentration; I&O; weigh daily. Nutritional support as indicated.
d. ROM exercises to prevent contractures, muscle atrophy; deep vein thrombosis prophylaxis; early referral to physical therapy (PT).
e. Skin care and position changes to prevent decubiti.

3. Goal: *provide for emotional relaxation.*
a. Identify grief reaction to changes in body image. Early referral to occupational therapy (OT) if indicated.
b. Encourage expression of feelings, concerns. Early referral to speech therapy if indicated.

4. Goal: *client safety.*
a. Identify existence of *homonymous hemianopia* (visual field blindness) and *agnosia* (disturbance in sensory information).
b. Use side rails and assist as needed.
c. Remind to walk slowly, take adequate rest periods, ensure good lighting, look where client is going.

5. Goal: *health teaching.*
a. Exercise routines.
b. Diet: self-feeding, but assist as needed.
c. Resumption of self-care activities.
d. Use of supportive devices; transfer techniques.
e. Involvement of family in rehabilitation activities.

F. Evaluation/outcome criteria:

1. No complications (e.g., pneumonia).
2. Regains functional independence—resumes self-care activities.
3. Return of control over body functions (e.g., bowel, bladder, speech).

VII. APHASIA: impaired ability to understand or use commonly accepted words or symbols; interferes with ability to speak, write, or read; language center—usually left hemisphere (85% of population). *Dysarthria* is motor impairment—inability to articulate words.

A. Types and pathophysiology:

1. *Receptive (sensory)*—lesion usually in Wernicke's area of temporal lobe; difficulty understanding spoken word (*auditory* aphasia) or written word (*visual* aphasia).
2. *Expressive (motor)*—difficulty expressing thoughts in speech or writing (*motor* aphasia); understands written and spoken words. Three types: *anomic*—fluent speech, but unable to

ADULT

name objects, qualities, and conditions; *fluent*—articulate and grammatically correct, but no content or meaning; *nonfluent*—unable to select, organize, and initiate speech (involves Broca's area of brain); may affect writing.

B. Risk factors:
1. Vascular disease of the brain (brain attack).
2. Alzheimer's disease (degeneration).
3. Tumor.
4. Trauma.

C. Analysis/nursing diagnosis:
1. *Impaired verbal communication* related to cerebral cortex disorder.
2. *Powerlessness* related to inability to express needs/concerns.
3. *Impaired social interaction* related to difficulty communicating.

D. Nursing care plan/implementation:
1. Goal: *assist with communication:* client does best when rested; small improvements will occur up to 1 year after injury (age is a factor).
2. *Strategies:*
   a. *Nonfluent*—allow time to respond; support efforts to speak; acknowledge frustration of client—anticipate needs when appropriate; use picture board or flash cards, pointing, to encourage communication; assess efforts to communicate with open-ended questions.
   b. *Fluent*—face the client, speak slowly and distinctly, not loudly; use gestures, repeat instructions as needed; involve family in techniques to improve communication; acknowledge frustration.

E. Evaluation/outcome criteria:
1. Communication reestablished.
2. Minimal frustration exhibited.
3. Participates in speech therapy.

ADULT

VIII. BACTERIAL MENINGITIS (see **Chapter 5, pp. 265–266**).

IX. ENCEPHALITIS (also includes aseptic meningitis): inflammation of the brain and its coverings due to direct viral invasion, which usually results in a lengthy coma.

A. Pathophysiology: brain tissue injury → release of enzymes that increase vascular dilation, capillary permeability → edema formation → increased intracranial pressure → depression of CNS function.

B. Risk factors:
1. Arboviruses.
2. Enteroviruses (poliovirus, echovirus).
3. Herpesvirus.
4. Varicella-zoster (chickenpox).
5. Postinfection complication (measles, mumps, smallpox).

C. Assessment:
1. *Subjective data:*
   a. Headache—severe.
   b. Fever—*sudden.*
   c. Nausea, vomiting.
   d. Sensitivity to light (photophobia).
   e. Difficulty concentrating.
2. *Objective data:*
   a. Altered level of consciousness.
   b. Nuchal rigidity.
   c. Tremors; facial weakness.
   d. Nystagmus.
   e. Elevated temperature.
   f. *Diagnostic test:* lumbar puncture—fluid cloudy; *increased* neutrophils, protein.
   g. Laboratory data: blood—slight to moderate leukocytosis (about 14,000).

D. Analysis/nursing diagnosis:
1. *Self-care deficit* related to altered level of consciousness.
2. *Risk for injury* related to coma.
3. *Sensory/perceptual alteration* related to brain tissue injury.
4. *Altered thought processes* related to increased intracranial pressure.

E. Nursing care plan/implementation:
1. Goal: *support physical and emotional relaxation.*
   a. Vital signs; neurological signs as ordered.
   b. Seizure precautions.
   c. *Position:* to maintain patent airway; prevent contractures; ROM.
   d. Medications as ordered:
      (1) *Analgesics* for headache and neck pain.
      (2) *Antipyretics* for fever.
      (3) *Antivirals.*
      (4) *Anticonvulsants* for seizures.
      (5) *Antibiotics* for infection in aseptic meningitis.
      (6) *Osmotic diuretics* (mannitol) to reduce cerebral edema.
      (7) *Corticosteroids* for inflammation.
   e. No isolation.
2. Goal: *health teaching:* self-care activities with residual motor and speech deficits; physical therapy.

F. Evaluation/outcome criteria:
1. Regains consciousness; is alert, oriented.
2. Performs self-care activities with minimal assistance.

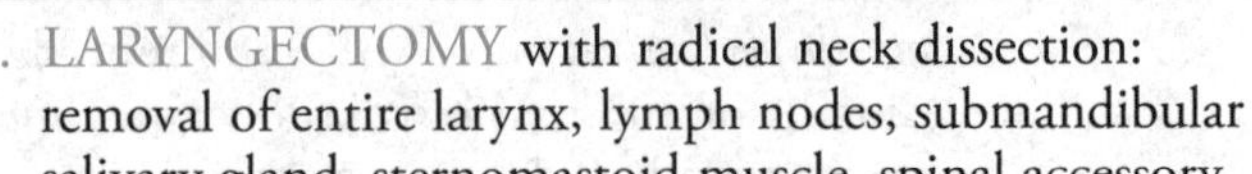

EYES, EARS, NOSE AND THROAT

I. LARYNGECTOMY with radical neck dissection: removal of entire larynx, lymph nodes, submandibular salivary gland, sternomastoid muscle, spinal accessory nerves, and jugular vein for cancer of the larynx that extends beyond the vocal cords. Permanent tracheostomy; new methods of speech will have to be learned.

Partial laryngectomy: removal of lesion on larynx. Client will be able to speak after operation, but quality of voice may be altered.

A. Assessment:

1. *Subjective data:*
   a. Feeling of lump in throat.
   b. *Pain:* Adam's apple; may radiate to ear.
   c. Dysphagia.
2. *Objective data:*
   a. Hoarseness: persistent (>2 weeks), progressive.
   b. Lymphadenopathy: cervical.
   c. Breath odor: foul.

B. Analysis/nursing diagnosis:

1. *Impaired verbal communication* related to removal of larynx.
2. *Body image disturbance* related to radical neck dissection.
3. *Ineffective airway clearance* related to copious amounts of mucus.
4. *Fear* related to diagnosis of cancer.
5. *Impaired swallowing* related to edema.
6. *Impaired social interaction* related to altered speech.

C. Nursing care plan/implementation:

1. *Preoperative care:*
   a. Goal: *provide emotional support and optimal physical preparation.*
      (1) Encourage verbalization of fears; answer all questions honestly, particularly about having no voice after surgery.
      (2) Referral: visit from person with laryngectomy (contact New Voice Club, Lost Chord, or International Association of Laryngectomees).
   b. Goal: *health teaching.*
      (1) Prepare for tracheostomy.
      (2) Other means to speak (esophageal "burp" speech, tracheoesophageal prosthesis or electronic artificial larynx).
2. *Postoperative care:*
   a. Goal: *maintain patent airway and prevent aspiration.*
      (1) *Position: semi-Fowler's* (elevate 30 to 45 degrees), preventing forward flexion of neck to reduce edema and keep airway open.
      (2) Observe for hypoxia:
         (a) *Early signs:* increased respiratory and pulse rates, apprehension, restlessness.
         (b) *Late signs:* dyspnea, cyanosis; swallowing difficulties—client should chew food well and swallow with water.
      (3) *Laryngectomy* tube care:
         (a) Observe for stridor (coarse, high-pitched inspiratory sound)—**report immediately.**
         (b) Have extra laryngectomy tube at bedside.
         (c) Suction with sterile equipment; 2 to 3 mL of sterile saline into stoma may be used to loosen secretions.
   b. Goal: *promote optimal physical and psychological function.*
      (1) Frequent mouth care.
      (2) *Wound:* exposed site; note color and amount of drainage.
      (3) *Tubes:* closed drainage system *(Hemovac, Jackson Pratt)* **(Fig. 6.2);** expect less than 100 up to 300 mL of serosanguineous drainage first postoperative day; drainage should decrease daily; observe patency.
      (4) Pain management—consider impact of impaired communication on assessment.
      (5) Post–drainage system removal—observe: skin flaps down, adherent to underlying tissue.
      (6) Use surgical *asepsis.*
      (7) Answer call bell *immediately;* use preestablished means of communication.
      (8) Reexplain all procedures while giving care.
      (9) Support head when lifting.

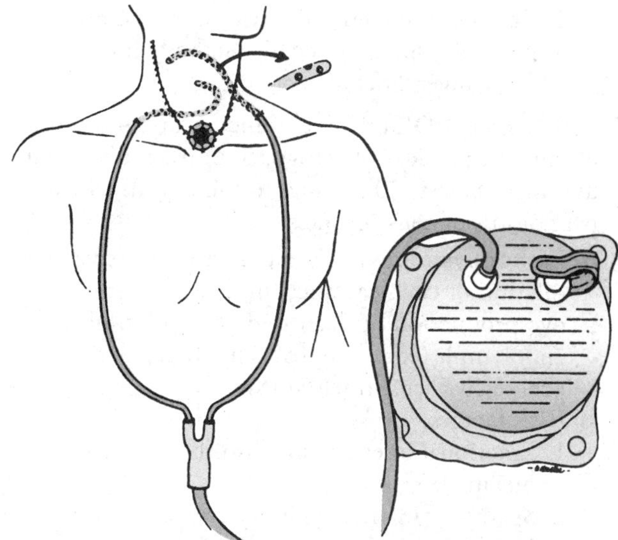

Figure 6.2 Closed drainage system for constant suction. Suction is maintained by a plastic container. The container serves as both suction source and receptacle for blood. It is emptied as required, and drainage tubes are left in the neck for approximately 3 days. (From De Weese, DD: *Saunders' Textbook of Otolaryngology.* Mosby, St. Louis, 1987. Out of Print.)

ADULT

c. Goal: *health teaching.*
(1) Referral: speech rehabilitation as soon as esophageal suture is healed.
(a) Information on laryngeal speech (International Association of Laryngectomees, American Cancer Society, American Speech and Hearing Association).
(b) *Esophageal speech* best learned in speech clinic—learn to burp column of air needed for speech; new voice sounds are natural but hoarse.
(2) *Stoma* care:
(a) Cover with scarf or shirt made of a porous material (material substitutes for nasal passage—warms and filters out particles).
(b) Use source of humidification ("mister" or commercial humidifier).
(c) *Caution* while bathing or showering, to decrease likelihood of aspiration.
(d) Swimming *not* recommended.
(e) Procedure for suctioning if cough ineffective.
(3) Simple ROM of neck; how to support head.
(4) Possible *contraindications:* use of talcum powder, tissues.

D. Evaluation/outcome criteria:
1. No surgical complications (e.g., no airway obstruction, infection, hemorrhage).
2. Learns alternative speech 30 to 60 days after surgery.
3. Demonstrates proper stoma care.
4. Resumes productive lifestyle (work, family).
5. Normal response to change in body image (e.g., anger, grief, denial).

ADULT

II. MÉNIÈRE'S DISEASE: chronic, recurrent disorder of inner ear; attacks of vertigo, tinnitus, and vestibular dysfunction; lasts 30 minutes to full day; usually no pain or loss of consciousness.

A. Pathophysiology: associated with excessive dilation of cochlear duct (unilateral) from overproduction or decreased absorption of endolymph (endolymphatic hydrops) → progressive sensorineural loss.

B. Risk factors:
1. Emotional or endocrine disturbance (diabetes mellitus).
2. Spasms of internal auditory artery.
3. Head trauma.
4. Allergic reaction.
5. High salt intake.
6. Smoking.
7. Ear infections.

C. Assessment:
1. *Subjective data:*
a. Tinnitus (constant or intermittent).
b. Headache; feeling of fullness or pressure in affected ear.
c. True vertigo: sudden attacks; room appears to spin.
d. Depression; irritability; withdrawal.
e. Nausea with sudden head motion.
2. *Objective data:*
a. Impaired hearing, especially *low* tones.
b. Change in gait; lack of coordination.
c. Vomiting with sudden head motion.
d. Nystagmus—during attacks.
e. *Diagnostic test:* caloric (cold water in ear canal)—may precipitate attack; audiometry—loss of hearing.

D. Analysis/nursing diagnosis:
1. *Risk for injury* related to vertigo, lack of coordination.
2. *Auditory sensory/perceptual alteration* related to progressive hearing loss.
3. *Anxiety* related to uncertainty of treatment.
4. *Risk for activity intolerance* related to sudden onset of vertigo.
5. *Sleep pattern disturbance* related to tinnitus.
6. *Ineffective individual coping* related to chronic disorder.

E. Nursing care plan/implementation:
1. Goal: *provide safety and comfort during attacks.*
a. Activity: bedrest during attack; side rails up; lower to chair or floor if attack occurs while standing; assist with ambulation (sudden dizziness common).
b. *Position:* recumbent; *affected ear uppermost* usually.
c. Identify prodromal symptoms (aura, ear pressure, increased tinnitus).
2. Goal: *minimize occurrence of attacks.*
a. Give medications as ordered:
(1) *Anticholinergics* (oral or transdermal scopolamine, atropine, glycopyrrolate [Robinul]) to minimize GI symptoms.
(2) *Antihistamines* (dimenhydrinate [Dramamine], diphenhydramine HCl [Benadryl]) to sedate vestibular system.
(3) *Antiemetics and antivertigo agents* (diazepam [Valium], meclizine HCl [Antivert]).
(4) *Diuretics* may help (hydrochlorothiazide) to decrease endolymphatic fluid.
b. *Diet: low* sodium (<2 gm/day).
c. *Avoid* precipitating stimuli: bright, glaring lights; noise; sudden jarring; turning head or eyes (stand in front of client when talking).

3. Goal: *health teaching.*
   a. *No* smoking (causes vasospasm) or alcoholic beverages (fluid retention, contraindicated with medications).
   b. Management of symptoms: play radio to mask tinnitus, particularly at night.
   c. Keep medication available at all times.
   d. Prepare for surgery if indicated (labyrinthectomy if hearing gone; or vestibular neurectomy to relieve vertigo and preserve hearing).

F. Evaluation/outcome criteria:
1. Decreased frequency of attacks.
2. Complies with treatment regimen and restrictions (e.g., low-sodium diet, no smoking).
3. Hearing preserved.

III. OTOSCLEROSIS: disease of the bone of otic capsule; insidious, progressive deafness; most common cause of conductive deafness; cause unknown.

A. Pathophysiology: formation of new spongy bone in labyrinth → fixation of stapes → prevention of sound transmission through ossicles to inner ear fluids.

B. Risk factors:
1. Heredity.
2. Women, puberty to 45 years.
3. Pregnancy.

C. Assessment:
1. *Subjective data:*
   a. Difficulty hearing—gradual loss in both ears.
2. *Diagnostic tests:*
   a. *Rinne* (tuning fork placed over mastoid bone)—*reduced* sound conduction by air and intensified by bone.
   b. *Weber* (tuning fork placed on top of head)—*increased* sound conduction to affected ear.
   c. *Audiometry—diminished* hearing ability.

D. Analysis/nursing diagnosis:
1. *Auditory sensory/perceptual alteration* related to hearing loss.
2. *Body image disturbance* related to hearing aid.
3. *Ineffective individual coping* related to grief reaction to loss.
4. *Impaired social interaction* related to hearing loss.

E. Nursing care plan/implementation, evaluation outcome criteria (see **IV. STAPEDECTOMY,** following).

IV. STAPEDECTOMY: removal of the stapes and replacing it with a prosthesis (steel wire, Teflon piston, or polyethylene); treatment for deafness due to otosclerosis, which fixes the stapes, preventing it from oscillating and transmitting vibrations to the fluids in the inner ear.

A. Analysis/nursing diagnosis:
1. *Sensory/perceptual alteration* related to edema and ear packing.
2. See **THE PERIOPERATIVE EXPERIENCE, p. 365,** for diagnoses relating to surgery.

B. Nursing care plan/implementation:
1. *Preoperative* health teaching.
   a. Important to keep head in position ordered by physician postoperatively.
   b. *Caution:* sneezing, blowing nose (keep mouth open), vomiting, coughing—all of which increase pressure in eustachian tubes (blow one side gently).
   c. Breathing exercises.
2. *Postoperative:*
   a. Goal: *promote physical and psychological equilibrium.*
      (1) *Position:* as ordered by physician—varies according to preference.
      (2) Activity: assist with ambulation; *avoid* rapid turning, which might increase vertigo.
      (3) Dressings: check frequently; may change cotton pledget in outer ear.
      (4) Give medications as ordered:
         (a) *Antiemetics.*
         (b) *Analgesics.*
         (c) *Antibiotics.*
      (5) Reassurance: reduction in hearing is normal; hearing may not immediately improve after surgery.
   b. Goal: *health teaching.*
      (1) Ear care: keep covered outdoors; keep outer ear plug clean, dry, and changed.
      (2) *Avoid:*
         (a) Water in ear for 6 weeks:
            (i) Use barrier when washing hair.
            (ii) Use two pieces of cotton; saturate outer piece with petroleum jelly.
         (b) Pressure or vibration from loud noise, flying, or heavy lifting until advised by physician.

C. Evaluation/outcome criteria:
1. Hearing improves—evaluate 1 month postoperatively (may require hearing aid).
2. Returns to work (usually 2 weeks after surgery).
3. Continues medical supervision.

V. DEAFNESS: (1) *Hard of hearing*—slight or moderate hearing loss that is serviceable for activities of daily living. (2) *Deaf*—hearing is nonfunctional for activities of daily living.

A. Risk factors:
1. *Conductive* hearing losses (transmission deafness):
   a. Impacted cerumen (wax).
   b. Foreign body in external auditory canal.
   c. Defects (thickening, scarring) of eardrum.
   d. Otosclerosis of ossicles.

2. *Sensorineural* hearing losses (perceptive or nerve deafness):
   a. Arteriosclerosis.
   b. Infectious diseases (mumps, measles, meningitis).
   c. Drug toxicities (quinine, streptomycin, neomycin SO_4).
   d. Tumors.
   e. Head traumas.
   f. High-intensity noises.
3. *Central* deafness:
   a. Tumors.
   b. Stroke (brain attack).
4. *Noise-induced or occupational noise* hearing loss:
   a. Blast injury.
   b. Firearms.
   c. Loud music.
5. *Aging* (presbycusis).

B. Assessment—*objective data:*
1. Facial expression: inattentive or strained.
2. Speech: excessive loudness or softness.
3. Frequent need to clarify content of conversation or inappropriate responses.
4. Tilting of head while listening.
5. Lack of response when others speak.
6. Audiological examinations:
   a. Pure tone air conduction test.
   b. Bone conduction test.
   c. Speech reception threshold.
   d. Word recognition.

C. Analysis/nursing diagnosis:
1. *Auditory/sensory/perceptual alteration* related to loss of hearing.
2. *Impaired social interaction* related to deafness.

D. Nursing care plan/implementation:
1. Goal: *maximize hearing ability and provide emotional support.*
   a. Gain person's attention before speaking; *avoid* startling.
   b. Provide adequate lighting so person can see who is speaking.
   c. Look at the person when speaking.
   d. Use nonverbal cues to enhance communication (e.g., writing, hand gestures, pointing).
   e. Speak slowly, distinctly; do *not* shout (excessive loudness distorts voice).
   f. If person does not understand, use different words; write it down.
   g. Use alternative communication system:
      (1) Speech (lip) reading.
      (2) Sign language.
      (3) Hearing aid.
      (4) Paper and pencil.
      (5) Flash cards.
   h. Supportive, nonstressful environment; alert staff to client's hearing impairment.
2. Goal: *health teaching.*
   a. Prepare for evaluative studies—audiogram.
   b. Referral: appropriate community resources: National Association of Hearing and Speech Agencies for *counseling services;* National Association for the Deaf to assist with *employment, education, legislation;* Alexander Graham Bell Association for the Deaf, Inc., serves as *information* center for those working with the client with hearing aid impairments; American Hearing Society provides educational information, employment services, *social clubs.*
   c. See **Table 11.10** for care of hearing aids.
   d. Safety precautions: when crossing street, driving.

E. Evaluation/outcome criteria:
1. Method of communication established.
2. Achieves independence (use of Dogs for Deaf, special telephones, visual signals).
3. Copes with lifestyle changes (minimal depression, anger, hostility).

VI. GLAUCOMA (acute and chronic): increased intraocular pressure; second most common cause of blindness.

A. Pathophysiology:
1. *Acute (closed-angle)*—impaired passage of aqueous humor into the circular canal of Schlemm due to closure of the angle between the cornea and the iris. ***Medical emergency;*** *requires surgery.*
2. *Chronic (open-angle)*—degenerative changes in trabecular meshwork; local obstruction of aqueous humor between the anterior chamber and the canal. *Most common; treated with medications (miotics, carbonic anhydrase inhibitors).*
3. *Secondary*—in some cases neovascularization (new vessels) may form; blocks passage of aqueous humor (uveitis, trauma, drugs, diabetes, retinal vein occlusion).
4. Untreated: imbalance between rate of secretion of intraocular fluids and rate of absorption of aqueous humor → increased intraocular pressures → decreased peripheral vision → corneal edema → halos and blurring of vision → blindness.

B. Risk factors—unknown, but associated with:
1. Emotional disturbances.
2. Hereditary factors.
3. Allergies.
4. Vasomotor disturbances.

C. Assessment:
1. *Subjective data:*
   a. *Acute* (closed-angle):
      (1) Pain: severe, in and around eyes.
      (2) Rainbow halos around lights.

(3) Blurring of vision.
(4) Nausea, vomiting.

b. *Chronic* (open-angle):
(1) Eyes tire easily.
(2) Loss of peripheral vision.
(3) Dull, morning headache.

2. *Objective data:*
a. Corneal edema.
b. Decreased peripheral vision.
c. Increased cupping of optic disk.
d. Tonometry—pressures greater than 22 mm Hg.
e. Pupils: dilated.
f. Redness of eye.

D. Analysis/nursing diagnosis:

1. *Visual sensory/perceptual alterations* related to increased intraocular pressure.
2. *Pain* related to sudden increase in intraocular pressure.
3. *Risk for injury* related to blindness.
4. *Impaired physical mobility* related to impaired vision.

E. Nursing care plan/implementation:

1. Goal: *reduce intraocular pressure.*
a. Activity: bedrest.
b. *Position:* semi-Fowler's.
c. Medications as ordered:
(1) *Miotics* (pilocarpine, carbachol); may not be effective with intraocular pressure (IOP) greater than 40 mm Hg.
(2) *Carbonic anhydrase inhibitors* (acetazolamide [Diamox]).
(3) *Anticholinesterase* (demecarium bromide [Humorsol]) to facilitate outflow of aqueous humor.
(4) *Ophthalmic beta blockers* (timolol) to decrease IOP.

2. Goal: *provide emotional support.*
a. Place personal objects within field of vision.
b. Assist with activities.
c. Encourage verbalization of concerns, fears of blindness, loss of independence.

3. Goal: *health teaching.*
a. *Prevent* increased IOP by *avoiding:*
(1) Anger, excitement, worry.
(2) Constrictive clothing.
(3) Heavy lifting.
(4) Excessive *fluid* intake.
(5) Atropine or other mydriatics that cause dilation.
(6) Straining at stool.
(7) Eye strain.
b. Relaxation techniques; stress management if indicated.
c. Prepare for surgical intervention, if ordered: laser trabeculoplasty, trabeculectomy (filtering), laser peripheral iridotomy.
d. Medications: purpose, dosage, frequency; *eyedrop instillation*—(1) wash hands; (2) head back, expose conjunctiva of lower lid, instill in center *without* touching eyelashes or eye; (3) close eyes gently, apply slight pressure to corner of eye to decrease systemic absorption; (4) wait at least 2 minutes before instilling a second eyedrop medication; have extra bottle in case of breakage or loss.
e. Activity: moderate exercise—walking.
f. Safety measures: eye protection (shield or glasses); Medic Alert band or tag; *avoid* driving 1 to 2 hours after instilling miotics.
g. Community resources as necessary.

F. Evaluation/outcome criteria:

1. Eyesight preserved if possible.
2. Intraocular pressure lowered (<22 mm Hg).
3. Continues medical supervision for life—reports reappearance of symptoms immediately.

VII. CATARACT: developmental or degenerative opacification of the crystalline lens.

A. Risk factors:

1. Aging (most common).
2. Trauma (x-rays, infrared or possibly ultraviolet exposure).
3. Systemic disease (diabetes).
4. Congenital defect.
5. Drug effects (corticosteroids).

B. Assessment:

1. *Subjective data*—vision: blurring, loss of acuity (sees best in low-light conditions); distortion; diplopia; photophobia.
2. *Objective data:*
a. Blindness: unilateral or bilateral (particularly in congenital cataracts).
b. Loss of red reflex; gray or cloudy white opacity of lens.

C. Analysis/nursing diagnosis:

1. *Visual sensory/perceptual alterations* related to opacity of lens.
2. *Risk for injury* related to accidents.
3. *Social isolation* related to impaired vision.

VIII. CATARACT REMOVAL: removal of opacified lens because of loss of vision; extracapsular cataract extraction followed by intraocular lens (IOL) insertion is procedure of choice.

A. Nursing care plan/implementation:

1. *Preoperative:*

a. Goal: *prepare for surgery* (ambulatory center). *Antibiotic* drops or ointment, *mydriatic* eyedrops as ordered; note dilation of pupils; *avoid* glaring lights; usually done under local anesthetic with sedation.
b. Goal: *health teaching.* Postoperative expectations: do *not* rub, touch, or squeeze eyes shut

after surgery; eye patches will be on; assistance will be given for needs; overnight hospitalization not required unless complications occur; mild iritis usually occurs.

2. *Postoperative:*
   a. Goal: *reduce stress on the sutures and prevent hemorrhage.*
      (1) Activity: ambulate as ordered, usually soon after surgery; generally discharged few hours after surgery.
      (2) *Position: flat* or *low Fowler's;* on *back* or turn to *nonoperative* side 3 to 4 weeks, because turning to operative side increases pressure.
      (3) *Avoid* activities that increase IOP: straining at stool, vomiting, coughing, brushing teeth, brushing hair, shaving, lifting objects over 20 lb, *bending,* or *stooping;* wear glasses or shaded lens during day, eye shield at night.
      (4) Provide mouthwash, hair care, personal items within easy reach, "step-in" slippers to *avoid* bending over.
   b. Goal: *promote psychological well-being.* With elderly, frequent contacts to prevent sensory deprivation.
   c. Goal: *health teaching.*
      (1) If intraocular lens not inserted, prescriptive glasses may be used (cataract glasses); explain about magnification, perceptual distortion, blind areas in peripheral vision; guide through activities with glasses; need to look through central portion of lens and turn head to side when looking to the side to decrease distortion.
      (2) Eye care: instillation of eyedrops (*mydriatics* and *carbonic anhydrase inhibitors*) to prevent glaucoma and adhesions if IOL not inserted; with IOL, steroid-antibiotic use (see **VI. GLAUCOMA, pp. 388–389**, for correct technique); eye shield at night to prevent injury for 1 month.
      (3) Signs/symptoms of *infection* (redness, pain, edema, drainage); iris *prolapse* (bulging or pear-shaped pupil); *hemorrhage* (sharp eye pain, half-moon of blood).
      (4) *Avoid:* heavy lifting; potential eye trauma.

B. Evaluation/outcome criteria:
1. Vision restored.
2. No complications (e.g., severe eye pain, hemorrhage).
3. Performs self-care activities (e.g., instills eyedrops).
4. Returns for follow-up ophthalmology care—recognizes symptoms requiring immediate attention.

IX. RETINAL DETACHMENT: separation of neural retina from underlying retinal pigment epithelium.

A. Risk factors:
1. Trauma.
2. Degeneration.

B. Assessment:
1. *Subjective data:*
   a. Flashes of light before eyes.
   b. Vision: blurred, sooty (*sudden* onset); sensation of floating particles; blank areas of vision.
2. *Objective data*—ophthalmic examination: retina is grayish in area of tear; bright red, horseshoe-shaped tear; B-mode ultrasonography.

C. Analysis/nursing diagnosis:
1. *Visual sensory/perceptual alteration* related to blurred vision.
2. *Anxiety* related to potential loss of vision.
3. *Risk for injury* related to blindness.

D. Nursing care plan/implementation:
1. *Preoperative:*
   a. Goal: *reduce anxiety and prevent further detachment.*
      (1) Encourage verbalization of feelings; answer all questions; reinforce physician's explanation of surgical procedures.
      (2) Activity: *bedrest;* eyes usually covered to promote rest and maintain normal position of retina; side rails up.
      (3) *Position:* according to location of retinal tear; involved area of eye should be in a *dependent* position.
      (4) Give medications as ordered: *cycloplegics* or *mydriatics* to dilate pupils widely and decrease intraocular movement.
      (5) Relaxing diversion: conversation, music.
   b. Goal: *health teaching.* Prepare for surgical intervention (often combination used):
      (1) *Cryopexy* or *cryotherapy*—supercooled probe is applied to the sclera, causing a scar, which pulls the choroid and retina together.
      (2) *Laser photocoagulation*—a beam of intense light from a carbon arc is directed through the dilated pupil onto the retina; seals hole if retina not detached.
      (3) *Scleral buckling*—the sclera is resected or shortened to enhance the contact between the choroid and retina; frequently combined with cryopexy.
      (4) *Banding or encirclement*—silicone band or strap is placed under the extraocular muscles around the globe.
      (5) *Pneumatic retinopexy*—instillation of expandable gas or oil to tamponade tear.

ADULT

2. *Postoperative:*
   a. Goal: *reduce intraocular stress and prevent hemorrhage.*

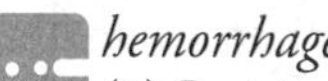

      (1) *Position: flat* or *low Fowler's;* sandbags may be used to position head; turn to nonoperative side if allowed, retinal tear dependent; special positions may be: *prone, side-lying,* or *sitting with face down* on table if gas or oil bubble injected; position may be restricted 4 to 8 days.
      (2) Activity: bedrest; decrease intraocular pressure by *not* stooping or bending and *avoiding* prone position.
      (3) Give medications as ordered:
         (a) *Cycloplegics* (atropine).
         (b) *Antibiotics.*
         (c) *Corticosteroids* to reduce eye movements and inflammation and prevent infection.
      (4) ROM—isometric, passive; elastic stockings to avoid thrombus related to immobility.
   b. Goal: *support coping mechanisms.*
      (1) Plan all care with client.
      (2) Encourage verbalization of feelings, fears.
      (3) Encourage family interaction.
      (4) Diversional activities.
   c. Goal: *health teaching.*
      (1) Eye care: eye patch or shield at night for about 2 weeks to prevent touching eye while asleep; dark glasses; *avoid* rubbing, squeezing eyes.
      (2) Limitations: *no* reading, needlework for 3 weeks, *no* physical exertion for 6 weeks; OK to watch TV, walk, except with bubble restrictions.
      (3) Medications: dosage, frequency, purpose, side effects: *avoid* nonprescription medications.
      (4) **Signs of redetachment:** flashes of light, increase in "floaters," blurred vision, acute eye pain.

E. Evaluation/outcome criteria:
1. Vision restored.
2. No further detachment—recognizes signs and symptoms.
3. No injury occurs—accepts limitations.

X. BLINDNESS: legally defined as vision less than 20/200 with the use of corrective lenses, or a visual field of no greater than 20 degrees; greatest incidence after 65 years.

A. Risk factors:
1. Glaucoma.
2. Cataracts.
3. Macular degeneration.
4. Diabetic retinopathy.
5. Atherosclerosis.
6. Trauma.

B. Analysis/nursing diagnosis:
1. *Visual sensory/perceptual alteration* related to blindness.
2. *Impaired social interaction* related to loss of sight.
3. *Risk for injury* related to visual impairment.
4. *Self-care deficit* related to visual loss.

C. Nursing care plan/implementation:
1. Goal: *promote independence and provide emotional support.*
   a. Familiarize with surroundings; encourage use of touch.
   b. Establish communication lines; answer questions.
   c. Deal with feelings of loss, overprotectiveness by family members.
   d. Provide diversional activities: radio, CDs, talking books, tapes.
   e. Encourage self-care activities; allow voicing of frustrations when activity is not done to satisfaction (spilling or misplacing something), to decrease anger and discouragement.
2. Goal: *facilitate activities of daily living.*
   a. *Eating:*
      (1) Establish routine placement for tableware (e.g., plate, glass).
      (2) Help person mentally visualize the plate as a clock or compass (e.g., "3 o'clock" or "east").
      (3) Take person's hand and guide the fingertips to establish spatial relationship.
   b. *Walking:*
      (1) Have person hold your forearm: walk a half-step in front.
      (2) Tell the person when approaching stairs, curb, incline.
   c. *Talking:*
      (1) Speak when approaching person; tell person before you touch him or her.
      (2) Tell the person who you are and what you will be doing.
      (3) *Do not avoid* words such as "see" or discussing the appearance of things.
3. Goal: *health teaching.*
   a. Accident prevention in the home.
   b. Referral: *community resources:*
      (1) Voluntary agencies:
         (a) American Foundation for the Blind—provides catalogs of devices for visually handicapped.
         (b) National Society for the Prevention of Blindness—comprehensive educational programs and research.

(c) Recording for the Blind, Inc.—provides recorded educational books on free loan.
(d) Lion's Club.
(e) Catholic charities.
(f) Salvation Army.
(2) Government agencies:
(a) Social and Rehabilitation Service—counseling and placement services.
(b) Veterans Administration—screening and pensions.
(c) State Welfare Department, Division for the Blind—vocational.

D. Evaluation/outcome criteria:
1. Acceptance of disability—participates in self-care activities, remains socially involved.
2. Regains independence with rehabilitation.

RESPIRATORY SYSTEM

I. PNEUMONIA: acute inflammation of lungs with exudate accumulation in alveoli and other respiratory passages that interferes with ventilation process.

A. Types:
1. *Typical/classic pneumonia: pneumococcal;* related to diminished defense mechanisms, immunocompromised, critically ill, history of smoking, general anesthesia/abdominal surgery, exposure to airborne pathogens, hospitalization, recent respiratory tract infection, viral influenza, increased age, and chronic obstructive pulmonary disease (COPD).
   a. *Lobar pneumonia*—occurs abruptly when an acute bacterial infection affects a large portion of a lobe; causes pleuritic pain, heavy sputum production.
   b. *Bronchopneumonia*—involves patchy infiltration over a general area.
   c. *Alveolar pneumonia*—caused by virus; diffuse bilateral infection without patchy infiltrates.
2. *Atypical pneumonia:* related to contact with specific organisms.
   a. *Mycoplasma pneumoniae* or *Legionella pneumophila,* if untreated, can lead to serious complications such as acute respiratory distress syndrome (ARDS), disseminated intravascular coagulation (DIC), thrombocytopenic purpura, renal failure, inflammation of the heart, neurological disorders, or possible death.
   b. *Pneumocystis* pneumonia in conjunction with AIDS.
3. *Aspiration pneumonia:*
   a. *Noninfectious:* aspiration of fluids (gastric secretions, foods, liquids, tube feedings) into the airways.
   b. *Bacterial aspiration pneumonia:* related to poor cough mechanisms due to anesthesia, coma (mixed flora of upper respiratory tract cause pneumonia).
4. *Hematogenous pneumonia bacterial infections:* related to spread of bacteria from the bloodstream.

B. Pathophysiology: caused by infectious or noninfectious agents, clotting of an exudate rich in fibrinogen, consolidated lung tissue.

C. Assessment:
1. *Subjective data:*
   a. *Pain* location: chest (affected side), referred to abdomen, shoulder, flank.
   b. Irritability, restlessness.
   c. Apprehensiveness.
   d. Nausea, anorexia.
   e. History of exposure.
2. *Objective data:*
   a. Cough:
      (1) Productive, rust-colored (blood) or yellowish sputum (greenish with atypical pneumonia).
      (2) Splinting of affected side when coughing.
   b. *Sudden* increased fever, chills.
   c. Nasal flaring, circumoral cyanosis.
   d. Respiratory distress: tachypnea.
   e. Auscultation:
      (1) Decreased breath sounds on *affected* side.
      (2) Exaggerated breath sounds on *unaffected* side.
      (3) Crackles, bronchial breath sounds.
      (4) Dullness on percussion over consolidated area.
      (5) Possible pleural friction rub.
   f. Chest retraction (air hunger in infants).
   g. Vomiting.
   h. Facial herpes simplex.
   i. *Diagnostic studies:*
      (1) Chest x-ray: haziness to consolidation.
      (2) Sputum culture: Gram stain and culture; specific organisms, usually pneumococcus.
      (3) Bronchoscopy if sputum results are inconclusive.
   j. Laboratory data:
      (1) Blood culture: organism specific except when viral.
      (2) WBC count: leukocytosis.
      (3) Sedimentation rate: *elevated.*
3. Factors contributing to the severity of pneumonia:
   a. *Demographics:*
      (1) Age—severity increased with age.
      (2) Gender.
      (3) Nursing home resident.

ADULT

b. *Comorbidities:*
   (1) Congestive heart failure (CHF).
   (2) Active cancer.
   (3) Liver disease.
   (4) Renal insufficiency.
   (5) Stroke with residual symptoms.
c. *Physical examination:*
   (1) Systolic BP less than 90; mean arterial pressure (MAP) less than 60.
   (2) Heart rate (HR) ≥125.
   (3) Respiratory rate ≥30.
   (4) Temperature (PO) ≥104°F or less than 95°F.
   (5) Altered level of consciousness (LOC).
d. *Laboratory results:*
   (1) Hematocrit (Hct) less than 30.
   (2) Na^+ less than 130.
   (3) BUN ≥30.
   (4) Arterial pH less than 7.35.
   (5) Pleural effusion on chest x-ray.
   (6) Glucose greater than 250 mg/dL.

D. Analysis/nursing diagnosis:
1. *Ineffective airway clearance* related to retained secretions.
2. *Activity intolerance* related to inflammatory process.
3. *Pain* related to continued coughing.
4. *Knowledge deficit* (learning need) related to proper management of symptoms.
5. *Risk for fluid volume deficit* related to tachypnea.

E. Nursing care plan/implementation:
1. Goal: *promote adequate ventilation.*
   a. Deep breathe, cough. Small-volume nebulizer treatment.
   b. Remove respiratory secretions, suction prn.
   c. High humidity with or without oxygen therapy.
   d. Intermittent positive-pressure breathing (IPPB); incentive spirometry, chest physiotherapy, as ordered and needed to loosen secretions.
   e. Use of *expectorants* as ordered.
   f. Change position frequently.
   g. Percussion with postural drainage.
2. Goal: *control infection.*
   a. Monitor vital signs; hypothermia for elevated temperature.
   b. Administer *antibiotics* as ordered to control infection—broad spectrum (e.g. penicillin, quinolones, aminoglycosides). *Note:* need cultures before starting on antibiotics.
3. Goal: *provide rest and comfort.*
   a. Planned rest periods.
   b. Adequate hydration by mouth, I&O; IVs as needed.
   c. *Diet: high* carbohydrate, *high* protein to meet energy demands and assist in the healing process.
   d. Mild *analgesics* for pain—*no* opioids.
4. Goal: *prevent potential complications.*
   a. Cross infection: use good hand-washing technique.
   b. *Sterile technique* when tracheobronchial suctioning to reduce risk of possible infection.
   c. Hyperthermia: tepid baths, hypothermia blanket.
   d. Respiratory insufficiency and acidosis: clear airway, promote expectoration of secretions.
   e. Assess cardiac and respiratory function.
   f. Keep ambulatory whenever possible.
5. Goal: *health teaching.*
   a. Proper disposal of tissues, cover mouth when coughing.
   b. Expected side effects of prescribed medications.
   c. Need for rest, limited interactions, increased caloric intake.
   d. Need to avoid future respiratory infections. *Immunization:* influenza each year for those at risk. Vaccine for pneumococcal pneumonia every 5 years.
   e. Correct dosage of antibiotics and the importance of taking entire prescription at prescribed times (times evenly distributed throughout the 24-hour period to maintain blood level of antibiotic) for increased effectiveness.

F. Evaluation/outcome criteria:
1. Adheres to medication regimen.
2. Has improved gas exchange as shown by improved pulmonary function tests.
3. No acid-base or fluid imbalance: normal pH.
4. Energy level: increased.
5. Sputum production: decreased, normal color.
6. Vital signs: stable.
7. Breath sounds: clear.
8. Cultures: negative.
9. Reports comfort level increased.

II. SEVERE ACUTE RESPIRATORY SYNDROME (SARS): viral respiratory illness caused by a coronavirus. Incubation period: 2 to 7 days, maybe as long as 10 to 14 days. Recommend limiting contact after infection until *10 days after fever* has gone.

A. Pathophysiology: little information is known about the SARS-associated coronavirus. May survive in the environment for several days—depends on temperature or humidity, and type of material or body fluid. Spread generally by respiratory droplets—up to 3 feet. May spread through air; other ways not known. Progresses to hypoxia → pneumonia → respiratory distress syndrome.

ADULT

B. Risk factors:
1. Weakened immune system.
2. Close contact (within 3 feet)—kissing, hugging, sharing utensils.

C. Assessment:
1. *Subjective data:*
   a. Headache.
   b. Feeling of discomfort; body aches; chills.
   c. Dyspnea.
2. *Objective data:*
   a. Temperature greater than 100.4°F (38.0°C), unless on antipyretics.
   b. Mild respiratory symptoms; dry cough.
   c. Diarrhea in 20%.
   d. Laboratory: reverse transcriptase–polymerase chain reaction (RT-PCR) of blood, stool, nasal secretions; serologic test for antibodies; viral culture (showing antibodies to virus more than 21 days after onset of illness).
   e. Additional laboratory findings:
      (1) Leukopenia.
      (2) Lymphopenia
      (3) Thrombocytopenia.
      (4) ↑ lactose dehydrogenase.
      (5) ↑ aspartate aminotransferase.
      (6) ↑ creatine kinase.
   f. Chest x-ray: focal interstitial infiltrates → generalized patchy infiltrates → areas of consolidation.

D. Analysis/nursing diagnosis:
1. *Ineffective breathing pattern* related to hypoxia and pneumonia.
2. *Risk for spread of infection* related to droplet or airborne transmission.
3. *Impaired gas exchange* related to pneumonia.

E. Nursing care plan/implementation, evaluation/outcome criteria (also see **I. PNEUMONIA, pp. 392–393**):
1. Goal: *infection control.*
   a. Standard precautions (e.g., strict hand hygiene).
   b. *Contact* precautions (e.g., gown and gloves) with eye protection.
   c. *Airborne* precautions (e.g., isolation room with negative pressure; use of an N95 filtering disposable respirator for those entering room, or surgical mask).
   d. Identify/isolate suspected SARS cases (*quarantine*).
2. Goal: *supportive care.*
   a. Empirical *antibiotic* therapy with broad coverage.
   b. *Isolation* (i.e., those without symptoms) for 10 days *after* becoming *afebrile.*

III. H1N1 INFLUENZA VIRUS **("swine flu"):** respiratory disease caused by a new strain of the type A influenza virus (novel H1N1 or 2009 H1N1 flu). Described initially as a possible pandemic, a technical term that refers to the geographical (global) *spread* of the disease, *not* severity. Called swine flu because it resembled a strain that circulates in pigs.

A. Pathophysiology:
1. Influenza A virus with two proteins, hemagglutinin (H1) and neuraminidase (N1); *human-to-human* transmission through respiratory secretions (*droplets*) from coughing or sneezing; touching something with the virus on the surface and then touching mouth, eyes, or nose. *Not* spread by food.
2. *Incubation* period: 1 day before symptoms occur and up to 7 days following illness onset.
3. *Infectious* (viral shedding): as long as symptomatic; a minimum of 7 days after onset up to 13 days. Young children may be contagious for longer periods.
4. Respiratory symptoms may progress to pneumonia → respiratory failure → death.

B. Risk factors:
1. Ages 6 months to 24 years; children younger than 5 years and *especially younger than 2 years.*
2. Pregnant women and women who are 2 weeks postpartum.
3. Persons 25 to 64 years with *chronic* conditions (e.g., asthma, diabetes, heart disease, kidney disease, and weakened immune system).
4. Residents of nursing homes and *chronic-care facilities.*

C. Assessment:
1. *Subjective data:* Classic flu:
   a. Fatigue
   b. Body aches; chills
   c. Sore throat
   d. Headache
   e. **Emergency** signs with *swine flu:*
      (1) Shortness of breath
      (2) Chest pain or abdominal pain
      (3) Sudden dizziness; confusion
2. *Objective data:* Classic flu:
   a. Fever above 100.4°F
   b. Cough
   c. Diarrhea; vomiting
   d. Runny nose
   e. **Emergency** signs with swine flu:
      (1) Severe or persistent vomiting
      (2) Difficulty breathing; rapid respiratory rate
      (3) Bluish or gray skin color (particularly in children)

Emergency Warning Signs in *Children* with Swine Flu:	Emergency Warning Signs in *Adults* with Swine Flu:
• Fast breathing or trouble breathing • Bluish or gray skin color • Not drinking enough fluids • Being so irritable that the child does not want to be held • Not waking up or not interacting • Severe or persistent vomiting • Flu-like symptoms improve but then return with fever and worse cough	• Difficulty breathing or shortness of breath • Pain or pressure in the chest or abdomen • Sudden dizziness • Confusion • Severe or persistent vomiting • Flu-like symptoms improve but then return with fever and worse cough

Source: www.flu.gov.

f. *Diagnostic tests:* viral culture, polymerase chain reaction (PCR), rapid antigen testing, and immunofluorescence. *"Rapid influenza diagnostic test"*—detects in 30 minutes, may not be conclusive.

D. Analysis/nursing diagnosis:

1. *Ineffective breathing pattern* related to hypoxia and pneumonia.
2. *Risk for spread of infection* related to droplet or airborne transmission.
3. *Risk for fluid volume deficit* related to persistent vomiting.

E. Nursing care plan/implementation:

1. Goal: *prevent spread of infection.*
   a. Stay home from work or school at least 24 hours **after** fever is gone without the use of a fever-reducing medicine; limit contact with others.
   b. Cover nose and mouth with tissue when coughing or sneezing.
   c. Wash hands after every sneeze or cough.
   d. Disinfect home surfaces to kill germs—virus can survive 2 to 8 hours; use hydrogen peroxide, iodophors, detergents, alcohol; heat.
2. Goal: *reduce risk of complications, alleviate symptoms.*
   a. Medications
      (1) *Antipyretic:* for fever 100°F or higher; acetaminophen or ibuprofen; aspirin if over 18 years of age.
      (2) *Antiviral:* treatment or prevention; stop spread of virus: oseltamivir (oral, Tamiflu)—take with food, nausea and vomiting may occur; zanamivir (inhaled)—do **not** take with history of asthma or lung disease; may cause dizziness, stuffy nose, sinusitis; peramivir (IV, reserved for critically ill); *neuraminidase inhibitors;* suspected or confirmed cases; most effective *within 48 hours;* 5 days of treatment.
      (3) Fluids, lozenges; cough suppressant for dry cough.
   b. *Fluids:* clear liquids (water, broth, sports drinks, ice chips, frozen popsicles); *avoid* alcohol and caffeine.
   c. Monitor for dehydration: urine color (dark yellow with dehydration); frequency of trips to bathroom. Look for tears with infants/toddlers; wet diapers.
3. Goal: *prevent occupational exposure.*
   a. Eliminate potential *exposures:* keep distance of 6 feet or more in community setting; restrict visitors who are ill; keep sick workers at home.
   b. *Respiratory hygiene* and cough etiquette. Encourage ill person to use tissues or wear a disposable face mask (use only once) or health-care provider should wear mask.
   c. *Respiratory protection* (personal protective equipment) in occupational health-care setting—N95 or higher filtering facepiece respirator; fit-tested (*not* recommended for children or people with facial hair); disposable, single use, do not share. Remove gloves and wash hands before and after touching respirator. Extended use of N95 increases risk of contact transmission. Usually reserved if assisting with an aerosol-generating procedure—intubation, extubation, bronchoscopy, nebulization.
   d. *Isolation;* standard (droplet) precautions—private room preferred; if not available at least 3-foot separation between patient beds with curtain between; share room with like diagnosis (cohorting). Caregiver wears mask—respirator not routinely necessary. Eye protection if within 6 feet of patient as treatments may cause splashing of respiratory secretions.
   e. Limit transport of patient; client wears mask outside of room.
   f. *Vaccination of staff*—may be required; *exempt:* with severe egg allergy; history of Guillain-Barré syndrome; religion prohibits vaccinations. May be required to wear mask if not vaccinated.
4. Goal: *health teaching—methods to prevent reinfection.*
   a. Hand-washing technique—soap, water, and friction for at least 20 seconds; alcohol-based (antibacterial) hand rub may be used.
   b. *Avoid* touching eyes, nose, or mouth.
   c. *Vaccination:* one dose of swine flu and seasonal flu vaccine for those 10 years of age and older—may be given on same day; two doses

of swine flu vaccine (separated 4 weeks, 21 days minimum) for children younger than 10 years.
   d. Pneumococcal vaccination if over 65 years, smoker, or history of chronic health problem.

F. Evaluation/outcome criteria:
1. No complications.
2. Temperature normal for 24 hours without medication.
3. Breath sounds clear; respirations unlabored.
4. Covers nose/mouth when coughing or sneezing.
5. Performs hand hygiene frequently.

IV. ATELECTASIS: collapsed alveoli in part or all of the lung.

A. Pathophysiology: due to compression (tumor), airway obstruction, decreased surfactant production, or progressive regional hypoventilation.

B. Risk factors:
1. Shallow breathing due to pain, abdominal distention, narcotics, or sedatives.
2. Decreased ciliary action due to anesthesia, smoking.
3. Thickened secretions due to immobility, dehydration.
4. Aspiration of foreign substances.
5. Bronchospasms.
6. Barotrauma; ↑ positive end-expiratory pressure (PEEP).

C. Assessment:
1. *Subjective data:*
   a. Restlessness.
   b. Pain.
2. *Objective data:*
   a. Tachypnea.
   b. Tachycardia.
   c. Dullness on percussion.
   d. Absent bronchial breathing.
   e. Crackles at bases as alveoli "pop" open on inspiration.
   f. Tactile fremitus in affected area.
   g. ↓ O_2 saturation.
   h. X-ray:
      (1) Patches of consolidation.
      (2) Elevated diaphragm.
      (3) Mediastinal shift.

D. Analysis/nursing diagnosis:
1. *Impaired gas exchange* related to shallow breathing.
2. *Pain,* acute, related to collapse of lung.
3. *Fear* related to altered respiratory status.

E. Nursing care plan/implementation:
1. Goal: *relieve hypoxia.*
   a. Frequent respiratory assessment.
   b. Respiratory hygiene measures, cough, deep breathe. Use bedside inspirometer q1h when awake.
   c. Oxygen as ordered.
   d. Monitor effects of respiratory therapy, ventilators, breathing assistance measures to ensure proper gas exchange.

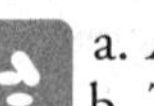

   e. *Position:* on *unaffected* side to allow for lung expansion.
   f. Prepare for possible needle decompression or chest tube insertion.
2. Goal: *prevent complications.*
   a. *Antibiotics* as ordered.
   b. Turn, cough, and deep breathe. Out of bed, ambulation.
   c. *Increase fluid* intake to liquefy secretions.
3. Goal: *health teaching.*
   a. Need to report signs and symptoms listed in assessment data for early recognition of problem.
   b. Importance of coughing and deep breathing to improve present condition and prevent further problems.

F. Evaluation/outcome criteria:
1. Lung expanded on x-ray.
2. Acid-base balance obtained and maintained.
3. No pain on respiration.
4. Activity level increased.

V. PULMONARY EMBOLISM: undissolved mass that travels in bloodstream and occludes a blood vessel; can be thromboembolus, fat, air, or catheter. Constitutes a **critical medical emergency.**

A. Pathophysiology: obstructs blood flow to lung → increased pressure on pulmonary artery and reflex constriction of pulmonary blood vessels → poor pulmonary circulation → pulmonary infarction.

B. Risk factors:
1. Thrombophlebitis.
2. Recent surgery.
3. Invasive procedures.
4. Immobility.
5. Obesity
6. Myocardial infarction, heart failure.
7. Smoking.
8. Varicose veins.
9. Hormone replacement therapy.

C. Assessment:
1. *Subjective data:*
   a. Chest *pain:* substernal, localized; type—crushing, sharp, stabbing with respirations.
   b. Sudden onset of profound dyspnea.
   c. Restless, irritable, anxious.
   d. Sense of impending doom.
2. *Objective data:*
   a. Respirations: either rapid, shallow or deep, gasping.
   b. *Elevated* temperature.

c. Auscultation: friction rub, crackles; diminished breath sounds.
d. Shock:
(1) Tachycardia.
(2) Hypotension.
(3) Skin: cold, clammy.
e. Cough: hemoptysis.
f. X-ray: area of density.
g. ECG changes that reflect right-sided failure.
h. Echocardiogram shows increased pulmonary dynamics.
i. Lung scan; pulmonary angiography.
j. Laboratory data:
(1) *Decreased* Pa_{CO_2}.
(2) *Elevated* WBC count.

D. Analysis/nursing diagnosis:
1. *Ineffective breathing pattern* related to shallow respirations.
2. *Impaired gas exchange* related to dyspnea.
3. *Pain* related to decreased tissue perfusion.
4. *Altered peripheral tissue perfusion* related to occlusion of blood vessel.
5. *Fear* related to emergency condition.
6. *Anxiety* related to sense of impending doom.

E. Nursing care plan/implementation:
1. Goal: *monitor for signs of respiratory distress.*
a. Auscultate lungs for areas of decreased/absent breath sounds.
b. *Elevate head of bed.*
c. Monitor arterial blood gases (ABGs).
d. Monitor pulse oximetry; administer oxygen, supplemental humidification as indicated.
e. Monitor blood coagulation studies (e.g., activated partial thromboplastin time [aPTT]).
f. Administer *anticoagulation* therapy, *thrombolytic* agents, morphine for *pain, vasopressor* medications.
g. Fluids: IV/PO as indicated.
h. Monitor signs: *Homans',* acidosis.
i. Ambulate as tolerated/indicated; change position.
j. Prepare for surgery if peripheral embolectomy is indicated.
2. Goal: *health teaching.*
a. Prevent further occurrence; importance of antiembolism stockings, intermittent pneumatic compression devices.
b. Decrease stasis.
c. If history of thrombophlebitis, *avoid* birth control pills.
d. Need to continue medication.
e. Follow-up care.

F. Evaluation/outcome criteria:
1. No complications; no further incidence of emboli.
2. Respiratory rate returns to normal.
3. Coagulation studies within normal limits (aPTT 25 to 41 seconds, ABGs within normal limits).
4. Reports comfort achieved.

VI. HISTOPLASMOSIS: infection found mostly in central United States. *Not transmitted from human to human but from dust and contaminated soil.* Progressive histoplasmosis, seen most frequently in middle-aged white men who have COPD, is characterized by cavity formation, fibrosis, and emphysema.

A. Pathophysiology: spores of *Histoplasma capsulatum* (from droppings of infected birds and bats) are inhaled, multiply, and cause fungal infections of respiratory tract. Leads to necrosis and healing by encapsulation.

B. Assessment:
1. *Subjective data:*
a. Malaise.
b. Chest pain, dyspnea.
2. *Objective data:*
a. Weight loss.
b. Nonproductive cough.
c. Fever.
d. Positive skin test for histoplasmosis.
e. Benign acute pneumonitis.
f. Chest x-ray: nodular infiltrate.
g. Sputum culture shows *Histoplasma capsulatum.*
h. Hepatomegaly, splenomegaly.

C. Analysis/nursing diagnosis:
1. *Ineffective airway clearance* related to pneumonitis.
2. *Ineffective breathing pattern* related to dyspnea.
3. *Pain,* acute, related to infectious process.
4. *Risk for infection* related to repeated exposure to fungal spores.
5. *Impaired gas exchange* related to chronic pulmonary disease.
6. *Knowledge deficit* (learning need) related to prevention of disease and potential side effects of medications.

D. Nursing care plan/implementation:
1. Goal: *relieve symptoms of the disease.*
a. Administer medications as ordered.
(1) Amphotericin B (IV) and ketoconazole.
(a) Monitor for drug side effects: local phlebitis, renal toxicity, hypokalemia, anemia, anaphylaxis, bone marrow depression.
(b) *Azotemia* (presence of nitrogen-containing compounds in blood) is monitored by biweekly BUN or creatinine levels.
BUN greater than 40 mg/dL or creatinine greater than 3.0 mg/dL necessitates *stopping* amphotericin B until values return to within normal limits.

ADULT

(2) Aspirin, diphenhydramine HCl (Benadryl), promethazine HCl (Phenergan), prochlorperazine (Compazine): used *to decrease systemic toxicity* of chills, fever, aching, nausea, and vomiting.

2. Goal: *health teaching.*
   a. Desired effects and side effects of prescribed medications; importance of taking medications for entire course of therapy (usually from 2 weeks to 3 months).
   b. Importance of follow-up laboratory tests to monitor toxic effects of drug.
   c. Identify source of contamination if possible and *avoid* future contact if possible.
   d. Importance of deep breathing, pursed-lip breathing, coughing (see **VIII. EMPHYSEMA, p. 401,** for specific care).
   e. Signs and symptoms of chronic histoplasmosis, COPD, drug toxicity, and drug side effects.

E. Evaluation/outcome criteria:
1. Complies with treatment plan.
2. Respiratory complications avoided.
3. Symptoms of illness decreased.
4. No further spread of disease.
5. Source of contamination identified and removed.

VII. TUBERCULOSIS: inflammatory, communicable disease that commonly attacks the lungs, although may occur in other body parts.

A. Pathophysiology: exposure to causative organism (*Mycobacterium tuberculosis*) in the alveoli in susceptible individual leads to inflammation. Infection spreads by lymphatics to hilus; antibodies are released, leading to fibrosis, calcification, or inflammation. Exudate formation leads to caseous necrosis, then liquefication of caseous material leads to cavitation.

B. Risk factors:
1. Persons who have inhaled the tubercle bacillus infectious particles called droplet nuclei.
2. Persons who have diseases or therapies known to suppress the immune system.
3. Immigrants from Latin America, Africa, Asia, and Oceania living in the United States for less than 1 year.
4. Americans living in those regions for a prolonged time.
5. Residents of U.S. metropolitan cities such as New York, Miami; those who live in poverty and are in overcrowded, poorly ventilated living conditions.
6. Men older than 65 years.
7. Women between ages 26 and 44 years and older than 65 years.
8. Children younger than 5 years.

ADULT

C. Assessment:
1. *Subjective data:*
   a. Loss of appetite, weight loss.
   b. Weakness, loss of energy.
   c. *Pain:* knifelike, chest.
   d. Though client may be symptom free, the disease is found on screening.
2. *Objective data:*
   a. Night sweats, chills.
   b. *Fever:* low grade, late afternoon.
   c. *Pulse:* increased.
   d. *Respiratory* assessment:
      (1) Productive persistent cough, hemoptysis.
      (2) Respirations: normal, increased depth.
      (3) Asymmetrical lung expansion.
      (4) Increased tactile fremitus.
      (5) Dullness to percussion.
      (6) Crackles following short cough.
   e. Hoarseness.
   f. Unexplained weight loss.
   g. *Diagnostic tests:*
      (1) *Positive tuberculin test (Mantoux)*—reaction to test begins approximately 12 hours after administration with area of redness and a central area of induration. The peak time is 48 hours. Determination of positive or negative is made. A reaction is positive when it measures *10 mm.* Contacts reacting from 5 to 10 mm may need to be treated prophylactically. This test is referred to as purified protein derivative (PPD) or intradermal skin test.
      (2) *Sputum:* three specimens tested positive for acid-fast bacilli (AFB) (smear and culture). Positive equals greater than 10 AFB per field.
      (3) *X-ray:* infiltration cavitation.
   h. Laboratory data: blood—*decreased* red blood cell (RBC) count, *increased* sedimentation rate.
   i. Classification of tuberculosis:

Class	Description
0	No TB exposure, not infected
1	TB exposure, no evidence of infection
2	TB infection, no disease
3	TB: current disease (persons with completed diagnostic evidence of TB—both a significant reaction to tuberculin skin test and clinical or x-ray evidence of disease)
4	TB: no current disease (persons with previous history of TB or with abnormal x-ray films but no significant tuberculin skin test reaction or clinical evidence)
5	TB: suspected (diagnosis pending) (used during diagnostic testing period of suspected persons, for no longer than 3 months)

D. Analysis/nursing diagnosis:

1. *Ineffective airway clearance* related to productive cough.
2. *Impaired gas exchange* related to asymmetrical lung expansion.
3. *Pain* related to unresolved disease process.
4. *Body image disturbance* related to feelings about tuberculosis.
5. *Social isolation* related to fear of spreading infection.
6. *Knowledge deficit* (learning need) related to medication regimen.

E. Nursing care plan/implementation:

1. Goal: *reduce spread of disease.*
   a. Administer medications: isoniazid (INH), rifampin, pyrazinamide, ethambutol, or streptomycin; or drug combinations such as Rifadin or Rifamate. Client will be treated as an outpatient; may need to go to clinic for directly observed therapy (DOT) to ensure compliance with this long-term medication regimen.
   b. The following may need to take 300 mg of INH daily for 1 year as *prophylactic* measure: positive skin test reactors, including contacts; persons who have diseases or are receiving therapies that affect the immune system; persons who have leukemia, lymphoma, or uncontrolled diabetes or who have had a gastrectomy.
   c. *Avoid direct contact with sputum.*
      (1) Use good hand-washing technique after contact with client, personal articles.
      (2) Have client cover mouth and nose when coughing and sneezing, and use disposable tissues to collect sputum.
   d. *Provide good circulation of fresh air.* (Changes of air dilute the number of organisms. This plus chemotherapy provide protection needed to prevent spread of disease.)
   e. Implement *airborne or droplet* precautions (see **Chapter 3, pp. 89–90, Table 3.5, p. 91, Tables 3.7 and 3.8**).
2. Goal: *promote nutrition.*
   a. *Increased protein, calories* to aid in tissue repair and healing.
   b. Small, frequent feedings.
   c. *Increased fluids,* to liquefy secretions so they can be expectorated.
3. Goal: *promote increased self-esteem.*
   a. Encourage client and family to express concerns regarding long-term illness and treatment protocol.
   b. Explain methods of disease prevention, and encourage contacts to be tested and treated if necessary.
   c. Encourage client to maintain role in family while home treatment is ongoing and to return to work and social contacts as soon as it is determined safe for progress of treatment plan.
4. Goal: *health teaching.*
   a. Desired effects and side effects of medications:
      (1) *INH* may affect memory and ability to concentrate. May result in peripheral neuritis, hepatitis, rash, or fever.
      (2) *Streptomycin* may cause eighth cranial nerve damage and vestibular ototoxity, causing hearing loss; may cause labyrinth damage, manifested by vertigo and staggering; also may cause skin rashes, itching, and fever.
      (3) Important for client to know that medication regimen must be adhered to for entire course of treatment.
      (4) Discontinuation of therapy may allow organism to flourish and make the disease more difficult to treat.
   b. Need for follow-up, long-term care, and contact identification.
   c. Importance of nutritious diet, rest, avoidance of respiratory infections.
   d. Identify community agencies for support and follow-up.
   e. Inform that this communicable disease must be reported.

F. Evaluation/outcome criteria:

1. Complies with medication regimen.
2. Lists desired effects and side effects of medications prescribed.
3. Gains weight, eats food high in protein and carbohydrates.
4. Sputum culture becomes negative.
5. Retains role in family.
6. No complications (i.e., no hemorrhage, bacillus not spread to others).

VIII. EMPHYSEMA: chronic disease with excessive inflation of the air spaces distal to the terminal bronchioles, alveolar ducts, and alveoli; characterized by increased airway resistance and decreased diffusing capacity. Emphysema and chronic bronchitis together constitute *chronic obstructive pulmonary disease (COPD).*

A. Pathophysiology: imbalance between proteases, which break down lung tissue, and α_1-antitrypsin, which inhibits the breakdown. Increased airway resistance during expiration results in air trapping and hyperinflation → increased residual volumes. Increased dead space → unequal ventilation → perfusion of poorly ventilated alveoli → hypoxia and carbon dioxide retention (hypercapnia).

ADULT

Chronic hypercapnia reduces sensitivity of respiratory center; chemoreception in aortic arch and carotid sinus become principal regulators of respiratory drive (respond to hypoxia).

B. Risk factors:
1. Smoking.
2. Air pollution: long-term exposure to environmental irritants, fumes, dust.
3. Antienzymes and α_1-antitrypsin deficiencies.
4. Destruction of lung parenchyma.
5. Family history and increased age.

C. Assessment:
1. *Subjective data:*
   a. Weakness, lethargy.
   b. History of repeated respiratory infections, shortness of breath.
   c. Long-term smoking.
   d. Irritability.
   e. Inability to accept medical diagnosis and treatment plan.
   f. Refusal to stop smoking.
   g. Dyspnea on exertion, dyspnea at rest **(Table 6.14).**
2. *Objective data:*
   a. *Increased* BP.
   b. *Increased* pulse. *Decreased* O_2 saturation.
   c. Nostrils: flaring.
   d. Cough: chronic, productive.
   e. Episodes of wheezing, crackles.
   f. Increased anterior-posterior diameter of chest (barrel chest).
   g. Use of accessory respiratory muscles, abdominal and neck.
   h. Asymmetrical thoracic movements, decreased diaphragmatic excursion.
   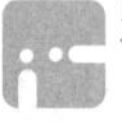
   i. *Position:* sits up, leans forward to compress abdomen and push up diaphragm, increasing intrathoracic pressure, producing more efficient expiration.
   j. Pursed lips for greater expiratory breathing phase (*"pink puffer"*).
   k. Weight loss due to hypoxia.
   l. Skin: ruddy color, nail clubbing; when combined with bronchitis: cyanosis (*"blue bloater"*).
   m. Respiratory: *early* disease—alkalosis; *late* disease—acidosis, respiratory failure.
   n. Spontaneous pneumothorax.
   o. Cor pulmonale (**emergency cardiac condition** involving right ventricular failure due to increased pressure within pulmonary artery).
   p. X-ray: hyperinflation of lung, flattened diaphragm; lung scan differentiates between ventilation and perfusion.
   q. Pulmonary function tests:
      (1) Prolonged rapid, forced exhalation.
      (2) *Decreased:* vital capacity (<4,000 mL); forced expiratory volume.
      (3) *Increased:* residual volume (may be 200%); total lung capacity.
   r. Laboratory data:
      (1) PaO_2 less than 80 mm Hg, pH less than 7.35.
      (2) $PaCO_2$ greater than 45 mm Hg.

   Note: In clients whose compensatory mechanisms are functioning, laboratory values may be out of the normal range, but if a 20:1 ratio of bicarbonate to carbonic acid is maintained, then appropriate acid-base balance also will be maintained. (Carbonic acid value can be

Table 6.14

Differentiating Between Causes of Dyspnea

	Asthma	Chronic Obstructive Pulmonary Disease	Pneumothorax	Pulmonary Edema	Pulmonary Emboli
Characteristics	• Episodic, acute • History of allergies • Recent cold or flu	• History of emphysema, bronchitis • Heavy smoker • Recent cold or respiratory infection	• Chest pain: sudden, sharp • *Sudden* onset; associated with coughing, air travel, strenuous exertion	• History of myocardial infarction • Rapid weight gain • Cough • Taking diuretics • Increasing need for pillows for sleep	• *Sudden* dyspnea • Sharp chest pain • Recent immobilization, surgery, or fracture of lower extremities • History of: thrombophlebitis, use of birth control pills, sickle cell anemia
Assessment Findings	• Wheezing • Hyperresonance • Chest may be silent with bronchospasms	• Use of pursed-lip breathing • Wheezing, crackles • "Barrel" chest • Uses accessory muscles to breathe	• Tracheal deviation • Asymmetrical chest motion • Diminished breath sounds	• Crackles • Pink, frothy sputum • Gallop (S_3) • Air hunger	• Tachycardia • Hypotension • Tachypnea • Pleural rub

ADULT

obtained by multiplying the P_{CO_2} value by 0.003.)

D. Analysis/nursing diagnosis:

1. *Impaired gas exchange* related to thick pulmonary secretions.
2. *Ineffective breathing pattern* related to hyperinflated alveoli.
3. *Ineffective airway clearance* related to pulmonary secretions.
4. *Altered nutrition, less than body requirements,* related to weight loss due to hypoxia.
5. *Infection* related to chronic disease process and decreased ciliary action.
6. *Activity intolerance* related to increased energy demands used for breathing.
7. *Sleep pattern disturbance* related to changes in body positions necessary for breathing.
8. *Anxiety* related to disease progression.
9. *Knowledge deficit* (learning need) related to disease, treatment, and self-care needs.

E. Nursing care plan/implementation:

1. Goal: *promote optimal ventilation.*
   a. Institute measures designed to decrease airway resistance and enhance gas exchange.
   b. *Position:* Fowler's or leaning forward to encourage expiratory phase.
   c. Oxygen with humidification, as ordered—no more than 2 L/min to prevent depression of hypoxic respiratory drive (see **Oxygen Therapy** in **Chapter 11, p. 835**). May need long-term oxygen therapy as disease progresses, to improve quality of life and reduce risk of complications.
   d. Intermittent positive-pressure breathing (IPPB) with nebulization as ordered. Small-volume nebulizer treatment.
   e. Assisted ventilation.
   f. Postural drainage, chest physiotherapy.
   g. Medications, as ordered:
      (1) *Bronchodilators* to increase airflow through bronchial tree: inhaled: beta_2-adrenergic agonists (albuterol, metaproterenol); anticholinergic agent: ipratropium (Atrovent); aminophylline, theophylline, terbutaline, isoproterenol (Isuprel).
      (2) *Antimicrobials* to treat infection (determined by sputum cultures and sensitivity): trimethoprim and sulfamethoxazole (Bactrim, Septra); doxycycline, erythromycin, amoxicillin, cephalosporins, and macrolides (condition deteriorates with respiratory infections).
      (3) *Corticosteroids* to decrease inflammation, mucosal edema, improve pulmonary function during exacerbation; *systemic:* prednisone, methylprednisolone sodium succinate (Solu-Medrol); *inhaled:* triamcinolone acetonide (Azmacort), beclomethasone (Beclovent, Vanceril), flunisolide (AeroBid).
      (4) *Expectorants* (increase water intake to achieve desired effect): glyceryl guaiacolate (Robitussin).
      (5) *Bronchial detergents*/liquefying agents (Mucomyst).
   h. Immunotherapy: helps ward off life-threatening influenza and pneumonia. Flu vaccination every October or November. Pneumococcal vaccination routinely one dose; revaccinate 5 years later if high risk.
2. Goal: *employ comfort measures and support other body systems.*
   a. Oral hygiene prn; frequently client is mouth breather.
   b. Skin care: waterbed, air mattress, foam pads to prevent skin breakdown.
   c. Active and passive ROM exercises to prevent thrombus formation; antiembolic stocking or woven elastic (Ace) bandages may be applied.
   d. Increase activities to tolerance.
   e. Adequate rest and sleep periods to prevent mental disturbances due to sleep deprivation and to reduce metabolic rate.
3. Goal: *improve nutritional intake.*
   a. *High-protein, high-calorie diet* to prevent negative nitrogen balance.
   b. Give small, frequent meals.
   c. Supplement diet with high-calorie drinks.
   d. *Push fluids* to 3,000 mL/day, unless contraindicated—helps moisten secretions.
4. Goal: *provide emotional support for client and family.*
   a. Identify factors that increase anxiety:
      (1) Fears related to mechanical equipment.
      (2) Loss of body image.
      (3) Fear of dying.
   b. Assist family coping:
      (1) Do *not* reinforce denial or encourage overconcern.
      (2) Give accurate, up-to-date information on client's condition.
      (3) Be open to questioning.
      (4) Encourage client–family communication.
      (5) Provide appropriate diversional activities.
5. Goal: *health teaching.*
   a. Breathing exercises, such as pursed-lip breathing and diaphragmatic breathing.
   b. Stress-management techniques.
   c. Methods to stop smoking.
   d. Importance of avoiding respiratory infections.

e. Desired effects and side effects of prescribed medications, possible interactions with over-the-counter drugs.
f. Purposes and techniques for effective bronchial hygiene therapy.
g. Rest/activity schedule that increases with ability.
h. Food selection for *high-protein, high-calorie* diet.
i. Importance of taking *2,500 to 3,000 mL fluid* per day (unless contraindicated by another medical problem).
j. Importance of medical follow-up.

F. Evaluation/outcome criteria:
1. Takes prescribed medication.
2. Participates in rest/activity schedule.
3. Improves nutritional intake, gains appropriate weight for body size.
4. No complications of respiratory failure, cor pulmonale.
5. No respiratory infections.
6. Acid-base balance maintained through compensatory mechanisms, acidosis prevented.

IX. ASTHMA: sometimes called reactive airway disease (RAD) or reversible obstructive airway disease (ROAD); a complex inflammatory process that causes increased airway resistance and, over time, airway tissue damage. Characterized by airway inflammation and hyperresponsiveness to a variety of stimuli such as allergens, cold air, dust, smoke, exercise, medications (e.g., aspirin), some food additives, and viral infections. *Immunologic* asthma occurs in childhood and follows other allergic disease. *Nonimmunologic* asthma occurs in adulthood and is associated with a history of recurrent respiratory tract infections.

A. Pathophysiology: triggers initiate the release of inflammatory mediators such as histamine, which produce airway obstruction through smooth muscle constriction, microvascular leakage, mucus plugging, and swelling. This process involves *six sequential steps:* (1) triggering—the allergic or antigenic stimuli activate the inflammatory (mast) cells; (2) these mast cells signal the systemic immune system to release proinflammatory substances; (3) migration of circulating inflammatory cells to regions of inflammation in the respiratory tract; (4) migrating cells are activated by the proinflammatory mediators; (5) this results in tissue damage; and (6) resolution. The airways of many clients with asthma are chronically inflamed.
1. *Immunologic,* or allergic asthma in persons who are atopic (hypersensitivity state that is subject to hereditary influences); immunoglobulin E (IgE) usually *elevated.*
2. *Nonimmunologic,* or nonallergic asthma in persons who have a history of repeated respiratory tract infections; age usually more than 35 years.
3. *Mixed,* combined immunologic and nonimmunologic; any age, allergen or nonspecific stimuli.

B. Risk factors:
1. History of allergies to identified or unidentified irritants; seasonal and environmental inhalants.
2. Recurrent respiratory infection.

C. Assessment:
1. *Subjective data:*
   a. History: upper respiratory infection (URI), rhinitis, allergies, family history of asthma.
   b. Increasing tightness of the chest → dyspnea (see **Table 6.14**).
   c. Anxiety, restlessness.
   d. Attack history:
      (1) *Immunologic:* contact with allergen to which person is sensitive; seen most often in children and young adults.
      (2) *Nonimmunologic:* develops in adults older than 35 years; aggravated by infections of the sinuses and respiratory tract.
2. *Objective data:*
   a. Peak flowmeter level drops.
   b. Respiratory assessment: increased rate, audible expiratory wheeze (also inspiratory when severe) on auscultation, hyperresonance on percussion, rib retractions, use of accessory muscles on inspiration.
   c. Tachycardia, tachypnea.
   d. Cough: dry, hacking, persistent.
   e. General appearance: pallor, cyanosis, diaphoresis, chronic barrel chest, elevated shoulders, flattened malar bones, narrow nose, prominent upper teeth, dark circles under eyes, distended neck veins, orthopnea.
   f. Expectoration of tenacious mucoid sputum.
   g. *Diagnostic tests:*
      (1) Forced vital capacity (FVC): *decreased.*
      (2) Forced expiratory volume in 1 second (FEV_1): *decreased.*
      (3) Peak expiratory flow rate: *decreased.*
      (4) Residual volume: *increased.*
   h. Laboratory data: blood gases—*elevated* PCO_2; *decreased* PO_2, pH.

Emergency note: Persons severely affected may develop *status asthmaticus,* a **life-threatening** asthmatic attack in which symptoms of asthma continue and do not respond to usual treatment. Could lead to respiratory failure and hypoxemia.

D. Analysis/nursing diagnosis:
1. *Ineffective airway clearance* related to tachypnea.
2. *Impaired gas exchange* related to constricted bronchioles.

3. *Anxiety* related to breathlessness.
4. *Activity intolerance* related to persistent cough.
5. *Knowledge deficit* (learning need) related to causal factors and self-care measures.

E. Nursing care plan/implementation:

1. Goal: *promote pulmonary ventilation.*

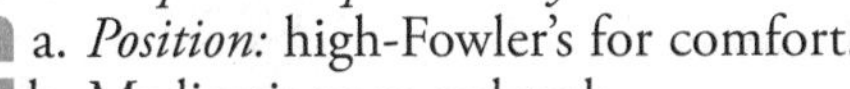

   a. *Position:* high-Fowler's for comfort.
   b. Medications as ordered:
      (1) *Rescue* medications: *corticosteroids* (e.g., prednisone, methylprednisolone [Medrol]; beta-adrenergic agonists, such as albuterol [Proventil, Ventolin], metaproterenol [Alupent, Metaprel]).
      (2) *Maintenance* medications: *nonsteroidal* anti-inflammatory drugs: cromolyn (Intal), nedocromil (Tilade); *corticosteroids:* beclomethasone (Vanceril), triamcinolone (Azmacort); *leukotriene inhibitors/receptor antagonists:* zafirlukast (Accolate), zileuton (Zyflo); *theophylline* (Theo-Dur, Slo-Bid, Uni-Dur, theophylline ethylenediamino [Aminophylline]); *anticholinergic:* ipratropium (Atrovent); beta agonists: salmeterol (Serevent); *mast cell stabilizers:* nedocromil sodium (Tilade).
      (3) *Antibiotics* to control infection.
   c. Oxygen therapy with increased humidity as ordered.
   d. Frequent monitoring for respiratory distress.
   e. Rest periods and gradual increase in activity.
2. Goal: *facilitate expectoration.*
   a. High humidity.
   b. *Increase fluid* intake.
   c. Monitor for dehydration.
   d. Respiratory therapy: IPPB.
3. Goal: *health teaching to prevent further attacks.*
   a. Identify and avoid all asthma triggers.
   b. Teach importance of peak flowmeter readings.
   c. Medications—when to use, how to use, side effects, withdrawals.
   d. Using a metered-dose inhaler:
      (1) Shake vigorously.
      (2) Position inhaler about 1 inch in front of mouth. Use 2 fingers to measure the 1-inch distance.
      (3) A spacer is recommended: connect spacer device, shake, press down the canister; place lips on the mouthpiece and take a slow deep breath through mouth. *Without* spacer: breathe out all the way, open mouth wide, and take a slow deep breath through mouth. Press down the canister and continue to breathe in.
      (4) Once lungs are full, hold breath for 10 seconds if possible.
      (5) Exhale normally through pursed lips.
      (6) Wait 1 to 2 minutes between puffs. Depending on the particular medication, may need to rinse mouth with water or mouthwash after each treatment.
   e. Methods to facilitate expectoration—increase humidity, postural drainage when appropriate, percussion techniques.
   f. Breathing techniques to increase expiratory phase.
   g. Stress-management techniques.
   h. Importance of recognizing early signs of asthma attack and beginning treatment immediately.
   i. Steps to take during an attack.

F. Evaluation/outcome criteria:

1. No complications.
2. Has fewer attacks.
3. Takes prescribed medications, avoids infections.
4. Adjusts lifestyle.
5. Pulmonary function tests return to normal.

X. BRONCHITIS: acute or chronic inflammation of bronchus resulting as a complication from colds and flu. *Acute bronchitis* is caused by an extension of upper respiratory infection, such as a cold, and can be given to others. It can also result from an irritation from physical or chemical agents. *Chronic bronchitis* is characterized by hypersecretion of mucus and chronic cough for 3 months per year for 2 consecutive years.

A. Pathophysiology: bronchial walls are infiltrated with lymphocytes and macrophages; lumen becomes obstructed due to decreased ciliary action and repeated bronchospasms. Hyperventilation of alveolar sacs occurs. Long-term condition results in respiratory acidosis, recurrent pneumonitis, emphysema, or cor pulmonale.

B. Risk factors:

1. Smoking.
2. Repeated respiratory infections.
3. History of living in area where there is much air pollution.

C. Assessment:

1. *Subjective data:*
   a. History: recurrent, chronic cough, especially when arising in the morning.
   b. Anorexia.
2. *Objective data:*
   a. *Respiratory:*
      (1) Shortness of breath.
      (2) Use of accessory muscles.
      (3) Cyanosis, dusky complexion: "blue bloater."
      (4) Sputum: excessive, nonpurulent.
      (5) Vesicular and bronchovesicular breath sounds; wheezing.
   b. Weight loss.
   c. Fever.

d. Pulmonary function tests:
   (1) *Decreased* forced expiratory volume.
   (2) PaO_2 less than 90 mm Hg; $PaCO_2$ greater than 40 mm Hg.
e. Laboratory data:
   (1) RBC count: *elevated* to compensate for hypoxia (polycythemia).
   (2) WBC count: *elevated* to fight infection.

D. Analysis/nursing diagnosis:
1. *Ineffective airway clearance* related to excessive sputum.
2. *Ineffective breathing pattern* related to need to use accessory muscles for breathing.
3. *Impaired gas exchange* related to shortness of breath.
4. *Activity intolerance* related to increased energy used for breathing.

E. Nursing care plan/implementation:
1. Goal: *assist in optimal respirations.*
   a. *Increase* fluid intake.
   b. IPPB, chest physiotherapy.
   c. Administer medications as ordered:
      (1) *Bronchodilators.*
      (2) *Antibiotics.*
      (3) *Bronchial detergents,* liquefying agents.
2. Goal: *minimize bronchial irritation.*
   a. *Avoid* respiratory irritants (e.g., smoke, dust, cold air, allergens).
   b. Environment: air-conditioned, increased humidity.
   c. Encourage nostril breathing rather than mouth breathing.
3. Goal: *improve nutritional status.*
   a. Diet: soft, *high* calorie.
   b. Small, frequent feedings.
4. Goal: *prevent secondary infections.*
   a. Administer *antibiotics* as ordered.
   b. *Avoid* exposure to infections, crowds.
5. Goal: *health teaching.*
   a. *Avoid* respiratory infections.
   b. Medications: desired effects and side effects.
   c. Methods to stop smoking.
   d. Rest and activity balance.
   e. Stress management.

F. Evaluation/outcome criteria:
1. Stops smoking.
2. Acid-base balance maintained.
3. Respiratory infections less frequent.

XI. ACUTE ADULT RESPIRATORY DISTRESS SYNDROME (ARDS) (formerly called by other names, including *shock lung*): noncardiogenic pulmonary infiltrations resulting in stiff, wet lungs and refractory hypoxemia in an adult who was previously healthy. Acute hypoxemic respiratory failure without hypercapnea.

A. Pathophysiology: damage to alveolar capillary membrane, increased vascular permeability creating noncardiac pulmonary edema, and impaired gas exchange; decreased surfactant production → atelectasis; severe hypoxia; refractory to ↑ FiO_2 → possible death.

B. Risk factors:
1. *Primary:*
   a. Shock, multiple trauma.
   b. Infections.
   c. Aspiration, inhalation of chemical toxins.
   d. Drug overdose.
   e. Disseminated intravascular coagulation (DIC).
   f. Emboli, especially fat emboli.
2. *Secondary:*
   a. Overaggressive fluid administration.
   b. Oxygen toxicity.
   c. Mechanical ventilation.

C. Assessment:
1. *Subjective data:*
   a. Restlessness, anxiety.
   b. History of risk factors.
   c. Severe dyspnea (see **Table 6.14**).
2. *Objective data:*
   a. Cyanosis.
   b. Tachycardia.
   c. Hypotension.
   d. Hypoxemia, acidosis.
   e. Crackles.
   f. X-ray—bilateral patchy infiltrates.
   g. Death if untreated.

D. Analysis/nursing diagnosis:
1. *Anxiety* related to serious physical condition.
2. *Ineffective breathing pattern* related to severe dyspnea.
3. *Impaired gas exchange* related to alveolar damage.
4. *Altered tissue perfusion* related to hypoxia.

E. Nursing care plan/implementation:
1. Goal: *assist in respirations.*
   a. May require mechanical ventilatory support to maintain respirations.
   b. May need to be transferred to ICU.
   c. May need oxygen to combat hypoxia.
   d. Suction prn.
   e. Monitor blood gas results to detect early signs of acidosis/alkalosis.
   f. If not on ventilator, assess vital signs and respiratory status every 15 minutes.
   g. Cough, deep breathe every hour.
   h. May need:
      (1) Rotation therapy and/or prone position.
      (2) Postural drainage, suction.
      (3) *Bronchodilator* medications.

ADULT

2. Goal: *prevent complications.*
   a. Decrease anxiety and provide psychological care:
      (1) Maintain a calm atmosphere.
      (2) Encourage rest to conserve energy.
      (3) Emotional support.
   b. Obtain fluid balance:
      (1) Slow IV flow rate.
      (2) *Diuretics:* rapid acting, low dose.
   c. Monitor:
      (1) Pulmonary artery and capillary wedge pressure cardiac output.
      (2) Central venous pressure (CVP), peripheral perfusion, arterial line BP.
      (3) I&O.
      (4) Assess for bleeding tendencies, potential for disseminated intravascular coagulation.
   d. Protect from infection:
      (1) *Strict aseptic* technique.
      (2) *Antibiotic* therapy.
      (3) Deep vein thrombosis prophylaxis.
   e. Provide physiological support:
      (1) Maintain nutrition.
      (2) Skin care.
3. Goal: *health teaching.*
   a. Briefly explain procedures as they are happening (emergency situation can frighten client).
   b. Give rationale for follow-up care.
   c. Identify risk factors as appropriate for prevention of recurrence.

F. Evaluation/outcome criteria:
1. Client survives and is alert.
2. Skin warm to touch.
3. Respiratory rate within normal limits.
4. Laboratory values and pressures within normal limits.
5. Urinary output greater than 30 mL/hr.

XII. PNEUMOTHORAX: presence of air within the pleural cavity; occurs spontaneously or as a result of trauma **(Fig. 6.3).**

A. Types:
1. *Closed* (spontaneous): rupture of a subpleural bulla, tuberculous focus, carcinoma, lung abscess, pulmonary infarction, severe coughing attack, or blunt trauma.
2. *Open* (traumatic): communication between atmosphere and pleural space because of opening in chest wall.
3. *Tension:* one-way leak; may occur during mechanical ventilation or cardiopulmonary resuscitation (CPR), or as a complication of any type of spontaneous or traumatic pneumothorax. Positive pressure within chest cavity resulting from accumulated air that cannot escape during expiration. Leads to collapse of lung, mediastinal shift, and compression of the heart and great vessels.

B. Pathophysiology: pressure builds up in the pleural space, lung on the affected side collapses, and the heart and mediastinum shift toward the unaffected lung.

C. Assessment:
1. *Subjective data:*
   a. *Pain:*
      (1) Sharp, aggravated by activity.
      (2) Location—chest; may be referred to shoulder, arm on affected side.

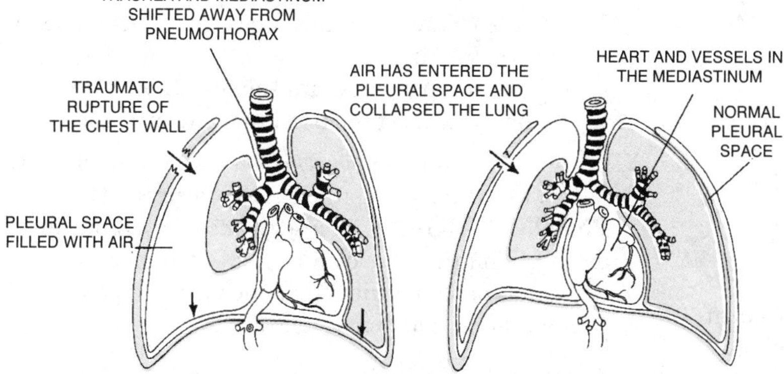
PNEUMOTHORAX
(OPEN —THE CHEST WALL INJURY PERMITS AIR TO FLOW IN AND OUT OF THE PLEURAL SPACE ON THE AFFECTED SIDE)
TRACHEA AND MEDIASTINUM SHIFTED AWAY FROM PNEUMOTHORAX
TRAUMATIC RUPTURE OF THE CHEST WALL
AIR HAS ENTERED THE PLEURAL SPACE AND COLLAPSED THE LUNG
HEART AND VESSELS IN THE MEDIASTINUM
NORMAL PLEURAL SPACE
PLEURAL SPACE FILLED WITH AIR
INHALATION: AIR ENTERS THE INJURED SIDE, CAUSING COLLAPSE OF THE LUNG AND SHIFT OF THE MEDIASTINUM AND HEART TOWARD THE UNAFFECTED SIDE
EXHALATION: THE AIR IS PARTIALLY FORCED FROM THE AFFECTED SIDE PLEURAL SPACE AND THE MEDIASTINUM SHIFT TOWARD THE AFFECTED SIDE

Figure 6.3 **Pneumothorax.** (From Venes, D [ed]: *Taber's Cyclopedic Medical Dictionary,* ed 21. FA Davis, Philadelphia, 2009.)

b. Restlessness, anxiety.
c. Dyspnea (see **Table 6.14**).

2. *Objective data:*
a. Cough.
b. Cessation of normal movements on affected side.
c. Absence of breath sounds on affected side.
d. Pallor, cyanosis.
e. Shock.
f. Tracheal deviation to unaffected side.
g. X-ray: air in pleural space.

D. Analysis/nursing diagnosis:

1. *Ineffective breathing pattern* related to collapse of lung.
2. *Impaired gas exchange* related to abnormal thoracic movement.
3. *Pain* related to trauma to chest area.
4. *Fear* related to emergency situation.

E. Nursing care plan/implementation:

1. Goal: *prevent damage until medical intervention available.*
a. Place sterile occlusive gauze dressing over wound.
b. Tape dressing on three sides to allow air to escape during expiration.
c. Place client on *affected side* to diminish possibility of tension pneumothorax.

2. Goal: *protect against injury during thoracentesis.*
a. Provide sterile equipment.
b. Explain procedure.
c. Monitor vital signs for shock.
d. Monitor for respiratory distress, mediastinal shift.

3. Goal: *promote respirations.*
a. *Position:* Fowler's.
b. Oxygen therapy as ordered.
c. Encourage slow breathing to improve gas exchange.
d. Careful administration of narcotics to prevent respiratory depression (*avoid* morphine).

4. Goal: *prepare client for closed chest drainage, physically and psychologically.*
a. Explain purpose of the procedure—to provide means for evacuation of air and fluid from pleural cavity; to reestablish negative pressure in pleural space; to promote lung reexpansion.
b. Explain procedure and apparatus (see Chest tubes section in **Table 11.5**).
c. Cleanse skin at tube insertion site; place client in *sitting position,* ensuring safety by having locked over-the-bed table for client to lean on, or have a nurse stay with client so appropriate position is maintained throughout the procedure.

5. Goal: *prevent complications with chest tubes.*
a. Observe for and **immediately report:** crepitations (air under skin, also called *subcutaneous emphysema*), labored or shallow breathing, tachypnea, cyanosis, tracheal deviation, or signs of hemorrhage.
b. Monitor for signs of infection.
c. Ensure that tubing stays intact.
d. *Monitor proper tube function.* Attach chest tube to a water-seal drainage apparatus and use wall suction for negative pressure. Monitor amount and color of tube drainage every 2 hours. Notify physician if bloody drainage exceeds 100 mL/hr. Chest drainage system should be at least 1 foot (30 cm) below the chest tube insertion site. Change dressing at tube insertion site every 48 hours. Air bubbles will continue in the water-seal chamber for 24 to 48 hours after insertion. Persistent air bubbles indicate an air leak between alveoli and pleural space. Fluctuation of fluid level is expected (when suction is off) because respiration changes the pleural pressure. If a clot forms in the tube, gently squeeze the tube, without occluding it, to move the clot, or follow specific orders as written. Make sure tube is free of kinks. When moving client, do *not* clamp tube; disconnect it from the wall suction. See key points for nursing intervention with chest tubes in **Table 11.5.**
e. Change position every 1 to 2 hours.
f. Arm and shoulder ROM.

6. Goal: *health teaching.*
a. How to prevent recurrence by avoiding overexertion; *avoid* holding breath.
b. Signs and symptoms of condition.
c. Methods to stop smoking.
d. Encourage follow-up care.

F. Evaluation/outcome criteria:

1. No complications noted.
2. Closed system remains intact until chest tubes are removed.
3. Lung reexpands, breath sounds heard, pain diminished, symmetrical thoracic movements.

XIII. HEMOTHORAX: *presence of blood* in pleural cavity related to trauma or ruptured aortic aneurysm (see **XII. PNEUMOTHORAX** for assessment, analysis/nursing diagnosis, nursing care plan/implementation, and evaluation/outcome criteria). **Table 6.15** compares pneumothorax and hemothorax.

XIV. CHEST TRAUMA

Flail chest: multiple rib fractures resulting in instability of the chest wall, with subsequent paradoxical breathing (portion of lung under injured chest wall

Table 6.15

Comparison of Pneumothorax and Hemothorax

	Pneumothorax (Free Air Between Visceral and Parietal Pleurae)	Hemothorax (Blood in Pleural Space)
Cause	*Spontaneous*—air enters without trauma; rupture of bleb (vesicle) on pleura; non–life threatening *Traumatic*—open chest wound: life threatening; closed chest wound—usually non–life threatening unless untreated *Tension*—air cannot escape via route of entry; causes atelectasis	Blunt trauma (assaults, falls) Penetrating trauma (knives, gunshot wounds)
Assessment Findings	Minimal to sudden onset; sharp chest pain; dyspnea; cough; hypotension; tachypnea; tachycardia; mediastinal shift (tracheal deviation)	Asymptomatic or pleuritic pain and dyspnea; decreased or absent breath sounds; often discovered during chest x-ray; in severe cases: shock

moves in on inspiration while remaining lung expands; on expiration, the injured portion of the chest wall expands while unaffected lung tissue contracts).

Sucking chest wound: penetrating wound of chest wall with hemothorax and pneumothorax, resulting in lung collapse and mediastinal shift toward unaffected lung.

A. Assessment:

1. *Subjective data:*
   a. Severe, sudden, sharp pain.
   b. Dyspnea.
   c. Anxiety, restlessness, fear, weakness.
2. *Objective data:*
   a. *Vital signs:*
      (1) *Pulse:* tachycardia, weak.
      (2) *BP:* hypotension.
      (3) *Respirations:* shallow, decreased expiratory force, tachypnea, stridor, accessory muscle breathing.
   b. Skin color: cyanosis, pallor.
   c. *Chest:*
      (1) Asymmetrical chest expansion (*paradoxical movement*).
      (2) Chest wound, rush of air through trauma site.
      (3) Crepitus over trauma site (from air escaping into surrounding tissues).
      (4) Lateral deviation of trachea, mediastinal shift.
   d. Pneumothorax: documented by absence of breath sounds, x-ray examination.
   e. Hemothorax: documented by needle aspiration by physician, x-ray examination.
   f. Shock; blood and fluid loss.
   g. Hemoptysis.
   h. Distended neck veins.

B. Analysis/nursing diagnosis:

1. *Ineffective airway clearance* related to shallow respirations.
2. *Impaired gas exchange* related to asymmetrical chest expansion.
3. *Pain* related to chest trauma.
4. *Fear* related to emergency situation.
5. *Risk for trauma* related to fractured ribs.
6. *Risk for infection* related to open chest wound.

C. Nursing care plan/implementation:

1. Goal: *restore adequate ventilation and prevent further air from entering pleural cavity:* **MEDICAL EMERGENCY.**
   a. In emergency situation: place air-occlusive dressing or hand over open wound as client exhales forcefully against glottis (*Valsalva maneuver* helps expand collapsed lung by creating positive intrapulmonary pressures); or place client's weight onto *affected* side. Administer oxygen.
   b. Assist with endotracheal tube insertion; client will be placed on volume-controlled ventilator. (See discussion of ventilators under **Oxygen Therapy** in **Chapter 11**.)
   c. Assist with thoracentesis and insertion of chest tubes with connection to water-seal drainage as ordered (see Chest tubes section in **Table 11.5**).
   d. Monitor vital signs to determine *early shock.*
   e. Monitor blood gases to determine *early acid-base imbalances.*
   f. Pain medications given with caution, so as not to depress respiratory center.

D. Evaluation/outcome criteria:

1. Respiratory status stabilizes, lung reexpands.
2. Shock and hemorrhage are prevented.
3. No further damage done to surrounding tissues.
4. Pain is controlled.

XV. THORACIC SURGERY: used for bronchogenic and lung carcinomas, lung abscesses, tuberculosis, bronchiectasis, emphysematous blebs, and benign tumors.

ADULT

A. Types:

1. *Thoracotomy*—incision in the chest wall, pleura is entered, lung tissue examined, biopsy secured. *Chest tube is needed postoperatively.*
2. *Lobectomy*—removal of a lobe of the lung. *Chest tube is needed postoperatively.*
3. *Pneumonectomy*—removal of an entire lung. *No chest tube is needed postoperatively.*

B. Analysis/nursing diagnosis:

1. *Risk for injury* related to chest wound.
2. *Impaired gas exchange* related to pain from surgical procedure.
3. *Ineffective airway clearance* related to decreased willingness to cough due to pain.
4. *Pain* related to surgical incision.
5. *Impaired physical mobility* related to large surgical incision and chest tube drainage apparatus.
6. *Knowledge deficit* (learning need) related to importance of coughing and deep breathing to prevent complications.

C. Nursing care plan/implementation:

1. *Preoperative care:*
   a. Goal: *minimize pulmonary secretions.*
      (1) Humidify air to moisten secretions.
      (2) Use IPPB, as ordered, to improve ventilation.
      (3) Administer *bronchodilators, expectorants,* and *antibiotics* as ordered.
      (4) Use postural drainage, cupping, and vibration to mobilize secretions.
   b. Goal: *preoperative teaching.*
      (1) Teach client to cough against a closed glottis to increase intrapulmonary pressure for improved expiratory phase.
      (2) Instruct in diaphragmatic breathing and coughing.
      (3) Encourage to stop smoking.
      (4) Instruct and supervise practice of postoperative arm exercises—flexion, abduction, and rotation of shoulder—to prevent ankylosis.
      (5) Explain postoperative use of chest tubes, IV, and oxygen therapy.
2. *Postoperative care:*
   a. Goal: *maintain patent airway.*
      (1) Auscultate chest for breath sounds; report diminished or absent breath sounds on unaffected side (indicates decreased ventilation → respiratory embarrassment).
      (2) Turn, cough, and deep breathe, every 15 minutes to 1 hour for first 24 hours and prn according to pulmonary congestion heard on auscultation.
   b. Goal: *promote gas exchange.*
      (1) Splint chest during coughing—support incision to help *cough up sputum (most important activity postoperatively).*

      (2) *Position:* high-Fowler's.
         (a) Turn client who has had a *pneumonectomy* to *operative* side (*avoid* extreme lateral positioning and mediastinal shift) to allow unaffected lung expansion and drainage of secretions; can also be turned onto back.
         (b) Client who has had a *lobectomy* or *thoracotomy* can be turned on *either* side or back because chest tubes will be in place.
   c. Goal: *reduce incisional stress and discomfort*—pad area around chest tube when turning on operative side to maintain tube patency and promote comfort.
   d. Goal: *prevent complications related to respiratory function.*
      (1) Maintain chest tubes to water-seal drainage system.
      (2) See Chest tubes section in **Table 11.5**.
      (3) Observe for *mediastinal shift* (trachea should always be midline; movement toward either side indicates shift).
         (a) Move client onto back or toward opposite side.
         (b) **MEDICAL EMERGENCY:** *Notify physician immediately.*
   e. Goal: *maintain fluid and electrolyte balance.*
      (1) Administer parenteral infusion *slowly* (risk of pulmonary edema due to decrease in pulmonary vasculature with removal of lung lobe or whole lung).
   f. Goal: *postoperative teaching.*
      (1) Prevent ankylosis of shoulder—teach passive and active ROM exercises of operative arm.
      (2) Importance of early ambulation, as condition permits.
      (3) Importance of stopping smoking.
      (4) Dietary instructions—nutritious diet to aid in healing process.
      (5) Importance of deep breathing, coughing exercises, to prevent stasis of respiratory secretions.
      (6) Importance of *increased fluids* in diet to liquefy secretions.
      (7) Desired and side effects of prescribed medications.
      (8) Importance of rest, *avoidance* of heavy lifting and work during healing process.
      (9) Importance of follow-up care; give names of referral agencies where client and family can obtain assistance.
      (10) Signs and symptoms of complications.

D. Evaluation/outcome criteria:

1. Client or significant other or both will be able to:
   a. Give rationale for activity restriction and demonstrate prescribed exercises.
   b. Identify name, dosage, side effects, and schedule of prescribed medications.
   c. State plans for necessary modifications in lifestyle, home.
   d. Identify support systems.
2. Wound heals without complications.
3. Obtains ROM in affected shoulder.
4. No complications of thoracotomy, such as:
   a. *Respiratory*—pulmonary insufficiency, respiratory acidosis, pneumonitis, atelectasis, pulmonary edema.
   b. *Circulatory*—hemorrhage, hypovolemia, shock, myocardial infarction.
   c. *Mediastinal shift.*
   d. *Renal failure.*
   e. *Gastric distention.*

XVI. TRACHEOSTOMY: opening into trachea, temporary or permanent. *Rationale:* airway obstruction due to foreign body, edema, tumor, excessive tracheobronchial secretions, respiratory depression, decreased gaseous diffusion at alveolar membrane, increased dead space (e.g., severe emphysema), or failure to wean from mechanical ventilator.

A. Analysis/nursing diagnosis:

1. *Ineffective airway clearance* related to increased secretions and decreased ability to cough effectively.
2. *Ineffective breathing pattern* related to physical condition that necessitated tracheostomy.
3. *Impaired verbal communication* related to inability to speak when tracheostomy tube cuff inflated.
4. *Fear* related to need for specialized equipment to breathe.

B. Nursing care plan/implementation:

1. *Preoperative care:*
   a. Goal: *relieve anxiety and fear.*
      (1) Explain purpose of procedure and equipment.
      (2) Demonstrate suctioning procedure.
      (3) Establish means of postoperative communication (e.g., paper and pencil, "magic slate," picture cards, and call bell). Specialized tubes such as a fenestrated tracheostomy tube or a tracheostomy button allow the individual to talk when the external opening is plugged.
      (4) Remain with client as much as possible.
2. *Postoperative care:*
   a. Goal: *maintain patent airway* **(Table 6.16).**
   b. Goal: *alleviate apprehension.*
      (1) Remain with client as much as possible.
      (2) Encourage client to communicate feelings using preestablished communication system.

   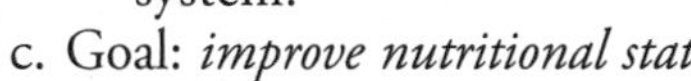

   c. Goal: *improve nutritional status.*
      (1) Provide nutritious foods/liquids the client can swallow.
      (2) Give supplemental drinks to maintain necessary calories.
   d. Goal: *health teaching.*
      (1) Explain all procedures.
      (2) Teach alternative methods of communication (best if done before the tracheostomy if it is not an emergency situation).
      (3) Teach self-care of tracheostomy as soon as possible.

Table 6.16

Tracheostomy Suctioning Procedure

1. Suction as necessary to facilitate respirations. Explain to client what to expect.
2. *Position:* semi-Fowler's to prevent forward flexion of neck, to facilitate respiration, to promote drainage, and to minimize edema.
3. Administer *mist* to tracheostomy because natural humidifying of oropharynx pathways has been eliminated.
4. Auscultate for moist, noisy respirations because nonproductive coughing may indicate need for suctioning.
5. Prevent hypoxia by administering *100% oxygen before suctioning* (unless contraindicated).
6. Use *strict aseptic technique* and sterile suctioning catheters with each aspiration; use sterile saline to clear catheter of secretions. Keep dominant hand gloved with sterile glove, nondominant hand with nonsterile glove to control thumb control of suction. Suction tracheostomy before nose or mouth.
7. *Do not apply suction when inserting* suction catheter to prevent injury to respiratory tract and prevent loss of oxygen. Insert catheter about 5 inches (12.5 cm).
8. If client coughs during suctioning, gently remove catheter to permit ejection and suction of mucus.
9. Apply suction intermittently for *no longer* than 5–10 seconds because prolonged suction decreases arterial oxygen concentration. Allow 2–3 minutes between attempts.
10. Cuff deflation: if high-volume, low-pressure cuffed tube is used, deflation not necessary. If other tracheostomy cuffed tube is used, deflate for 5 minutes every hour to prevent damage to trachea.
11. Use caution not to dislodge tube when changing dressing or ties that secure tube.

C. Evaluation/outcome criteria:
1. Airway patent.
2. Acid-base balance maintained.
3. No respiratory infection/obstruction.

CARDIOVASCULAR SYSTEM

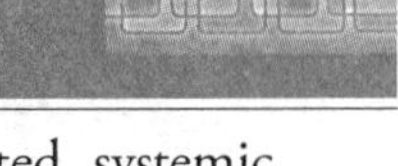

I. HYPERTENSION: sustained, elevated, systemic arterial blood pressure; diastolic elevation more serious, reflecting pressure on arterial wall during resting phase of cardiac cycle **(Table 6.17).**

A. Pathophysiology: increased peripheral resistance leading to thickened arterial walls and left ventricular hypertrophy.

B. Risk factors:
1. Black race (2:1).
2. Use of birth control pills.
3. Overweight.
4. Smoking.
5. Stress.
6. Excessive sodium intake or saturated fat.
7. Lack of activity.
8. Genetics, heredity.

C. Classifications:
1. *Essential* (primary or idiopathic): occurs in 90% to 95% of clients; etiology unknown; diastolic pressure is ≥90 mm Hg, and other causes of hypertension are absent. *Benign* hypertension (diastolic pressure ≤ 120 mm Hg) considered controllable; asymptomatic until complications develop.
2. *Secondary:* occurs in remaining 5% to 10%; usually renal, endocrine, neurogenic, or cardiac in origin.
3. *Malignant hypertension* (diastolic > 140 to 150 mm Hg); uncontrollable. May arise from both types.
4. *Labile* (prehypertensive): a fluctuating blood pressure; increases during stress, otherwise normal or near normal.

D. Assessment:
1. *Subjective data:*
   a. Early-morning headache, usually occipital.
   b. Light-headedness, tinnitus.

Table 6.17

Imbalances in Blood Pressure: Comparative Assessment of Hypotension and Hypertension

	Hypotension	Hypertension
Common Causes		
	Angina pectoris Myocardial infarction Acute and chronic pericarditis Valvular defects Heart failure	Essential hypertension Iron-deficiency anemia Pernicious anemia Arteriosclerosis obliterans Polycythemia vera
Assessment		
Behavior	Anxiety, apprehension, decreasing mentation, confusion	Nervousness, mood swings, irritability, difficulty with memory, depression, confusion
Neurological	Essentially noncontributory	Decreased vibratory sensations, increased/decreased reflexes, Babinski reflex, changes in coordination
Head/neck	Distended neck veins, worried expression	Bruits over carotids, distended neck veins, epistaxis, diplopia, ringing in ears, dull occipital headaches on arising
Skin	Pale, cool, moist	Dry, pale, glossy, flaky, cold; decreased or absent hair
GI	Anorexia, nausea, vomiting, constipation	Anorexia, flatulence, diarrhea, constipation
Respiratory	Dyspnea, orthopnea, paroxysmal nocturnal dyspnea, tachypnea, moist crackles, cough	Dyspnea, orthopnea, crackles
Cardiovascular	Tires easily Blood pressure—*decreased* systolic, *decreased* systolic/diastolic Pulse—increased/decreased/weak, thready, irregular, arrhythmias	Decreased exercise tolerance, weakness, palpitations Blood pressure—increased systolic and/or diastolic Decreased or absent pedal pulses
Renal	Oliguria	Oliguria, nocturia, proteinuria
Extremities	Dependent edema	Tingling, numbness, or cold hands and feet, dependent edema, ulcers of legs or feet

c. Palpitations.
d. Fatigue, insomnia.
e. Forgetfulness, irritability.
f. Altered vision: white spots, blurring, or loss.

2. *Objective data:*
   a. Epistaxis (nosebleeds).
   b. Elevated blood pressure: systolic greater than 120 mm Hg, diastolic greater than 90 mm Hg; narrowed pulse pressure. Rise in diastolic from sitting to standing with *essential;* fall in BP from sitting to standing with *secondary.*
   c. Retinal changes; papilledema.
   d. Shortness of breath on slight exertion.
   e. Cardiac, cerebral, and renal changes.
   f. *Laboratory data:* urinalysis, ECG, chest x-ray to rule out complications of hypertension.

E. Analysis/nursing diagnosis:

1. *Knowledge deficit* (learning need) regarding condition, treatment plan, and self-care and discharge needs.
2. *Risk for decreased cardiac output* related to ventricular hypertrophy, vasoconstriction, or myocardial ischemia.
3. *Risk for injury* related to complications of hypertension.
4. *Impaired adjustment* related to required lifestyle changes.
5. *Activity intolerance* related to weakness, fatigue.

F. Nursing care plan/implementation:

1. Goal: *provide for physical and emotional rest.*
   a. Rest periods before/after eating, visiting hours; *avoid* upsetting situations.
   b. Give *tranquilizers, sedatives,* as ordered.
2. Goal: *provide for special safety needs.*
   a. Monitor blood pressure: both arms; standing, sitting, lying positions.
   b. Limit/prevent activities that increase pressure (anxiety, anger, frustration, upsetting visitors, fatigue).
   c. Assist with ambulation; change position gradually to prevent dizziness and light-headedness (postural hypotension).
   d. Monitor for electrolyte imbalance when on low-sodium diet, diuretic therapy; I&O to prevent fluid depletion and arrhythmias from potassium loss.
   e. Observe for signs of hemorrhage, shock, stroke, which may occur following surgery.
3. Goal: *health teaching* (client and family).
   a. Procedures to decrease anxiety; relaxation techniques, stress management.
   b. Side effects of hypotensive drugs: initial therapy includes *diuretics* and *beta blockers;* if response inadequate may use *angiotensin-converting enzyme (ACE) inhibitors, adrenergic blockers, vasodilators, calcium channel blockers* (faintness, nausea, vomiting, hypotension, sexual dysfunction) (see **Chapter 8** for specific pharmacological actions).

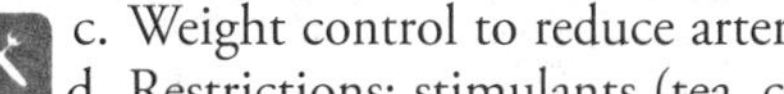

   c. Weight control to reduce arterial pressure.
   d. Restrictions: stimulants (tea, coffee, tobacco), sodium, calories, fat.
   e. *Lifestyle adjustments:* daily exercise needed; reduce occupational and environmental stress; importance of rest.
   f. Blood pressure measurement: daily, same conditions, both arms, position preference of physician; use of self-monitoring cuff; check at least twice per week.
   g. Signs, symptoms, complications of disease (headache, confusion, visual changes, nausea/vomiting, convulsions).
   h. Causes of intermittent hypotension: alcohol, hot weather, exercise, febrile illness, hot bath.

G. Evaluation/outcome criteria:

1. Blood pressure within normal range for age (diastolic less than 90 mm Hg)—stable.
2. Minimal or no pathophysiological or therapeutic complications (e.g., visual changes, stroke, drug side effects).
3. Reduces weight to reasonable level for height, bone structure.
4. Takes prescribed medications regularly, even after symptoms have resolved.
5. Complies with restrictions: no smoking; restricted sodium, fat.
6. Exercises regularly—program compatible with personal and health-care goals.

II. CARDIAC ARRHYTHMIAS (DYSRHYTHMIAS):

any variations in normal rate, rhythm, or configuration of waves on ECG **(Fig. 6.4).**

A. Pathophysiology:

1. Dysfunction of sinoatrial (SA) node, atria, atrioventricular (AV) node, or ventricular conduction.
2. Primary heart problem or secondary systemic problem.

B. Risk factors:

1. Myocardial infarction.
2. Drug toxicity.
3. Stress.
4. Cardiac surgery.
5. Hypoxia.
6. Congenital.

C. Assessment: see **Table 6.18** for specific dysrhythmias.

D. Analysis/nursing diagnosis:

1. *Decreased cardiac output* related to abnormal ventricular function.
2. *Altered tissue perfusion* related to inadequate cardiac functioning.

(text continues on page 415)

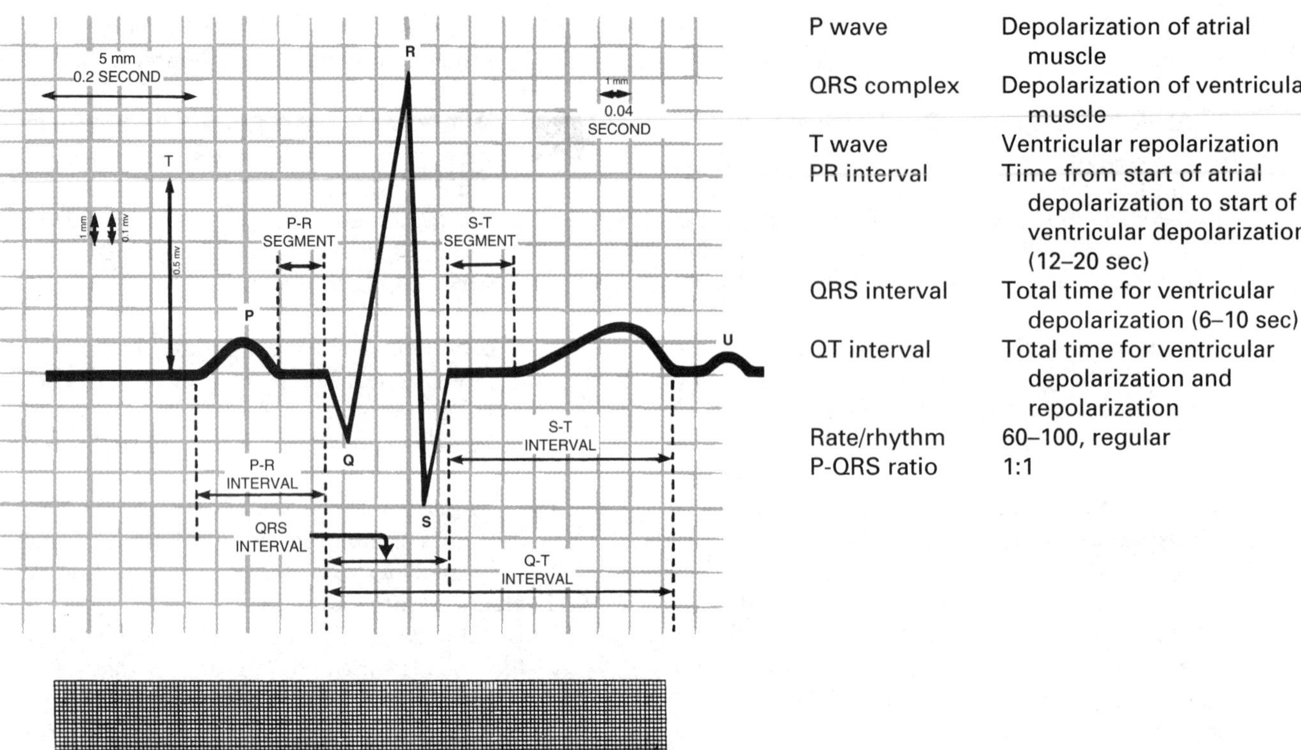

Figure 6.4 Interpretation of normal cardiac cycle. (From Venes, D [ed]: *Taber's Cyclopedic Medical Dictionary,* ed 21. FA Davis, Philadelphia, 2009.)

Table 6.18

Comparison of Selected Cardiac Dysrhythmias

Dysrhythmia	Description	Etiology	Symptoms/Consequences	Treatment
Dysrhythmias of Sinus Node				
Sinus dysrhythmia	Phasic shortening, then lengthening of P-P and R-R intervals	Respiratory variation in impulse initiation by SA node	Usually none	Usually none Atropine if rate *below* 40 beats/min
Sinus tachycardia	• P waves present followed by QRS complex • Rhythm regular • Heart rate 100–150 beats/min	• Increased metabolic demands • Decreased oxygen delivery • Heart failure • Shock • Hemorrhage • Anemia	• May produce palpitations • Prolonged episodes may lead to decreased cardiac output	Treat underlying cause Occasionally sedatives
Sinus bradycardia	• P waves present followed by QRS complex • Rhythm regular • Heart rate <60 beats/min	• Physical fitness • Parasympathetic stimulation (sleep) • Brain lesions • Sinus dysfunction • Digitalis excess	Very low rates may cause decreased cardiac output: light-headedness, faintness, chest pain	• Atropine if cardiac output is decreased • Pacemaker • Treat underlying cause if necessary

Table 6.18

Comparison of Selected Cardiac Dysrhythmias—cont'd

Dysrhythmia	Description	Etiology	Symptoms/Consequences	Treatment
Atrial Dysrhythmias				
Premature atrial beats	• Early P wave • QRS complex may or may not be normal • Rhythm irregular	Stress Ischemia Atrial enlargement Caffeine Nicotine	• May produce palpitations • Frequent episodes may decrease cardiac output • Is sign of chamber irritability	Sedation Eliminate nicotine and caffeine May require no other treatment
Atrial tachycardia	• P wave present (may merge into previous T wave), QRS complex usually normal; rapid heart rate (usually >150 beats/min)	• Sympathetic stimulation • Chemical stimuli (caffeine, nicotine) • Drug toxicity • Fluid-electrolyte imbalance • Thoracic surgery	Palpitations Possible anxiety Hypotension	• Usually none if short burst (<1 min) • Prolonged episodes may require carotid artery pressure, vagal stimulation, verapamil, digitalis, beta blockers, calcium channel blockers
Atrial fibrillation	• Rapid, irregular P waves (>350/min) • Ventricular rhythm irregularly irregular • Ventricular rate varies, may increase to 120–150/min if untreated	• Rheumatic heart disease • Mitral stenosis • Atrial infarction • Coronary atherosclerotic heart disease • Hypertensive heart disease • Thyrotoxicosis	• Hypotension • Palpitations • Pulse deficit • Decreased cardiac output if rate is rapid • Promotes thrombus formation in atria	Digitalis Cardizem Amiodarone Anticoagulation Cardioversion
Atrial flutter	• "Sawtooth" or "picket fence" P waves (220–350 beats/min) • Ratio of atrial to ventricular rate constant (3:1, 4:1, etc.)	Heart failure Mitral valve disease Pulmonary embolus	Occasional palpitations Chest pain	Cardioversion Anticoagulation medications if cardioversion unsuccessful
Ventricular Dysrhythmias				
Premature ventricular beats (PVBs)	• Early, wide, bizarre QRS complex, not associated with a P wave • Rhythm irregular	• Stress • Acidosis • Ventricular enlargement • Electrolyte imbalance • Myocardial infarction • Digitalis toxicity • Hypoxemia • Hypercapnia	Same as for premature atrial beats	Check Mg^{++}, K^{+} levels **MEDICATIONS:** Procainamide Disopyramide (Norpace) Lidocaine Mexiletine Sodium bicarbonate Potassium • Oxygen • Treat heart failure
Ventricular tachycardia	• No P wave before QRS complex; QRS complex wide and bizarre; ventricular rate >100, usually 140–240	• PVBs striking during vulnerable period • Hypoxemia • Drug toxicity • Electrolyte imbalance • Bradycardia	Decreased cardiac output: hypotension, loss of consciousness, respiratory arrest	**MEDICATIONS:** Lidocaine Procainamide Amiodarone • Cardioversion • Electrolytes
Ventricular fibrillation	• Chaotic electrical activity • No recognizable QRS complex	Myocardial infarction Electrocution Freshwater drowning Drug toxicity	No cardiac output Absent pulse or respiration Cardiac arrest	• Defibrillation **MEDICATIONS:** Epinephrine Lidocaine Sodium bicarbonate Bretylium Magnesium sulfate • CPR

Continued

Table 6.18

Comparison of Selected Cardiac Dysrhythmias—cont'd

Dysrhythmia	Description	Etiology	Symptoms/Consequences	Treatment
Pulseless electrical activity (PEA)	Organized ECG rhythm	• Electromechanical dissociation • Escape rhythms	Pulseless Minimal or no perfusion	• CPR • Epinephrine • Fluid challenge
Ventricular standstill	• Can be distinguished from ventricular fibrillation only by ECG • P waves *may* be present • No QRS complex • "Straight line"	• Myocardial infarction • Chronic diseases of conducting system	Same as for ventricular fibrillation	• CPR • Pacemaker • Intracardiac epinephrine
Impulse Conduction Deficits				
First-degree atrioventricular [AV] block	• P-R interval prolonged, >0.20 sec	• Rheumatic fever • Digitalis toxicity • Degenerative changes of coronary atherosclerotic heart disease • Infections (e.g., Lyme carditis) • Decreased oxygen in AV node	Warns of impaired conduction	• Usually none as long as it occurs as an isolated deficit • Atropine if P-R interval >0.26 sec or bradycardia
Bundle branch block	• Same as normal sinus rhythm (NSR) except QRS complex duration >0.10 sec	• Hypoxia • Acute myocardial infarction • Heart failure • Coronary atherosclerotic heart disease • Pulmonary embolus • Hypertension	Same as first-degree AV block	Usually none unless severe blockage of left posterior division (see text)
Second-degree AV blocks	• P waves usually occur regularly at rates consistent with SA node initiation (not all P waves followed by QRS complex; P-R interval may lengthen before nonconducted P wave or may be consistent; QRS complex may be widened)	• Acute myocardial infarction • Same as first-degree AV block	• Serious dysrhythmia that may lead to decreased heart rate and cardiac output, hypotension	• May require temporary pacemaker • If symptomatic (e.g., hypotension, dizziness), atropine 1 mg
Complete third-degree AV block	• Atria and ventricles beat independently • P waves have no relation to QRS complex • Ventricular rate may be as low as 20–40 beats/min	• Digitalis toxicity • Infectious disease • Coronary artery disease • Myocardial infarction	Very low rates may cause decreased cardiac output: light-headedness, fainting, chest pain	• Pacemaker • Isoproterenol to increase heart rate • Epinephrine if isoproterenol ineffective

From Phipps, W, Long, B, Woods, N, and Cassmeyer, V (eds): *Medical-Surgical Nursing,* ed. 5. Mosby, St. Louis, 2007.

ADULT

3. *Knowledge deficit* (learning need) regarding cause/treatment of condition, self-care, and discharge needs.
4. *Anxiety* related to dependence, fear of death.

E. Nursing care plan/implementation:

1. Goal: *provide for emotional and safety needs.*
   a. Document ECG tracing for presence of life-threatening arrhythmia.
   b. Encourage discussion of fears, feelings (client and significant other).
   c. *Bedrest:* restricted activities; quiet environment; limit visitors.
   d. Oxygen, if ordered.
   e. Check vital signs frequently for shock, heart failure (HF), drug toxicity.
   f. Prepare for cardiac emergency: CPR.
   g. Give cardiac medications; check laboratory tests for digitalis and potassium levels, to prevent drug toxicity.
2. Goal: *prevent thromboemboli.*
   a. Apply antiembolic stockings (TED hose); segmental compression device.
   b. Give *anticoagulants* as ordered. (Check for bleeding—gums, urine; monitor *laboratory tests*—Lee-White clotting time and activated partial thromboplastin time with heparin; prothrombin time or international normalized ratio [INR] with warfarin [Coumadin].)
   c. Encourage flexion and extension of feet.
3. Goal: *prepare for cardioversion with atrial fibrillation if indicated* (usually if pulse greater than 140 beats/min, symptomatic, or no conversion after 3 days of drug therapy and anticoagulated).
   a. Give Cardizem or amiodarone as ordered at least 24 hours before.
   b. NPO 8 hours before.
   c. *Hold* digoxin morning of cardioversion per order.
   d. Give *conscious sedation* medications as ordered.
4. Goal: *provide for physical and emotional needs with pacemaker insertion.*
   a. *General concerns:*
      (1) Report excessive bleeding/infection at insertion site—hematoma may contribute to wound infection.
      (2) Encourage verbalization of feelings.
      (3) Report prolonged hiccups, which may indicate pacemaker failure.
      (4) Know pacing mode: fixed-rate or demand (most common); type of insertion (temporary or permanent), sensitivity.
   b. *Temporary pacemaker:*
      (1) Limit excessive activity of extremity if antecubital insertion, to prevent displacement; subclavian insertion increases catheter stability.
      (2) Secure wires to chest to prevent tension on catheter.
      (3) Do *not* defibrillate over insertion site, to avoid electrical hazards.
      (4) Electrical safety (grounding; disconnect electric beds/call lights; use battery-operated equipment).
      (5) Check settings.
   c. *Permanent pacemaker:*
      (1) Limit activity of shoulder for 48 to 72 hours after insertion of transvenous catheter to prevent dislodgement; *avoid* extending arms over head for 8 weeks.
      (2) Postinsertion ROM (passive) at least once per shift after 48 hours to prevent frozen shoulder.
      (3) If defibrillation is required, place paddles at least 4 inches from pulse generator.
      (4) Check site.
   d. *Health teaching* following permanent pacemaker:
      (1) Explain procedure: duration, equipment, purpose, type of pacemaker.
      (2) Medic Alert bracelet; pacemaker information card.
      (3) Daily pulse taking on arising (report variation of ± 5 beats).
      (4) Signs, symptoms of *malfunction* (vertigo, syncope, dyspnea, slowed speech, confusion, fluid retention); *infection* (fever, heat, pain, skin breakdown at insertion site).
      (5) **Restrictions:** limit vigorous arm and shoulder motion for 6 to 8 weeks; contact sports; electromagnetic interferences (few)—TV/radio transmitters, improperly functioning microwave oven (maintain distance of 3 feet), certain cautery machines; may trigger airport metal-detector alarm.

F. Evaluation/outcome criteria:

1. Regular cardiac rhythm, monitors own radial pulse.
2. No complications (e.g., pacemaker malfunction).
3. Returns for regular follow-up of pacemaker function.
4. Tolerates physical or sexual activity.
5. Wears identification bracelet; carries pacemaker identification card.
6. Reports anxiety is reduced to manageable level.

III. CARDIAC ARREST: sudden unexpected cessation of heartbeat and effective circulation leading to inadequate perfusion and sudden death.

A. Risk factors:

1. Myocardial infarction.
2. Multiple traumas.

ADULT

3. Respiratory arrest.
4. Drowning.
5. Electrical shock.
6. Drug reactions.
7. Multisystem failure.

B. Assessment—*objective data:*

1. Unresponsive to stimuli (i.e., verbal, painful).
2. Absence of breathing, carotid pulse.
3. Pale or bluish: lips, fingernails, skin.
4. Pupils: dilated.

C. Analysis/nursing diagnosis:

1. *Decreased cardiac output* related to heart failure.
2. *Impaired gas exchange* related to breathlessness.
3. *Altered tissue perfusion* related to pulselessness.

D. Nursing care plan/implementation:

1. Goal: *prevent irreversible cerebral anoxic damage:* initiate CPR within 4 to 6 minutes; continue until relieved; document assessment factors, effectiveness of actions; presence or absence of pulse at 1 minute and every 4 to 5 minutes.
2. Goal: *establish effective circulation, respiration* (see **Cardiovascular Emergencies, Table 6.44,** for complete protocols).

E. Evaluation/outcome criteria:

1. Carotid pulse present; check after 1 minute and every few minutes thereafter.
2. Responds to verbal stimuli.
3. Pupils constrict in response to light.
4. Return of spontaneous respiration; adequate ventilation.

IV. ARTERIOSCLEROSIS: loss of elasticity, thickening, hardening of arterial walls; symptoms depend on organ system involved; common type—atherosclerosis. Atherosclerosis (coronary heart disease [CHD]) precedes angina pectoris and myocardial infarction.

A. Pathophysiology:

1. Atherosclerotic plaque, discrete lumpy thickening of arterial wall; cholesterol-lipid-calcium deposits in lining.
2. Narrows lumen, can occlude vessel.

B. Risk factors:

1. Increased serum cholesterol (low-density lipids ≥160 mg/dL).
2. Hypertension.
3. Cigarette smoking.
4. Diabetes mellitus.
5. Family history of premature CHD.

See following sections **V. ANGINA PECTORIS** and **VI. MYOCARDIAL INFARCTION** for nursing implications.

V. ANGINA PECTORIS: transient paroxysmal episodes of substernal or precordial pain. Types: *stable* (follows an event, same severity); *unstable* (at rest or minimal exertion, recent onset, increasing severity); *Prinzmetal's variant* (at rest, caused by coronary spasms).

A. Pathophysiology:

1. Insufficient blood flow through coronary arteries. Oxygen demand exceeds supply.
2. Temporary myocardial ischemia.

B. Risk factors:

1. Cardiovascular:
   a. Atherosclerosis.
   b. Thromboangiitis obliterans.
   c. Aortic regurgitation.
   d. Hypertension.
2. Hormonal:
   a. Hypothyroidism.
   b. Diabetes mellitus.
3. Blood disorders:
   a. Anemia.
   b. Polycythemia vera.
4. *Lifestyle choices:*
   a. Smoking.
   b. Obesity.
   c. Cocaine use.
   d. Inactivity.

C. Assessment:

1. *Subjective data:*
   a. *Pain—typical* (**Table 6.19**).
      (1) *Type:* squeezing, pressing, burning.
      (2) *Location:* retrosternal, substernal, left of sternum, radiates to left arm (**Fig. 6.5**).
      (3) *Duration:* short, usually 3 to 5 minutes, less than 30 minutes.
      (4) *Cause:* emotional stress, overeating, physical exertion, exposure to cold; may occur at rest.
      (5) *Relief:* rest, nitroglycerin.
   b. *Note: Atypical* complaints by women include jaw and upper back pain and persistent gastric upset.
   c. Dyspnea.
   d. Palpitations.
   e. Dizziness; faintness.
   f. Epigastric distress; indigestion; belching.
2. *Objective data:*
   a. Tachycardia.
   b. Pallor.
   c. Diaphoresis.
   d. ECG changes during attack.

D. Analysis/nursing diagnosis:

1. *Altered cardiopulmonary tissue perfusion* related to insufficient blood flow.
2. *Pain* related to myocardial ischemia.
3. *Activity intolerance* related to onset of pain.

E. Nursing care plan/implementation:

1. Goal: *provide relief from pain.*

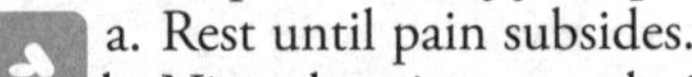

   a. Rest until pain subsides.
   b. Nitroglycerin or amyl nitrite, beta-adrenergic blockers, as ordered.

Table 6.19

Comparison of Physical Causes of Chest Pain

Characteristic	Myocardial Infarction	Pericarditis	Gastric Disorders	Angina Pectoris	Dissecting Aneurysm	Pulmonary Embolism
Onset	Gradual or sudden	Sudden	Gradual or sudden	Gradual or sudden	Abrupt, without prodromal symptoms	Gradual or sudden
Precipitating factors	Can occur at rest or after exercise or emotional stress	Breathing deeply, rotating trunk, recumbency, swallowing or yawning	Inflammation of stomach or esophagus; hypersecretion of gastric juices; some medications	Usually after: physical exertion, emotional stress, eating, exposure to cold, or defecation; unstable angina occurs at rest	Hypertension	Immobility or prolonged bedrest following: surgery, trauma, hip fracture, HF, malignancy, oral contraceptives
Location	Substernal, anterior chest, or midline; rarely back; radiates to jaw or neck	Precordial; radiates to neck or left shoulder and arm	Xiphoid to umbilicus	Substernal, anterior chest; poorly localized	Correlates with site of intimal rupture; anterior chest or back; between shoulder blades	Pleural area, retrosternal area
Quality	Crushing, burning, stabbing, squeezing or vicelike	Pleuritic, sharp	Aching, burning, cramplike, gnawing	Squeezing, feeling of heavy pressure; burning	Sharp, tearing or ripping sensation	Sharp, stabbing
Intensity	Asymptomatic to severe; increases with time	Mild to severe	Mild to severe	Mild to moderate	Severe and unbearable; maximal from onset	Aggravated by breathing
Duration	30 min to 1–2 hr; may wax and wane	Continuous	Periodic	Usually 2–10 min; average 3–5 min	Continuous; does not abate once started	Variable
Relief	Narcotics	Sitting up, leaning forward	Physical and emotional rest, food, antacids, H_2-receptor antagonists	Nitroglycerin, rest	Large, repeated doses of narcotics	O_2; sitting up; morphine
Associated symptoms	Nausea, fatigue, heartburn; peripheral pulses equal	Fever, dyspnea, nausea, anorexia, anxiety	Nausea, vomiting, dysphagia, anorexia, weight loss	Belching, indigestion, dizziness	Syncope, loss of sensations or pulses, oliguria; discrepancy between BP in arms; decrease in femoral or carotid pulse	Dyspnea, tachypnea, diaphoresis, hemoptysis, cough, apprehension

c. Identify precipitating factors: large meals, heavy exercise, stimulants (coffee, smoking), sex when fatigued, cold air.
d. Vital signs: hypotension.
e. Assist with ambulation; dizziness, flushing occurs with nitroglycerin.

2. Goal: *provide emotional support.*
   a. Encourage verbalization of feelings, fears.
   b. Reassurance; positive self-concept.
   c. Acceptance of limitations.
3. Goal: *health teaching.*
   a. Pain: alleviation, differentiation of angina from myocardial infarction, precipitating factors (see **Table 6.19**).
   b. Medication: frequency, expected effects (headache, flushing); carry fresh nitroglycerin; loses potency after 6 months ("stings" under tongue when potent); may use nitroglycerin paste—instruct how to apply.

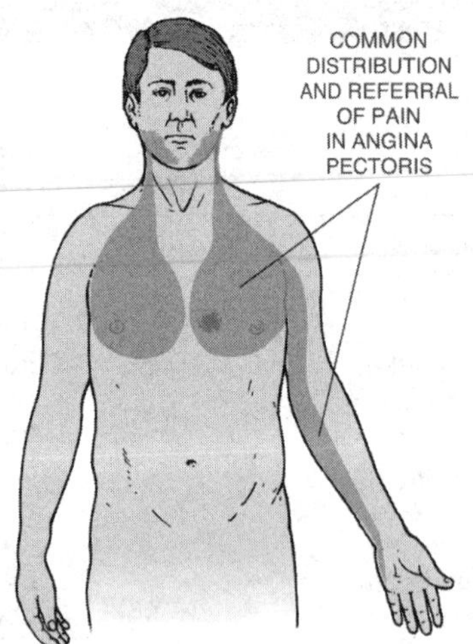

Figure 6.5 Angina pectoris. (From Venes, D [ed]: *Taber's Cyclopedic Medical Dictionary,* ed 21. FA Davis, Philadelphia, 2009.)

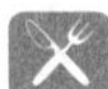

c. *Diet:* restricted calories if weight loss indicated; restricted fat, cholesterol, gas-producing foods; small, frequent meals.
d. *Diagnostic tests* if ordered (e.g., thallium stress test, cardiac catheterization; interventional [stents]; see **pp. 421–422** and **Chapter 11, pp. 829–830**).
e. Exercise: regular, graded, to promote coronary circulation.
f. Prepare for coronary artery bypass graft (CABG) surgery, if necessary.
g. Behavior modification to assist with lifestyle changes (e.g., stress reduction, stop smoking).

F. Evaluation/outcome criteria:
1. Relief from pain.
2. Fewer attacks.
3. No myocardial infarction.
4. Alters lifestyle; stress management; complies with limitations.
5. No smoking.

VI. MYOCARDIAL INFARCTION (MI, HEART ATTACK): localized area of necrotic tissue in myocardium from cessation of blood flow; leading cause of death in North America.

A. Pathophysiology:
1. Coronary occlusion due to thrombosis, embolism, or hemorrhage adjacent to atherosclerotic plaque.
2. Insufficient blood flow from cardiac hypertrophy, hemorrhage, shock, or severe dehydration.

B. Risk factors:
1. Age (35 to 70 years).
2. Men more than women until menopause.
3. Lifestyle: obesity, smoking, sedentary, amphetamine or cocaine use.
4. Stress or type A personality.
5. High levels of low-density lipoproteins, and high serum triglyceride levels.
6. Chronic illness (diabetes, hypertension).

C. Assessment:
1. *Subjective data:*
   a. *Pain* (see **Table 6.19**).
      (1) *Type:* sudden, severe, crushing, heavy tightness. May be absent in elderly or those who have diabetes.
      (2) *Location:* substernal; radiates to one or both arms, jaw, neck. May be confused with indigestion.
      (3) *Duration:* greater than 30 minutes.
      (4) *Cause:* unrelated to exercise; frequently occurs when sleeping (rapid-eye-movement [REM] stage).
      (5) *Relief:* oxygen, *narcotics; not* relieved by rest or nitroglycerin.
   b. Nausea.
   c. Shortness of breath.
   d. Apprehension, fear of impending death.
   e. History of cardiac disease (family); occupational stress.
2. *Objective data:*
   a. *Vital signs:* shock; rapid (>100), thready pulse; fall in blood pressure; S_3 gallop; tachypnea, shallow respirations; elevated temperature within 24 hours (100° to 103°F).
   b. Skin: ashen or clammy; diaphoretic.
   c. Emotional: restless.
   d. Laboratory data: *increased*—WBC count (12,000 to 15,000/microL), troponin T and I levels, serum enzymes (creatine kinase-MB [CK-MB]; lactate dehydrogenase (LDH): $LDH_1 > LDH_2$—"flipped LDH"); *changes*—ECG (*elevated* ST segment, inverted T wave, arrhythmia).

D. Analysis/nursing diagnosis:
1. *Decreased cardiac output* related to myocardial damage.
2. *Impaired gas exchange* related to poor perfusion, shock.
3. *Pain* related to myocardial ischemia.
4. *Activity intolerance* related to pain or inadequate oxygenation.
5. *Fear* related to possibility of death.

E. Nursing care plan/implementation:
1. Goal: *reduce pain, discomfort.*
   a. *Narcotics*—morphine; note response. *Avoid* IM.
   b. Humidified oxygen 2 to 4 L/min; mouth care—oxygen is drying.
   c. *Position:* semi-Fowler's to improve ventilation.
2. Goal: *maintain adequate circulation,* stabilize heart rhythm.
   a. Monitor vital signs and urine output; observe for cardiogenic shock.

ADULT

b. Monitor ECG for arrhythmias.

c. Give medications as ordered: *antiarrhythmics*—lidocaine HCl, amiodarone, atropine, beta blockers, procainamide (Pronestyl), bretylium (Bretylol); propranolol (Inderal); verapamil; *anticoagulants*—heparin sodium, bishydroxy-coumarin or dicoumarin; *thrombolytic agents*—streptokinase (tPA), APSAC/anistreplase (Eminase), reteplase followed by IV heparin or a glycoprotein IIB/IIIA inhibitor (Integrilin).

d. *Diagnostic tests*—echocardiogram, prepare for cardiac catheterization, possible interventional cardiology (stents), possible CABG surgery.

e. Recognize heart failure: edema, cyanosis, dyspnea, cough, crackles.

f. Check laboratory data—normal; troponin; *serum enzymes* (CK 20 to 220 IU/L depending on gender; CK-MB 0 to 12 IU/L; LDH <115 IU/L; $LDH_1 < LDH_2$); *blood gases* (pH 7.35 to 7.45; P_{CO_2} 35 to 45 mEq/L; P_{O_2} 80 to 100 mm Hg; HCO_3 22 to 26); *electrolytes* (K^+ 3.5 to 5.0 mEq/L; Mg^{++} 1.3 to 2.1 mg/dL); *clotting time* (aPTT 25 to 41 seconds; *prothrombin time* [PT] 11 to 15 seconds).

g. CVP—zero level at right atrium; fluctuates with respiration; normal range 5 to 15 cm H_2O; note trend; increases with heart failure.

h. ROM of lower extremities; TED hose/antiembolic stockings.

3. Goal: *decrease oxygen demand/promote oxygenation, reduce cardiac workload.*
   a. O_2 as ordered.
   b. Activity: bedrest (24 to 48 hours) with bedside commode; planned rest periods; control visitors.
   c. *Position:* semi-Fowler's to facilitate lung expansion and decrease venous return.
   d. Anticipate needs of client: call light, water.
   e. Assist with feeding, turning.
   f. Environment: quiet, comfortable.
   g. Reassurance; stay with client who is anxious.
   h. Give medications as ordered: cardiotonics, calcium channel blockers, vasodilators, vasopressors.
4. Goal: *maintain fluid, electrolyte, nutritional status.*
   a. IV (keep vein open); CVP; vital signs.
   b. Urine output—30 mL/hr.
   c. Laboratory data within *normal* limits (Na^+ 135 to 145 mEq/L; K^+ 3.5 to 5.0 mEq/L; Mg^{++} 1.3 to 2.1 mg/dL).
   d. Monitor ECG—*hyperkalemia:* peaked T wave; *hypokalemia:* depressed T wave.
   e. *Diet:* progressive *low* calorie, *low* sodium, *low* cholesterol, *low* fat, without caffeine.
5. Goal: *facilitate fecal elimination.*

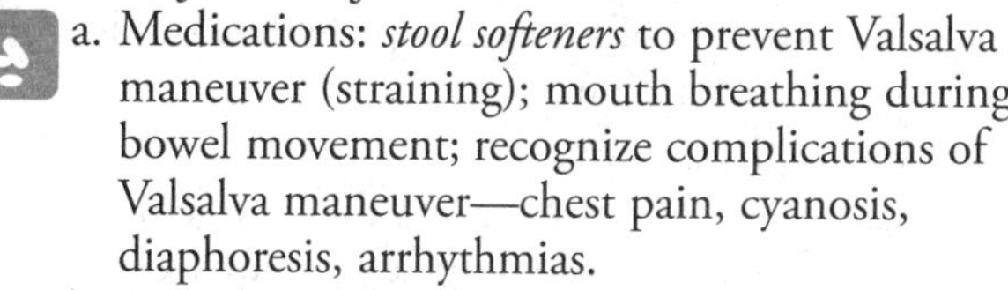

   a. Medications: *stool softeners* to prevent Valsalva maneuver (straining); mouth breathing during bowel movement; recognize complications of Valsalva maneuver—chest pain, cyanosis, diaphoresis, arrhythmias.
   b. Bedside commode if possible.
6. Goal: *provide emotional support.*
   a. Recognize fear of dying: denial, anger, withdrawal.
   b. Encourage expression of feelings, fears, concerns.
   c. Discuss rehabilitation, lifestyle changes: prevent cardiac invalid syndrome by promoting self-care activities, independence.
7. Goal: *promote sexual functioning.*
   a. Encourage discussion of concerns regarding activity, inadequacy, limitations, expectations, use of drugs for erectile dysfunction—include partner (usually resume activity 5 to 8 weeks after uncomplicated MI or when client can climb two flights of stairs).
   b. Identify need for referral for sexual counseling.
8. Goal: *health teaching.*
   a. Diagnosis and treatment regimen.
   b. *Caution* about when to *avoid* sexual activity: after heavy meal, alcohol ingestion; when fatigued, tense, under stress; with unfamiliar partners; in extreme temperatures.
   c. Information about sexual activity: less fatiguing positions (side to side; noncardiac partner on top); vasodilators, if ordered, before intercourse; select comfortable, familiar environment.
   d. Referral to available community resources for information, support groups (e.g., American Heart Association, Stop Smoking Clinics).
   e. Medications: administration, importance, untoward effects, pulse taking.
   f. Control risk factors: rest, diet, exercise, no smoking, weight control, stress-reduction techniques.
   g. Need for follow-up care for regulation of medications, evaluating risk factors.
   h. Prepare for angioplasty or coronary bypass if planned.

F. Evaluation/outcome criteria:

1. No complications: stable vital signs; relief of pain.
2. Adheres to prescribed medication regimen, demonstrates knowledge about medications.
3. Activity tolerance is increased, participates in program of progressive activity.
4. Reduction or modification of risk factors. Plans to alter lifestyle (e.g., loses weight, quits smoking).

VII. CARDIAC VALVULAR DEFECTS: alteration in the structure of a valve; impede flow of blood or permit regurgitation.

A. Pathophysiology:

1. *Stenosis*—narrowing of valvular opening due to adherence, thickening, and rigidity of valve cusp from fibrosis, scarring, and calcification.
2. *Insufficiency* (incompetence)—incomplete closure of valve due to contraction of chordae tendineae, papillary muscles; or to calcification, scarring of leaflets. Results in regurgitation.
3. *Mitral stenosis:*
   a. Most common residual cardiac lesion of rheumatic fever.
   b. Affects *women* younger than 45 years more often than men.
   c. Narrowing of mitral valve.
   d. Interferes with filling of left ventricle.
   e. Produces pulmonary hypertension, right ventricular failure.
4. *Mitral insufficiency* (incompetence):
   a. Leaking/regurgitation of blood back into left atrium.
   b. Results from rheumatic fever, bacterial endocarditis; less common.
   c. Affects *men* more often.
   d. Produces pulmonary congestion, right ventricular failure.
5. *Aortic stenosis:*
   a. Fusion of valve flaps between left ventricle and aorta.
   b. Congenital or acquired from atherosclerosis or from rheumatic fever and bacterial endocarditis; seen in *men* more often; pulmonary circulation congested, cardiac output decreased.
6. *Aortic insufficiency:*
   a. Incomplete closure of valve between left ventricle and aorta (regurgitation).
   b. Left ventricular failure leading to right ventricular heart failure.

B. Risk factors:

1. Congenital abnormality.
2. History of rheumatic fever.
3. Atherosclerosis.

C. Assessment: see **Table 6.20.**

D. Analysis/nursing diagnosis:

1. *Decreased cardiac output* related to inadequate ventricular filling.
2. *Fluid volume excess* related to compensatory response to decreased cardiac output.
3. *Impaired gas exchange* related to pulmonary congestion.
4. *Activity intolerance* related to impaired cardiac function.
5. *Fatigue* related to poor oxygenation.

E. Nursing care plan/implementation:

1. Goal: *reduce cardiac workload.*
2. Goal: *promote physical comfort and psychological support.*
3. Goal: *prevent complications.*
4. Goal: *prepare for surgery* (commissurotomy, valvuloplasty [valvotomy], or valvular replacement, depending on defect and severity of condition).
5. See section **X. CARDIAC SURGERY, pp. 422–425,** for specific nursing actions.

F. Evaluation/outcome criteria:

1. Relief of symptoms.
2. Increase in activity level.
3. No complications following surgery.

Table 6.20

Comparison of Symptomatology for Valvular Defects

Assessment *Subjective Data*	Mitral Stenosis	Mitral Insufficiency	Aortic Stenosis	Aortic Insufficiency
Fatigue	✓	✓	✓	✓
Shortness of breath	✓			
Orthopnea	✓		✓	✓
Paroxysmal nocturnal dyspnea	✓		✓	✓
Cough	✓	✓		
Dyspnea on exertion		✓	✓	✓
Palpitations		✓	✓	
Syncope on exertion			✓	
Angina			✓	✓
Weight loss		✓		

Table 6.20

Comparison of Symptomatology for Valvular Defects—cont'd

Assessment *Objective Data*	Mitral Stenosis	Mitral Insufficiency	Aortic Stenosis	Aortic Insufficiency
Vital signs				
Blood pressure:				
Low or normal	✓	✓		
Normal or elevated			✓	✓
Pulse:				
Weak, irregular	✓	✓		
Rapid, "waterhammer"				✓
Respirations:				
Increased, shallow	✓			
Cyanosis	✓			
Jugular vein distention	✓			
Enlarged liver	✓		✓	
Dependent edema	✓		✓	
Murmur	✓	✓	✓	✓

VIII. CARDIAC CATHETERIZATION: a diagnostic procedure to evaluate cardiac status. Introduces a catheter into the heart, blood vessels; analyzes blood samples for oxygen content, ejection fraction, cardiac output, pulmonary artery blood flow; done before heart surgery; frequently combined with angiography to visualize coronary arteries; also provides access for specialized cardiac techniques (e.g., internal pacing and percutaneous transluminal coronary angioplasty [PTCA]).

A. Approaches

1. *Right-heart* catheterization—venous approach (antecubital or femoral) → right atrium → right ventricle → pulmonary artery.
2. *Left-heart* catheterization—retrograde approach: right brachial artery or percutaneous puncture of femoral artery → ascending aorta → left ventricle.
   a. Transseptal: femoral vein → right atrium → septum → left atrium → left ventricle.
   b. Angiography/arteriography: done during left-heart catheterization.

B. Precatheterization

1. **Assessment:**
   a. *Subjective data:*
      (1) Allergies: iodine, seafood.
      (2) Anxiety.
      (3) Comfort.
   b. *Objective data:*
      (1) Vital signs: baseline data.
      (2) Distal pulses: mark for reference after catheterization.
2. **Analysis/nursing diagnosis:**
   a. *Anxiety* related to fear of unknown.
   b. *Knowledge deficit* (learning need) related to limited exposure to information or sudden need for procedure.
3. **Nursing care plan/implementation:**
   a. Goal: *provide for safety, comfort.*
      (1) Signed informed consent.
      (2) NPO (except for medications 6 to 8 hours before).
      (3) Have client urinate before going to lab.
      (4) Give *sedatives,* as ordered, 30 minutes before procedure (e.g., midazolam HCl [Versed] IV, diazepam [Valium] PO).
      (5) Possible shaving of insertion site.
   b. Goal: *health teaching.*
      (1) Procedure: length (1 to 3 hours).
      (2) Expectations (strapped to table for safety, must lie still, awake but mildly sedated).
      (3) Sensations (hot, flushed feeling in head with dye injection; thudding in chest from premature beats during catheter manipulation; desire to cough, particularly with right-heart angiography and contrast-medium injection).
      (4) Alert physician to unusual sensations (coolness, numbness, paresthesia).

C. Postcatheterization

1. **Assessment** (potential complications):
   a. *Subjective data:*
      (1) Puncture site: increasing pain, tenderness.

(2) Palpitations, chest pain.
(3) Affected extremity: tingling, numbness, pain from hematoma or nerve damage.

b. *Objective data:*
(1) Vital signs: shock, respiratory distress (related to pulmonary emboli, allergic reaction).
(2) Puncture site: bleeding (hematoma).
(3) ECG: arrhythmias, signs of MI.
(4) Affected extremity: color, temperature, peripheral pulses.

2. **Analysis/nursing diagnosis:**
a. *Decreased cardiac output* related to arrhythmias or MI.
b. *Altered tissue perfusion* related to bleeding following procedure.
c. *Pain* related to puncture site tenderness.

3. **Nursing care plan/implementation:**
a. Goal: *prevent complications.*
(1) Bedrest: depends on size of catheter and closure procedure—Perclose dissolvable suture, 30 minutes; Angioseal (collagen plug), 2 hours; compression pump or 15-minute manual compression followed by sandbag, 4 to 5 hours; 12 to 24 hours with sheath or antiplatelet drip (abciximab [ReoPro]).
(2) Vital signs: record q15 min for 1 hour, q30 min for 3 hours or until stable; check BP on opposite extremity.
(3) Puncture site: observe for bleeding, swelling, or tenderness; check pulse distal to insertion site to determine patency of artery; report complaints of coolness, numbness, or paresthesia in extremity.
(4) ECG: monitor, document rhythm.
(5) Give medications as ordered: *sedatives;* mild *narcotics; antiarrhythmics; antiplatelet* (Plavix, aspirin) or *low-molecular-weight heparin* (enoxaparin [Lovenox]) with stent insertion.

b. Goal: *provide emotional support.*
(1) Explanations: brief, accurate; client anxious to learn results of test.
(2) Counseling: refer as indicated.

c. Goal: *health teaching.*
(1) Late complications: infection.
(2) Prepare for surgery if indicated.
(3) Follow-up medical care.
(4) Limitations following PTCA procedure (see section **IX** below): *no* lifting greater than 10 lb and *no* vigorous exertion for 1 to 2 weeks; return to normal work and sexual activity in 2 to 3 days.

4. **Evaluation/outcome criteria:** no complications (e.g., cardiac arrest, hematoma at insertion site).

IX. PERCUTANEOUS TRANSLUMINAL CORONARY ANGIOPLASTY (PTCA): A balloon-tipped catheter is threaded to site of coronary occlusion and inflated repeatedly until blood flow increases distal to the obstruction. It is a nonsurgical alternative to bypass surgery for coronary artery occlusion **(Fig. 6.6);** recommended for clients with poorly controlled angina, mild or no symptoms, multiple- or single-vessel disease with a noncalcified, discrete, and proximal lesion that can be reached by the catheter; costs less and requires shorter hospitalization and rehabilitation period; successful in 90% of clients; approximately 30% restenose by 3 months (see **VIII. CARDIAC CATHETERIZATION, p. 421,** for nursing process). **Rotational atherectomy** may also be done; a high-speed drill pulverizes plaque into small particles. An **intravascular stent,** steel mesh or coiled spring, may be placed in the coronary artery; the stent acts as a mechanical scaffold to reopen the blocked artery. The client receives low-molecular-weight heparin and/or platelet therapy following the procedure and after discharge.

X. CARDIAC SURGERY: done to alter the structure of the heart or vessels when congenital or acquired disorders interfere with cardiac functioning: septal defects; transposition of great vessels; tetralogy of Fallot; pulmonary/aortic stenosis; coronary artery bypass; valve replacement.

Cardiopulmonary bypass (open-heart surgery): blood from cardiac chambers and great vessels is diverted into a pump oxygenator; allows full visualization of heart during surgery; maintains perfusion and body functioning.

A. Preoperative

1. **Assessment:** see specific conditions for preoperative signs and symptoms (i.e., valvular defects, angina, MI); (see also **THE PERIOPERATIVE EXPERIENCE, pp. 365–367**). Establish complete baseline: daily weight; vital signs—integrity of all pulses, BP both arms; CVP or pulmonary artery pressures; neurological status; emotional status; nutritional and elimination patterns; *laboratory values* (urine, electrolytes, enzymes, coagulation studies, cholesterol); pulmonary function studies; echocardiogram, chest x-ray.

2. **Analysis/nursing diagnosis** (see also **VI. MYOCARDIAL INFARCTION, pp. 418, 419**):
a. *Decreased cardiac output* related to myocardial damage.
b. *Activity intolerance* related to poor cardiac function.
c. *Knowledge deficit* (learning need) related to insufficient time for teaching.

d. *Anxiety* related to fear of unknown.
e. *Fear* related to possible death.
f. *Risk for spiritual distress* related to possible death.

3. **Nursing care plan/implementation:**
   a. Goal: *provide emotional and spiritual support.*
      (1) Arrange for religious consultation if desired.
      (2) Provide opportunity for family visit morning of surgery.
      (3) Encourage verbalization/questions: fear, depression, despair frequently occur.
      (4) Involve family during explanations.
   b. Goal: *health teaching.*
      (1) Diagnostic procedures, treatments, specifics for surgery (i.e., internal mammarian artery or leg incision with use of saphenous vein in coronary artery bypass graft surgery) **(Fig. 6.7).**

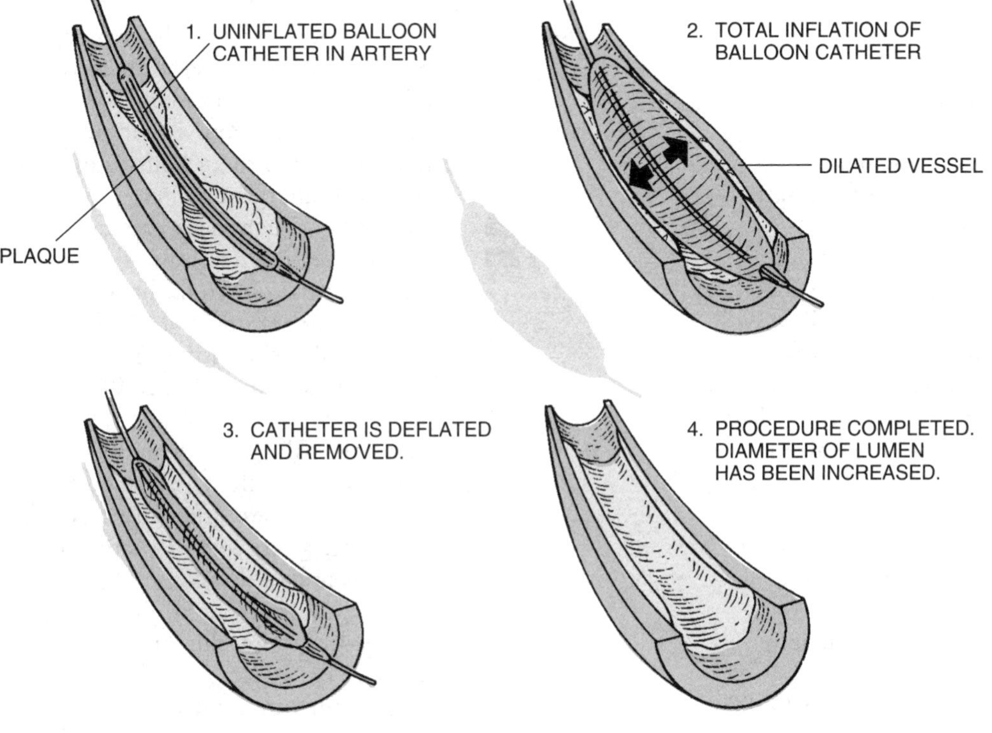

Figure 6.6 Arterial balloon angioplasty. (From Venes, D [ed]: *Taber's Cyclopedic Medical Dictionary,* ed 21. FA Davis, Philadelphia, 2009.)

ADULT

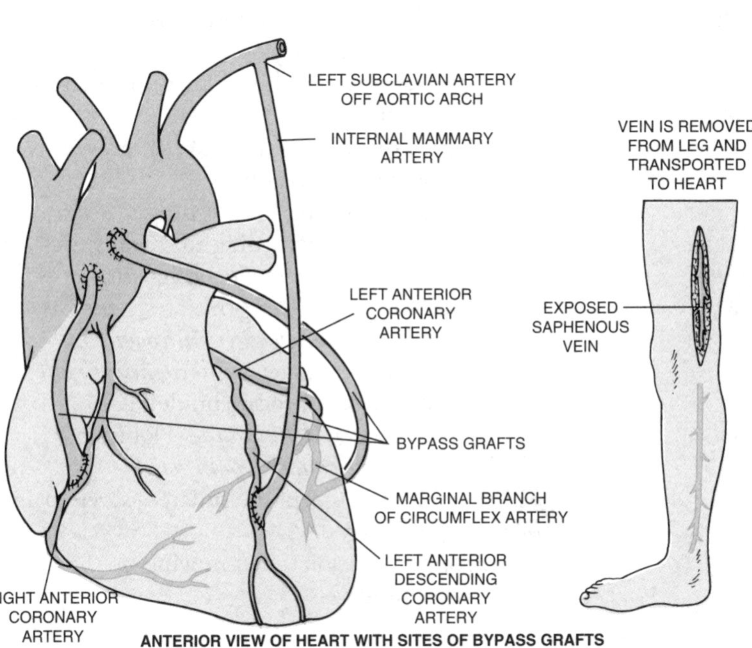

Figure 6.7 Bypass. Anterior view of heart with sites of bypass graft. (From Venes, D [ed]: *Taber's Cyclopedic Medical Dictionary,* ed 21. FA Davis, Philadelphia, 2009.)

(2) Postoperative regimen: turn, cough, deep breathe, ROM, equipment used, medication for pain.
(3) Tour ICU; meet personnel.
(4) Alternative method of communication while intubated.

4. **Evaluation/outcome criteria:**
   a. Displays moderate anxiety level.
   b. Verbalizes/demonstrates postoperative expectations.
   c. Quits smoking before surgery.

B. Postoperative

1. **Assessment:**
   a. *Subjective data:*
      (1) Pain.
      (2) Fatigue—sleep deprivation.
   b. *Objective data:*
      (1) *Neurological:* level of consciousness; pupillary reactions; movement of limbs (purposeful, spontaneous).
      (2) *Respiratory:* rate changes (*increases* occur with obstruction, pain; *decreases* occur with CO_2 retention); depth (shallow with pain, atelectasis); symmetry; skin *color;* patency/*drainage* from chest tubes, *sputum* (amount, color); endotracheal tube placement (bilateral breath sounds); arterial blood gases, O_2 saturation.
      (3) *Cardiovascular:*
         (a) BP—*hypotension* may indicate: heart failure, tamponade, hemorrhage, arrhythmias, or thrombosis; *hypertension* may indicate: anxiety, hypervolemia.
         (b) Pulse: radial, apical, pedal; rate (>100 may indicate: shock, fever, hypoxia, arrhythmias); rhythm, quality. Check pacing wires.
         (c) CVP and PA catheter (*elevated* in cardiac failure); temperature (normal postoperative: 98.6° to 101.6°F oral).
      (4) *GI:* nausea, vomiting, distention.
      (5) *Renal:* urine—minimum output (30 mL/hr); color
      Specific gravity (<1.010 occurs with *overhydration,* renal tubular damage; >1.020 present with *dehydration,* oliguria, blood in urine).

2. **Analysis/nursing diagnosis:**
   a. *Decreased cardiac output* related to decreased myocardial contractility or postoperative hypothermia.
   b. *Pain* (acute) related to incision.
   c. *Ineffective airway clearance* related to effects of general anesthesia.
   d. *Altered tissue perfusion* related to postoperative bleeding or thromboemboli.
   e. *Fluid volume deficit* related to blood loss.
   f. *Risk for infection* related to wound contamination.
   g. *Altered thought processes* related to anesthesia or stress.
   h. *Altered role performance* related to uncertainty about future.

3. **Nursing care plan/implementation:**
   a. Goal: *provide constant monitoring to prevent complications.*
      (1) *Respiratory:*
         (a) Observe for respiratory distress: restlessness, nasal flaring, *Cheyne-Stokes* respiration, dusky/cyanotic skin; assisted or controlled ventilation via endotracheal tube common 6 to 24 hours; supplemental O_2 after extubation.
         (b) Suctioning; cough, deep breathe.
         (c) Elevate *head of bed* at least 30 degrees.
         (d) Position chest tube to facilitate drainage; suction maintains patency—do not "milk" chest tube. (See also Chest tube section in **Table 11.5**.)
      (2) *Cardiovascular:*
         (a) Vital signs: BP greater than 80 to 90 mm Hg systolic; *CVP:* range 5 to 15 cm H_2O unless otherwise ordered; pulmonary artery line (PA catheter): mean pressure 4 to 12 mm Hg; I&O: report less than 30 mL/hr of urine from indwelling urinary catheter.
         (b) ECG; premature ventricular contractions (PVCs) occur most frequently following aortic valve replacement and bypass surgery.
         (c) Peripheral pulses if leg veins used for grafting.
         (d) Activity: turn q2h; ROM; progressive, early ambulation.
      (3) Inspect dressing for bleeding.
      (4) Medications according to therapeutic directives—*cardiotonics* (digoxin); *coronary vasodilators* (nitrates); *antibiotics* (penicillin); *analgesics; anticoagulants* (with valve replacements); *antiarrhythmics* (amiodarone, procainamide HCl [Pronestyl]); *dobutamine* [Dobutrex].
   b. Goal: *promote comfort, pain relief.*
      (1) Medicate: morphine sulfate—severe pain lasts 2 to 3 days.
      (2) Splint incision when moving or coughing.

ADULT

(3) Mouth care: frequent, especially if intubated; keep lips moist.
(4) *Position:* use pillows to prevent tension on chest tubes, incision.

c. Goal: *maintain fluid, electrolyte, nutritional balance.*
(1) I&O; urine specific gravity.
(2) Measure chest drainage—should *not* exceed 200 mL/hr for first 4 to 6 hours.
(3) Give fluids as ordered; maintain IV patency, central line care.
(4) *Diet:* clear fluids → solid food if no nausea, GI distention; sodium intake *restricted, low* fat; give H_2 blocker as ordered.

d. Goal: *promote emotional adjustment.*
(1) Anticipate behavior disturbances (depression, disorientation often occur 3 days postoperatively) related to medications, fear, sleep deprivation.
(2) Calm, oriented, supportive environment, as personalized as possible.
(3) Encourage verbalization of feelings (family and client).
(4) Encourage independence to avoid "cardiac cripple" role.

e. Goal: *promote early mobilization.*
(1) Out of bed within 24 hours postoperative to prevent deep vein thrombosis (DVT).
(2) In chair three times daily by postoperative day 2.

f. Goal: *health teaching.*
(1) Alterations in lifestyle; activity, diet, work; resumption of sexual activity usually when client can climb two flights of stairs.
(2) Refer to available community resources for cardiac rehabilitation (e.g., American Heart Association, Mended Hearts).
(3) Drug regimen: purpose, side effects.
(4) Potential complications: dyspnea, pain, palpitations common postoperatively.

4. **Evaluation/outcome criteria:**
a. No complications; incision heals; no dysrhythmias; pacing wires discontinued.
b. Activity level increases—no signs of overexertion (e.g., fatigue, dyspnea, pain).
c. Relief of symptoms.
d. Returns for follow-up medical care.
e. Takes prescribed medications; knows purposes and side effects.

XI. MINIMALLY INVASIVE DIRECT CORONARY ARTERY BYPASS (MIDCAB): a variation of CABG for clients for whom sternotomy and cardiopulmonary bypass is contraindicated or unnecessary. The left internal mammary artery is anastomosed to the left anterior descending coronary artery through a thoracic incision without bypass. Small incision and minimal recovery time.

XII. HEART FAILURE (HF): inability of the heart to meet the peripheral circulatory demands of the body; cardiac decompensation; combined right and left ventricular heart failure.

A. Pathophysiology: increased cardiac workload or decreased effective myocardial contractility → decreased cardiac output (forward effects). Left ventricular failure → pulmonary congestion; right atrial and right ventricular failure → systemic congestion → peripheral edema (backward effects). Compensatory mechanisms in HF include tachycardia, ventricular dilation, and hypertrophy of the myocardium; develops in 50% to 60% of clients with heart disease.

B. Risk factors:
1. Decreased myocardial contractility:
a. Myocarditis.
b. MI.
c. Tachyarrhythmias.
d. Bacterial endocarditis.
e. Acute rheumatic fever.
2. Increased cardiac workload:
a. Elevated temperature.
b. Physical/emotional stress.
c. Anemia.
d. Hyperthyroidism (thyrotoxicosis).
e. Valvular defects.
f. Uncontrolled hypertension.

C. Assessment:
1. *Subjective data:*
a. Shortness of breath.
(1) Orthopnea (sleeps on two or more pillows).
(2) Paroxysmal nocturnal dyspnea (sudden breathlessness during sleep).
(3) Dyspnea on exertion (climbing stairs).
b. Apprehension; anxiety; irritability.
c. Fatigue; weakness.
d. Reported weight gain; feeling of puffiness.
2. *Objective data* (**Table 6.21**):
a. *Vital signs:*
(1) *BP:* decreasing systolic; narrowing pulse pressure.
(2) *Pulse:* pulsus alternans (alternating strong-weak-strong cardiac contraction), increased.
(3) *Respirations:* crackles, *Cheyne-Stokes.*
b. Edema: dependent, pitting (1^+ to 4^+ mm).
c. Liver: enlarged, tender.
d. Neck veins: distended.
e. Chest x-ray:
(1) Cardiac enlargement.
(2) Dilated pulmonary vessels.
(3) Diffuse interstitial lung edema.

ADULT

Table 6.21

Left Ventricular Compared with Right Ventricular Heart Failure

Left Ventricular Failure	Right Ventricular Failure
Pulmonary crackles	Jugular venous distention
Tachypnea	Peripheral edema
S_3 gallop	Perioral and peripheral cyanosis
Cardiac murmurs	Congestive hepatomegaly
Paradoxical splitting of S_2	Ascites
	Hepatojugular reflux

D. Analysis/nursing diagnosis:

1. *Decreased cardiac output* related to decreased myocardial contractility.
2. *Activity intolerance* related to generalized weakness and inadequate oxygenation.
3. *Fatigue* related to edema and poor oxygenation.
4. *Altered tissue perfusion* related to peripheral edema and inadequate blood flow.
5. *Fluid volume excess* related to compensatory mechanisms.
6. *Impaired gas exchange* related to pulmonary congestion.
7. *Anxiety* related to shortness of breath.
8. *Sleep pattern disturbance* related to paroxysmal nocturnal dyspnea.

E. Nursing care plan/implementation:

1. Goal: *provide physical rest/reduce emotional stimuli.*
   a. *Position: sitting* or *semi*-Fowler's until tachycardia, dyspnea, edema resolved; change position frequently; pillows for support.
   b. Rest: planned periods; limit visitors, activity, noise. Chair and commode privileges.
   c. Support: stay with client who is anxious; have family member who is supportive present; administer *sedatives/tranquilizers* as ordered.
   d. Warm fluids if appropriate.
2. Goal: *provide for relief of respiratory distress; reduce cardiac workload.*
   a. Oxygen: low flow rate; encourage deep breathing (5 to 10 minutes q2h); auscultate breath sounds for congestion, pulmonary edema.
   b. *Position:* elevating head of bed 20 to 25 cm (8 to 10 inches) alleviates pulmonary congestion.
   c. Medications as ordered:
      (1) *Digitalis* preparations.
      (2) *ACE inhibitors*—captopril, enalapril.
      (3) *Inotropic agent*—dobutamine, dopamine.
      (4) *Diuretics*—thiazides, furosemide, metolazone.
      (5) *Tranquilizers*—phenobarbital, diazepam (Valium), chlordiazepoxide HCl (Librium).
      (6) *Vasodilators*—hydralazine, isosorbide.
3. Goal: *provide for special safety needs.*
   a. Skin care:
      (1) Inspect, massage, lubricate bony prominences.
      (2) Use foot cradle, heel protectors; sheepskin.
   b. Side rails up if hypoxic (disoriented).
   c. Vital signs: monitor for signs of fatigue, pulmonary emboli.
   d. ROM: active, passive; elastic stockings, DVT prophylaxis.
4. Goal: *maintain fluid and electrolyte balance, nutritional status.*
   a. Urine output: 30 mL/hr minimum; estimate insensible loss in client who is diaphoretic. Monitor: BUN, serum creatinine, and electrolytes, B-type natriuretic peptide (BNP).
   b. Daily weight; same time, clothes, scale.
   c. IV: IV infusion pump to avoid circulatory overloading; strict I&O.
   d. *Diet:*
      (1) *Low* sodium as ordered.
      (2) Small, frequent feedings.
      (3) Discuss food preferences with client.
5. Goal: *health teaching.*
   a. Diet restrictions; meal preparation.
   b. Activity restrictions, if any; planned rest periods.
   c. Medications: schedule (e.g., diuretic in early morning to limit interruption of sleep), purpose, dosage, side effects (importance of daily pulse taking, daily weights, intake of *potassium*-containing foods).
   d. Refer to available *community resources* for dietary assistance, weight reduction, exercise program.

F. Evaluation/outcome criteria:

1. Increase in activity level tolerance—fatigue decreased.
2. No complications—pulmonary edema, respiratory distress.
3. Reduction in dependent edema.

XIII. PULMONARY EDEMA: sudden transudation of fluid from pulmonary capillaries into alveoli. **Life-threatening condition.**

A. Pathophysiology: increased pulmonary capillary permeability; increased hydrostatic pressure (pulmonary hypertension); decreased blood colloidal osmotic pressure; fluid accumulation in alveoli → decreased compliance → decreased diffusion of gas → hypoxia, hypercapnia.

B. Risk factors:
1. Left ventricular failure.
2. Pulmonary embolism.
3. Drug overdose.
4. Smoke inhalation.
5. CNS damage.
6. Fluid overload.
7. Valvular disorders.

C. Assessment:
1. *Subjective data:*
   a. Anxiety.
   b. Restlessness at onset, progressing to agitation.
   c. Stark fear.
   d. Intense dyspnea, orthopnea, fatigue.
2. *Objective data:*
   a. *Vital signs:*
      (1) *Pulse:* tachycardia; gallop rhythm.
      (2) *Respirations:* tachypnea, moist, bubbling, wheezing, labored, ↓ O_2 saturation.
      (3) *Temperature:* normal to subnormal.
   b. Skin: pale, cool, diaphoretic, cyanotic.
   c. Auscultation: crackles, wheezes.
   d. Cough: productive of large quantities of pink, frothy sputum.
   e. Right ventricular heart failure: distended (bulging) neck veins, peripheral edema, hepatomegaly, ascites.
   f. Mental status: restless, confused, stuporous.
   g. Arterial blood gases: hypoxia; pulse oximetry: *decreased* O_2 saturation.
   h. Chest x-ray: haziness of lung fields, cardiomegaly. Echocardiogram.

D. Analysis/nursing diagnosis:
1. *Decreased cardiac output* related to decreased myocardial contractility.
2. *Impaired gas exchange* related to pulmonary congestion.
3. *Altered tissue perfusion* related to inadequate blood flow.
4. *Anxiety,* severe, related to difficulty breathing.
5. *Fear* related to life-threatening situation.

E. Nursing care plan/implementation:
1. Goal: *promote physical, psychological relaxation measures to relieve anxiety.*
   a. Slow respirations: morphine sulfate 3 to 10 mg IV/SQ/IM, as ordered, to reduce respiratory rate, sedate, and produce vasodilation.
   b. Remain with client.
   c. Encourage slow, deep breathing; assist with coughing.
   d. Work calmly, confidently, unhurriedly.
   e. Frequent rest periods.
2. Goal: *improve cardiac function, reduce venous return, relieve hypoxia.*
   a. O_2: slow respiratory rate, provide uniform ventilation via nasal cannula, ventimask, 100% non-rebreather mask, or intubation, depending on O_2 need. Possibly PEEP. Small-volume nebulizer treatment with *ipratropium (Atrovent) or albuterol (Proventil).*
   b. Give aminophylline, as ordered, to lower venous pressure and increase cardiac output.
   c. IV: D_5W.
   d. *Position: high Fowler's,* extremities in dependent position, to reduce venous return and facilitate breathing.
   e. Medications as ordered: digitalis; *diuretics*—furosemide (Lasix); *inotropic agents* —dobutamine (Dobutrex), dopamine; nitroglycerin, nitroprusside.
   f. Vital signs; auscultate breath sounds.
   g. *Diet: low* sodium; fluid *restriction* as ordered.
3. Goal: *health teaching* (include family or significant other).
   a. Medications.
      (1) Side effects.
      (2) Potassium supplements if indicated.
      (3) Pulse taking.
   b. Exercise; rest.
   c. *Diet: low* sodium.
   d. *Signs of complications*: edema; weight gain of 2 to 3 lb (0.9 to 1.4 kg) in a few days; dyspnea.

F. Evaluation/outcome criteria:
1. No complications; vital signs stable; clear breath sounds.
2. No weight gain; weight loss if indicated.
3. Alert, oriented, calm.

XIV. SHOCK: a critically severe deficiency in nutrients, oxygen, and electrolytes delivered to body tissues, plus deficiency in removal of cellular wastes; results from: cardiac failure, insufficient blood volume, or increased vascular bed size.

A. Types, pathophysiology, and risk factors:
1. *Hypovolemic* (hemorrhagic, hematogenic)—markedly decreased **volume** of blood (hemorrhage or plasma loss from intestinal obstruction, burns, physical trauma, or dehydration) → *decreased* venous return, cardiac output → *decreased* tissue perfusion.
2. *Cardiogenic*—failure of cardiac muscle **pump** (myocardial infarction) → generally decreased cardiac output → pulmonary congestion, hypoxia → inadequate circulation; high mortality rate.
3. *Distributive:*
   a. *Neurogenic*—massive **vasodilation** from reduced vasomotor, vasoconstrictor tone (e.g., spinal shock, head injuries, anesthesia, pain); interruption of sympathetic nervous system; blood volume is normal but inadequate for

vessels → decreased venous return → tissue hypoxia.

b. *Vasogenic* (anaphylactic, septic, systemic inflammatory response syndrome [SIRS], endotoxic)—severe reaction to foreign protein (insect bites, drugs, toxic substances, aerobic, gram-negative organisms) → histamine release **vasodilation,** venous stasis → diminished venous return.

B. Assessment: varies, depending on degree of shock **(Table 6.22).**

1. *Subjective data:*
   a. Anxiety; restlessness.
   b. Dizziness; fainting.
   c. Thirst.
   d. Nausea.
2. *Objective data:*
   a. *Vital signs:*
      (1) *BP*—hypotension (postural changes in early shock; systolic less than 70 mm Hg in late shock).
      (2) *Pulse*—tachycardia, thready; irregular *(cardiogenic shock);* could be slow if conduction system of heart damaged.
      (3) *Respirations*—increased depth, rate; wheezing *(anaphylactic shock),* O_2 saturation ↓ 90%.
      (4) *Temperature*—decreased (elevated in *septic shock*).
   b. Skin:
      (1) Pale (or mottled), cool, clammy (warm to touch in *septic shock*).
      (2) Urticaria (*anaphylactic shock*).
   c. Level of consciousness: alert, oriented → acute alteration in mental status → unresponsive.
   d. CVP:
      (1) *Below* 5 cm H_2O with *hypovolemic* shock, also *anaphylactic* or *septic* shock.
      (2) *Above* 15 cm H_2O with *cardiogenic* shock.
   e. Urine output: *decreased* (<30 mL/hr).
   f. Capillary refill: slowed; normally nailbed "pinks up" within 2 seconds after blanching (nailbed pressure).

C. Analysis/nursing diagnosis:

1. *Altered tissue perfusion* related to vasodilation or decreased myocardial contractility.
2. *Impaired gas exchange* related to ventilation-perfusion imbalance.
3. *Decreased cardiac output* related to loss of circulating blood volume or diminished cardiac contractility; peripheral vasodilation.
4. *Altered urinary elimination* related to decreased renal perfusion.
5. *Fluid volume deficit* related to blood loss.
6. *Anxiety* related to severity of condition.

D. Nursing care plan/implementation: Goal: *promote venous return, circulatory perfusion.*

1. *Position:* foot of bed *elevated* 20 degrees (12 to 16 inches), knees straight, trunk horizontal, head slightly elevated; *avoid* Trendelenburg position.
2. Ventilation: monitor respiratory effort, loosen restrictive clothing; O_2 as ordered.
3. Fluids:
   a. Maintain IV infusions—with sepsis, may receive 2 to 6 L to keep CVP greater than 12 mm Hg to prevent end organ hypoxia and organ failure. Mean arterial pressure greater than 60 mm Hg.
   b. Give blood, plasma expanders as ordered (exception—***stop* blood immediately** in anaphylactic shock).
4. *Vital signs:*
   a. CVP (*decreased* with hypovolemia) arterial line, PA catheter (*increased* pulmonary artery wedge pressure indicating cardiac failure). Check central venous O_2 ($_{scv}O_2$).
   b. Urine output (insert catheter for hourly output).
   c. Monitor ECG (increased rate, dysrhythmias).
5. Medications (depending on type of shock) as ordered:
   a. *Adrenergics*—dobutamine, norepinephrine (Levophed), isoproterenol (Isuprel), dopamine (Intropin) (*cardiogenic, neurogenic, septic* shock).
   b. *Antiarrhythmics* (*cardiogenic* shock).
   c. *Cardiac glycosides* (*cardiogenic* shock).
   d. *Adrenocorticoids* (*anaphylactic* shock).
   e. *Antibiotics* (*septic* shock).

Table 6.22

Signs of Hypovolemic Shock

Blood Loss (% of Total)	Assessment Data
800–1500 mL (15%–30%)	Restlessness Pulse >100 Systolic pressure unchanged Diastolic pressure ↑ Urine output ↓
2000 mL (30%–40%)	Mental status ↓ Pulse >120 Respirations > 30 Systolic pressure ↓
>2500 mL (>40%)	Cold, clammy skin Pulse >120 Respirations >30 Narrowed pulse pressure (= systolic minus diastolic)

f. *Vasodilators*—nitroprusside (*cardiogenic* shock).
g. *Antihistamines*—epinephrine, vasopressin, Benadryl IV, methlyprednisone.

6. Mechanical support: military (or medical) antishock trousers (MAST) or pneumatic antishock garment (PASG); used to promote internal autotransfusion of blood from legs and abdomen to central circulation; at lower pressures may control bleeding and promote hemostasis; do *not* remove (deflate) suddenly to examine underlying areas or BP will drop precipitously; *compartment syndrome* may result with prolonged use and high pressure; controversial.

E. Evaluation/outcome criteria:

1. Vital signs stable, within normal limits.
2. Alert, oriented.
3. Urine output greater than 30 mL/hr.

XV. DISSEMINATED INTRAVASCULAR COAGULATION (DIC): diffuse or widespread coagulation initially within arterioles and capillaries leading to hemorrhage.

A. Pathophysiology: activation of coagulation system from tissue injury → fibrin microthrombi form throughout the vascular system → microinfarcts, tissue necrosis → red blood cells, platelets, prothrombin, other clotting factors trapped in capillaries, destroyed in process → excessive clotting → release of fibrin split products → inhibition of platelet clotting → profuse bleeding.

B. Risk factors:

1. Obstetric complications (50% of cases).
2. Neoplastic disease.
3. Low perfusion states (e.g., burns, hypothermia); hypovolemia.
4. Infections, sepsis.

C. Assessment—*objective data:*

1. Skin, mucous membranes: petechiae, ecchymosis.
2. Extremities (fingers, toes): cyanosis.
3. Bleeding: venipuncture sites, wound, oral, rectal, vaginal.
4. Urine output: oliguria → anuria.
5. Level of consciousness: ↓ LOC progressing to coma.
6. Laboratory data: *prolonged*—prothrombin time (PT) greater than 15 seconds; *decreased*—platelets, fibrinogen level.

D. Analysis/nursing diagnosis:

1. *Altered tissue perfusion* related to peripheral microthrombi.
2. *Risk for injury* (death) related to bleeding.
3. *Risk for impaired skin integrity* related to ischemia.
4. *Altered urinary elimination* related to renal tubular necrosis.

E. Nursing care plan/implementation: Goal: *prevent and detect further bleeding.*

1. Carry out nursing measures designed to alleviate underlying problem (e.g., shock, birth of fetus, surgery/irradiation for cancer, antibiotics for infection).
2. Medications: heparin sodium IV, 1,000 units/hr, if ordered, to reverse abnormal clotting (controversial). Possible human recombinant activated protein C.
3. IVs: blood to lessen shock; platelets, cryoprecipitate, fresh plasma to restore clotting factors, fibrinogen.
4. Observe: vital signs, CVP (normal 5 to 15 mm Hg), PA pressure (normal 20 to 30 systolic and 8 to 12 diastolic), and I&O for signs of shock or fluid overload from frequent infusions; specimens for occult blood (urine, stool).
5. *Precautions: avoid* IM injections if possible; pressure 5 minutes to venipuncture sites; *no* rectal temperatures.

F. Evaluation/outcome criteria:

1. Clotting mechanism restored (*increased* platelets, *normal* PT).
2. Renal function restored (urine output >30 mL/hr).
3. Circulation to fingers, toes; no cyanosis.
4. No irreversible damage from renal, cerebral, cardiac, or adrenal hemorrhage.

XVI. PERICARDITIS: inflammation of parietal or visceral pericardium or both; acute or chronic condition; may occur with or without effusion. Cardiac tamponade may result.

A. Pathophysiology: fibrosis or accumulation of fluid in pericardium → compression of cardiac pumping → decreased cardiac output → increased systemic, pulmonic venous pressure.

B. Risk factors:

1. Bacterial, viral, fungal infections.
2. Tuberculosis.
3. Collagen diseases.
4. Uremia.
5. Transmural MI.
6. Trauma.

C. Assessment:

1. *Subjective data:*
   a. *Pain:*
      (1) *Type*—sharp, moderate to severe.
      (2) *Location*—wide area of pericardium, may radiate: right arm, jaw/teeth.
      (3) *Precipitating factors*—movement, deep inspiration, swallowing.
   b. Chills; sweating.
   c. Apprehension; anxiety.
   d. Fatigue.

ADULT

e. Abdominal pain.
f. Shortness of breath.

2. *Objective data:*
a. *Vital signs:*
(1) *BP: decreased* pulse pressure; pulsus paradoxus—abnormal drop in systolic BP of greater than 8 to 10 mm Hg during inspiration.
(2) *Pulse:* tachycardia.
(3) *Temperature: elevated;* erratic course; low grade.
b. Pericardial friction rub.
c. *Increased* CVP; distended neck veins; dependent pitting edema; liver engorgement.
d. Restlessness.
e. Laboratory data: *elevated* aspartate aminotransferase (AST, or serum glutamic-oxaloacetic transaminase [SGOT]), WBC count; CT or magnetic resonance imaging (MRI)—pericardial thickening; troponin, LDH.
f. Serial ECGs: *increased* ST segment; echocardiogram: pericardial fluid.

D. Analysis/nursing diagnosis:
1. *Decreased cardiac output* related to impaired cardiac muscle contraction.
2. *Pain* related to pericardial inflammation.
3. *Anxiety* related to unknown outcome.
4. *Fatigue* related to inadequate oxygenation.

E. Nursing care plan/implementation:
1. Goal: *promote physical and emotional comfort.*
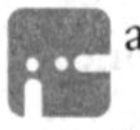
a. *Position:* semi-Fowler's (upright or sitting); bedrest.
b. Vital signs: q2–4h and prn; apical and radial pulse; notify physician if heart sounds *decrease* in amplitude or if pulse pressure *narrows,* indicating cardiac tamponade; see **i** below.
c. O_2 as ordered.
d. Medications as ordered:
(1) *Analgesics*—aspirin, morphine sulfate, meperidine or codeine.
(2) *Nonsteroidal anti-inflammatory agents*—indomethacin, ketorolac [Toradol].
(3) *Antimicrobial.*
(4) *Digitalis and diuretics,* if heart failure present.
e. Assist with aspiration of pericardial sac (pericardiocentesis) if needed: medicate as ordered; *elevate* head 60 degrees; monitor ECG; have defibrillator and pacemaker available.
f. Prepare for pericardiectomy (excision of constricting pericardium) as ordered.
g. Continual emotional support.
h. Enhance effects of analgesics: positioning; turning; NPO.
i. Monitor for:
Signs of cardiac tamponade: tachycardia; tachypnea; hypotension; pallor; narrowed pulse pressure; pulsus paradoxus; distended neck veins; ECG changes.

2. Goal: *maintain fluid, electrolyte balance.*
a. Parenteral fluids as ordered; strict I&O.
b. Assist with feedings; *low-sodium* diet may be ordered.

F. Evaluation/outcome criteria:
1. Relief of pain, dyspnea.
2. No complications (e.g., cardiac tamponade).
3. Return of normal cardiac functioning.

XVII. CHRONIC ARTERIAL OCCLUSIVE DISEASE:
arteriosclerosis obliterans most common occlusive disorder of the arterial system (aorta, large and medium-size arteries); frequently involves the femoral, iliac, and popliteal arteries (Buerger's disease).

A. Pathophysiology: fatty deposits in intimal, medial layer of arterial walls; plaque formation → narrowed arterial lumens; decreased distensibility → decreased blood flow; ischemic changes in tissues.

B. Risk factors:
1. Age (>50).
2. Sex (men).
3. Diabetes mellitus.
4. Hyperlipidemia—obesity.
5. Cigarette smoking.
6. Hypertension.
7. Family history.

C. Assessment:
1. *Subjective data:*
a. *Pain:*
(1) *Type*—cramplike.
(2) *Location*—foot, calf, thigh, buttocks.
(3) *Duration*—variable, may be relieved by rest.
(4) *Precipitating causes*—exercise (intermittent claudication), but occasionally may occur when at rest.
b. Tingling, numbness in toes, feet.
c. Persistent coldness of one or both lower extremities.

2. *Objective data:*
a. Lower extremities:
(1) Pedal pulses—absent or diminished.
(2) Skin—shiny, glossy; dry, cold, chalky white, decreased/absent hair, ulcers, gangrene.
b. Laboratory data: *increased* serum cholesterol, triglycerides, complete blood count (CBC), platelets.
c. Arteriography—indicates location, nature of occlusion. *Noninvasive:* ultrasound, segmental limb pressure, exercise testing.

D. Analysis/nursing diagnosis:
1. *Altered tissue perfusion* related to peripheral vascular disease.
2. *Risk for activity intolerance* related to pain and sensory changes.
3. *Pain* related to ischemia.
4. *Risk for impaired skin integrity* related to poor circulation.
5. *Risk for injury* related to numbness of extremities.

E. Nursing care plan/implementation:
1. Goal: *promote circulation; decrease discomfort.*

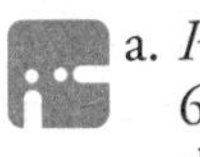

   a. *Position: elevate head* of bed on blocks (3 to 6 inches), because gravity aids perfusion to thighs, legs; elevating legs increases pain.
   b. Comfort: keep warm: *avoid* chilling or use of heating pads, which may burn skin; apply bed socks.
   c. Circulation: check pedal pulses, skin color, temperature four times daily.

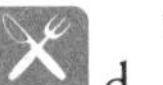

   d. Medications:
      (1) *Vasodilators.*
      (2) *Antiplatelet*—acetylsalicylic acid (ASA), ticlopidine, dipyridamole.
      (3) *Dihydropyridines*—nifedipine, amlodipine.
      (4) *Xanthine derivatives*—pentoxifylline.
2. Goal: *prevent infection, injury.*
   a. Skin care: use bed cradle, sheepskin, heel pads; mild soap; dry thoroughly; lotion; do *not* massage, to prevent release of thrombus.
   b. Foot care: wear properly fitting shoes, slippers when out of bed; inspect for injury or pressure areas; nail care by podiatrist.
3. Goal: *health teaching.*
   a. Skin care; inspect daily.
   b. Activity: balance exercise, rest to increase collateral circulation; walk only until painful.
   c. Exercises: walking, Buerger-Allen exercises (gravity alternately fills and empties blood vessels).
   d. *Diet: low*-fat, heart-healthy diet to slow disease progression.
   e. Lifestyle choices: *avoid* smoking.
   f. Recognize and report signs of occlusion (e.g., pain, cramping, numbness in extremities; color changes—white or blue; temperature changes—cool to cold).

F. Evaluation/outcome criteria:
1. Decreased pain.
2. Skin integrity preserved; no loss of limb.
3. Quits smoking.
4. Does exercises to increase collateral circulation.

XVIII. ANEURYSMS (thoracic or abdominal aortic): localized or diffuse dilations/outpouching of a vessel wall, usually an artery; exerts pressure on adjacent structures; affects primarily men over age 60; greater than 6 cm in diameter, 50% will rupture; resected surgically, reconstructed with synthetic or vascular graft.

A. Risk factors:
1. Atherosclerosis.
2. Trauma.
3. Syphilis.
4. Congenital weakness.
5. Local infection.
6. Cigarette smoking.
7. Uncontrolled hypertension.

B. Assessment:
1. *Subjective data:*
   a. *Pain:*
      (1) Constant, boring, neuralgic, intermittent—low back, abdominal.
      (2) Angina—sudden onset may mean rupture or dissection, which is an **emergency** condition.
   b. Dyspnea; orthopnea—pressure on trachea or bronchus.
2. *Objective data:*
   a. *Vital signs:*
      (1) Radial pulses differ.
      (2) Tachycardia.
      (3) Hypotension following rupture leading to shock.
   b. Pulsating mass: abdominal, chest wall pulsation; edema of chest wall (*thoracic* aneurysm); periumbilical (*abdominal* aneurysm); audible bruit over aorta.
   c. Skin: cyanosis, mottled below level of aneurysm.
   d. Veins: dilated, superficial—neck, chest, arms.
   e. Cough: paroxysmal, brassy.
   f. Diaphoresis, pallor, fainting following rupture.
   g. Peripheral pulses:
      (1) Femoral present.
      (2) Pedal weak or *absent.*
   h. Stool: bloody from irritation.

C. Analysis/nursing diagnosis:
1. *Risk for injury* related to possible aneurysm rupture.
2. *Pain* related to pressure on lumbar nerves.
3. *Anxiety* related to risk of rupture.

D. Nursing care plan/implementation:
1. Goal: *provide **emergency** care before surgery for dissection or rupture.*
   a. Vital signs: frequent, depending on severity (systolic BP <100 mm Hg and pulse >100 with rupture).

   b. IVs: may have 2 to 4 sites; lactated Ringer's solution may be ordered.
   c. Urine output: monitored every 15 to 30 minutes.

d. O_2: usually via nasal prongs.
e. Medications as ordered: *antihypertensives* to prevent extension of dissection.
f. Transport to operating room quickly.
g. See **THE PERIOPERATIVE EXPERIENCE, pp. 365–368,** for general preoperative care.

2. Goal: *prevent complications postoperatively.*
a. *Position:* initially flat in bed; *avoid* sharp flexion of hip and knee, which places pressure on femoral and popliteal arteries; turn gently side to side; note erythema on back from pooled blood.
b. *Vital signs:* CVP; hourly peripheral pulses distal to graft site, including neurovascular check of lower extremities; absent pulses for 6 to 12 hours indicates occlusion; check with Doppler blood flow detector.
c. *Urine output:* hourly from indwelling catheter.
(1) Immediately report anuria or oliguria (<30 mL/hr).
(2) Check color for hematuria.
(3) Monitor daily blood urea nitrogen (BUN) and creatinine.
d. Observe *for signs of atheroembolization* (patchy areas of ischemia); report change in color, motor ability, or sensation of lower extremities.
e. Observe for *signs of bowel ischemia* (decreased/absent bowel sounds, pain, guaiac-positive diarrhea, abdominal distention); may have nasogastric tube.
f. Measure abdominal girth; increase seen with graft leakage.

3. Goal: *promote comfort.*
a. *Position:* alignment, comfort; prevent heel ulcers.
b. Medication: *narcotics.*

4. Goal: *health teaching.*
a. Minimize recurrence: *avoid* trauma, infection, smoking, high-cholesterol diet, obesity.
b. Regular medical supervision.

E. Evaluation/outcome criteria:
1. Surgical intervention before rupture.
2. No loss of renal function.

XIX. RAYNAUD'S PHENOMENON: a primary vasospastic disease that affects digits of both hands (rarely feet).

A. Pathophysiology: constriction of small arteries and arterioles from vasospasm or obstruction → spasm → hypoxia → hyperthermia as spasm stops.

B. Risk factors:
1. Cigarette smoking.
2. Caffeine.
3. Cold temperature.
4. Emotional upsets (stress reaction).
5. Autoimmune conditions:
a. Systemic lupus erythematosus (SLE).
b. Rheumatoid arthritis (RA).
c. Scleroderma.
6. Women between teenage years and age 40.

C. Assessment:
1. *Subjective data:*
a. Numbness and sensations of cold. Pain.
b. During "red phase": throbbing, paresthesia, tingling in one or more digits.
2. *Objective data:*
a. Intermittent *episodes of classic color changes,* occurring in *sequence* in digits: pallor (arterial spasm starts) → bluish (cyanosis from hypoxia) → redness (hyperthermia, as arterial spasm stops); ↓ capillary refill.
b. Skin and subcutaneous tissue: atrophy.
c. Nails: brittle.

D. Analysis/nursing diagnosis:
1. *Pain* (acute/chronic) related to vasospasm/altered perfusion of affected tissues and ischemia of tissues.
2. *Altered peripheral tissue perfusion* related to vasospastic disease.
3. *Risk for injury* related to numbness.

E. Nursing care plan/implementation:
1. Goal: *maintain warmth in extremities.*
a. Use wool gloves (when handling cold objects or touching refrigerator/freezer), wool socks and insulated shoes in cold weather.
b. *Avoid* prolonged exposure to cold material, environment.
2. Goal: *increase hydrostatic pressure, and therefore circulation.*
a. Vigorous exercise of arms.
b. Meds: *vasodilators,* including calcium channel blockers, nitrates.
3. Goal: *health teaching:*
a. *Avoid* smoking.
b. Biofeedback for stress management.
c. Identify and *avoid* precipitating factors (e.g., cold, stress).

F. Evaluation/outcome criteria:
1. Severity and frequency of attacks are reduced.
2. Tissue perfusion is maintained.
3. Verbalization of less numbness and tingling. Relief from discomfort.

XX. VARICOSE VEINS: abnormally lengthened, tortuous, dilated superficial veins (saphenous); result of incompetent valves, especially in lower extremities; process is *irreversible.*

A. Pathophysiology: dilated vein → venous stasis → edema, fibrotic changes, pigmentation of skin, lowered resistance to trauma.

B. Risk factors:
1. Heredity.
2. Obesity.
3. Pregnancy.
4. Chronic disease (heart, liver).
5. Occupations requiring long periods of standing.

C. Assessment:
1. *Subjective data:*
   a. Dull aches; heaviness in legs.
   b. Pain; muscle cramping.
   c. Fatigue in lower extremities, increased with hot weather, high altitude, history of risk factors.
2. *Objective data:*
   a. Nodular protrusions along veins.
   b. Edema.
   c. *Diagnostic tests:* Trendelenburg test; phlebography; Doppler flowmeter.

D. Analysis/nursing diagnosis:
1. *Altered tissue perfusion* related to venous valve incompetence.
2. *Pain* related to edema and muscle cramping.
3. *Risk for activity intolerance* related to leg discomfort.
4. *Body image disturbance* related to disfigurement of leg.

E. Nursing care plan/implementation:
1. Goal: *promote venous return from lower extremities.*
   a. Activity: walk every hour.
   b. Discourage prolonged sitting, standing, sitting with crossed legs.
   c. *Position:* elevate legs q2–3h; elastic stockings or Ace wraps. Compression stockings.
2. Goal: *provide for safety.*
   a. Assist with early ambulation.
   b. *Surgical asepsis* with wounds, leg ulcers.
   c. Observe for hemorrhage—if occurs: *elevate* leg, apply pressure, notify physician.
   d. Observe for allergic reactions if sclerosing drugs used; have *antihistamine* available.
3. Goal: *health teaching.*
   a. Weight-reducing techniques, dietary approaches if indicated.
   b. Preventive measures: leg elevation; *avoiding* prolonged standing, sitting, high chairs, tight girdles, constrictive clothing; wear support hose.
   c. Expectations for *Trendelenburg test:*
      (1) While client is lying down, *elevate* leg 65 degrees for approximately 1 minute to empty veins.
      (2) Apply tourniquet high on upper thigh (do *not* constrict deep veins).
      (3) Client stands with tourniquet in place.
      (4) Filling of veins is observed.
      (5) Normal response is slow filling from below in 20 to 30 seconds, with no change in rate when tourniquet is removed.
      (6) Incompetent veins distend very quickly with backflow.
   d. Prepare for sclerotherapy or vein ligation and stripping.

F. Evaluation/outcome criteria:
1. Relief or control of symptoms.
2. Activity without pain.

XXI. VEIN LIGATION AND STRIPPING: surgical intervention for advancing varicosities, stasis ulcerations, and cosmetic needs of client. Procedure involves ligation of the saphenous vein at the groin, where it joins the femoral vein; saphenous stripping from the groin to the ankle; legs are wrapped with a pressure bandage. Frequently done as outpatient surgery.

A. See preceding section on **varicose veins** for *assessment* data and *nursing diagnosis* of the client requiring surgery.

B. Nursing care plan/implementation:
1. Goal: *prevent complications* after discharge.
   a. *Position: elevate* legs as instructed.
   b. Activity: *No* chair sitting to prevent venous pooling, thrombus formation. *Avoid* standing in one place.
   c. Bleeding: report to physician.
2. Goal: *health teaching* to prevent recurrence.
   a. Weight reduction.
   b. *Avoid* constricting garments.
   c. Change positions frequently.
   d. Wear support hose/stockings to enhance venous return.
   e. *No* crossing legs at knees.

C. Evaluation/outcome criteria:
1. No complications—hemorrhage, infection, nerve damage, deep vein thrombosis.
2. No recurrence of varicosities.
3. Adequate circulation to legs: strong pedal pulses.
4. Resumes daily activities; free of pain.

XXII. DEEP VEIN THROMBOSIS (THROMBOPHLEBITIS): formation of a blood clot in an inflamed vein, secondary to phlebitis or partial obstruction; may lead to venous insufficiency and pulmonary embolism. Deep vein thrombosis (DVT) is most serious form.

A. Pathophysiology: endothelial inflammation → formation of platelet plug (blood clot) → slowing of blood flow → increase in procoagulants in local area → initiation of clotting mechanisms.

B. Risk factors:
1. Immobility/stasis—prolonged sitting, bedrest, obesity, pregnancy.
2. Venous disease; history DVT.

3. Age—increased incidence in elderly.
4. Gender—more often women.
5. Hypercoagulability of blood.
6. Intimal damage—IVs, drug abuse.
7. Fractures.
8. Oral contraceptives (related to estrogen content).

C. Assessment:

1. *Subjective data:*
   a. Calf stiffness, soreness.
   b. Severe pain: walking, dorsiflexion of foot (*Homans' sign*—may be unreliable).
2. *Objective data:*
   a. Vein: redness, heat, hardness, threadiness.
   b. Limb: swollen, pale, cold.
   c. *Vital signs:* low-grade fever.
   d. *Diagnostic tests:* venogram, impedance plethysmography (electrical resistance to blood flow), ultrasonography.

D. Analysis/nursing diagnosis:

1. *Altered peripheral tissue perfusion* related to venous stasis.
2. *Pain* related to inflammation.
3. *Activity intolerance* related to leg pain.
4. *Risk for injury* related to potential pulmonary emboli.

E. Nursing care plan/implementation:

1. Goal: *provide rest, comfort, and relief from pain.*
   a. Bedrest until therapeutic level of heparin reached (5 to 7 days with traditional heparin; after 24 hours with low-molecular-weight heparin).
   b. *Position:* as ordered; usually extremity *elevated;* watch for pressure points.
   c. Apply warm, moist heat to affected area as prescribed (cold may also be ordered).
   d. Assess progress of affected area: swelling, pain, soreness, temperature, color.
   e. Administer *analgesics* as ordered.
2. Goal: *prevent complications.*
   a. Observe for signs of embolism (pain at site of embolism); allergic reaction (anaphylactic shock) with streptokinase.
   b. *Precautions: no* rubbing or massage of limb.
   c. Medications: *anticoagulants* (sodium heparin, enoxaparin, warfarin [Coumadin]); streptokinase (Varidase), tissue plasminogen activator **(Table 6.23).**
   d. Bleeding: hematuria, epistaxis, ecchymosis. Check INR levels.
   e. Skin care, to relieve increased redness/maceration from hot or cold applications.
   f. ROM: unaffected limb.
3. Goal: *health teaching.*
   a. *Precautions:* tight garters, girdles; sitting with legs crossed; oral contraceptives.
   b. *Preventive* measures: walking daily, swimming several times weekly if possible, wading, rest periods with legs *elevated,* elastic stockings (may remove at bedtime).
   c. Medication side effects: *anticoagulants*—pink toothbrush, hematuria, easily bruised.
      (1) Carry Medic Alert card/bracelet.
      (2) **Contraindicated** drugs—aspirin, glutethimide (Doriden), chloramphenicol (Chloromycetin), neomycin, phenylbutazone (Butazolidin), barbiturates.
   d. Prepare for surgery (thrombectomy, vein ligation).

F. Evaluation/outcome criteria:

1. No complications (e.g., embolism).
2. No recurrence of symptoms.
3. Free of pain—ambulates without discomfort.

XXIII. PERIPHERAL EMBOLISM: fragments of thrombi, globules of fat, clumps of tissue, calcified plaques, or air moves in the circulation and lodges in

Table 6.23

Nursing Responsibilities with Anticoagulant Therapy

	Heparin	Warfarin (Coumadin)	Low-Molecular-Weight Heparin (LMWH)
Monitor	PTT (25–38 sec) (2–3 times baseline)	PT (11–15 sec) (1½–2½ times baseline) INR: 2–3.5	Anti–factor Xa, CBC, platelets
Inspect	Ecchymosis, bleeding gums, petechiae, hematuria	Bleeding, ecchymosis	Bleeding, hemorrhage, unusual bruising
Administer	With an infusion pump; **never** mix with other drugs; **never** aspirate; **avoid** massaging site	Same time every day; PO	Subcutaneous twice daily
Avoid	Salicylates and other anticoagulants, e.g., antacids, corticosteroids, penicillin, phenytoin	Same as heparin	Warfarin, platelet aggregation inhibitors (e.g., ASA, NSAIDs, dextran)
Antidote	Protamine sulfate	Vitamin K	Protamine sulfate

ADULT

vessel, obstructing blood flow; thrombic emboli most common; may be venous or arterial.

GASTROINTESTINAL SYSTEM

I. GENERAL NUTRITIONAL DEFICIENCIES

A. Assessment:

1. *Subjective data:*
   a. Mental irritability or confusion.
   b. History of poor dietary intake.
   c. History of lack of adequate resources to provide adequate nutrition.
   d. Lack of knowledge about proper diet, food selection, or preparation.
   e. History of eating disorders.
   f. Paresthesia (burning and tingling): hands and feet.
2. *Objective data:*
   a. *Appearance:* listless; *posture:* sagging shoulders, sunken chest, poor gait.
   b. *Muscle:* weakness, fatigue, wasted appearance.
   c. *GI:* indigestion, vomiting, enlarged liver, spleen.
   d. *Cardiovascular:* tachycardia on minimal exertion; bradycardia at rest; enlarged heart, elevated BP.
   e. *Hair:* brittle, dry, thin, sparse; lack of natural shine; color changes; can be easily plucked out.
   f. *Skin:* dryness (xerosis), scaly, dyspigmentation, petechiae, lack of fat under skin.
   g. *Mouth:*
      (1) *Teeth:* missing, abnormally placed, caries.
      (2) *Gums:* bleed easily, receding.
      (3) *Tongue:* swollen, sore.
      (4) *Lips:* red, swollen, angular fissures at corners.
   h. *Eyes:* pale conjunctivae, corneal changes.
   i. *Nails:* brittle, ridged.
   j. *Nervous system:* abnormal reflexes.
   k. Laboratory data: blood—*decreased* albumin, iron-binding capacity, lymphocyte, hemoglobin, and hematocrit.
   l. Anthropometric measurements document nutritional deficiencies.

B. Analysis/nursing diagnosis:

1. *Altered nutrition, less than body requirements,* related to poor dietary intake.
2. *Knowledge deficit* (learning need) related to nutritional requirements.
3. *Altered health maintenance* related to inability to provide own nutritional care.
4. *Ineffective individual coping* related to eating disorders.
5. *Ineffective family coping, disabling,* related to inadequate resources or knowledge to provide appropriate family nutrition.

C. Nursing care plan/implementation:

1. Goal: *prevent complications of specific deficiency.*
   a. Identify etiology of nutritional deficiency.
   b. Recognize signs of nutritional deficiencies (see **Chapter 9, Table 9.6**).
   c. Identify foods high in deficient nutrient (see **Chapter 9**).
   d. Evaluate economic resources to purchase appropriate foods.
   e. Identify community resources for assistance.
   f. Monitor progress for potential additional illnesses.
2. Goal: *health teaching.*
   a. Effects of nutritional deficiencies on health.
   b. Foods to include in diet to avoid deficits.

D. Evaluation/outcome criteria:

1. Complications do not occur.
2. Client gains weight.
3. Client selects appropriate foods to alleviate deficiency.

II. CELIAC DISEASE

(gluten enteropathy, nontropical sprue): immune to gluten, causing impaired absorption and digestion of nutrients through the small bowel. Affects adults and children and is characterized by inability to digest and use sugars, starches, and fats.

A. Pathophysiology: intolerance to the gliadin fraction of grains causing degeneration of the epithelial surface of the intestine, atrophy of the intestinal villi, and impaired absorption of essential nutrients.

B. Risk factors:

1. Possible genetic or familial factors.
2. Hypersensitivity response.
3. History of childhood celiac disease.

C. Assessment:

1. *Subjective data:* family history.
2. *Objective data:*
   a. Loss: weight, fat deposits, musculature.
   b. Anemia.
   c. Vitamin deficiencies.
   d. Abdomen distended with flatus.
   e. *Stools*: diarrhea, foul smelling, bulky, fatty, float in commode.
   f. Skin condition known as *dermatitis herpetiformis.*
   g. History of acute attacks of fluid and electrolyte imbalances.
   h. *Diagnostic tests:* stool for fat; barium enema; antibody tests, including endomysial antibody (EMA); blood studies of: iron, folate, proteins, minerals, and clotting factors; small bowel biopsy.

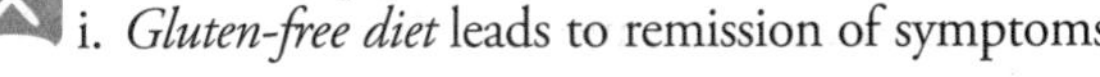
   i. *Gluten-free diet* leads to remission of symptoms.

ADULT

D. Analysis/nursing diagnosis:

1. *Altered nutrition, less than body requirements,* related to inability to digest and use sugars, starches, and fats.
2. *Diarrhea* related to intestinal response to gluten in diet.
3. *Fluid volume deficit* related to loss through excessive diarrhea.
4. *Knowledge deficit* (learning need) related to dietary restrictions to control symptoms.

E. Nursing care plan/implementation:

1. Goal: *prevent weight loss.*

   a. *Diet: high* in calories, protein, vitamins, and minerals, and gluten free.
      (1) *Avoid:* wheat, rye, oats, barley.
      (2) All other foods permitted.
   b. Daily weights to monitor weight changes.
2. Goal: *health teaching.*
   a. Nature of disease.
   b. Dietary restrictions and allowances.
   c. Complications of noncompliance.

F. Evaluation/outcome criteria:

1. No further weight loss.
2. Normal stools.
3. Fluid/electrolyte balance obtained and maintained.

III. HEPATITIS: inflammation of the liver.

A. Pathophysiology:

1. Infection with *hepatitis A* (formerly called infectious hepatitis), *hepatitis B* (formerly called serum hepatitis), *hepatitis C* (single-stranded RNA virus of the *Flaviviridae* family; usually asymptomatic), *delta hepatitis* (infection caused by a defective RNA virus that requires hepatitis B virus to multiply), or *hepatitis E* (major etiological agent of the enterically transmitted non-A, non-B hepatitis worldwide) → inflammation, necrosis, and regeneration of liver parenchyma. Hepatocellular injury impairs clearance of urobilinogen → elevated urinary urobilinogen; and, as injury increases → conjugated bilirubin not reaching the intestines → decreased urine and fecal urobilinogen → increased serum bilirubin → jaundice.
2. Failure of liver to detoxify products → increased toxic products of protein metabolism → gastritis and duodenitis.

B. Risk factors:

1. Exposure to virus.
2. Exposure to carriers of virus.
3. Exposure to hepatotoxins such as dry-cleaning agents.
4. Nonimmunized.

C. Assessment:

1. *Subjective data:*
   a. Anorexia, nausea.
   b. Malaise, dull ache in right upper quadrant, abdominal pain.
   c. Repugnance to: food, cigarette smoke, strong odors, alcohol.
   d. Headache.
2. *Objective data:*
   a. Fever.
   b. Liver: enlarged (hepatomegaly), tender, smooth.
   c. *Skin:* icterus in sclerae of eyes, jaundice; rash; pruritus; petechiae, bruises.
   d. Urine: normal, dark.
   e. Stool: normal, clay colored, loose.
   f. Vomiting, weight loss.
   g. Lymph nodes: enlarged.
   h. Laboratory data:
      (1) Blood—leukocytosis.
      (2) *Increased* AST (SGOT), alanine aminotransferase (ALT, or serum glutamic-pyruvic transaminase [SGPT]), and bilirubin levels, alkaline phosphatase.
      (3) Urine—*increased* urobilinogen.
   i. See **Table 6.24** for comparison of hepatitis A, B, C, and D.

D. Analysis/nursing diagnosis:

1. *Pain* related to inflammation of liver.
2. *Impaired skin integrity* related to pruritus.
3. *Activity intolerance* related to fatigue.
4. *Risk for infection* to others related to incubation/infectious period.
5. *Altered nutrition, less than body requirements,* related to repugnance of food.
6. *Social isolation* related to isolation precautions.

E. Nursing care plan/implementation:

1. Goal: *prevent spread of infection to others.*
   a. Isolation according to type
      (1) *Hepatitis A:*
         (a) *Contact* precautions (see **Chapter 3, pp. 90, 92, 93, Tables 3.3, 3.7, and 3.8**).
         (b) Private room preferred.
         (c) Gown/gloves for direct contact with feces.
         (d) Hand washing when in direct contact with feces.
      (2) *Hepatitis B: blood and body fluid* precautions.
         (a) *Needle/dressing* precautions.
         (b) Private room not necessary.
         (c) Gown: only if enteric precautions also necessary.
         (d) Hand washing: use gloves when in direct contact with blood.
      (3) *Hepatitis C: blood and body fluid precautions*—same as hepatitis B, except when in countries with

ADULT

Table 6.24

Etiology, Incidence, and Epidemiological and Clinical Comparison of Hepatitis A, Hepatitis B, Hepatitis C, and Delta Hepatitis

	Hepatitis A	Hepatitis B	Hepatitis C	Delta Hepatitis
Incubation	2–6 wk	4 wk to 6 mo	Variable: 14–160 days; average, 50 days	Same as hepatitis B
Communicable	Until 7–9 days after jaundice occurs	Several months—as long as virus present in blood	As long as virus present in blood	As long as virus present in blood
Transmission	Fecal-oral; blood; sexual	Parenteral; sexual; perinatal	Percutaneous, via contaminated blood, parenteral drug abuse; some fecal-oral forms; sexual; perinatal	Parenteral; blood
Sources	Crowding; contaminated: food, milk, or water	Contaminated: needles, syringes, surgical instruments	Persons who have received 15 or more blood transfusions; IV drug users; persons traveling to contaminated areas	Contaminated needles, syringes
Portal of entry	GI tract; asymptomatic carriers	Integumentary: blood plasma or transfusions	Blood	Integumentary: blood
HB antigen	Not present	Present	Not present	Present as with hepatitis B
Incidence	Sporadic epidemics; increased in children <15	Increased in ages 15–29, particularly in heroin addiction; occupational hazard for: laboratory workers, nurses, physicians	All age groups; higher in adults because of exposure to risk factors	Same as hepatitis B
Immunity	*Preexposure:* immune globulin, 0.02 mL/kg	*Preexposure:* hepatitis B vaccine	None; immune globulin may be given	None
	Postexposure: within 2 wk of exposure, as above	*Postexposure:* immune globulin with high amounts of anti-HBs (HBIG); hepatitis B vaccine		
Prevention	Hand washing, use of gloves; hepatitis A vaccine	Care when handling products contaminated by blood, use of gloves; hepatitis B vaccine	Same as hepatitis B	Same as hepatitis B
Severity	Mild	Mild to moderate	Mild to moderate	Moderate to severe
Fever	Common	Uncommon	Uncommon	Uncommon
Nausea/vomiting	Common	Common	Common	Common

fecal-oral form, then use hepatitis A precautions also.

(4) *Delta:* same as hepatitis B.

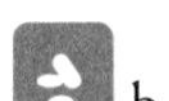

b. Passive immunity for contacts.

(1) *Hepatitis A:* hepatitis A vaccine (Havrix, VAQTA), immune serum globulin (ISG), administered before and after exposure.

(2) *Hepatitis B:* hepatitis B immune globulin (HBIG) (Recombivax HB, Energix-B) or ISG.

(3) *Hepatitis C:* prophylaxis not as effective; ISG may be given.

(4) *Delta:* same as for hepatitis B.

2. Goal: *promote healing.*

a. *Diet* as tolerated:

(1) NPO with parenteral infusions, when in acute stage.

(2) *High* protein, *high* carbohydrate, *low* fat, offered in frequent small meals.

(3) Push fluids, if not contraindicated; I&O.

b. Medications:
(1) *Antiviral* for clients with persistently elevated ALT levels.
(2) Interferon for initial treatment of hepatitis C.

3. Goal: *monitor for worsening of disease process, failure to respond to prescribed treatment.*
   a. Observe urine—dark due to presence of bile and stool, clay colored.
   b. Observe sclerae, laboratory tests for increasing jaundice.
   c. Mental confusion, unusual somnolence may indicate decreased liver function.
   d. Weigh daily—increase indicates fluid retention and possible ascites.
4. Goal: *health teaching.*
   a. Diet and fluid intake to promote liver regeneration.
   b. Importance of rest and limited activity to reduce metabolic workload of liver.
   c. Personal hygiene practices to prevent contamination.
   d. *Avoid:* alcohol, blood donations, and contact with communicable infections.
   e. Follow-up case referral; may take 6 months for full recovery.
   f. Teach contacts about available immunizations.
5. Goal: *promote comfort.*
   a. Bedrest to combat fatigue and reduce metabolic needs until hepatomegaly subsides; *semi-Fowler's* or *supine* positioning.
   b. Oral hygiene q1–2h to decrease nausea.
   c. ROM exercises to maintain muscle strength.
   d. *Measures to reduce pruritus:*
      (1) Mild, oil-based lotion to reduce itching.
      (2) Nails cut short, cotton gloves, long-sleeved clothing to prevent skin injury from scratching.
      (3) Environment: cool and dry.
      (4) Cool wet soaks to skin.
      (5) Diversional activities.
      (6) Medications as ordered:
         (a) *Emollients* to relieve dry skin.
         (b) *Topical corticosteroids* to reduce inflammation.
         (c) *Antihistamines* to reduce itch.
         (d) *Tranquilizers and sedatives* to allow rest and prevent exhaustion.

F. Evaluation/outcome criteria:
1. Tolerates food; nausea and vomiting decreased.
2. Signs of infection/inflammation absent.
3. No complications, hemorrhage, liver damage, ascites.
4. No jaundice noted.

ADULT

IV. PANCREATITIS: inflammatory disease of the pancreas that may result in autodigestion of the pancreas by its own enzymes.

A. Pathophysiology: proteolytic enzymes within the pancreas are activated by endotoxins, exotoxins, ischemia, anoxia, or trauma. Pancreatic enzymes begin process of autodigestion of pancreas and surrounding tissues; also activate other enzymes that digest cellular membranes. Autodigestion leads to: edema, hemorrhage, vascular damage, coagulation necrosis, and fat necrosis.

B. Risk factors:
1. Obesity.
2. Alcoholism, alcohol consumption.
3. Biliary tract disease.
4. Abdominal trauma.
5. Surgery.
6. Drugs.
7. Metabolic disease.
8. Intestinal disease.
9. Obstruction of the pancreatic ducts.
10. Infections.
11. Carcinoma.
12. Adenoma.
13. Hypercalcemia.

C. Assessment:
1. *Subjective data:*
   a. *Pain:*
      (1) Sudden onset; severe, widespread, constant, and incapacitating.
      (2) Location—epigastrium, right upper quadrant (RUQ) and left upper quadrant (LUQ) of abdomen; radiates to back, flanks, and substernal area.
   b. Nausea.
   c. History of risk factors.
   d. Dyspnea.
2. *Objective data:*
   a. *Elevated:* temperature, pulse, respirations, BP (unless in shock).
   b. *Decreased* breath sounds related to atelectasis/pleural effusion.
   c. *Increased* crackles, cyanosis.
   d. Hemorrhage, shock.
   e. Vomiting.
   f. Fluid and electrolyte imbalances, dehydration.
   g. *Decreased* bowel sounds; abdominal tenderness with guarding.
   h. *Stools:* bulky, pale, foul smelling, steatorrhea (excessive fat in stools).
   i. *Skin:* pale, moist, cold; may be jaundiced.
   j. Muscle rigidity.
   k. Supine position leads to increased pain.
   l. Fluid accumulation in the abdomen.

m. Laboratory data:
  (1) *Elevated:*
    (a) Amylase, serum, and urine.
    (b) Serum lipase, AST (SGOT).
    (c) Alkaline phosphatase.
    (d) Bilirubin, glucose; serum and urine.
    (e) Urine protein, WBC count.
    (f) Leukocytes.
    (g) BUN.
    (h) LDH (liver function).
  (2) *Decreased:*
    (a) Serum calcium.
    (b) Protein.

n. Ultrasound for gallstones, CT scan.

D. Analysis/nursing diagnosis:

1. *Altered nutrition, less than body requirements,* related to nausea and vomiting.
2. *Pain* related to inflammatory and autodigestive processes of pancreas.
3. *Fluid volume deficit* related to inflammation, decreased intake, and vomiting.
4. *Ineffective breathing pattern* related to pain and pleural effusion.
5. *Knowledge deficit* (learning need) related to risk factors and disease management.

E. Nursing care plan/implementation:

1. Goal: *control pain.*
   a. Medications: *analgesics*—meperidine (*not* morphine or codeine due to spasmodic effect).
   b. *Position:* sitting with knees flexed.
2. Goal: *rest injured pancreas.*
   a. NPO.
   b. Nasogastric (NG) tube to low suction.
   c. Medications:
     (1) *Antiulcers.*
     (2) *Antibiotics.*
     (3) *Antiemetics.*
     (4) *Antispasmodics.*
     (5) *Anticholinergics.*
     (6) *Histamine$_2$ receptors* (cimetidine).
3. Goal: *prevent fluid and electrolyte imbalance.*
   a. Monitor: vitals, CVP.
   b. IVs, fluids, blood, albumin, plasma.
4. Goal: *prevent respiratory and metabolic complications.*
   a. Cough, deep breathe, change position.
   b. Monitor: blood sugar as ordered.
   c. Monitor calcium levels: *Chvostek's* and *Trousseau's signs* positive when calcium deficit exists (see **ENDOCRINE SYSTEM, IV. THYROIDECTOMY, p. 473,** for description of tests).

5. Goal: *provide adequate nutrition.*
   a. *Low-fat diet.*
   b. Bland, small, frequent meals.
   c. Vitamin supplements.
   d. *Avoid* alcohol.
6. Goal: *prevent complications.*
   a. Monitor for signs of:
     (1) Peritonitis.
     (2) Perforation.
     (3) Respiratory complications.
     (4) Hypotension, shock.
     (5) DIC.
     (6) ARDS.
     (7) Hemorrhage from ulcers, varices.
     (8) Anemia.
     (9) Encephalopathy.
7. Goal: *health teaching.*
   a. Food selections for low-fat, bland diet.
   b. Necessity of vitamin therapy.
   c. Importance of avoiding alcohol.
   d. Signs and symptoms of recurrence.
   e. Importance of rest, to prevent relapse.
   f. Desired effects and side effects of prescribed medications:
     (1) *Narcotics* for pain.
     (2) *Antiemetics* for nausea and vomiting.
     (3) *Pancreatic hormone and enzymes* to replace enzymes not reaching duodenum.

F. Evaluation/outcome criteria:

1. Pain is relieved.
2. No complications (e.g., peritonitis, respiratory).
3. States dietary allowances and restrictions.
4. Takes medications as ordered; states purposes, side effects.

V. CIRRHOSIS: chronic inflammation and fibrosis (irreversible scarring) of the liver in which some liver cells (hepatocytes) undergo necrosis and others undergo proliferative regeneration.

A. Pathophysiology: progressive destruction of hepatic cells → loss of normal metabolic function of the liver and formation of scar tissue. Regeneration and proliferation of fibrous tissue → obstruction of the portal vein → increased portal hypertension, ascites, liver failure, and eventual death.

B. Risk factors:

1. Alcohol abuse most common cause.
2. Nutritional deficiency with decreased protein intake.
3. Hepatotoxins.
4. Virus.
5. Hepatitis B and C.

C. Assessment:

1. *Subjective data:*
   a. Chronic feeling of malaise.
   b. Anorexia, nausea.
   c. Abdominal pain.
   d. Pruritus.

2. *Objective data:*
   a. *GI:*
      (1) Malnutrition, weight loss.
      (2) Vomiting.
      (3) Flatulence.
      (4) Ascites.
      (5) Enlarged liver and spleen.
      (6) Glossitis.
      (7) Fetid breath (sweet, musty odor).
   b. *Blood*—coagulation defects, possible esophageal varices, portal hypertension, bleeding from gums and injection sites.
   c. *Skin and hair*—edema, jaundice, spider angioma (telangiectasias); palmar erythema, decreased pubic and axillary hair.
   d. *Reproductive*—menstrual abnormalities, gynecomastia, testicular atrophy, impotence.
   e. *Neurological deficits*—memory loss, hepatic coma, decreased level of consciousness: flapping tremor, grimacing.
   f. Laboratory data:
      (1) *Decreased:* albumin, potassium, magnesium, blood urea nitrogen (BUN).
      (2) *Elevated:* prothrombin time, globulins, ammonia, AST (SGOT), bromsulphalein (BSP), alkaline phosphate, uric acid, blood sugar.
   g. *Diagnostic tests:*
      (1) Celiac angiography, hepatoportography.
      (2) Liver biopsy.
      (3) Paracentesis.

D. Analysis/nursing diagnosis:
1. *Altered nutrition, less than body requirements,* related to decreased intake, nausea, and vomiting.
2. *Risk for injury* related to decreased prothrombin production.
3. *Activity intolerance* related to fatigue.
4. *Fatigue* related to anorexia and nutritional deficiencies.
5. *Self-esteem disturbance* related to physical body changes.
6. *Risk for impaired skin integrity* related to pruritus.

E. Nursing care plan/implementation:
1. Goal: *provide for special safety needs.*
   a. Monitor vitals (including neurological) frequently for hemorrhage from esophageal varices (may have *Sengstaken-Blakemore* or *Linton* tube inserted).
   b. Prepare client for *LeVeen shunt* surgery for portal hypertension as needed.
   c. Assist with *paracentesis* performed for ascites; monitor vitals to prevent shock during procedure.
2. Goal: *relieve discomfort caused by complications.*
   a. *Position: semi-Fowler's* or *Fowler's* to decrease pressure on diaphragm due to ascites.
   b. Deep breathing q2h to prevent respiratory complications.
   c. Skin care, topical medications to relieve pruritus; nail care to decrease possibility of further skin injury.
   d. Frequent oral hygiene related to nausea, vomiting, and fetid breath.
3. Goal: *improve fluid and electrolyte balance.*
   a. IV fluids and vitamins.
   b. I&O, hourly urines during acute attacks.
   c. Daily: girths, weights to monitor fluid balance.
   d. *Diuretics* as ordered to decrease edema.
   e. May receive *serum albumin* to promote adequate vascular volume, prevent azotemia and encephalopathy, and promote diuresis (observe carefully, because albumin could escape quickly through cell walls and cause increase in ascites).
4. Goal: *promote optimum nutrition within dietary restrictions.*
   a. NPO during acute episodes.
   b. Small, frequent meals when able to eat.
   c. *Low protein* (to decrease the amount of nitrogenous materials in the intestines) and *sodium* (to decrease fluid retention).
   d. *Moderate carbohydrate* (to meet energy demands) and *fat* (to make diet more palatable to clients who are anorexic).
5. Goal: *provide emotional support.*
   a. Quiet environment during acute episodes to decrease external stimuli.
   b. Refer to *community agencies* for assistance for client (e.g., Alcoholics Anonymous; for family, Al-Anon/Alateen).
6. Goal: *health teaching.*
   a. *Avoid* alcohol, exposure to infections.
   b. Dietary allowances, restrictions (see **Chapter 9,** Sodium-restricted diet, **p. 694,** and purine-restricted diet, **p. 699**).
   c. Drugs: names, purposes.
   d. Signs, symptoms of disease; complications.
   e. Stress-management techniques.

F. Evaluation/outcome criteria:
1. No complications.
2. Nutritional status improves; lists dietary restrictions.
3. No alcohol consumption.
4. Lists signs and symptoms of progression of disease and complications.
5. Complies with discharge plan, becomes involved with an alcohol treatment program.

VI. ESOPHAGEAL VARICES: **life-threatening hemorrhage** from tortuous dilated, thin-walled veins in submucosa of lower esophagus. May rupture when chemically or mechanically irritated, or when pressure is increased because of sneezing, coughing, use of the Valsalva maneuver, or excessive exercise.

A. Pathophysiology: portal hypertension related to cirrhosis of the liver → distended branches of the azygos vein and inferior vena cava where they join the smaller vessels of the esophagus.

B. Risk factors for hemorrhage:

1. Exertion that increases abdominal pressure.
2. Trauma from ingestion of coarse foods.
3. Acid pepsin erosion.

C. Assessment:

1. *Subjective data:*
   a. Fear.
   b. Dysphagia.
   c. History: alcohol ingestion, liver dysfunction.
2. *Objective data:*
   a. Hematemesis.
   b. Hemorrhage: sudden, often fatal.
   c. *Decreased* BP; *increased* pulse, respirations.
   d. Melena (occult blood in stool).
   e. Diagnostic endoscopy.

D. Analysis/nursing diagnosis:

1. *Fluid volume deficit* related to blood loss.
2. *Risk for injury* related to hemorrhage.
3. *Fear* related to massive blood loss.
4. *Ineffective individual coping* related to complications of cirrhosis.

E. Nursing care plan/implementation:

1. Goal: *provide safety measures related to hemorrhage.*
   a. Recognize signs of shock; vitals q15 min.
   b. Assist with insertion of *Sengstaken-Blakemore* (or Minnesota) or *Linton tube* (tube is large and uncomfortable for client during insertion); explain procedure briefly to decrease fear and attempt to gain client's cooperation.
   c. While tube is in place, observe for respiratory distress; if present, *deflate the balloon by releasing pressure; do not cut the tube.*
   d. Deflate the balloon as ordered to prevent necrosis.
   e. NG tube to low gastric suction; monitor for amount of bright-red blood; irrigate only as ordered using tepid, *not* iced, solutions.
   f. Vitamin K as ordered to control bleeding.
2. Goal: *promote fluid balance.*
   a. IV fluids, expanders.
   b. Fresh blood as ordered to avoid increased ammonia; aids in coagulation.
3. Goal: *prevent complications of hepatic coma.*
   a. *Saline cathartics* as ordered to remove old blood from GI tract.
   b. *Antibiotics* as ordered to prevent infection.
   c. Reduce portal hypertension; give propranolol (Inderal), vasopressin (Pitressin).
4. Goal: *provide emotional support.*
   a. Stay with client.
   b. Calm atmosphere.
5. Goal: *health teaching.*
   a. Explain use of tube to client and family.
   b. Bland diet instructions.
   c. Recognize signs of bleeding.
   d. *Avoid* straining at stool.
   e. *Avoid* aspirin because of increased bleeding tendency.

F. Evaluation/outcome criteria:

1. Survives acute bleeding episode.
2. Further episodes prevented by avoiding irritants, especially alcohol.
3. Improves nutritional status.
4. Recognizes symptoms of complications (e.g., bleeding).
5. Demonstrates knowledge of medications by avoiding aspirin.

VII. DIAPHRAGMATIC (HIATAL) HERNIA: protrusion of part of stomach through diaphragm and into thoracic cavity **(Fig. 6.8).** *Types:* sliding (most common); paraesophageal "rolling."

A. Pathophysiology: weakening of the musculature of the diaphragm, aggravated by increased intra-abdominal pressure → protrusion of the abdominal organs through the esophageal hiatus → reflux of gastric contents → esophagitis.

B. Risk factors:

1. Congenital abnormality.
2. Penetrating wound.
3. Age (middle-aged or elderly).
4. Women more than men.
5. Obesity.
6. Ascites.
7. Pregnancy.
8. History of constipation.

C. Assessment:

1. *Subjective data:*
   a. Pressure: substernal.
   b. *Pain:* epigastric, burning.
   c. Eructation, heartburn after eating.
   d. Dysphagia.
   e. Symptoms aggravated when recumbent.
2. *Objective data:*
   a. Cough, dyspnea.
   b. Tachycardia, palpitations.
   c. *Bleeding:* hematemesis, melena, signs of anemia due to gastroesophageal irritation, ulceration, and bleeding.

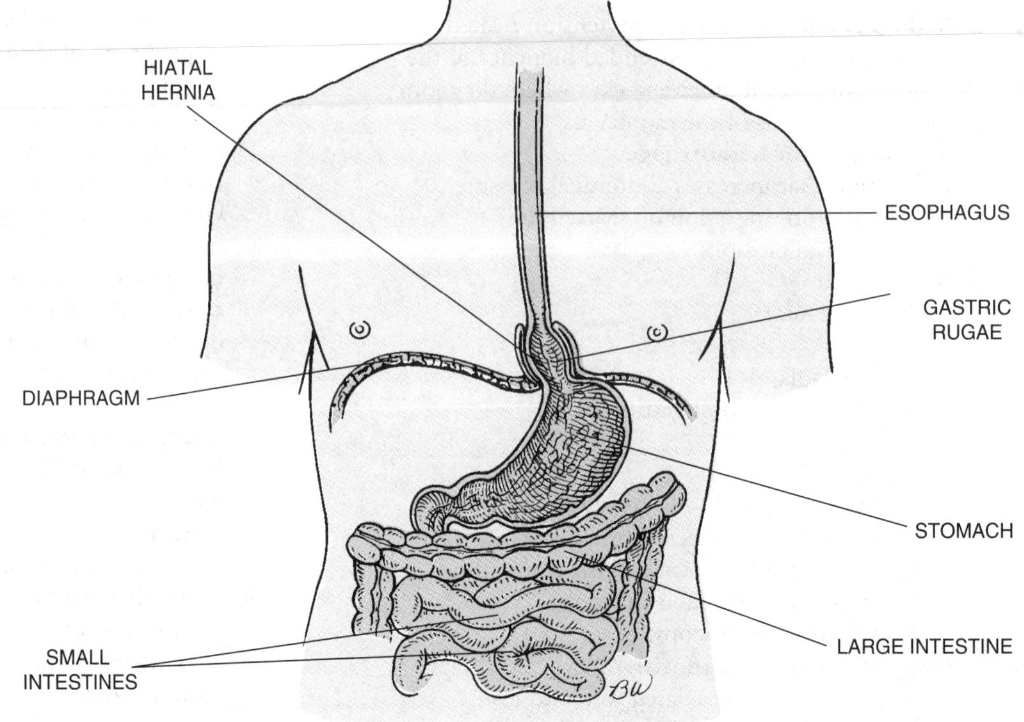

Figure 6.8 Hiatal hernia. (From Venes, D [ed]: *Taber's Cyclopedic Medical Dictionary,* ed 21. FA Davis, Philadelphia, 2009.)

d. *Diagnostic tests:*
   (1) Chest x-rays, showing protrusion of abdominal organs into thoracic cavity.
   (2) Barium swallow (upper GI series) to show presence of hernia.
   (3) Endoscopy.

e. Symptoms parallel those of gastroesophageal reflux disease (GERD).

D. Analysis/nursing diagnosis:

1. *Pain* related to irritation of lining of GI tract.
2. *Altered nutrition, less than body requirements,* related to dysphagia.
3. *Sleep pattern disturbance* related to increase in symptoms when recumbent.
4. *Risk for aspiration* related to reflux of gastric contents.
5. *Activity intolerance* related to dyspnea.
6. *Anxiety* related to palpitations.

E. Nursing care plan/implementation:

1. *Presurgical:*
   a. Goal: *promote relief of symptoms.*
      (1) *Diet:*
         (a) Small, frequent feedings of *soft, bland* foods, to reduce abdominal pressure and reflux.
         (b) Fluid when swallowing solids may push food into stomach; *hot* fluid may work best.
         (c) *Avoid* eating 2 hours before bedtime.
         (d) *High*-protein, *low*-fat foods to decrease heartburn.
      (2) *Positioning: head elevated* to increase movement of food into stomach. Symptoms may decrease if head of bed at home is elevated on 8-inch blocks.
      (3) Weight reduction to decrease abdominal pressure.
      (4) Medications as ordered:
         (a) 30 mL *antacid* 1 hour *after* meals and at bedtime.
         (b) *Avoid* anticholinergic drugs, which decrease gastric emptying.

2. *Postsurgical:*
   a. Goal: *provide for postoperative safety needs.*
      (1) Respiratory: deep breathing, coughing, splint incision area.
      (2) *Nasogastric (NG) tube:* check patency.
         (a) Drainage: should be small amount.
         (b) Color: dark brown 6 to 12 hours after surgery, changing to greenish-yellow.
         (c) Do *not* disturb tube placement to *avoid* traction on suture line.

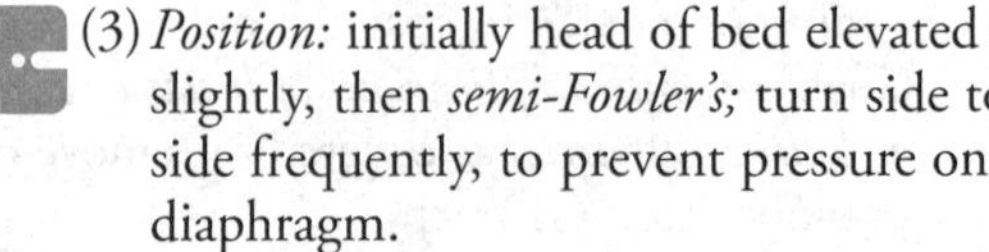

      (3) *Position:* initially head of bed elevated slightly, then *semi-Fowler's;* turn side to side frequently, to prevent pressure on diaphragm.

(4) Maintain closed chest drainage if indicated (see **Table 11.5**).
(5) Check for return of bowel sounds.

b. Goal: *promote comfort and maintain nutrition.*

(1) IVs for hydration and electrolytes.
(2) Initiate feeding through *gastrostomy* tube if present.

(a) Usually attached to intermittent, low suction after surgery.
(b) Aspirate gastric contents before feeding—delay if 75 mL or more is present; report these findings to physician.

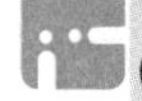

(c) Feed in *high Fowler's* or sitting position; keep head elevated for 30 minutes after eating.
(d) Warm feeding to room temperature; dilute with H_2O if too thick.
(e) Give 50 mL H_2O before feeding; 200 to 500 mL feeding by gravity over 10 to 15 minutes; follow with 50 mL H_2O.
(f) Give frequent mouth care.

c. Goal: *health teaching.*

(1) *Avoid* constricting clothing and activities that increase intra-abdominal pressure (e.g., lifting, bending, straining at stool).

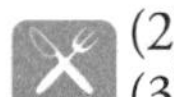

(2) Weight reduction.
(3) Dietary needs: small, frequent, soft, bland meals.
(4) Chew thoroughly.
(5) Upright position for at least 1 hour after meals.

F. Evaluation/outcome criteria:

1. Obtains relief from symptoms; is comfortable.
2. Receives adequate, balanced nutrition.
3. Describes dietary changes, recommended positioning, and activity limitations to prevent recurrence.

VIII. GASTROESOPHAGEAL REFLUX DISEASE (GERD): inappropriate relaxation of the lower esophageal sphincter (LES) in response to unknown stimulus.

A. Pathophysiology: gastric volume or intra-abdominal pressure elevated, or LES tone decreased → frequent episodes of acid reflux → breakdown of mucosal barrier → esophageal inflammation, hyperemia, and erosion → fibrotic tissue formation → esophageal stricture → impaired swallowing.

B. Risk factors:

1. Hiatal hernia.
2. Diet—foods that lower pressure of LES (fatty foods, chocolate, cola, coffee, tea).
3. Smoking.
4. Drugs (calcium channel blockers, NSAIDs, theophylline).
5. Elevated intra-abdominal pressure (obesity, pregnancy, heavy lifting).

C. Assessment:

1. *Subjective data:*
   a. Heartburn (pyrosis)—substernal or retrosternal; may mimic angina; 20 minutes to 2 hours after eating.
   b. Regurgitation—sour or bitter taste not associated with belching or nausea.
   c. Dysphagia or odynophagia (difficult or painful swallowing)—severe cases.
   d. Belching, feeling bloated.
   e. Nocturnal cough.
2. *Objective data:*
   a. Hoarseness, wheezing.
   b. *Diagnostic tests:* 24-hour pH monitoring; barium swallow with fluoroscopy; endoscopy.

D. Analysis/nursing diagnosis:

1. *Pain* related to acid reflux and esophageal inflammation.
2. *Knowledge deficit* (learning need) related to modifications needed to control reflux.

E. Nursing care plan/implementation:

1. Goal: *promote comfort and reduce reflux episodes.*
   a. Medications as ordered:
      (1) *Antacids* to neutralize gastric acid.
      (2) *Histamine$_2$ (H_2) receptor antagonists* (cimetidine, ranitidine, famotidine) to reduce gastric acid secretion and support tissue healing.
      (3) *Proton pump inhibitor* (omeprazole [Prilosec]) to inhibit gastric enzymes and suppress gastric acid secretion.
   b. *Diet: avoid* strong stimulants of acid secretion (caffeine, alcohol); *avoid* foods that reduce LES competence (fatty foods, onions, tomato-based foods); *increase* protein; *restrict* spicy, acidic foods until healing occurs.
   c. Activity: *avoid* heavy lifting, straining, constrictive clothing, bending over.
   d. *Position: elevate head* of bed 6 to 12 inches for sleeping. Reflux more likely on right side.
2. Goal: *health teaching.*
   a. Weight reduction if indicated.
   b. Smoking cessation.
   c. Diet modification: *avoid* overeating—eat 4 to 6 small meals.
   d. Medication administration.
   e. Potential complications if uncontrolled (hemorrhage, aspiration).

F. Evaluation/outcome criteria:

1. No heartburn reported.
2. Changes diet as instructed.
3. No complications of continued reflux.

IX. PEPTIC ULCER DISEASE: circumscribed loss of mucosa, submucosa, or muscle layer of the gastrointestinal tract caused by a decreased resistance of gastric mucosa to acid-pepsin injury. *Peptic ulcer disease* is a chronic disease and may occur in the distal esophagus, stomach, upper duodenum, or jejunum. *Gastric ulcers,* located on the lesser curvature of the stomach, are larger and deeper than duodenal ulcers and tend to become *malignant. Duodenal ulcers* are located on the first part of the duodenum and are more common than gastric ulcers. *Esophageal ulcers* occur in the esophagus. *Stress ulcers,* an acute problem, occur after a major insult to the body.

A. Pathology: failure of the body to regenerate mucous epithelium at a sufficient rate to counterbalance the damage to tissue during the breakdown of protein; decrease in the quantity and quality of the mucus; poor local mucosal blood flow, along with individual susceptibility to ulceration. A *peptic ulcer* is a hole in the lining of the stomach, duodenum, or esophagus. This hole occurs when the lining of these organs is corroded by the acidic digestive juices secreted by the stomach cells. Excess acid is still considered to be significant in ulcer formation. The leading cause of ulcer disease is currently believed to be infection of the stomach by *Helicobacter pylori (H. pylori).* Another major cause of ulcers is chronic use of nonsteroidal anti-inflammatory drugs (NSAIDs). Cigarette smoking is also an important cause of ulcers.

B. Risk factors:

1. *Gastric ulcers.*
   a. Infection with *H. pylori.*
   b. Decreased resistance to acid-pepsin injury.
   c. Increased histamine release → inflammatory reaction.
   d. Ulcerogenic drugs (aggravate preexisting conditions).
   e. Cigarette smoking.
   f. Increased alcohol and caffeine use (aggravates preexisting conditions).
   g. Gastric ulcer is thought to be a risk for gastric cancer.
   h. Difficulty coping with stressful situations.
2. *Duodenal ulcers.*
   a. Infection with *H. pylori.*
   b. Elevated gastric acid secretory rate.
   c. Elevated gastric acid levels postprandially (after eating).
   d. Increased rate of gastric emptying → increased amount of acid in duodenum → irritation and breakdown of duodenal mucosa.
   e. Ulcerogenic medication use (aggravates preexisting conditions).
   f. Cigarette smoking.
   g. Alcohol and caffeine use (aggravates preexisting condition).
   h. Difficulty coping with stressful situations.
3. *Stress ulcers.*
   a. Severe trauma or major illness.
   b. Severe burns *(Curling's ulcer);* develop in 72 hours with majority of persons with burns over more than 35% of the body surface.
   c. Head injuries or intracranial disease *(Cushing's ulcer).*
   d. Medications in large doses: corticosteroids, salicylates, ibuprofen, indomethacin, phenylbutazone (Butazolidin).
   e. Shock.
   f. Sepsis.

C. Assessment:

1. *Subjective data:*
   a. *Gastric ulcers.*
      (1) *Pain:*
         (a) *Type:* gnawing, aching, burning.
         (b) *Location:* epigastric, left of midline, localized.
         (c) *Occurrence:* periodic pain, often 2 hours after eating.
         (d) *Relief: antacids;* may be aggravated, *not* relieved, by food.
         (e) Some clients report no discomfort at all.
      (2) Weakness.
      (3) History of risk factors as above.
   b. *Duodenal ulcers.*
      (1) *Pain:*
         (a) *Type:* gnawing, aching, burning, hungerlike, boring.
         (b) *Location:* right epigastric, localized; steady pain near midline of back may indicate perforation.
         (c) *Occurrence:* 1 to 3 hours after eating, worse at end of day or during the night; initial attack occurs spring or fall; history of remissions and exacerbations.
         (d) *Relief:* food, *antacids,* or both.
         (e) Some clients report no discomfort at all.
      (2) Nausea.
      (3) History of risk factors (see **IX. B.**).
   c. *Stress ulcers.*
      (1) *Pain:* often painless until serious complication (hemorrhage, perforation) occurs.
      (2) History of risk factors as above.
2. *Objective data:*
   a. *Gastric ulcer.*
      (1) Vomiting blood (hematemesis).
      (2) Melena (tarry stools).
      (3) Weight loss.
      (4) X-ray (upper GI series) confirms "crater" (punched-out appearance, clean base).

(5) Endoscopy confirms presence of ulcer; biopsy for cytology.
(6) Monitor for blood loss: CBC, stool for occult blood.
(7) Orthostatic hypotension.
(8) *Laboratory data:* positive for *H. pylori.*

b. *Duodenal ulcer.*
(1) Eructation.
(2) Vomiting blood (hematemesis).
(3) Regurgitation of sour liquid into back of mouth.
(4) Constipation.
(5) X-ray (upper GI series) confirms ulcer craters and niches, as well as outlet deformities: round or oval funnel-like lesion extending into musculature.
(6) Endoscopy for direct visualization.
(7) Monitor for blood loss: CBC, stool for occult blood.
(8) Orthostatic hypotension.
(9) *Laboratory data:* positive for *H. pylori.*

c. *Stress ulcer.*
(1) GI bleeding.
(2) Multiple, superficial erosions affecting large area of gastric mucosa.

D. Analysis/nursing diagnosis (all types):
1. *Pain* related to erosion of gastric lining.
2. *Ineffective individual coping* related to inability to change lifestyle.
3. *Altered nutrition, less than body requirements,* related to inadequate intake.
4. *Knowledge deficit* (learning need) regarding preventive measures.
5. *Risk for injury* related to possible hemorrhage or perforation.

E. Nursing care plan/implementation (all types):
1. Goal: *promote comfort.*

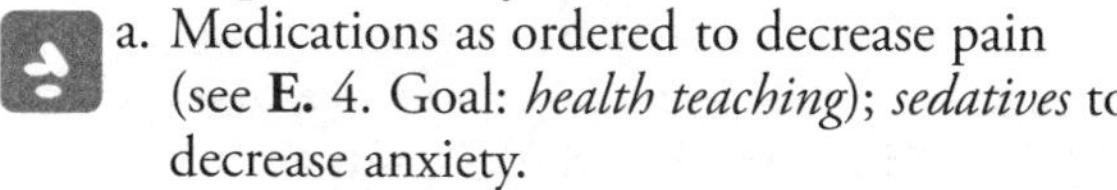

a. Medications as ordered to decrease pain (see **E.** 4. Goal: *health teaching*); *sedatives* to decrease anxiety.
b. Prepare for *diagnostic tests.*
(1) X-rays; upper GI series (barium swallow); lower GI (barium enema).
(2) Endoscopy.
(3) Gastric analysis, to determine amount of hydrochloric acid in GI tract.

2. Goal: *prevent/recognize signs of complications.*
a. Monitor vitals for shock.
b. Check stool for occult blood/ hemorrhage.
c. Palpate abdomen for perforation (rigid, boardlike); arterial bleeding.

3. Goal: *provide emotional support.*
a. Stress-management techniques.
b. Restful environment.
c. Prepare for surgery, if necessary.

4. Goal: *health teaching.*
a. Medications:
(1) *Antibiotics.* Sometimes antibiotics work best if given in combination with omeprazole (Prilosec), H_2 blockers, or bismuth (Pepto-Bismol). *Caution:* use of antibiotic treatment can cause allergic reactions, diarrhea, and severe antibiotic-induced colitis.
(a) Tetracycline.
(b) Amoxicillin.
(c) Metronidazole (Flagyl).
(d) Clarithromycin (Biaxin).
(2) *Histamine antagonists: given with meals/bedtime* to block the action of histamine-stimulated gastric secretions (basal and stimulated); inhibit pepsin secretion and reduce the volume of gastric secretions.
(a) Cimetidine (Tagamet) inhibits gastrin release; can be given PO, IV, or IM; *cannot* be given within 1 hour of antacid therapy.
(b) Ranitidine (Zantac) has greater reduction of acid secretion, longer duration, less frequent administration (twice daily versus 4 times a day), and fewer side effects than cimetidine.
(c) Nizatidine (Axid).
(d) Famotidine (Pepcid).
(3) *Proton pump inhibitors* (gastric acid inhibitors): superior in treating esophageal ulcers; equal to other H_2 receptors for gastric and duodenal ulcers.
(a) Omeprazole (Prilosec).
(b) Lansoprazole (Prevacid).
(c) Pantoprazole.
(4) *Antiulcers: give 1 to 3 hours after meals and at bedtime* to decrease pain by lowering acidity; monitor for:
(a) Diarrhea (seen most often with magnesium carbonate and magnesium oxide [Maalox, Mylanta]).
(b) Constipation (seen most often with calcium carbonate [Tums] or aluminum hydroxide [Amphojel]).
(c) Electrolyte imbalance (seen with systemic antacid, soda bicarbonate).
(d) Best 1 to 3 hours *after meals.*
(e) Liquids more effective than tablets; if taking tablets, chew slowly.
(5) *Sucralfate* (Carafate) and misoprostol (Cytotec): *given 1 hour before meals and at bedtime.*
(a) Locally active topical agent that forms a protective coat on mucosa, prevents

further digestive action of both acid and pepsin.
(b) Must *not* be given within 30 minutes of antacids.
(6) *Anticholinergic*—when used, given *before* meals to decrease gastric acid secretion and delay gastric emptying.
(7) Important: *avoid aspirin* (could increase bleeding possibility).

b. *Diet:*
(1) Change diet only to relieve symptoms; diet may not influence ulcer formation.
(2) *Avoid* foods that increase acidity—caffeine and alcohol in moderation.
(3) *Plan:*
(a) Small, frequent meals (to prevent exacerbations of symptoms related to an empty stomach).
(b) Weight control.

c. Complications—signs and symptoms:
(1) Gastric ulcers may be premalignant.
(2) Perforation.
(3) Hemorrhage.
(4) Obstruction.

d. *Lifestyle changes:*
(1) Decrease:
(a) Smoking.
(b) Noise.
(c) Rush.
(d) Confusion.
(2) Increase:
(a) Communication.
(b) Mental/physical rest.
(c) Compliance with medical regimen.

F. Evaluation/outcome criteria:
1. *Avoids* foods/liquids that cause irritation.
2. Takes prescribed medications.
3. Pain decreases.
4. No complications.
5. States signs and symptoms of complications.
6. Participates in stress-reduction activities.
7. Stops smoking.

X. GASTRIC SURGERY: peformed when ulcer medical regimen is unsuccessful, ulcer is determined to be precancerous, or complications are present.

A. Types:
1. *Subtotal gastrectomy:* removal of a portion of the stomach.
2. *Total gastrectomy:* removal of the entire stomach.
3. *Antrectomy:* removal of entire antrum (lower) portion of the stomach.
4. *Pyloroplasty:* repair of the pyloric opening of the stomach.
5. *Vagotomy:* interruption of the impulses carried by the vagus nerve, which results in reduction of gastric secretions and decreased physical activity of the stomach (being done less often).
6. Combination of vagotomy and gastrectomy.

B. Analysis/nursing diagnosis:
1. *Pain* related to surgical incision.
2. *Ineffective breathing pattern* related to high surgical incision.
3. *Risk for trauma* related to possible complications postgastrectomy.
4. *Knowledge deficit* (learning need) regarding medication regimen and factors that aggravate condition.
5. *Fear* related to possible precancerous lesion.
6. *Ineffective individual coping* related to adjustments in lifestyle needed to lessen symptoms.

C. Nursing care plan/implementation:
1. Goal: *promote comfort in the postoperative period.*
a. *Analgesics:* to relieve pain and allow client to cough, deep breathe to prevent pulmonary complications.
b. *Position: semi-Fowler's* to aid in breathing.
2. Goal: *promote wound healing.*
a. Keep dressings dry.
b. NG tube to low intermittent suction (Levin) or low continuous suction (Salem sump).
(1) Check drainage from NG tube; normally bloody first 2 to 3 hours postsurgery, then brown to dark green.
(2) Excessive bright-red blood drainage: take vital signs; report vital signs, color and volume of drainage to physician **immediately.**
(3) Irrigate gently with saline in amount ordered; do ***not*** irrigate against resistance; may not be done in early postoperative period.
(4) Tape tube securely to face, but prevent obstructed vision.
(5) Frequent mouth and nostril care.
3. Goal: *promote adequate nutrition and hydration.*
a. Administer parenteral fluids as ordered.
b. Accurate I&O.
c. Check bowel sounds, at least q4h; NPO 1 to 3 days; bowel sounds normally return in 21 to 36 hours; oral fluids as ordered when bowel sounds present—usually 30 mL, then *small* feedings, then *bland* liquids to *soft* diet.
d. Observe for nausea and vomiting due to suture line edema, food intake (too much, too fast).
4. Goal: *prevent complications.*
a. Check dressing q4h for bleeding.
b. *Vitamin* B_{12} and iron replacement as indicated to avoid pernicious anemia and iron-deficiency anemia.
c. *Avoid* dumping syndrome.

D. Evaluation/outcome criteria:

1. Hemorrhage, dumping syndrome avoided.
2. Healing begins.
3. Adjust lifestyle to prevent recurrence/marginal ulcer.

XI. DUMPING SYNDROME: hypoglycemic-type episode; occurs postoperatively after gastric resection (may also occur after vagotomy, antrectomy, or gastroenterostomy), when food and fluids that are more hyperosmolar than the jejunal secretions pass *quickly* into jejunum, producing fluid shifts from bloodstream to jejunum. This is a mild problem for about 20% of clients and will disappear in a few months to a year. Symptoms cause serious problem for about 7% of clients. This discomfort may occur during a meal or up to 30 minutes after the meal and last from 20 to 60 minutes. The reaction is greatest after the ingestion of sugar.

A. Assessment:

1. *Subjective data:*
   a. Feeling of fullness, weakness, faintness.
   b. Palpitations.
   c. Nausea.
   d. Discomfort during or after eating.
2. *Objective data:*
   a. Diaphoresis.
   b. Diarrhea.
   c. Fainting.
   d. Symptoms of hypoglycemia.

B. Analysis/nursing diagnosis:

1. *Altered nutrition, more than body requirements,* related to body's inability to properly digest high-carbohydrate, high-sodium foods.
2. *Diarrhea* related to food passing into jejunum too quickly.
3. *Risk for injury* related to hypoglycemia.
4. *Knowledge deficit* (learning need) related to dietary restrictions.

C. Nursing care plan/implementation:

1. Goal: *health teaching.*

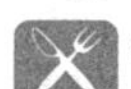

   a. *Include:*
      (1) *Increased fat, protein* to delay emptying.
      (2) Rest after meals.
      (3) Small, frequent meals.
      (4) Fluids *between* meals.

   b. *Avoid:*
      (1) Foods high in *salt, carbohydrate.*
      (2) Large meals.
      (3) Stress at mealtime.
      (4) Fluids at mealtime.

D. Evaluation/outcome criteria:

1. No complications.
2. Client heals.
3. No further ulcers.
4. Incorporates health teaching into lifestyle and prevents syndrome.

XII. CHOLECYSTITIS/CHOLELITHIASIS: inflammation of gallbladder due to bacterial infection, presence of cholelithiasis (stones, cholesterol, calcium, or bile in the gallbladder), or choledocholithiasis (stone in the common bile duct) and/or obstruction. *Acute* cholecystitis is abrupt in onset, but the client usually has a history of several attacks of fatty food intolerance. The client with *chronic* cholecystitis has a history of several attacks of moderate severity and has usually learned to avoid fatty foods to decrease symptoms.

A. Pathophysiology: calculi from increased concentration of bile salts, pigments, or cholesterol due to metabolic or hemolytic disorders, biliary stasis → precipitation of salts into stones, or inflammation causing bile constituents to become altered.

B. Risk factors:

1. Adult women.
2. Obesity.
3. Pregnancy or previous pregnancies.
4. Use of birth control pills or hormone replacement therapy.
5. High-fat, low-fiber diets.
6. Rapid weight loss.
7. History of Crohn's disease.
8. Genetics.
9. Age: increased risk over 40.
10. Certain drugs to lower lipids; clofibrate (Atromid-S).
11. Other diseases: cirrhosis of liver.

C. Assessment:

1. *Subjective data:*
   a. *Pain:*
      (1) *Type*—severe colic, radiating to the back under the scapula and to the right shoulder.
      (2) Positive *Murphy's sign*—a sign of gallbladder disease consisting of pain on taking a deep breath when pressure is placed over the location of the gallbladder.
      (3) *Location*—right upper quadrant, epigastric area, flank **(Fig. 6.9).**
      (4) *Duration*—spasm of duct attempting to dislodge stone lasts until dislodged or relieved by medication, or sometimes by vomiting.
   b. GI—anorexia, nausea, feeling of fullness, indigestion, intolerance of fatty foods.
2. *Objective data:*
   a. *GI*—belching, vomiting, clay-colored stools.
   b. *Vital signs*—*increased* pulse, fever.
   c. *Skin*—chills, jaundice.
   d. *Urine*—dark amber.
   e. Laboratory data—*elevated:*
      (1) WBC count.
      (2) Alkaline phosphatase.

ADULT

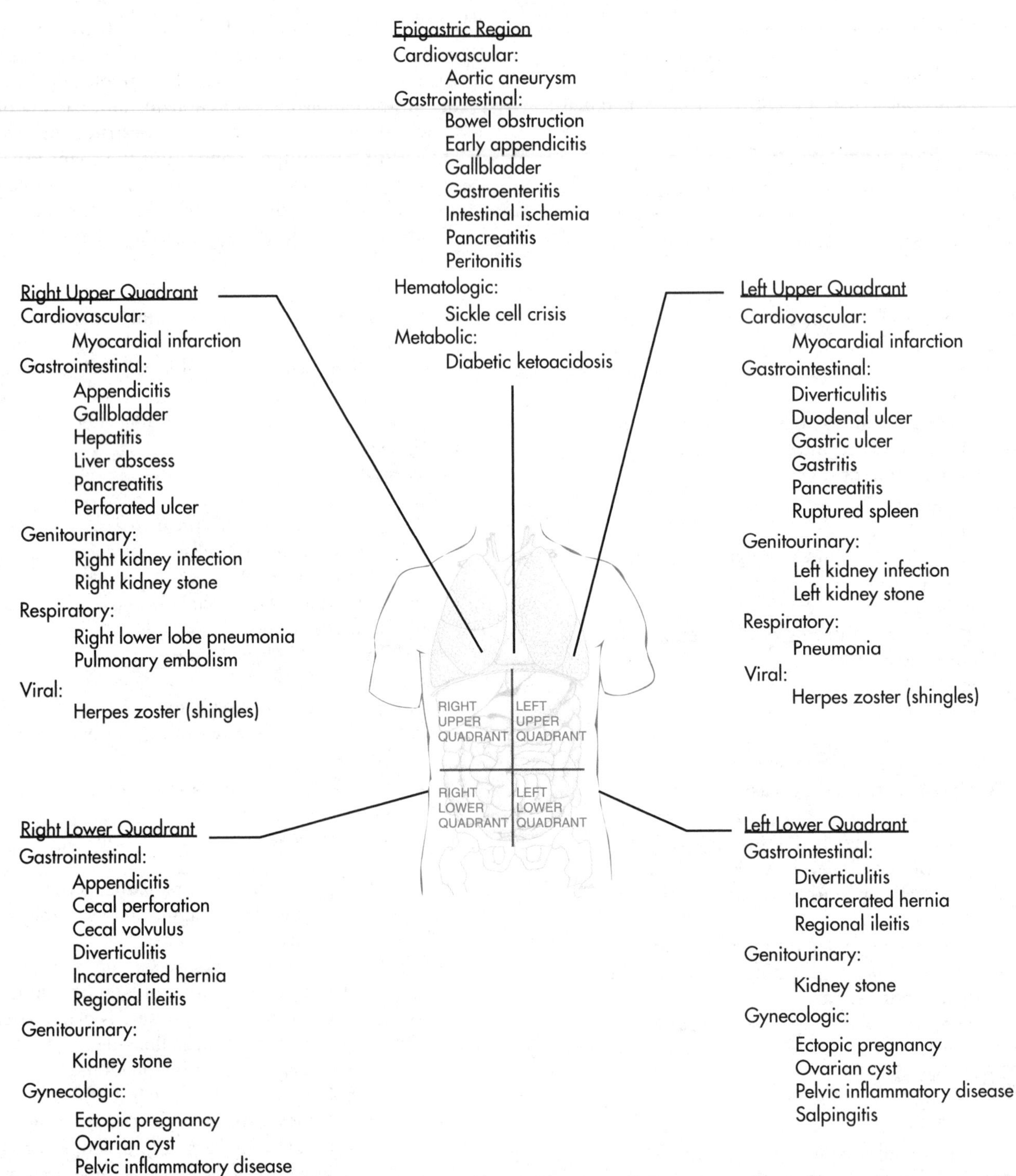

Figure 6.9 Abdominal pain by location. (Modified from Caroline, NL: *Emergency Care in the Streets,* ed 5. Boston, Little, Brown, 1995, p 641; and from Venes, D [ed]: *Taber's Cyclopedic Medical Dictionary,* ed 20. FA Davis, Philadelphia, 2005.)

ADULT

(3) Serum amylase, lipase.
(4) AST (SGOT).
(5) Bilirubin.

f. *Diagnostic studies:*
(1) Ultrasound.
(2) Cholangiography.
(3) Computed tomography (CT) scan.
(4) Endoscopic retrograde cholangiopancreatography (ERCP).

D. Analysis/nursing diagnosis:

1. *Pain* related to obstruction of bile duct due to cholelithiasis.

2. *Altered nutrition, more than body requirements,* related to ingestion of fatty foods.
3. *Altered nutrition, less than body requirements,* related to hesitancy to eat due to anorexia and nausea.
4. *Risk for fluid volume deficit* related to episodes of vomiting.
5. *Knowledge deficit* (learning need) related to dietary restrictions.

E. Nursing care plan/implementation:

1. Nonsurgical interventions:
   a. Goal: *promote comfort.*
      (1) Medications as ordered: meperidine, *antibiotics, antispasmodics, electrolytes.*
      (2) *Avoid* morphine due to spasmodic effect.
      (3) NG tube to low suction.
      (4) *Diet: fat free* when able to tolerate food.
      (5) Lithotripsy: gallstones fragmented by shock waves.
      (6) Oral dissolution therapy: ursodeoxycholic acid (ursodiol [Actigall]).
   b. Goal: *health teaching:*
      (1) Signs, symptoms, and complications of disease.
      (2) Fat-free diet.
      (3) Desired effects and side effects of prescribed medications.
      (4) Prepare for possible removal of gallbladder (cholecystectomy) if conservative treatment unsuccessful.
2. Surgical interventions:
   a. *Preoperative*—Goal: *prevent injury* (see **I. PREOPERATIVE PREPARATION, p. 365**).
   b. *Postoperative*—Goal: *promote comfort* (see **III. POSTOPERATIVE EXPERIENCE, p. 369**).
      (1) *Laparoscopic laser cholecystectomy*—tiny incisions/puncture wounds; gallbladder is removed using a video-guided system with a camera; client is discharged that day or next day, able to resume normal diet and work activities in a few days.
      (2) *Endoscopic retrograde cholangiopancreatography (ERCP)* with papillotomy—removes stones from bile duct. No incision; done under sedation, not anesthesia.
      (3) *Open-incision cholecystectomy.*
         (a) Promote tube drainage:
            (i) NG tube to low suction.
            (ii) *T-tube* to closed-gravity drainage, to preserve patency of edematous common duct and ensure bile drainage; usual amount 500 to 1,000 mL/24 hr; dark brown drainage.
            (iii) Provide enough tubing to allow turning without tension.
            (iv) Empty and record bile drainage q8h.
         (b) *Position: low Fowler's* to *semi-Fowler's* to facilitate T-tube drainage.
         (c) Dressing: dry to protect skin (because bile excoriates skin).
         (d) Clamp T-tube as ordered.
            (i) Observe for: abdominal distention, pain, nausea, chills, or fever.
            (ii) Unclamp tube and notify physician if symptoms appear.
   c. Goal: *prevent complications.*
      (1) IV fluids with vitamins.
      (2) Cough, turn, and deep breathe with open incision, particularly with removal of gallbladder (prone to respiratory complication because of high incision).
      (3) Early ambulation to prevent vascular complications and aid in expelling flatus.
      (4) Monitor for jaundice: skin, sclerae, urine, stools.
      (5) Monitor for signs of hemorrhage, infection.
   d. Goal: *health teaching.*
      (1) *Diet:* fat free for 6 weeks.
      (2) Signs of complications of food intolerance, pain, infection, hemorrhage.

F. Evaluation/outcome criteria:

1. No complications.
2. Able to tolerate food.
3. Plans follow-up care.
4. Possible weight reduction.

XIII. OBESITY—more calories consumed than expended leading to fat accumulation. Most common nutritional/metabolic disease in the United States.

A. Definition: *Women*—more than 45% above ideal body weight. *Men*—more than 35% above ideal body weight. Determined by **body mass index** (BMI) formula: divide weight in kilograms by height in meters squared (or divide weight in pounds by height in inches squared) and multiply by 703:

$$\frac{\text{Wt (lb)}}{\text{Ht (in}^2)} \times 703 \qquad \text{or:} \qquad \frac{\text{Wt (kg)}}{\text{Ht (m}^2)} \times 703$$

B. Risk factors:

1. Genetics (e.g., ↓ BMI), hormonal.
2. Environmental (e.g., ↓ physical activity).
3. Diet (e.g., ↑ fat, calories).
4. Some medications (e.g., tricyclic antidepressants [TCAs], insulin, sulfonylurea agents).

C. Comorbidity:

1. Cardiovascular disease; hypertension.
2. Type 2 diabetes.

ADULT

3. Gallbladder disease.
4. Arthritis.
5. Cancer (colorectal, breast, prostate).
6. Stroke.
7. Emotional distress.
8. Surgical risk.

D. Assessment:
1. *Overweight*—BMI 25.0 to 29.9 kg/m^2.
2. *Obese*—BMI ≥30.0 kg/m^2.
3. *Morbid obesity*—BMI greater than 40 kg/m^2.

E. Analysis/nursing diagnosis:
1. *Altered nutrition, more than body requirements,* related to genetics, environmental, or dietary factors.
2. *Chronic low self-esteem/body image disturbance* related to view of self in contrast to societal values; control, sex, and love issues (see also **Chapter 10, Body Image Disturbance, p. 720**).
3. *Activity intolerance* related to imbalance between oxygen supply and demand, and to sedentary lifestyle.

F. Nursing care plan/implementation—Goal: *decrease weight, initially 10% from baseline.*

1. Modify eating pattern (quality vs. quantity); ↓ portion size; modify composition: ↓ calories, fat, and cholesterol; ↓ daily kcal by 500 to 1,000.
2. Increase activity—moderate activity 30 minutes daily.
3. Behavioral therapy—change eating behaviors; motivation and readiness to lose weight.
4. Weight-loss drugs in combination with lifestyle changes.
5. Surgery—gastric stapling, bariatric (Roux-en-Y).

G. Evaluation/outcome criteria:
1. Weight loss of 1 to 2 lb/wk for 6 months.
2. Reduction in kcal by 500 to 1,000/day.
3. Increased daily physical activity.
4. Expressed commitment to lose weight.

XIV. APPENDICITIS: obstruction of appendiceal lumen and subsequent bacterial invasion of appendiceal wall; **acute emergency.**

A. Pathophysiology: when obstruction is partial or mild, inflammation begins in mucosa with slight appendiceal swelling, accompanied by periumbilical pain. As the inflammatory process escalates and/or obstruction becomes more complete, the appendix becomes more swollen, the lumen fills with pus, and mucosal ulceration begins. When inflammation extends to the peritoneal surface, pain is referred to the right lower abdominal quadrant. *Danger:* rigidity over the entire abdomen is usually indicative of ruptured appendix; the client is then prone to peritonitis.

B. Risk factors:
1. Men more than women.
2. Most frequently seen between ages 10 and 30 years.

C. Assessment:
1. *Subjective data:*
   a. *Pain:* generalized, then right lower quadrant at McBurney's point, with rebound tenderness.
   b. Anorexia, nausea.
2. *Objective data:*
   a. *Vital signs: elevated temperature,* shallow respirations.
   b. Either diarrhea or constipation.
   c. Vomiting, fetid breath odor.
   d. Splinting of abdominal muscles, flexion of knees onto abdomen.
   e. Laboratory data:
      (1) WBC count *elevated* (>10,000).
      (2) Neutrophil count *elevated* (>75%).
   f. *Diagnostic studies:*
      (1) Ultrasound.
      (2) CT scan.

D. Analysis/nursing diagnosis:
1. *Pain* related to inflammation of appendix.
2. *Risk for trauma* related to ruptured appendix.
3. *Knowledge deficit* (learning need) related to possible surgery.

E. Nursing care plan/implementation:
1. Goal: *promote comfort.*
   a. *Preoperative:*
      (1) Explain procedures.
      (2) Assist with diagnostic work-up.
   b. *Postoperative:*
      (1) Relieve pain related to surgical incision.
      (2) Prevent infection: wound care, dressing technique.
      (3) Prevent dehydration: IVs, I&O, fluids to solids by mouth as tolerated.
      (4) Promote ambulation to prevent postoperative complications.

F. Evaluation/outcome criteria:
1. No infection.
2. Tolerates fluid; bowel sounds return.
3. Heals with no complications.

XV. HERNIA: protrusion of the intestine through a weak portion of the abdominal wall.

A. Types:
1. *Reducible:* visceral contents return to their normal position, either spontaneously or by manipulation.
2. *Irreducible, or incarcerated:* contents cannot be returned to normal position.
3. *Strangulated:* blood supply to the structure within the hernia sac becomes occluded (usually a loop of bowel).

4. Most common hernias: umbilical, femoral, inguinal, incisional, and hiatal.

B. Pathophysiology: weakness in the wall may be either congenital or acquired. Herniation occurs when there is an increase in intra-abdominal pressure from: coughing, lifting, crying, straining, obesity, or pregnancy.

C. Assessment:
1. *Subjective data:*
   a. Pain, discomfort.
   b. History of feeling a lump.
2. *Objective data:*
   a. Soft lump, especially when straining or coughing.
   b. Sometimes alteration in normal bowel pattern.
   c. Swelling.

D. Analysis/nursing diagnosis:
1. *Activity intol*erance related to pain and discomfort.
2. *Risk for trauma* related to lack of circulation to affected area of bowel.
3. *Pain* related to protrusion of intestine into hernia sac.

E. Nursing care plan/implementation:
1. Goal: *prevent postoperative complications.*
   a. Monitor bowel sounds.
   b. Prevent postoperative scrotal swelling with inguinal hernia by applying ice and support to scrotum.
2. Goal: *health teaching.*
   a. Prevent recurrence with correct body mechanics.
   b. Gradual increase in exercise.

F. Evaluation/outcome criteria: healing occurs with no further hernia recurrence.

XVI. DIVERTICULOSIS: A *diverticulum* is a small pouch or sac composed of mucous membrane that has protruded through the muscular wall of the intestine. The presence of several of these is called *diverticulosis.* Inflammation of the diverticula is called *diverticulitis.*

A. Pathophysiology: weakening in a localized area of muscular wall of the colon (especially the sigmoid colon), accompanied by increased intraluminal pressure.

B. Risk factors:
1. Diverticulosis:
   a. Age: seldom before 35 years; 60% incidence in older adults.
   b. History of constipation.
   c. Diet history: low in vegetable fiber, high in carbohydrate.
2. Diverticulitis: highest incidence between ages 50 and 60 years.

C. Assessment:
1. *Subjective data: pain:* cramplike; left lower quadrant of abdomen.
2. *Objective data:*
   a. Constipation or diarrhea, flatulence.
   b. Fever.
   c. Rectal bleeding.
   d. *Diagnostic procedures:*
      (1) Palpation reveals tender colonic mass.
      (2) Barium enema (done only in absence of inflammation) reveals presence of diverticula.
      (3) Sigmoidoscopy/colonoscopy.

D. Analysis/nursing diagnosis:
1. *Constipation* related to dietary intake.
2. *Pain* related to inflammatory process of intestines.
3. *Risk for fluid volume deficit* related to episodes of diarrhea or bleeding.
4. *Risk for injury* related to bleeding.
5. *Knowledge deficit* (learning need) related to prevention of constipation.

E. Nursing care plan/implementation:
1. Goal: *bowel rest during acute episodes.*
   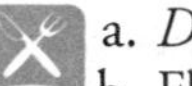
   a. *Diet: soft, liquid.*
   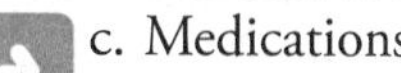
   b. Fluids, IVs if oral intake not adequate.
   c. Medications:
      (1) *Antibiotics:* ciprofloxacin (Cipro), metronidazole (Flagyl), cephalexin (Keflex), doxycycline (Vibramycin).
      (2) *Antispasmodics:* chlordiazepoxide (Librax), dicyclomine (Bentyl), Donnatal, hyoscyamine (Levsin).
   d. Monitor stools for signs of bleeding.
2. Goal: *promote normal bowel elimination.*
   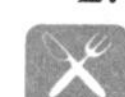
   a. *Diet:* bland, *high* in vegetable fiber if no inflammation.
      (1) *Include:* fruits, vegetables, whole-grain cereal, unprocessed bran.
      (2) *Avoid:* foods difficult to digest (corn, nuts).
   b. *Bulk-forming* agents as ordered: methylcellulose, psyllium.
   c. Monitor: abdominal distention, acute bowel symptoms.
3. Goal: *health teaching.*
   a. Methods to avoid constipation.
   b. Foods to include/avoid in diet.
   c. Relaxation techniques.
   d. Signs and symptoms of complications of chronic inflammation: abscess, obstruction, fistulas, perforation, or hemorrhage.

F. Evaluation/outcome criteria:
1. Inflammation decreases.
2. Bowel movements return to normal.
3. Pain decreases.
4. No perforation, fistulas, or abscesses noted.

XVII. ULCERATIVE COLITIS: inflammation of mucosa and submucosa of the large intestine. Inflammation leads to ulceration with bleeding. Involved areas are continuous. Disease is characterized by remissions and exacerbations.

A. Pathophysiology: Currently believed to be an autoimmune disease. The body's immune system is called on to attack the inner lining of the large intestine, causing inflammation and ulceration. Edema and hyperemia of colonic mucous membrane → superficial bleeding with increased peristalsis, shallow ulcerations, abscesses; bowel wall thins and shortens and becomes at risk for perforation. Increased rate of flow of liquid ileal contents → decreased water absorption and diarrhea.

B. Risk factors:

1. Highest occurrence in young adults (ages 20 to 40 years).
2. Genetic predisposition: higher in whites, Jews.
3. Autoimmune response.
4. Infections.
5. More common in urban areas (upper-middle incomes and higher educational levels).
6. Nonsmokers/ex-smokers.
7. Genetic, inherited, or familial tendencies.
8. Chronic ulcerative colitis is a risk factor for colon cancer.

C. Assessment:

1. *Subjective data:*
   a. Urgency to defecate, particularly when standing.
   b. Loss of appetite, nausea.
   c. Colic-like abdominal pain.
   d. History of intolerance to dairy products.
   e. Emotional depression.
2. *Objective data:*
   a. *Diarrhea:* 10 to 20 stools/day; can be chronic or intermittent, episodic or continual; stools contain blood, mucus, and pus.
   b. Weight loss and malnutrition, dehydration.
   c. Fever.
   d. Rectal bleeding.
   e. Laboratory data: *decreased:* RBC count, potassium, sodium, calcium, bicarbonate related to excessive diarrhea.
   f. Lymphadenitis.
   g. *Diagnostic tests:*
      (1) Sigmoidoscopy/colonoscopy for visualization of lesions.
      (2) Barium enema.

D. Analysis/nursing diagnosis:

1. *Diarrhea* related to increased flow rate of ileal contents.
2. *Self-esteem disturbance* related to progression of disease and increased number and odor of stools.
3. *Pain* (acute) related to inflammatory process.
4. *Fluid volume deficit* related to frequent episodes of diarrhea.
5. *Knowledge deficit* (learning need) related to methods to control symptoms.
6. *Social isolation* related to continual diarrhea episodes.

E. Nursing care plan/implementation:

1. Goal: *prevent disease progression and complications.*
   a. Administer medications:
      (1) *Salicylates:* sulfasalazine (Azulfidine), olsalazine (Dipentum), mesalamine (Asacol, Pentasa). All given PO in high doses. Mesalamine (Rowasa) is given in enema or suppository form.
      (2) *Corticosteroids:* prednisone, PO or IV. Hydrocortisone (Cortenema) is given by enema.
      (3) *Immunosuppressants:* azathioprine (Imuran), and 6-mercaptopurine (Purinthol), cyclosporine (Sandimmune), and methotrexate (Rheumatrex).
      (4) *Nicotine.*
      (5) *Sedatives and tranquilizers to produce rest and comfort.*
      (6) *Absorbents:* kaolin/pectin (Kaopectate).
      (7) *Anticholinergics* and *antispasmotics to relieve cramping and diarrhea:* atropine sulfate, phenobarbital, diphenoxylate/atropine sulfate (Lomotil).
      (8) *Anti-infective* agents *to relieve bacterial overgrowth in bowel* and *limit secondary infections:* metronidazole (Flagyl).
      (9) *Potassium supplements to relieve deficiencies* related to excessive diarrhea.
      (10) Calcium folate and vitamin B_{12} when malabsorption is present.
2. Goal: *reduce psychological stress.*
   a. Provide quiet environment.
   b. Encourage verbalization of concerns.
3. Goal: *health teaching.*
   a. *Diet:*
      (1) *Avoid:* coarse-residue, high-fiber foods (e.g., raw fruits and vegetables), whole milk, cold beverages (because of inflammation).
      (2) *Include:* bland, *high*-protein, *high*-vitamin, *high*-mineral, *high* calorie foods.
      (3) Parenteral hyperalimentation for severely ill.
      (4) Force fluids by mouth.
   b. Monitor for colon cancer, especially 8 to 10 years after incidence.
4. Goal: *prepare for surgery if medical regimen unsuccessful.*
   a. Possible surgical procedures:
      (1) Permanent ileostomy *(J pouch).*

(2) Continent ileostomy *(Kock pouch)*.
(3) Total colectomy, anastomosis with rectum.
(4) Total colectomy, anastomosis with anal sphincter.

F. Evaluation/outcome criteria:

1. Fluid balance is obtained and maintained.
2. Alterations in lifestyle are managed.
3. Stress-management techniques are successful.
4. Complications such as fistulas, obstruction, perforation, and peritonitis are avoided.
5. Client is prepared for surgery if medical regimen is unsuccessful or complications develop.

XVIII. CROHN'S DISEASE: a chronic inflammatory disease causing ulcerations in the small and large intestines. The immune system seems to react to a variety of substances and/or bacteria in the intestines, causing inflammation, ulceration, and bowel injury. Called Crohn's *colitis* when only large intestine is involved; Crohn's *enteritis* when only small intestine is involved; *terminal ileitis* when lowest part of small intestine is involved; Crohn's *enterocolitis* or *ileocolitis* when both small and large intestines are involved.

A. Pathophysiology: *one of two conditions called "inflammatory bowel disease"* (ulcerative colitis is the other) that affects all layers of the ileum, the colon, or both, causing patchy, shallow, longitudinal mucosal ulcers; possible correlation with autoimmune disease and adenocarcinoma of the bowel. Small, scattered, shallow crater-like areas cause scarring and stiffness of the bowel → bowel becomes narrow → obstruction, then pain, nausea, and vomiting.

B. Risk factors:

1. Age: 15 to 20, 55 to 60 years.
2. Whites, especially Jews.
3. Familial predisposition.
4. Possible virus involvement.
5. Possible psychosomatic involvement.
6. Possible hormonal or dietary influences.

C. Assessment:

1. *Subjective data:*
   a. Abdominal pain.
   b. Anorexia.
   c. Nausea.
   d. Malaise.
   e. History of isolated, intermittent, or recurrent attacks.
2. *Objective data:*
   a. Diarrhea.
   b. Weight loss, vomiting.
   c. Fever, signs of infection.
   d. Fluid/electrolyte imbalances.
   e. Malnutrition, malabsorption.
   f. Occult blood in feces.

D. Analysis/nursing diagnosis, Nursing care plan/implementation, Evaluation/outcome criteria (see **XVII. ULCERATIVE COLITIS, p. 452**).

XIX. INTESTINAL OBSTRUCTION: blockage in movement of intestinal contents through small or large intestine.

A. Pathophysiology:

1. *Mechanical causes*—physical impediments to passage of intestinal contents (e.g., adhesions, hernias, neoplasms, inflammatory bowel disease, foreign bodies, fecal impactions, congenital or radiational strictures, intussusception, or volvulus).
2. *Paralytic causes*—passageway remains open, but peristalsis ceases (e.g., after abdominal surgery, abdominal trauma, hypokalemia, myocardial infarction, pneumonia, spinal injuries, peritonitis, or vascular insufficiency).

B. Assessment:

1. *Subjective data: pain* related to:
   a. *Proximal loop obstruction:* upper abdominal, sharp, cramping, intermittent pain.
   b. *Distal loop obstruction:* poorly localized, cramping pain.
2. *Objective data:*
   a. Bowel sounds: initially loud, high pitched; then when smooth muscle atony occurs, bowel sound absent.
   b. Increased peristalsis above level of obstruction in attempt to move intestinal contents through the obstructed area.
   c. Obstipation (no passage of gas or stool through obstructed portion of bowel; no reabsorption of fluids).
   d. Distention.
   e. Vomiting:
      (1) *Proximal loop obstruction:* profuse nonfecal vomiting.
      (2) *Distal loop obstruction:* less frequent fecal-type vomiting.
   f. Urinary output: *decreased.*
   g. Temperature: *elevated;* pulse: *tachycardia;* BP: *hypotension* → shock if untreated.
   h. Dehydration, hemoconcentration, hypovolemia.
   i. Laboratory data:
      (1) Leukocytosis.
      (2) *Decreased:* sodium (<138 mEq/L), potassium (<3.5 mEq/L).
      (3) *Increased:* bicarbonate (>26 mEq/L), BUN (>18 mg/dL).
      (4) *pH:* If obstruction is at gastric outlet, pH will be *elevated,* indicating *metabolic alkalosis;* if obstruction is distal duodenal or proximal jejunal, the pH will *drop* and *metabolic acidosis* occurs.

ADULT

C. Analysis/nursing diagnosis:
1. *Fluid volume deficit* related to vomiting.
2. *Pain* related to increased peristalsis above the level of obstruction.
3. *Altered nutrition, less than body requirements,* related to vomiting.
4. *Risk for trauma* related to potential perforation.

D. Nursing care plan/implementation:
1. Goal: *obtain and maintain fluid balance.*
   a. Nursing care of client with nasogastric tube (see **Table 11.5, pp. 841–842**).
      (1) *Miller-Abbott tube:* dual lumen, balloon inflated with air after insertion. *Caution:* do *not* tape tube to face until tube reaches point of obstruction.
      (2) *Cantor tube:* has mercury in distal sac, which helps move tube to point of obstruction. *Caution:* do *not* tape tube to face until tube reaches point of obstruction.
   b. Nothing by mouth, IV therapy, strict I&O.
   c. Take daily weights (early morning), monitor CVP for hydration status.
   d. Monitor abdominal girth for signs of distention and urinary output for signs of retention or shock.
2. Goal: *relieve pain and nausea.*
   a. Medications as ordered:
      (1) *Analgesics, antiemetics.*
      (2) If problem is paralytic: medical treatment includes neostigmine *to stimulate peristalsis.*
   b. Observe for bowel sounds, flatus (tape intestinal tube to face once peristalsis begins).
   c. Skin and frequent mouth care.
3. Goal: *prevent respiratory complications.*
   a. Encourage coughing and deep breathing.
   b. *Semi-Fowler's* or position of comfort.
4. Goal: *postoperative nursing care* (if treated surgically) (see **III. POSTOPERATIVE EXPERIENCE, p. 369**).

E. Evaluation/outcome criteria:
1. Fluid balance obtained and maintained.
2. Shock prevented.
3. Obstruction resolved.
4. Pain decreased.
5. Fluids tolerated by mouth.
6. Complications such as perforation and peritonitis avoided.

XX. FECAL DIVERSION—*stomas:* performed because of disease or trauma; may be temporary or permanent.

A. Types (Table 6.25).
1. *Temporary*—fecal stream rerouted to allow GI tract to heal or to provide outlet for stool when obstructed.
2. *Permanent*—intestine cannot be reconnected. Rectum and anal sphincter removed (abdominal perineal resection). Often performed for cancer of the colon and/or rectum.
3. *Continent ileostomy*—pouch is created inside the wall of the intestine. The pouch serves as a reservoir similar to a rectum. The pouch is emptied on a regular basis with a small tube.

Table 6.25

Comparison of Ileostomy and Colostomy

	Ileostomy	Colostomy
Procedure	Surgical formation of a fistula, or stoma, between the abdominal wall and *ileum:* continent ileostomy (*Kock* pouch) may be constructed	Surgical formation of an artificial opening between the surface of the abdominal wall and *colon* *Single barrel*—only one loop of bowel is opened to the abdominal surface *Double barrel*—two loops of bowel, a proximal and distal portion, are open to the abdominal wall; feces will be expelled from the proximal loop, mucus will be expelled from the distal loop; client may expel some excreta from rectum as well
Reasons performed	Unresponsive ulcerative colitis: complications of ulcerative colitis (e.g., hemorrhage, carcinoma [suspected])	*Single barrel:* colon or rectal cancer *Double barrel:* relieve obstruction
Results	Permanent stoma	*Single barrel:* permanent stoma *Double barrel:* temporary stoma
Discharge	Green liquid, nonodorous	Consistency of feces dependent on diet and portion of the bowel used as the stoma; from brown odorous liquid to normal stool consistency
Nursing care	See **FECAL DIVERSION, pp. 454–456**	See **Tables 11.6, Emptying Colostomy Appliance,** and **11.7, Changing Colostomy Appliance**

4. *Ileoanal anastomosis (J pouch, S reservoir,* or *ileoperistaltic reservoir)*—the large intestine is removed and the small intestine is inserted into the rectum and attached just above the anus. The muscles of the rectum remain intact and the normal route of stool elimination is maintained.

B. Analysis/nursing diagnosis:

1. *Bowel incontinence* related to lack of sphincter in newly formed stoma.
2. *Altered health maintenance* related to knowledge of ostomy care.
3. *Body image disturbance* related to stoma.
4. *Fear* related to medical condition requiring stoma.
5. *Fluid volume deficit* related to increased output through stoma.

C. Nursing care plan/implementation:

1. *Preoperative period:*
   a. Goal: *prepare bowel for surgery.*
      (1) Administer neomycin as ordered to *reduce* colonic bacteria.
      (2) Administer cathartics, enemas as ordered to *cleanse* the bowel of feces.
      (3) Administer *low-residue* or *liquid diet* as ordered.
   b. Goal: *relieve anxiety and assist in adjustment to surgery.*
      (1) Provide accurate, brief, and reassuring explanations of procedures; allow time for questions.
      (2) Referral: have enterostomal nurse visit to discuss ostomy management and placement of stoma appliance.
      (3) Referral: offer opportunity for a visit with an Ostomy Association Visitor.
   c. Goal: *health teaching.*
      (1) Determine knowledge of surgery and potential impact.
      (2) Begin teaching regarding ostomy.
2. *Postoperative period:*
   a. Goal: *maintain fluid balance.*
      (1) Monitor I&O because large volume of fluid is lost through stoma.
      (2) Administer IV fluids as ordered.
      (3) Monitor losses through NG tube.
   b. Goal: *prevent other postoperative complications.*
      (1) Monitor for signs of intestinal obstruction.
      (2) Maintain sterility when changing dressings; *avoid* fecal contamination of incision.
      (3) Observe appearance of stoma: rosy pink, raised **(Fig. 6.10).**
   c. Goal: *initiate ostomy care.*
      (1) *Protect skin around stoma:* use commercial preparation to toughen skin and use protective barrier wafer (Stomahesive) or paste (Karaya or substitute) to keep drainage (which can cause excoriation) off the skin.
      (2) *Keep skin around stoma clean and dry;* empty appliance frequently. Check for drainage in appliance at least twice during each shift. If drainage present (diarrhea-type stool):
         (a) Unclip bottom of bag.
         (b) Drain into bedpan.
         (c) Use a squeeze-type bottle filled with warm water to rinse inside of appliance.
         (d) Clean clamp, if soiled.
         (e) Put a few drops of deodorant in appliance if not odor-proof.

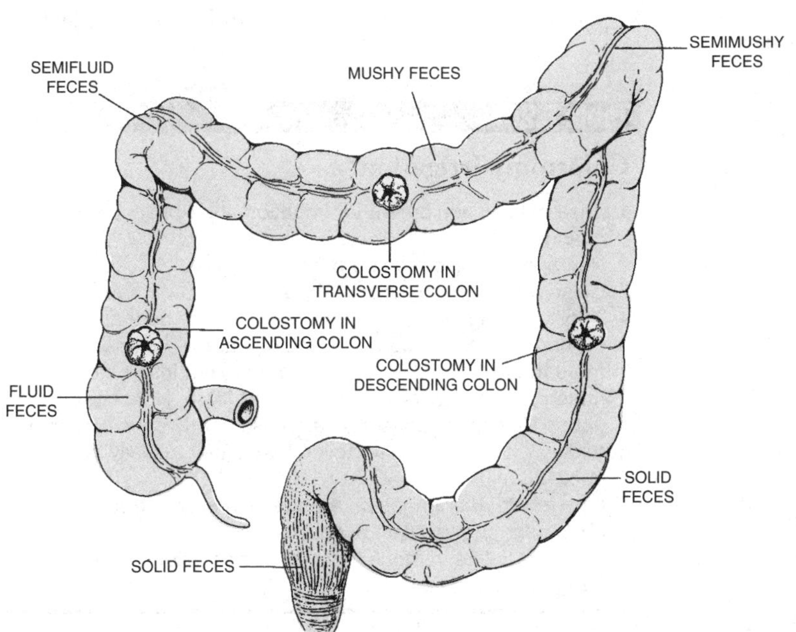

Figure 6.10 Colostomy sites. (From Venes, D [ed]: *Taber's Cyclopedic Medical Dictionary,* ed 21. FA Davis, Philadelphia, 2009.)

(f) Fasten bottom of appliance securely (fold bag over clamp two or three times before closing).
(g) Check for leakage under appliance every 2 to 4 hours.

(3) *Change appliance* when drainage leaks around seal, or approximately every 2 to 3 days. Initially, size of stoma will be large due to edema. Pouch opening should be slightly larger than stoma so it will not constrict. Stoma will need to be measured for each change until swelling subsides to ensure appropriate fit.
(a) Gather equipment: gloves, skin prep packet, colostomy appliance measured to fit stoma properly (use stoma measuring guide), skin barrier, warm water and soap, face cloth/towel, plastic bag for disposal of old equipment.
(b) Remove old appliance carefully, pulling from area with least drainage to area with most drainage.
(c) Wash skin area (*not* stoma) with soap and water. Be careful *not to:* irritate skin, put soap on stoma, irritate stoma; do *not* put anything dry onto stoma. *Remember:* bowel is very fragile; working near bowel increases peristalsis so that feces and flatulence may be expelled.
(d) Observe skin area for potential breakdown.
(e) Use packet of skin prep on the skin around the stoma. Do *not* put this solution onto stoma, because it will cause irritation. Allow skin prep solution to dry on skin before applying colostomy appliance.
(f) Apply skin barrier you have measured and cut to size.
(g) Put appliance on so that bottom of appliance is easily accessible for emptying (e.g., if client is *out* of bed most of the time, put the bottom facing the feet; if client is *in* bed most of the time, have bottom face the side). Picture-frame the adhesive portion of the appliance with 1-inch tape.
(h) Put a few drops of deodorant in appliance if not odor-proof.
(i) Use clamp to fasten bottom of appliance.
(j) Talk to client (or communicate in best way possible during and after procedure). *This is a very difficult alteration in body image.*
(k) Use good hand-washing technique.

(4) Use deodorizing drops in appliance and provide adequate room ventilation to decrease odors. *Caution:* deodorizing drops must be safe for mucous membranes. *No* pinholes in pouch.
(5) If continent ileostomy (a *Kock pouch*) has been constructed, the client does not have to wear an external pouch. The stool is stored intra-abdominally. The client drains the pouch several times daily, when there is a feeling of fullness, using a catheter. The stoma is flat and on the right side of the abdomen.

d. Goal: *promote psychological comfort.*
(1) Support client and family—accept feelings and behavior.
(2) Recognize that such a procedure may initiate the grieving process.

e. Goal: *health teaching.*
(1) Self-care management skills related to ostomy appliance, skin care, and irrigation, if indicated **(Table 6.26).**

(2) *Diet:* adjustments to control character of feces; *avoid* foods that increase flatulence.
(3) Signs of complications of infection, obstruction, or electrolyte imbalance.
(4) Community referral for follow-up care.

D. Evaluation/outcome criteria:
1. Demonstrates self-care skill for independent living.
2. Makes dietary adjustments.
3. Ostomy functions well.
4. Adjusts to alteration in bowel elimination pattern.

XXI. HEMORRHOIDS: enlarged vein/veins in mucous membrane of rectum. Hemorrhoids can be *internal* or *external.* Bleeding internal hemorrhoids can be painful and are best treated by: rubber band ligation, injection

Table 6.26

Colostomy Irrigation*

1. Assemble all equipment for irrigation and appliance change.
2. Remove and discard old pouch.
3. Clean the peristomal skin.
4. Apply the irrigating sleeve; place in toilet or bedpan.
5. Fill container with 500–1,000 mL of warm water, *never* more than 1,000 mL. Clear air from tubing. Insert lubricated tubing 2–4 inches into stoma. Do *not* force. Hold container about 18 inches above stoma. Infuse gently over 7–10 min.
6. Allow stool to empty into toilet. Evacuation usually occurs in 20–25 min.
7. If no return after irrigation, ambulate, gently massage abdomen, or give client a warm drink.
8. Once complete, remove the sleeve, and follow guidelines for applying appliance.

*Colostomy irrigation is seldom used with newer colostomies.

ADULT

sclerotherapy, infrared coagulation, or surgery (scalpel, cautery, or laser). Laser surgery is usually done on an outpatient basis and causes minimal discomfort. High-fiber diets can minimize constipation and prevent hemorrhoids.

A. Pathophysiology: venous congestion and interference with venous return from hemorrhoidal veins → increase in pelvic pressure, swelling, and distortion.

B. Risk factors:

1. Straining to expel constipated stool.
2. Pregnancy.
3. Intra-abdominal or pelvic masses.
4. Interference with portal circulation.
5. Prolonged standing or sitting.
6. History of low-fiber, high-carbohydrate diet, which contributes to constipation.
7. Family history of hemorrhoids.
8. Enlarged prostate.

C. Assessment:

1. *Subjective data:* discomfort, anal pruritus, pain.
2. *Objective data:*
   a. Bleeding, especially on defecation.
   b. Narrowing of stool.
   c. Grapelike clusters around anus (pink, red, or blue).
   d. *Diagnostic test:*
      (1) Visualization for external hemorrhoids.
      (2) Digital examination or proctoscopy for internal hemorrhoids.

D. Analysis/nursing diagnosis:

1. *Pain* related to defecation.
2. *Constipation* related to dietary habits and pain at time of defecation.
3. *Knowledge deficit* (learning need) related to foods to prevent constipation.

E. Nursing care plan/implementation:

1. Goal: *reduce anal discomfort.*
   a. Sitz baths, as ordered; perineal care to prevent infection.
   b. Hot or cold compresses as ordered to reduce inflammation and pruritus.
   c. Topical medications as ordered:
      (1) *Anti-inflammatory:* hydrocortisone cream (Anusol).
      (2) *Astringents:* witch hazel–impregnated pads.
      (3) *Topical anesthetics:* pramoxine (Procto-Foam); dibucaine (Nupercainal).
   d. *Bulk laxatives:* psyllium (Metamucil), Konsyl, polycarbophil (FiberCon).
2. Goal: *prevent complications related to surgery.*
   a. Encourage postoperative ambulation.
   b. *Pain* relief until packing removed.
   c. Monitor for: bleeding, infection, pulmonary emboli, phlebitis.
   d. Facilitate bowel evacuation: stool softeners, laxatives, suppositories, oil enemas as ordered.
   e. Monitor for: syncope/vertigo during first postoperative bowel movement.

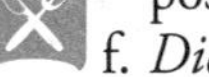

   f. *Diet:*
      (1) *Low* residue (postoperative)—until healing has begun.
      (2) *High* fiber to prevent constipation after healing.
   g. Increase fluid intake.
3. Goal: *health teaching*—methods to avoid constipation.

F. Evaluation/outcome criteria:

1. No complications.
2. Client has bowel movement.
3. Incorporates knowledge of correct foods into lifestyle.

GENITOURINARY SYSTEM

I. PYELONEPHRITIS (PN): acute or chronic inflammation due to bacterial infection of the parenchyma and renal pelvis; 95% of cases caused by gram-negative enteric bacilli (*Escherichia coli*); occurs more frequently in women.

A. Pathophysiology: inflammation of renal medulla or lining of the renal pelvis → nephron destruction; hypertrophy of nephrons needed to maintain urine output → impaired sodium reabsorption (salt wasting); inability to concentrate urine; progressive renal failure; hypertension (two thirds of all cases).

B. Risk factors:

1. Urinary obstruction (tumors, prostate).
2. Cystitis.
3. Neurogenic bladder.
4. Pregnancy.
5. Catheterization, cystoscopy.

C. Assessment:

1. *Subjective data:*
   a. *Pain:* flank—one or both sides; back; dysuria; headache.
   b. *Loss of appetite;* weight loss.
   c. *Night sweats;* chills.
   d. *Urination:* frequency, urgency.
2. *Objective data:*
   a. Fever; shaking chills.
   b. Laboratory data:
      (1) *Blood*—polymorphonuclear leukocytosis greater than 11,000/mm^3.
      (2) *Urine*—leukocytosis, hematuria, white blood cell casts, proteinuria (<3 gm in 24 hours), positive cultures; specific gravity—normal *or increased* with acute PN, *decreased* with chronic PN; cloudy; foul smelling.
   c. Intravenous pyelogram (IVP)—may manifest structural changes.

ADULT

D. Analysis/nursing diagnosis:
1. *Altered urinary elimination* related to kidney disease.
2. *Pain* related to dysuria and kidney damage.
3. *Hyperthermia* related to inflammation.
4. *Risk for fluid volume excess* related to renal failure.

E. Nursing care plan/implementation:
1. Goal: *combat infection, prevent recurrence, alleviate symptoms.*

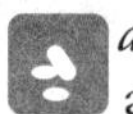

   a. Medications:
      (1) *Antibiotics, urinary antiseptics,* and/or sulfonamides appropriate for causative organism; also reduce pain.
      (2) *Analgesics* for pain—phenazopyridine (Pyridium); stronger if calculi present.
      (3) *Antipyretics* for fever—acetaminophen (Tylenol).
   b. *Fluids:* 1,500 to 2,000 mL/day to flush kidneys, relieve dysuria, reduce fever, prevent dehydration.
   c. Observe hydration status: I&O (output minimum 1,500 mL/24 hr); daily weight; urine—check each voiding for protein, blood, specific gravity; vital signs q4h to monitor for hypertension, tachycardia; skin turgor.
   d. *Hygiene:* meticulous perineal care; cleanse with soap and water; antibiotic ointment may be used around urinary meatus with retention catheter.
   e. Cooling measures: tepid sponging.
   f. *Diet:* sufficient calories and protein to prevent malnutrition; sodium supplement as ordered. *Acid-ash* to prevent renal calculus.
2. Goal: *promote physical and emotional rest.*
   a. Activity: bedrest or as tolerated—depends on whether anemia or fever is present; encourage activities of daily living as tolerated.
   b. Emotional support: encourage expression of fears (possible renal failure, dialysis); provide diversional activities; include family in care; answer questions.
3. Goal: *health teaching.*
   a. Medications: take regularly to maintain blood level; side effects.
   b. *Personal care:* perineal hygiene; *avoid* urethral contamination (by wiping perineum front to back); *avoid* tub baths.
   c. Possible recurrence with pregnancy.
   d. Monitoring daily weight.

F. Evaluation/outcome criteria:
1. Normal renal function (minimum 1,500 mL urine/24 hr).
2. Blood pressure within normal range.
3. No recurrence of symptoms.
4. Laboratory findings within normal limits.

II. ACUTE GLOMERULONEPHRITIS (see **Chapter 5, pp. 292–294**).

III. ACUTE RENAL FAILURE (ARF): broadly defined as rapid onset of oliguria accompanied by a rising BUN and serum creatinine; usually reversible.

A. Pathophysiology: acute renal ischemia → tubular necrosis → decreased urine output. *Oliguric phase* (<400 mL/24 hr)—waste products are retained → metabolic acidosis → water and electrolyte imbalances → anemia. *Recovery phase*—diuresis → dilute urine → rapid depletion of sodium, chloride, and water → dehydration.

B. Types and risk factors:
1. *Prerenal*—due to factors *outside* of kidney; usually circulatory collapse—cardiovascular disorders, hypovolemia, peripheral vasodilation, renovascular obstruction, severe vasoconstriction.
2. *Intrarenal*—parenchymal disease from ischemia or *nephrotoxic damage;* nephrotoxic agents—poisons, such as lead (carbon tetrachloride); heavy metals (mercury); antibiotics (gentamicin); incompatible blood transfusion; alcohol myopathies; obstetric complications; acute renal disease—acute glomerulonephritis, acute pyelonephritis.
3. *Postrenal*—obstruction in *collecting system:* renal or bladder calculi; tumors of bladder, prostate, or renal pelvis; gynecological or urological surgery in which ureters are accidentally ligated.

C. Assessment:
1. *Subjective data:*
   a. Sudden decrease or cessation of urine output (<400 mL/24 hr).
   b. Anorexia, nausea, vomiting from azotemia.
   c. Sudden weight gain from fluid accumulation.
   d. Headache.
2. *Objective data:*
   a. *Vital signs* (vary according to cause and severity):
      (1) *BP*—usually *elevated.*
      (2) *Pulse*—tachycardia, irregularities.
      (3) *Respirations*—*increased* rate, depth, crackles.
   b. *Neurological:* decreasing mentation, unresponsive to verbal or painful stimuli, psychoses, convulsions.
   c. *Halitosis;* cracked mucous membranes; uremic odor.
   d. *Skin:* dry, rashes, purpura, itchy, pale.
   e. Laboratory data:
      (1) Blood: *increased*—potassium, BUN, creatinine, WBC count; *decreased*—pH, bicarbonate, hematocrit, hemoglobin.
      (2) Urine: **oliguric renal failure**—*decreased* volume; specific gravity fixed or ↑; *increased*—protein, casts, red and white

ADULT

blood cells, sodium. **Non-oliguric renal failure**—up to 2 L/day, ↓ specific gravity, dilute, isomolar.

D. Analysis/nursing diagnosis:

1. *Altered urinary elimination* related to kidney malfunction.
2. *Fluid volume excess* related to decreased urine output.
3. *Altered nutrition, less than body requirements,* related to anorexia.
4. *Altered oral mucous membrane* related to stomatitis.
5. *Altered thought processes* related to uremia.

E. Nursing care plan/implementation:

1. Goal: *maintain fluid and electrolyte balance and nutrition.*
   a. Monitor: daily weight (should not vary more than ±1 lb); vital signs—include CVP; blood chemistries (BUN 6 to 20 mg/dL; creatinine 0.6 to 1.5 mg/dL).
   b. *Fluids:* IV as ordered; blood: plasma, packed cells, electrolyte solutions to replace losses; restricted to 400 mL/24 hr if hypertension present or during oliguric phase to prevent fluid overload.
   c. *Diet*, as tolerated: *high* carbohydrate, *low* protein, may be *low* potassium and *low* sodium; hypertonic glucose (total parenteral nutrition [TPN]) if oral feedings not tolerated; intravenous L-amino acids and glucose.
   d. Control hyperkalemia: infusions of hypertonic glucose and insulin to force potassium into cells; calcium gluconate (IV) to reduce myocardial irritability from K^+; sodium bicarbonate (IV) to correct acidosis; polystyrene sodium sulfonate (Kayexalate) or other exchange resins, orally or rectally (enema), to remove excess K^+; continuous renal replacement therapy, peritoneal or hemodialysis.
   e. Medications—*diuretics* (mannitol, furosemide [Lasix]) to increase renal blood flow and diuresis.
2. Goal: *use assessment and comfort measures to reduce occurrence of complications.*
   a. *Respiratory:* monitor rate, depth, breath sounds, arterial blood gases; encourage deep breathing, coughing, turning; use incentive spirometer or nebulizer as indicated.
   b. Frequent oral care to prevent stomatitis.
   c. Observe for signs of:
      (1) *Infection*—elevated temperature, localized redness, swelling, heat, or drainage.
      (2) *Bleeding*—stools, gums, venipuncture sites.
3. Goal: *maintain continual emotional support.*
   a. Same caregivers, consistency in procedures.
   b. Give opportunities to express concerns, fears.
   c. Allow family interactions.
4. Goal: *health teaching.*
   a. Preparation for dialysis (indications: uremia, uncontrolled hyperkalemia, or acidosis). **Continuous renal replacement therapy** (CRRT) may be used in ARF with fluid overload or rapidly developing azotemia and metabolic acidosis. Continuous ultrafiltration (8 to 24 hours) of extracellular fluid and uremic toxins. Client's BP powers system. Arterial and venous access required.
   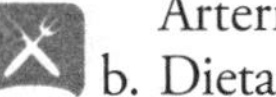
   b. Dietary *restrictions: low sodium, fluid restriction.*
   c. Disease process; treatment regimen.

F. Evaluation/outcome criteria:

1. Return of kidney function—normal creatinine level (<1.5 mg/dL), urine output.
2. Resumes normal life pattern (about 3 months after onset).

IV. CHRONIC RENAL FAILURE: as a result of progressive destruction of kidney tissue, the kidneys are no longer able to maintain their homeostatic functions; considered irreversible.

A. Pathophysiology: destruction of glomeruli → reduced glomerular filtration rate → retention of metabolic waste products; decreased urine output; severe fluid, electrolyte, acid-base imbalances → uremia. Clinical picture includes:

1. Ammonia in skin and alimentary tract by bacterial interaction with urea → inflammation of mucous membranes.
2. Retention of phosphate → decreased serum calcium → muscle spasms, tetany, and increased parathormone release → demineralization of bone.
3. Failure of tubular mechanisms to regulate blood bicarbonate → metabolic acidosis → hyperventilation.
4. Urea osmotic diuresis → flushing effect on tubules → decreased reabsorption of sodium → sodium depletion.
5. Waste product retention → depressed bone marrow function → decreased circulating RBCs → renal tissue hypoxia → decreased erythropoietin production → further depression of bone marrow → anemia.

B. Risk factors:

1. Diabetic retinopathy.
2. Chronic glomerulonephritis.
3. Chronic urinary obstruction, ureteral stricture, calculi, neoplasms.
4. Chronic pyelonephritis.
5. Hypertensive nephrosclerosis.
6. Congenital or acquired renal artery stenosis.
7. Systemic lupus erythematosus.

C. Assessment:

1. *Subjective data:* excessive fatigue, weakness.

2. *Objective data:*
   a. Skin: bronze colored, uremic frost.
   b. Ammonia breath.
   c. See also **III. ACUTE RENAL FAILURE, p. 458;** symptoms gradual in onset.

D. Analysis/nursing diagnosis:

1. In addition to the following, see **III. ACUTE RENAL FAILURE, p. 459.**
2. *Fatigue* related to severe anemia.
3. *Risk for impaired skin integrity* related to pruritus.
4. *Ineffective individual coping* related to chronic illness.
5. *Body image disturbance* related to need for dialysis.
6. *Noncompliance* related to denial of illness.

E. Nursing care plan/implementation:

1. Goal: *maintain fluid, electrolyte balance and nutrition* (see also **III. ACUTE RENAL FAILURE, p. 459**).

   a. *Diet: low* sodium; foods *high* in: calcium, vitamin B complex, vitamins C and D, and iron (to reduce edema, replace deficits, and promote absorption of nutrients).
   b. Medications: given to control BP, regulate electrolytes, control fluid volume; supplemental vitamins if deficient; *electrolyte modifier* (aluminum hydroxide [Alu-Cap, Amphojel]), calcium carbonate to bind phosphate.
   c. I&O; intake should be equivalent to previous daily output to prevent fluid retention.
2. Goal: *employ comfort measures that reduce distress and support physical function.*
   a. *Activity:* bedrest; facilitate ventilation; turn, cough, deep breathe q2h; ROM—active and passive, to prevent thrombi.
   b. *Hygiene:* mouth care to prevent stomatitis and reduce discomfort from mouth ulcers; perineal care.
   c. *Skin care:* soothing lotions to reduce pruritus.
   d. Encourage communication of concerns.
3. Goal: *health teaching.*
   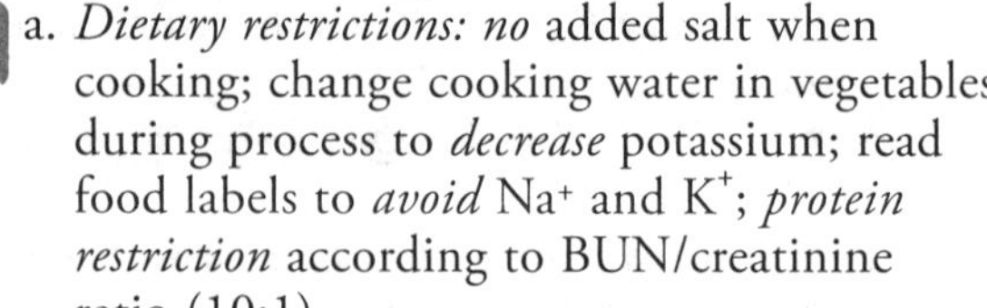
   a. *Dietary restrictions: no* added salt when cooking; change cooking water in vegetables during process to *decrease* potassium; read food labels to *avoid* Na^+ and K^+; *protein restriction* according to BUN/creatinine ratio (10:1).
   b. Importance of daily weight: same scale, time, clothing.
   c. Prepare for dialysis; transplantation.

F. Evaluation/outcome criteria:

1. Acceptance of chronic illness (no indication of indiscretions, destructive behavior, suicidal tendency).
2. Compliance with dietary restriction—no signs of protein excess (e.g., nausea, vomiting) or fluid sodium excess (e.g., edema, weight gain).

V. DIALYSIS: diffusion of solute through a semipermeable membrane that separates two solutions; direction of diffusion depends on concentration of solute in each solution; rate and efficiency depend on concentration gradient, temperature of solution, pore size of membrane, and molecular size; two methods available **(Table 6.27).**

A. *Indications:* acute poisonings; acute or chronic renal failure; hepatic coma; metabolic acidosis; extensive burns with azotemia.

Table 6.27

Comparison of Hemodialysis and Peritoneal Dialysis

	Hemodialysis	Peritoneal Dialysis
Process	Rapid—uses either *external* AV shunt (acute renal failure) or *internal* AV fistula (chronic renal failure); typical treatment is 3–4 hr, 3 days/wk; also used for barbiturate overdoses to remove toxic agent quickly	**Intermittent**—up to 36 hr for hospitalized clients; outpatient 4–8 hr, 5–6 times per week; dwell time 30–45 min for manual dialysis or 10–20 min for automatic cycler; either rigid stylet catheter or surgically inserted soft catheter; advantage for clients who cannot tolerate rapid fluid and electrolyte changes **Continuous**—two methods: (1) four cycles in 24 hr; dwell time is 4–5 hr during the day and 8–12 hr overnight; no need for machinery, electricity, or water source; surgically inserted soft catheter; closely resembles normal renal function; (2) automated cycler infuses and removes dialysate; generally done while client sleeps; built-in alarms for client safety.
Vascular access	Required	Not necessary; therefore suitable for clients with vascular problems
Heparinization	Required: systemic or regional	Little or no heparin necessary; therefore suitable for clients with bleeding problems
Complications (other than fluid and electrolyte imbalances, which are common to all)	Dialysis dysequilibrium syndrome (preventable) Mechanical dysfunctions of dialyzer	Peritonitis Hypoalbuminemia Bowel or bladder perforation Plugged or dislodged catheter

B. *Goals:*

1. *Reduce level of nitrogenous waste.*
2. *Correct acidosis, reverse electrolyte imbalances, remove excess fluid.*

C. *Hemodialysis:* circulation of client's blood through a compartment formed of a semipermeable membrane (polysulfone, polyacrylonitrile) surrounded by dialysate fluid.

1. Types of venous access for hemodialysis:
   a. External shunt **(Fig. 6.11).**
      (1) Cannula is placed in a large vein and a large artery that approximate each other.
      (2) External shunts, which provide easy and painless access to bloodstream, are prone to infection and clotting and cause erosion of the skin around the insertion area.
         (a) Daily cleansing and application of a sterile dressing.
         (b) Prevention of physical trauma and avoidance of some activities, such as swimming.

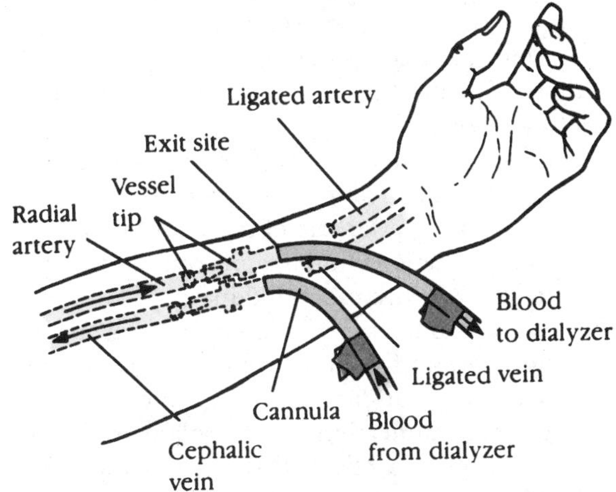

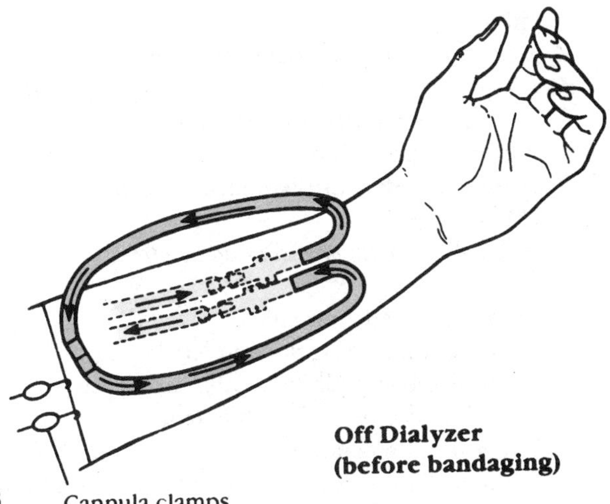

Figure 6.11 AV shunt (cannulae).

   b. Arteriovenous fistulas or graft **(Fig. 6.12).**
      (1) Large artery and vein are sewn together (anastomosed) below the surface of the skin (fistula) or subcutaneous graft using the saphenous vein, synthetic prosthesis, or bovine xenograft to connect artery and vein.
      (2) Purpose is to create one blood vessel for withdrawing and returning blood.
      (3) *Advantages:* greater activity range than AV shunt and no protective asepsis.
      (4) *Disadvantage:* necessity of two venipunctures with each dialysis.
   c. Vein catheterization.
      (1) Femoral or subclavian vein access is immediate.
      (2) May be short- or long-term duration.
2. **Complications during hemodialysis:**
   a. *Dysequilibrium syndrome*—rapid removal of urea from blood → reverse osmosis, with water moving into brain cells → cerebral edema → possible headache, nausea, vomiting, confusion, and convulsions; usually occurs with initial dialysis treatments; shorter dialysis time and slower rate minimizes.
   b. *Hypotension*—results from excessive ultrafiltration or excessive antihypertensive medications.
   c. *Hypertension*—results from volume overload (water and/or sodium), causing *dysequilibrium syndrome* or anxiety.
   d. *Transfusion reactions* (see **Chapter 8, Table 8.2**).
   e. *Arrhythmias*—due to hypotension, fluid overload, or rapid removal of potassium.
   f. *Psychological problems:*
      (1) Clients react in varying ways to dependence on hemodialysis.
      (2) Nurse needs to identify client reactions and defense mechanisms and to employ

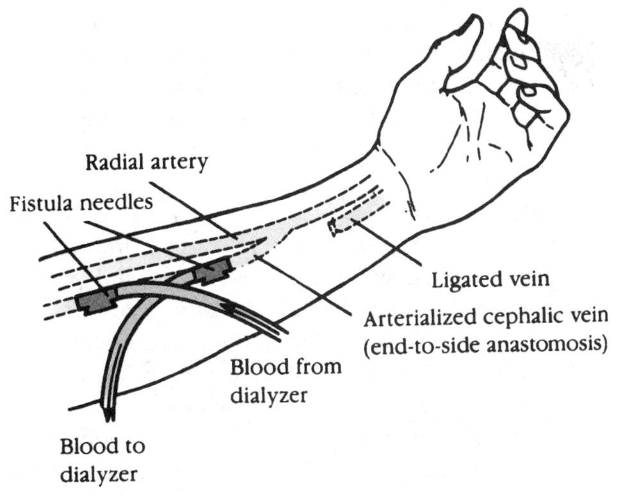

Figure 6.12 AV fistula.

supportive behaviors (e.g., include client in care; continual repetition and reinforcement); do *not* interpret client's behavior—for example, do *not* say, "You're being hostile" or "You're acting like a child"; answer questions honestly regarding quality and length of life with dialysis and/or transplantation; encourage independence as much as possible.

3. Commonly used medications:
   a. *Antihypertensives* (ACE inhibitors, beta blockers, diuretics).
   b. *Phosphorus binders* (calcium acetate, calcium carbonate, Renagel).
   c. *B-complex vitamins* with vitamin *C* and *folic acid.*
   d. *Synthetic erythropoietin* (Aranesp, Epogen).
   e. Iron.
   f. Activated vitamin *D.*

D. *Intermittent peritoneal dialysis:* involves introduction of a dialysate solution into the abdomen, where the peritoneum acts as the semipermeable membrane between the solution and blood in abdominal vessels. *Procedure:*
1. Area around umbilicus is prepared and anesthetized with local anesthetic, and a catheter is inserted into the peritoneal cavity through a trocar; the catheter is then sutured into place to prevent displacement.
2. Warmed dialysate is then allowed to flow into the peritoneal cavity. *Inflow time:* 5 to 10 minutes; 2 L of solution are used in each cycle in the adult; solutions contain glucose, Na^+, Ca^{++}, Mg^{++}, K^+, Cl^-, and lactate or acetate.
3. When solution bottle is empty, dwell time (exchange time) begins. *Dwell time:* 10 to 20 minutes; processes of diffusion, osmosis, and filtration begin to move waste products from bloodstream into peritoneal cavity.
4. Draining of the dialysate begins with the unclamping of the outflow clamp. *Outflow time:* usually 10 minutes; returns less than 2 L usually result from incomplete peritoneal emptying; turn side to side to increase return; multiple exchanges in 24 hours depending on client need.

E. *Continuous ambulatory peritoneal dialysis (CAPD):* functions on the same principles as peritoneal dialysis, yet allows greater freedom and independence for clients on dialysis. *Procedure:*
1. Dialysis solution is infused into peritoneum three times daily and once before bedtime.
2. *Dwell time*—≥4 hours for each daily exchange, and overnight for the fourth (8 to 12 hours).
3. Indwelling peritoneal catheter is connected to solution bag at all times—serves to fill and drain peritoneum; concealed in cloth pouch, strapped to the body during dwell time; client can move about doing usual activities.

F. *Continuous cycling peritoneal dialysis (CCPD):* same principles as CAPD, except uses an automated system to infuse and remove dialysate; reduces nursing care needs with clients who are hospitalized. Cumbersome equipment inhibits nighttime mobility. *Procedure:*
1. Long exchanges without an automated cycler during the day, and short exchanges with a cycler at night.
2. *Dwell time*—6 to 8 hours while sleeping.
3. Automatic alarms to prevent malfunction with home use.

VI. KIDNEY TRANSPLANTATION: placement of a donor kidney (from sibling, parent, cadaver) into the iliac fossa of a recipient and the anastomosis of its ureter to the bladder of the recipient; indicated in end-stage renal disease.

A. *Criteria for recipient:* irreversible kidney function; under 70 years of age; patent and functional lower urinary tract; and good surgical risk, free of serious cardiovascular complications. *Contraindicated* in those with another life-threatening condition.

B. *Donor selection:*
1. Sibling or parent—survival rate of kidney is greater; preferred for transplantation.
2. Cadaver—greater rate of rejection following transplantation, although majority of transplantations are with cadaver kidneys.

C. Bilateral nephrectomy: necessary for clients with rapidly progressive glomerulonephritis, malignant hypertension, or chronic kidney infections; prevents complications in transplanted kidney (see **VII. NEPHRECTOMY** for nursing care, **p. 464**).

D. Analysis/nursing diagnosis:
1. *Altered urinary elimination* related to kidney failure.
2. *Fear* related to potential transplant rejection.
3. *Risk for infection* related to immunosuppression.
4. *Body image disturbance* related to immunosuppression.

E. Nursing care plan/implementation:
1. *Preoperative:*
   a. Goal: *promote physical and emotional adjustment.*
      (1) Informed consent.
      (2) Laboratory work completed—histocompatibility, CBC, urinalysis, blood type and crossmatch.
      (3) Skin preparation.
   b. Goal: *encourage expression of feelings:* origin of donor, fear of complications, rejection.

c. Goal: *minimize risk of organ rejection:* give medications: begin *immunosuppression* (azathioprine, corticosteroids, cyclosporine); *antibiotics* if ordered.

d. Goal: *health teaching.*
   (1) Nature of surgery; placement of kidney.
   (2) Postoperative expectations: deep breathing, coughing, turning, early ambulation; *reverse isolation.*
   (3) Medications: *immunosuppressive* therapy: purpose, effect.

2. *Postoperative:*
   a. Goal: *promote uncomplicated recovery of recipient.*
      (1) Vital signs; CVP; I&O—urine output usually immediate with living donor; with cadaver kidney may not work for a week or more and dialysis will be needed within 24 to 48 hours. Report less than 100 mL/hr **immediately.**
      (2) *Isolation:* strict *reverse* isolation with immunosuppression; wear face mask when out of room.
      (3) *Position:* back to *nonoperative* side; *semi-Fowler's* to promote gas exchange.
      (4) Indwelling catheter care: *strict* asepsis; characteristics of urine—report gross hematuria, heavy sediment; clots; perineal care; bladder spasms may occur after removal of catheter.
      (5) Activity: ambulate 24 hours after surgery; *avoid* prolonged sitting.
      (6) Weigh daily.
      (7) Medications: *immunosuppressives; analgesics* as ordered (pain decreases significantly after 24 hours).
      (8) Drains: irrigate *only* on physician order; *meticulous* catheter care.
      (9) *Diet:* regular after return of bowel sounds; liberal amounts of protein; *restrict* fluids, sodium, potassium *only if* oliguric.
   b. Goal: *observe for signs of rejection*—most dangerous complication.
      (1) Three classifications:
         (a) **Hyperacute**—occurs within 5 to 10 minutes up to 48 hours after transplantation (rare).
         (b) **Acute**—most common 7 to 14 days; varies depending on living (1 week to 6 months) or cadaver (1 week to 2 years) donor.
         (c) **Chronic**—occurs several months to years.
      (2) **Assessment:**
         (a) *Subjective data:*
            (i) Lethargy, anorexia.
            (ii) Tenderness over graft site.
         (b) *Objective data:*
            (i) Laboratory data: **Urine:** *decreased*—output, creatinine clearance, sodium; *increased*—protein. **Blood:** *increased*—BUN, creatinine.
            (ii) Rapid weight gain; more than 3 lb/day.
            (iii) *Vital signs:* BP, temperature—*elevated.*
   c. Goal: *maintain immunosuppressive therapy.*
      (1) Azathioprine (*Imuran*)—an antimetabolite that interferes with cellular division. *Side effects:*
         (a) Gastrointestinal bleeding (give PO form with food).
         (b) Bone marrow depression; leukopenia; anemia.
         (c) Development of malignant neoplasms.
         (d) Infection.
         (e) Liver damage.
      (2) Prednisone—believed to affect lymphocyte production by inhibiting nucleic acid synthesis: anti-inflammatory action helps prevent tissue damage if rejection occurs. *Side effects:*
         (a) Stress ulcer with bleeding (give with food).
         (b) *Decreased* glucose tolerance (hyperglycemia).
         (c) Muscle weakness.
         (d) Osteoporosis.
         (e) Moon facies.
         (f) Acne and striae.
         (g) Depression and hallucinations.
      (3) Cyclosporine (Neoral, Sandimmune)—polypeptide antibiotic used to prevent rejection of kidney, liver, or heart allografts; PO dose given with *room-temperature chocolate milk or orange juice* in a glass dispenser. *Side effects:*
         (a) Nephrotoxicity (*increased* BUN, creatinine).
         (b) Hypertension.
         (c) Tremor.
         (d) Hirsutism, gingival hyperplasia.
         (e) *GI*—nausea, vomiting, anorexia, diarrhea, abdominal pain.
         (f) Infections—pneumonia, septicemia, abscesses, wound.
      (4) Additional drugs may include cyclophosphamide (Cytoxan), antithymocyte globulin (ATG), antilymphocyte globulin, muromonab-CD3 (OKT3), tacrolimus (Prograf), and mycophenolate mofetil (CellCept).

d. Goal: *health teaching.*
   (1) Signs of rejection (see Goal **b.**).
   (2) Drugs: side effects of immunosuppression (see Goal **c.**).
   (3) *Self-care activities:* temperature, blood pressure, I&O, urine specimen collection.
   (4) Avoidance of infection.
   (5) See also goals of care, under **III. POSTOPERATIVE EXPERIENCE, pp. 370, 374–375.**

F. Evaluation/outcome criteria:
1. No signs of rejection (e.g., no weight gain, oliguria).
2. No depression.
3. Client resumes role responsibilities.

VII. NEPHRECTOMY (radical or partial): removal of kidney through flank, retroperitoneal, abdominal, thoracic, or thoracic-abdominal approach; indicated with malignant tumors, severe trauma, or under certain conditions before renal transplantation (see **VI. KIDNEY TRANSPLANTATION, pp. 462–464**).

A. Analysis/nursing diagnosis:
1. *Pain* related to surgical incision.
2. *Risk for infection* related to wound contamination.
3. *Risk for fluid volume excess.*
4. *Risk for aspiration* related to vomiting.
5. *Constipation* related to paralytic ileus.
6. *Anxiety* related to possible loss of function in remaining kidney.
7. *Dysfunctional grieving* related to perceived loss.

B. Nursing care plan/implementation:
1. *Preoperative:* Goal: *optimize physical and psychological functioning* (see **I. PREOPERATIVE PREPARATION, pp. 365–367**).
2. *Postoperative:* Goal: *promote comfort and prevent complications.*
   a. Observe for signs of:
      (1) *Paralytic ileus*—abdominal distention, absent bowel sounds, vomiting (common complication following renal surgery).
      (2) *Hemorrhage.*
   b. Fluid balance: daily weight—maintain within 2% of preoperative level.

C. Evaluation/outcome criteria:
1. No complications (e.g., hemorrhage, paralytic ileus, wound infection).
2. Acceptance of loss of kidney.

VIII. RENAL CALCULI (UROLITHIASIS): formation of calculi (stones) in renal calyces or pelvis that pass to lower regions of urinary tract—ureters, bladder, or urethra; occurs after age 30, with greatest incidence in *men,* particularly over age 50.

A. Pathophysiology: organic crystals form (most consist of calcium salts or magnesium and ammonium phosphate (struvite) → obstruction, infection; increased backward pressure in kidney → hydronephrosis → atrophy, fibrosis of renal tubules.

B. Risk factors (in over 50% of cases, cause is idiopathic):
1. Urinary tract infection.
2. Urinary stasis—obstruction.
3. Metabolic factors—excessive intake of vitamin D or C, calcium carbonate.

C. Assessment (depends on size, shape, location of stone):
1. *Subjective data:*
   a. *Pain:* occasional, dull, in loin or back when stones are in calyces or renal pelvis; *excruciating* in flank area (renal colic), radiating to groin when stones are ureteral.
   b. Nausea associated with pain.
2. *Objective data:*
   a. Pallor, sweating, syncope, shock, and vomiting due to pain.
   b. Palpable kidney mass with hydronephrosis.
   c. Fever and pyuria with infection.
   d. Laboratory data:
      (1) Urinalysis: abnormal—pH (acidic or alkaline); RBCs (injury); WBCs (infection); *increased*—specific gravity; casts; crystals; other organic substances, depending on type of stone (i.e., calcium, struvite, uric acid, or cystine); *positive* culture.
      (2) Blood: *increased* calcium, phosphorus, total protein, alkaline phosphatase, creatinine, uric acid, BUN.
   e. *Diagnostic tests:*
      (1) IVP: reveals nonopaque stones, degree of obstruction.
      (2) X-ray; radiopaque stones seen.
      (3) Ultrasound may also be used.

D. Analysis/nursing diagnosis:
1. *Pain* related to passage of stone.
2. *Altered urinary elimination* related to potential obstruction.
3. *Urinary retention* related to obstruction of urethra.

E. Nursing care plan/implementation:
1. Goal: *reduce pain and prevent complications.*
   a. Medication: *narcotics, antiemetics, antibiotics.*
   b. Fluids: 3 to 4 L/day; IVs if nauseated, vomiting.
   c. Activity: ambulate to promote passage of stone, except bedrest during acute attack (colic).
   d. Reduce spasms: warm soaks to affected flank.
   e. Observe for signs of:
      (1) *Obstruction*—decreased urinary output, increased flank pain.
      (2) *Passage of stone* (90% will pass <5-mm size)—cessation of pain; filter urine with gauze.

f. Monitor: hydration status—I&O, daily weight; vital signs—particularly temperature for sign of infection; urine—color, odor.

2. Goal: *health teaching.*
   a. Importance of *fluids:* minimum 3,000 mL/day; 2 glasses during night.
   b. *Diet:* modify according to stone type (see **Chapter 9**).
      (1) *Calcium oxalate and calcium phosphate stones—low* calcium, phosphorus, and oxalate (e.g., *avoid* tea, cocoa, cola, beans, spinach, acidic fruits).
      (2) *Magnesium and ammonium phosphate—low* phosphorus.
      (3) *Uric acid stones—low* purine.
      (4) *Cystine stones—low* protein.
   c. *Acid-ash diet* with calcium oxalate and calcium phosphate stones, magnesium and ammonium phosphate (struvite) stones.
   d. *Alkaline-ash diet* with uric acid and cystine stones (see **Common Therapeutic Diets** in **Chapter 9, pp. 699–701**).
   e. Signs of urinary infection: dysuria, frequency, hematuria; seek immediate treatment.
   f. Prepare for removal if indicated; 20% of stones require additional treatment: *cytoscopy* for small stones; *cystolitholapaxy* for soft stones; *lithotripsy* or *surgical removal* (nephroscopic, pyelolithotomy, or nephrolithotomy).

F. Evaluation/outcome criteria:
1. Relief from pain.
2. No signs of urinary obstruction (e.g., increased flank pain, decreased urine output).
3. No recurrence of lithiasis (adheres to diet and fluid regimen).

IX. LITHOTRIPSY. *Laser lithotripsy*—newer treatment using laser and a ureteroscope; constant water irrigation because of heat. *Extracorporeal shock wave*—a noninvasive mechanical procedure used to break up renal calculi so they can pass spontaneously, in most cases. The trunk of the client is submerged in distilled water. In addition to being strapped to a frame, the client may also receive *sedation* and *analgesia* for pain from sound waves. The procedure takes 30 to 45 minutes, and remaining still is important. An underwater electrode generates shock waves that fragment the stone so it can be excreted in the urine a few days after the procedure. A degree of renal colic may occur, requiring *narcotics* for up to 3 days. ***Nursing measures*** should encourage ambulation and promote diuresis through *forcing* fluids. *Percutaneous lithotripsy*—nephrostomy tract above kidney region; nephroscope used to retrieve calculi. Urinary drainage from incision for 3 to 4 days is normal. May be required for large fragments remaining after extracorporeal lithotripsy. ***Nursing measures*** include: dressing changes to prevent infection and prevent skin breakdown, and administration of *antibiotics* and *narcotics* for pain.

X. BENIGN PROSTATIC HYPERPLASIA (BPH): bladder outlet obstruction resulting from an enlargement of the prostate gland.

A. Pathophysiology: prostate enlarges, bulges upward, blocks flow of urine from bladder into urethra → obstruction → hydroureter, hydronephrosis.

B. Risk factors:
1. Changes in estrogen and androgen levels.
2. Men older than 50.

C. Assessment:
1. *Subjective data—urination:*
   a. Difficulty starting stream.
   b. Smaller, less forceful.
   c. Dribbling.
   d. Frequency.
   e. Urgency.
   f. Nocturia.
   g. Retention (incomplete emptying).
   h. Inability to void after ingestion of alcohol or exposure to cold.
2. *Objective data:*
   a. Catheterization for residual urine: 25 to 50 mL after voiding.
   b. Enlarged prostate on rectal examination.
   c. Laboratory data:
      (1) Urine—*increased* RBC, WBC counts.
      (2) Blood—*increased* creatinine, prostate-specific antigen (PSA).

D. Analysis/nursing diagnosis:
1. *Urinary retention* related to incomplete emptying.
2. *Altered urinary elimination* related to obstruction.
3. *Urinary incontinence* related to urgency, pressure.
4. *Anxiety* related to potential surgery.
5. *Body image disturbance* related to threat to masculine identity.

E. Nursing care plan/implementation:
1. Goal: *relieve urinary retention.*
   a. Catheterization: release maximum of 1,000 mL initially; *avoid* bladder decompression, which results in hypotension, bladder spasms, ruptured blood vessels in bladder; empty 200 mL every 5 minutes.
   b. Patency: irrigate intermittently or continually, as ordered.
   c. *Fluids:* minimum 2,000 mL/24 hr.
2. Goal: *health teaching.*
   a. Preparation for surgery (cystostomy, prostatectomy):
      (1) Expectations—indwelling catheter (will feel urge to void).

(2) *Avoid* pulling on catheter (this increases bleeding and clots).
(3) Bladder spasms common 24 to 48 hours after surgery, particularly with transurethral resection and suprapubic approaches.
(4) Threatening nature of procedure (possibility of impotence with perineal prostatectomy).

b. See also **I. PREOPERATIVE PREPARATION, pp. 365–367.**

XI. PROSTATECTOMY: surgical procedure to relieve urinary retention and frequency caused by benign prostatic hyperplasia or cancer of the prostate.

A. Types

1. *Transurethral resection (TUR)*—removal of obstructive prostatic tissue surrounding urethra by an electrical wire (resectoscope) introduced through the urethra; hypertrophy may recur, and TUR repeated; little risk of impotence. Laser also being used.
2. *Suprapubic*—low midline incision is made directly over the bladder; bladder is opened and large mass of prostatic tissue is removed through incision in urethral mucosa.
3. *Retropubic*—removal of hypertrophied prostatic tissue high in pelvic area through a low abdominal incision; bladder is not opened; client may remain potent.
4. *Perineal*—removal of prostatic tissue low in pelvic area is accomplished through an incision made between the scrotum and the rectum; usually results in impotency and incontinence.

B. Nursing care plan/implementation:

1. *Preoperative* (see **X. BENIGN PROSTATIC HYPERPLASIA, p. 465**).
2. *Postoperative:*

a. Goal: *promote optimal bladder function and comfort.*

(1) Urinary drainage: sterile closed-gravity system—maintain external traction as ordered.
(2) Reinforce purposes, sensations to expect.
(3) Bladder irrigation to control bleeding, keep clots from forming.
(4) Suprapubic catheter care (suprapubic prostatectomy)—closed-gravity drainage system; observe character, amount, flow of drainage.
(5) *After removal:*
(a) Observe for urinary drainage q4h for 24 hours.
(b) Skin care.
(c) Report excessive drainage to physician.
(6) Dressings: keep dry, clean; reinforce if necessary (may need to change suprapubic dressing if urinary drainage); notify physician of *excessive bleeding.*
(7) Observe for signs of:
(a) *Bladder distention*—distinct mound over pubis, slow drip in collecting bottle; irrigate catheter as ordered.
(b) *Increased bleeding*—expect and report frank bleeding (if *venous* bleeding, increase traction on catheter); if bright-red drainage, and clots (*arterial* bleeding), may need surgical control; cool, clammy, pale skin and increased pulse rate indicate *shock.*

b. Goal: *assist in rehabilitation.* Emotional support: *fears* of incontinence, loss of masculine identity, impotence.

c. Goal: *health teaching.*

(1) Expectations: mild incontinence, dribbling for a while (several months) after surgery; need to void as soon as urge is felt; *push fluids.*
(2) Exercises: perineal (Kegel) 1 to 2 days after surgery—buttocks are tightened for a count of ten, 20 to 50 times daily.
(3) *Avoid:*
(a) Long auto trips, vigorous exercise, heavy lifting (anything heavier than 10 lb), and sexual intercourse for about 3 weeks or until medical permission, because they may increase tendency to bleed.
(b) Alcoholic beverages for 1 month, because this may cause burning on urination; caffeine, because it causes diuresis.
(c) Tub baths, because of increase chance of infection.
(4) Medications: *stool softeners* or mild *cathartics* to decrease straining.

C. Evaluation/outcome criteria:

1. Relief of symptoms.
2. No complications (e.g., hemorrhage, impotence).

XII. URINARY DIVERSION: *Incontinent*—ileal conduit: anastomosis of ureters to a small portion of the ileum; stoma is called *urostomy;* urine flow is constant; requires external collection device. *Continent—Kock pouch, Indiana pouch:* segment of small bowel or colon is used to create a pouch; holds urine without leakage; requires self-catheterization.

A. Indications:

1. Congenital anomalies of bladder.
2. Neurogenic bladder.
3. Mechanical obstruction to urine flow (e.g., bladder cancer).
4. Chronic progressive pyelonephritis.
5. Trauma to lower urinary tract.

ADULT

B. Analysis/nursing diagnosis:

1. *Altered urinary elimination* related to surgical diversion.
2. *Risk for impaired skin integrity* related to leakage of urine.
3. *Risk for infection* related to contamination of stoma.
4. *Constipation* related to absence of peristalsis.
5. *Body image disturbance* related to stoma.

C. Nursing care plan/implementation:

1. *Preoperative:* optimal bowel and stoma site preparation.

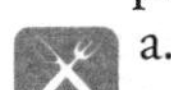

   a. *Diet: low* residue 2 days followed by clear liquids for 24 hours.
   b. Medications:
      (1) Neomycin (for bowel sterilization).
      (2) Cathartics (GoLYTELY), enemas.
   c. Site selection: appliance faceplate (incontinent diversion) must bond securely; *avoid* areas of pressure from clothing (waistline); usual site is right or left lower abdominal quadrant.
   d. See also **I. PREOPERATIVE PREPARATION, pp. 365–367.**

2. *Postoperative:*
   a. Goal: *prevent complications and promote comfort.*
      (1) Observe for signs of:
         (a) *Paralytic ileus* (common complication)—keep NG tube patent.
         (b) *Stoma necrosis*—dusky or cyanotic color (**emergency** situation).
      (2) Skin care: check for leakage around ostomy bag.
      (3) Urinary drainage—stents or catheter in stoma; blood in urine in immediate postoperative period; mucus normal.
      (4) See **III. POSTOPERATIVE EXPERIENCE, pp. 370, 374–375.**
   b. Goal: *health teaching.*
      (1) Self-care activities:
         (a) *Peristomal skin care*—prevent irritation, breakdown; proper cleansing—soap and water; adhesive remover, if needed.
         (b) *Appliance application and emptying;* pouch opening 2 to 3 mm larger than stoma; do *not* remove each day; change appliance every 3 to 5 days or when leaking.

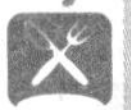

         (c) *Odor control*—dilute urine, hygiene, *acid-ash diet; avoid* asparagus, tomatoes.
         (d) *Use of night drainage system if necessary* for uninterrupted sleep.
      (2) Signs *of complications:* change in urine color, clarity, quantity, smell; stomal color change (normal is bright pink or red).

D. Evaluation/outcome criteria:

1. Acceptance of new body image.
2. Regains independence.
3. Demonstrates confidence in management of self-care activities.

ENDOCRINE SYSTEM

I. DIABETES: heterogeneous group of diseases involving the disruption of the metabolism of carbohydrates, fats, and protein. If uncontrolled, serious vascular and neurological changes occur.

A. Types:

1. *Type 1:* formerly called *insulin-dependent diabetes mellitus (IDDM);* and also formerly called "juvenile-onset diabetes." Insulin is needed to prevent ketosis; onset usually in youth but may occur in adulthood; prone to ketosis, unstable diabetes.
2. *Type 2:* formerly called *non–insulin-dependent diabetes mellitus (NIDDM);* and also *formerly* called "maturity-onset diabetes" or "adult-onset diabetes." May be controlled with diet and oral hypoglycemics or insulin; client less apt to have ketosis, except in presence of infection. May be further classified as *obese type 2* or *nonobese type 2.*
3. *Type 3: gestational diabetes mellitus (GDM):* glucose intolerance during pregnancy in women who were not known to have diabetes before pregnancy; will be reclassified after birth; may need to be treated or may return to prepregnancy state and need no treatment.
4. *Type 4:* diabetes secondary to another condition, such as pancreatic disease, other hormonal imbalances, or drug therapy such as receiving glucocorticoids.

B. Pathophysiology:

1. *Type 1*—absolute deficiency of insulin due to destruction of pancreatic beta cells by the interaction of genetic, immunological, hereditary, or environmental factors.
2. *Type 2*—relative deficiency of insulin due to:
   a. An islet cell defect resulting in a slowed or delayed response in the release of insulin to a glucose load; or
   b. Reduction in the number of insulin receptors from continuously elevated insulin levels; or
   c. A postreceptor defect; or
   d. A major peripheral resistance to insulin induced by hyperglycemia. These factors lead to deprivation of insulin-dependent cells → a marked decrease in the cellular rate of glucose uptake, and therefore elevated blood glucose.

C. Risk factors:

1. Obesity.
2. Family history of diabetes.

3. Age 45 or older.
4. Women whose babies at birth weighed more than 9 lb.
5. History of autoimmune disease.
6. Members of high-risk ethnic group (African American, Latino, or Native American).
7. History of gestational diabetes mellitus.
8. Hypertension.
9. Elevated high-density lipoprotein (HDL).

D. Assessment:

1. *Subjective data:*
   a. *Eyes:* blurry vision.
   b. *Skin:* pruritus vulvae.
   c. *Neuromuscular:* paresthesia, peripheral neuropathy, lethargy, weakness, fatigue, increased irritability.
   d. *GI:* polydipsia (increased thirst).
   e. *Reproductive:* impotence.
2. *Objective data:*
   a. *Genitourinary:* polyuria, glycosuria, nocturia (nocturnal enuresis in children).
   b. *Vital signs:*
      (1) *Pulse* and *temperature:* normal or elevated.
      (2) *BP:* normal or decreased, unless complications present.
      (3) *Respirations: increased* rate and depth (*Kussmaul's* respirations).
   c. *GI:*
      (1) Polyphagia, dehydration.
      (2) Weight loss, failure to gain weight.
      (3) Acetone breath.
   d. *Skin:* cuts heal slowly; frequent infections, foot ulcers, vaginitis.
   e. *Neuromuscular:* loss of strength, peripheral neuropathy.
   f. Laboratory data:
      (1) *Elevated:*
         (a) Blood sugar greater than 126 mg/dL fasting or 200 mg/dL 1 to 2 hours after eating.
         (b) Glucose tolerance test.
         (c) Glycosuria (>170 mg/100 mL).
         (d) Potassium (>5 mg/dL) and chloride (>145 mg/dL).
         (e) Hemoglobin A_{1c} greater than 7%.
      (2) *Decreased:*
         (a) pH (<7.4).
         (b) $Paco_2$ (<32).
   g. Long-term pathological considerations:
      (1) *Cataract formation and retinopathy:* thickened capillary basement membrane, changes in vascularization and hemorrhage, due to chronic hyperglycemia.
      (2) *Nephropathy:* due to glomerulosclerosis, arteriosclerosis of renal artery and pyelonephritis, progressive uremia.
      (3) *Neuropathy:* due to reduced tissue perfusion; affecting motor, sensory, voluntary, and autonomic functions.
      (4) *Arteriosclerosis:* due to lesions of the intimal wall.
      (5) *Cardiac:* angina, coronary insufficiency, myocardial infarction.
      (6) *Vascular changes:* occlusions, intermittent claudication, loss of peripheral pulses, arteriosclerosis.

E. Analysis/nursing diagnosis:

1. *Altered nutrition, less than body requirements,* related to inability to metabolize nutrients and weight loss.
2. *Altered nutrition, more than body requirements,* related to excessive glucose intake.
3. *Risk for injury* related to complications of uncontrolled diabetes.
4. *Body image disturbance* related to long-term illness.
5. *Knowledge deficit* (learning need) related to management of long-term illness and potential complications.
6. *Ineffective individual coping* related to inability to follow diet/medication regimen.
7. *Sexual dysfunction* related to impotence from diabetes and treatment.

F. Nursing care plan/implementation:

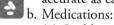

1. Goal: *obtain and maintain normal sugar balance.*
   a. Monitor: vital signs; blood glucose before meals, at bedtime, and as symptoms demand (urine testing for glucose levels is not as accurate as capillary blood testing).
   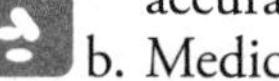
   b. Medications:
      (1) *Oral hypoglycemics:*
         (a) Sulfonylureas; tolbutamide (Orinase), chlorpropamide (Diabenese), tolazamide (Tolinase), acetohexamide (Dymelor), glimepiride (Amaryl), glyburide (DiaBeta and Micronase), and glipizide (Glucocotrol).
         (b) Others: metformin (Glucophage) increases body's sensitivity to insulin. Acarbose (Precose) inhibits cells of the small intestine from absorbing complex carbohydrates.
      (2) *Insulin* (biosynthetic human insulin): *bolus insulin*—released in response to meals; *basal insulin*—released between meals, at nighttime.
         (a) Rapid-acting bolus analogue of human insulin (Lispro, Aspart).
         (b) Short-acting bolus (crystalline, regular) (Humulin R).
         (c) Intermediate-acting basal (Lente and NPH).

ADULT

(d) Slow acting (protamine zinc).
(e) Long, extended-acting basal (Ultralente).
(f) Long-acting basal analogue (Glargine).
(3) Methods of administration:
(a) Subcutaneous injection.
(b) Prefilled injectable insulin pens (Novopen and Novolin).
(c) Continuous subcutaneous insulin infusion therapy (insulin pumps).

c. *Diet,* as ordered.
(1) Carbohydrate, 50% to 60%; protein, 20%; fats, 30% (saturated fats limited to 10%, unsaturated fats, 90%).
(2) Calorie reduction in adults who are obese; enough calories to promote normal growth and development for children or adults who are not obese.
(3) Limit refined sugars.
(4) Add vitamins, minerals as needed for well-balanced diet.

d. Monitor for signs of *acute* (hypoglycemia, ketoacidosis) or *chronic* (circulatory compromise, neuropathy, nephropathy, retinopathy) complications.

2. Goal: *health teaching:*
a. *Diet:* foods allowed, restricted, substitutions.
b. Medications: administration techniques, importance of using room-temperature insulin and rotating injection sites to prevent tissue damage.
c. Desired and side effects of prescribed insulin type; onset, peak, and duration of action of prescribed insulin.
d. Blood glucose testing techniques.
e. Signs of complications **(Table 6.28).**
f. Importance of health maintenance:
(1) Infection prevention, especially foot and nail care.
(2) Routine checkups.
(3) Maintain stable balance of glucose by carefully monitoring glucose level and making necessary adjustments in diet and activity level; seeking medical attention when unable to maintain balance; regular exercise program.

Table 6.28

Comparison of Diabetic Complications

	Hypoglycemia	Ketoacidosis
Pathophysiology	Major metabolic complication when too little food or too-large dose of insulin or hypoglycemic agents administered; interferes with oxygen consumption of nervous tissue	Major metabolic complication in which there is insufficient insulin for metabolism of carbohydrates, fats, and proteins; seen most frequently with clients who are insulin dependent; precipitated in the person with known diabetes by stressors (such as infection, trauma, major illness) that increase insulin needs
Risk factors	Too little food Emotional or added stress Vomiting or diarrhea Added exercise	Insufficient insulin or oral hypoglycemics Noncompliance with dietary instructions Major illness/infections Therapy with steroid administration Trauma, surgery Elevated blood sugar: >200 mg/dL
Assessment	**Behavioral change:** *Subjective data*—nervous, irritable, anxious, confused, disoriented *Objective data*—abrupt mood changes, psychosis **Visual:** *Subjective data*—blurred vision, diplopia *Objective data*—dilated pupils **Skin:** *Objective data*—diaphoresis, pale, cool, clammy, goosebumps (piloerection), tenting **Vitals:** *Subjective data—palpitations* **Gastrointestinal:** *Subjective data*—hunger, nausea *Objective data*—diarrhea, vomiting	**Behavioral change:** *Subjective data*—irritable, confused *Objective data*—drowsy **Visual:** *Objective data*—eyeballs: soft, sunken **Skin:** *Objective data*—loss of turgor, flushed face, pruritus vulvae **Vitals:** *Objective data*— tachycardia; thready; respirations: *Kussmaul's;* BP: hypovolemic shock **Gastrointestinal:** *Subjective data*—increased thirst and hunger, abdominal pain, nausea *Objective data*—vomiting, diarrhea, dry mucous membrane; lips, tongue: red, parched; breath: fruity

Continued

Table 6.28

Comparison of Diabetic Complications—cont'd

	Hypoglycemia	Ketoacidosis
	Neurological: *Subjective data*—headache; lips/tongue: tingling, numbness *Objective data*—fainting, yawning; speech: incoherent; convulsions; coma **Musculoskeletal:** *Subjective data*—weak, fatigue *Objective data*—trembling Blood sugar: <80 mg/dL	**Neurological:** *Subjective data*—headache; irritability; confusion; lethargy, weakness **Musculoskeletal** *Subjective data*—fatigue; general malaise **Renal:** *Objective data*—polyuria Blood sugar: >130 mg/dL
Analysis/nursing diagnosis	*Risk for injury* related to deficit of needed glucose *Knowledge deficit* (learning need) related to proper dietary intake or proper insulin dosage *Altered nutrition, less than body requirements*, related to glucose deficiency	*Risk for injury* related to glucose imbalance *Knowledge deficit* (learning need) related to proper balance of diet and insulin dosage
Nursing care plan/ implementation	Goal: *provide adequate glucose to reverse hypoglycemia:* administer simple sugar STAT, PO or IV, glucose paste absorbed in mucous membrane; monitor blood sugar levels; identify events leading to complication Goal: *health teaching:* how to prevent further episodes (see I. **DIABETES, Health Teaching, p. 469**); importance of careful monitoring of balance between glucose levels and insulin dosage	Goal: *promote normal balance of food and insulin:* **regular** insulin as ordered; IV saline, as ordered; bicarbonate and electrolyte replacements, as ordered; potassium replacements once therapy begins and urine output is adequate Goal: *health teaching:* diet instructions, desired effects and side effects of prescribed insulin or hypoglycemic agent (onset, peak, and duration of action); importance of recognizing signs of imbalance
Evaluation/outcome criteria	Adheres to diet and correct insulin dosage Adjusts dosage when activity is increased Glucose level: 80–120 mg/dL	Accepts prescribed diet Takes medication (correct dose and time) Serious complications avoided Glucose level: 80–120 mg/dL

ADULT

G. Evaluation/outcome criteria:

1. Optimal blood-glucose levels achieved.
2. Ideal weight maintained.
3. Adequate hydration.
4. Carries out self-care activities: blood testing, foot care, exchange diets, medication administration, exercise.
5. Recognizes and treats hyperglycemic or hypoglycemic reactions.
6. Seeks medical assistance appropriately.

II. NONKETOTIC HYPERGLYCEMIC HYPEROSMOLAR COMA (NKHHC): profound hyperglycemia and dehydration without ketosis or ketoacidosis; seen in type 2 diabetes; brought on by infection or illness. This condition may lead to impaired consciousness and seizures. The client is *critically ill.* Mortality rate is over 50%.

A. Pathophysiology: hyperglycemia greater than 1,000 mg/dL causes osmotic diuresis, depletion of extracellular fluid, and hyperosmolarity related to infection or another stressor as the precipitating factor. Client unable to replace fluid deficits with oral intake.

B. Risk factors:

1. Old age.
2. History of non–insulin-dependent diabetes.
3. Infections: pneumonia, pyelonephritis, pancreatitis, gram-negative infections.
4. Kidney failure: uremia and peritoneal dialysis or hemodialysis.
5. Shock:
   a. Lactic acidosis related to bicarbonate deficit.
   b. Myocardial infarction.
6. Hemorrhage:
   a. GI.
   b. Subdural.
   c. Arterial thrombosis.

7. Medications:
   a. Diuretics.
   b. Glucocorticoids.
8. Tube feedings.

C. Assessment:

1. *Subjective data:*
   a. Confusion.
   b. Lethargy.
2. *Objective data:*
   a. Nystagmus.
   b. Dehydration.
   c. Aphasia.
   d. Nuchal rigidity.
   e. Hyperreflexia.
   f. Laboratory data:
      (1) Blood glucose level greater than 1,000 mg/dL.
      (2) Serum sodium and chloride—normal to *elevated.*
      (3) BUN greater than 60 mg/dL (higher than in ketoacidosis because of more severe gluconeogenesis and dehydration).
      (4) Arterial pH—slightly *depressed.*

D. Analysis/nursing diagnosis:

1. *Risk for injury* related to hyperglycemia.
2. *Altered renal peripheral tissue perfusion* related to vascular collapse.
3. *Ineffective airway clearance* related to coma.

E. Nursing care plan/implementation:

1. Goal: *promote fluid and electrolyte balance.*
   a. IVs: fluids and electrolytes, sodium chloride solution used initially to combat dehydration. Rate of infusion will be determined by: BP assessment, cardiovascular status, balance between fluid input and output, and laboratory values.
   b. Monitor I&O because of the high volume of fluid replaced in the critical stage of this condition.
   c. Administer nursing care for the problem that precipitated this serious condition.
   d. *Diet:* Food by mouth when client is able.
2. Goal: *prevent complications.*
   a. Administer *regular* insulin (initial dose usually 5 to 15 units) and food, as ordered.
   b. Uncontrolled condition leads to: cardiovascular disease, renal failure, blindness, and diabetic gangrene.

F. Evaluation/outcome criteria:

1. Blood sugar returns to normal level of 80 to 120 mg/dL.
2. Client is alert to time, place, and person.
3. Primary medical problem resolved.
4. Client recognizes and reports signs of imbalance.

III. HYPERTHYROIDISM (also called *thyrotoxicosis; Graves' disease):* spectrum of symptoms of accelerated metabolism caused by excessive amounts of circulating thyroid hormone. *Graves' disease* is most common cause of hyperthyroidism. The three components of *Graves' disease* are: (1) *hyperthyroidism,* (2) *ophthalmopathy* (protrusion of the eyes), and (3) *skin lesions* (dermopathy). *Graves' disease* is triggered by: stress, smoking, radiation of the neck, some medications (interleukin-2), and infections. *Treatment* of hyperthyroidism is accomplished by antithyroid medications, radioactive iodine administration (capsule given once), or surgery. Clients may need to take supplemental thyroid hormone (levothyroxine) after treatment.

A. Pathophysiology: diffuse hyperplasia of thyroid gland → overproduction of thyroid hormone and increased blood serum levels. Hormone stimulates mitochondria to increase energy for cellular activities and heat production. As metabolic rate increases, fat reserves are utilized, despite increased appetite and food intake. Cardiac output is increased to meet increased tissue metabolic needs, and peripheral vasodilation occurs in response to increased heat production. Neuromuscular hyperactivity → accentuation of reflexes, anxiety, and increased alimentary tract mobility. *Graves' disease* is caused by stimulation of the gland by immunoglobulins of the IgG class.

B. Risk factors:

1. Possible autoimmune response resulting in increase of a gamma globulin called *long-acting thyroid stimulator* (LATS).
2. Occurs in third and fourth decade.
3. Affects women more than men.
4. Emotional trauma, infection, increased stress.
5. Overdose of medications used to treat hypothyroidism.
6. Use of certain weight-loss products.
7. Radiation of neck.

C. Assessment:

1. *Subjective data:*
   a. Nervousness, mood swings.
   b. Palpitations.
   c. Heat intolerance.
   d. Dyspnea.
   e. Weakness.
2. *Objective data:*
   a. *Eyes:* exophthalmos, characteristic stare, lid lag.
   b. *Skin:*
      (1) Warm, moist, velvety.
      (2) Increased sweating; increased melanin pigmentation.
      (3) Pretibial edema with thickened skin and hyperpigmentation.
   c. *Weight:* loss of weight *despite* increased appetite.

d. *Muscle:* weakness, tremors, hyperkinesia.
e. *Vital signs:* BP—*increased* systolic pressure, *widened pulse pressure*; *tachycardia.*
f. *Goiter:* thyroid gland noticeable and palpable.
g. *Gynecological:* abnormal menstruation.
h. GI: frequent bowel movements.
i. Activity pattern: overactivity leads to fatigue, which leads to depression, which stimulates client into overactivity, and pattern continues. *Danger:* total exhaustion.
j. Laboratory data:
   (1) *Elevated:* serum thyroxine (T_4) (>11 mcg/100 mL), free T_4 or free T_4 index, triiodothyronine (T_3) level (>35%) and free T_3 level.
   (2) *Elevated:* radioactive iodine uptake (RAIU) by thyroid.
   (3) *Elevated:* basal metabolic rate (BMR).
   (4) *Decreased:* WBC count caused by *decreased* granulocytosis (<4,500).

D. Analysis/nursing diagnosis:
1. *Altered nutrition, less than body requirements,* related to elevated basal metabolic rate.
2. *Risk for injury* related to exophthalmos and tremors.
3. *Activity intolerance* related to fatigue from overactivity.
4. *Fatigue* related to overactivity.
5. *Anxiety* related to tachycardia.
6. *Sleep pattern disturbance* related to excessive amounts of circulating thyroid hormone.

E. Nursing care plan/implementation:
1. Goal: *protect from stress:* private room, restrict visitors, quiet environment.
2. Goal: *promote physical and emotional equilibrium.*
   a. Environment: quiet, cool, well ventilated.
   b. Eye care:
      (1) Sunglasses to protect from photophobia, dust, wind.
      (2) Protective drops (methylcellulose) to soothe exposed cornea.

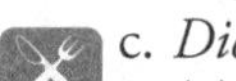

   c. *Diet:*
      (1) *High:* calorie, protein, vitamin B.
      (2) 6 meals/day, as needed.
      (3) Weigh daily.
      (4) *Avoid* stimulants (coffee, tea, colas, tobacco).
3. Goal: *prevent complications.*
   a. Medications as ordered:
      (1) Propylthiouracil to block thyroid synthesis; hyperthyroidism returns when therapy is stopped.
      (2) Methimazole (Tapazole) to inhibit synthesis of thyroid hormone.
      (3) Iodine preparations: used in combination with other medications when hyperthyroidism not well controlled; saturated solution of potassium iodide (SSKI) or *Lugol's* solution; more palatable if diluted with water, milk, or juice; give through a *straw* to prevent staining teeth. Takes 2 to 4 weeks before results are evident.
      (4) Propranolol (Inderal), atenolol (Tenormin), metoprolol (Lopressor) given to counteract the increased metabolic effect of thyroid hormones, but do not alter their levels. Relieve the symptoms of tachycardia, tremors, and anxiety.
   b. Monitor for *thyroid storm (crisis)*—**medical emergency:** acute episode of thyroid overactivity caused when increased amounts of thyroid hormone are released into the bloodstream and metabolism is markedly increased.
      (1) **Risk factors** for thyroid storm: client with uncontrolled hyperthyroidism (usually *Graves' disease*) who undergoes severe sudden stress, such as:
         (a) Infection.
         (b) Surgery.
         (c) Beginning labor to give birth.
         (d) Taking inadequate antithyroid medications before thyroidectomy.
      (2) **Assessment:**
         (a) *Subjective data*—thyroid storm:
            (i) Apprehension.
            (ii) Restlessness.
         (b) *Objective data*—thyroid storm:
            (i) *Vital signs: elevated* temperature (106°F), hypotension, *extreme* tachycardia.
            (ii) Marked respiratory distress, pulmonary edema.
            (iii) Weakness and delirium.
            (iv) **If untreated, client could die of heart failure.**
      (3) Medications—thyroid storm:
         (a) Propylthiouracil or methimazole (Tapazole) *to decrease synthesis of thyroid hormone.*
         (b) Sodium iodide IV; Lugol's solution orally *to facilitate thyroid hormone synthesis.*
         (c) Propranolol (Inderal) *to slow heart rate.*
         (d) Aspirin *to decrease temperature.*
         (e) Steroids *to combat crisis.*
         (f) Diuretics, digitalis *to treat heart failure.*
4. Goal: *health teaching.*
   a. Stress-reduction techniques.
   b. Importance of medications, their desired effects and side effects.

c. Methods to protect eyes from environmental damage.
d. Signs and symptoms of thyroid storm (see **E. 3. b.**).

5. Goal: *prepare for additional treatment as needed.*
   a. *Radioactive iodine therapy:* ^{131}I, a radioactive isotope of iodine to decrease thyroid activity.
      (1) ^{131}I dissolved in water and given by mouth.
      (2) Hospitalization necessary only when large dose is administered.
      (3) *Minimal precautions* needed for usual dose.
         (a) Sleep alone for several nights.
         (b) Flush toilet several times after use.
      (4) Effectiveness of therapy seen in 2 to 3 weeks; single dose controls 90% of clients.
      (5) Monitor for signs of hypothyroidism.
   b. Surgery (see **IV. THYROIDECTOMY,** following).

F. Evaluation/outcome criteria:
1. Complications avoided.
2. Compliance with medical regimen.
3. No further weight loss.
4. Able to obtain adequate sleep.

IV. THYROIDECTOMY: partial removal of thyroid gland (for hyperthyroidism) or total removal (for malignancy of thyroid).

A. Risk factor: unsuccessful medical treatment of hyperthyroidism.

B. Analysis/nursing diagnosis:
1. *Risk for injury* related to possible trauma to parathyroid gland during surgery.
2. *Ineffective breathing pattern* related to neck incision.
3. *Pain* related to surgical incision.
4. *Altered nutrition, less than body requirements,* related to difficulty in swallowing because of neck incision.
5. *Impaired verbal communication* related to possible trauma to nerve during surgery.
6. *Risk for altered body temperature* related to thyroid storm.

C. Nursing care plan/implementation: *Prepare for surgery* (see **I. THE PREOPERATIVE PREPARATION, pp. 365–367**). *Postoperative:*
1. Goal: *promote physical and emotional equilibrium.*
   a. *Position: semi-Fowler's* to reduce edema.
   b. *Immobilize* head with pillows/sandbags.
   c. Support head during position changes to *avoid* stress on sutures, *prevent flexion* or *hyperextension* of neck.
2. Goal: *prevent complications of hypocalcemia and tetany,* due to accidental trauma to parathyroid gland during surgery; signs of tetany indicate necessity of *calcium gluconate IV.*
   a. Check *Chvostek's sign*—tapping face in front of ear produces spasm of facial muscles.
   b. Check *Trousseau's sign*—compression of upper arm (usually with BP cuff) elicits carpal (wrist) spasm.
   c. Monitor for *respiratory distress* (due to laryngeal nerve injury, edema, bleeding); keep tracheostomy set/suction equipment at bedside.
   d. Monitor for elevated temperature, indicative of *thyroid storm* (see **Objective Assessment Data** for **Thyroid Storm, p. 472**).
   e. Monitor vital signs, check dressing and beneath head, shoulders for bleeding q1h and prn for 24 hours; *hemorrhage* is possible complication; if swallowing is difficult, loosen dressing. If client still complains of tightness when dressing is loosened, look for further signs of hemorrhage.
   f. Check voice postoperatively as soon as responsive after anesthesia and every hour (assess for possible *laryngeal nerve damage*); crowing voice sound indicates laryngeal nerves on both sides have been injured; *respiratory distress possible from swelling.*
      (1) *Avoid* unnecessary talking to lessen hoarseness.
      (2) Provide alternative means of communication.
3. Goal: *promote comfort measures.*
   a. *Narcotics* as ordered.
   b. Offer iced fluids.
   c. Ambulation and *soft diet,* as tolerated.
4. Goal: *health teaching.*
   a. How to support neck to prevent pressure on suture line: place both hands behind neck when moving head or coughing.
   b. Signs of hypothyroidism; needs supplemental thyroid hormone if total thyroidectomy.
   c. Signs and symptoms of hemorrhage and respiratory distress.
   d. Importance of adequate rest and nutritious diet.
   e. Importance of voice rest in early recuperative period.

D. Evaluation/outcome criteria:
1. No respiratory distress, hemorrhage, laryngeal damage, tetany.
2. Preoperative symptoms relieved.
3. Normal range of neck motion obtained.
4. States signs and symptoms of possible complications.

V. HYPOTHYROIDISM (MYXEDEMA): deficiency of circulating thyroid hormone; often a final consequence of *Hashimoto's thyroiditis* and *Graves' disease.*

A. Pathophysiology: atrophy, destruction of gland by endogenous antibodies or inadequate pituitary thyrotropin production → insidious slowing of body processes, personality changes, and generalized, interstitial nonpitting (mucinous) edema—myxedema; pronounced involvement in systems with high protein turnover (e.g., cardiac, GI, reproductive, hematopoietic).

B. Risk factors:

1. Total thyroidectomy; inadequate replacement therapy.
2. Inherited autosomal recessive gene coding for disorder.
3. Hypophyseal failure.
4. Dietary iodine deficiencies.
5. Irradiation of thyroid gland.
6. Overtreatment of hyperthyroidism.
7. Chronic lymphocytic thyroiditis.
8. Postpartum thyroiditis.
9. Viral thyroiditis.
10. Medications, such as amiodarone HCl (Cordarone), used to treat abnormal heart rhythms.

C. Assessment:

1. *Subjective data:*
   a. Weakness, fatigue, lethargy.
   b. Headache.
   c. Slow memory, psychotic behavior.
   d. Loss of interest in sexual activity.
2. *Objective data:*
   a. Depressed basal metabolic rate (BMR).
   b. Cardiomegaly, bradycardia, hypotension, anemia.
   c. Menorrhagia, amenorrhea, infertility.
   d. Dry skin, brittle nails, coarse hair, hair loss.
   e. Slow speech, hoarseness, thickened tongue.
   f. Weight gain: edema, generalized interstitial; peripheral nonpitting; periorbital puffiness.
   g. Intolerance to cold.
   h. Hypersensitive to narcotics and barbiturates.
   i. *Laboratory data:*
      (1) *Elevated:* thyroid-releasing hormone (TRH), thyroid-stimulating hormone (TSH), cholesterol (>220 mg/dL), lipids (>850 mg/dL), protein (>8 gm/dL).
      (2) *Normal-low:* serum thyroxine (T_4), serum triiodothyronine (T_3).
      (3) *Decreased:* radioactive iodine uptake (RAIU).

D. Analysis/nursing diagnosis:

1. *Risk for injury* related to hypersensitivity to drugs.
2. *Altered nutrition, more than body requirements,* related to decreased BMR.
3. *Activity intolerance* related to fatigue.
4. *Constipation* related to decreased peristalsis.
5. *Decreased cardiac output* related to hypotension and bradycardia.
6. *Risk for impaired skin integrity* related to dry skin and edema.
7. *Social isolation* related to lethargy.

E. Nursing care plan/implementation:

1. Goal: *provide for comfort and safety.*
   a. Monitor for infection or trauma; may precipitate *myxedema coma,* which is manifested by: unresponsiveness, bradycardia, hypoventilation, hypothermia, and hypotension.
   b. Provide warmth; prevent heat loss and vascular collapse.
   c. Administer thyroid medications as ordered: levothyroxine (Synthroid)—most common drug used; liothyronine sodium (Cytomel); dosage adjusted according to symptoms.
2. Goal: *health teaching.*
   a. *Diet: low* calorie, *high* protein.
   b. Signs and symptoms of hypothyroidism and hyperthyroidism.
   c. Lifelong medications, dosage, desired effects and side effects.
   d. Medication dosage adjustment: *take one third to one half the usual dose of narcotics and barbiturates.*
   e. Stress-management techniques.
   f. Exercise program.

F. Evaluation/outcome criteria:

1. No complications noted. Most common complications: atherosclerotic coronary heart disease, acute organic psychosis, and myxedema coma.
2. Dietary instructions followed.
3. Medication regimen followed.
4. Thyroid hormone balance obtained and maintained.

VI. CUSHING'S DISEASE: an endogenous overproduction of adrenocorticotropic hormone (ACTH) that can be caused by pituitary-dependent adenomas. **Cushing's syndrome:** condition marked by chronic excessive circulating cortisol with or without pituitary involvement. One of the most common causes of Cushing's syndrome is the administration of cortisone-like medications for treatment of a variety of conditions.

A. Pathophysiology:

1. Excess glucocorticoid production, leading to:
   a. *Increased* gluconeogenesis → raised serum glucose levels → glucose in urine, increased fat deposits in face and trunk.
   b. *Decreased* amino acids → protein deficiencies, muscle wasting, poor antibody response, and lack of collagen.

ADULT

B. Risk factors:
1. Adrenal hyperplasia.
2. Excessive hypothalamic stimulation.
3. Tumors: adrenal, hypophyseal, pituitary, bronchogenic, or gallbladder.
4. Excessive steroid therapy.

C. Assessment:
1. *Subjective data:*
   a. Headache, backache.
   b. Weakness, decreased work capacity.
   c. Mood swings.
2. *Objective data:*
   a. Hypertension, weight gain, pitting edema.
   b. Characteristic fat deposits, truncal and cervical obesity (*buffalo hump*).
   c. Pendulous abdomen, purple striae, easy bruising.
   d. Moon facies, acne.
   e. Hyperpigmentation.
   f. Impotence.
   g. Virilization in women: hirsutism, breast atrophy, and amenorrhea.
   h. Pathological fractures, reduced height.
   i. Slow wound healing.
   j. Laboratory data:
      (1) Urine: *elevated* 17-ketosteroids (>12 mg/24 hr) and glucose (>120 mg/dL).
      (2) Plasma: *elevated* 17-hydroxycorticosteroids, cortisol (>10 mcg/dL). Cortisol *does not decrease during the day* as it should.
      (3) Serum: *elevated*—glucose, RBC, WBC counts; *diminished*—potassium, chlorides, eosinophils, lymphocytes.
   k. X-rays and scans to determine tumors metastasis.

D. Analysis/nursing diagnosis:
1. *Body image disturbance* related to changes in physical appearance.
2. *Activity intolerance* related to backache and weakness.
3. *Risk for injury* related to infection and bleeding.
4. *Knowledge deficit* (learning need) related to management of disease.
5. *Pain* related to headache.

E. Nursing care plan/implementation:
1. Goal: *promote comfort.*
   a. Assist with preparation of diagnostic work-up.
   b. Explain procedures.
   c. Protect from trauma.
2. Goal: *prevent complications;* monitor for:
   a. Fluid balance—I&O, daily weights.
   b. Glucose metabolism—blood, urine for sugar and acetone.
   c. Hypertension—vital signs.
   d. Infection—skin care, urinary tract; check temperature.
   e. Mood swings—observe behavior.
3. Goal: *health teaching.*

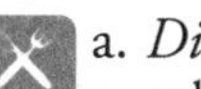

   a. *Diet: increased* protein, potassium; *decreased* calories, sodium.

   b. Medications:
      (1) *Cytotoxic agents:* aminoglutethimide (Cytadren), trilostane (Modrastane), mitotane (Lysodren)—to decrease cortisol production.
      (2) *Replacement hormones* as needed.
   c. Signs and symptoms of progression of disease as noted in assessment.
   d. Preparation for adrenalectomy if medical regimen unsuccessful.

F. Evaluation/outcome criteria:
1. Symptoms controlled by medication.
2. No complications—adrenal steroids within normal limits.
3. If adrenalectomy necessary, see **VIII. ADRENALECTOMY**.

VII. PHEOCHROMOCYTOMA: a rare, typically benign neuroendocrine tumor of the adrenal medulla. Appears to have a familial basis; common in middle age—rare after 60 years.

A. Pathophysiology: catecholamine-secreting tumor → increased epinephrine and norepinephrine (paroxysm) → hypertensive retinopathy and nephropathy, myocarditis → cerebral hemorrhage and cardiac failure.

B. Risk factors for paroxysm:
1. Voiding.
2. Smoking.
3. Drugs (i.e., histamine, anesthesia, atropine, steroids, fentanyl).
4. Bending, straining, exercising (displacing abdominal organs) → increased abdominal pressure.

C. Assessment:
1. *Subjective data:*
   a. Apprehension.
   b. Pounding headache.
   c. Nausea.
   d. Pain with vomiting.
   e. Visual disturbances.
   f. Palpitations.
   g. Heat intolerance.
2. *Objective data:*
   a. Hypertension: rapid onset, abrupt cessation; postural hypotension.
   b. Profuse diaphoresis with acute attack.
   c. Pulse: rapid, dysrhythmia.
   d. Pupils: dilated.
   e. Extremities: cold, tremors.

f. Laboratory data:
   (1) Hyperglycemia, glycosuria.
   (2) ↑ Urinary catecholamines: single-voided, 2- to 4-hour specimen and 24-hour urine, greater than 14 mg/100 mL.
   (3) Direct assay of catecholamines—epinephrine greater than 0.2 mg/L; norepinephrine 0.5 mg/L.
   (4) ↑ BMR.

g. X-ray, CT, and MRI—used to localize tumor before surgery.

D. Analysis/nursing diagnosis:

1. *Anxiety* related to excessive physiological stimulation of sympathetic nervous system.
2. *Fluid volume deficit* related to excessive gastric losses, hypermetabolic state, diaphoresis.
3. *Risk for decreased cardiac output* related to excessive secretion of catecholamines as evidenced by hypertension.
4. *Risk for injury* related to excessive release of epinephrine and norepinephrine.
5. *Altered nutrition, greater than body requirements,* related to elevated glucose.

E. Nursing care plan/implementation:

1. Goal: *prevent paroxysmal hypertension.*
   a. Rest: reduce stress, ↓ environmental stimulation.
   b. Give *sedatives, alpha-adrenergic blocker* (phenoxybenzamine) for hypertension and *antidysrhythmics* as ordered.
   c. Diet: *high* vitamin, *high* calorie, mineral, calcium; *restrict* caffeine.
   d. Monitor vital signs (especially BP in sitting and supine positions).
2. Goal: *prepare for surgical removal of tumor* (see **VIII. ADRENALECTOMY**, following).

F. Evaluation/outcome criteria:

1. No paroxysmal hypertension.
2. See **VIII. ADRENALECTOMY.**

VIII. ADRENALECTOMY: surgical removal of adrenal glands because of tumors or uncontrolled overactivity; also bilateral adrenalectomy may be performed to control metastatic breast or prostate cancer.

A. Risk factors:

1. Pheochromocytoma.
2. Adrenal hyperplasia.
3. Cushing's syndrome.
4. Metastasis of prostate or breast cancer.
5. Adrenal cortex or medulla tumors.

B. Assessment:

1. *Objective data:* validated evidence of:
   a. Benign lesion (unilateral adrenalectomy) or malignant tumor (bilateral adrenalectomy).
   b. Adrenal hyperfunction that cannot be managed medically.
   c. Bilateral excision for metastasis of breast and sometimes metastasis of prostate cancer.

C. Analysis/nursing diagnosis:

1. *Knowledge deficit* (learning need) related to planned surgery.
2. *Risk for physical injury* related to hormone imbalance.
3. *Risk for decreased cardiac output* related to possible hypotensive state resulting from surgery.
4. *Risk for infection* related to decreased normal resistance.
5. *Altered health maintenance* related to need for self-administration of steroid medications, orally or by injection.

D. Nursing care plan/implementation:

1. Goal: *preoperative: reduce risk of postoperative complications.*
   a. Prescribed *steroid* therapy, given 1 week before surgery, is gradually decreased; will be given again postoperatively.
   b. *Antihypertensive* drugs are *discontinued* because surgery may result in severe hypotension.
   c. *Sedation* as ordered.
   d. General preoperative measures (see **I. PREOPERATIVE PREPARATION, pp. 365–367**).
2. Goal: *postoperative: promote hormonal balance.*
   a. Administer *hydrocortisone* parenteral therapy as ordered; rate indicated by fluid and electrolyte balance, blood sugar, and blood pressure.
   b. Monitor for signs of *addisonian (adrenal) crisis* (see **IX. ADDISON'S DISEASE, p. 477**).
3. Goal: *prevent postoperative complications.*
   a. Monitor vital signs until stability is regained; if on *vasopressor* drugs such as metaraminol (Aramine):
      (1) Maintain flow rate as ordered.
      (2) Monitor BP q5–15 min, notify physician of significant elevations in BP (dose needs to be *decreased*) or drop in BP (dose needs to be *increased*). *Note:* readings that are normotensive for some may be hypotensive for clients who have been hypertensive.
   b. NPO—attach *nasogastric tube* to intermittent suction; abdominal distention is common side effect of this surgery.
   c. Respiratory care:
      (1) Turn, cough, and deep breathe.
      (2) Splint flank incision when coughing.
      (3) Administer *narcotics* to reduce pain and allow client to cough; flank incision is close to diaphragm, making coughing very painful.

(4) Auscultate breath sounds q2h; decreased or absent sounds could indicate *pneumothorax.*
(5) Sudden chest pain and dyspnea should be reported ***immediately*** (*spontaneous pneumothorax*).

d. *Position: flat* or *semi*-Fowler's.
e. Mouth care.
f. Monitor dressings for bleeding; reinforce prn.
g. Ambulation, as ordered.
(1) Check BP q15 min when ambulation is first attempted.
(2) Place elastic stockings on lower extremities to enhance stability of vascular system.
h. *Diet*—once NG tube removed, diet as tolerated.

4. Goal: *health teaching.*
a. *Signs and symptoms of adrenal crisis:*
(1) Pulse: rapid, weak, or thready.
(2) Temperature: elevated.
(3) Severe weakness and hypotension.
(4) Headache.
(5) Convulsions, coma.
b. Importance of maintaining steroid therapy schedule to ensure therapeutic serum level.
c. Weigh daily.
d. Monitor blood glucose levels daily.
e. Report undesirable side effects of steroid therapy or adrenal crisis to physician.
f. *Avoid* persons with infections, due to decreased resistance.
g. Daily schedule: include adequate rest, moderate exercise, good nutrition.

E. Evaluation/outcome criteria:

1. Adrenal crisis avoided.
a. Vital signs within normal limits.
b. No neurological deficits noted.
2. Healing progresses: no signs of infection or wound complications.
3. Adjusts to alterations in physical status.
a. Complies with medication regimen.
b. Avoids infections.
c. Incorporates good nutrition, periods of rest and activity into daily schedule.

IX. ADDISON'S DISEASE: chronic primary adrenal corticotropic insufficiency. A hormonal (endocrine) disorder involving destruction of the adrenal glands, which then are unable to produce sufficient adrenal hormones (cortisol) necessary for the normal body functions.

A. Pathophysiology:

1. Atrophy of adrenal gland is most common cause of adrenal insufficiency; manifested by *decreased* adrenal cortical secretions.
a. Deficiency in mineralocorticoid secretion (*aldosterone*) → increased sodium excretion → dehydration → hypotension → decreased cardiac output and resulting decrease in heart size.
b. Deficiency in glucocorticoid secretion (*cortisol*) → decrease in gluconeogenesis → hypoglycemia and liver glycogen deficiency, emotional disturbances, diminished resistance to stress. Cortisol deficiency → failure to inhibit anterior pituitary secretion of ACTH and melanocyte-stimulating hormone → increased levels of ACTH and hyperpigmentation.
c. Deficiency in androgen hormone → less axillary and pubic hair in women (testes supply adequate sex hormone in men, so no symptoms are produced).

B. Risk factors:

1. Autoimmune processes.
2. Infection.
3. Malignancy.
4. Vascular obstruction.
5. Bleeding.
6. Environmental hazards.
7. Congenital defects.
8. Bilateral adrenalectomy.
9. Tuberculosis.

C. Assessment:

1. *Subjective data:*
a. Muscle weakness, fatigue, lethargy.
b. Dizziness, fainting.
c. Nausea, food idiosyncrasies, anorexia.
d. Abdominal pain/cramps.
2. *Objective data:*
a. *Vital signs: decreased BP*, orthostatic hypotension, *widened* pulse pressure.
b. Pulse—*increased*, collapsing, irregular.
c. Temperature—*subnormal.*
d. Vomiting, diarrhea, and weight loss.
e. Tremors.
f. Skin: poor turgor, excessive pigmentation (*bronze tone*).
g. Laboratory data:
(1) Blood:
(a) *Decreased:* sodium (<135 mEq/L); glucose (<60 mg/dL), chloride (<98 mEq/L), bicarbonate (<23 mEq/L).
(b) *Increased:* hematocrit, potassium (>5 mEq/L).
(2) Urine: *decreased* (or absent) 17-ketosteroids, 17-hydroxycorticosteroids (<5 mg/24 hr).
h. *Diagnostic tests:*
(1) CT scan, MRI.
(2) ACTH stimulation test (cortisol levels are measured *before* and *after* administration of synthetic ACTH).

ADULT

D. Analysis/nursing diagnosis:

1. *Fluid volume deficit* related to decreased sodium.
2. *Altered renal tissue perfusion* related to hypotension.
3. *Decreased cardiac output* related to aldosterone deficiency.
4. *Risk for infection* related to cortisol deficiency.
5. *Activity intolerance* related to muscle weakness and fatigue.
6. *Altered nutrition, less than body requirements,* related to nausea, anorexia, and vomiting.

E. Nursing care plan/implementation:

1. Goal: *decrease stress.*
   a. Environment: quiet, nondemanding schedule.
   b. Anticipate events for which extra resources will be necessary.
2. Goal: *promote adequate nutrition.*
   a. *Diet: acute phase—high* sodium, *low* potassium; *nonacute phase—increase* carbohydrates and protein.
   b. *Fluids: force,* to balance fluid losses; monitor I&O, daily weights.
   c. Administer lifelong exogenous replacement therapy as ordered:
      (1) *Glucocorticoids*—prednisone, hydrocortisone.
      (2) *Mineralocorticoids*—fludrocortisone (Florinef).
3. Goal: *health teaching.*
   a. Take medications *with* food or milk.
   b. May need antacid therapy to prevent GI disturbances.
   c. Side effects of steroid therapy.
   d. *Avoid* stress; may need adjustment in medication dosage when stress is increased.
   e. Signs and symptoms of *addisonian (adrenal) crisis:* very serious condition characterized by severe hypotension, shock, coma, and vasomotor collapse related to strenuous activity, infection, stress, omission of prescribed medications. **If untreated, could quickly lead to death.**
4. Goal: *prevent serious complications if addisonian crisis evident.*
   a. Complete bedrest; *avoid* stimuli.
   b. High dose of hydrocortisone IV or cortisone IM.
   c. Treat shock—IV saline.
   d. I&O, vital signs q15 min to 1 hour or prn until crisis passes.

F. Evaluation/outcome criteria:

1. No complications occur.
2. Medication regimen followed, is adequate for client's needs.
3. Adequate nutrition and fluid balance obtained.

ADULT

HEMATOLOGICAL SYSTEM

I. IRON-DEFICIENCY ANEMIA (hypochromic microcytic anemia): inadequate production of red blood cells due to lack of heme (iron); common in infants, women who are pregnant and premenopausal.

A. Pathophysiology: decreased dietary intake, impaired absorption, or increased utilization of iron decreases the amount of iron bound to plasma transferrin and transported to bone marrow for hemoglobin synthesis; decreased hemoglobin in erythrocytes decreases amount of oxygen delivered to tissues.

B. Risk factors:

1. *Excessive menstruation.*
2. *Gastrointestinal bleeding*—peptic ulcer, hookworm, tumors.
3. *Inadequate diet*—anorexia, fad diets, cultural practices.
4. *Poor absorption*—stomach, small intestine disease.

C. Assessment:

1. *Subjective data:*
   a. Fatigue: increasing.
   b. Headache.
   c. Change in appetite; difficulty swallowing due to pharyngeal edema/ulceration; heartburn.
   d. Shortness of breath on exercise.
   e. Extremities: numbness, tingling.
   f. Flatulence.
   g. Menorrhagia.
2. *Objective data:*
   a. *Vital signs:*
      (1) *BP—increased* systolic, widened pulse pressure.
      (2) *Pulse*—tachycardia.
      (3) *Respirations*—tachypnea.
      (4) *Temperature*—normal or subnormal.
   b. Skin/mucous membranes: pale, dry; tongue—smooth, shiny, bright red; cheilosis (cracked, painful corners of mouth).
   c. Sclerae: pearly white.
   d. Nails: brittle, spoon shaped, flattened.
   e. Laboratory data: *decreased*—hemoglobin (<10 g/dL blood), serum iron (<65 mcg/dL blood); *increased* total iron-binding capacity.

D. Analysis/nursing diagnosis:

1. *Altered nutrition, less than body requirements,* related to inadequate iron absorption.
2. *Altered tissue perfusion* related to reduction in red cells.

3. *Risk for activity intolerance* related to profound weakness.
4. *Impaired gas exchange* related to decreased oxygen-carrying capacity.

E. Nursing care plan/implementation:

1. Goal: *promote physical and mental equilibrium.*
   a. *Position:* optimal for respiratory excursion; deep breathing; turn frequently to prevent skin breakdown.
   b. Rest: balance with activity, as tolerated; assist with ambulation.
   c. Medication (*hematinics*):
      (1) Oral iron therapy (ferrous sulfate)—give *with* meals.
      (2) Intramuscular therapy (iron dextran)—use second needle for injection after withdrawal from ampule; use *Z-track method:* inject 0.5 mL of air before withdrawing needle, to prevent tissue necrosis; use 2- to 3-inch needle; rotate sites; do *not* rub site or allow wearing of constricting garments after injection.
   d. Keep warm: *no* hot water bottles, heating pads, due to decreased sensitivity.
   e. *Diet: high* in protein, iron, vitamins (see **Chapter 9**); assistance with feeding, if needed; nonirritating foods with mouth or tongue soreness.
2. Goal: *health teaching.*
   a. Dietary regimen.
   b. Iron therapy: explain purpose, dosage, side effects (black or green stools, constipation, diarrhea); take *with* meals.
   c. Activity: exercise to tolerance, with planned rest periods.

F. Evaluation/outcome criteria:

1. Hemoglobin and hematocrit levels return to normal range.
2. Tolerates activity without fatigue.
3. Selects foods appropriate for dietary regimen.

II. HEMOLYTIC ANEMIA (normocytic normochromic anemia): premature destruction (hemolysis) of erythrocytes; occurs extravascularly (autoimmune) or intravascularly (dialysis, heart valves).

A. Risk factors—autoimmune hemolytic anemia:

1. *Warm reacting* (idiopathic): women, lupus, rheumatoid arthritis, myeloma.
2. *Cold reacting* (e.g., Raynaud's): older women, Epstein-Barr virus.
3. *Drug induced:* methyldopa, penicillin, quinine.

B. Assessment:

1. *Subjective data:*
   a. Fatigue; physical weakness.
   b. Dizziness.
   c. Shortness of breath.
   d. Diaphoresis on slight exertion.
2. *Objective data:*
   a. Skin: pallor, jaundice.
   b. Posture: drooping.
   c. Laboratory data:
      (1) *Decreased* hematocrit.
      (2) *Increased* reticulocyte count; bilirubin.
      (3) Direct Coombs' test *positive.*

C. See **I. IRON-DEFICIENCY ANEMIA** for **Analysis/nursing diagnosis, Nursing care plan/implementation,** and **Evaluation/outcome criteria.**

III. PERNICIOUS ANEMIA (megaloblastic macrocytic anemia) lack of intrinsic factor found in gastric mucosa, which is necessary for vitamin B_{12} (extrinsic factor) absorption; slow developing, usually after age 50; may be an autoimmune disorder.

A. Pathophysiology: atrophy or surgical removal of glandular mucosa in fundus of stomach → degenerative changes in brain, spinal cord, and peripheral nerves from lack of vitamin B_{12}.

B. Risk factors:

1. Partial or complete gastric resection.
2. Prolonged iron deficiency; veganism.
3. Heredity.

C. Assessment:

1. *Subjective data:*
   a. Hands, feet: tingling, numbness.
   b. Weakness, fatigue.
   c. Sore tongue, anorexia.
   d. Difficulties with memory, balance.
   e. Irritability, mild depression.
   f. Shortness of breath.
   g. Palpitations.
2. *Objective data:*
   a. Skin: pale, flabby, jaundiced.
   b. Sclerae: icterus (yellow).
   c. Tongue: smooth, glossy, red, swollen.
   d. *Vital signs:*
      (1) *BP*—normal or elevated.
      (2) *Pulse*—tachycardia.
   e. Nervous system:
      (1) Decreased vibratory sense in lower extremities.
      (2) Loss of coordination.
      (3) *Babinski reflex* present (flaring of toes with stimulation of sole of foot).
      (4) Positive *Romberg's sign* (loses balance when eyes closed).
      (5) Increased or diminished reflexes.
   f. Laboratory data: *decreased*—hemoglobin, RBCs, platelets, gastric secretions (achlorhydria); *Schilling test* (radioactive vitamin B_{12} urine test).

ADULT

D. Analysis/nursing diagnosis:
1. *Altered nutrition, less than body requirements,* related to B_{12} deficiency.
2. *Impaired physical mobility* related to numbness of extremities.
3. *Fatigue* related to decreased oxygen-carrying capacity.
4. *Altered oral mucous membrane* related to changes in gastric mucosa.
5. *Altered thought processes* related to progressive neurological degeneration.

E. Nursing care plan/implementation:
1. *Goal: promote physical and emotional comfort.*
   a. Activity: bedrest or activity as tolerated—restrictions depend on neurological or cardiac involvement.
   b. Comfort: keep extremities warm—light blankets, loose-fitting socks.

   c. Medication: vitamin B_{12} therapy as ordered.
   d. *Diet:*
      (1) Six small feedings.
      (2) *Soft* or *pureed.*
      (3) Organ meats, fish, eggs.
   e. Mouth care: before and after meals, to increase appetite and relieve mouth discomfort.
2. Goal: *health teaching.*
   a. Medication:
      (1) Lifelong therapy.
      (2) Injection techniques; rotation of sites.
   b. Diet.
   c. Rest; exercise to tolerance.

F. Evaluation/outcome criteria:
1. No irreversible neurological or cardiac complications.
2. Takes vitamin B_{12} for the rest of life—uses safe injection technique.
3. Returns for follow-up care.

IV. POLYCYTHEMIA VERA: abnormal increase in circulating red blood cells (myeloproliferative disorder); considered to be a form of malignancy; occurs more frequently among middle-aged Jewish men.

A. Pathophysiology: unknown causes → massive increases of erythrocytes, myelocytes (bone marrow leukocytes), and thrombocytes → increased blood viscosity/volume and tissue/organ congestion; increased peripheral vascular resistance; intravascular thrombosis usually develops in middle age, particularly in Jewish men; in contrast, *secondary* polycythemia occurs as a compensatory response to tissue hypoxia associated with prolonged exposure to high altitude, chronic lung disease, and heart disease.

B. Assessment:
1. *Subjective data:*
   a. Headache; dizziness; ringing in ears.
   b. Weakness; loss of interest.
   c. Feelings of abdominal fullness.
   d. Shortness of breath; orthopnea.
   e. Pruritus, especially after bathing.
   f. Pain: gouty-arthritic.
2. *Objective data:*
   a. Skin: mucosal erythema, ruddy complexion (reddish purple).
   b. Ecchymosis; gingival (gum) bleeding.
   c. Enlarged liver, spleen.
   d. Hypertension.
   e. Laboratory data:
      (1) *Increased*—hemoglobin, hematocrit, RBCs, leukocytes, platelets, uric acid.
      (2) *Decreased* bone marrow iron.

C. Analysis/nursing diagnosis:
1. *Altered tissue perfusion* related to capillary congestion.
2. *Risk for injury* related to dizziness, weakness.
3. *Fluid volume excess* related to mass production of red blood cells.
4. *Risk for impaired skin integrity* related to pruritus.
5. *Ineffective breathing pattern* related to shortness of breath, orthopnea.

D. Nursing care plan/implementation:
1. Goal: *promote comfort and prevent complications.*
   a. Observe for signs of bleeding, thrombosis—stools, urine, gums, skin, ecchymosis.
   b. Reduce occurrence: *avoid* prolonged sitting, knee gatch.
   c. Assist with ambulation.
   d. *Position: elevate* head of bed.
   e. Skin care: cool-water baths to decrease pruritus; may add bicarbonate of soda to water.
   f. Fluids: *force,* to reduce blood viscosity and promote urine excretion; 1,500 to 2,500 mL/24 hr.
   g. *Diet: avoid* foods high in iron, to reduce RBC production.
   h. Assist with venesection (phlebotomy), as ordered; 350 to 500 mL blood every other day until Hct low-normal.
2. Goal: *health teaching.*
   a. *Diet:* foods to *avoid* (e.g., liver, egg yolks); fluids to be *increased.*
   b. Signs/symptoms of complications: infections, hemorrhage.
   c. *Avoid:* falls, bumps; hot baths/showers (worsens pruritus).
   d. Drugs: *myelosuppressive* agents (busulfan [Myleran], cyclophosphamide [Cytoxan], chlorambucil, radioactive phosphorus); purpose; side effects.
   e. Procedures: venesection (phlebotomy) if ordered.

E. Evaluation/outcome criteria:
1. Acceptance of chronic disease.
2. Reports at prescribed intervals for follow-up.
3. Remission: reduction of bone marrow activity, blood volume and viscosity (RBC count <6,500,000/mm^3; hemoglobin (Hgb) <18 g/dL; Hct <45%; WBC <10,000/mm^3).
4. No complications (e.g., thrombi, hemorrhage, gout, CHF, leukemia).

V. LEUKEMIA (ACUTE AND CHRONIC): a neoplastic disease involving the leukopoietic tissue in either the bone marrow or lymphoid areas; acute leukemia occurs in children, young adults; chronic forms occur in later adult life.

A. Types:
1. *Acute nonlymphocytic (ANLL)*—also known as acute myelogenous leukemia (AML); seen generally in older age (>60 years).
2. *Acute lymphocytic (ALL)*—common in children 2 to 10 years.
3. *Chronic lymphocytic (CLL)*—generally affects the elderly.
4. *Chronic myelogenous (CML)*—also known as chronic granulocytic leukemia (CGL); more likely to occur between 25 and 60 years.

B. Pathophysiology: displacement of normal marrow cells by proliferating leukemic cells (abnormal, immature leukocytes) → normochromic anemia, thrombocytopenia.

C. Risk factors:
1. Viruses.
2. Genetic abnormalities.
3. Exposure to chemicals.
4. Radiation.
5. Treatment for other types of cancer (e.g., alkylating agents).

D. Assessment:
1. *Subjective data:*
   a. Fatigue, weakness.
   b. Anorexia, nausea.
   c. *Pain:* joints, bones (acute leukemia).
   d. Night sweats, weight loss, malaise.
2. *Objective data:*
   a. Skin: pallor due to anemia; jaundice.
   b. Fever: frequent infections; mouth ulcers.
   c. Bleeding: petechiae, purpura, ecchymosis, epistaxis, gingiva.
   d. Organ enlargement: spleen, liver.
   e. Enlarged lymph nodes; tenderness.
   f. Bone marrow aspiration: increased presence of blasts.
   g. Laboratory data:
      (1) WBC count—abnormally low (<1,000/mm^3) or extremely high (>200,000/mm^3); differential is important.
      (2) RBC count—normal to severely *decreased.*
      (3) Hgb—low or normal.
      (4) Platelets—usually low.

E. Analysis/nursing diagnosis:
1. *Risk for infection* related to immature or abnormal leukocytes.
2. *Activity intolerance* related to hypoxia and weakness.
3. *Fatigue* related to anemia.
4. *Altered tissue perfusion* related to anemia.
5. *Anxiety* related to diagnosis and treatment.
6. *Altered oral mucous membrane* related to susceptibility to infection.
7. *Fear* related to diagnosis.
8. *Ineffective individual or family coping* related to potentially fatal disease.

F. Nursing care plan/implementation:
1. Goal: *prevent, control, and treat infection.*
   a. *Protective isolation* if indicated.
   b. Observe for early signs of infection:
      (1) Inflammation at injection sites.
      (2) Vital sign changes.
      (3) Cough.
      (4) Obtain cultures.
   c. Give *antibiotics* as ordered.
   d. Mouth care: clean q2h, examine for new lesions, *avoid* trauma.
2. Goal: *assess and control bleeding, anemia.*
   a. Activity: *restrict,* to prevent trauma.
   b. Observe for hemorrhage: vital signs; body orifices, stool, urine.
   c. Control localized bleeding: ice, pressure at least 3 to 4 minutes after needle sticks, positioning.
   d. Use soft-bristle or foam-rubber toothbrush to prevent gingival bleeding.
   e. Give blood/blood components as ordered; observe for transfusion reactions.
3. Goal: *provide rest, comfort, nutrition.*
   a. Activity: 8 hours sleep or rest; daily nap.
   b. Comfort measures: flotation mattress, bed cradle, sheepskin.
   c. *Analgesics:* without delay.
      (1) Mild pain (acetaminophen [Tylenol], tramadol 50 mg without aspirin).
      (2) Severe pain (codeine, meperidine HCl [Demerol]).
   d. *Diet:* bland.
      (1) *High* in protein, minerals, vitamins.
      (2) *Low* roughage.
      (3) Small, frequent feedings.
      (4) Favorite foods.
   e. Fluids: 3,000 to 4,000 mL/day.

4. Goal: *reduce side effects from therapeutic regimen.*
   a. Nausea: *antiemetics,* usually half-hour *before* chemotherapy.
   b. *Increased* uric acid level: force fluids.
   c. Stomatitis: *antiseptic anesthetic* mouthwashes.
   d. Rectal irritation: meticulous toileting, sitz baths, topical relief (e.g., Tucks).
5. Goal: *provide emotional/spiritual support.*
   a. Contact clergy if client desires.
   b. Allow, encourage client-initiated discussion of death (developmentally appropriate).
   c. Allow family to be involved in care.
   d. If death occurs, provide privacy for family, listening, sharing of grief.
6. Goal: *health teaching.*
   a. Prevent infection.
   b. Limit activity.
   c. Control bleeding.
   d. Reduce nausea.
   e. Mouth care.
   f. Chemotherapy: regimen; side effects.

G. Evaluation/outcome criteria:

1. Alleviate symptoms; obtain remission.
2. Prevent complications (e.g., infection).
3. Ventilates emotions—accepts and deals with anger.
4. Experiences peaceful death (e.g., pain free).

VI. IDIOPATHIC THROMBOCYTOPENIC PURPURA (ITP): potentially fatal disorder characterized by spontaneous increase in platelet destruction; possible autoimmune response; seen predominantly in 2- to 4-year-olds and girls/women ≥10 years old. Remissions occur spontaneously or following splenectomy; in contrast, *secondary thrombocytopenia* (STP) is caused by viral infections, drug hypersensitivity (i.e., *quinidine, sulfonamides*), lupus, or bone marrow failure; treat cause.

A. Assessment:

1. *Subjective data:*
   a. Spontaneous skin hemorrhages—lower extremities.
   b. Menorrhagia.
   c. Epistaxis.
2. *Objective data:*
   a. Bleeding: GI, urinary, nasal; following minor trauma, dental extractions.
   b. Petechiae; ecchymosis.
   c. *Tourniquet test*—positive, demonstrating increased capillary fragility.
   d. Laboratory data:
      (1) *Decreased* platelets (<100,000/mm³).
      (2) *Increased* bleeding time.

B. Analysis/nursing diagnosis:

1. *Risk for injury* related to hemorrhage.
2. *Altered tissue perfusion* related to fragile capillaries.
3. *Impaired skin integrity* related to skin hemorrhages.

C. Nursing care plan/implementation:

1. Goal: *prevent complications from bleeding tendencies.*
   a. *Precautions:*
      (1) Injections—use small-bore needles; rotate sites; apply direct pressure.
      (2) *Avoid* bumping, trauma.
      (3) Use swabs for mouth care.
   b. Observe for signs of bleeding, petechiae following blood pressure reading, ecchymosis, purpura.
   c. Administer *steroids* (e.g., prednisone) with ITP to increase platelet count; give platelets for count below 20,000 to 30,000/mm³ with STP; high-dose *immunoglobulins.*
2. Goal: *health teaching.*
   a. *Avoid* traumatic activities:
      (1) Contact sports.
      (2) Violent sneezing, coughing, nose blowing.
      (3) Straining at stool.
      (4) Heavy lifting.
   b. *Signs of decreased platelets*—petechiae, ecchymosis, gingival bleeding, hematuria, menorrhagia.
   c. Use Medic Alert tag/card.
   d. *Precautions:* self-medication; particularly *avoid* aspirin-containing drugs.
   e. Prepare for splenectomy if drug therapy unsuccessful (prednisone, cyclophosphamide, azathioprine [Imuran]).

D. Evaluation/outcome criteria:

1. Returns for follow-up.
2. No complications (e.g., intracranial hemorrhage).
3. Platelet count greater than 200,000/mm³.
4. Skin remains intact.
5. Resumes self-care activities.

VII. SPLENECTOMY: removal of spleen following rupture due to acquired hemolytic anemia, trauma, tumor, or idiopathic thrombocytopenic purpura.

A. Analysis/nursing diagnosis:

1. *Risk for fluid volume deficit* related to hemorrhage.
2. *Risk for infection* related to impaired immune response.
3. *Pain* related to abdominal distention.
4. *Ineffective breathing pattern* related to high abdominal incision.

B. Nursing care plan/implementation:

1. Goal: *prepare for surgery.*
   a. Give whole blood, as ordered.
   b. Insert nasogastric tube to decrease postoperative abdominal distention, as ordered.
2. Goal: *prevent postoperative complications.*
   a. Observe for:
      (1) *Hemorrhage*—bleeding tendency with thrombocytopenia due to decreased platelet count.

(2) *Gastrointestinal distention*—removal of enlarged spleen may result in distended stomach and intestines, to fill void.

b. Recognize 101°F temperature as normal for 10 days.

c. Incision: splint when coughing, to prevent high incidence of atelectasis (common complication), pneumonia with upper abdominal incision.

3. Goal: *health teaching.*
   a. Increased risk of infection postsplenectomy.
   b. Report signs of infection immediately.

C. Evaluation/outcome criteria:

1. No complications (e.g., respiratory, subphrenic abscess or hematoma, thromboemboli, infection).
2. Complete and permanent remission—occurs in 60% to 80% of clients.

IMMUNOLOGICAL SYSTEM

I. LYME DISEASE: a spirochetal illness (syndrome); most common tick-borne infectious disease in United States; prevalent Northeast, upper Midwest, and coastal northern California. Reporting is mandatory. With *early* treatment, recovery is usually quick and complete.

A. Stages:

1. *Stage I.* Rash (erythema migrans) at site of tick bite; bull's-eye or target pattern; may appear as hives or cellulitis; common in moist areas (groin, armpit, behind knees). Flu-like symptoms may occur (joint pain, chills, fever).
2. *Stage II.* If untreated, may progress to cardiac problems (10% of clients) or neurological disturbances—Bell's palsy (10% of clients); occasionally meningitis, encephalitis, and eye damage may result.
3. *Stage III.* From 4 weeks to 1 year after the tick bite, "arthritis," primarily large joint, develops in half the clients. If untreated, chronic neurological problems may develop.

B. Assessment (depends on stage): History is important—where do they live or work? Recent travel? Outdoor activities (gardening, hiking, camping, clearing brush)? Knowledge of tick bite and how removed? Pets?

1. *Subjective data:*
   a. Malaise (stage I).
   b. Headache (stage I).
   c. Joint, neck, or back pain (stages I and III).
   d. Weakness (stages II and III).
   e. Chest pain (stage II).
   f. Light-headedness (stage II).
   g. Numbness, pain in arms or legs (stage III).
2. *Objective data:*
   a. Rash—erythema migrans (stage I); at least 5 cm/lesion.
   b. Dysrhythmias; heart block (stage II).
   c. Facial paralysis (stage II).
   d. Conjunctivitis, iritis, optic neuritis (stage II).
   e. Laboratory data: Lyme titer—*elevated* (stages II and III). Often inconclusive.
   f. *Diagnostic tests:* isolation of *Borrelia burgdorferi* in tissue or body fluid; diagnostic levels of IgM or IgG antibodies in serum or CSF.

C. Analysis/nursing diagnosis:

1. *Anxiety* related to diagnosis.
2. *Pain* related to joint inflammation.
3. *Fatigue* related to viral illness.
4. *Impaired physical mobility* related to joint pain.
5. *Altered thought processes* related to neurological deficit.
6. *Decreased cardiac output* related to dysrhythmias.
7. *Knowledge deficit* (learning need) related to treatment and course of disease.

D. Nursing care plan/implementation:

1. Goal: *minimize irreversible tissue damage and complications.*

   a. Medications according to presenting symptoms: *stage I—oral antibiotics* for 21 days (doxycycline, amoxicillin, cefotaxime); *stages II and III*—oral (see stage I) or *intravenous antibiotics* for 21 to 28 days (ceftriaxone).
   b. If hospitalized, monitor vital signs q4h for increased temperature, signs of heart failure; check level of consciousness and cranial nerve functioning.
   c. Note treatment response: worsening of symptoms during first 24 hours: *redder* rash, *higher* fever, *greater* pain *(Jarisch-Herxheimer reaction).*
2. Goal: *alleviate pain, promote comfort.*

   a. Medications: *salicylates, nonsteroidal anti-inflammatory agents,* or other *analgesic,* as ordered; observe for side effects (GI irritation).
   b. Rest: give instructions on relaxation techniques; create a quiet environment.
3. Goal: *maintain physical and psychological well-being.*
   a. Activity: ROM at regular intervals; *medicate for pain* before exercise; encourage proper posture to reduce joint stress; rest periods between activities and treatments.
   b. Referral: occupational or physical therapy as appropriate.
   c. Reassurance: give psychological support; encourage discussion of feelings.

4. Goal: *health teaching.*
   a. Information on disease. Transmission from tick not likely if removed before 48 hours of attachment.
   b. Instructions for home IV antibiotics with heparin lock, if ordered.
   c. Side effects of antibiotics (drug specific); importance of completing therapy.
   d. Signs of disease recurrence (later stages of disease: less severe attacks).
   e. Preventing subsequent infections: wear proper clothing and tick repellent on clothing (20% to 30% DEET); conduct "tick checks" of self, children, and pets; proper tick removal (use tweezers, steady, gentle traction).
   f. Start vaccination series (LYMErix); three injections at 0, 1, and 12 months.

E. Evaluation/outcome criteria:
1. Achieves reasonable comfort.
2. Regains normal physiological and psychological functioning—no irreversible complications; vital signs within normal limits.
3. Resumes previous activity level; returns to work.
4. Adheres to follow-up care recommendations.
5. Knows ways to minimize risk of reinfection.

II. ACQUIRED IMMUNODEFICIENCY SYNDROME (AIDS): the terminal stage of the disease continuum caused by human immunodeficiency virus (HIV), a retrovirus; typically progresses from asymptomatic seronegative status to asymptomatic seropositive status to subclinical immune deficiency to lymphadenopathy (early AIDS) to AIDS-related complex (middle stage with combination of symptoms) to AIDS; hallmarks of HIV infection include opportunistic infections: *Pneumocystis jiroveci (carinii)* pneumonia (PCP); cytomegalovirus (CMV); *Mycobacterium tuberculosis;* hepatitis B; herpes simplex or zoster; candidiasis; may take 7 to 10 years before signs and symptoms occur.

A. High-risk populations:
1. Men, homosexual or bisexual (71%).
2. Injection drug users (IDU)/heterosexual (10%).
3. IDU/homosexual (9%).
4. People who have hemophilia and are recipients of multiple transfusion (1%).
5. Heterosexual (5%).
6. Undetermined/other (4%).

B. Pathophysiology: abnormal response to foreign antigen stimulation (acquired immunity) → deficiency in cell-mediated immunity—T lymphocytes, specifically helper T cells (CD4 cells) and hyperactivity of the humoral system (B cells).

C. Assessment:
1. *Subjective data:*
   a. Fatigue: prolonged; associated with headache or light-headedness.
   b. Unexplained weight loss: greater than 10%.
2. *Objective data:*
   a. Fever: prolonged or night sweats longer than 2 weeks.
   b. Lymphadenopathy.
   c. Skin or mucous membrane lesions: purplish-red, nodules *(Kaposi's sarcoma).*
   d. Cough: persistent, heavy, dry.
   e. Diarrhea: persistent.
   f. Tongue/mouth "thrush"; oral hairy leukoplakia.
   g. *Diagnostic tests* (with permission of client): enzyme-linked immunosorbent assay (ELISA); Western blot test.
   h. Laboratory data: *decreased*—CD4 T lymphocytes, hematocrit, WBCs, platelets. *Seropositive*—syphilis, hepatitis B; ELISA—*positive;* Western blot test—*positive* (mean time for seroconversion is 6 weeks after infection).

D. Analysis/nursing diagnosis:
1. *Risk for infection* related to immunocompromised state.
2. *Fatigue* related to anemia.
3. *Altered nutrition, less than body requirements,* related to anorexia.
4. *Impaired skin integrity* related to nonhealing viral lesions, Kaposi's sarcoma.
5. *Diarrhea* related to infection or parasites.
6. *Risk for activity* intolerance related to shortness of breath.
7. *Ineffective airway clearance* related to pneumonia.
8. *Visual sensory/perception alteration* related to retinitis.
9. *Risk for altered body temperature* (fever) related to opportunistic infections.
10. *Social isolation* related to stigma attached to AIDS.
11. *Powerlessness* related to inability to control disease progression.
12. *Altered thought processes* related to dementia.
13. *Ineffective individual coping* related to poor prognosis.
14. *Risk for violence, self-directed,* related to anger, panic, or depression.

E. Nursing care plan/implementation:
1. Goal: *reduce risk of infection; slow disease progression.*
   a. Observe signs of opportunistic infections: weight loss, diarrhea, skin lesions, sore throat.
   b. Monitor vital signs (including temperature).

ADULT

c. Note secretions and excretions: changes in color, consistency, or odor indicating infection.
d. *Diet:* monitor fluid and electrolytes; strict measurement; encourage adequate dietary intake (*high* calorie, *high* protein, *low* bulk); 5 to 10 times recommended dietary allowance (RDA) for water-soluble vitamins (B complex, C); favorite foods from home; enteral feedings. Six small meals/day.
e. *Protective isolation,* if indicated, for severe immunocompromise.
f. *Antiviral* medications, as ordered: nucleoside reverse transcriptase inhibitors (e.g., zidovudine [Retrovir]); nonnucleoside reverse transcriptase inhibitors (e.g., nevirapine [Viramune]); protease inhibitors (e.g., indinavir sulfate [Crixivan]); drug toxicity and numerous side effects likely (rash, GI upset); large number of pills and tight administration schedule; costly; potential for drug resistance.

2. Goal: *prevent the spread of disease.*
a. Frequent hand washing, even after wearing gloves.
b. *Avoid* exposure to blood, body fluids of client; wear gloves, gowns; proper disposal of needles, IV catheters (see **Chapter 3, Table 3.4, p. 91**).

3. Goal: *provide physical and psychological support.*
a. Oral care: frequent.
b. Cooling bath: 1:10 concentration of isopropyl alcohol with tepid water; *avoid* plastic-backed pads if client has night sweats.
c. Encourage verbalization of fears, concerns without condemnation; may suffer loss of job, lifestyle, significant other.
d. Determine status of support network: arrange contact with support group.
e. Observe for severe emotional symptoms (suicidal tendencies).
f. Address issues surrounding death to ensure quality of life: advance directive prepared and on file; "code blue" status; reassurance of comfort and pain control.

4. Goal: *health teaching.*
a. *Avoidance* of environmental sources of infection (kitty litter, bird cages, tub bathing).
b. Precautions following discharge: risk-reducing behaviors; condoms (latex), limit number of sexual partners, *avoid* exposure to blood or semen during intercourse.
c. Family counseling; availability of community resources.
d. Information on disease progression and life span.
e. Stress-reduction techniques: visualization, guided imagery, meditation.
f. Expected side effects with drug therapy; importance of compliance.

F. Evaluation/outcome criteria:
1. Relief of symptoms (e.g., afebrile, gains weight).
2. Resumes self-care activities; returns to work; improved quality of life.
3. Accepts diagnosis; participates in support group.
4. Progression of disease slows; improved survival probability.
5. Retains autonomy, self-worth.
6. Permitted to die with dignity.

III. ANIMAL-BORNE DISEASES **(Table 6.29).**

IV. BIOTERRORISM **(Table 6.30).**

INTEGUMENTARY SYSTEM

I. BURNS: wounds caused by exposure to excessive heat, chemicals, fire, steam, radiation, or electricity; most often related to carelessness or ignorance; 10,000 to 12,000 deaths annually; survival best at ages 15 to 30 years and in burns covering less than 20% of total body surface.

A. Pathophysiology:
1. *Emergent phase* (injury to 72 hours): shock due to pain, fright, or terror → fatigue, failure of vasoconstrictor mechanisms → hypotension.

ADULT

Table 6.29

Infectious Diseases: Animal-Borne

Disease	Caused by	Onset	Symptoms	Treatment
Avian influenza (bird flu) Highly infectious virus affecting millions of birds across Asia (especially Hong Kong, Thailand, Vietnam).	• Poultry—birds excrete the virus → people inhale fecal dust • Human-to-human transmission rare	24–72 hr	• Eye infection • Fever, sore throat, cough • In fatal cases: viral pneumonia, severe respiratory problems	• Antiviral drug (Tamiflu, Relenza) • No vaccine

Continued

Table 6.29

Infectious Diseases: Animal-Borne—cont'd

Disease	Caused by	Onset	Symptoms	Treatment
Lyme disease (see **pp. 483–484**)				
Mad cow disease (bovine spongiform encephalopathy [BSE]) Causes **variant Creutzfeldt-Jakob disease (VCJD)**: a CNS degenerative brain disorder that has killed >100 in past decade, mostly in Britain.	• Eating meat from cattle (brain, spinal cord, eyes, bone marrow, spleen), or eating contaminated tissue from cattle that ate these parts (have been fed offal)	5 or more years	• ↓ Memory • Speech abnormalities • Hallucinations • Incontinence • Difficulty in dressing	• None • Fatal • Lasts for several months
Monkey pox Related to smallpox. Fatal in 10% of cases. Found in midwestern U.S. (Illinois, Indiana, Missouri, Wisconsin).	• Animal bites by or bodily fluids from rats, mice, squirrels, prairie dogs, or imported west African rodent pets • *Can* be transmitted human-to-human	7–18 days	• Lymphadenopathy • Fever • Headache • Fatigue • Rash → blisters over entire body	• None
Rabies Viral disease. 7,000 cases/yr in U.S.	• Bite from infected cat, dog, or wild animal (raccoon, skunk, fox)	Within 24 hr	• Fever • Hypersalivation • Dysphagia • Partial paralysis • Hallucinations • Excitation	• *Postexposure prophylaxis* (PEP): immune globulin for 1 mo; rabies vaccine • No effective therapy after symptoms appear
Salmonella Bacterial disease; kills approx. 1,000/yr; 40,000 cases/yr.	• Drinking contaminated water or eating contaminated chicken or eggs • Can be transmitted by reptiles (snakes, turtles, lizards), chicks, ducklings	Hours to 7 days	• Severe diarrhea • Fever • Abdominal pain	• No treatment, as resolved in 5–7 days • Antibiotics if infection spreads from intestines
Tularemia (see **Table 6.30 Bioterrorism)**				
West Nile virus Fatal in 10% of cases; first found in Uganda.	• Mosquitoes	3–14 days	• Flu-like (fever, headache, body aches)	• IV fluids • Prevention of pneumonia as secondary infection

For more information, go to the Centers for Disease Control and Prevention (CDC) Web site: www.cdc.gov.

ADULT

Capillary dilation, increased permeability → plasma loss to blisters, edema → hemoconcentration → hypovolemia → hypotension → decreased renal perfusion → potential shutdown.

2. *Acute phase* (3 to 5 days): interstitial-to-plasma fluid shift → hemodilution → hypervolemia → diuresis.

B. Assessment:

1. *Subjective data:* how the burn occurred.
2. *Objective data:*
   a. Extent of body surface involved: *"rule of nines"*—head and both upper extremities, 9% each; front and back of trunk, 18% each; lower extremities, 18% each; and perineum, 1%. Requires adjustment for variation in size of head and lower extremities according to age.
   b. *Location*—facial, perineal, and hand and foot burns have potentially more complications because of poor vascularization.
   c. *Depth* of burn **(Table 6.31):**
      (1) *First degree (superficial)*—epidermal tissue only; not serious unless large areas involved.
      (2) *Second degree (shallow or deep partial thickness)*—epidermal and dermal tissue, hospitalization required if more than 10% of body surface involved (major burn).
      (3) *Third degree (full thickness)*—destruction of all skin layers; requires immediate hospitalization; involvement of 10% of body surface considered major burn.
      (4) *Fourth degree (deep penetrating)*—muscles (fascia), bone.

(text continues on page 489)

Table 6.30

Recognizing Bioterrorism Agents and Associated Syndromes

Disease	Pathophysiology	Transmission and Incubation	Signs/Symptoms	Treatment
Anthrax—Greek word for "coal" • **Cutaneous** • **GI** • **Inhaled** (most lethal)	• Caused by *Bacillus anthracis,* a bacterium that is commonly found in grazing animals • Forms spores that live in soil for years • Man-made form more potent and resistant to treatment	• Contact with spores through break in skin • Eating contaminated meat • Inhaling spores • *Not* spread from person to person • Incubation: 1–6 days (inhalation can take up to 42 days)	***Cutaneous:*** Skin sores that turn black after a few days ***GI:*** Nausea, loss of appetite, bloody diarrhea, fever, followed by bad stomach pain ***Inhaled:*** Cold or flu-like symptoms; cough, fatigue, chest discomfort → shortness of breath (SOB) → severe pneumonia → severe respiratory distress: diaphoresis, stridor, cyanosis, shock; death in 24–36 hours	• Ciprofloxacin or doxycycline plus one or two additional *antimicrobials* (e.g., rifampin, vancomycin, penicillin, ampicillin, clindamycin [60-day treatment]) • Isolation not required • Standard precautions
Botulism—a neuroparalytic illness	• A potent neurotoxin produced from *Clostridium botulinum,* an anaerobic, spore-forming bacterium • Characterized by: symmetrical, descending flaccid paralysis of motor and autonomic nerves • **Always** begins with cranial nerves	• Foodborne; ingestion of toxin produced in food (home-canned is most frequent) • Fatal in 5% of cases	**Vision:** double, blurred **Eyelids:** drooping **Speech:** slurred **Mouth:** dry **Muscles:** weakness, symmetrical flaccid paralysis **Swallowing:** dysphagia If untreated, → descending paralysis of respiratory muscles, arms and legs; death from respiratory failure	• Botulinum antitoxin from CDC • If survive, have SOB and fatigue for years
Plague • **Pneumonic** • **Bubonic** • **Septicemic**	• Caused by bacterium *Yersinia pestis (Y. pestis);* found in rodents and their fleas • Easily destroyed by sunlight and drying • Will survive up to 1 hr	***Pneumonic:*** • Infects lungs • Airborne transmission • Spreads person to person ***Bubonic:*** • Most common form • Infected flea bites the skin • Does *not* spread person to person ***Septicemic:*** • Often complication of pneumonic or bubonic • Does *not* spread from person to person	***Pneumonic:*** Fever Headache Weakness Signs of pneumonia for 2–4 days (SOB, chest pain, cough, bloody or watery sputum) → respiratory failure → shock ***Bubonic:*** Swollen lymph glands (buboes) Fever Headache Chills Weakness ***Septicemic:*** Fever Chills Prostration Abdominal pain Shock Bleeding into skin and organs	• Give *antibiotics* within 24 hr of symptoms—streptomycin, gentamicin, tetracyclines, chloramphenicol • Prophylactic antibiotics for 7 days • Close-fitting surgical mask to protect against infection

Continued

Table 6.30

Recognizing Bioterrorism Agents and Associated Syndromes—cont'd

Disease	Pathophysiology	Transmission and Incubation	Signs/Symptoms	Treatment
Smallpox—Latin word for "spotted" • **Variola major** (severe and most common) • **Variola minor**	• An acute contagious disease caused by variola virus (a member of the orthopoxvirus family)	• Aerosolized; droplets • Direct face-to-face, prolonged contact • Incubation: 7–21 days—not contagious at this time • Lethal in 20%–40% of cases if unvaccinated	*Prodrome* 2–4 days (sometimes contagious): flu-like—malaise, fever (101°–104°F), headache, body aches, sometimes vomiting *Early rash* about 4 days (most contagious): small red spots on tongue and mouth; erythema spreads from face/arms to legs, then centrally *Pustular rash:* macules (bellybutton center)→ papules → pustular vesicles → scabs	• No specific treatment • Smallpox vaccine effective if given within 3 days of exposure • Cidofovir possibly effective • Ribavirin • Victim of attack should be undressed, shower with soap • For visible contamination, use 0.5% diluted household bleach
Tularemia ("rabbit fever")	• A bacterial zoonosis • Caused by *Francisella tularensis,* one of the most infectious pathogenic bacteria • Survives for weeks at low temperatures in: *water*, moist soil, hay, straw, and decaying animal carcasses	• Infects humans through: skin, mucous membranes, *GI* tract, and lungs • Abrupt onset • Lower fatality rate than plague or anthrax • Aerosol release would be likely in terrorist attack • Incubation: 1–14 days • *Not* transmitted person to person	Skin and oral ulcers Fever (sudden) Chills Headache Rigor Generalized body aches (low back) Coryza Sore throat, dry or slightly productive cough Substernal pain or tightness Atypical *pneumonia* *Pleuritis* Hilar lymphadenopathy	Medications: • Streptomycin (drug of choice) • Gentamicin (an alternative) • Doxycycline and ciprofloxacin in mass casualty • Isolation not recommended • In hospitals, standard precautions are recommended
Viral hemorrhagic fever (VHF) (multisystem syndrome) • **Ebola** (severe, often fatal) • **Lassa** • **Hantavirus pulmonary syndrome**	• Four distinct RNA viruses: arenaviruses, filoviruses, bunyaviruses, and flaviviruses • Often animal or insect host, except for ***Ebola*** (host unknown) • Damaged vascular system → bleeding	• Infected host or vector initially transmits to human; then human to human with **Ebola** or **Lassa.** ***Ebola:*** • 2–21 days; abrupt onset ***Lassa:*** • Spread through contact with body fluids • 1–3 wk ***Hantavirus:*** • Carried by rodents (mice) • Aerosolization of virus shed in urine, droppings and saliva • *No* person-to-person transmission • 1–5 wk after exposure	***VHF:*** marked fever, fatigue, dizziness, muscle aches, loss of strength, exhaustion. Bleeding: under skin, organs, mouth, eyes, ears (rarely fatal) ***Ebola:*** fever, headache, red eyes, hiccups, joint/muscle aches, sore throat → diarrhea, vomiting, stomach pain ***Lassa:*** 80% may have no symptoms or mild. May be varied; fever, retrosternal pain, sore throat, back pain, cough, abdominal pain, vomiting, diarrhea, conjunctivitis, facial bleeding ***Hantavirus:*** *Early*—fatigue, fever, muscle aches, headache, nausea, vomiting, abdominal pain *Late*—4–10 days; cough, SOB, chest tightness, feeling of suffocation	***Ebola:*** • Supportive therapy—fluids, electrolytes, O_2 ***Lassa:*** • Ribavirin • Supportive care ***Hantavirus:*** • No specific cure • Early admission to ICU—intubation and ventilator support

For more information, see www.bioterrorism.uab.edu

Table 6.31

Burn Characteristics According to Depth of Injury

Classification	Tissue Damage	Appearance	Pain	Clinical Course
Superficial (first degree)	Epidermis	Mild to fiery red erythema; no blisters	Very painful	Ordinarily heals in 3–7 days
Partial thickness; superficial or deep (second degree)	Epidermis and dermis	• *Superficial:* mottled, moist, pink or red; may or may not blanch with pressure; usually blisters • *Deep:* dry-white or deep red	• *Superficial:* extreme pain and hypersensitivity to touch • *Deep:* may or may not be painful	Healing takes 10–18 days; if infection develops in deep burn, it converts to full-thickness burn • *Deep:* often grafted
Full thickness (third degree)	All layers of skin and subcutaneous tissue	Charred, leathery or pale and dry	Usually absent	Heals only with grafting or scarring
*Fourth degree	All layers of skin, subcutaneous tissue, muscle, and bone	Black	Same as full thickness	Same as full thickness

*Used in some classification systems. May require several days after a severe burn to determine fourth degree.

d. Indications of airway burns (e.g., singed nasal hair, progressive hoarseness, sooty expectoration); edema may occur in 1 hour; increased mortality rate.
e. Poorer prognosis—*infants,* due to immature immune system and effects of fluid loss; *elderly,* due to degenerative diseases and poor healing.
f. Medical history—presence of hypertension, diabetes, alcohol abuse, or chronic obstructive pulmonary disease increases complication rate.

C. Analysis/nursing diagnosis:

1. *Impaired skin integrity* related to thermal injury.
2. *Pain* (depending on type of burn) related to exposure of sensory receptors.
3. *Fluid volume excess or deficit* related to hemodynamic changes.
4. *Risk for infection* related to destruction of protective skin.
5. *Impaired gas exchange* related to airway injury.
6. *Body image disturbance* related to scarring, disfigurement.
7. *Ineffective individual or family coping* related to traumatic experience.

D. Nursing care plan/implementation:

1. Goal: *alleviate pain, relieve shock, and maintain fluid and electrolyte balance.*
   a. Medications: give *opioid analgesic* and *anxiolytics* incrementally.
   b. *Fluids:* IV therapy (see **Chapter 8**); colloids, crystalloids, or 5% dextrose according to burn formula.
   c. Monitor hydration status:
      (1) Insert indwelling catheter.
      (2) Note: color, odor, and amount of urine hourly.
      (3) *Strict* intake and output; hourly for 36 hours with large burns.
      (4) Check hematocrit: normal: men greater than 40%; women greater than 37%. *Increased* Hct with intravascular fluid depletion.
      (5) Weigh daily.
2. Goal: *prevent physical complications.*
   a. *Vital signs:* hourly; central venous pressure (CVP) for signs of shock or fluid overload with clients who are at-risk.
   b. Assess respiratory function (particularly with head, neck burns); patent airway; breath sounds.
   c. Give medications as ordered—*tetanus booster; antibiotics* to treat documented infection; *sedatives* and *analgesics; antipyretics*—**avoid** aspirin; H_2 blockers.
   d. *Isolation:* protective; contact isolation (hand washing, protective clothing).
   e. *Positioning:* turn q2h; prevent contractures.
      (1) *Head and neck burns*—use pillows under shoulders only for hyperextension of neck.
      (2) *Hand burns*—splints.
      (3) *Arm and hand burns*—keep arms at *90-degree angle* from body and slightly above shoulders.
      (4) *Ankle and foot burns*—splints; *elevate* to prevent edema.
      (5) Splints to maintain functional positions.
      (6) ROM exercises according to therapy guidelines; usually several times per day; active exercises most beneficial.

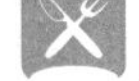

   f. *Diet:* begin oral fluids at once; food as tolerated—*high* protein, *high* calorie for energy and tissue repair (promote positive nitrogen balance); enteral feedings if protein and calorie goals not met.

g. Observe for: constriction (circumferential or chest wall burns); check peak inspiratory pressure in client who is intubated—report increased pressure; check pulses in burned extremities every 1 to 2 hours for 24 hours—report loss of pulses.

3. Goal: *promote emotional adjustment and provide supportive therapy.*
   a. Care by same personnel as much as possible, to develop rapport and trust.
   b. Involve client in care plans.
   c. Answer questions clearly, accurately.
   d. Encourage family involvement and participation.
   e. Provide diversional activities and change furnishings or room adornments when possible, to prevent perceptual deprivation related to immobility.
   f. Point out signs of progress (e.g., decreased edema, healing) because client and family tend to become discouraged and cannot see progress.
   g. Encourage self-care to highest level tolerated.
   h. Anticipate psychological changes:
      (1) *Acute period*—severe anxiety: medicate with *anxiolytics* as ordered; maintain eye contact; explain procedures.
      (2) *Intermediate period*—reactions associated with pain, dependency, depression, anger; give medications to decrease *pain;* explain procedures; have open, nonjudgmental attitude; use consistent approaches to care; contract with client regarding division of responsibilities; encourage self-care.
      (3) *Recuperative period*—grief process reactivated. Anxiety, depression, anger, bargaining, as client tries to cope with altered body image, leaving security of hospital, finances. Encourage verbalization; refer to support group to assist adaptation.

4. Goal: *promote wound healing*—wound care:
   a. *Open method*—exposure of burns to air; useful in burns of *face;* thin layer (2 to 4 mm) topical *antimicrobial* ointment applied.
   b. *Closed method*—dressings applied to burned areas, changed 1 to 3 times/day; give PO *pain* medication 30 minutes *before* change; *IV pain* medication *during* dressing change; tubbing facilitates removal.
   c. *Multiple dressing change*—common approach; dressings changed twice daily to q4h depending on wound condition.
   d. *Topical antimicrobial therapies* **(Table 6.32).**
   e. *Tubbing and débridement.*
      (1) Hydrotherapy—body-temperature bath water; loosens dressings so some float off;

Table 6.32

Topical Antimicrobials Used in Burn Care

Agent	Advantages	Disadvantages	Nursing Implications
Silver sulfadiazine 1% (Silvadene)	• Broad-spectrum antimicrobial • Antifungal • Nonstaining • Relatively painless • No systemic metabolic abnormalities	• Less eschar penetration than mafenide acetate (Sulfamylon) • Decreased granulocyte formation; transient leukopenia • Macular rash	Check for allergy to sulfa
Mafenide acetate (Sulfamylon) cream or solution	• Eschar penetration • Effective with *Pseudomonas* • Topical of choice for electrical burns • Suitable for open or closed method of treatment (cream) • Used for gram-negative organisms	• Severe pain and burning sensation (lasts 30 min) • Metabolic acidosis • Carbonic anhydrase inhibitor • Ineffective against fungi • May cause hypersensitivity rash	• Administer pretreatment analgesic • Monitor for metabolic acidosis and hyperventilation • Check for allergy to sulfa; observe for rash
Silver nitrate	• Low cost • Broad spectrum • Effective with *Candida*	• Continuous wet soaks • Superficial penetration • Black staining of sheets • Stinging • Electrolyte imbalances (low sodium, low chloride, low calcium, low potassium), alkalosis	• Check serum electrolytes daily • Rewet dressing to keep moist
Petroleum- and mineral oil–based (e.g., Bacitracin, Neosporin, Polysporin)	• Bactericidal, gram-positive and gram-negative organisms • Painless • Prevents drying of wound	Limited ability to penetrate eschar	Apply in thin layer (1 mm) Reapply as needed.

soak 20 to 30 minutes; encourage limb exercises; do *not* leave unattended; loss of body heat may occur, with chilling and poor perfusion resulting.

(2) Removal of eschar *(débridement)*—done with forceps and curved scissors; medicate for *pain* before; use *sterile technique;* only loose eschar removed, to prevent bleeding; examine wound for: infection, color change, decreased granulation—report changes **immediately.** Chemical débridement also done; agent digests necrotic tissue.

f. Wound coverage, to decrease chances of infection:

(1) Temporary and semipermanent wound coverings **(Table 6.33).**

(2) *Autograft*—client donates skin for wound coverage.

(a) Types—free grafts (unattached to donor site) and pedicle grafts (attached to donor site).

(b) Procedure—general anesthesia; donor sites shaved and prepared; graft applied to granulation bed; face, hands, and arms grafted first.

(c) *Post–skin-graft care:*

(i) Sheet grafts: roll cotton-tipped applicator over graft to remove excess exudate; maintain dressings; *aseptic technique;* mesh grafts: irrigate as ordered.

(ii) Third to fifth day—graft takes on pink appearance if it has taken.

(iii) Padding, then splints applied to immobilize grafted extremities.

(iv) Pressure garments worn up to 18 months to decrease hypertrophic scarring.

5. Goal: *health teaching.*

a. Mobility needs: exercise; physical therapy; occupational therapy; splints, braces.

b. Community resources: mental health practitioner or psychotherapist if needed for problems with self-image or sexual role; referrals as needed.

c. Techniques to camouflage appearance: slacks, turtlenecks, long sleeves, wigs, makeup.

Table 6.33
Wound Coverings

Example	Advantages	Disadvantages	Nursing Implication
Biological			
Xenograft	Promotes healing of clean wound; relieves pain; readily available; reduces water and heat loss	Easily digested by wound collagenase; allergic reactions	Overlap edges slightly; trim away when skin underneath has healed
Homograft–cadaver skin	Reduces water and heat loss; relieves pain; used with antimicrobial mesh; may be left in place until rejection occurs	May harbor disease	Observe for signs of infection
Amnion	Relieves pain; reduces water and heat loss; has bacteriostatic properties	Limited shelf life; requires special preparation for use; may harbor diseases	Change cover dressing q48h; leave on wound until it sloughs
Biosynthetic (Temporary)			
Biobrane	Protects from microbial penetration; decreases pain; promotes healing in partial-thickness burn	Not effective for preparing a granulation bed	Must be secured to skin with sutures, closure straps, tape, or staples; wrap with gauze; after 48 hr, check for adherence; once adherence has occurred, may be left open to air; check for signs of infection
Biosynthetic (Semipermanent)			
Integra Artificial Skin	Postexcisional treatment of life-threatening full or deep partial-thickness burns when autograft not available	Infection rate lower than autograft	Maintain integrity of covering; 18–20 days before thin autograft applied. *Avoid* hydrotherapy; observe for infection.

E. Evaluation/outcome criteria:
1. Return of vital signs to preburn levels.
2. Minimal to no hypertrophic scarring.
3. Free of infection; demonstrates wound care.
4. Maintains functional mobility of limbs; no contractures.
5. Adjusts to changes in body image; no depression.
6. Regains independence; returns to work, social activities.

MUSCULOSKELETAL SYSTEM

I. IMMOBILITY: Impaired physical mobility or limitation of physical movement may be accompanied by a number of complications that can involve any or all of the major systems of the body. Regardless of the cause of immobilization, there are a number of conditions that arise primarily as a complication of immobility. These are discussed in **Table 6.34.**

A. Types of immobility:
1. *Physical*—physical restriction due to limitation in movement or physiological processes (e.g., breathing).
2. *Intellectual*—lack of action due to lack of knowledge (e.g., mental retardation, brain damage).
3. *Emotional*—immobilized when highly stressed (e.g., after loss of loved person or diagnosis of terminal illness).
4. *Social*—decreased social interaction due to separation from family when hospitalized or when alone, as in old age.

B. Risk factors:
1. Pain, trauma, injury.
2. Loss of body function or body part.
3. Chronic disease.
4. Emotional, mental illness; neglect.
5. Malnutrition.
6. Bedrest, traction, surgery, medications.

C. Assessment:
1. *Subjective data: psychological/social effects* of immobility:
   a. Decreased motivation to learn; decreased retention.
   b. Decreased problem-solving abilities.
   c. Diminished drives; decreased hunger.
   d. Changes in body image, self-concept.
   e. Exaggerated emotional reactions, inappropriate to situation or person; aggression, apathy, withdrawal.
   f. Deterioration of time perception.
   g. Fear, anxiety, feelings of worthlessness related to change in role activities (e.g., when no longer employed).
2. *Objective data: physical effects* of immobility:
   a. *Cardiovascular.*
      (1) Orthostatic hypotension.
      (2) Increased cardiac load.
      (3) Thrombus formation.
   b. *Gastrointestinal.*
      (1) Anorexia.
      (2) Diarrhea.
      (3) Constipation.
   c. *Metabolic.*
      (1) Tissue atrophy and protein catabolism.
      (2) BMR reduced.
      (3) Fluid/electrolyte imbalances.
   d. *Musculoskeletal.*
      (1) Demineralization (osteoporosis).
      (2) Contractures and atrophy.
      (3) Skin breakdown.
   e. *Respiratory.*
      (1) Decreased respiratory movement.
      (2) Accumulation of secretions in respiratory tract.
      (3) O_2/CO_2 level imbalance.
   f. *Urinary.*
      (1) Calculi.
      (2) Bladder distention, stasis.
      (3) Infection.
      (4) Frequency.

D. Analysis/nursing diagnosis:
1. *Impaired physical mobility* related to specific client condition.
2. *Impaired skin integrity* related to physical immobilization.
3. *Urinary retention* related to incomplete emptying of bladder.
4. *Constipation* related to inactivity.
5. *Risk for disuse syndrome* related to lack of range of motion.
6. *Bathing/hygiene self-care deficit* related to musculoskeletal impairment.
7. *Sensory/perceptual alteration* related to complications of immobility.
8. *Body image disturbance* related to physical limitations.

E. Nursing care plan/implementation:
1. Goal: *prevent physical, psychological hazards.*
   a. Apply nursing measures to promote venous flow, muscle strength, endurance, joint mobility, skin integrity.
   b. Assess and counteract *psychological* impact of immobility (e.g., feelings of helplessness, hopelessness, powerlessness).
   c. Help maintain accurate sensory processing to prevent and lessen *sensory disturbances.*
   d. Help adapt to *altered body image* due to increased dependency, sensory deprivation,

(text continues on page 499)

ADULT

Table 6.34

Complications of Immobilization

Disorder	Pathophysiology	Assessment	Analysis/Nursing Diagnosis	Nursing Care Plan/ Implementation	Evaluation/Outcome Criteria
Orthostatic hypotension	A decrease in BP >30/15 caused by failure of vasomotor responses to compensate for change from a recumbent to an upright position	• *Subjective data:* weakness; dizziness • *Objective data:* decreased BP >30/15 measured 2 min after moving from a supine to a sitting or standing position; loss of muscle tone and strength; client may faint	• *Decreased cardiac output* related to orthostatic hypotension • *Risk for injury* related to vertigo • *Activity intolerance* related to dizziness	• *Prevent trauma resulting from sudden decrease in BP* 1. Change position gradually 2. Elastic stockings 3. Leg exercises 4. Dangle before getting up 5. Tilt table 6. Sitting and lying BP 7. Monitor side effects of drugs • *Health teaching* 1. Explain signs and symptoms to client 2. Encourage client to dangle before standing 3. Encourage slow movement from sitting to standing 4. Exercises to maintain muscle tone	• Client tolerates increased activity • No trauma occurs • BP remains within normal limits
Cardiac overload	When the body is recumbent, some of the total blood volume that would be in the legs as a result of gravity is redistributed to other parts of the body, thereby increasing the circulating volume and increasing the workload of the heart; heart rate, which is decreased because blood is prevented from entering the thoracic vessels by pressure from the Valsalva maneuver, increases when normal breathing resumes	• *Subjective data:* fear; apprehension • *Objective data: Valsalva* maneuver (pressure against the closed glottis when breath is held) 10–20 times/hr, when trying to move in bed; tachycardia; decreased exercise tolerance	• *Risk for injury* related to increased workload of heart • *Activity intolerance* related to increased workload of heart • *Fear* related to tachycardia	• *Prevent injury and further ischemic damage to cardiac tissue* by decreasing workload of heart 1. Out of bed in chair when possible 2. *Semirecumbent* position when in bed; pillows between legs when side-lying 3. Exercises: passive and active ROM, isometric 4. Encourage participation in self-care 5. Turn every 2 hr, dangle 6. *Avoid* Valsalva, fatigue 7. Minimize constipation 8. Encourage slow, deep breathing when moving in bed • *Health teaching* 1. Exhale while turning; do *not* hold breath 2. Measures to conserve energy	• No complications noted • Client tolerates increased activity • Heart rate within normal limit

Continued

Table 6.34

Complications of Immobilization—cont'd

Disorder	Pathophysiology	Assessment	Analysis/Nursing Diagnosis	Nursing Care Plan/ Implementation	Evaluation/Outcome Criteria
Thrombus formation	Mass of blood constituents formed in the heart or blood vessels due to pooling of blood from lack of activity; increased viscosity related to dehydration or possible external pressure	• *Subjective data:* discomfort over involved vessel • *Objective data:* increased RBC count; venous stasis; hypercoagulability	• *Altered peripheral tissue perfusion* related to obstructed vessel • *Risk for injury* related to emboli	• *Prevent injury* by reducing risk factors and venous stasis 1. *Position:* change q1–2h 2. Do *not* gatch bed (causes pressure against leg vessels) 3. *Increase* fluid intake 4. Monitor coagulation laboratory values 5. *Medications: anticoagulation* therapy, as prescribed for clients at risk (immobilized, trauma, low pelvic surgery) 6. Ambulate as soon as possible • *Health teaching* 1. How to recognize signs of thrombophlebitis/thromboemboli 2. Leg exercise program to strengthen muscles for improved tone, to prevent pooling of blood in vessels 3. Precautions necessary when on anticoagulation therapy 4. Side effects of anticoagulation therapy (bleeding from gums, body fluids, obvious bleeding)	No thromboemboli *Note:* If *Homans'* sign present (discomfort behind knee on forced dorsiflexion of the foot) see **Nursing care for client with thromboemboli, pp. 372, 434**
Respiratory congestion related to decreased respiratory movements	Decreased thoracic movement due to: restriction against bed or chair, lack of position change, restrictive clothing or binders/bandages, or abdominal distention	• *Subjective data:* dyspnea; pain • *Objective data:* trauma; immobilization of thorax or abdomen, due to position in bed; inability to cough or deep breathe; abdominal distention	• *Ineffective breathing pattern* related to splinting to reduce pain • *Ineffective airway clearance* related to retained secretions • *Impaired physical mobility* related to trauma	• *Prevent complications related to respiratory status* 1. Maintain a clear airway, assist with ventilation prn 2. Remove or minimize causes of dyspnea 3. Conserve client's energy (periods of rest and activity—client able to cough more effectively when rested) 4. Incentive spirometry • *Promote comfort* 1. Maintain hydration and nutrition 2. *Position:* change q2h; out of bed in chair when possible (chest expansion greater when sitting in chair)	No respiratory complications or excess secretions noted

				• *Health teaching* 1. Methods to allay anxieties precipitated by dyspnea 2. Effective breathing and coughing exercises	
Respiratory congestion related to pooled secretions	Inability of cilia to move normal secretions out of bronchial tree due to: ineffective coughing, lack of thoracic expansion, or effects of medications	• *Subjective data:* dyspnea; pain • *Objective data:* dehydration; *drugs—anticholinergic, CNS depressants,* anesthesia; inadequate coughing; stationary position	• *Ineffective airway clearance* related to pooled secretions • *Impaired gas exchange* related to ineffective coughing	• *Prevent atelectasis, infection, stasis of air, and secretions in lungs* 1. Maintain patent airway; cough; suction; change position 2. See nursing care plan for *Respiratory congestion related to decreased respiratory movements* (above) • *Health teaching* 1. Effective coughing techniques 2. Importance of adequate hydration	• No respiratory complications • Client coughs and removes secretions
Oxygen/carbon dioxide imbalance	Imbalance in oxygen and carbon dioxide levels related to pulmonary congestion, ineffective breathing patterns, trauma, or effects of medications	• *Subjective data:* confusion, irritable, restless, dyspnea • *Objective data:* hypoxia, hypercapnia, cyanosis	• *Impaired gas exchange* related to immobilization	• *Promote improved respirations* 1. Change position frequently 2. Increase humidification 3. Monitor side effects of administered medication, especially *narcotics, barbiturates* 4. See nursing care plan for *Respiratory congestion related to decreased respiratory movements* **(p. 494)**	• No respiratory complications • Respiratory rate and depth are adequate for maintaining balance of oxygen and carbon dioxide
Malnutrition of adult who is immobilized	Lack of adequate dietary intake to maintain healthy tissue related to lack of food; lack of knowledge about food; problems with ingestion, digestion, or absorption; or psychosocial factors that influence client's motivation to eat	• *Subjective data:* anorexia, nausea; diet history validating lack of adequate nutritional intake; mental irritability • *Objective data:* 1. Recent weight loss of >10% 2. *Decreased:* healing ability, GI motility, absorption, secretion of digestive enzymes 3. *Appearance:* listlessness, muscle weakness; posture—sagging shoulders, sunken chest 4. Anthropometric data (measurement of size, weight, and body proportions): <85% of standard 5. *Cardiovascular:* tachycardia (>100 beats/min) on minimal exertion; bradycardia at rest	• *Altered nutrition, less than body requirements,* related to decreased appetite • *Knowledge deficit* (learning need) related to nutrition requirements	• *Improved nutritional intake* to maintain basal metabolism requirements and replace losses from catabolism 1. Provide balanced or prescribed diet, *soft* or *ground food* if cannot chew or is edentulous 2. *Increase* fluid intake 3. Attain/maintain normal weight 4. Feed, assist with feeding, or place foods within client's reach • *Promote comfort* 1. Mouth care; to facilitate mastication of food → improved digestion and absorption 2. Relieve constipation (see nursing care plan for **Constipation, p. 496**) 3. Observe for stomatitis, bleeding, changes in skin texture, color 4. Medications: monitor nausea and vomiting side effects of prescribed medications; administer *antiemetics* as ordered to control nausea and vomiting	• No complications • Client obtains/maintains normal weight • No tissue breakdown

Continued

Table 6.34

Complications of Immobilization—cont'd

Disorder	Pathophysiology	Assessment	Analysis/Nursing Diagnosis	Nursing Care Plan/ Implementation	Evaluation/Outcome Criteria
		6. *Hair:* brittle, dry, thin 7. *Skin:* dry, scaly 8. Lack of financial resources: sociocultural influences 9. *Decreased* blood values: serum albumin, iron-binding capacity, lymphocyte levels, hematocrit, and hemoglobin		5. Ambulate to alleviate flatulence and distention 6. Alleviate pain and discomfort by: distractions, increased social interactions, pleasant environment, back rubs, and administration of prn pain medications, as ordered • *Health teaching* 1. Diet and elimination 2. See **Chapter 9** for foods *high in protein and carbohydrate*	
Constipation	Waste material in the bowel is too hard to pass easily; or bowel movements are so infrequent that client has discomfort	• *Subjective data:* discomfort, pain, distress, and pressure in the rectum; reported decrease in normal elimination pattern • *Objective data:* immobilization; hard formed stool, possible palpable impaction; decreased bowel sounds; bowel elimination less frequent than usual	• *Constipation* related to decreased water and fiber intake • *Knowledge deficit* (learning need) related to dietary and exercise requirements to prevent constipation	• *Promote normal pattern of bowel elimination* 1. Administer: *stool softeners* or *bulk cathartics* as ordered; oil retention, soap suds enemas as ordered 2. Encourage change of position and activity as tolerated 3. Provide *high-bulk* diet 4. *Increase fluid* intake 5. Provide for privacy 6. Encourage regular time for evacuation • *Health teaching* 1. Dietary instructions regarding *increased fiber* 2. Exercise program as tolerated 3. *Increase* fluids	• Client has normal bowel elimination pattern • No impactions • Increases fluid and fiber in diet
Osteoporosis	Metabolic bone disorder in which there is a generalized loss of bone density due to an imbalance between bone formation and bone resorption; immobilization can cause calcium losses of 200–300 mg/day	• *Subjective data:* backache • *Objective data:* demineralization of bone seen on x-ray; kyphosis; spontaneous fracture of bone (hip, spine, wrist); collapsed vertebrae; loss of height; stooped posture	*Pain* related to bone fractures or body structural changes	• *Prevent injury related to decreased bone strength* 1. *Position:* correct body alignment, firm mattress 2. Encourage self-care activities: plan maximum activity allowed by physical condition; muscle exercises against resistance as tolerated 3. Rest/activity pattern: encourage ROM exercise; *avoid* fatigue	• No fractures • No renal calculi • Incorporates dietary improvements in daily menu selection • Participates in exercise program on a regular basis • Regular bone density tests (1–2 years for ages 40–65+)

	Risk factors: women, family history; postmenopause, thin and/or small frame, anorexia or bulimia, diet low in calcium; use of corticosteroids and anticonvulsants; inactive lifestyle; cigarette smoking, excessive use of alcohol			4. *Weight-bearing* positions, tilt table 5. *Diet: high* protein, *high vitamin D, calcium* rich 6. *Increase* fluids to prevent renal calculi (calcium from bones could cause kidney stones) • *Health teaching* 1. Dietary instructions: foods to include for high-protein, high–vitamin D, high-calcium diet 2. Exercise program 3. Sign and symptoms of renal calculi 4. *Avoid* smoking, alcohol	
Contractures	Abnormal shortening of muscle tissue, rendering the muscle highly resistant to stretching; related to lack of active or passive ROM, or improper support and positioning of joints affected by arthritis or injury	• *Subjective data:* pain • *Objective data:* muscles—fixed, shortened, decreased tone; resistance of muscles to stretch; decreased ROM in affected limb	• *Impaired physical mobility* related to muscle weakness and contractures • *Pain* related to injury • *Self-care deficit* related to immobility	• *Prevent deformities* 1. Active or passive ROM 2. *Positioning:* functional, correct alignment 3. Footboard to prevent footdrop 4. *Avoid* knee gatch • *Health teaching* 1. Importance of ROM 2. Correct anatomical positions	ROM maintained No deformities noted
Skin breakdown	Presence of risk factors that could lead to skin breakdown, such as: immobility, inadequate nutrition, lack of position changes	• *Subjective data:* fatigue; pain; inability to turn on own • *Objective data:* interruption of skin integrity, especially over: ears, occiput, heels, sacrum, scrotum, elbows, trochanter, ischium, scapula; immobilization; malnutrition	• *Impaired skin integrity* related to lack of frequent position change	• *Prevent skin breakdown* 1. Change *position* q1–2h and prn, out of bed when possible 2. Protect from infection 3. Increase *dietary* intake: *protein, carbohydrates* 4. Increase *fluids* • *Assess for/reduce contributing factors known to cause decubitus ulcers:* incontinence, stationary position, malnutrition, obesity, sensory deficits, emotional disturbances, paralysis • *Promote healing* 1. Wash gently, pat dry—to *avoid* skin abrasion 2. Clean, dry, wrinkle-free bed linens and pads	No skin breakdown

Continued

Table 6.34

Complications of Immobilization—cont'd

Disorder	Pathophysiology	Assessment	Analysis/Nursing Diagnosis	Nursing Care Plan/ Implementation	Evaluation/Outcome Criteria
				3. Massage skin with lotion that does *not contain alcohol* (alcohol dries skin) 4. Protect with: wafer barrier, alternating mattress, sheepskin pads, protectors, flotation devices 5. *No* "doughnuts" or rubber rings (interfere with circulation of tissue within center of ring)	
Urinary stasis	Immobility leads to inability to completely empty the bladder, which increases risk for urinary tract infection and renal calculi	• *Subjective data:* pain, due to infection or renal calculi • *Objective data:* difficulty in urinating due to position or lack of privacy; infection related to catheter insertion or stasis of urine; hematuria	*Altered urinary elimination* related to inability to empty bladder	• *Prevent urinary infections, stasis, and renal calculi* 1. Increase activity as allowed 2. Check for distended bladder 3. *Increase* fluids, I&O 4. *Diet: acid-ash* to increase acidity, thereby preventing infection 5. *Avoid* catheterization; use intermittent catheterization instead of Foley whenever possible or *Credé's maneuver* to empty bladder (manual exertion of pressure on the bladder to force urine out) 6. Bladder training	No urinary infections or evidence of renal calculi; bladder emptied, no urinary stasis

and changes in status and power that accompany immobility.

e. Offer counseling when sexual expression is impaired.

2. Goal: *health teaching:* how to prevent physical problems related to immobility (e.g., anticonstipation diet, range of motion, skin care); teach activities while immobile that encourage independence and provide sensory stimulation.

F. Evaluation/outcome criteria:

1. Minimal contractures, skin breakdown, muscle atrophy, or loss of strength.
2. Interest in self and environment; positive self-image.
3. Returns to optimal level of physical activity.

II. FRACTURES: disruptions in the continuity of bone as the result of trauma or various disease processes, such as *Cushing's* syndrome or osteoporosis, that weaken the bone structure.

A. Types (Fig. 6.13):

1. *Open or compound*—fractured bone extends *through skin* and mucous membranes; increased potential for infection.

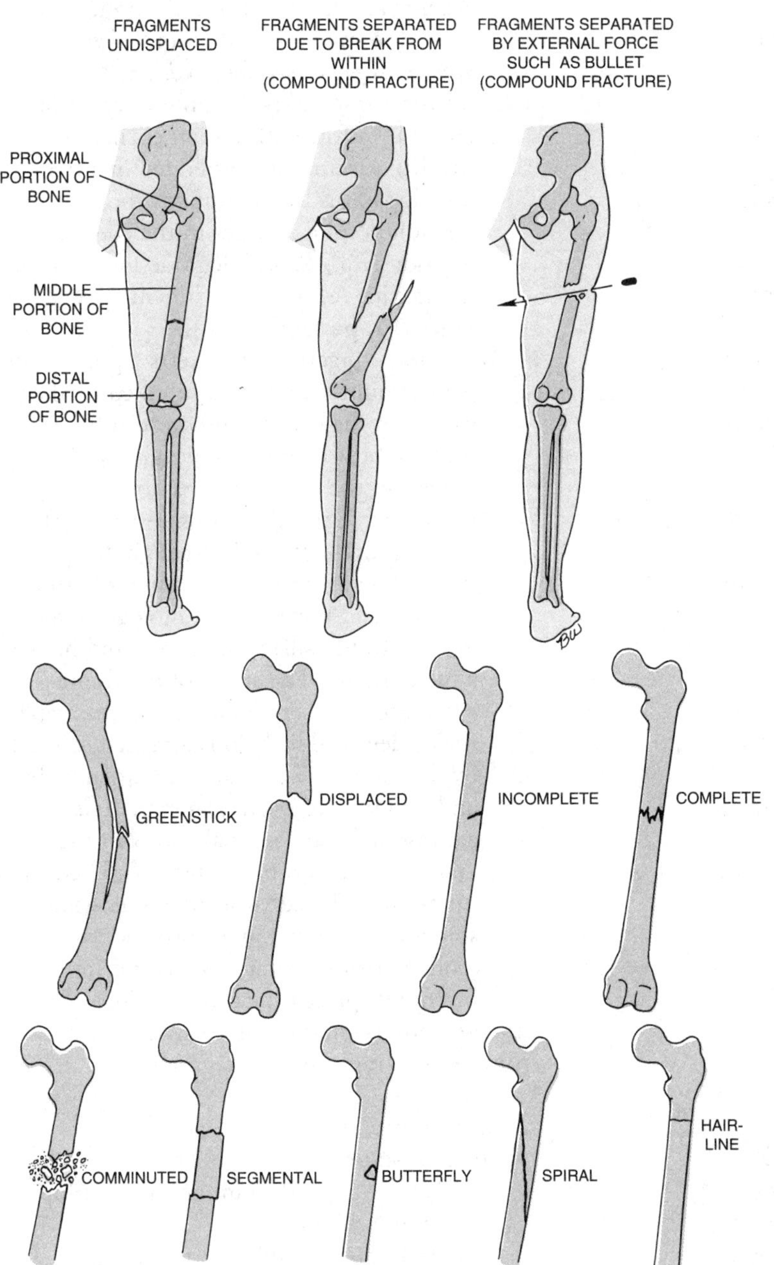

Figure 6.13 Types of fractures and terminology. (From Venes, D [ed]: *Taber's Cyclopedic Medical Dictionary,* ed 21. FA Davis, Philadelphia, 2009.)

2. *Closed or simple*—fractured bone *does not* protrude through skin.
3. *Complete*—fracture extends through *entire bone,* disrupting the periosteum on both sides of the bone, producing two or more fragments.
4. *Incomplete*—fracture extends *only partway* through bone; bone continuity is not totally interrupted.
5. *Greenstick* or *willow-hickory stick*—fracture of *one* side of bone; *other side merely bends;* usually seen only in children.
6. *Impacted or telescoped*—fracture in which bone fragments are *forcibly driven into* other or adjacent bone structures.
7. *Comminuted*—fracture having *more than one* fracture line and with bone fragment broken into *several pieces.*
8. *Depressed*—fracture in which bone or bone fragments are driven *inward,* as in skull or facial fractures.
9. See also **VI. TOTAL HIP REPLACEMENT, p. 510.**

B. Methods used to reduce/immobilize fractures: reduction or setting of the bone—restores bone alignment as nearly as possible.

1. *Closed reduction*—manual traction or manipulation. Usually done under anesthesia to reduce pain and muscle spasm. Maintenance of reduction and immobilization is accomplished by casting (fiberglass or plaster of Paris).
2. *Open reduction*—operative procedure utilized to achieve bone alignment; pins, wires, nails, or rods may be used to secure bone fragments in position; prosthetic implants may also be used.
3. *Traction reduction*—force is applied in two directions: to obtain alignment, and to reduce or eliminate muscle spasm. Used for fractures of long bones. May be:
   a. Continuous—used with fractures or dislocations of bones or joints.
   b. Intermittent—used to reduce flexion contractures or lessen pain and muscle spasm.
   c. Applied as follows:
      (1) *Skin*—traction applied to skin by using a commercial foam-rubber *Buck's* traction splint or by using adhesive, plastic, or a moleskin strip bound to the extremity by elastic bandage; exerts indirect traction on bone or muscles (e.g., *Bryant's, Buck's* extension, head, pelvic, *Russell's*) (**Fig. 6.14, parts *A* through *E***).
      (2) *Skeletal*—direct traction applied to bone using pins (*Steinmann*), wires (*Kirchner*). Pin is inserted through the bone in or close to the involved area and usually protrudes through skin on both sides of the extremity. Skeletal traction for fractured vertebrae accomplished with tongs (e.g., *Crutchfield* tongs, *Gardner-Wells* tongs) (see **Fig. 6.14, parts *F* through *H***).
   d. Specific types of traction:
      (1) *Cervical*—direct traction applied to cervical vertebrae using a head halter or *Crutchfield, Gardner-Wells,* or *Vinke* tongs that are inserted into the skull (see **Fig. 6.14, parts *C* and *G***). Traction is increased with weights until vertebrae move into position and alignment is regained. After reduction is obtained, weights are decreased to the amount needed to maintain reduction. *Weight amount is prescribed by physician.*
      (2) *Balanced suspension*—countertraction produced by a force other than client's body weight; extremity is suspended in a traction apparatus that maintains the line of traction despite changes in the client's position (e.g., *Russell's* leg traction, *Thomas'* splint with *Pearson's* attachment) (see **Fig. 6.14, parts *E* and *F***).
      (3) *Running*—traction that exerts a pull in one plane; countertraction is supplied by the weight of the client's body or can be increased through use of weights and pulleys in the opposite direction (e.g., *Buck's* extension, *Russell's* traction) (see **Fig. 6.14, parts *B* through *E***).
      (4) *Halo*—an apparatus that employs both a plastic and metal frame; molded frame extends from axilla to iliac crest and houses a metal frame. The struts of the frame extend to skull and attach to round metal (halo) device. The halo is attached to skull by four pins—two located anterolaterally and two located posterolaterally. They are inserted into external cortex of the cranium (see **Fig. 6.14, part *H***). Used to immobilize the cervical spine following spinal fusion, give some correction to scoliosis before spinal fusion, and immobilize nondisplaced fracture of spine.
4. *Immobilization*—maintains reduction and promotes healing of bone fragments. Achieved by:
   a. *External fixation:*
      (1) Casts—types:
         (a) *Spica*—applied to immobilize hip or shoulder joints.
         (b) Body cast—applied to trunk.
         (c) Arm or leg cast—joints above and below site included in cast.

SKIN

A. Bryant's traction

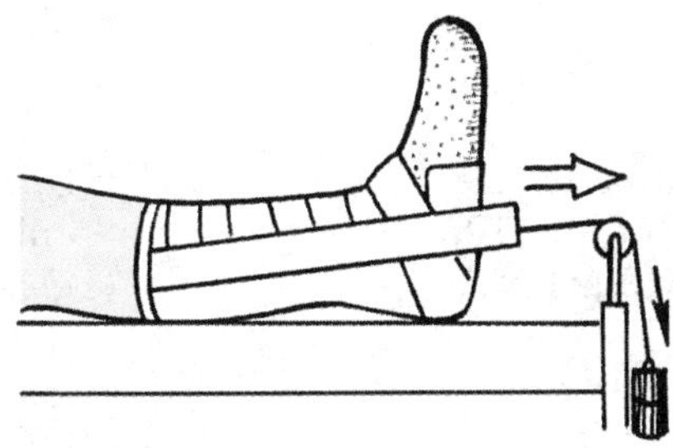

B. Buck's traction

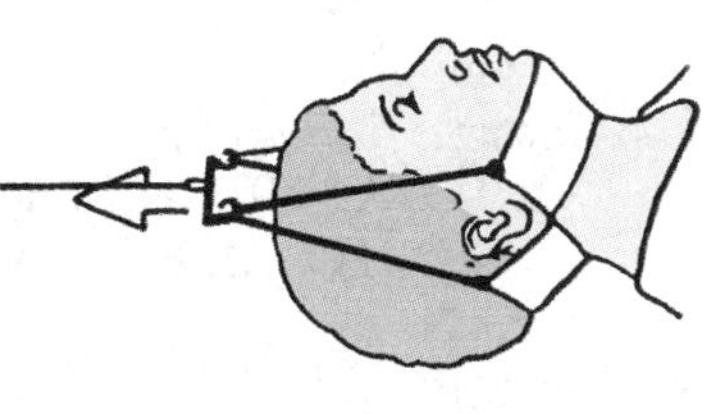

C. Head halter traction

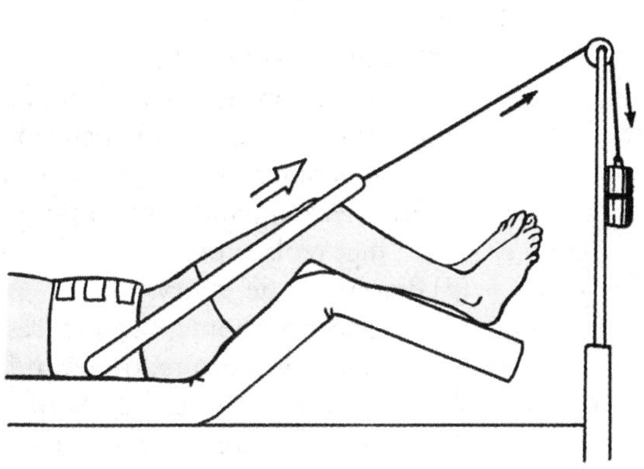

D. Pelvic traction

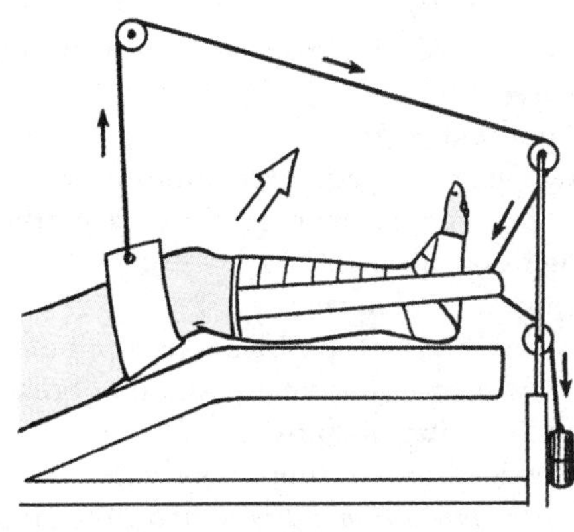

E. Russell's traction

SKELETAL

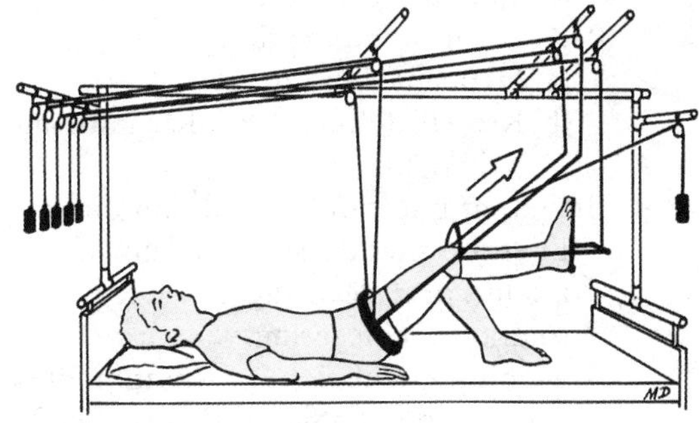

F. Balanced suspension traction

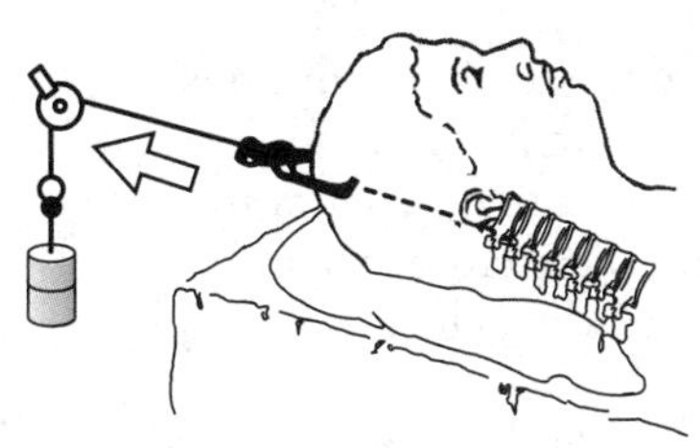

G. Crutchfield tongs

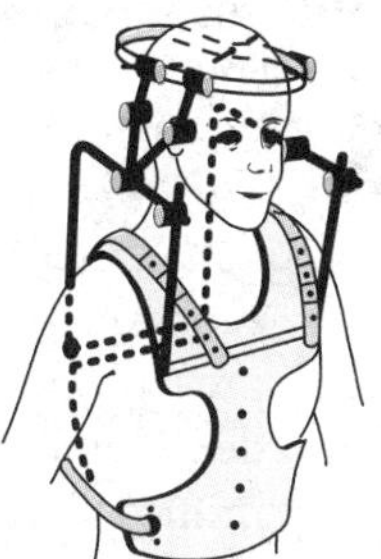

H. Halo vest

Figure 6.14 **Types of skin and skeletal traction.**

(2) Splints, continuous traction.
(3) External fixation devices (*Charnley*)—multiple pins/rods through limb above and below fracture site, attached to external metal supports. Client able to become ambulatory.

b. *Internal fixation*—pins, wires, nails, rods (see **VI. TOTAL HIP REPLACEMENT, p. 510,** and **VII. TOTAL KNEE REPLACEMENT, p. 512**).

C. Assessment:

1. *Subjective data:*
   a. Pain, tenderness.
   b. Tingling, numbness.
   c. Nausea.
   d. History of traumatic event.
   e. Muscle spasm.
2. *Objective data:*
   a. Function: abnormal or lost.
   b. Deformities.
   c. Ecchymosis, increased heat over injured part.
   d. Localized edema.
   e. Crepitation (grating sensations heard or felt as bone fragments rub against each other).
   f. Signs of shock.
   g. Indicators of anxiety.
   h. X-ray: *fracture*—positive interruption of bone; *dislocation*—abnormal position of bone.

D. Analysis/nursing diagnosis:

1. *Pain* related to interruption in bone.
2. *Impaired physical mobility* related to fracture treatment modality.
3. *Risk for injury* related to complications of fractures.
4. *Knowledge deficit* (learning need) regarding cast care, crutch walking, traction.
5. *Constipation* related to immobilization.
6. *Risk for impaired skin integrity* related to immobility or friction from materials used to immobilize the fracture during healing.

E. Nursing care plan/implementation:

1. Goal: *promote healing and prevent complications of fractures* **(Table 6.35).**
   a. *Diet: high* protein, iron, vitamins to improve tissue repair; *moderate* carbohydrates to prevent weight gain; *no* increase in calcium to prevent kidney stones (decalcification and demineralization occur when client is immobilized).
      (1) Encourage *increased fluid intake,* to prevent kidney stones.
      (2) Prevent or correct constipation through *increasing bulk foods, fruits, and fruit juices,* or using prescribed *stool softeners, laxatives,* or *cathartics* as necessary.
   b. Provide activities to reduce perceptual deprivation—reading, handcrafts, music, special interests/hobbies that can be done while maintaining correct position for healing.
2. Goal: *prevent injury or trauma in relation to:*
   a. *Fracture care:*
      (1) Maintain affected part in optimum alignment.
      (2) Maintain skin integrity; check all bony prominences for evidence of pressure q4h and prn, depending on amount of pressure.
      (3) Monitor: circulation in, sensation of, and motion of (CSM) affected part q15 min for first 4 hours; q1h until 24 hours; q4h and prn, depending on amount of edema **(Table 6.36).**
      (4) Maintain mobility in unaffected limb and unaffected joints of affected limb by active and passive ROM; prevent footdrop by using ankle-top sneakers.
   b. *Skin traction:*
      (1) Maintain correct alignment:
         (a) If tape or moleskin is used, shave extremity and apply benzoin to improve adherence of strip and reduce itching.
         (b) Check apparatus for slippage, bunching; replace prn.
      (2) Prevent tissue injury:
         (a) Check all bony prominences for evidence of pressure: q15 min for first 4 hours; q1h until 24 hours, q4h and prn, depending on amount of edema.
         (b) Nonadhesive (e.g., *Bryant's*) traction may be removed q8h to check skin.
   c. *Skeletal traction:*
      (1) Maintain affected part in optimum alignment:
         (a) Ropes on pulleys.
         (b) Weights hang free.
         (c) *Elevate* head of bed as prescribed.
         (d) Check knots routinely.
      (2) Maintain skin integrity:
         (a) Frequent skin care.
         (b) Keep bed linens free of crumbs and wrinkles.
      (3) Prevent infection: special skin care to pin insertion sites three times daily. Keep area around pins clean and dry. Use prescribed solution for cleansing.
      (4) Monitor circulation in, sensation of, and motion of affected part (see **E. 2. a. Fracture care** (see above), and **Table 6.36, p. 506**).
      (5) Maintain mobility in unaffected limb and unaffected joints; prevent footdrop of affected limb.

(text continues on page 506)

ADULT

Table 6.35

Complications of Fractures

Complication	Assessment	Analysis/Nursing Diagnosis	Nursing Care Plan/Implementation	Evaluation/Outcome Criteria
Shock (see **pp. 427–428**)				
Thrombophlebitis (see **pp. 433–434**)				
Fat emboli: serious, potentially life-threatening complication in which pressure changes in interior of fracture force molecules of fat from marrow into systemic circulation; may cause problems in respiratory or nervous system; seen most frequently on *third day* after multiple fractures, fractures of long bones, or comminuted fracture	• *Subjective data:* dyspnea, severe chest pain; confusion, agitation; decrease in level of consciousness; numbness; feeling faint; history of diabetes, obesity • *Objective data:* cyanosis; pupillary changes; muscle twitching; petechiae—chest, buccal cavity, axilla, conjunctiva, soft palate; extremities—pallor, cold; shock; vomiting	• *Risk for injury* related to fat emboli • *Altered tissue perfusion* related to fat emboli	1. *Position:* high Fowler's to relieve respiratory symptoms 2. Administer oxygen **STAT,** to relieve anoxia and reduce surface tension of fat globules 3. Institute respiratory support measures, as ordered—IPPB, respiratory assistive devices: **be prepared for CPR** in event of respiratory failure 4. Monitor vital signs, cardiac monitor, q15 min during acute episode and prn (shock/cardiac failure possible) 5. Obtain baseline data and monitor level of consciousness, neurological signs q15 min during acute episode and prn (neurological involvement possible) 6. Administer parenteral fluids, as ordered: IV alcohol, blood and fluid replacements 7. Administer medications as ordered: *corticosteroids; digitalis; aminophylline; heparin* sodium 8. **DO NOT RUB ANY LEG CRAMPS, BUT REPORT IMMEDIATELY**	• Client alert • Pain relieved • Respiratory, cardiac, and neurological systems have no permanent damage
Nerve compression: pressure on nerve in affected area from edema, dislocation of bone, or immobilization apparatus; if pressure not relieved, permanent paralysis can result	• *Subjective data:* discomfort, pain, referred pain; burning, tingling, "stinging sensation"; numbness, altered sensation, inability to distinguish touch • *Objective data:* limited movement; muscle weakness; paralysis; reflexes—diminished, irritable, or absent; color changes related to impaired circulation	• *Pain* related to pressure on nerve • *Potential for physical injury* related to pressure on nerve • *Impaired tissue perfusion* related to impaired circulation • *Impaired physical mobility* related to joint contracture, numbness	1. Monitor for potential signs q1h for first 48 hr; neurovascular assessment q12h and prn as condition indicates (circulation, sensation, and motion [*CSM*]) 2. *Elevate* affected limb; *flex* hand or foot of affected extremity; passive and active ROM exercises 3. **Be prepared to cut cast or remove constrictions if signs of impairment exist** 4. Begin active ROM exercises to unaffected extremities 5. Use footboard to prevent footdrop 6. Encourage use of trapeze if applicable 7. Isometric exercises, as ordered 8. Ambulation, weight bearing as ordered, support casts	• Sensation, motor function are normal • No complications noted

Continued

ADULT

Table 6.35

Complications of Fractures—cont'd

Complication	Assessment	Analysis/Nursing Diagnosis	Nursing Care Plan/Implementation	Evaluation/Outcome Criteria
Avascular necrosis/circulatory impairment: interference with normal circulation to affected area due to interruption of blood vessel, pressure on the vessel from dislocation, edema, or immobilization devices; results of impaired circulation lead to discomfort and, if not corrected, necrosis of tissue and bone due to lack of oxygen supply	• *Subjective data:* tenderness; pain, especially on passive motion • *Objective data:* edema, swelling in affected area; decreased color, temperature, mobility; bleeding from wound	• *Risk for altered peripheral tissue perfusion* related to vessel damage	1. Monitor for potential signs q1h for first 48 hr; blanching, coolness, edema; palpate pulse above and below injury, report absent pulse or major discrepancies **STAT** 2. *Elevate* affected limb to decrease edema 3. Report to physician if signs persist 4. Be prepared to assist with bivalving of casts, or cut cast to relieve pressure 5. Monitor size of drainage stains on casts; measure accurately and report if size increases	• Circulation adequate to limb, to prevent tissue damage
Infection	• *Subjective data:* pain • *Objective data: elevated* temperature and pulse: erythema—discoloration of surrounding skin; edema—*sudden,* local induration; drainage—thin, watery, foul-smelling exudate; crepitus (may be indicative of **gas gangrene**); with cast—warm area, foul smell	• *Risk for injury* related to tissue destruction • *Altered peripheral tissue perfusion* related to swelling	1. Monitor vital signs, drainage 2. Ensure client has had prophylactic tetanus toxoid 3. May have prophylactic **antibiotics** ordered if wound was contaminated at time of injury 4. Instruct client *not* to touch open wound or pin sites or put anything inside cast (could interrupt skin integrity and become potential source of infection)	• No infection or heals with no serious complications
Delayed union/nonunion: failure of bone to heal within normal time related to lack of use, inadequate circulation, other complicating medical conditions such as diabetes or poor nutrition	• *Subjective data:* pain • *Objective data:* lack of callus formation on x-ray: poor alignment	• *Risk for injury* related to poor healing of bone fracture • *Impaired physical mobility* related to lower-limb fractures • *Dressing/grooming bathing/hygiene, self-care deficit* related to upper-limb fracture	1. Maintain immobilization and alignment of affected limb 2. Maintain adequate nutrition 3. *Avoid* trauma to affected limb 4. Monitor for circulatory or infection complication 5. Dietary instructions regarding foods containing *calcium* and *protein* necessary for bone healing	• Bone heals • No complications noted • Pain decreased • Ambulation and self-care return to preinjury status

Skin breakdown (related to cast)	• *Subjective data:* pain • *Objective data:* temperature and pulse *elevated;* erythema; edema—cast edges, exposed distal portion of limb, limb area within cast; drainage and foul odor from break in skin (may be under cast and stain through or exit at ends of cast); crepitus (crackling sound could indicate **gas gangrene**); *hyperactive reflexes*	• *Impaired skin integrity* related to cast trauma	1. If open wound: verify tetanus administration; monitor site through cast window, change dressing daily and prn 2. Apply lotion or cornstarch to exposed skin (*no* powder) 3. Petal-tape edges of cast to reduce irritation 4. Inspect skin for irritation, edema, odor, drainage—q2h initially, then q3h 5. Instruct client *not* to place any object under cast because skin abrasions may lead to decubitus ulcers 6. Promote drying of cast by leaving it uncovered and exposed to air for 48 hr; use *no* plastic 7. Prevent indenting casts with fingertips or hard surface: place on pillows; use palms of hands when positioning affected limb 8. *Avoid* excessive padding of Thomas' splint in groin area—padding traps moisture, may lead to skin breakdown	• No skin breakdown
Duodenal distress (with spica cast): *spica* cast incorporates the trunk and affected limb and can cause respiratory or abdominal distress when edema is present under the cast or cast is too tight to allow for normal body functions	• *Subjective data:* anorexia, nausea, abdominal pain • *Objective data:* duodenal distress, vomiting, distention, cast too tight	• *Ineffective breathing* related to pressure from cast • *Pain* related to abdominal distress from pressure • *Fear* related to cast constriction	1. Place on firm mattress; use bedboards if necessary to reduce muscle spasm 2. Maintain warmth by covering uncasted areas 3. *Avoid* turning for first 8 hr; when turning: use enough personnel to logroll; do *not* use bar between legs as turning device; support chest with pillows 4. Monitor for signs of respiratory distress: increased respirations, apprehension 5. Monitor for signs of duodenal distress: vomiting, distention; *if these signs occur:* place in *prone* position; have cast bivalved; may need NG tube; monitor for fluid imbalance 6. Protect cast with nonabsorbent material during elimination	• Complications avoided or detected early enough to prevent serious damage

Table 6.36

Assessing Injured Limb: CSM

C	**Circulation** Is it warm to touch? Are both limbs equal in size? Are peripheral pulses present? Is there adequate capillary refill?
S	**Sensation** Does the client feel pain? Can the client distinguish different sensations (e.g., painful stimuli vs. soft touch)? Is the client aware of the position of the limb?
M	**Motion** Can the client move extremities that are not immobilized? Can the client do this independently? Can the client do this on command?

d. *Running traction* (see **Fig. 6.14, p. 501**):
   (1) Keep well centered in bed.
   (2) *Elevate head of bed only* to point of countertraction.
   (3) *No* turning from side to side—will cause rubbing of bony fragments.
   (4) Check distal circulation frequently.
   (5) Frequent back care to prevent skin breakdown.
   (6) Fracture bedpan for toileting.
   (7) *Avoid* excessive padding of splints in groin area to prevent tissue trauma.

e. *Balanced suspension traction* (see **Fig. 6.14, part *F*, p. 501**):
   (1) Maintain alignment and countertraction:
      (a) Ropes on pulleys.
      (b) Weights hang free.
      (c) *Elevate* head of bed as prescribed.
      (d) Check knots routinely.
   (2) May move client, but turn only slightly (*no more than 30 degrees* to *unaffected* side).
   (3) Heel of affected leg must remain *free* of the bed.
   (4) *20-degree angle* between thigh and bed.
   (5) Check for pressure from sling to popliteal area.
   (6) Provide foot support to prevent footdrop.
   (7) Maintain *abduction* of extremity.
   (8) Check for signs of infection at pin insertion sites; cleanse three times daily as ordered.
   (9) If tape or moleskin is used, shave extremity and apply benzoin to improve adherence of strip and reduce itching.

f. *Cervical traction* (see **Fig. 6.14, p. 501**):
   (1) May be placed on specialized bed (e.g., *Stryker frame*).

   (2) *Position:* maintain body alignment.
   (3) Keep tongs free from bed, and keep weights hanging freely to allow traction to function properly.

g. *Halo traction:*
   (1) Several times a day, check screws to the head and screws that hold the upper portion of the frame, to determine correct position.
   (2) Pin sites cleansed three times daily with *bacteriostatic* solution to prevent infection.
   (3) Monitor for signs of infection.
   (4) *Position* as any other client in body cast, except *no* pressure to rest on halo—pillows may be placed under abdomen and chest when client is prone.
   (5) Institute ROM exercises to prevent contractures.
   (6) Turn frequently to prevent development of pressure areas.
   (7) Allow client to verbalize about having screws placed in skull.
   (8) Postapplication nursing care same as pin insertion for other traction.

h. *External fixation devices:*
   (1) Pin care same as for skeletal traction.
   (2) Teach clothing adjustment.
   (3) Teach to adjust for size of apparatus.

i. *Internal fixation devices:*
   (1) Monitor for signs of infection/allergic reaction to materials used for maintenance of reduction (drainage, pain, increased temperature).
   (2) Position as ordered to prevent dislocation.

j. *Casts:*
   (1) Support drying cast on *firm pillow; avoid* finger imprints on cast.
   (2) *Elevate* limb to reduce edema.
   (3) Prevent complications of fractures as listed.
   (4) Closely monitor *circulation* (blanching, swelling, decreased temperature); *sensation* (absence of feeling; pain or burning); and *motion* (inability to move digits of affected limb).
   (5) **Be prepared to notify physician or cut cast if circulatory impairment occurs.**
   (6) Protect skin integrity: *avoid* pressure of edges of cast; petal prn.
   (7) Monitor for signs of infection if skin integrity impaired.

3. Goal: *provide care related to ambulation with crutches.*
   a. Teach appropriate gait **(Table 6.37).**

b. Measure crutches correctly (**Table 6.38**).
   (1) Subtract 16 inches from total height; top of crutch should be 2 inches below the axilla.
   (2) Complete extension of the elbows should be possible *without* pressure of axilla bar into the axilla.

Table 6.37

Teaching Crutch Walking

A. When only *one* leg can bear weight:
1. *Swing-to gait:* crutches forward; swing body to crutches.
   a. Move both crutches forward.
   b. Move both legs to meet the crutches.
   c. Continue pattern.
2. *Swing-through gait:* crutches forward; swing body through crutches.
   a. Move both crutches forward.
   b. Move both legs farther ahead than crutches.
   c. Continue pattern.
3. *Three-point gait:* crutches and affected extremity forward; swing forward, placing nonaffected foot ahead of or between crutches.
   a. Both crutches and affected limb move at same time.
   b. Move both crutches and affected leg (e.g., left) ahead 6 inches.
   c. Move unaffected leg (e.g., right) to same place as left and crutches.
   d. Continue pattern.

B. When *both* legs can move separately and bear some weight:
1. *Four-point gait:* right crutch forward, left foot forward; swing weight to right side while bringing left crutch forward, then right foot forward; gait simulates normal walking.
   a. Move right crutch forward 4–6 inches.
   b. Move left foot forward same distance as right crutch.
   c. Move left crutch forward ahead of left foot.
   d. Move right foot forward to meet right crutch.
   e. Continue pattern.
2. *Two-point gait:* same as four-point gait but faster; one crutch and opposite leg moving forward at same time.
   a. Opposite crutch and limb move together.
   b. Move right crutch and left leg ahead 6 inches.
   c. Move left crutch and right leg ahead.
   d. Continue pattern.

C. When client is *unable* to walk: *tripod gait:* crutches forward at a wide distance; drag legs to point just behind crutches, balance, and repeat.

Table 6.38

Measuring Crutches Correctly

1. Have client lie on a flat surface. Measure from anterior fold of axilla to 4 inches lateral to heel.
2. Have client stand. Measure from 1–2 inches below axilla to 2 inches in front of and 6 inches to the side of the foot.
3. Hand placement on bar of crutch: have client stand upright, support body weight with hand on bar (*not* putting weight on axilla). Elbow flexion should be *30 degrees*.
4. Slightly pad the shoulder rests of the crutches for general comfort.
5. Make sure there are nonskid rubber tips on the crutches.

   (3) Handgrip should be adjusted so that complete wrist extension is possible.
   (4) Instruct in correct body alignment:
      (a) Head erect.
      (b) Back straight.
      (c) Chest forward.
      (d) Feet 6 to 8 inches apart, wide base for support.

4. Goal: *provide safety measures related to possible complications following fracture* (see **Table 6.35**).
5. Goal: *health teaching.*
   a. Explain and show apparatus before application, if possible.
   b. Pin care at least once daily to prevent granulation and cellulitis.
   c. Correct position for rest/sleep and prevention of injury with halo traction—*no* pressure on halo.
   d. Purpose of cast: to immobilize, to support body tissues, to prevent or correct deformities.
   e. Teach signs and symptoms of *complications* to report related to cast care (i.e., numbness, odor, crack/break in cast; extremity cold, bluish).
   f. Isometric exercises for use with affected joint.
   g. *Safety measures with crutches:*
      (1) Weight-bearing on hands, *not* axilla.
      (2) Position crutches 4 inches to side and 4 inches to front.
      (3) Use short strides, looking ahead, not at feet.
      (4) Prevent injury: if client begins to fall, throw crutches to side to prevent falling on them; body should be relaxed.
      (5) Check for environmental hazards: rugs, water spills.

F. Evaluation/outcome criteria:
1. No injury or complications related to apparatus or immobilization (e.g., infection, tissue injury, altered circulation/sensation, dislocation).
2. Bone remains in correct alignment and begins to heal.
3. Demonstrates elevated limb position to relieve edema with casted extremity.
4. Lists complications related to circulation or neurological impairment and infection.
5. Begins to use affected part.
6. Demonstrates correct technique for ambulation with crutches—no pressure on axilla, uses strength of arms and wrists.
7. No falls while using crutches.

III. COMPARTMENT SYNDROME: an accumulation of fluid in the muscle compartment, resulting in an increase in pressure that reduces blood flow to the tissues. Can lead to neuromuscular deficit, amputation, and death.

A. Pathophysiology: inability of the fascia surrounding the muscle group to expand to accommodate the increased volume of fluid → compartment pressure increases → venous flow impaired → arterial flow continues, increasing capillary pressure → fluid pushed into the extravascular space → intracompartment pressure further increased → prolonged or severe ischemia → muscle and nerve cells destroyed, contracture, loss of function, necrotic tissue, infection, release of potassium, hydrogen, and myoglobin into bloodstream.

B. Risk factors:
1. Fractures.
2. Burns.
3. Crushing injuries.
4. Restrictive bandages.
5. Cast.
6. Prolonged lithotomy positioning.
7. Ischemic injury (arterial or venous injury).

C. Assessment:
1. *Subjective data:*
   a. Severe, unrelenting pain, unrelieved by narcotics and associated with passive stretching of muscle.
   b. Paresthesias.
2. *Objective data:*
   a. Edema; tense skin over limb.
   b. Paralysis.
   c. Decreased or absent peripheral pulses.
   d. Poor capillary refill.
   e. Limb temperature change (colder).
   f. Ankle-arm pressure index (API) *decreased;* 0.4 indicates ischemia (see **Chapter 11, Doppler ultrasonography, p. 828**).
   g. Urine output—*decreased* (developing acute tubular necrosis); reddish-brown color.

D. Analysis/nursing diagnosis:
1. *Pain* related to tissue swelling and ischemia.
2. *Risk for injury* related to neuromuscular deficits.
3. *Impaired physical mobility* related to contracture and loss of function.
4. *Risk for infection* related to tissue necrosis.
5. *Altered urinary elimination* related to acute tubular necrosis from myoglobin accumulation.
6. *Body image disturbance* related to limb disfigurement.

E. Nursing care plan/implementation:
1. Goal: *recognize early indications of ischemia.*
   a. Assess *neurovascular* status frequently (q1h): skin temperature, capillary refill, peripheral pulses, mobility, and sensation.
   b. Listen to client complaints; report suspected complications.
   c. Report nonrelief of pain with narcotics.
   d. Recognize unrelenting pain with passive muscle stretching.
2. Goal: *prevent complications.*
   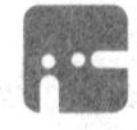
   a. *Elevate* injured extremity initially; if ischemia suspected, keep extremity at *heart level* to prevent compensatory increase in blood flow.
   b. *Avoid* tight bandages, splints, or casts.
   c. Monitor intravenous infusion for signs of infiltration.
   d. Prepare client for fasciotomy (incision of skin and fascia to release tight compartment).

F. Evaluation/outcome criteria:
1. Relief from pain; normal perfusion restored.
2. Neurovascular status within normal limits.
3. Retains function of limb; no contractures or infection.
4. Compartment pressure returns to normal (<20 mm Hg).
5. No systemic complications (e.g., normal cardiac and renal function, acid-base balance within normal limits).

IV. OSTEOARTHRITIS: joint disorder characterized by degeneration of articular cartilage and formation of bony outgrowths at edges of weight-bearing joints.

A. Pathophysiology: excessive friction combined with risk factors → thinning of articular cartilage, narrowing of joint space, and loss of joint stability; cartilage erodes, producing shallow pits on articular surface and exposing bone in joint space. Bone responds by becoming denser and harder.

B. Risk factors:
1. Aging (>50).
2. Rheumatoid arthritis.
3. Arteriosclerosis.
4. Obesity.
5. Trauma.
6. Family history.

C. Assessment:
1. *Subjective data:*
   a. Pain; tender joints.
   b. Fatigability, malaise.
   c. Anorexia.
   d. Cold intolerance.
   e. Extremities: numbness, tingling.
2. *Objective data:*
   a. *Joints:*
      (1) Enlarged.
      (2) Stiff, limited movement.
      (3) Swelling, redness, and heat around affected joint.
      (4) Shiny stretched skin over and around joint.
      (5) Subcutaneous nodules.
   b. Weight loss.
   c. Fever.
   d. Crepitation (creaking or grating of joints).
   e. Deformities, contractures.

ADULT

f. Cold, clammy extremities.
g. Laboratory data: *decreased* Hgb, *elevated* WBC count.
h. *Diagnostic tests:* x-ray, thermography, arthroscopy.

D. Analysis/nursing diagnosis:
1. *Pain* related to friction of bones in joints.
2. *Bathing/hygiene self-care deficit* related to decreased mobility of involved joints.
3. *Risk for injury* related to fatigability.
4. *Impaired physical mobility* related to stiff, limited movement.
5. *Impaired home maintenance management* related to contractures.

E. Nursing care plan/implementation:
1. Goal: *promote comfort: reduce pain, spasms, inflammation, swelling.*
   a. Medications as prescribed.
      (1) *Nonsteroidal antiinflammatory agents:* aspirin (Ecotrin), acetaminophen (Tylenol), ibuprofen (Motrin), indomethacin (Indocin), corticosteroids, nabumetone (Relafen), naproxen (Naprosyn).
      (2) *Antimalarials:* chloroquine (Aralen), hydroxychloroquine (Plaquenil), to relieve symptoms.
   b. Heat to reduce muscle spasms, stiffness.
   c. Cold to reduce swelling and pain.
   d. Prevent contractures:
      (1) Exercise.
      (2) Bedrest on firm mattress during attacks.
      (3) Splints to maintain proper alignment.
   e. *Elevate* extremity to reduce swelling.
   f. Rest.
   g. Assistive devices to decrease weight-bearing of affected joints (canes, walkers).
2. Goal: *health teaching to promote independence.*
   a. Encourage self-care with assistive devices for activities of daily living (ADLs).
   b. Activity, as tolerated, with ambulation-assistive devices.
   c. Scheduled rest periods.
   d. Correct body posture and body mechanics.
3. Goal: *provide for emotional needs.*
   a. Accept feelings of frustration regarding long-term debilitating disorder.
   b. Provide diversional activities appropriate for age and physical condition to promote comfort and satisfaction.

F. Evaluation/outcome criteria:
1. Remains independent as long as possible.
2. No contractures.
3. States comfort has increased.
4. Uses methods that are successful in pain control.

V. RHEUMATOID ARTHRITIS: chronic, systemic, collagen inflammatory disease; etiology unknown; may be autoimmune, viral, or genetic; affects primarily women ages 20 to 40 years; present in 2% to 3% of total population; follows a course of exacerbations and remissions.

A. Pathophysiology: synovitis with edema → proliferation of various blood material (formation of pannus) → destruction and fibrosis of cartilage (fibrous ankylosis); calcification of fibrous tissue (osseous ankylosis) **(Fig. 6.15).**

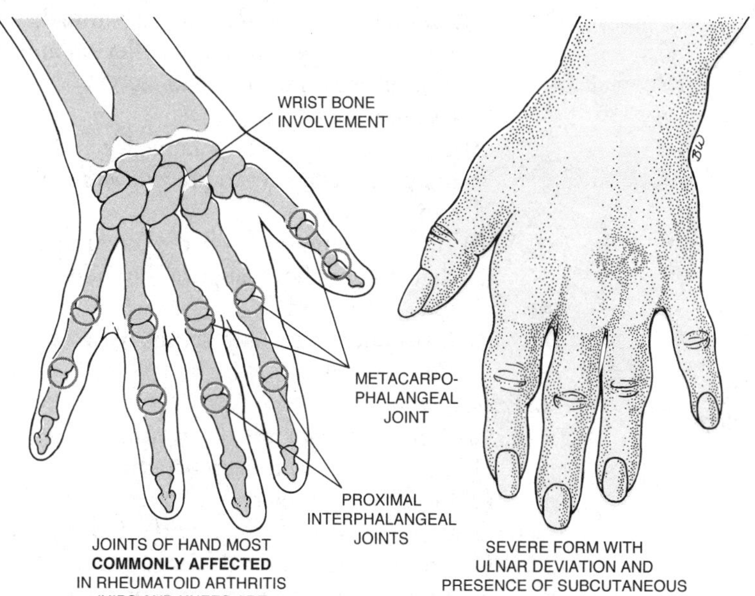

Figure 6.15 Rheumatoid arthritis. (From Venes, D [ed]: *Taber's Cyclopedic Medical Dictionary,* ed 21. FA Davis, Philadelphia, 2009.)

B. Assessment:

1. *Subjective data:*
   a. Joints: pain; morning stiffness; swelling.
   b. Easily fatigues; malaise.
   c. Anorexia; weight loss.
2. *Objective data:*
   a. Subcutaneous nodules over bony prominences.
   b. Bilateral symmetrical involvement of joints: crepitation, creaking, grating.
   c. Deformities: contractures, muscle atrophy.
   d. Laboratory data: blood: *decreased*—hemoglobin/hematocrit; RBCs; *increased*—WBCs (12,000 to 15,000), sedimentation rate (>20 mm/hr), rheumatoid factor. Positive antinuclear antibody titer.

C. Analysis/nursing diagnosis:

1. *Pain* related to joint destruction.
2. *Impaired physical mobility* related to joint contractures.
3. *Risk for injury* related to the inflammatory process.
4. *Body image disturbance* related to joint deformity.
5. *Self-care deficit* related to musculoskeletal impairment.
6. *Risk for activity intolerance* related to fatigue and stiffness.
7. *Altered nutrition, less than body requirements,* related to anorexia and weight loss.
8. *Self-esteem disturbance* related to chronic illness.

D. Nursing care plan/implementation:

1. Goal: *prevent or correct deformities.*
   a. Activity:
      (1) Bedrest during exacerbations.
      (2) Daily ROM—active and passive exercises *even* in acute phase, 5- to 10-minute periods; *avoid* fatigue and persistent pain.
      (3) Heat or pain medication before exercise.
   b. Medications: *aspirin* (high dosages); *nonsteroidals; steroids; antacids* given for possible GI upset with ASA, steroids; *disease-modifying antirheumatics* (methotrexate, hydroxychloroquine, sulfasalazine).
   c. *Fluids:* at least 1,500 mL liquid daily to avoid renal calculi; milk for GI upset.
2. Goal: *health teaching.*
   a. Side effects of medications: tarry stools (GI bleeding); tinnitus (ASA).
   b. Psychosocial aspects: possible need for early retirement; financial hardship; loss of libido; unsatisfactory sexual relations.
   c. Prepare for joint repair or replacement if indicated.

E. Evaluation/outcome criteria:

1. Remains as active as possible; limited loss of mobility; performs self-care activities.
2. No side effects from drug therapy (e.g., GI bleeding).
3. Copes with necessary lifestyle changes; complies with treatment regimen.

VI. TOTAL HIP REPLACEMENT: femoral head and acetabulum are replaced by a prosthesis, which is cemented into the bone with plastic cement. Performed to replace a joint with limited and painful function due to bony alkalosis and deformity, caused by degenerative joint disease or when vascular supply to femoral head is compromised from a fracture. *Goal of the surgery:* restore or improve mobilization of hip joint and prevent complications of extended immobilization.

A. Risk factors:

1. Rheumatoid arthritis.
2. Osteoarthritis.
3. Complications of femoral neck fractures—avascular necrosis and malunion **(Table 6.39).**
4. Congenital hip disease.

B. Analysis/nursing diagnosis:

1. *Risk for injury* related to implant surgery.
2. *Knowledge deficit* (learning need) regarding joint replacement surgery.
3. *Impaired physical mobility* related to major hip surgery.
4. *Pain* related to surgical incision.
5. *Risk for impaired skin integrity* related to immobility.

C. Nursing care plan/implementation:

1. *Preoperative:*
   a. Goal: *prevent deep vein thrombosis or pulmonary emboli.*
      (1) Antiembolic stockings.
      (2) *Increase* fluid intake.
   b. Goal: *prevent infection: antibiotics* as ordered, given prophylactically (Cefazolin).
   c. Goal: *health teaching.*
      (1) *Isometric exercises*—gluteal, abdominal, and quadriceps-setting; dorsiflexion and plantar flexion of the feet.
      (2) Use of trapeze.
      (3) Explain position of operative leg and hip postoperatively to prevent *adduction* and flexion.
      (4) Transfer techniques—bed to chair and chair to crutches; dangle at bedside first time out of bed.
      (5) Assist client with skin scrubs with antibacterial soap.
2. *Postoperative:*
   a. Goal: *prevent respiratory complications.*
      (1) Turn, cough, and deep breathe.
      (2) Incentive spirometry.
   b. Goal: *prevent complications of shock or infection.*
      (1) Check dressings for drainage q1h for first 4 hours; then q4h and prn; may have

ADULT

Table 6.39

Fractures of the Hip

Risk	Types	Assessment	Surgical Intervention
• Osteoporosis • Age >60 • Women (white) • While postmenopausal • Immobility/sedentary lifestyle	Intracapsular (femoral neck; *within* hip joint and capsule)	• Slight trauma • Pain: groin and hip • Lateral rotation, shortening of leg, minimal deformity	Total hip replacement
	Extracapsular (*outside* hip joint; also called *intertrochanteric*)	• Direct trauma • Severe pain • External rotation, shortening of leg, obvious deformity	• Internal fixation with nail (*open reduction*) • Possible total hip replacement
	Subtrochanteric (below lesser trochanter)	• Direct trauma • Leg pain near fracture site • External rotation, shortening of leg, deformity • Presence of hematoma	• Internal fixation with nail (open reduction) • Closed reduction

Hemovac or other drainage tubes inserted in wound to keep dressing dry.

(2) Monitor I&O and vital signs hourly for 4 hours, then q4h and prn.

c. Goal: *prevent contractures, muscle atrophy:* initiate exercises as soon as allowed: isometric quadriceps, dorsiflexion and plantar flexion of foot, and flexion and extension of the ankle—sequential compression device while in bed.

d. Goal: *promote early ambulation and movement.*

(1) Use trapeze.

(2) Transfer technique (pivot on unaffected leg); crutches/walker.

(3) Initiate progressive ambulation as ordered; ensure *maximum extension* of leg when walking.

(4) Administer *anticoagulation* therapy as ordered (warfarin immediately postoperatively) to prevent deep vein thrombosis and pulmonary emboli.

(5) Recognize early side effects of medications and report appropriately.

e. Goal: *prevent constipation.*

(1) *Increase* fluid intake.

(2) Use fracture bedpan.

f. Goal: *prevent dislocation of prosthesis.*

(1) Maintain *abduction* of the affected joint (prevent external rotation); *elevate* head of bed, turn according to physician's order. When turning to unaffected side, turn with abduction pillow between legs to maintain abduction.

(2) *Buck's extension* or *Russell's traction* may be applied (temporary skin traction).

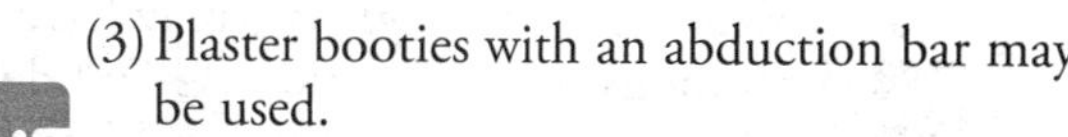

(3) Plaster booties with an abduction bar may be used.

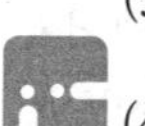

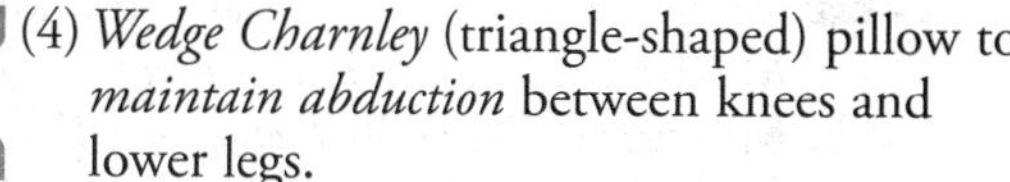

(4) *Wedge Charnley* (triangle-shaped) pillow to *maintain abduction* between knees and lower legs.

(5) Provide periods throughout day when client lies *flat* in bed to *prevent hip flexion* and strengthen hip muscles.

(6) Report signs of dislocation: *anteriorly*—knee flexes, leg turns outward, leg looks longer than other, femur head may be felt in groin area; *posteriorly*—leg turns inward, appears shorter than other, greater trochanter elevated.

g. Goal: *promote comfort.*

(1) Initiate skin care; monitor pressure points for redness; back care q2h.

(2) Alternating pressure mattress; sheepskin when sitting in chair.

h. Goal: *health teaching.*

(1) Exercise program with written list of activity restrictions.

(2) Methods to *prevent* hip adduction.

(3) *Avoid* sitting for more than 1 hour: stand, stretch, and walk frequently to *prevent* hip flexion contractures.

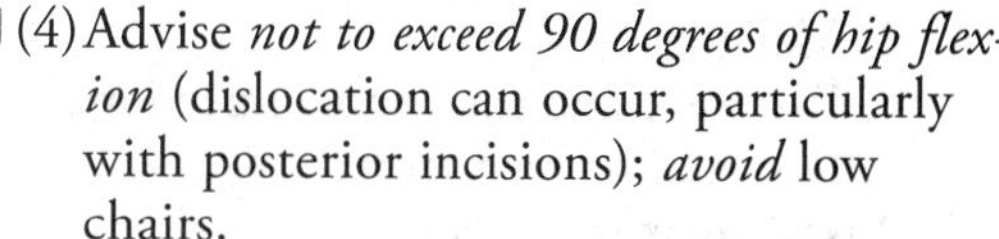

(4) Advise *not to exceed 90 degrees of hip flexion* (dislocation can occur, particularly with posterior incisions); *avoid* low chairs.

(5) Teach alternative methods of usual self-care activities to prevent hip dislocation (e.g., *avoid:* bending from waist to tie shoes, sitting up straight in a low chair, using a low toilet seat).

ADULT

(6) *Avoid* crossing legs, driving a car for 6 weeks.
(7) Wear support hose for 6 weeks to enhance venous return and avoid thrombus formation.

D. Evaluation/outcome criteria:

1. Participates in postoperative nursing care plan to prevent complications.
2. Reports pain has decreased.
3. Ambulates with assistive devices.
4. Complications of immobility avoided.
5. Able to resume self-care activities.

VII. TOTAL KNEE REPLACEMENT: both sides of the joint are replaced by metal or plastic implants.

A. Analysis/nursing diagnosis (see **VI. TOTAL HIP REPLACEMENT, p. 510**).

B. Nursing plan/implementation:

1. See **VI. TOTAL HIP REPLACEMENT, pp. 510–512.**
2. Goal: *achieve active flexion beyond 70 degrees.*
   a. *Immediately postoperatively:* may have continuous passive motion (CPM) device for flexion-extension of affected knee. Maximum flexion *110 degrees.*
   b. Monitor drainage in *Hemovac* (q15 min for first 4 hours, q1h until 24 hours; q4h and prn while Hemovac in place).
   c. Analgesics as ordered for pain.
   d. While dressings are still on: quadriceps-setting exercises for approximately 5 days (consult with physical therapist for specific instructions).
   e. After dressings removed: active flexion exercises.
   f. *Avoid* pressure on heel.

C. Evaluation/outcome criteria:

1. No complications of infection, hemorrhage noted.
2. ROM of knee increases with exercises.

VIII. AMPUTATION: surgical removal of a limb as a result of trauma or circulatory impairment (gangrene). The amount of tissue amputated is determined by the severity of disease or trauma and the ability of the remaining tissue to heal.

A. Risk factors:

1. Atherosclerosis obliterans.
2. Uncontrolled diabetes mellitus.
3. Malignancy.
4. Extensive and intractable infection.
5. Result of severe trauma.

B. Assessment *(preoperative):*

1. *Subjective data:* pain in affected part.
2. *Objective data:*
   a. Soft tissue damage.
   b. Partial or complete severance of a body part.
   c. Lack of peripheral pulses.
   d. Skin color changes, pallor → cyanosis → gangrene.
   e. Infection, hemorrhage, or shock.

C. Analysis/nursing diagnosis:

1. *Impaired physical mobility* related to lower-limb amputation.
2. *Body image disturbance* related to loss of body part.
3. *Pain* related to interruption of nerve pathways.
4. *Anxiety* related to potential change in lifestyle.
5. *Knowledge deficit* (learning need) related to rehabilitation goals.

D. Nursing care plan/implementation:

1. Goal: *prepare for surgery, physically and emotionally.*
   a. Validate that client and family are aware that amputation of body part is planned.
   b. Validate that informed consent is signed.
   c. Allow time for grieving.
   d. If time allows, prepare client for postoperative phase (e.g., teach arm-strengthening exercises if lower limb is to be amputated; teach alternative methods of ambulation).
   e. Provide time to discuss feelings.
   f. Prepare surgical site to decrease possibility of infection (e.g., shave, scrub as ordered).
   g. Discuss postoperative expectations.
2. Goal: *promote healing postoperatively.*
   a. Monitor *respiratory status* q1–4h and prn: rate, depth of respiration; auscultate for signs of congestion; and question client about chest pain (*pulmonary emboli* common complication).
   b. Monitor for hemorrhage; keep tourniquet at bedside.
   c. Medicate for pain as ordered—client may have phantom limb pain.
   d. Support stump on pillow for first 24 hours; **remove pillow** after 24 hours to prevent contracture.
   e. *Position: turn client on to stomach* to prevent hip contracture.
   f. ROM exercises for joint above amputation to prevent joint immobilization; strengthening exercises for arms, nonaffected limbs, abdominal muscles.
   g. *Stump care:*
      (1) Early postoperative dressings changed prn.
      (2) As incision heals, bandage is applied in cone shape to prepare stump for prosthesis.
      (3) Inspect for blisters, redness, abrasions.
      (4) Remove stump sock daily and prn.
   h. Assist in rehabilitation program.

E. Evaluation/outcome criteria:

1. Begins rehabilitation program.
2. No hemorrhage, infection.
3. Adjusts to altered body image.

ADULT

IX. GOUT: disorder of purine metabolism; genetic disease believed to be transmitted by a dominant gene, characterized by recurrent attacks of acute pain and swelling of one joint (usually the great toe).

A. Pathophysiology: urate crystals and infiltrating leukocytes appear to damage the intracellular phagolysosomes, resulting in leakage of lysomal enzymes into the synovial fluid, causing tissue damage and joint inflammation.

B. Risk factors:
1. Men.
2. Age (>50).
3. Genetic/familial tendency.
4. Prolonged hyperuricemia (elevated serum uric acid).
5. Obesity.
6. Moderate to heavy alcohol intake.
7. Hypertension.
8. Abnormal kidney function.

C. Assessment:
1. *Subjective data:*
   a. *Pain:* excruciating
   b. Fatigue
   c. Anorexia.
2. *Objective data:*
   a. *Joint:* erythema (redness), hot, swollen, difficult to move; skin stretched and shiny over joint.
   b. Subcutaneous nodules, tophi (deposits of urate) on hands and feet.
   c. Weight loss.
   d. Fever.
   e. Sensory changes, with cold intolerance.
   f. Laboratory data:
      (1) Serum uric acid: *increased significantly* (6.5 mg/100 mL in women, 7.5 mg/100 mL in men) in chronic gout; only *slightly increased* in acute gout.
      (2) WBC count: 12,000 to 15,000/mm^3.
      (3) Erythrocyte sedimentation rate: >20 mm/hr.
      (4) 24-hour urinary uric acid: slightly *elevated.*
      (5) Proteinuria (chronic gout).
      (6) Azotemia (presence of nitrogen-containing compounds in blood) in chronic gout.
   g. *Diagnostic tests:* arthrocentesis, x-rays.

D. Analysis/nursing diagnosis:
1. *Pain* related to inflammation and swelling of affected joint.
2. *Impaired physical mobility* related to pain.
3. *Knowledge deficit* (learning need) related to diet restrictions and increased fluid needs.
4. *Altered urinary elimination* related to kidney damage.

E. Nursing care plan/implementation:
1. Goal: *decrease discomfort.*

   a. Administer antigout medications as ordered:
      (1) Treatment of *acute* attacks: colchicine, phenylbutazone (Butazolidin), indomethacin (Indocin), allopurinol (Zyloprim), naproxen (Naprosyn), corticosteroids (prednisone).
      (2) *Preventive therapy:* probenecid (Benemid), sulfinpyrazone (Anturane). These drugs are *not* used during acute attacks.

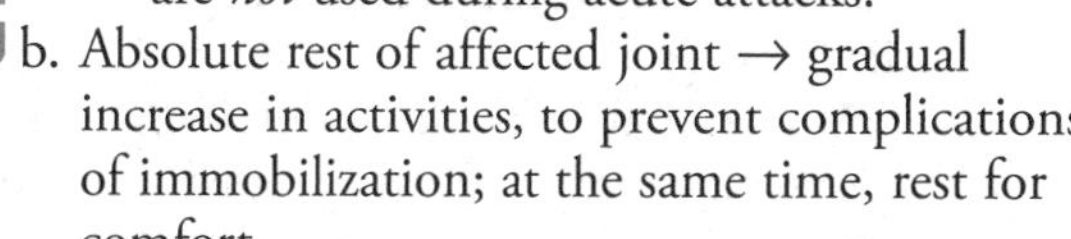

   b. Absolute rest of affected joint → gradual increase in activities, to prevent complications of immobilization; at the same time, rest for comfort.
2. Goal: *prevent kidney damage.*
   a. *Increase* fluid intake to 2,000 to 3,000 mL/day.
   b. Monitor urinary output.
3. Goal: *health teaching.*

   a. Need for *low-purine diet* during acute attack (see **Purine-restricted diet, Common Therapeutic Diets, Chapter 9, p. 699**).
   b. Importance of *increased fluid in diet.*
   c. Signs and symptoms of increased progression of disease.
   d. Dosage and side effects of prescribed medications.

F. Evaluation/outcome criteria:
1. Swelling decreased.
2. Discomfort alleviated.
3. Mobility returned to status before attack.
4. Laboratory values return to normal.

X. LUPUS ERYTHEMATOSUS (LE): chronic inflammatory disease of connective tissue; may affect or involve any organ; vague etiology, but genetic factors, viruses, hormones, and drugs are being investigated; occurs primarily in women ages 18 to 35 years. Two forms: discoid lupus erythematosus (DLE) affects skin only, and systemic lupus erythematosus (SLE) affects multiple organs.

A. Pathophysiology: possible toxic effects from immune complexes deposited in tissue (antibody-antigen trapping in organ capillaries)—fibrinoid necrosis of collagen in connective issue, small arterial walls (kidneys and heart particularly) → cellular death, obstructed blood flow.

B. Assessment:
1. *Subjective data:*
   a. Pain: joints.
   b. Anorexia; weight loss.
   c. Photophobia; sensitivity to sun.
   d. Weakness.
   e. Nausea, vomiting.
2. *Objective data:*
   a. Fever.
   b. Rash: butterfly distribution across nose, cheeks.

c. Lesions: raised, red, scaling plaques—coinlike (discoid).
d. Ulceration: oral or nasopharyngeal.
e. Laboratory data:
(1) Blood: *increased* LE cells; *decreased*—RBCs, WBCs, thrombocytes. Positive antinuclear antibody (ANA) titer.
(2) *Urine*—hematuria, proteinuria (nephritis).

C. Analysis/nursing diagnosis:
1. *Risk for injury* related to possible autoimmune disorder.
2. *Pain* related to joint inflammation.
3. *Risk for activity intolerance* related to extreme fatigue, anemia.
4. *Body image disturbance* related to chronic skin eruptions.
5. *Altered nutrition, less than body requirements,* related to anorexia, nausea, vomiting.
6. *Altered oral mucous membrane* related to ulcerations.

D. Nursing care plan/implementation:
1. Goal: *minimize or limit immune response and complications.*
a. Activity: rest; 8 to 10 hours' sleep; unhurried environment; assist with stressful activities; ROM to prevent joint immobility and stiffness.
b. Skin care: hygiene; *topical steroid* cream as ordered for inflammation, pruritus, scaling.
c. Mouth care: several times daily if stomatitis present; *soft, bland, or liquid diet* to prevent irritation.
d. *Diet: low* sodium if edematous; *low* protein with renal involvement.
e. Observe for signs of complications:
(1) *Cardiac/respiratory* (tachycardia, tachypnea, dyspnea, orthopnea).
(2) *GI* (diarrhea, abdominal pain, distention).
(3) *Renal* (increased weight, oliguria, *decreased* specific gravity).
(4) *Neurological* (ptosis, ataxia).
(5) *Hematological* (malaise, weakness, chills, epistaxis); **report immediately.**
f. Medications, as ordered:
(1) *Analgesics.*
(2) *Anti-inflammatory* agents (aspirin, prednisone) and *immunosuppressive drugs* (azathioprine [Imuran], cyclophosphamide [Cytoxan]) to control inflammation.
(3) *Antimalarials* for skin and joint manifestations.
2. Goal: *health teaching.*
a. Disease process: diagnosis, prognosis, effects of treatment.
b. *Avoid* precipitating factors:
(1) Sun (aggravates skin lesions; thus, cover body as much as possible).
(2) Altering dosage of medications.
(3) Pregnancy (requires medical clearance).
(4) Fatigue, stress.
(5) Infections.
c. Medications: side effects of immunosuppressives and corticosteroids.
d. Regular exercise: walking, swimming; but *avoid* fatigue.
e. Wear Medic Alert bracelet.

E. Evaluation/outcome criteria:
1. Attains a state of remission.
2. No organ involvement (e.g., no cardiac, renal complications).
3. Keeps active within limitations.
4. Continues follow-up medical care—recognizes symptoms requiring immediate attention.

NEUROMUSCULAR SYSTEM

I. MULTIPLE SCLEROSIS: progressive neurological disease, common in northern climates, characterized by demyelination of brain and spinal cord leading to degenerative neurological function; chronic remitting and relapsing disease; cause unknown. Visual problems are often the first indication of multiple sclerosis. *Classifications of multiple sclerosis:* relapsing-remitting, primary progressive, secondary progressive, and progressive-relapsing. Exacerbations aggravated by fatigue, chilling, and emotional distress.

A. Pathophysiology: multiple foci (patches) of nerve degeneration throughout brain, spinal cord, optic nerve, and cerebrum cause nerve impulses to be interrupted (blocked) or distorted (slowed). Researchers suggest that, in genetically susceptible people, the disease results from an abnormal autoimmune response to some agent, perhaps a virus or environmental trigger.

B. Risk factors:
1. Northern climate.
2. Onset age: 20 to 40 years.
3. Two to three times more common in women than men.

C. Assessment:
1. *Subjective data:*
a. Extremities: weak, numb, decreased sensation.
b. Emotional: instability, apathy, irritability, mood swings, fatigue.
c. Eyes: diplopia (double vision), spots before eyes (scotomas), potential blindness.
d. Difficulty in swallowing.
e. Pain.
2. *Objective data:*
a. Nystagmus (involuntary rhythmic movements of eyeball) and decreased visual acuity.

ADULT

b. Inappropriate outbursts of laughing or crying (sometimes related to ingestion of hot food).
c. Disorders of speech.
d. Susceptible to infections.
e. Tremors to severe muscle spasms and contractures.
f. Changes in muscular coordination; *gait:* ataxic, spastic.
g. Changes in bowel habits (e.g., constipation).
h. Urinary frequency and urgency.
i. Incontinence (urine and feces).
j. Sexual dysfunction.
k. Cognitive changes/depression.
l. *Laboratory tests:* cerebrospinal fluid has presence of gamma globulin IgG.
m. *Diagnostic tests:*
(1) Neurological examination.
(2) Positive *Lhermitte's* sign (electric shock–like sensation along spine on flexion of the head).
(3) Positive *Babinski* reflex.
(4) MRI detects plaques.

D. Analysis/nursing diagnosis:
1. *Impaired physical mobility* related to changes in muscular coordination.
2. *Self-esteem disturbance* related to chronic, debilitating disease.
3. *Altered health maintenance* related to spasms and contractures.
4. *Risk for impaired skin integrity* related to contractures.
5. *Constipation* related to immobility.
6. *Impaired swallowing* related to tremors.
7. *Visual sensory/perceptual alteration* related to nystagmus and decreased visual acuity.

E. Nursing care plan/implementation:
1. Goal: *maintain normal routine as long as possible.*
a. Maintain mobility—encourage walking as tolerated; active and passive ROM; splints to decrease spasticity.
b. *Avoid* fatigue, infections.
c. Frequent position changes to prevent skin breakdown and contractures; *position at night: prone,* to minimize flexor spasms of knees and hips.
d. Bowel/bladder training program to minimize incontinence.
e. *Avoid* stressful situations.
2. Goal: *decrease symptoms*—medications as ordered:
a. Methylprednisolone (high dose, IV) plus sodium succinate, followed by gradual tapering of steroids to treat at *initial* diagnosis.
b. Methylprednisolone (Solu-Medrol), prednisone (Deltasone), and dexamethasone (Decadron) used to treat *acute relapses.*
c. Methotrexate (Rheumatrex) (low dose) used *to delay progression of impairment.*
d. Interferon beta-1b (Betaseron) reduces *number* of lesions and *frequency of relapses.*
e. Glatiramer (Copaxone) *to reduce number of relapses.*
f. Baclofen (Lioresal) for *alleviating spasticity* 5 mg three times daily, increased by 5 mg every 3 days; not to exceed 80 mg/day (20 mg four times daily). Optimal effect between 40 and 80 mg; sudden withdrawal of medication may cause *hallucinations* and *rebound spasticity.*
g. Diazepam (Valium), dantrolene (Dantrium) to relieve *muscle spasm.*
h. Carbamazepine (Tegretol) or amitriptyline HCl (Elavil) for *dysesthesias* or *neuralgia.*
i. Ciprofloxacin (Cipro) to treat *bladder dysfunction.*
j. Psyllium hydrophilic mucilloid (Metamucil) to treat *bowel dysfunction.*
k. Phenytoin (Dilantin) to treat *sensory symptoms.*
l. Analgesics to treat *pain.*
3. Goal: *health teaching to prevent complications.*
a. Signs and symptoms of disease; measures to prevent exacerbations.
b. Teach to monitor respiratory status to prevent infections.
c. Referral: importance of *physical therapy* to prevent contractures.
d. Referral: possible counseling or community support group for assistance in accepting long-term condition.
e. Teach special skin care to prevent decubitus ulcers.
f. Teach use of assistive devices to maintain independence.
4. Goal: *provide psychosocial support.*
a. Answer questions of client and family members.
b. Provide referrals to appropriate agencies.
c. Monitor for signs of suicide (higher incidence of suicide in clients with MS than the general population).
d. Encourage communication.

F. Evaluation/outcome criteria:
1. Establishes daily routine; adjusts to altered lifestyle.
2. Injuries prevented; no falls.
3. Urinary and bowel routines established; incontinence decreased.
4. Infections avoided.
5. Symptoms minimized by medications.

II. MYASTHENIA GRAVIS: chronic neuromuscular disease characterized by weakness and easy fatigability of facial, oculomotor, pharyngeal, and respiratory muscles. The muscle weakness increases during periods of activity and improves after periods of rest.

A. Pathophysiology: inadequate acetylcholine or excessive or altered cholinesterase, leading to impaired transmission of nerve impulses to muscles at myoneural junction.

B. Risk factors:

1. Possible autoimmune reaction.
2. Thymus tumor.
3. Young women and older men, but can occur at any age.

C. Assessment:

1. *Subjective data:*
   a. Diplopia (double vision).
   b. Severe generalized fatigue.
2. *Objective data:*
   a. Muscle weakness: hands and arms affected first.
   b. Ptosis (drooping of eyelids), expressionless facies.
   c. Hypersensitivity to narcotics, barbiturates, tranquilizers.
   d. Abnormal speech pattern, with high-pitched nasal voice.
   e. Difficulty chewing/swallowing food.
   f. Decreased ability to cough and deep breathe, vital capacity.
   g. Positive *Tensilon test* (administration of edrophonium chloride, 10 mg IV, produces relief of symptoms within 30 seconds).
   h. Positive *Prostigmin test* (1.5 mg subcutaneous neostigmine methylsulfate, produces relief of symptoms within 15 minutes; increased muscle strength within 30 minutes).

D. Analysis/nursing diagnosis:

1. *Ineffective breathing pattern* related to weakness.
2. *Risk for injury* related to muscle weakness.
3. *Activity intolerance* related to severe fatigue.
4. *Bathing/dressing self-care deficit* related to progressive disease.
5. *Impaired physical mobility* related to decrease in strength.
6. *Anxiety* related to physical symptoms and disease progression.
7. *Knowledge deficit* (learning need) related to medication administration and expected effectiveness.

E. Nursing care plan/implementation:

1. Goal: *promote comfort.*
   a. Passive and active ROM, as tolerated, to increase strength.
   b. Mouth care: before and after meals.
   c. *Diet:* as tolerated, *soft,* pureed, or *tube* feedings.
   d. Skin care to prevent decubiti.
   e. Eye care: remove crusts; patch affected eye prn.
   f. Monitor respiratory status—suction airway prn.
2. Goal: *decrease symptoms.*
   a. Administer medications as ordered:
      (1) Anticholinesterase (neostigmine [Prostigmin], pyridostigmine [Mestinon]) to elevate concentration of acetylcholine at myoneural junction.
      (2) Give *before* meals to aid in chewing, *with* milk or food to *decrease GI symptoms;* may be given parenterally.
3. Goal: *prevent complications.*
   a. Respiratory assistance if breathing pattern not adequate.
   b. Monitor for choking/increased oral secretion.
   c. **Avoid:** narcotics, barbiturates, tranquilizers.
4. Goal: *promote increased self-concept.*
   a. Encourage independence when appropriate.
   b. Encourage communication; provide alternative methods when speech pattern impaired.
5. Goal: *health teaching.*
   a. Medication information:
      (1) Adjust dosage to maintain muscle strength.
      (2) Medication must be taken at prescribed time to avoid:
         (a) *Myasthenic crisis* (too little medication).
         (b) *Cholinergic crisis* (too much medication).
   b. *Signs and symptoms of crisis:* dyspnea, severe muscle weakness, respiratory distress, difficulty in swallowing.
   c. Importance of *avoiding upper respiratory infections.*
   d. Determine methods to conserve energy, to maintain independence as long as possible, while avoiding overexertion.
   e. *Refer* to Myasthenia Gravis Foundation and other *community agencies* for assistance in reintegration into the community and plans for follow-up care.

F. Evaluation/outcome criteria:

1. Independence maintained as long as possible.
2. Respiratory arrest avoided.
3. Infection avoided.
4. Medication regimen followed and crisis avoided.

III. PARKINSON'S DISEASE: progressive disease of the brain occurring generally in later life; characterized by stiffness of muscles and by tremors.

A. Pathophysiology: depigmentation of the substantia nigra of basal ganglia → decreased dopamine (neurotransmitter necessary for proper muscle movement) → decreased and slowed

ADULT

voluntary movement, masklike facies, and difficulty initiating ambulation. Decreased inhibitions of alpha-motoneurons → increased muscle tone → rigidity of both flexor and extensor muscles and tremors at rest.

B. Risk factors:

1. Age older than 40; most often 50 to 60 years.
2. Affects men and women equally.
3. Cause unknown; possibly connected to arteriosclerosis or viral infection.
4. Drug-induced parkinsonian syndromes have been linked to:
   a. Phenothiazines.
   b. Reserpine (Serpasil).
   c. Butyrophenones (haloperidol).

C. Assessment:

1. *Subjective data:*
   a. Insomnia.
   b. Depression.
   c. Defects in judgment related to emotional instability; dementia (memory loss).
2. *Objective data:*
   a. Limbs, shoulders: stiff, offer resistance to passive ROM.
   b. Loss of coordination, muscular weakness with rigidity.
   c. Shuffling gait: difficulty in initiating gait, then propulsive, trunk bent forward.
   d. Tremors: pill-rolling of fingers, to-and-fro head movements.
   e. Loss of postural reflexes.
   f. Weight loss, constipation.
   g. Difficulty in maintaining social interactions because of impaired speech, lack of facial affect, drooling.
   h. Facies: wide-eyed, decreased eye blinking, decreased facial expression.
   i. Akinesia (abnormal absence of movement).
   j. Excessive salivation, drooling.
   k. Speech: slowed, slurred.
   l. Judgment defective (e.g., poor decision making); intelligence intact.
   m. Heat intolerance.

D. Analysis/nursing diagnosis:

1. *Impaired physical mobility* related to loss of coordination.
2. *Altered health maintenance* related to defective judgment.
3. *Risk for injury* related to altered gait.
4. *Dressing/grooming self-care deficit* related to muscular rigidity.
5. *Sleep pattern disturbance* related to insomnia.
6. *Body image disturbance* related to tremors and drooling.
7. *Social isolation* related to altered physical appearance.
8. *Altered nutrition, less than body requirements,* related to lack of appetite.
9. *Impaired swallowing* related to excessive drooling.
10. *Constipation* related to dietary changes.

E. Nursing care plan/implementation:

1. Goal: *promote maintenance of daily activities.*
   a. ROM exercises, skin care, physical therapy.
   b. Encourage ambulation; discourage sitting for long periods.
   c. Assist with meals—*high-protein, high-calorie; soft diet;* small, frequent feedings; encourage increased *fluids.*
   d. Encourage compliance with medication regimen:
      (1) *Dopamine agonists:*
         (a) Levodopa: given in increasing doses until symptoms are relieved; given *with food* to decrease GI symptoms. *Side effects:* nausea, vomiting, anorexia, postural hypotension, mental changes, cardiac arrhythmias. Levodopa (L-Dopa) helps *restore dopamine deficiency* in striated muscles: 500 to 1,000 mg/day in divided doses; increase by 100 to 750 mg/day every 3 to 7 days until response reached; usual maintenance dose should *not* exceed 18 gm/day.
         (b) Carbidopa-levodopa (Sinemet): 25/250 mg/day in 3 to 4 divided doses. Limits the metabolism of levodopa peripherally and provides more levodopa for the brain.
      (2) *Anticholinergics:* effective in *lessening muscle rigidity.*
         (a) Benztropine mesylate (Cogentin): 0.5 to 6 mg/day in 1 to 2 divided doses.
         (b) Biperiden (Akineton): 2 mg 3 to 4 times daily, *not* to exceed 16 mg/day.
         (c) Trihexyphenidyl (Artane): 1 to 2 mg day; increased by 2 mg every 3 to 5 days; usual maintenance dose: 5 to 15 mg/day in 3 to 4 divided doses.
      (3) *Antihistamines:* have mild central anticholinergic properties.
2. Goal: *protect from injury.*
   a. Monitor BP, side effects of medications (e.g., orthostatic hypotension).
   b. Monitor for GI disturbances.
   c. *Avoid* pyridoxine (vitamin B_6): it cancels effect of levodopa.
   d. Levodopa *contraindicated* with:
      (1) Glaucoma (causes increased intraocular pressure).
      (2) Monoamine oxidase (MAO) inhibitors (causes possible hypertensive crisis).

ADULT

3. Goal: *health teaching.*
   a. Teach client and family about medications: dosage range, side effects, not discontinuing medications abruptly.
   b. Exercise program to maintain ROM and normal body posture; also to get adequate rest to prevent fatigue.
   c. *Dietary adjustment and precautions* regarding cutting food in small pieces to prevent choking, taking fluid with food for easier swallowing.
   d. Importance of adding *roughage* to *diet* to prevent constipation.
   e. Assist client and family to adjust to this chronic debilitating illness.

F. Evaluation/outcome criteria:
1. Activity level maintained.
2. Symptoms relieved by medications; no drug interactions.
3. Complications avoided.

IV. AMYOTROPHIC LATERAL SCLEROSIS (ALS; Lou Gehrig's disease): progressive degeneration of motor neurons within the brain, spinal cord, or both, leading to death within 2 to 7 years, usually from infection (pneumonia) or consequences of respiratory or bulbar paralysis. There are three types of ALS: classic sporadic, familial, and Mariana Islands (Guam).

A. Pathophysiology: myelin sheaths destroyed, replaced by scar tissue; involves lateral tracts of spinal cord, eventually medulla and ventral tracts.

B. Risk factors:
1. Affects men more than women.
2. Usually in middle age.
3. Viral infection possible causal agent.
4. Possible familial or genetic component.

C. Assessment:
1. *Subjective data:*
   a. Early symptoms: fatigue, awkwardness.
   b. Dysphagia, dysarthria; speech slurred—may sound drunk.
   c. Alert, no sensory loss.
2. *Objective data:*
   a. Symptoms depend on which motor neurons affected.
   b. Decreased fine finger movement.
   c. Progressive muscular weakness, atrophy, especially lower limbs at onset of disease; later arms, hands, and shoulders.
   d. Spasticity of flexor muscles; one side of body becomes more involved than other.
   e. Progressive respiratory difficulties → diaphragmatic paralysis.
   f. Progressive disability of upper and lower extremities.
   g. Fasciculations (muscle twitching visible under skin).
   h. *Diagnostic tests:*
      (1) Electromyography (EMG).
      (2) Nerve conduction velocities (NCVs).

D. Analysis/nursing diagnosis:
1. *Ineffective airway clearance* related to difficulty in coughing.
2. *Ineffective breathing pattern* related to progressive respiratory difficulties and eventually respiratory paralysis.
3. *Altered health maintenance* related to inability to perform self-care activities.
4. *Impaired physical mobility* related to progressive muscular weakness.
5. *Self-care deficits: bathing/hygiene and dressing/grooming.*
6. *Powerlessness* related to lifestyle of progressive physical helplessness.
7. *Impaired swallowing* related to disease progression.

E. Nursing care plan/implementation:
1. Goal: *maintain independence as long as possible.*
   a. Assistance with ADLs; splints, prosthetic devices to support weak limbs and maintain mobility.
   b. Skin care to prevent decubiti.
   c. *Soft/liquid diet* to aid in swallowing, prevent choking; suction prn; *head of bed elevated* when eating.
   d. Respiratory assistance as needed; ventilators as disease progresses and diaphragm becomes involved.
   e. Arrange long-term care arrangements if home maintenance no longer feasible.
   f. Emotional support, when client is alert; continue involving client in decisions regarding care.
   g. Medications: riluzole (Rilutek) has some effect in reducing disease progression; other drugs offer temporary relief of symptoms.
2. Goal: *health teaching.*
   a. Skin care to prevent decubitus ulcer.
   b. Explain ramifications of disease so client and family can make decisions regarding future care, whether client will remain at home as disease progresses or enter a long-term care facility.
   c. How to use suction apparatus to clear airway.
   d. Care of nasogastric or gastrostomy feeding tube.

F. Evaluation/outcome criteria:
1. Obtains physical and emotional support.
2. Complications avoided in early stage of disease.
3. Remains in control of ADLs as long as possible.
4. Skin breakdown avoided.
5. Peaceful death.

ADULT

V. GUILLAIN-BARRÉ SYNDROME: an uncommon, acquired autoimmune disease resulting in demyelination of the cranial and peripheral nerves and a *progressive ascending* paralysis that is usually reversible; develops in hours or up to 10 days. Also known as **acute inflammatory polyradiculoneuropathy**; incidence 1.6/100,000. Client is often completely paralyzed, yet sensation and mentation remain intact.

A. Pathophysiology: macrophages attack normal myelin of the peripheral nerves → demyelination and blocked conduction of impulses to muscles → progressive symmetrical and bilateral muscle weakness from distal lower extremities to proximal upper extremities, trunk, and neck.

B. Risk factors:
1. Viral infection 1 to 3 weeks before paralysis in 50% of cases.
2. Gastroenteritis.
3. Immunizations.
4. May be linked to cytomegalovirus and Epstein-Barr virus.

C. Assessment:
1. *Subjective data:*
   a. Pain, tingling in legs and back (paresthesias).
   b. Reports falling.
   c. Dyspnea.
2. *Objective data:*
   a. Footdrop; unable to walk.
   b. Gradual, progressive facial weakness; dysphagia; dysarthria.
   c. Flaccid paralysis; absent superficial and deep tendon reflexes (DTRs).
   d. Respiratory muscle paralysis → respiratory failure.
   e. Postural hypotension; arterial hypertension, heart block, tachycardia.
   f. Laboratory data: ↑ CSF protein.
   g. *Diagnostic tests*: lumbar puncture; electrophysiologic studies (*EEG:* abnormal; *EMG:* slowed neural conduction).

D. Analysis/nursing diagnosis:
1. *Impaired physical mobility* related to progressive muscular weakness.
2. *Ineffective breathing pattern* related to progressive respiratory difficulties and eventual respiratory paralysis.
3. *Anxiety* related to disease progression.
4. *Self-care deficits: bathing/hygiene and dressing/grooming.*

E. Nursing care plan/implementation:
1. Goal: *prevent complications during recovery from paralysis.*
   a. Respiratory:
      (1) Observe for signs of failure: ↓ forced vital capacity, oximetry.
      (2) Prepare for mechanical ventilation if needed.
      (3) Tracheostomy care and ventilator weaning as indicated.
   b. Prepare for IV plasma exchanges.
      (1) 2 to 3 hours daily over 4 to 5 days; 200 to 250 mL/kg body weight of albumin exchanged.
      (2) *Monitor* for: hypotension, arrhythmias, vascular access problems.
   c. IV immune globulin also may be given. Complications include: hypotension, dyspnea, fever, transient hematuria.
2. Goal: *monitor for signs of autoimmune dysfunction.*
   a. Acute periods of ↑ BP alternating with ↓ BP.
   b. Arrhythmias: give *antiarrhythmic* medications.
3. Goal: *prevent tachycardia.*
   a. Medication: propranolol.
   b. ECG monitoring (continuous) to detect alteration in cardiac rate and pattern.
4. Goal: *assess cranial nerve function.*
   a. Check *gag* and *swallowing* reflex.
   b. Check ability to clear secretions.
   c. Check *voice.*
5. Goal: *maintain adequate ventilation.*
   a. Monitor respiratory rate and depth.
   b. Perform serial vital capacities and ABGs.
   c. Observe for ventilatory insufficiency.
   d. Prevent pneumonia, atelectasis.
6. Goal (in acute phase): *check for progression of muscular weakness*—check individual muscle groups q2h.
7. Goal: *maintain nutrition.*
   a. NG tube—balanced *liquid* diet; mouth care.
   b. Check gag and swallowing reflex before starting *soft, pureed* foods.
8. Goal: *prevent injury and complications.*
   a. *Eye* care: artificial tears or ointment, due to lack of blinking or poor eyelid closure.
   b. *Mobility:*
      (1) ROM.
      (2) Prevent DVT, contractures: use splints, high-top sneakers, footboards, heel and elbow protectors.
      (3) Antiembolic stockings.
   c. *Elimination:*
      (1) Observe for urinary retention and constipation.
      (2) *Avoid* enemas if possible (prevent further autonomic response).
9. Goal: *support communication.*
   a. Develop two methods:
      (1) To indicate immediate needs.
      (2) For basic conversation.

F. Evaluation/outcome criteria:

1. Complete reversal of paralysis.
2. Complications avoided: maintains respiratory function, able to swallow, no complications from immobility.
3. After onset and plateau period, recovery may take 3 to 12 months.

VI. SPINAL CORD INJURIES: trauma from hyperextension, hyperflexion, axial compression, lateral flexion, or shearing of the spine.

A. Types:

1. *C1 and C2 injury level*—resulting deficit:
   a. Phrenic nerve involvement.
   b. Diaphragmatic paralysis.
   c. Respiratory difficulties (require permanent ventilatory support).
   d. Possible quadriplegia.
   e. Possible death.
2. *C4 through T1 injury level*—resulting deficit: possible quadriplegia.
3. *Thoracic-lumbar injury level*—resulting deficit: possible paraplegia.

B. Pathophysiology: trauma → vertebral dislocation or fractures → cord trauma, compression, or severance of the cord.

C. Risk factors:

1. Motor vehicle accidents.
2. Diving, surfing, contact sports.
3. Falls.
4. Gunshot wounds.

D. Assessment:

1. *Subjective data:*
   a. Pain *at* the level of injury.
   b. Numbness/weakness, loss of sensation *below* level of injury.
   c. Psychological distress related to severity of injury and its effects.
2. *Objective data:*
   a. Symptoms depend on extent of injury to spinal cord/spinal nerves.
   b. Paralysis: motor, sphincter.
      (1) Initially a period of *flaccid paralysis* and loss of reflexes, called *spinal* or *neural shock*.
      (2) *Incomplete injuries* may lead to loss of voluntary movement and sensory deficits below injury level (symptoms vary depending on injury).
      (3) *Complete injury* leads to loss of function and all voluntary movement below level of injury.
   c. Respiratory distress.
   d. Alterations in temperature control.
   e. Alterations in bowel and bladder function.
   f. Involved muscles become spastic and hyperreflexic within days or weeks.

ADULT

E. Analysis/nursing diagnosis:

1. *Ineffective breathing pattern* related to high-level injury.
2. *Impaired physical mobility* related to injuries affecting lower limbs.
3. *Fear* related to uncertain future health status.
4. *Anxiety* related to loss of control over own activities of daily living.
5. *Bathing/hygiene self-care deficit* related to injuries above T1.
6. *Impaired home maintenance management* related to possible quadriplegia and paraplegia.
7. *Risk for altered body temperature* related to absence of sweating below level of injury.
8. *Risk for injury* related to equipment necessary for daily activities.
9. *Tactile sensory/perceptual alterations* related to injury level.
10. *Body image disturbance* related to permanent change in physical status.

F. Nursing care plan/implementation:

1. Goal: *maintain patent airway.*
   a. Suction, cough, tracheostomy care, prn.
   b. Oxygen, ventilator care.
   c. Monitor blood gas levels.
2. Goal: *prevent further damage.*
   a. Immobilize spine.
   b. Firm mattress, *Stryker frame, Foster frame, CircO-electric* bed, traction, braces (see **II. FRACTURES, pp. 499, 500, 502, 506**).
   c. Skeletal traction via tongs: *Crutchfield, Gardner-Wells* (see **II. FRACTURES, pp. 499, 500, 501**).
   d. *Halo* traction (see **II. FRACTURES, pp. 499, 500, 501, 506**).
3. Goal: *relieve edema: anti-inflammatory medications, corticosteroids.*
4. Goal: *relieve discomfort: analgesics, sedatives, muscle relaxants.*
5. Goal: *promote comfort:*
   a. Maintain fluid intake: PO/IV, I&O.
   b. Increase nutritional intake.
   c. Prevent contractures and decubiti.
   d. Assist client to deal with psychosocial issues (e.g., role changes).
   e. Begin rehabilitation plan.
6. Goal: *prevent complications.*
   a. Monitor for *spinal shock* during *initial* phase of injury (see **VII. SPINAL SHOCK, p. 521**).
   b. Monitor for *hyperreflexia* with severed spinal cord injuries (see **VIII. AUTONOMIC DYSREFLEXIA, pp. 521–522**).
7. Goal: *health teaching.*
   a. Self-care techniques for highest level of independence; include significant others in teaching.

b. How to use ambulation assistive devices (battery-operated wheelchair controlled by mouthpiece or hand controls, depending on level of paralysis).
c. Identify community resources for follow-up care and career counseling.
d. Signs and symptoms of autonomic hyper-reflexia (see **VIII. AUTONOMIC DYSREFLEXIA, pp. 521–522**).
e. Methods to prevent skin breakdown, infections of respiratory, urinary tract.
f. Bowel, bladder program.

G. Evaluation/outcome criteria:

1. Complications avoided.
2. Accomplishes self-care to greatest level for injury.
3. Participates in rehabilitation plan.
4. Grieves over loss and begins to integrate self into society.

VII. SPINAL SHOCK: temporary flaccid paralysis and areflexia following a severe injury to the spinal cord.

A. Pathophysiology: squeezing or shearing of the spinal cord due to fractures or dislocation of vertebrae; interruption of sensory tracts; loss of conscious sensation; interruption of motor tracts; loss of voluntary movement; loss of facilitation; loss of reflex activity; loss of muscle tone; loss of stretch reflexes, leading to bowel and bladder retention. If injury between *T1 and L2,* leads to loss of sympathetic tone and *decrease* in *blood pressure. Afferent* impulses are unable to ascend from below the injured site to the brain, and *efferent* impulses are unable to descend to points below the site.

B. Risk factors:

1. Automobile/motorcycle accidents.
2. Athletic accidents (e.g., diving in shallow water).
3. Gunshot wounds.

C. Assessment:

1. *Subjective data:*
   a. Loss of sensation below level of injury.
   b. Inability to move extremities.
   c. Pain at level of injury.
2. *Objective data:*
   a. *Neurological* examination:
      (1) *Absent:* pinprick, pressure, and vibratory sensations below level of injury; reflexes below level of injury.
      (2) Muscles: flaccid.
   b. *Vital signs:*
      (1) *BP decreased* (loss of vasomotor tone below level of injury).
      (2) *Bradycardia.*
      (3) *Elevated temperature.*
      (4) *Respirations:* may be *depressed;* possible respiratory failure if diaphragm involved.
   c. Absence of sweating below level of injury.
   d. Urinary retention.
   e. Abdominal distention: retention of feces, paralytic ileus.
   f. Skin: cold, clammy.

D. Analysis/nursing diagnosis:

1. *Decreased cardiac output* related to loss of vasomotor tone below level of injury.
2. *Ineffective breathing pattern* related to injuries involving diaphragm.
3. *Impaired physical mobility* related to loss of voluntary movement of limbs.
4. *Urinary retention* related to loss of stretch reflexes.
5. *Fear* related to serious physical condition.
6. *Risk for injury* related to potential organ damage if shock continues.

E. Nursing care plan/implementation:

1. Goal: *prevent injury related to shock.*
   a. Maintain patent airway: intubation and mechanical ventilation may be necessary with cervical spinal injuries due to involvement of diaphragm.
   b. Monitor vital signs; *profound hypotension* and *bradycardia* are **most dangerous** *aspects* of spinal shock.
   c. Administer blood/IV fluids as ordered.
   d. Nutrition and hydration:
      (1) NPO in *acute* stage: maintain nutrition by IV infusions as ordered.
      (2) When allowed to eat: *high-protein, high-calorie, high-vitamin diet.*
   e. Maintain proper *position* to prevent further injury.
      (1) Backboard is necessary to transport from place of injury.
      (2) Support head in neutral alignment and prevent flexion.
      (3) Skeletal traction will be applied once diagnosis is made.
   f. Monitor urinary output q1h; may have Foley catheter while in shock; later, intermittent catheterization will be used as needed.
   g. Relieve bowel distention; use lubricant containing *anesthetic,* as necessary, when checking for or removing impaction.

F. Evaluation/outcome criteria:

1. Complications are avoided.
2. Body functions are maintained.

VIII. AUTONOMIC DYSREFLEXIA (autonomic hyperreflexia): a group of symptoms in which many spinal cord autonomic responses are activated simultaneously. This may occur when cord lesions are *above the sixth thoracic* vertebra; it is *most commonly* seen with *cervical* and *high thoracic* cord injuries; may occur up to 6 years after injury.

A. Pathophysiology: pathological reflex condition, which is an acute **medical emergency** characterized by extreme hypertension and exaggerated autonomic responses to stimuli.

B. Risk factors:
1. Distention of bladder or rectum.
2. Stimulation of skin (e.g., decubitus ulcers, wrinkled clothing).
3. Stimulation of pain receptors.

C. Assessment:
1. *Subjective data:*
   a. Severe, pounding headache.
   b. Blurred vision; sees spots in front of eyes.
   c. Nausea.
   d. Restlessness.
   e. Feels flushed.
2. *Objective data:*
   a. *Severe hypertension* (systolic BP may reach 300 mm Hg).
   b. *Bradycardia* (30 to 40 beats/min); fever.
   c. Profuse diaphoresis *above* level of injury.
   d. Flushing of skin *above* level of injury.
   e. Pale skin *below* level of injury.
   f. Pilomotor spasm (gooseflesh); chills.
   g. Nasal congestion.
   h. Distended bladder, bowel.
   i. Skin breakdown.
   j. Seizures.

D. Analysis/nursing diagnosis:
1. *Dysreflexia* related to high spinal cord injury.
2. *Risk for injury* related to complications of hypertension, stroke.
3. *Visual sensory/perceptual alteration* related to blurred vision.
4. *Urinary retention* related to inability to empty bladder due to spinal injury.
5. *Constipation* related to inability to establish successful bowel training program.
6. *Impaired skin integrity* related to immobility.

E. Nursing plan/implementation:
1. Goal: *decrease symptoms to prevent serious side effects.*
   a. *Elevate head of bed;* this lowers BP in persons with high spinal cord injuries.
   b. Identify and correct source of stimulation if possible; notify physician.
   c. Monitor vital signs (BP) q15 min and prn; uncontrolled hypertension can lead to stroke, blindness, death.
   d. Give medications as ordered: nitrates, nifedipine (Procardia), or hydralazine (Apresoline).
2. Goal: *maintain patency of catheter.*
   a. Monitor output; *palpate* for distended bladder.
   b. Check for tubing kinks; *irrigate* catheter prn.
   c. Insert new catheter **immediately** if blocked. Do *not* use Credé's maneuver (see **Table 6.34, p. 498**) or tap the bladder; it could exacerbate the response.
   d. Culture if infection suspected.
3. Goal: *promote regular bowel elimination.*
   a. Bowel training program.
   b. Administer *suppository/enemas/laxatives* as ordered and prn.
   c. When checking for and removing impaction, first use *anesthetic ointment* (e.g., dibucaine [Nupercainal] ointment) to decrease irritation.
4. Goal: *prevent decubitus ulcers.*
   a. Meticulous skin care.
   b. *Position change* q1–2h.
   c. Flotation pads, alternating pressure mattress on bed and wheelchair.
5. Goal: *health teaching.*
   a. How to recognize risk factors that could initiate this condition.
   b. Methods to prevent situations that increase risk (e.g., bowel program, bladder program, skin care, position change schedule).

F. Evaluation/outcome criteria:
1. BP remains within normal limits.
2. No complications occur.

IX. HERNIATED/RUPTURED DISK

(ruptured nucleus pulposus): strain or injury to a weakened cartilage between vertebrae can result in herniation of the nucleus, causing pressure on nerve roots in spinal canal, pain, and disability.

A. Pathophysiology: pulpy substance of disk interior (nucleus pulposus) bulges or ruptures through the outer annulus fibrosus → irritation and pressure on nerve endings in the spinal ligaments → muscle spasm and distortion of the joints of vertebral arches.

B. Risk factors:
1. Strain as result of poor body mechanics.
2. Trauma.
3. History of back injuries.
4. Degenerative disk (spondylosis).

C. Assessment:
1. *Lumbar injuries* (90% of herniations):
   a. *Subjective data:*
      (1) *Pain:* low back, radiating to buttocks, posterior thigh, and calf; relieved by recumbency; aggravated by sneezing, coughing, and flexion; sciatic pain continues even when back pain subsides.
      (2) Numbness, tingling.
   b. *Objective data:*
      (1) Muscle weakness—leg and foot.
      (2) Inability to flex leg.
      (3) Sensory loss, leg and foot.
      (4) Alterations in posture: leans to side, unable to stand up straight.

(5) Edema: leg and foot.
(6) Positive *Lasègue's sign:* straight leg raising with hip flexed and knee extended will produce sciatic pain.

2. *Cervical injuries* (10% of herniations):
   a. *Subjective data:*
      (1) *Pain*—upper extremities, radiating to hands and fingers; aggravated by coughing, sneezing, and straining.
      (2) Tingling, burning sensation in upper extremities and back of neck.
   b. *Objective data:*
      (1) Upper extremities: weakness and atrophy.
      (2) Neck: restricted movement.
      (3) *Diagnostic tests* for both lumbar and cervical injuries.
         (a) Spine x-rays.
         (b) CT scan.
         (c) MRI.
         (d) Myelography (less preferred than CT scan or MRI).
         (e) Electromyography.
         (f) *Neurological* examination: special attention to *sensory* status, including pain, touch, and temperature identification; and to *motor* status, including strength, gait, and reflexes.

D. Analysis/nursing diagnosis:

1. *Pain* related to pressure on nerve roots.
2. *Fear* related to disease progression and/or potential surgery.
3. *Knowledge deficit* (learning need) related to correct body mechanics.
4. *Impaired physical mobility* related to continued pain.
5. *Sleep pattern disturbance* related to difficulty finding comfortable position.

E. Nursing care plan/implementation:

1. Goal: *relieve pain and promote comfort.*
   a. Bedrest with bedboard.
   b. *Position—avoid* twisting.
      (1) *Lumbar disk: William's* (*head elevated* 30 degrees, knee gatch *elevated* to flatten the lumbosacral curve). Can be duplicated at home with pillow placement.
      (2) *Cervical: low Fowler's.*
   c. Medications as ordered:
      (1) *Analgesics.*
      (2) *Muscle relaxants.*
      (3) *Anti-inflammatory.*
      (4) *Stool softeners.*
   d. Moist heat.
   e. Fracture bedpan.
   f. Gradual increase in activity.
   g. Brace application for support.
   h. Traction application prn for comfort.
   i. Prepare for surgery if medical regimen unsuccessful.
2. Goal: *health teaching.*
   a. Correct body mechanics, keep back straight.
   b. Exercise program as symptoms decrease.

F. Evaluation/outcome criteria:

1. Reports pain decreased.
2. Mobility increased, normal body posture attained.

X. LAMINECTOMY: excision of dorsal arch of vertebrae with or without spinal fusion of two or more vertebrae with a bone graft from iliac crest, to stabilize spine.

A. Analysis/nursing diagnosis:

1. *Pain* related to edema of surgical procedure.
2. *Impaired physical mobility* related to pain and discomfort resulting from surgery.

B. Nursing care plan/implementation:

1. Goal: *relieve anxiety.*
   a. Answer questions, explain routines.
   b. See **THE PERIOPERATIVE EXPERIENCE, p. 365.**
2. Goal: *prevent injury postoperatively.*
   a. Monitor vital signs:
      (1) *Neurological* signs (e.g., check sensation and motor strength of limbs).
      (2) *Respiratory* status (risk for **respiratory depression** with cervical laminectomy).
   b. Monitor I&O (**urinary retention** common, especially with cervical laminectomy); may need catheterization. Encourage *fluids.*
   c. Monitor bowel sounds (**paralytic ileus** common with lumbar laminectomy).
   d. Monitor dressing for possible bleeding.
   e. Bed *position* as ordered:
      (1) *For lumbar laminectomy: head of bed flat; supine* with *slight flexion* of legs; with pillow between knees for turning and side-lying position.
      (2) *For cervical laminectomy: head of bed elevated,* neck immobilized with collar or sandbags.
   f. Encourage deep breathing to prevent respiratory complications. Use of inspirometer q1h when awake.
   g. Prevent strain or flexion at surgical site: *logrolling* with spinal fusion.
   h. Some surgical interventions that require small incisions (microsurgery) have no specific postoperative positions.
3. Goal: *promote comfort.*
   a. Administer *analgesics* if sciatic-type pain continues after lumbar surgery (arm pain after cervical surgery), due to edema from trauma of surgery.

ADULT

4. Goal: *prepare for early discharge.*
   a. Clients having microsurgery for repair of herniated disk will usually be discharged from the hospital 1 day postoperative; teaching regarding allowed and restricted activities must be done early.
5. Goal: *health teaching.*
   a. How to *turn and move* from side to side in one motion, *sit up,* and *get out of bed without twisting spine;* to get out of bed: raise head of bed while in side-lying position, then put feet over edge of bed, and stand.
   b. Proper positioning and *ambulation* techniques.
   c. Correct posture, *body mechanics,* activities to prevent further injury; increase activities according to tolerance.
   d. Referral: physiotherapy; encourage compliance for full rehabilitation.

C. Evaluation/outcome criteria:

1. No respiratory, bowel, or bladder complications noted.
   a. Lung sounds clear.
   b. Bowel sounds present; able to pass gas and feces.
   c. Urinary output adequate.
2. Regains mobility.
3. Comfort level increases: reports leg and back pain decreased.
4. Demonstrates protective positioning and mbulation techniques.

ONCOLOGICAL DISORDERS

I. THE CLIENT WITH CANCER: Cancer is a multisystem stressor. Regardless of the specific type of cancer, certain aspects of the disease and of nursing care are the same. The following principles apply universally and should be referred to when studying individual kinds of cancer.

A. Pathophysiology: result of altered cellular mechanisms. Several theories about causation, but current thinking is multiple causation. Alterations result in a progressive, uncontrolled multiplication of cells, with selective ability to invade and metastasize.

B. Risk factors:

1. Heredity (e.g., retinoblastoma).
2. Familial susceptibility (e.g., breast).
3. Acquired diseases (e.g., ulcerative colitis).
4. Virus (e.g., Burkitt's lymphoma).
5. Environmental factors:
   a. Tobacco.
   b. Alcohol.
   c. Radiation.
   d. Occupational hazards.
   e. Drugs (e.g., immunosuppressive, cytotoxic).
   f. Asbestos.
6. Age.
7. Air pollution.
8. Diet (e.g., high animal protein).
9. Chronic irritation.
10. Precancerous lesions (e.g., gastric ulcers).
11. Stress.

C. Assessment:

1. Specific symptoms depend on the anatomical and functional characteristics of the organ or structure involved.
2. *Mechanical effects:*
   a. *Pressure*—tumors growing in confined areas such as bone produce pain early, whereas tumors growing in expandable areas such as the abdomen may be undetected for some time.
   b. *Obstruction*—tumors that compress tubular structures such as the esophagus, bronchi, or lymph channels may cause symptoms such as swallowing difficulties, shortness of breath, edema. Symptoms depend on location of tumor and on the particular organ or structure receiving pressure.
   c. *Interruptions of blood supply*—compression of blood vessels or diversion of blood supply may cause necrosis or ulceration or may precipitate hemorrhage.
3. *Systemic effects:*
   a. Anorexia, weakness, weight loss.
   b. Metabolic disturbances—*malabsorption syndrome.*
   c. Fluid and electrolyte imbalances.
   d. Hormonal imbalances—increased antidiuretic hormone (ADH), adrenocorticotropic hormone (ACTH), thyrotropin (TSH), or parathyroid hormone (PTH).
   e. *Diagnostic tests:*
      (1) *Biopsy*—excision of part of tumor mass.
      (2) *Needle biopsy*—aspiration of cells from subcutaneous masses or organs such as liver.
      (3) *Exfoliative cytology*—scraping of any endothelium (cervix, mucous membranes, skin) and applying to slide.
      (4) *X-rays*—detect tumor growth in GI, respiratory, and renal systems.
      (5) *Endoscopy*—visualization of body cavity through endoscope.
      (6) *Computed tomography (CT)*—visualization of a body part whereby layers of tissue can be seen utilizing the very narrow beams of this type of x-ray equipment.
      (7) *Magnetic resonance imaging (MRI)*—a scanning device using a magnetic field for visualization.

(8) *Positron emission tomography (PET)*—a scanning device in which radioactive glucose is injected prior to scanning. Areas of high glucose uptake, such as rapidly dividing cancer cells, are dramatically displayed in the scan imagery; useful in detecting early cancers.

f. Laboratory data:
(1) *Blood and urine tests*—refer to **Appendix A** for normal values.
(2) *Alkaline phosphatase*—greatly *increased* in osteogenic carcinoma (>92 units/L).
(3) *Calcium*—*elevated* in multiple myeloma bone metastases (>10.5 mg/dL).
(4) *Sodium*—*decreased* in bronchogenic carcinoma (<135 mEq/L).
(5) *Potassium*—*decreased* in extensive liver carcinoma (<3.5 mEq/L).
(6) *Serum gastrin*—measures gastric secretions. *Decreased* in gastric carcinoma. Normal value 0 to 180 ng/L.
(7) *Neutrophilic leukocytosis*—tumors.
(8) *Eosinophilic leukocytosis*—brain tumors, Hodgkin's disease.
(9) *Lymphocytosis*—chronic lymphocytic anemia.

D. Analysis/nursing diagnosis:

1. *Pain* related to diagnostic procedures, pressure, obstruction, interruption of blood supply, or potential side effects of drugs.
2. *Anxiety* related to fear of diagnosis or disease progression, treatment, and its known or expected side effects.
3. *Altered nutrition, less than body requirements,* related to anorexia.
4. *Risk for injury* related to radioactive contamination of excreta.
5. *Body image disturbance* related to loss of body parts, change in appearance as a result of therapy.
6. *Powerlessness* related to diagnosis and own perception of its meaning.
7. *Self-esteem disturbance* related to impact of cancer diagnosis.
8. *Risk for infection* related to immunosuppression from radiation and chemotherapy.
9. *Altered urinary elimination* related to dehydration.
10. *Risk for injury* related to normal tissue damage from radiation source.
11. *Fluid volume deficit* related to nausea and vomiting.
12. *Diarrhea* related to radiation of bowel.
13. *Constipation* related to dehydration.

E. Nursing care plan/implementation—general care of the client with cancer:

1. Goal: *promote psychosocial comfort* (see also **Chapter 10**).
   a. Assist with diagnostic work-up by providing psychological support and information about specific disease, diagnostic tests, diagnosis, and treatment options.
   b. Reduce anxiety by listening, making *referrals* for special problems (peer support groups, self-help groups such as Reach to Recovery), supplying information, or correcting misinformation, as appropriate.
   c. Stress-management techniques (see **Orientation, Chapter 1, pp. 11–12**).
   d. Nursing management related to client who is depressed (see **Chapter 10**).
2. Goal: *minimize effects of complications.*
   a. Anorexia/anemia:
      (1) *Decrease anemia* by:
         (a) Providing well-balanced, *iron-rich, small, frequent* meals.
         (b) Administering supplemental vitamins and iron as ordered.
         (c) Administering packed red blood cells as ordered.
         (d) Maintaining hyperalimentation as ordered.
         (e) Monitoring red blood cell count.
      (2) *Enhance nutrition* by providing nutritional supplements and a *diet high in protein;* necessary because of increased metabolism related to metastatic process. *Consult* with dietitian for suggestions of best food for individual client.
   b. Hemorrhage: monitor platelet count and maintain platelet infusions as ordered. Teach client to monitor for any signs of bleeding.
   c. Infection: observe for signs of sepsis (changes in vital signs, temperature of skin, mentation, urinary output or pain); monitor laboratory values (WBCs); administer *antibiotics* as ordered.
   d. Pain and discomfort: alleviate by frequent position changes, diversions, conversations, guided imagery, relaxation, back rubs, and *narcotics* as ordered.
   e. Assist in adjusting to altered body image by encouraging expression of fears and concerns. Do *not* ignore client's questions, and give honest answers; be available.
   f. Fatigue. Encourage periods of rest and a decrease in daily exertion.

3. Goal: *general health teaching.*
   a. Self-care skills to maintain independence (e.g., client who has a colostomy should know how to manage the colostomy before going home).
   b. Importance of follow-up care and routine physical examinations to monitor for general health and possible signs of further disease.
   c. Dietary instructions, adjustments necessary to maintain nutrition during and after treatment.
   d. Health maintenance programs: teach hazards of the use of tobacco and alcohol. *Avoid* high-fat, low-roughage diet.
   e. Risk factors: family history, stress, age, diet, occupation, environment.
   f. Access to information: clients should have telephone numbers for facility where questions can be answered and symptoms reported 24 hours a day.

F. **General surgical intervention:** surgery may be *diagnostic, curative* (when the lesion is localized or with minimal metastases to the lymph nodes), *palliative* (to decrease symptomatology), or *reconstructive.* (See also **THE PERIOPERATIVE EXPERIENCE, pp. 365–367,** and specific types of cancer, following.)

1. **Nursing care plan/implementation**—*preoperative:*
   a. Goal: *prevent respiratory complications.*
      (1) Coughing and deep-breathing techniques.
      (2) *No* smoking for 1 week before surgery.
   b. Goal: *counteract nutritional deficiencies.*
      (1) *Diet:*
         (a) *High* protein, *high* carbohydrate for tissue repair.
         (b) Vitamin and mineral supplements.
         (c) Hyperalimentation as ordered.
      (2) Blood transfusions may be needed if counts are low.
   c. Goal: *reduce apprehension.*
      (1) Clarify postoperative expectations.
      (2) Explain care of ostomies or tubes.
      (3) Answer client's questions honestly.
2. *Postoperative:*
   a. Goal: *prevent complications.*
      (1) Monitor respiratory status and hemodynamic status.
      (2) Wound care; active and passive exercises as allowed; respiratory hygiene; coughing, deep breathing, and turning; fluids (see **III. POSTOPERATIVE EXPERIENCE, pp. 369–375**).
   b. Goal: *alleviate pain and discomfort.*
      (1) Encourage early ambulation, depending on surgical procedure.
      (2) Administer prescribed medications as needed.
      (3) Administer *stool softeners* and enemas as ordered.
   c. Goal: *health teaching.*
      (1) Involve client, significant others, and family members in rehabilitation program.
      (2) Prepare for further therapies, such as radiation or chemotherapy.
      (3) Referral: *support groups,* as appropriate: Reach to Recovery, Ostomy Associates, Laryngectomy Association.
      (4) Develop skills to deal with disease progression if cure not realistic or metastasis evident.

G. **Chemotherapy:** used as single treatment or in combination with surgery and radiation, for early or advanced diseases. Used to cure, increase survival time, or decrease specific life-threatening complications. Antineoplastic agents' primary mode of action involves interfering with the supply and utilization of building blocks of nucleic acids, as well as interfering with intact molecules of DNA or RNA, which are needed for replication and cell growth. *Bone marrow, hair follicles,* and the *gastrointestinal tract are three areas of the body* in *which cells are actively dividing;* this is why most side effects are related to these areas of the body. Most often antineoplastic agents are used in combination.

1. *Types: alkylating* agents, *antimetabolites, antitumor antibiotics, antimiotic* agents, *plant alkaloids, enzymes, hormones,* and *biotherapy* (e.g., bacille Calmette-Guérin [BCG], interferon) (see **Chapter 8, Table 8.11, p. 625**).
2. *Major problem:* lacks specificity, thus affecting normal as well as malignant cells.
3. *Major side effects:* bone marrow depression, stomatitis, nausea and vomiting, gastrointestinal ulcerations, diarrhea, and alopecia (see **Chapter 8, Table 8.12, p. 626**).
4. *Routes of administration:* oral, intramuscular, intravenous (*Hickman or Groshong catheter*), subclavian lines, portacaths, peripheral, intraarterial (may have infusion pump for continuous or intermittent flow rate), intracavitary (e.g., bladder through cystoscopy). (See **6. Nursing precautions with chemotherapy** following for information about administration of IV chemotherapeutic agents.)
5. **Nursing care plan/implementation:**
   a. Goal: *assist with treatment of specific side effects.*
      (1) *Nausea and vomiting—antiemetic* drugs (e.g., prochloroperazine, ondansetron [Zofran]) as ordered and scheduled; small, frequent, *high-calorie, high-potassium, high-protein* meals; chopped or blended

ADULT

foods for ease in swallowing; include milk and milk products when tolerated for *increased calcium;* carbonated drinks; frequent mouth care; *antacid* therapy as ordered; rest after meals; *avoid* food odors during preparation of meals; pleasant environment during meals; appropriate distractions; IV therapy; *nasogastric* tube for control of severe nausea or as route for *tube feeding* if unable to take food by mouth; *hyperalimentation.*

(2) *Diarrhea—low-residue diet; increased potassium; increased* fluids; atropine SO_4–diphenoxylate HCl (Lomotil) or kaolin-pectin (Kaopectate) as ordered; *avoid* hot or cold foods/liquids.

(3) *Stomatitis* (painful mouth)—soft toothbrushes or sponges (toothettes); mouth care q2–q4; viscous lidocaine HCl (Xylocaine) as ordered *before* meals. Oral salt-and-soda mouth rinses; *avoid* commercial mouthwashes that contain high level of alcohol, which could be very irritating to mucous membranes. *Avoid* hot foods/liquids; include *bland* foods at cool temperatures; remove dentures if sores are under dentures; moisten lips with lubricant.

(4) *Skin care*—monitor: wounds that do not heal, infections (client receives frequent sticks for blood tests and therapy); *avoid* sunlight; use sunblock, especially if receiving doxorubicin (Adriamycin).

(5) *Alopecia*—be gentle when combing or lightly brushing hair; use wigs, nightcaps, scarves; provide frequent linen changes. Advise client to have hair cut short before treatment with drugs known to cause alopecia (bleomycin, cyclosphosphamide, dactinomycin, daunorubicin hydrochloride, doxorubicin hydrochloride, 5-fluorouracil, ICRF-159, hydroxyurea, methotrexate, mitomycin, VP 16–213, vincristine). Other techniques may be used, depending on client's age and protocol in clinical agency.

(6) *Extravasation*—infiltration of chemotherapeutic agents into surrounding tissues. Document and treat according to agency protocols for administered drug.

b. Goal: *health teaching.*

(1) Orient client and family to purpose of proposed drug regimen and anticipated side effects.

(2) Advise that frequent checks on hematological status will be necessary (client will receive frequent IV sticks, laboratory tests).

(3) Advise client/family on increased risk for infection (*avoid* uncontrolled crowds and individuals with upper respiratory tract infections or childhood diseases).

(4) Monitor injection site for signs of extravasation (infiltration); site must be changed if leakage suspected, and guidelines to neutralize must be followed according to drug protocol.

6. **Nursing precautions with chemotherapy:**
   a. Nurse should wear gloves and mask when preparing chemotherapy drugs for administration. Mixing of drug into IV bag done under laminar flow hood.
   b. Drugs are toxic substances, and nurses must take every precaution to handle them with care.
   c. When expelling air bubbles from syringes, care must be taken that the drugs are not sprayed into the atmosphere.
   d. Contaminated needles and syringes should be disposed of intact (to prevent aerosol generation) in plastic-lined box according to environmental standards. Disposable equipment should be used whenever possible.
   e. If skin becomes contaminated with a drug, wash under running water.
   f. Nurses should know the half-life and excretion route of the drugs being administered and take the special precautions necessary. For example, while the drug is actively being excreted, use gloves when touching client, stool, urine, dressings, vomitus, etc.
   g. If the nurse is in the early phase of pregnancy, she should seek specific information about risks to her unborn child before caring for the client receiving chemotherapeutic agents.

H. **Radiation therapy:** used in high doses to kill cancer cells, or palliatively for pain relief. *Side effects of radiation therapy* depend on site of therapy (side effects are also variable in each individual): nausea, vomiting, stomatitis, esophagitis (*Candida*), dry mouth, diarrhea, depression of bone marrow, suppression of immune response, decreased life span, and sterility.

1. **External radiation:** cobalt or linear accelerator machine.
   a. *Procedure:* daily treatments, Monday through Friday, for prescribed number of times according to size and location of tumor (length of treatment schedule is usually 4 to 6 weeks). Client remains alone in room during treatment. (Nurse, therapist, family members cannot stay in room with client due to radiation exposure during treatment.) Client instructed to lie still so exactly same area is

irradiated each treatment. Marks (tattoos or via permanent-ink markers) are made on skin to delineate area of treatment; marks must *not* be removed during entire treatment course.

b. **Nursing care plan/implementation:**
   (1) Goal: *prevent tissue breakdown.*
      (a) Do *not* wash off site identification marks (tattoos cannot be removed); dosage area is carefully calculated and must be exact for each treatment.
      (b) Assess skin daily and teach client to do same (most radiation therapy is done on outpatient basis, so client needs skills to manage independently).
      (c) Keep skin dry; cornstarch usually the only topical application allowed; 100% aloe (no alcohol) for redness.
      (d) *Contraindications:*
         (i) Talcum powders, due to potential radiation dosage alteration.
         (ii) Lotions, due to increased moistening of skin.
         (iii) Products containing alcohol, due to increased dryness.
      (e) Reduce skin friction by *avoiding* constricting bedclothes or clothing, and by using electric shaver.
      (f) Dress areas of skin breakdown with nonadherent dressing and paper tape.
   (2) Goal: *decrease side effects of therapy.*
      (a) Provide meticulous oral hygiene.
      (b) If diarrhea occurs, may need IV infusions, *antidiarrheal* medications; monitor bowel movements (possible adhesions from surgery and radiation treatments).
      (c) Monitor vital signs, particularly respiratory function, and BP (sloughing of tissue puts client at *risk for hemorrhage*).
      (d) Monitor hematological status—bone marrow depression can cause *fatal toxicosis and sepsis.*
      (e) Institute *reverse isolation* as necessary to prevent infections (reverse isolation usually instituted if less than 50% neutrophils).
   (3) Goal: *health teaching.*
      (a) Instruct client to *avoid:*
         (i) Strong sunlight; must wear sunblock lotion, protective clothing over radiation site.
         (ii) Extremes in temperature to the area (hot-water bottles, ice caps, spas).
         (iii) Synthetic, nonporous clothes or tight constrictive clothing over area.
         (iv) Eating 2 to 3 hours before treatment and 2 hours after, to decrease nausea; give small, frequent meals *high* in protein and carbohydrates and *low* in residue.
         (v) Strong alcohol-based mouthwash; use daily salt-and-soda mouthwash.
         (vi) Fatigue, an overwhelming problem. Need to pace themselves, nap; may need someone to drive them to therapy; can continue with usual activities as tolerated.
         (vii) Crowds and persons with upper respiratory infections or any other infections.
      (b) Provide appropriate birth control information for clients of childbearing age.

2. **Internal radiation: sealed** (radium, iridium, cesium):
   a. Used for localized masses (e.g., mouth, cervix, breast, testes). Due to exposure from radiation source, precautions must be taken while it is in place. Health-care personnel and family must adhere to *principles of time, distance, and shielding to decrease exposure* (*shortest* amount of time possible, stay as *far away* as possible from the source of radiation, and wear *protective* lead apron, gloves). If source of radiation accidentally falls out, it should be picked up only with *forceps.* Radiation officer should be notified **immediately.** Client should be in *private* room, and bed should be in the center of the room, if possible, to protect others. Unless the walls are lead lined, radiation will penetrate them; placing the bed in *center of room* will decrease exposure. Once the source of radiation has been removed, there is no exposure from client, excretions, or linens.
   b. **Nursing care plan/implementation:**
      (1) Goal: *assist with cervical radium implantation* (cervical radium is used here as the most common example of internal radiation source).
         (a) *Before insertion*—give douche, enema, perineal prep; insert Foley catheter, as ordered.
         (b) *After implantation*—check position of applicator q24h.
            (i) Keep client on bedrest in *flat position* to *avoid* displacing applicator (may turn to side for eating).
            (ii) Notify physician if temperature elevates, nausea and/or vomiting occur (indicates *radiation reaction or infection*).
            (iii) *After removal* of implant (48 to 144 hours)—bathe, douche, and remove catheter as ordered.

ADULT

(2) Goal: *health teaching.*
(a) Explain that nursing care will be limited to essential activities in postinsertion period.
(b) Signs and symptoms of complications so client can notify staff if something unusual happens (bleeding, radiation source falls out, fever, etc.).

c. **Nursing precautions for sealed internal radiation:**
(1) **Never handle radium directly**—if applicators should accidentally be removed, pick up applicator by strings with long-handled forceps and **notify radiation officer.**
(2) Linen must remain in client's room and *not* be sent to laundry until source of radiation has been accounted for and returned to its container.
(3) **Time, distance,** and **shielding** are factors that increase or decrease potential effects on personnel. Need to minimize exposure of nursing staff, client's family, and other health professionals. Nurses who may be pregnant should *not* care for clients with internal radiation because of possible damage to the fetus from radiation exposure. Children under 16 should *not* be allowed to visit while internal radiation is in use.

3. **Internal radiation: unsealed** (radioisotope/radionuclide):
a. Source of radiation is given orally or intravenously or instilled into a cavity as a liquid.
b. **Nursing care plan/implementation:** Goal: *reduce radiation exposure of others.*
(1) *Isolate* client and tag room with radioactivity symbol.
(2) *Rotate* personnel to avoid overexposure (*principles of time, distance, and shielding*). Staff should use good hand-washing technique. Client should be in a room with running water. (Nurse who may be pregnant should *not* care for client while radiation source still active.)
(3) Encourage family to maintain telephone contact or use intercom, to decrease exposure to others.
(4) Plan independent diversional activities.
c. ***Specific nursing precautions*** (post in chart, on client's door):
(1) *Radioactive iodine* (^{131}I): half-life 8.1 days; excreted in urine, saliva, perspiration, vomitus, feces.
(a) Wear gloves and isolation gowns when handling client, *excreta,* or dressings directly.
(b) Collect paper plates, eating utensils, dressings, and linen in impermeable bags; label and dispose according to agency protocol.
(c) Collect excreta in shielded container and send to laboratory daily to monitor excretion rate and disposal.
(2) *Radioactive phosphorus* (^{32}P): half-life 14 days; injected into cavity or given IV or orally.
(a) If injected into cavity, turn client q10–15 min for 2 hours to ensure distribution.
(b) No radiation hazard unless leakage from instillation site or from client's *excreta,* which are collected in *lead-lined containers* and brought to the radioisotope laboratory for disposal. Linen is collected in container, marked *radioactive,* and brought to the radioisotope laboratory for special handling.
(c) Seepage will stain linens *blue;* wear gloves when handling contaminated linens, dressings. Excreta disposed of as in **(b).**
(3) *Radioactive gold* (^{198}Au): half-life 2.7 days; usually injected into pleural or abdominal cavity.
(a) May seep from instillation site or drainage tubes in cavity; stains *purple.*
(b) Turn client q15 min for 2 hours, as in **(2)(a).**
(c) Same precautions regarding handling excreta as in **(1)(a)** and **(2)(b).**

4. **Precautions for nurses:**
a. Use *principles of time, distance,* and *shielding* when caring for clients who are having active radiation therapy treatments.
b. Nurses who may be pregnant should *not* accept an assignment caring for clients who have active radiation in place.
c. *Always* use gloves, gowns to protect skin and clothing.
d. Wear detection badge to determine exposure to energy source.

I. Immunotherapy: it has been hypothesized that clinical malignancy may occur as a result of failure of the immunological surveillance system of the body to fight off cancer cells as they develop. The goal of immunotherapy is to immunize clients against their own tumors.
1. *Nonspecific* immunotherapy—encourages a host immune response by use of an unrelated agent. Bacille Calmette-Guérin (BCG) vaccine and *Corynebacterium parvum* are the two agents used for this type of immunotherapy.

2. *Specific* immunotherapy—uses substances that are antigenically related to the tumor that stimulate a specific host immune response.
3. *Side effects*—malaise, chills, nausea, vomiting, diarrhea; local reaction at site of injection, such as pruritus, scabbing.
4. **Nursing care plan/implementation:**
   a. Goal: *decrease discomfort associated with side effects of therapy.*
      (1) Identify measures to lessen symptoms of side effects (see **E. Nursing care plan/implementation—general care of the client with cancer, pp. 525–526**).
      (2) Know type of immunotherapy being used, adverse and desirable effects of therapy.
      (3) Administer fluids, encourage rest.
      (4) Administer *acetaminophen* as ordered to decrease flu-like symptoms.
      (5) Administer *antiemetics* as ordered for nausea.
      (6) Monitor for respiratory distress.
      (7) Administer *analgesics* as ordered for pain.
   b. Goal: *health teaching.*
      (1) Comfort measures to decrease side effects of therapy.
      (2) Expected and side effects of therapy.
      (3) Investigational nature of therapy.
      (4) Care of site of administration.
      (5) Answer questions honestly.

J. Palliative care: when treatment has been ineffective in control of the disease, the nurse must plan palliative, terminal care. Cure is not possible for such clients in an advanced phase of malignancy. Symptoms increase in severity; clients and family have many special problems.

1. General problems of clients with terminal cancer:
   a. *Cachexia:* progressive weakness, wasting, and weight loss.
   b. *Anemia:* leukopenia, thrombocytopenia, hemorrhage.
   c. *Gastrointestinal disturbances:* anorexia, constipation.
   d. *Tissue breakdown* leading to decubiti, seeping wounds.
   e. *Urine:* retention, incontinence, renal calculi, tumor obstruction of ureters.
   f. *Hypercalcemia* occurs in 10% to 30% of clients.
   g. *Pain* due to: tumor growth, obstruction, vertebral compression, or secondary to complications (e.g., decubiti, stiffened joints, stomatitis). Also neuropathy, due to prolonged use of neurotoxic chemotherapeutic agents such as vincristine.
   h. *Fatigue:* major and debilitating problem.
2. **Nursing care plan/implementation:**
   a. Goal: *make client as comfortable as possible;* involve nursing staff, family, support personnel, clergy, volunteers, support groups. Hospice is **very** valuable program.
      (1) *Nutrition:* obtain nutritional consultation; *high-calorie, high-protein diet;* small, frequent meals; blenderized or strained; commercial nutritional supplements (Ensure, Vivonex, Sustacal).
      (2) Prevent tissue breakdown and vascular complications: frequent turning, massage, air mattress, active and passive ROM exercises.
      (3) *GI tract* disturbances: observe for toxic reactions to therapy, particularly vomiting and diarrhea; administer medications: *antiemetics, antidiarrheal* agents as ordered.
      (4) Relieve pain.
         (a) Use supportive measures such as massage, relaxation techniques, guided imagery; and drugs for *pain* relief: administer codeine, fentanyl, aspirin–oxycodone HCl (Percodan), pentazocine (Talwin), morphine, methadone, as ordered.
         (b) Methods of administration: oral, injected, rectal, analgesic patches, or pumps (IV or SQ).
         (c) Monitor for side effects of narcotics: depressed respiratory status, constipation, anorexia.
   b. Goal: *assist client to maintain self-esteem and identity.*
      (1) Encourage self-care.
      (2) Spend time with client; isolation is a great fear for the client who is dying.
   c. Goal: *assist client with psychological adjustment*—see nursing care for clients who are grieving, clients who are dying (see **Chapter 10**).

K. Evaluation/outcome criteria:

1. Tolerates treatment modality—complications of surgery are avoided or minimized; tolerates chemotherapy; completes radiation therapy.
2. Side effects of treatment are managed by effective nursing care and health teaching.
3. Maintains good nutritional status.
4. Uses effective coping mechanisms or seeks appropriate assistance to deal with psychosocial concerns.
5. Makes choices for follow-up care based on accurate information.
6. Finds methods to control pain and minimize discomfort.

7. Participates in decisions regarding continuation of therapy (living will, health-care proxy, do-not-resuscitate [DNR] decisions).
8. Dignity maintained until death and during dying.

II. LUNG CANCER

A. Pathophysiology: *squamous cell carcinoma:* undifferentiated, pleomorphic in appearance; accounts for 45% to 60% of all lung cancer; *small cell (oat cell) carcinoma:* small, dark cells located between cells of mucosal surfaces; characterized by early metastasis and poor prognosis; *large cell (giant cell) carcinoma:* located in the peripheral areas of the lung, has poor prognosis; *adenocarcinoma:* found in men and women; not necessarily related to smoking.

B. Risk factors:

1. Heavy cigarette smoking, 20-year smoking history.
2. Exposure to certain industrial substances, such as asbestos.
3. Increased incidence in women during the last decade of life.

C. Assessment:

1. *Subjective data:*
   a. Dyspnea.
   b. *Pain:* on swallowing; dull and poorly localized chest pain, referred to shoulders.
   c. Anorexia.
   d. History of cigarette smoking over a period of years; recurrent respiratory infections with chills and fever, especially pneumonia or bronchitis.
2. *Objective data:*
   a. Wheezing; dry to productive persistent cough; hemoptysis, hoarseness.
   b. Weight loss.
   c. Positive diagnosis: cytology report of cells from bronchoscopy.
   d. Chest pain.
   e. Signs of metastasis.

D. Analysis/nursing diagnosis:

1. *Ineffective breathing pattern* related to pain.
2. *Impaired gas exchange* related to tumor growth.
3. *Pain* related to disease progression.
4. *Fear* related to uncertain future.
5. *Powerlessness* related to inability to control symptoms.
6. *Knowledge deficit* (learning need) related to disease and treatment.

E. Nursing care plan/implementation:

1. Goal: *make client aware of diagnosis and treatment options.*
   a. Allow time to talk and to discuss diagnosis.
   b. Client makes informed decision regarding treatment.
2. Goal: *prevent complications related to surgery* for client who is diagnosed early and for whom surgery is an option: wedge or segmental resection, laser therapy, lobectomy, or pneumonectomy are usual procedures.
   a. See **Nursing care plan/implementation for the client having thoracic surgery, p. 408.**
   b. Monitor vital signs, including accurate respiratory assessment for *respiratory congestion, blood loss, infection.*
   c. Assist client to deep breathe, cough, change position.
3. Goal: *assist client to cope with alternative therapies* when surgery is deemed not possible.
   a. *Radiation:* megavoltage x-ray, cobalt—usual form of radiation (see **Nursing care plan/implementation for the client having radiation therapy, p. 528**).
   b. *Chemotherapy:*
      (1) Cisplatin and VP-16 with irradiation has become standard form of induction chemotherapy. Cyclophosphamide (Cytoxan), doxorubicin (Adriamycin), CCNU, methotrexate, vincristine sulfate (Oncovin) are the other drugs given for lung cancer.
      (2) See **Nursing care plan/implementation for the client having chemotherapy, pp. 526–527.**
4. Goal: *health teaching.*
   a. Encourage client to stop smoking to offer best possible air exchange.
   b. Encourage *high-protein, high-calorie diet* to counteract weight loss.
   c. *Force fluids,* to liquefy secretions so they can be expectorated.
   d. Encourage adequate rest and activity to prevent problems of immobility.
   e. Desired effects and side effects of medications prescribed for therapy and pain relief.
   f. Coping mechanisms for maximal comfort and advanced disease (see **Palliative care, p. 530**).

F. Evaluation/outcome criteria:

1. Copes with disease and treatment.
2. Side effects of treatment are minimized by proper nursing management.
3. Acid-base balance is maintained by careful management of respiratory problems.
4. Client is aware of the seriousness of the disease.

III. COLON AND RECTAL CANCER

A. Risk factors:

1. Men, middle age, personal or family history of colon and rectal cancer, personal or family history of polyps in the rectum or colon, ulcerative colitis.

2. Diet high in beef and low in fiber.
3. *Gardner's syndrome* (multiple colonic adenomatous polyps, osteomas of the mandible or skull, multiple epidermoid cysts, or soft tissue tumors of the skin).

B. Assessment:

1. *Subjective data:*
   a. Change in bowel habits.
   b. Anorexia.
   c. Weakness.
   d. Abdominal cramping or vague discomfort with or without pain.
   e. Chills.
2. *Objective data:*
   a. Diarrhea (pencil-like or ribbon-shaped feces) or constipation.
   b. Weight loss.
   c. Rectal bleeding; anemia.
   d. Fever.
   e. Digital examination reveals palpable mass if lesion is in ascending or descending colon.
   f. Signs of intestinal obstruction: constipation, distention, pain, vomiting, fecal oozing.
   g. *Diagnostic tests:*
      (1) Digital examination.
      (2) Slides of stool specimen, for occult blood.
      (3) Proctoscopy.
      (4) Sigmoidoscopy, colonoscopy.
      (5) Barium enema.
   h. Laboratory data: occult blood, blood serotonin *increased,* carcinoembryonic antigen (CEA); *positive* radioimmunoassay of serum or plasma indicates presence of carcinoma or adenocarcinoma of colon; positive result after resection indicates return of tumor.

C. Analysis/nursing diagnosis:

1. *Constipation or diarrhea* related to presence of mass.
2. *Altered health maintenance* related to care of stoma.
3. *Sexual dysfunction* related to possible nerve damage during radical surgery.
4. *Body image disturbance* related to colostomy.

D. Nursing care plan/implementation (see also **Nursing care plan/implementation—general care of the client with cancer, pp. 525–526**):

1. *Radiation:* to reduce tumor or for palliation.
2. *Chemotherapy:* to reduce tumor mass and metastatic lesions.
   a. *Antitumor antibiotics*—mitomycin C, doxorubicin HCl (Adriamycin).
   b. *Alkylating agents*—methyl-CCNU.
   c. *Antimetabolites*—5-fluorouracil (5-FU).
   d. *Steroids* and *analgesics* for symptomatic relief.
3. Prepare client for surgery (colostomy) if necessary.

E. Evaluation/outcome criteria:

1. Return of peristalsis and formed stool following resection and anastomosis.
2. Adjusts to alteration in bowel elimination route following abdominoperineal resection (e.g., no depression, resumes lifestyle).
3. Demonstrates self-care skills with colostomy.
4. Makes dietary adjustments that affect elimination as indicated.
5. Identifies alternative methods of expressing sexuality, if needed.

IV. BREAST CANCER

A. Risk factors:

1. Women older than age 50.
2. Family history of breast cancer.
3. Never bore children, or bore first child after age 30.
4. Had breast cancer in other breast.
5. Menarche before age 11.
6. Menopause after age 50.
7. Exposure to endogenous estrogens.
8. Exposure to ionizing radiation.
9. High alcohol and fat intake may increase risk.

B. Assessment:

1. *Subjective data:*
   a. Burning, itching of nipple.
   b. Reported painless lump.
2. *Objective data:*
   a. Firm, nontender lump or mass.
   b. Asymmetry of breast.
   c. Nipple—retraction, discharge.
   d. Alteration in breast skin—redness, dimpling, ulceration.
   e. Palpation reveals lump.
   f. *Diagnostic tests:* mammography, needle biopsy, core biopsy, excisional biopsy—level of estrogen-receptor protein predicts response to hormonal manipulation of metastatic disease and may represent a prognostic indicator for primary cancer; carcinoembryonic antigen (CEA) useful with metastatic disease of the breast.

C. Analysis/nursing diagnosis:

1. *Risk for injury* related to surgical intervention.
2. *Body image disturbance* related to effects of surgery, radiation, or chemotherapy.
3. *Altered sexuality patterns* related to loss of breast.

D. Nursing care plan/implementation (see also **Nursing care plan/implementation—general care of the client with cancer, pp. 525–526**):

1. Goal: *assist through treatment protocol.*
   a. *Radiation*—primary treatment modality; adjunctive, external, or implantation to primary lesion site or nodes.

ADULT

b. *Chemotherapy* usually given in combinations.
   (1) *Cytotoxic* agents to destroy tumor and control metastasis.
   (2) *Alkylating* agents: cyclophosphamide (Cytoxan).
   (3) *Antitumor antibiotics:* doxorubicin (Adriamycin).
   (4) *Antimetabolites:* fluorouracil (5-FU); methotrexate (Amethopterine, MTX).
   (5) *Plant alkaloids:* vincristine sulfate (Oncovin).
   (6) *Hormones* to control metastasis, provide palliation: androgens, fluoxymesterone (Halotestin), testosterone (Teslac), diethylstilbesterol (estrogen).
   (7) *Antiestrogens:* tamoxifen (Nolvadex) may be used after initial treatment.
   (8) *Cortisols:* cortisone, prednisolone (Delta-Cortef), prednisolone acetate (Meticortelone), prednisone (Deltasone, Deltra).

c. *Surgery.*
   (1) *Preoperative:*
      (a) Goal: *prepare for surgery—types:*
         (i) *Lumpectomy* (with or without radiation)—used when lesion is small; section of breast is removed with clear margin around lesion (often accompanied by radiation therapy and then radium interstitial implant).
         (ii) *Simple mastectomy*—breast removed, no alteration in nodes.
         (iii) *Modified radical mastectomy*—breast, some axillary nodes, subcutaneous tissue removed; pectoralis minor muscle removed.
         (iv) *Radical mastectomy*—breast, axillary nodes, and pectoralis major and minor muscles removed.
         (v) Reconstructive surgery—done at time of initial mastectomy or (most often) later, when other adjuvant therapy has been completed.
      (b) Goal: *promote comfort.*
         (i) Allow client and family to express fears, feelings.
         (ii) Provide correct information about diagnostic tests, operative procedure, postoperative expectations.
         (iii) Client may be hospitalized for 24 hours or less. Have telephone number available for questions. Make appropriate community referrals.
   (2) *Postoperative:*
      (a) Goal: *facilitate healing.*
         (i) Observe pressure dressings for bleeding; will appear under axilla and toward the back.
         (ii) Report if dressing becomes saturated; reinforce dressing as need; monitor drainage from Hemovac or suction pump.
         (iii) *Position: semi-Fowler's* to facilitate venous and lymphatic drainage; use pillows to *elevate affected* arm *above right atrium,* to prevent edema if nodes removed.
      (b) Goal: *prevent complications.*
         (i) Monitor vital signs for shock.
         (ii) Use gloves when emptying drainage.
         (iii) Maintain joint mobility—flexion and extension of fingers, elbow, shoulder.
         (iv) ROM as ordered to prevent ankylosis.
         (v) If skin graft done, check donor site and limit exercises.
      (c) Goal: *facilitate rehabilitation.*
         (i) Encourage client, significant others, and family to look at incision.
         (ii) Involve client in incisional care, as tolerated.
         (iii) *Refer* to Reach to Recovery program of the American Cancer Society
         (iv) Exercise program, hydrotherapy for clients who are postmastectomy, to reduce lymphedema.
      (d) Goal: *health teaching.*
         (i) How to avoid injury to affected area; how to prevent lymphedema.
         (ii) Exercises to gain full ROM.
         (iii) Availability of prosthesis, reconstructive surgery.
         (iv) Correct breast self-examination (BSE) technique (client is at risk for breast cancer in remaining breast) **(Fig. 6.16).** Best time for examination: *women who are premenopausal,* seventh day of cycle; *women who are postmenopausal,* same day each month.

E. Evaluation/outcome criteria:
1. Identifies feelings regarding loss.
2. Demonstrates postmastectomy exercises.
3. Gives rationale for avoiding fatigue and avoiding constricting garments on affected arm; necessity for avoiding injury (cuts, bruises, burns) while carrying out activities of daily living.

ADULT

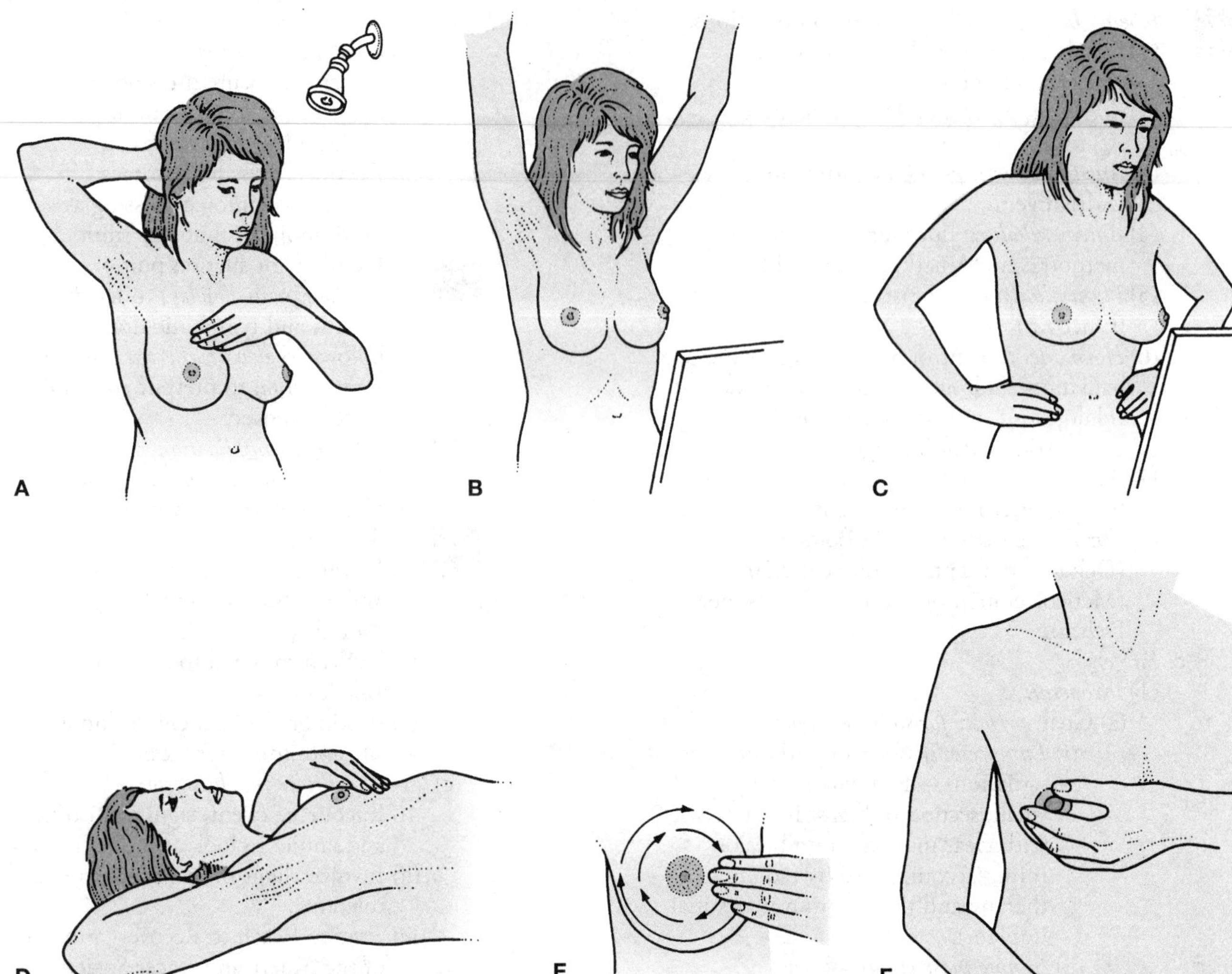

Figure 6.16 Breast self-examination. *(A)* Examine breasts during bath or shower because flat fingers glide easily over wet skin. Use right hand to examine left breast and left hand to examine the right breast. *(B)* Sit or stand before a mirror. Inspect breasts with hands at sides, then raised overhead. Look for changes in contour or dimpling of skin. *(C)* Place hands on hips and press down firmly to flex chest muscles. *(D)* Lie down with one hand under head and pillow or folded towel under that scapula. *(E)* Palpate that breast with the other hand using concentric circle method. It usually takes three circles to cover all breast tissue. Include the tail of the breast and the axilla. Repeat with other breast. *(F)* End in a sitting position. Palpate the areola areas of both breasts, and inspect and squeeze nipples to check for discharge.

4. Describes signs and symptoms of infection.
5. Demonstrates correct BSE technique.

V. UTERINE CANCER (endometrial): originates from epithelial tissues of the endometrium; second only to cervical cancer as cause of pelvic cancer. Slow growing; metastasizes late; responsive to therapy with early diagnosis; Papanicolaou (Pap) test not as effective—more effective to have endometrial tissue sample **(Table 6.40** and **Table 6.41). Table 6.42** discusses cervical cancer.

A. Risk factors:
1. History of infertility (nulliparity).
2. Failure of ovulation.
3. Prolonged estrogen therapy.
4. Obesity.
5. Menopause after age 52.
6. Diabetes.

B. Assessment:
1. *Subjective data:*
   a. History of risk factor(s).
   b. Pain (late symptom).
2. *Objective data:*
   a. Obese.
   b. Abnormal cells obtained from aspiration of endocervix or endometrial washings.
   c. Postmenopausal uterine bleeding.
   d. Abnormal menses; intermenstrual or unusual discharge.

C. **Analysis/nursing diagnosis:**
   1. *Pain* related to surgery.
   2. *Risk for injury* related to surgery.
   3. *Body image disturbance* related to loss of uterus.

Table 6.40

Papanicolaou (Pap) Smear Classes

Class	Recommended Actions
I Normal	
II Atypical cells, nonmalignant	Treat vaginal infections; repeat Pap smears
III Suspicious cells	Biopsy; dilation and curettage
IV Abnormal cells; suspicious of malignancy	Biopsy: dilation and curettage, conization
V Malignant cells present	See **Table 6.41**

Table 6.41

Uterine Cancer: Recommended Treatment, by Stage of Invasion

Stage of Invasion	Recommended Treatment
0 (In situ) Atypical hyperplasia	Cryosurgery, conization
I Uterus is of normal size	Hysterectomy
II Uterus slightly enlarged, but tumor is undifferentiated	Radiation implant, x-ray; hysterectomy 4–6 wk postradiation
III Uterus enlarged, tumor extends outside uterus	Radiation implant, total hysterectomy 4–6 wk postradiation
IV Advanced metastatic disease	Radiation, chemotherapy; progestin therapy to reduce pulmonary lesions

D. **Nursing care plan/implementation** (see also **Nursing care plan/implementation—general care of the client with cancer, pp. 525–526**):
   1. Goal: *assist client through treatment protocol.*
      a. *Radiation*—external, internal, or both with client who is a poor surgical risk.
      b. *Chemotherapy*—to reduce tumors and produce remission of metastasis. Antineoplastic drugs: dacarbazine (DTIC), doxorubicin (Adriamycin), medroxyprogesterone acetate (Provera), megestrol acetate (Megace).
   2. Goal: *prepare client for surgery—types:*
      a. *Subtotal hysterectomy:* removal of the uterus; cervical stump remains.
      b. *Total hysterectomy:* removal of entire uterus, including cervix (abdominally [approximately 70%] or vaginally).
      c. *Total hysterectomy with bilateral salpingo-oophorectomy:* removal of entire uterus, fallopian tubes, and ovaries.
   3. Goal: *reduce anxiety and depression:* allow for expression of feelings, concerns about femininity, role, relationships.
   4. Goal: *prevent postoperative complications.*
      a. Catheter care—temporary bladder atony may be present as a result of edema or nerve trauma, especially when vaginal approach is used.
      b. Observe for abdominal distention and hemorrhage:
         (1) Auscultate for bowel sounds.
         (2) Measure abdominal girth.
         (3) Use rectal tube to decrease flatus.
      c. *Decrease pelvic congestion* and prevent venous stasis.
         (1) *Avoid* high Fowler's position.
         (2) Antiembolic stockings as ordered.

Table 6.42

International System of Staging for Cervical Carcinoma

Stage	Location	Prognosis	Treatment
0	In situ	Highly curable	Conization
I	Cervix	Cure rate decreases as stage progresses	Radiation
II	Cervix to upper vagina		Radiation
III	Cervix to pelvic wall or lower third of vagina		Surgeries: 1. Panhysterectomy, wide vaginal excision with removal of lymph nodes; ileal conduit
IV	Cervix to true pelvis, bladder, or rectum		2. Pelvic exenteration: a. Anterior: removal of vagina and bladder; ileal conduit b. Posterior: removal of rectum and vagina; colostomy c. Total: both anterior and posterior 3. Chemotherapy

ADULT

(3) Institute passive leg exercises.
(4) Apply abdominal support as ordered.
(5) Encourage early ambulation.

5. Goal: *support coping mechanisms* to prevent psychosocial response of depression: allow for verbalization of feelings.
6. Goal: *health teaching* to prevent complications of hemorrhage, infection, thromboemboli.
   a. *Avoid:*
      (1) Douching or coitus until advised by physician.
      (2) Strenuous activity and work for 2 months.
      (3) Sitting for long time and wearing constrictive clothing, which tend to increase pelvic congestion.
   b. Explain hormonal replacement if applicable; correct dosage, desired and side effects of prescribed medications.
   c. Explain:
      (1) Menstruation will no longer occur.
      (2) Importance of reporting symptoms (e.g., fever, increased or bloody vaginal discharge, and hot flashes).

E. Evaluation/outcome criteria:
1. Adjusts to altered body image.
2. No complications—hemorrhage, shock, infection, thrombophlebitis.

VI. PROSTATE CANCER: malignant neoplasm, usually adenocarcinoma; most common cause of cancer in men.

A. Risk factors:
1. Men older than age 50.
2. Familial history.
3. Geographic distribution, environmental (e.g., industrial exposure to cadmium).
4. Hormonal factors (testosterone).
5. Diet (high fat).

B. Assessment:
1. *Subjective data:*
   a. Difficulty in starting urinary stream (hesitancy); urgency.
   b. Pain due to metastasis in lower back, hip, legs; perianal or rectal discomfort.
   c. Symptoms of cystitis; frequency, urgency.
2. *Objective data:*
   a. Urinary: smaller, less forceful stream; terminal dribbling; frequency, nocturia; *retention* (inability to void after ingestion of alcohol or exposure to cold).
   b. *Diagnostic tests:* digital rectal examination (DRE); transrectal ultrasonography (TRUS). Needle biopsy or tissue specimen reveals positive cancer cells.
   c. Laboratory data: *increased:*
      (1) Prostate-specific antigen (PSA)—over 4 ng/mL.
      (2) Urine RBCs (hematuria).
      (3) Gleason score for prostate cancer grading system (range: 2 to 10).

C. Analysis/nursing diagnosis:
1. *Altered urinary elimination* related to incontinence.
2. *Altered sexuality pattern* related to nerve damage and erectile dysfunction.
3. *Anxiety* related to diagnosis.
4. *Pain* related to metastasis to bone.

D. Nursing care plan/implementation (see also **Nursing care plan/implementation—general care of the client with cancer, pp. 525–526**):
1. Goal: *assist client through decisions about treatment protocol* (varies by stage: 0 to IV).
   a. *Radiation*—alone or in conjunction with surgery. Types: external beam radiation, 3-D conformal (focal), radioactive seed implants (brachytherapy).
   b. *Surgery*—cryosurgery; radical retropubic prostatectomy (see **XI. PROSTATECTOMY, p. 466**).
   c. Other options: hormones (*luteinizing hormone–releasing hormone agonists* [Lupron, Zoladex, Casodex, Nilandron]), *antiandrogen* (flutamide [Eulexin]); drugs in conjunction with orchiectomy, to limit production of androgens (*androgen deprivation therapy*).
   d. **Watchful waiting**—recommended with small contained tumor; older men; where surgery is contraindicated for other serious health problems.

E. Evaluation/outcome criteria (see **XI. PROSTATECTOMY, p. 466**).

VII. BLADDER CANCER: bladder is most common site of urinary tract cancer.

A. Risk factors:
1. Contact with certain dyes.
2. Cigarette smoking.
3. Excessive coffee intake.
4. Prolonged use of analgesics with phenacetin.
5. Three times more common in men.

B. Assessment:
1. *Subjective data:*
   a. Frequency, urgency.
   b. *Pain:* flank, pelvic; dysuria.
2. *Objective data:*
   a. Painless hematuria (initially).
   b. *Diagnostic tests:*
      (1) Cystoscopy, intravenous pyelogram (*IVP*)—mass or obstruction.
      (2) Bladder biopsy, urine cytology—malignant cells.
   c. Laboratory data: urinalysis—*increased* RBCs (>4.8 × 10^{12}/L—men, >4.3 × 10^{12}/L—women).

ADULT

C. Analysis/nursing diagnosis:
1. *Risk for injury* related to surgical intervention.
2. *Altered urinary elimination* related to surgery.

D. Nursing care plan/implementation (see also **Nursing care plan/implementation—general care of the client with cancer, pp. 525–526**):
1. Goal: *assist client through treatment protocol.*
   a. *Radiation:* cobalt, radioisotopes, radon seeds; often before surgery to slow tumor growth.
   b. *Chemotherapy:*
      (1) *Antitumor antibiotics:* doxorubicin HCl (Adriamycin), mitomycin.
      (2) *Antimetabolites:* 5-fluorouracil (5-FU).
      (3) *Alkylating* agents: thiotepa.
      (4) *Sedatives, antispasmodics.*
2. Goal: *prepare client for surgery*—types:
   a. *Transurethral fulguration or excision:* used for small tumors with minimal tissue involvement.
   b. *Segmental resection:* up to half the bladder may be resected.
   c. *Cystectomy with urinary diversion:* complete removal of the bladder; performed when disease appears curable.
3. Goal: *assist with acceptance of diagnosis and treatment.*
4. Goal: *prevent complication during postoperative period.*
   a. *Transurethral fulguration or excision:*
      (1) Monitor for clots, bleeding, spasms.
      (2) Maintain patency of Foley catheter.
   b. *Urinary diversion with stoma:*
      (1) Protect skin, ensure proper fit of appliance—because constantly wet with urine (see also **Ileal conduit, pp. 466–467** and **Ostomies and stoma care, pp. 454–456**).
      (2) Prevent infection by increasing *acidity* of urine and increasing *fluid* intake.
      (3) *Health teaching.*
         (a) Self-care of stoma and appliance.
         (b) Expected and side effects of medications.
         (c) Importance of follow-up visits for early detection of metastasis.

E. Evaluation/outcome criteria:
1. Accepts treatment plan.
2. Uses prescribed measures to decrease side effects of surgery, radiation, chemotherapy.
3. Plans follow-up visits for further evaluation.
4. Maintains dignity.

VIII. LARYNGEAL CANCER

A. Risk factors:
1. Eight times more common in men.
2. Occurs most often after age 60.
3. Cigarette smoking.
4. Alcohol.
5. Chronic laryngitis, vocal abuse.
6. Family predisposition to cancer.

B. Assessment:
1. *Subjective data:*
   a. Dysphagia—pain in areas of Adam's apple; radiates to ear.
   b. Dyspnea.
2. *Objective data:*
   a. Persistent hoarseness.
   b. Cough and hemoptysis.
   c. Enlarged cervical nodes.
   d. General debility and weight loss.
   e. Foul breath.
   f. Diagnosis made by history, laryngoscopy with biopsy and microscopic study of cells.

C. Analysis/nursing diagnosis:
1. *Impaired verbal communication* related to removal of larynx.
2. *Body image disturbance* related to radical surgery.
3. *Ineffective airway clearance* related to increased secretions through tracheostomy.

D. Nursing care plan/implementation (see also **Nursing care plan/implementation—general care of the client with cancer, pp. 525–526**): treatment primarily surgical (see **Laryngectomy, pp. 384–386**); radiation therapy may also be indicated.

E. Evaluation/outcome criteria: see **Laryngectomy, p. 386.**

IX. ADDITIONAL TYPES OF CANCER
(Table 6.43).

EMERGENCY NURSING PROCEDURES

I. PURPOSE—to initiate assessment and intervention procedures that will speed total care of the client toward a successful outcome.

II. EMERGENCY NURSING PROCEDURES for adults are detailed in **Table 6.44, pp. 542–552.**

III. LEGAL ISSUES (see **Chapter 3**).

Table 6.43

Selected Cancer Problems

	Assessment			
	Subjective Data	*Objective Data*	**Risk Factors**	**Specific Treatment**
GASTROINTESTINAL TRACT				
Oral cancer	Difficulty chewing, swallowing, moving tongue or jaws; history of heavy smoking, alcohol use, or chewing tobacco	Sore that bleeds and does not heal; persistent red or white patch; diagnosis by biopsy; early detection: dental checks	Heavy smoking and drinking, user of chewing tobacco, men >age 40 (affects twice as many men as women)	• Surgery, with reconstructive surgery useful for cure and palliatively (see **F. General surgical intervention, p. 526**) • *Radiation* using simulated computer localization to avoid destruction of normal tissue (see care of client having radiation therapy, **pp. 527–529**)
Esophageal cancer	Dysphagia—difficulty in swallowing; discomfort described as: lump in throat, pressure in chest, pain; fatigue, lethargy, apathy, depression; anorexia	Weight loss; regurgitation, vomiting; diagnostic tests—*barium swallow,* esophagoscopy, biopsy	Over age 50, alcoholism, use of tobacco; increasing risk in nonwhite women, in people with achalasia (inability to relax lower esophagus with swallowing) or hiatal hernias	• *Surgery:* resection with anastomosis, or removal with gastrostomy • *Radiation:* best form of therapy • *Chemotherapy:* antineoplastic drugs *ineffective;* medications to reduce symptoms of pain, discomfort, and anxiety (see nursing care plan/implementation for client with cancer **[p. 525]**; having radiation therapy **[pp. 527–529]**; having chemotherapy **[pp. 526–527]**; having surgery **[p. 526]**
Stomach cancer	Vague feeling of fullness, pressure, or epigastric pain following ingestion of food; anorexia, nausea, meat intolerance; malaise	Eructation, regurgitation, vomiting; melena, hematemesis, anemia; jaundice, diarrhea, ascites; big belly, upper gastric area; often palpable mass	Men, lower socioeconomic classes, colder climates, early exposure to dietary carcinogens, blood group A, pernicious anemia, atrophic achlorhydric gastritis	• *Surgery:* gastrectomy (see gastric surgery, **p. 446**, care) • *Radiation: not* as useful because dosage needed would cause side effects unlikely to be tolerated by client • *Chemotherapy* alone or in conjunction with surgery: *antitumor antibiotics, antimetabolites, nitrosoureas, hematinics* (see nursing care plan for client having chemotherapy, **pp. 526–527**)
Pancreatic cancer	Anorexia, nausea; pain in upper abdomen, radiating to back; dyspnea	Jaundice, vomiting, weight loss; determination of solid mass in area of pancreas by *computed tomography* and *ultrasound;* tissue identification by thin-needle *percutaneous biopsy*	Excessive use of alcohol; exposure to dry-cleaning chemicals, gasoline; coffee and decaffeinated coffee; possibly diabetes and chronic pancreatitis	• *Surgery:* removal (must then have supplemental *pancreatic enzymes;* some clients become diabetic, type 1) or bypass to relieve obstruction (see nursing care plan/implementation for client with diabetes, **pp. 468–469**) • *Chemotherapy:* pain relief, antiemetics, insulin, pancrelipase, 5-fluorouracil cyclophosphamide (5-FU), Cytoxan, carmustine (BCNU), methotrexate, vincristine, mitomycin-C (see nursing care plan/implementation for client having chemotherapy, **pp. 526–527**) • *Radiation:* intraoperative high dose to pancreatic tumors with external high beam; palliative radiation therapy for pain (see nursing care plan/implementation for client having radiation therapy, **pp. 527–529**; see nursing care plan/implementation for client with cancer, **p. 525**)

ADULT

Table 6.43

Selected Cancer Problems—cont'd

	Assessment: Subjective Data	Assessment: Objective Data	Risk Factors	Specific Treatment
SKIN				
Skin cancer: basal cell	Reported painless lesion	Scaly plaques, papules that ulcerate; pale, waxy, pearly nodule or red, sharply outlined patch; unusual skin condition, change in size or color, or other darkly pigmented growth or mole	Exposure to: sun, coal tar, pitch, arsenic compounds, creosote, radium; fair complexion	• *Surgery:* electrodesiccation (dehydration of tissue by use of needle electrode); cryosurgery (destruction of tissue by application of extreme cold; see care of cancer client, **p. 525**). • *Radiation therapy (see care of client having radiation therapy,* **pp. 527–529**) • *Prevention: avoid* sun from 10 a.m. to 3 p.m.; use protective clothing, sunblock lotion
NERVOUS SYSTEM				
Brain	*Headache:* steady, intermittent, severe (may be intensified by physical activity); nausea; lethargy, easy fatigability; forgetfulness, disorientation, impaired judgment; visual disturbances; blackouts	Vomiting, may be projectile; sight loss, auditory changes; signs of increased intracranial pressure; seizures; paresthesia; behavior changes. • *Diagnostic studies*—CT scan, arteriography, cytology of cerebrospinal fluid	None known for primary tumors; brain is common site for metastasis	• *Surgery:* craniotomy with excision of lesion; ventricular shunt to allow for drainage of fluid (see nursing care plan/implementation for craniotomy, **pp. 380–381**) • *Radiation:* cobalt (local or entire CNS); total brain radiation causes alopecia, which may be permanent (see nursing care plan/implementation for client having radiation therapy, **pp. 527–529**); could be used alone, with surgery, or with chemotherapy • *Chemotherapy: antineoplastic alkylating agents:* nitrosoureas (cross blood-brain barrier to reduce tumor)—carmustine (BCNU), lomustine (CCNU), semustine (methyl-CCNU); *cerebral diuretics* to reduce edema; *anticonvulsants; analgesics; sedatives* (see nursing care plan/implementation for client having chemotherapy, **pp. 526–527**)
ENDOCRINE				
Thyroid cancer	Painless nodule; dysphagia; difficulty breathing	Enlarged thyroid, thyroid nodule; palpable thyroid, lymph nodes; hoarseness; hypofunctional nodule seen on *isotopic imaging scanning; needle biopsy* for cytology studies	Radiation exposure in childhood	• *Surgery:* total thyroidectomy, possible radical neck dissection (see **IV. THYROIDECTOMY, p. 473**) • *Radiation:* external, or with radioactive iodine (^{131}I) (see care of client having radiation therapy, **pp. 527–529**) • *Chemotherapy:* chlorambucil, doxorubicin, vincristine (Leukeran, Adriamycin, Oncovin, respectively) (see care of client having chemotherapy, **pp. 526–527**)
BLOOD AND LYMPH TISSUES				
Hodgkin's disease	Fatigue; generalized pruritus; anorexia	Painless enlargement of lymph nodes, especially in cervical area; fever, night sweats; hepatosplenomegaly; anemia; peak age of	For young adults from 15 to 35 yr old, not clearly defined, some relationship to socioeconomic status; men-women ratio	*Staging and treatment:* • *Stage I*—involvement of a single node or a single node region; excision of lesion, and total nodal radiation (see care of client having radiation therapy, **pp. 527–529**)

Continued

ADULT

Table 6.43

Selected Cancer Problems—cont'd

	Assessment			
	Subjective Data	*Objective Data*	**Risk Factors**	**Specific Treatment**
		incidence, 15–35; • *Diagnostic tests*—biopsy shows presence of *Reed-Sternberg cells; x-rays, scans, laparotomy*	is 1.5:1; increased frequency among White persons	• *Stage II*—involvement of two or more lymph node regions on same side of diaphragm; excision of lesion and radiation (see care of client having radiation therapy, **pp. 527–529**) • *Stage III*—involvement of lymph node regions on both sides of the diaphragm, which may include the spleen; combination of radiation and chemotherapy • *Stage IV*—involvement of one or more extralymphatic organs or tissues, with or without lymphatic involvement; treated with chemotherapy alone, radiation therapy alone, or both • Presence or absence of symptoms of night sweats, significant fever, and weight loss; treated with *chemotherapy,* MOPP—Mustargen (mechlorethamine HCl, alkylating agent), Oncovin (vincristine, plant alkaloid), procarbazine (antineoplastic); prednisone (corticosteroid) (see care of client having chemotherapy, **pp. 526–527**)
Non-Hodgkin's lymphoma	Night sweats	Nontender lymphadenopathy, enlarged liver and spleen, weight loss, fever	Ages 50–60 yr	• Stage I—rarely observed, but remission possible with radiation therapy • Stage II—radiation therapy • Stage III and IV— combination chemotherapy, with or without radiation therapy
Multiple myeloma	Weakness; history of frequent infections, especially pneumonias; severe bone pain on motion; neurological symptoms, paralysis	• Fractures of long bones; deformity of: sternum, ribs, vertebrae, pelvis; hepatosplenomegaly; anemia and bleeding tendencies *Elevated* uric acid	Exposure to ionizing radiation; middle-aged or older women	• *Surgery:* relieve spinal cord compression; orthopedic procedures to relieve or support bone problems (see nursing care plan/implementation for clients with internal fixation for fractures, **p. 506**; client with spinal cord injuries when paralysis occurs, **pp. 520–521**) • *Radiation:* for some lesions (see nursing care plan/implementation for clients having radiation therapy, **pp. 527–529**) • *Chemotherapy: alkylating agents; antitumor antibiotics; plant alkaloids; hormones*—melphalan and prednisone (see nursing care plan/implementation for clients having chemotherapy, **pp. 526–527**)
URINARY ORGANS				
Kidney cancer	Fatigue; abdominal or flank pain; night sweats	Painless, gross hematuria; firm, nontender, palpable kidney; weight loss; fever of unknown origin (FUO); testicular enlargement. *Complications*: hypertension; *nephrotic syndrome;* metastasis to lung, brain, liver, bones	More common among men than women, Whites than Blacks; lymphoma; smoking; exposure to chemicals used in leather manufacturing; radiation exposure; possible familial influence;	• *Surgery:* stereotactic surgery; gamma knife (for brain metastasis); nephrectomy (see Nursing care plan/implementation for pre/postoperative care, **pp. 365–367, 369–375**) • *Radiation:* irradiation of *metastatic* sites when tumor is radiosensitive (see Nursing care plan/implementation for client having radiation therapy, **pp. 527–529**)

Table 6.43

Selected Cancer Problems—cont'd

	Assessment			
	Subjective Data	*Objective Data*	**Risk Factors**	**Specific Treatment**
		(e.g., scapula or pelvis); vena cava involvement *Laboratory and diagnostic tests:* CT scans (chest, abdomen, pelvis) with contrast; MRI; bone scan; urinalysis—presence of red cells and albumin; CBC—*decrease* in red cells and leukocytes, *reduction* in serum albumin, *elevation* of alpha globulin and calcium	common site of metastasis from lung	• *Chemotherapy:* plant alkaloids—vincristine (Oncovin); antitumor antibiotics—dactinomycin (Actinomycin D), doxorubicin (*Adriamycin*), gemcitabine (*Gemzar*); alkylating agents—cyclophosphamide (Cytoxan); IL-2; interferon alpha (see Nursing care plan/implementation for client having chemotherapy, **pp. 526–527**) • *Clinical trials:* Avastin, bone marrow transplant, Bay 43
GENITAL ORGANS				
Testicular cancer	Aching or dragging sensation in groin, usually painless	Gynecomastia; enlargement, swelling, lump, hardening of testes; young adult men early diagnosis—monthly testicular self-examination (see **Fig. 6.17**)	Second most common malignancy among men ages 25–40 yr; possibly exposure to chemical carcinogens; trauma, orchitis; gonadal dysgenesis; cryptorchidism (undescended testicles)	*Surgery:* orchiectomy (see Nursing care plan/implementation for the preoperative and postoperative client, **pp. 365–367, 368–369, 369–375**). *Radiation:* see nursing care plan/implementation for client having radiation therapy, **pp. 527–529**) *Chemotherapy:* cisplatin, bleomycin, etoposide, steroids (see nursing care plan/implementation for client having chemotherapy, **pp. 526–527**)
Cervical cancer	Vague pelvic or low back discomfort, pressure, or pain	Intermenstrual, postcoital, or postmenopausal bleeding, vaginal discharge—serosanguineous and malodorous hypermenorrhea; abdominal distention with urinary frequency; abnormal Pap test (see **Table 6.40**); recommended guidelines by American Cancer Society: *Pap test* annually; after three consecutive normal tests, physician may recommend less frequent testing; pelvic/uterine examination every 3 yr	Early age at first intercourse; multiple sex partners; low socioeconomic status; exposure to herpes simplex virus type 2	*Staging* (see **Table 6.42**) • *Stage 0*—carcinoma in situ; no distinct tumor observable; stage may last for 8–10 yr; cure rate 100% following treatment of wedge or cone resection of cervix during childbearing years, or simple hysterectomy • *Stage I*—malignant cells infiltrate cervical mucosa; lesion bleeds easily; cure rate 80% with treatment of hysterectomy • *Stage II*—neoplasm spreads through cervical muscular layers, involves upper third of vaginal mucosa; cure rate 50% with treatment of radical hysterectomy • *Stage III*—neoplasm involves lower third of vagina; cure rate 25% with pelvic exenteration • *Stage IV*—involves metastasis to bladder, rectum, and surrounding tissues; considered incurable • *Radiation:* external or internal or both, in conjunction with surgery or alone, depending on stage of disease or condition of client (see nursing care plan/implementation for client having radiation therapy, **pp. 527–529**) • *Chemotherapy:* progestin, *antineoplastics,* megestrol (Megace), medroxyprogesterone (Curretab, Provera); *alkylating agents*—dacarbazine (DTIC)

Testicular self-examination

To help detect abnormalities early, every male should examine his testes once a month. Instruct the client to follow this procedure:

1 If possible, take a warm bath or shower before beginning; the scrotum, which tends to contract when cold, will be relaxed, making the testes easier to examine.

2 With one hand, lift the penis and check the scrotum (the sac containing the testes) for any change in shape, size, or color. The left side of the scrotum normally hangs slightly lower than the right.

3 Next, check the testes for lumps and masses. Locate the crescent-shaped structure at the back of each testis. This is the epididymis, which should feel soft.

4 Use the thumb and first two fingers of your left hand to squeeze the spermatic cord gently; it extends upward from the epididymis, above the left testis. Then repeat on the right side, using your right hand. Check for lumps and masses by palpating along the entire length of the cord.

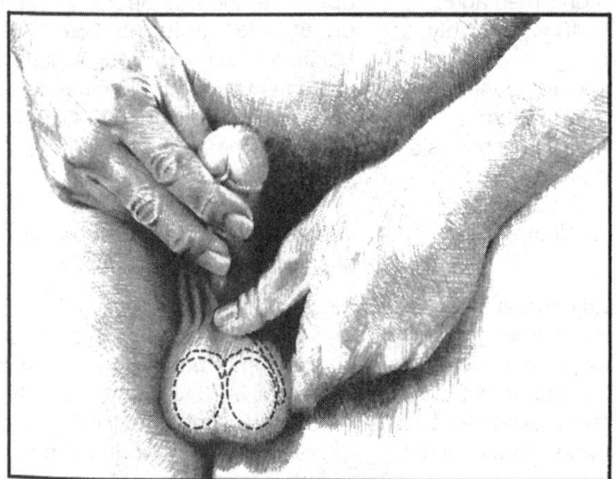

5 Next, examine each testis. To do so, place the index and middle fingers on its underside and the thumb on top, then gently roll the testis between the thumb and fingers. A normal testis is egg-shaped, rubbery-firm, and movable within the scrotum; it should feel smooth, with no lumps. Both testes should be the same size.

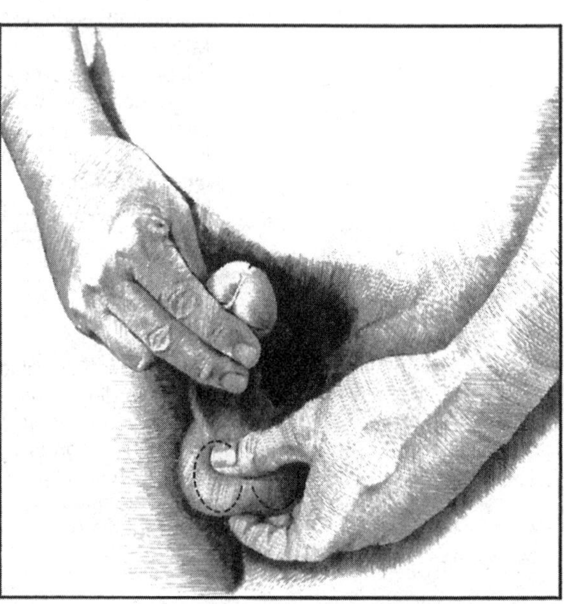

6 Promptly report any lumps, masses, or changes to the physician.

Figure 6.17 Testicular self-examination. (From Morton, PG: *Health Assessment in Nursing.* FA Davis, Philadelphia, 1993, p 451.)

ADULT

Table 6.44

Nursing Care of the Adult in Medical and Surgical Emergencies

Condition	Assessment: Signs and Symptoms	Prehospitalization Nursing Care	In-hospital Nursing Care
Cardiovascular Emergencies			
Myocardial infarction—ischemia and necrosis of cardiac muscle secondary to insufficient or obstructed coronary blood flow	*Prehospital*: • Chest pain: viselike, choking, unrelieved by rest or nitroglycerin • *Skin:* ashen, cold, clammy • *Vital signs:* pulse—rapid, weak, thready; increased rate and depth of respirations; dyspnea • *Behavior:* restless, anxious	1. If coronary suspected, call physician, paramedic service, or emergency ambulance 2. Calm and reassure client that help is coming 3. Place in *semi-Fowler's* position 4. Keep client warm but not hot	1. Rapidly assess hemodynamic and respiratory status 2. Place on cardiac monitor to determine treatment 3. Place on O_2 4. Start IV as ordered—usually D_5W per microdrip to establish lifeline for emergency drug treatment 5. Relieve pain—morphine SO_4 IV as needed, aspirin, nitroglycerin

Table 6.44

Nursing Care of the Adult in Medical and Surgical Emergencies—cont'd

Condition	Assessment: Signs and Symptoms	Prehospitalization Nursing Care	In-hospital Nursing Care
	In hospital: • *C/V:* blood pressure and pulse pressure *decreased* • *Heart sounds:* soft; S_3 may be present • *Respirations:* fine basilar crackles • *Laboratory:* ECG consistent with tissue necrosis (Q waves) and injury (ST-segment *elevation*); serum enzymes *elevated* (CK-MB, troponin)		6. Draw blood for electrolytes, enzymes, as ordered 7. Take 12-lead ECG 8. Once client is stable, transfer to coronary care unit (CCU)
Cardiac arrest—cardiac standstill or ventricular fibrillation secondary to rapid administration or overdose of anesthetics or narcotic drugs, obstruction of the respiratory tract (mucus, vomitus, foreign body), acute anxiety, cardiac disease, dehydration, shock, electric shock, or emboli	• Cyanosis, gasping • *Respirations:* rapid, shallow, absent • *Pulse:* weak, thready, >120 beats/min, absent • Muscle: twitching • *Pupils:* dilated • *Skin:* cold, clammy • Loss of consciousness	**CPR** 1. *Position:* flat on back 2. Check for no breathing or no normal breathing (only gasping) while checking for unresponsiveness 3. Activate the emergency response system: call 9-1-1. Get automated external defibrillator (AED) or send someone else to get; use within 5 min 4. Take 10 sec to check pulse 5. If no pulse, begin chest compressions—30 compressions at a rate of 100/min. Depress sternum at least 2 inches 6. After 30 compressions, open airway and give 2 breaths (**CAB—compressions, airway, breathing**) within 10 sec 7. Use AED when available	1. If monitored, note rhythm; call for help and note time 2. **Immediate** countershock if rhythm is ventricular fibrillation or ventricular tachycardia 3. If countershock unsuccessful, begin CPR, as in **prehospital care**
		• *No heartbeat:* *One- or two-person lay rescuer* 1. *CPR:* 100 chest compressions per minute, with two rescue breaths between every 30 compressions (no difference in ratio for one or two persons); 2. Check pulse at neck after 5 cycles or 2 min 3. *Provide early defibrillation* with AED within 5 min of arrest if indicated 4. *If heartbeat returns:* assist respiration and monitor pulse; continue CPR until help arrives	*Two-person rescue* *First person:* begins CPR as described in **prehospital care** *Second person:* 1. Pages arrest team 2. Brings defibrillator to bedside and countershocks, if indicated by rhythm; defibrillate within 3 min of arrest if indicated 3. Brings emergency cart to bedside 4. Suctions airway, if indicated due to vomitus or secretions 5. Bags client with 100% O_2 6. Assists with intubation when arrest team arrives 7. Establishes intravenous line if one is not available

Continued

ADULT

Table 6.44

Nursing Care of the Adult in Medical and Surgical Emergencies—cont'd

Condition	Assessment: Signs and Symptoms	Prehospitalization Nursing Care	In-hospital Nursing Care
Shock—cellular hypoxia and impairment of cellular function secondary to: trauma, hemorrhage, fright, dehydration, cardiac insufficiency, allergic reactions, septicemia, impairment of nervous system, poisons	**Early shock** • *Sensorium:* conscious, apprehensive, and restless; some slurring of speech • *Pupils:* dull but reactive to light • *Pulse:* rate <140/min; amplitude full to mildly decreased • *Blood pressure:* normal to slightly decreased • *Neck veins:* normal to slightly flat in supine position; may be full in septic shock or grossly distended in cardiogenic shock • *Skin:* cool, clammy, pale • *Respirations:* rapid, shallow • *GI:* nausea, vomiting, thirst • *Renal:* urine output 20–40 mL/hr	1. Check breathing—clear airway if necessary; if no breathing, give artificial respirations; if breathing is irregular or labored, raise head and shoulders 2. Control bleeding by placing pressure on the wound or at pressure points (proximal artery) 3. Make comfortable and reassure 4. Cover lightly to prevent heat loss, but do *not* bundle up 5. If neck or spine injury is suspected—do *not* move, unless victim in danger of more injury	1. Check vital signs rapidly—pulse, pupils, respirations 2. Check airway; clear if necessary; draw ABGs; Po_2 should be maintained above 60 mm Hg; elevated Pco_2 indicates need for intubation and ventilatory assistance 3. Control gross bleeding 4. Prepare for insertion of intravenous line and central lines—if abdominal injuries present 5. Peripheral line should be placed in upper extremity if fluids being lost in abdomen
		If client unconscious or has wounds of the lower face and jaw—place on *side* to promote drainage of fluids; position client on *back* unless otherwise indicated	1. Draw blood for specimens: Hgb, Hct, CBC, glucose, CO_2, sodium amylase, BUN, K^+; type and crossmatch, blood gases, CPK-MB, troponin, prothrombin times 2. Prepare infusion of crystalloid replacement—NS usual choice; may include Ringer's lactate or half-normal saline
	Severe or late shock • *Sensorium:* confused, disoriented, apathetic, unresponsive; slow, slurred speech, often incoherent • *Pupils:* dilating, dilated, slow or nonreactive to light • *Pulse:* rate >150 beats/min, thready, weak • *Blood pressure:* 80 mm Hg or unobtainable • *Neck veins:* flat in a supine position—no filling; full to distended in septic *or* cardiogenic shock	1. *Raise* feet 6–8 inches unless client has head or chest injuries; if victim becomes less comfortable, lower feet 2. If client complains of thirst, do *not* give fluids unless client is more than 6 hr away from professional medical help; under **no** conditions give water to clients: who are unconscious, having seizures or vomiting, appearing to need general anesthetic, or with a stomach, chest, or skull injury 3. Be calm and confident; reassure client help is on the way	1. Assess and intervene as for early shock; then obtain information as to onset and past history. **Treat underlying cause** STAT. 2. Catheterize and monitor client urine output as ordered 3. Take 12-lead ECG 4. Insert nasogastric tube and assess aspirate for volume, color, and blood; save specimen if poison or drug overdose suspected 5. *If CVP low* (<12)—infuse 200–300 mL over 5–10 min. *If CVP rises* sharply—fluid restriction necessary; if remains low—hypovolemia present 6. *If client febrile*—blood cultures and wound cultures will be ordered 7. *If urine output* scanty or absent—give mannitol as ordered

ADULT

Table 6.44

Nursing Care of the Adult in Medical and Surgical Emergencies—cont'd

Condition	Assessment: Signs and Symptoms	Prehospitalization Nursing Care	In-hospital Nursing Care
	• *Skin:* cold, clammy, mottled; circumoral cyanosis, dusky, cyanotic • *Eyes:* sunken—vacant expression *Renal:* urine output <20 mL/hr		 8. *If systolic BP* <90 mm Hg—give vasopressors (Levophed, vasopressin)
Respiratory Emergencies			
Choking—obstruction of airway secondary to aspiration of a foreign object	• Gasping, wheezing; looks panicky, but can still breathe, talk, cough • *Cough:* weak, ineffective; breathing sounds like high-pitched crowing; • *Color*—white, gray, blue • Difficulty speaking; clutches throat	Do not interfere if coughing; do *not* slap on back; watch closely; call for assistance • ***Victim standing/sitting and conscious:*** Perform *obstructive airway maneuver* (formerly called Heimlich maneuver): stand behind victim, wrap arms around waist, place fist against abdomen, and with your other hand, press it into the victim's abdomen with a quick upward thrust until the obstruction is relieved or the victim becomes unconscious • ***Victim lying down:*** Roll the victim onto his or her back; straddle the victim's thighs; place heel of hand in the middle of abdomen; place other hand on top of the first; stiffen arms and deliver 6–10 abdominal thrusts • ***Unconscious victim:*** *Lay rescuers*—proceed to CPR. No abdominal thrusts or blind finger sweeps *EMS responders*—Try to ventilate; if unsuccessful, deliver abdominal thrusts using technique described for obstructive airway; probe mouth for foreign objects; keep repeating above procedure until ventilation occurs; as victim becomes more deprived of air, muscles will relax and maneuvers that were previously unsuccessful will begin to work; when successful in removing obstruction, give two breaths; check pulse; start CPR if indicated • On ***obese or pregnant*** victims—use chest thrusts instead of abdominal thrusts ***You are victim and alone:*** Place your two fists for abdominal thrusts; bend over back of chair, sink, etc. and exert hard, repeated pressure on abdomen to force object up; push fingers down your throat to encourage regurgitation	As in ***prehospital care***; when probing mouth for foreign object, turn *head to side,* unless client has neck injury; in event of neck injury, *raise* the arm opposite you and roll the head and shoulders as a unit, so that head ends up supported on the arm

Continued

Table 6.44

Nursing Care of the Adult in Medical and Surgical Emergencies—cont'd

Condition	Assessment: Signs and Symptoms	Prehospitalization Nursing Care	In-hospital Nursing Care
Acute respiratory failure—sudden onset of an abnormally low PaO_2 (<60 mm Hg) or high PCO_2 (>60 mm Hg) secondary to: lung disease or trauma, peripheral or central nervous system depression, cardiac failure, severe obesity, airway obstruction, environmental abnormality	• *Hypoxia* *Sensorium:* acute apprehension *Respiration:* dyspnea; shallow, rapid respirations *Skin:* circumoral cyanosis; pale, dusky skin and nailbeds *C/V:* slight hypertension and tachycardia, or hypotension and bradycardia • *Hypercapnia* *Sensorium:* decreasing mentation; headache *Skin:* flushed, warm, moist *C/V:* hypertension; tachycardia	If you suspect respiratory distress, call physician; calm and reassure client; place in a chair or *semisitting* position; keep warm but not hot; phone for ambulance; *if respirations cease* or client becomes unconscious: clear airway and commence respiratory resuscitation; check pulse: initiate CPR if necessary; continue resuscitation until help arrives	Check client's ability to speak; maintain airway by placing in *high Fowler's position;* check vital signs: BP, pulse rate and rhythm, temperature, skin color, rate and depth of respirations; place on O_2, pulse oximetry, **STAT** ABG • *Prepare for intubation if:* 1. Client has flail chest 2. Client is comatose without gag reflex 3. Client has respiratory arrest; open airway, ambu bag with 100% O_2 via face mask until intubation 4. $Paco_2$ >55 mm Hg 5. Pao_2 <60 mm Hg 6. F_iO_2 >50% using nasal cannula, catheter, or mask 7. Respiratory rate >36 • *After intubation:* 1. Check bilateral lung sounds 2. Observe for symmetrical lung expansion 3. Maintain humidified oxygen at lowest F_iO_2 possible to achieve Pao_2 of 60 mm Hg 4. Monitor exhaled CO_2 with caprometer. • *Improve ventilation (decrease Pco_2) by:* 1. Frequent suctioning—oral and above cuff of ET tube 2. IPPB indicated if tidal volume decreases 3. Administer *drugs* as ordered: sympathomimetics, xanthines, antibiotics, and steroids 4. Monitor: arterial blood gases, electrolytes, Hct, Hgb, and WBCs 5. Bronchoscopy may be indicated for thick, tenacious secretions **Do not:** 1. Administer sedatives 2. Correct acid-base problems without monitoring electrolytes 3. Overcorrect $Paco_2$ 4. Leave client alone while oxygen therapy is initiated. Once client is stable, transfer to ICU
Near-drowning—asphyxiation or partial asphyxiation due to immersion or submersion in a fluid or liquid medium	*Conscious victim:* • Acute anxiety, panic; increased rate of respirations • Pale, dusky skin	*Conscious victim:* 1. Try to talk victim out of panic so can find footing and way to shore 2. Utilize devices such as poles, rings, clothing to extend to victim; do *not* let victim who is panicked grab you; do *not* attempt swimming rescue unless specially trained	*Nonsymptomatic near-drowning victim:* 1. Draw blood for arterial blood gases with client breathing room air 2. PA and lateral chest x-ray 3. Auscultate lungs 4. Admit to hospital for further evaluation if: a. Pao_2 <80 mm Hg b. pH <7.35

Table 6.44

Nursing Care of the Adult in Medical and Surgical Emergencies—cont'd

Condition	Assessment: Signs and Symptoms	Prehospitalization Nursing Care	In-hospital Nursing Care
		3. If you suspect head or neck injury—handle carefully, floating victim back to shore with body and head as straight as possible; do *not* turn head or bend back	c. Pulmonary infiltrates present, or auscultation reveals crackles d. Victim inhaled fluids containing: choline, hydrocarbons, sewage, or hypotonic or freshwater
	Unconscious victim: • Shallow or no respirations • Weak or no pulse	*Unconscious victim:* 1. *If victim not breathing:* as soon as you have firm support, begin resuscitation 2. Tilt head back, bring jaw forward, pinch nostril shut, give two quick breaths	
		On shore: 1. Check breathing 2. *Lay* victim flat on back; cover and keep warm 3. Calm and reassure victim 4. Do *not* give food or water 5. Get to medical assistance as soon as possible 6. *If unconscious and not breathing:* begin sequence for CPR; compress water from abdomen *only* if interfering with ventilation attempts 7. *If airway obstructed:* reposition head; attempt to ventilate; *if EMS responder:* perform 6–10 abdominal thrusts; sweep mouth deeply; attempt to ventilate; repeat until successful 8. Once ventilation established, check pulse; *if absent*, begin chest compressions as in CPR, one-person or two-person rescue 9. Continue CPR until victim revives or help arrives 10. If victim revives, cover and keep warm; reassure victim help is on the way 11. Rescue personnel can further assist emergency department personnel by: a. Documenting prehospital resuscitation methods used b. Immobilizing victims suspected of cervical spine injuries c. Using a sterile container to take a sample of immersion fluid d. Taking on-scene arterial blood gas sample for later analysis	*Symptomatic near-drowning victim:* 1. Provide basic or advanced cardiac life support 2. Provide clear airway and adequate ventilation by: a. Suctioning airway b. Inserting artificial airway and attaching it to ventilator as indicated c. Inserting nasogastric tube to suction to minimize aspiration of vomitus 3. Monitor ECG continuously 4. Start IV infusion D_5W at keep-open rate for *freshwater near-drowning;* D_5NS in *saltwater near-drowning* 5. Assist with insertion of *CVP* and *pulmonary artery (PA) catheter* to guide subsequent infusion rates 6. Administer drugs as ordered: anticonvulsants; steroids, antibiotics, stimulants, antiarrhythmics 7. Provide rewarming if hypothermia present 8. Insert *Foley* to assess kidney function because freshwater near-drowning causes renal tubular necrosis due to RBC hemolysis 9. Transfer to ICU when stabilized

Continued

ADULT

Table 6.44

Nursing Care of the Adult in Medical and Surgical Emergencies—cont'd

Condition	Assessment: Signs and Symptoms	Prehospitalization Nursing Care	In-hospital Nursing Care
Systemic Injuries			
Multiple traumas	• *Sensorium:* alert; disoriented, stuporous, comatose • *Respirations:* increased rate, depth; shallow; asymmetrical; paradoxical breathing; mediastinal shift; gasping, blowing *C/V:* signs of shock (see **pp. 427–429, 544–545**) • *Abdomen:* contusions; pain; abrasions; open wounds; rigidity; increasing distention • *Skeletal system:* pain; swelling; deformity; inappropriate or no movement • *Neurological:* pupils round, equal, react to light; ipsilateral dilation and unresponsive; fixed and dilated bilaterally • Bilateral movement and sensation in all extremities • Progressive contralateral weakness • Loss of voluntary motor function See *Sensorium* (above) for level of consciousness	1. Do *not* move client unless you must, to prevent further injury; send for help 2. Check breathing—give mouth-to-mouth resuscitation if indicated 3. Check for bleeding 4. Control bleeding by applying pressure on wound or on pressure points (artery proximal to wound) 5. Use tourniquet *only* if above pressure techniques fail to stop severe bleeding 6. Check for shock (pulse, pupils, skin color) and other injuries 7. Fractures: keep open-fracture area clean 8. Do *not* try to set bone 9. If client must be moved—splint broken bones with splints that extend past the limb joints; tie splints on snugly but not so tight as to cut off circulation 10. Check peripheral pulses 11. If head or back injury suspected—keep body *straight;* move only with help 12. Reassure client that help is on the way	1. Assess vital functions; ECG monitoring, continuous pulse oximetry 2. Establish airway; ventilate with ambu bag, ventilator 3. Draw arterial blood gases 4. Control bleeding 5. Prepare infusions of blood, crystalloids 6. Assess for other injuries: head injuries—suspect cervical neck injury with all head injuries 7. Place sandbags to immobilize head and neck 8. Do mini-neurological examination: level of consciousness, pupils, bilateral movement, and sensation 9. Get history—time of injury; any loss of consciousness; any drug ingestion 10. Stop bleeding on or about head 11. Apply ice to contusions and hematomas 12. Check for bleeding from nose, pharynx, ears 13. Check for cerebrospinal fluid from ears or nose 14. Assist with spinal tap if ordered 15. Keep accurate I&O 16. Protect from injury if restless, seizures; orient to time, place, person 17. Administer steroids, diuretics, as ordered 18. *Check for signs of increasing intracranial pressure:* slowing pulse and respiration, widened pulse pressure, decreasing mentation
Spinal injuries			1. Assess and support vital functions as above 2. Immobilize—*no* flexion or extension allowed 3. *If in respiratory distress*—nasotracheal intubation or tracheostomy to *avoid* hyperextending neck 4. *Check for level of injury and function*, asking client to: a. Lift elbow to shoulder height (C5) b. Bend elbow (C6) c. Straighten elbow (C7) d. Grip your hand (C8-T1) e. Lift leg (L3) f. Straighten knee (L4, L5) g. Wiggle toes (L5) h. Push toes down (S1)

Table 6.44

Nursing Care of the Adult in Medical and Surgical Emergencies—cont'd

Condition	Assessment: Signs and Symptoms	Prehospitalization Nursing Care	In-hospital Nursing Care
			5. *If client is comatose:* a. Rub sternum with knuckles b. If all extremities move, severe injury unlikely c. If one side moves and other does not, potential hemiplegia d. If arms move and legs do not, lower spinal cord injury 6. Administer steroids as ordered 7. Assist with application of skull tongs—*Vinke* or *Crutchfield* 8. Maintain IV infusions 9. Insert *Foley* as indicated 10. Assist with dressing of open wounds
Chest injuries			1. Note color and pattern of respirations, position of trachea 2. Auscultate lungs and palpate chest for: crepitus, pain, tenderness, and position of trachea 3. Place gauze soaked in petroleum jelly, if available, over open pneumothorax (sucking chest wound) to seal hole and decrease respiratory distress 4. Assist with tracheostomy if indicated 5. Prepare for insertion of chest tubes if pneumothorax or hemothorax present
Abdominal injuries			1. Observe for rigidity 2. Check for hematuria 3. Auscultate for bowel sounds 4. Assist with paracentesis to confirm bleeding in abdominal cavity 5. Prepare for exploratory laparotomy 6. Insert nasogastric tube—to detect presence of upper GI bleeding 7. Monitor vital signs • *If organs protruding:* 1. *Flex* client's knees 2. Cover intestines with sterile towel soaked in saline 3. Do *not* attempt to replace organs
Fractures			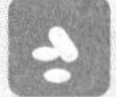 1. Administer tetanus toxoid as ordered 2. Observe for pain, peripheral pulses, pallor, loss of sensation and/or movement 3. Assist with wound cleansing, casting, x-rays, reduction 4. Prepare for surgery if indicated 5. Monitor vital signs

Continued

ADULT

Table 6.44

Nursing Care of the Adult in Medical and Surgical Emergencies—cont'd

Condition	Assessment: Signs and Symptoms	Prehospitalization Nursing Care	In-hospital Nursing Care
Burns—tissue trauma secondary to scalding fluid or flame, chemicals, or electricity	• *Superficial (first degree):* Erythema and tenderness Usually sunburn	Relieve pain by applying cold, wet towel or cold water (*not* iced)	1. Cleanse thoroughly with mild detergent and water 2. Apply gauze or sterile towel 3. Administer sedatives and narcotics as ordered 4. Arrange for follow-up care, or prepare for admission if burn ambulatory care impractical
	• *Partial thickness (second degree):* Swelling, blisters; moisture due to escaping plasma	1. Douse with cold water until pain relieved 2. Blot skin dry and cover with clean towel 3. Do *not:* break blisters, remove pieces of skin, or apply antiseptic ointments 4. If arm or leg burned, keep *elevated* 5. Seek medical attention if *second-degree* burns: a. Cover 10% of body surface b. Involve hands, feet, or face	1. Check tetanus immunization status 2. Administer sedatives or narcotics as ordered 3. Assess respiratory and hemodynamic status; oxygen or ventilatory assist as indicated, intravenous infusions as ordered to combat shock 4. Remove all clothing from burn area 5. Using *aseptic technique*, cleanse burns as indicated
	• *Full thickness (third degree):* White, charred areas	1. Do *not* remove charred clothing 2. Cover burned area with clean towel, sheet 3. *Elevate* burned extremities 4. Apply cold pack to hand, face, or feet 5. Sit client up with face or chest wound to assist respirations 6. Maintain airway 7. Observe for shock 8. Do *not*: a. Put ice water on burns or immerse wounds in ice water—may increase shock b. Apply ointments 9. Calm and reassure victim 10. Get medical help promptly 11. *If* client conscious, not vomiting, and medical assistance is more than 6 hr away: may give sips of weak solution of salt, soda, and water	1. Do *not* break blebs or attempt débridement 2. Assist with application of dressings as ordered 3. Maintain frequent checks of vital signs, urine output 4. Provide psychological support—explain procedures, orient, etc. 5. Assist with application of splints as ordered 6. Administer tetanus immune globulin or toxoid as ordered 7. Assist with transfer to hospital unit
	Fourth degree: Black	Same as full thickness.	
	Chemical burns	1. Flush with copious amounts of water 2. Get rid of clothing over burned area	1. Flush with copious amounts of water 2. Administer sedation or narcotics as ordered
	Burns of the eye: Acid	1. Flush eye with water for at least 15 min 2. Pour water from inside to outside of eye to *avoid contaminating unaffected eye* 3. Cover—seek medical attention **at once**	1. Irrigate with water: *never* use neutralizing solution 2. Instill 0.5% tetracaine as ordered 3. Apply patch

ADULT

Table 6.44

Nursing Care of the Adult in Medical and Surgical Emergencies—cont'd

Condition	Assessment: Signs and Symptoms	Prehospitalization Nursing Care	In-hospital Nursing Care
	Alkali (laundry detergent or cleaning solvent)	1. Do *not* allow client to rub eye 2. Flush eye with water for at least 30 min 3. Cover—seek medical attention **at once**	As above for acid
Abdominal Emergencies			
Aortic aneurysm—rupture or dissection	• Primarily men >age 60 • Sudden onset of excruciating pain: abdominal, lumbosacral, groin, or rectal • Orthopnea, dyspnea • Fainting, hypotension; if dissecting, marked hypertension may be present • Palpable, tender, pulsating mass in umbilical area • Femoral pulse present; dorsalis pedis—weak or absent	1. Notify physician 2. Lay client flat, or raise head if in respiratory distress 3. Cover to keep warm but *not* hot 4. Institute shock measures (see **pp. 544–545**) 5. Calm; reassure that help is on the way.	1. Assess respiratory and hemodynamic status 2. Institute shock measures (see **pp. 544–545**) if indicated 3. Evaluate and compare peripheral pulses 4. Assist with x-rays 5. Assist with emergency preoperative treatment
Blunt injuries—spleen	• Left upper quadrant pain, tenderness and moderate rigidity; left shoulder pain (*Kehr's sign*) • Hypotension; weak, thready pulse; increased respirations (shock)	1. Lay client *flat* 2. Institute shock measures (see **pp. 544–545**).	1. Assess respiratory and hemodynamic status a. Maintain airway and ventilation as indicated b. Institute infusions of colloid or crystalloids as ordered c. Insert both CVP and arterial monitoring lines d. Insert *Foley* catheter 2. Prepare for splenectomy
Eye and Ear Emergencies			
Chemical burns	*See* **Burns, p. 550**	*See* **Burns**	*See* **Burns**
Blunt injuries secondary to flying missiles (e.g., balls, striking face against car dashboard)	• Decreased visual acuity, diplopia, blood in anterior chamber • Pain, conjunctiva reddened, edema of eyelids	1. Prevent victim from rubbing eye 2. Cover with patch to protect eye 3. Seek medical help **immediately**	1. Test visual acuity of each eye using *Snellen* or *Jaeger* chart 2. Assist with *fluorescein* administration—to facilitate identifying breaks in cornea
Sharp ocular trauma—secondary to small or larger foreign bodies	• Reports feeling as if something were hitting eye • Pain, tearing, reddened conjunctiva • Blurring of vision Foreign object may be visible	1. Keep victim from rubbing eye 2. Cover very lightly—do *not* apply pressure	1. Check visual acuity in both eyes 2. Check pupils 3. Instill 1% tetracaine HCl as ordered to relieve pain 4. Administer antibiotic drops or ointment as ordered 5. Apply eye patch 6. Provide instructions for subsequent care and follow-up
Foreign bodies in ears—beans, peas, candy, foxtails, insects	• Decreased hearing; pulling, poking at ear and ear canal; buzzing, discomfort	1. Do *not* attempt to remove object 2. Seek medical assistance	1. Inspect ear canal 2. Assist with sedating (especially children)—restraint may be necessary

Continued

ADULT

Table 6.44

Nursing Care of the Adult in Medical and Surgical Emergencies—cont'd

Condition	Assessment: Signs and Symptoms	Prehospitalization Nursing Care	In-hospital Nursing Care
			3. Assist with procedures to remove object: a. Forceps or curved probe for *fox-tails, irregularly shaped* objects b. 10F or 12F catheter with tip cut squarely off and attached to suction to remove *round* object 4. Irrigate external auditory canal to flush out *insects*, materials that do not absorb water; do *not* irrigate if danger of perforation

Questions

Select the one answer that is best for each question, unless otherwise directed.

1. Which action by the nurse is correct for droplet precautions?
 1. Tests N95 respirator for fit prior to use in client room.
 2. Wears a surgical mask when within 3 feet of client.
 3. Wears eye protection upon entering the client's room.
 4. Uses sterile gloves when bathing the client.

2. What health teaching should be included for a client being discharged home from an emergency department with an infection?
 1. Take an extra antibiotic tablet as needed if the temperature is over 38.5°C.
 2. If chills occur after 24 hours, check temperature and call provider if over 38.5°C.
 3. Do not take acetaminophen for 24 hours after starting antibiotic.
 4. Use cooling measures for temperature over 37°C.

3. Following a head injury, a client has no cough or gag reflex. The correct nursing action for feeding this client is to:
 1. Position the head of bed 90 degrees for meals.
 2. Give only solid foods.
 3. Give only thick liquids.
 4. Use a feeding tube.

4. Which technique is correct for reducing swelling after a traumatic injury to the ankle?
 1. Apply intermittent ice during the first 24 hours.
 2. Apply continuous heat during the first 48 hours.
 3. Perform range of motion every 4 hours on the ankle.
 4. Position the foot below the level of the heart.

5. A nurse tells a client that the most effective treatment for a rash from lupus erythematosus is:
 1. Getting sun exposure 15 minutes each day.
 2. Washing with soap and water.
 3. Taking an antimalarial drug.
 4. Getting a varicella vaccine booster.

6. Following an auto accident, a client's vital signs and hematocrit will be monitored for 24 hours for signs of internal bleeding. During this time, the client should receive:
 1. High-carbohydrate clear liquids orally.
 2. High-protein liquids via nasogastric tube.
 3. Intravenous total parenteral nutrition.
 4. Nothing by mouth.

7. Postoperatively, a client's fingers are cold and pale. Which action should a nurse take?
 1. Apply warm blankets.
 2. Check oxygen saturation on finger.
 3. Encourage deep breathing.
 4. Check blood sugar.

8. A client with cancer has anorexia and loss of weight. Which intervention should a nurse perform *first?*
 1. Giving TPN through a central line.
 2. Starting liquid nutrition through a gastric port.
 3. Starting liquid nutrition through a duodenal port.
 4. Giving megestrol and a diet of choice with nutritional supplements.

9. A client, who is nondiabetic and receiving 5% dextrose in one-half normal saline (D_5 ½NS) running at 125 mL/hr, has a blood sugar of 130 mg/dL on the morning chemistry panel. The client is concerned. It is most important for the nurse to:
 1. Provide diabetic teaching to the client who is newly diagnosed.
 2. Check another blood sugar and ask the physician about insulin.
 3. Explain the consequences of stress and IV fluids on blood sugar level.
 4. Keep the client NPO.

10. A nurse is planning care for a client admitted with chest pain after myocardial ischemia. Which outcome should the nurse document for this problem?
 1. Client states that pain is decreased to a tolerable level.
 2. Client agrees to rest and take pain medication.

QUESTIONS

3. Client rates pain 0 on scale of 1 (least) to 10 (worst).
4. Pain medication is administered within 5 minutes.

11. A woman who has received radiation therapy says that she feels like she is voiding through her vagina. This client may be experiencing:
1. Extreme stress due to a diagnosis of cancer.
2. Altered perineal sensations as a side effect of radiation therapy.
3. The development of a vesicovaginal fistula.
4. Rupture of the bladder.

12. The correct nursing action for a client who has a nephrostomy tube would include:
1. Attaching tube to suction prn with low urine output.
2. Changing the bandage and drainage bag daily.
3. Irrigating, if ordered, with no more than 10 mL sterile NS.
4. Clamping and unclamping the tube at hourly intervals.

13. Following perineal surgery, a client is at risk for a wound infection related to incontinence. The correct management of this problem is to:
1. Insert a continuous indwelling catheter per order.
2. Assist to the toilet and protect the skin with cream.
3. Limit oral fluid intake.
4. Give a loop diuretic, such as furosemide, as ordered.

14. A client comes to an emergency department with complaints of low abdominal pain and hematuria. The client is afebrile. The nurse should *first* ask the client if:
1. There is a family history of bladder cancer.
2. There had been recent trauma to the bladder or lower abdomen.
3. This could be recurrence of glomerulonephritis.
4. The client had ever had pyelonephritis.

15. A client with diabetes has a blood sugar of 300 mg/dL and an Na^+ of 133. What nursing intervention is indicated to manage the sodium with this client?
1. Pad the side rails to protect from injury during a possible seizure.
2. Notify dietary department to send salt tablets.
3. Encourage the client to drink water.
4. Monitor Na^+ return to normal with lowering of blood sugar.

16. The nursing *priorities* for the care of a client with acute glomerulonephritis are:
Select all that apply.
1. Performing range of motion.
2. Encouraging a diet high in protein.
3. Maintaining strict I&O.
4. Teaching intermittent self-catheterization for urine retention.
5. Monitoring daily weight.
6. Recording BP at least q4h.

17. A nurse is caring for a client with a left hemisphere stroke. The appropriate nursing actions for this client are:
Select all that apply.
1. Place food and the television on the left side of the bedside table.
2. Assist the client out of bed on the right side.
3. Raise the left side rail and place the television on the right side.
4. Talk into the client's right ear and place food on the right side.
5. Teach the client to pivot on the left leg in and out of bed.

18. A nurse notes that a client, who experienced a head injury 24 hours ago has returned to the emergency department with slurred speech and is disoriented to time and place. The *first* nursing action should be to:
1. Continue to assess hourly as ordered.
2. Report the change to the physician.
3. Repeat a neurologic assessment in 15 minutes.
4. Notify the operating room of the need for surgery.

19. Which assessment finding should indicate to a nurse that a client has progression of intermittent claudication?
1. The distance a client can walk before leg pain starts.
2. Presence of pedal edema in the legs after sitting 20 minutes.
3. Changes in strength of peripheral pulses in the affected leg.
4. Changes in skin temperature and color of the feet.

20. Which assessment findings should *alert* a nurse to early alcohol withdrawal in a client 2 days after surgery? *Select all that apply.*
1. Auditory hallucinations.
2. Decreased blood pressure.
3. Depression.
4. Diaphoresis.
5. Tachycardia
6. Dilated pupils

21. An older adult attending a community health fair asks about receiving the necessary vaccines for the swine flu. The nurse tells the client that, to prevent the spread of swine flu, the client should receive:
1. Just the seasonal flu and the pneumonia vaccines.
2. The novel H1N1 vaccine instead of the seasonal vaccine.
3. The seasonal and novel H1N1 vaccines the same day.
4. The novel H1N1 and seasonal vaccines a week apart.

22. A client, who had been playing golf in 110°F outside temperature, is admitted to an emergency department with hyperthermia. A nursing assessment would reveal:
Select all that apply.
1. Absence of sweating.
2. Decrease in body temperature.
3. Increase in sweating.
4. Increased blood pressure.
5. Tachycardia.
6. Flushed appearance.

23. A client comes to an emergency department reporting chest pain; vital signs are: BP 110/68 mm Hg, P 110 and irregular, R 24, and pulse oximetry 88%. Which interventions should a nurse perform *first?* Prioritize the nurse's actions by placing each intervention in the correct sequence.

_______ Give morphine 10 mg as ordered.
_______ Start O_2 6 L per mask.
_______ Give nitroglycerin (NTG) sublingual gr 1/150.
_______ Run an ECG strip.

24. A nurse should recognize the signs of deep vein thrombosis (DVT) if a client reports:
Select all that apply.
1. Leg feeling cool with no pain.
2. Numbness of legs with diaphoresis.
3. Sudden swelling of one leg with dependent edema.
4. Dizziness and blurred vision.
5. Pain behind the knee with dorsiflexion of foot.

25. What nursing action is appropriate if a client has a K^+ of 8 mEq/L?
1. No change is required in treatment.
2. Restrict intake of K^+ and/or give sodium polystyrene sulfonate (Kayexalate).
3. Restrict fluids to reduce K^+.
4. Give insulin, glucose, calcium, and/or bicarbonate STAT, as ordered.

26. Which client has the *greatest* need for K^+ replacement?
1. A client in renal failure with a postdialysis serum K^+ of 3.4.
2. A client with a large NG output who is receiving Kayexalate with a serum K^+ of 5.5.
3. A client with cardiac disease who is about to receive furosemide with a K^+ of 3.5.
4. A client with cardiac disease who is about to receive spironolactone with a K^+ of 3.5.

27. A nurse knows that the choice of a topical antimicrobial for a client with burns is most influenced by:
1. The bactericidal and fungicidal effectiveness of the agent.
2. The form of the agent, whether it is a liquid or cream.
3. The presence and extent of eschar formation.
4. The ability of the agent to deliver uniform absorption.

28. Which condition should a community health nurse report to the health department?
1. Confirmation of acid-fast bacilli.
2. Pruritic eruptions from *Sarcoptes scabiei* (scabies).
3. *Borrelia burgdorferi* (Lyme disease).
4. *Microsporum* species (ringworm) in a child who is in preschool.

29. Which client can be safely discharged to make room for clients suffering from a salmonella outbreak from a local food chain?
1. An 18-year-old diagnosed 1 day ago with type 1 diabetes, who lives in the college dormitory.
2. A 61-year-old with osteoarthritis who lives in a nursing home.
3. A client who is 48 hours post-MI, with a WBC of 9,000/mm³ and a CK-MB of 25 ng/mL.
4. A 70-year-old man with anemia and a Hct of 39% and O_2 saturation of 90%.

30. What should a nurse monitor *first* when caring for a client who is undergoing treatment for pheochromocytoma?
1. Pulse rate.
2. Blood sugar.
3. Blood pressure.
4. ECG changes

31. Which aspect of care is most important for a client with diabetic neuropathy?
1. Teach the client to inspect the feet using a mirror.
2. Teach the client to wash feet, then pat dry.
3. Have client moisturize feet with lotion to prevent dryness.
4. Teach the client to cut toenails straight across.

32. A client with diabetic ketoacidosis has been treated with an insulin drip for the past 3 hours. For which imbalance is this client at *greatest* risk?
1. Hypovolemia.
2. Hypokalemia.
3. Hyponatremia.
4. Hypoglycemia.

33. Which symptom would a nurse most likely observe in a client with cholecystitis?
1. Black stools.
2. Nausea after a high-fat meal.
3. Temperature of 104°F.
4. Colicky left upper quadrant pain.

34. If a client's bowel sounds are absent, a nurse should listen for at least:
1. 30 seconds.
2. 60 seconds.
3. 2 minutes.
4. 3 minutes.

35. What should be the *first* nursing action if an NG tube is not draining?
1. Irrigate the tube.
2. Reposition the client.
3. Determine tube placement.
4. Remove the tube and reinsert.

36. A nurse is observing a client for possible complications of postoperative peritonitis. Which manifestations are *most* indicative of peritonitis? *Select all that apply.*
1. Hyperactive bowel sounds.
2. Localized or diffuse pain.
3. Abdominal rigidity.
4. Shallow respirations.
5. Temperature over 102°F.

37. A nurse would know that a client was experiencing chronic renal failure (CRF) if which signs or symptoms were present?
1. Nausea and vomiting.
2. Asterixis and ascites.
3. Kussmaul's breathing and drowsiness.
4. Pruritus and anemia.

38. A client has returned to the unit from surgery after having an arteriovenous (A-V) fistula created in the left arm. The client's teaching should include:
Select all that apply.
1. Protecting site by wearing an elastic sleeve.
2. Squeezing a ball to increase vessel size.
3. Expecting fistula to be used for the next dialysis treatment.
4. Avoiding BP or drawing of blood samples from left arm.
5. Ensuring clothing fits loosely over left arm.

39. After a cystectomy and construction of an ileal conduit, which complication should a nurse instruct a client to take special precautions to prevent?
1. Paralytic ileus.
2. Urinary calculi.
3. Pyelonephritis.
4. Mucus in the urine.

40. A nurse should teach a client with a Kock pouch urinary diversion to prevent urinary tract infection by:
1. Avoiding people with upper respiratory infections (URI).
2. Maintaining a daily fluid intake of 2 liters.
3. Using sterile technique to change the appliance.
4. Irrigating the stoma daily.

41. A client who is scheduled for surgery to correct a retinal detachment should be positioned:
1. On the side opposite of the retinal detachment.
2. Upright with face down.
3. On the side of the retinal detachment.
4. Prone with face supported by pillow ring.

42. A client has been admitted with mild symptoms of novel H1N1. Which family member is at *greatest* risk for developing the infection?
1. The elderly grandmother.
2. A 6-year-old daughter.
3. The healthy 45-year-old spouse.
4. The 13-year-old son with asthma.

43. Which respiratory change would a nurse see most often in a client with increased intracranial pressure?
1. Nasal flaring and retractions.
2. Slow, irregular respirations.
3. Rapid, deep respirations.
4. Paradoxical chest movements.

44. Leakage of spinal fluid is a potential neurosurgical complication. How should a nurse assess for this complication?
1. Check for urine specific gravity greater than 1.030.
2. Monitor for urine output greater than 5–10 L/day.
3. Test all nasal and ear drainage for glucose.
4. Test all spinal fluid from lumbar punctures for glucose.

45. A client is admitted to an ICU with a possible brain attack (stroke). Assessment findings consistent with a brain attack include:
Select all that apply.
1. Pronator drift.
2. Facial droop.
3. Slurred speech.
4. Weakness of affected extremity.
5. Crackles in lungs.
6. Decreased urine output.

46. Which is the most common treatment for a client in addisonian crisis?
1. IV normal saline and glucocorticoids.
2. IV lactated Ringer's and packed cells.
3. IV 5% dextrose in normal saline and dopamine.
4. IV total parenteral nutrition (TPN) and insulin coverage.

47. When a client is on chemotherapy, for which manifestations of bone marrow depression should a nurse continuously assess?
1. Night sweats and fatigue.
2. Loss of skin turgor and weight loss.
3. Low urine output and elevated BUN levels.
4. Ecchymosis, weakness, and fatigue.

48. A client is admitted to a hospital in the terminal stage of illness. At this time, a nurse, who is planning end-of-life care, should recognize that the client is most likely to fear:
1. The terminal diagnosis.
2. Further chemotherapy.
3. Being socially inadequate.
4. Dying alone and in pain.

49. A complication of Buck's extension traction would be noted by a nurse if:
1. Redness and purulent drainage appeared at the pin site.
2. Toes of affected leg became dusky in color.
3. Skin over the fracture site was flushed.
4. Dorsiflexion developed in the affected foot.

50. Due to the extent of a client's fracture, a hip prosthesis is inserted. A nurse knows that the *most serious* complication of implant surgery is:
1. Infection.
2. Phlebitis.
3. Urinary retention.
4. Narcotic addiction.

51. A client returns from an operating room. The client's IV is running at 150 mL/hr; pulse is 90 and full; respirations are moist and wheezy. A nurse's *initial* action should be to:
 1. Speed up the IV and call the physician.
 2. Check the electrolyte levels.
 3. Report the IV rate to the charge nurse.
 4. Slow down the IV and call the physician.

52. During the first 24 hours after an above-the-knee amputation for vascular disease, nursing *priority* for stump care would be:
 1. Inspecting for redness and pressure points.
 2. Elevating to reduce edema.
 3. Cleansing with soap and water.
 4. Initiating fitting for prosthesis.

53. What are the *emergency* nursing actions for a client with a head injury due to a fall from a third-floor roof?
 1. Assess respirations, assess circulation, and assess level of consciousness.
 2. Stabilize C-spine, determine responsiveness, and begin chest compressions.
 3. Stabilize C-spine, assess airway, and assess respirations.
 4. Assess airway, assess respirations, and assess circulation.

54. As a nurse is assisting a client out of bed, which objective sign should indicate to the RN that the client is experiencing hypotension?
 1. Pupil response is sluggish to light.
 2. Orientation level changes.
 3. Pulse rate increases 20 beats per minute.
 4. Increased muscle rigidity in legs.

55. Which group is considered high risk for acquiring the human immunodeficiency virus (HIV)?
 1. Women in menopause.
 2. Men who are 65 plus years of age.
 3. People who engage in oral sex.
 4. Children of women with multiple partners.

56. Victims of a disastrous earthquake have been transported to an emergency department. Which victim should the nurse assess *first?*
 1. A victim with second-degree burns on 25% of the body.
 2. A victim with facial lacerations.
 3. A victim with a Glasgow Coma Scale score of 15 who is hyperventilating.
 4. A victim with no heartbeat.

57. A client with a tracheotomy just pulled out the tracheal tube. Which action by a RN is correct?
 1. Call the respiratory therapist to reinsert the tracheal tube.
 2. Get a hemostat to open the tracheotomy, and then try to reinsert the tube.
 3. Give 100% O_2 by mask over the stomal opening.
 4. Place mouth to stoma and ventilate every 5 seconds.

58. A client with COPD is scheduled for abdominal surgery. Arterial blood gases before surgery were: pH 7.36, Pco_2 54, Po_2 70. After surgery the ABGs were pH 7.35, Pco_2 60, Po_2 65 on 2 L of O_2. Which action should a nurse take?
 1. Suction the client.
 2. Have the client cough and deep breathe.
 3. Administer sodium bicarbonate, per order.
 4. Position the client in high Fowler's.

59. Which symptom(s) would be expected if a pacemaker suddenly malfunctioned?
 1. Pulse rate higher than set.
 2. Shortness of breath, dizziness.
 3. Atrial fibrillation, hypotension.
 4. Premature ventricular contractions (PVCs).

60. What signs will a nurse observe in a client who is experiencing right-sided heart failure? *Select all that apply.*
 1. Bilateral ankle edema.
 2. Jugular venous distention (JVD).
 3. Crackles on auscultation.
 4. Enlarged liver.
 5. Sacral edema.

61. When assessing a client for signs of early septic shock, a nurse should observe for:
 1. Cool, clammy skin.
 2. Warm, flushed skin.
 3. Decreased systolic blood pressure.
 4. Disseminated intravascular coagulation (DIC).

62. An indicator of a worsening hypovolemic shock related to GI bleeding would be:
 1. Decreased level of consciousness (LOC).
 2. Complaints of abdominal pain with hematemesis.
 3. Deepening, rapid respirations.
 4. Increasingly rapid, thready pulse.

63. A 50-year-old client is being seen in the outpatient clinic with complaints of a fever, cough, muscle soreness, and fatigue. The nurse would be concerned that the client had novel H1N1 flu if the complaints included: *Select all that apply.*
 1. Persistent cough.
 2. Shortness of breath.
 3. Persistent vomiting.
 4. Temperature of 104°F.
 5. Diarrhea.

64. A client's vital signs are: BP 80/60 mm Hg, P 120, R 30, T 100.4°F. A nurse should know that these findings most likely indicate:
 1. Neurogenic shock from increased intracranial pressure.
 2. Hypovolemic shock from fluid volume deficits.
 3. Septic shock from gram-negative sepsis.
 4. Cardiogenic shock from MI.

65. A nurse should expect that a client with a severe loss of potassium (hypokalemia) from diarrhea will have:
1. Fatigue, tetany, cardiac standstill.
2. Kussmaul's respirations, thirst, furrowed tongue.
3. Muscle weakness, cramps, cardiac irritability.
4. Confusion, pitting edema, irregular pulse.

66. Which finding should indicate to a nurse that a client has recovered from respiratory acidosis?
1. Increasing respiratory rate.
2. Increasing serum creatinine.
3. Decreasing respiratory rate.
4. Increasing serum bicarbonate.

67. The goal of care for a client with liver failure is to lower the blood ammonia level. Which actions would prevent increased ammonia? *Select all that apply.*
1. Prevent gastrointestinal bleeding.
2. Reduce dietary protein intake.
3. Avoid diarrhea and vomiting.
4. Decrease bacterial flora in the intestines.
5. Prevent ascites.

68. If a bowel obstruction occurs from inflammatory bowel disease at the transverse colon, a nurse will initially hear bowel sounds that are:
1. Increased RLQ; decreased LLQ.
2. Decreased RLQ; decreased LLQ.
3. Absent RLQ; absent LLQ.
4. Decreased RLQ; increased LLQ.

69. Identify the appropriate actions in the prevention of thrombophlebitis in a client on bedrest. *Select all that apply.*
1. Elevate the knee gatch of the bed.
2. Encourage exercises that dorsiflex and plantar flex the ankle.
3. Apply sequential compression devices bilaterally.
4. Prevent dehydration.
5. Periodically elevate the feet and lower legs above level of heart.
6. Apply warm, moist packs bilaterally to lower legs.

70. Which nursing actions should be completed before a physician performs a thoracentesis? *Select all that apply.*
1. Assessing the client for any allergy to local anesthetics.
2. Teaching the client to do pursed-lip breathing during the procedure.
3. Placing the client in an upright sitting position leaning forward, if able.
4. Placing the client in a prone position with the affected lung on a pillow.
5. Making sure that the consent form is signed and in the chart.
6. Telling the client not to expect discomfort.

71. A nurse should evaluate the effects of coumadin, used in the treatment of deep vein thrombosis, by looking at the results of which laboratory tests?
1. Prothrombin time (PT).
2. Lee-White clotting time.
3. Partial thromboplastin time (PTT).
4. Fibrinogen clotting time (FCT).

72. Which client should be the *first priority* for a telephone advice RN? A client who reports:
1. Headache, vomiting, and fever.
2. Ankle swelling and shortness of breath.
3. Productive cough.
4. Palpitations.

73. To promote maximum ventilation in a client who is postoperative, a nurse should:
1. Auscultate breath sounds bilaterally.
2. Give humidified oxygen via cannula.
3. Maintain placement of airway until the client is awake.
4. Position the client on the side, with the neck extended.

74. A nurse gets a report that a client will be admitted with an ejection fraction of 58%. Which history and physical finding should the nurse anticipate?
1. Inspiratory wheezing in upper lobes, bilaterally.
2. O_2 saturation that increases from 90% to 99% when head of bed is lowered to a flat position.
3. Crackles in the lung bases that clear with deep breathing.
4. A client is unable to walk up two flights of stairs without dyspnea.

75. Management of a BUN of 71 and a creatinine of 2.7 in a client with diabetic ketoacidosis (DKA) is correctly accomplished with:
1. Rehydration.
2. Fluid restriction.
3. Dialysis.
4. Bladder catheterization.

76. A nurse notes that a client has a total bilirubin of 1.0 mg/dL. The nurse should:
1. Record this normal finding.
2. Check urine for blood.
3. Check the stool for guaiac.
4. Assess the sclerae for yellow coloration.

77. Ten hours after beginning an insulin drip on a client with diabetic ketoacidosis, the following laboratory results are returned: Na^+ 130, K^+ 4.4, Cl^- 100, bicarb 15, BUN 60, creatinine 2.5, glucose 100. Which action should a nurse take?
1. Administer potassium.
2. Continue the insulin.
3. Administer salt tablets.
4. Restrict fluids.

78. A client is admitted with diabetic ketoacidosis (DKA). Five months ago, the hemoglobin A_{1c} ($HgbA_{1c}$) was 9.4%; currently it is 10.3%. Based on this information, a nurse should:
1. Record this expected finding.
2. Recheck the $HgbA_{1c}$ after the DKA is resolved.
3. Provide diabetic teaching.
4. Ask the physician about longer-acting insulin.

79. Seizure precautions should be applied to clients who have:
1. A serum sodium of less than 125 mg/dL.
2. An $HgbA_{1c}$ over 8%.
3. An anion gap less than 12.
4. Chronic peripheral neuropathies.

80. Which techniques are effective in communicating with a client who has complete loss of vision? *Select all that apply.*
1. Raise the voice when talking.
2. Avoid using the words "see" and "look."
3. Talk very softly, since hearing is overly sensitive.
4. Face the client when talking.
5. Touch the client's hand before speaking.
6. Avoid using phrases such as "over there."

81. A client with mild hypertension asks a nurse for suggestions to control blood pressure. What should a nurse recommend?
1. Follow a regular exercise program.
2. Attend a stress-reduction support group.
3. Avoid use of tobacco and limit alcohol intake.
4. Increase intake of fruits and vegetables.

82. A nurse is checking a client's third cranial nerve. How should physical assessment be performed?
1. Sweep a piece of cotton briskly across the cornea.
2. Ask the client to follow the examiner's finger with the eyes.
3. Use a Snellen chart to check visual acuity.
4. Check pupillary reaction using a penlight.

83. A nurse should assess for hypercalcemia by checking a client for:
1. Chvostek's sign.
2. Trousseau's sign.
3. Deep tendon reflex.
4. Babinski reflex.

84. The mother of a 2-year-old child is concerned her child may have novel H1N1. The nurse tells the mother that she should *immediately* report:
1. Loss of appetite.
2. Fever for 2 days.
3. Vomiting
4. Lack of alertness.

85. Which nursing intervention should a nurse complete *first* for a client experiencing addisonian crisis?
1. Maintain a quiet, nonstressful environment.
2. Take measures to avoid exertion by the client.
3. Administer hormone replacement as prescribed.
4. IV administration of fluid, glucose, and electrolytes.

86. A nurse knows that the serum sodium level of a client with a head trauma should be above 140 to:
1. Keep cerebral perfusion pressure up.
2. Prevent cerebral vasodilation.
3. Lower the seizure threshold.
4. Prevent cerebral edema.

87. A client is admitted with diabetic ketoacidosis. A nurse's *first* priority should be to give:
1. IV bicarbonate.
2. IV normal saline.
3. IV albumin.
4. Insulin subcutaneously.

88. A client with diabetic ketoacidosis (DKA) has been receiving IV insulin for 6 hours. Laboratory findings are: Na^+ 131, K^+ 3.7, Cl^- 102, HCO_3 22, and glucose 170. Which action should a nurse take?
1. Administer 3% sodium chloride at 200 mL/hr.
2. Expect the insulin drip to be discontinued.
3. Give potassium IV.
4. Administer D_5 ¼NS with the insulin drip.

89. A client, who is malnourished, is admitted with a serum calcium of 7.5. A nurse should:
1. Administer glucocorticoids, as ordered.
2. Check urine for ketones.
3. Check the serum albumin lab result.
4. Administer Neutra-Phos, as ordered.

90. Following a thyroidectomy, a nurse assesses for complications related to damage or removal of the parathyroid. The nurse should assess for:
1. Hypertension.
2. Numbness around the mouth.
3. Polyuria.
4. Muscle weakness.

91. A 19-year-old victim of trauma is admitted to an emergency department with a blood pressure of 80/50 mm Hg, and a heart rate of 130 bpm. Which action should a nurse take *first?*
1. Give 1 liter of D_5W IV as fast as possible.
2. Give 1 liter NS IV as fast as possible.
3. Start an additional large-bore IV as saline lock.
4. Calculate the anion gap before selecting IV fluid.

92. A client with CHF has: 2+ pedal edema, jugular venous distention (JVD), bilateral basilar crackles, urine output of 1.2 L/24 hr, blood pressure of 145/88 mm Hg, Na^+ of 129. A nurse should plan to:
1. Restrict fluids.
2. Give salt tablets PO.
3. Change IV to NS.
4. Give 3% sodium chloride IV.

93. A client is scheduled for outpatient bariatric surgery. Deep vein thrombosis (DVT) is best prevented by:
1. Early ambulation.
2. Postoperative low-dose heparin.
3. Alternating compression leg wraps.
4. Range-of-motion exercises to wrist.

94. Following general anesthesia for a hip replacement, an elderly client's vital signs are: P 80, R 14, blood pressure 110/78 mm Hg; O_2 Sat 100% on 40% mask; pain 2/10. The client is shivering and complains of being cold. The *first* nursing priority should be to:
1. Remove the oxygen.
2. Check the temperature.
3. Apply warm blankets.
4. Give pain medication.

95. Which finding is consistent with a client developing fluid overload?
1. Pulse over 100.
2. Pulmonary crackles that clear with deep breathing.
3. Concentrated urine.
4. Oxygen saturation less than 92% on 40% O_2 via facemask.

96. What is the best nursing action to prevent pressure sores during a long surgical procedure?
1. Pad bony prominences before surgery begins.
2. Turn the client every 2 hours.
3. Perform range of motion on the affected joints.
4. Provide an alternating pressure mattress.

97. A client with diabetes and hypertension has returned from surgery. Which nursing intervention will most likely reduce the risk of wound infection?
1. Monitor blood sugar and keep it under 200 postoperatively.
2. Place the client in contact isolation postoperatively.
3. Administer prophylactic antibiotics 48 hours preoperatively, as ordered.
4. Administer glucocorticoid stress hormone replacements postoperatively, as ordered.

98. A client asks a nurse what to expect with a condition of uncomplicated gallstones. The best response would be:
1. "There may be blood in the stools, with increased mucus."
2. "There may be RLQ cramping, with pain relieved after eating a fatty meal."
3. "You may feel fatigue because of low hemoglobin level."
4. "Most clients do not notice any effects."

99. A nurse is caring for a 32-year-old client who is 1 day post–gastric bypass. Vital signs are: T 37.9°C, P 100, R 18, BP 130/80 mm Hg, pain 2/10, O_2 Sat 92% on room air. The nurse should *first:*
1. Notify the physician for antibiotic orders.
2. Have the client use the incentive spirometer.
3. Increase intravenous fluids.
4. Administer pain medication.

100. One day after surgery for intestinal resection, a client has no bowel sounds. Which action should a nurse take?
1. Take the vital signs and notify the physician.
2. Record this expected finding.
3. Check rectally for impacted stool.
4. Perform abdominal massage.

101. A client with gallstones asks a nurse what might have caused the condition. The nurse knows the risk of developing this condition is greater in:
1. African Americans.
2. Men.
3. Significant recent weight loss.
4. Drinking a lot of coffee.

102. A client is in a rehabilitation unit 2 weeks after a right middle cerebral artery infarct. Which is the best activity plan?
1. Passive range of motion should be performed on the right arm and leg several times a day.
2. The client should know how to get up from the right side of the bed.
3. Maintain bed rest with all rails up until the client can lift both legs off the mattress.
4. Immobilize joints on the left side of the body into a position of flexion contracture.

103. A client with a vertebrobasilar stroke is being managed for dysphagia. Which intervention will be most helpful?
1. Eliminate distractions when giving directions.
2. Keep the head of the bed flat after meals.
3. Provide a thin liquid diet.
4. Provide nutrition through a feeding tube.

104. Which intervention will be most helpful to a client with aphasia?
1. Encourage use of gestures in communication.
2. Use many adjectives and adverbs when describing desired activity.
3. Speak loudly when giving directions.
4. Chew food thoroughly before swallowing.

105. The nursing assistant asks the nurse if a N95 respirator should be worn when caring for the client with H1N1. The correct response by the nurse is:
1. Droplet precautions require a direct caregiver to wear a respirator.
2. There is an N95 in the client's room for use by the nursing staff.
3. The N95 is usually reserved if treatment produces an aerosol spray of sputum.
4. The respirator should be worn if the nurse has cold symptoms.

Answers/Rationales/Tips

1. CORRECT ANSWER: 2. Answer 1 is incorrect because the N95 respirator *is not required* whenever the nurse enters the client's room. It is important if a respiratory is used that it properly fit, not be shared or reused. **Answer 2 is correct because a medical-surgical mask is indicated if the nurse will be within 3 feet of the client. Answer 3** is incorrect because eye protection is needed when there is a *potential for sputum* to be sprayed during a procedure such as suctioning. **Answer 4** is incorrect because the gloves do *not* have to be sterile.

■ **TEST-TAKING TIP:** *Think: infection is spread by droplets; a very* basic *precaution is a surgical mask.*

Content Area: Adult Health, Infectious Disease; ***Integrated Process:*** Nursing Process, Implementation; ***Cognitive Level:*** Application; ***Client Need/Subneed:*** Safe, Effective Care Environment/Safety and Infection Control, Preventive Measures

2. CORRECT ANSWER: 2. Answer 1 is incorrect because antibiotics are taken on a routine schedule, *not* prn for symptom management. **Answer 2 is correct because chilling is an indication that the hypothalamus "thermostat" has been reset at a higher level, and the body feels cold until metabolism increases the temperature to the new "fever" level. Twenty-four hours after antibiotics have been started, the client should be feeling better. Chilling and fever may indicate that the antibiotic is not effective against the organism. Answer 3** is incorrect because it is generally *safe* to take acetaminophen with an antibiotic, even in the first 24 hours. **Answer 4** is incorrect because fever does not usually require cooling *until over 38.3°C* (101°F). Antipyretics are the preferred treatment. A cool cloth on the forehead will not cool internal tissues.

■ **TEST-TAKING TIP:** *Only one option indicates a worsening of the client's condition.*

Content Area: Adult Health, Infection Control; ***Integrated Process:*** Teaching and Learning; ***Cognitive Level:*** Application; ***Client Need/Subneed:*** Physiological Integrity/Reduction of Risk Potential/Vital Signs Changes/Abnormalities

3. CORRECT ANSWER: 4. Answer 1 is incorrect because having the elevated head reduces the risk of aspiration, but this client is not able to swallow and should not receive meals. **Answer 2** is incorrect because solid food is easier to swallow than thin liquids, but this client is not able to swallow and should not have either. **Answer 3** is incorrect because thick liquids are easier to swallow than thin liquids, but this client cannot swallow and should not have any liquids. **Answer 4 is correct because this client is at great risk for aspiration. The feeding tube bypasses the junction of the esophagus and trachea, where the aspiration could most likely occur.**

■ **TEST-TAKING TIP:** *Three options require oral intake. Only one option is different. Choose the option that is different.*

Content Area: Adult Health, Neurological; ***Integrated Process:*** Nursing Process, Implementation; ***Cognitive Level:*** Application; ***Client Need/Subneed:*** Physiological Integrity/Reduction of Risk Potential/Potential for Complications of Diagnostic Tests/Treatments/Procedures

4. CORRECT ANSWER: 1. Answer 1 is correct because intermittent ice causes vasoconstriction and reduces swelling. Answer 2 is incorrect because heat would cause vasodilation and make swelling *worse.* **Answer 3** is incorrect because an injured joint needs to rest. Range of motion would be *painful* and disruptive to initial healing. **Answer 4** is incorrect because positioning the foot lower than the heart would *increase* swelling.

■ **TEST-TAKING TIP:** *Think of the effect of each option on blood flow, which affects swelling the first 24 hours.*

Content Area: Adult Health, Musculoskeletal; ***Integrated Process:*** Nursing Process, Implementation; ***Cognitive Level:*** Comprehension; ***Client Need/Subneed:*** Physiological Integrity/Reduction of Risk Potential/Potential for Complications of Diagnostic Tests/Treatments/Procedures

5. CORRECT ANSWER: 3. Answer 1 is incorrect because lupus rashes *worsen* with sunlight exposure. **Answer 2** is incorrect because soap and water washing does *not help* manage the rash. **Answer 3 is correct because antimalarial drugs are one of the first lines of treatment for lupus. Topical steroids are *also* often used for skin rashes. Answer 4** is incorrect because a varicella vaccine booster is *not related* to the management of lupus rashes.

■ **TEST-TAKING TIP:** *Eliminate the obvious (sunlight and soap, which is drying). Only one option appears to do something to treat the rash.*

Content Area: Adult Health, Integumentary; ***Integrated Process:*** Nursing Process, Implementation; ***Cognitive Level:*** Application; ***Client Need/Subneed:*** Physiological Integrity/Pharmacological and Parenteral Therapies/Expected Effects/Outcomes

6. CORRECT ANSWER: 4. Answer 1 is incorrect because the client should not have any foods or fluid externally to avoid surgical delays, aspiration risk, or leakage of ingested substances out of damaged viscera. **Answer 2** is incorrect because the client should not have any food or fluid internally to avoid surgical delays, aspiration risk, or leakage of ingested substances out of damaged viscera. **Answer 3** is incorrect because the risks of TPN are not warranted in this client who may only be NPO for a day or two. **Answer 4 is correct because, if internal bleeding is present, the client will need to go to surgery. Keep the client NPO to avoid surgical delays, aspiration risk, or leakage of ingested substances out of damaged viscera.**

■ **TEST-TAKING TIP:** *Three options involve ingestion of food or fluid. Choose the option that is different.*

Content Area: Adult Health, Hematological; ***Integrated Process:*** Nursing Process, Implementation; ***Cognitive Level:*** Application; ***Client Need/Subneed:*** Physiological Integrity/Reduction of Risk Potential/Potential for Alterations in Body Systems

7. CORRECT ANSWER: 1. Answer 1 is correct because decreased blood flow can cause fingers to be pale and cool, such as one might see with Raynaud's phenomenon. Symptoms lessen when covered. **Answer 2** is incorrect because oxygen saturation readings would be inaccurate if checked on a digit with poor blood flow. **Answer 3** is incorrect because the problem is related to hypothermia, *not* hypoventilation. **Answer 4** is incorrect because the fingers are cool and pale because of poor local blood flow. This is *unrelated* to blood sugar.

■ **TEST-TAKING TIP:** *Only one intervention will directly affect* cold *fingers.*

Content Area: Adult Health, Circulation; ***Integrated Process:*** Nursing Process, Implementation; ***Cognitive Level:*** Application; ***Client Need/Subneed:*** Physiological Integrity/Basic Care and Comfort/Non-pharmacological Comfort Interventions

8. CORRECT ANSWER: 4. **Answer 1** is incorrect because TPN may be necessary, but it is not the first strategy to try. The gastrointestinal system should be used for nutrition when functional. **Answer 2** is incorrect because light nutrition via a feeding tube may be necessary, but is not the first strategy to try in a client who is able to swallow. **Answer 3** is incorrect because, although administration of enteral feedings via a tube is a reasonable strategy to manage malnutrition, less invasive strategies should be tried first. **Answer 4 is correct because malnutrition in cancer clients is complicated and often difficult to manage. While megestrol stimulates appetite, nutritional supplements provide nutrients.**

■ **TEST-TAKING TIP:** *Only one option focuses on oral intake. The other three are more invasive or aggressive.*

Content Area: Adult Health, Oncological; ***Integrated Process:*** Nursing Process, Implementation; ***Cognitive Level:*** Application; ***Client Need:*** Physiological Integrity/Basic Care and Comfort/Nutrition and Oral Hydration

9. CORRECT ANSWER: 3. **Answer 1** is incorrect because this slight elevation in blood sugar may reflect a neuroendocrine response to stress or may be a result of the intravenous sugar. Additional testing would be required to determine *if* the client is prediabetic. **Answer 2** is incorrect because insulin is *not* required for this slight elevation in blood glucose. **Answer 3 is correct because this slight elevation in blood sugar may reflect a neuroendocrine response to stress or may be a result of the intravenous sugar. Additional testing would be required to determine if the client is prediabetic.** **Answer 4** is incorrect because NPO status in *not* indicated.

■ **TEST-TAKING TIP:** *Choose the option that best addresses the client's concern: information.*

Content Area: Adult Health, Endocrine; ***Integrated Process:*** Nursing Process, Implementation; ***Cognitive Level:*** Application; ***Client Need/Subneed:*** Physiological Integrity/Reduction of Risk Potential/Potential for Alterations in Body Systems

10. CORRECT ANSWER: 3. **Answer 1** is incorrect because often "tolerable pain" is not a reasonable outcome. This pain is a result of ischemia, so any continued pain may mean ongoing damage to the heart. **Answer 2** is incorrect because the expected outcome needs to reflect resolution of the problem. A client could agree to rest and even take pain medicine, yet the ischemia could be ongoing. **Answer 3 is correct because continuing chest pain indicates continued ischemia. Treatment should be given until the pain is gone.** **Answer 4** is incorrect because the expected outcome needs to reflect resolution of the problem, not completion of an intervention. Giving pain medications may not resolve the problem, and additional interventions would be required.

■ **TEST-TAKING TIP:** *Look for the option that indicates the problem is resolved—no pain.*

Content Area: Adult Health, Cardiology; ***Integrated Process:*** Nursing Process, Planning; ***Cognitive Level:*** Analysis; ***Client Need/Subneed:*** Physiological Integrity/Physiological Adaptation/Alterations in Body Systems

11. CORRECT ANSWER: 3. **Answer 1** is incorrect because stress would *not* be associated with this sensation. **Answer 2** is incorrect because, while sensations might be affected, her reported symptoms could be a real problem that should be investigated. **Answer 3 is correct because radiation damages tissue, and the healing process may not effectively keep the vagina and bladder separate. Bladder contraction could send urine through a fistula, to come out the vagina.** **Answer 4** is incorrect because rupture of the bladder would cause signs associated with *sepsis.*

■ **TEST-TAKING TIP:** *Look for an option that best explains the description of "voiding through." A fistula is an abnormal opening.*

Content Area: Adult Health, Oncological; ***Integrated Process:*** Nursing Process, Analysis; ***Cognitive Level:*** Application; ***Client Need/Subneed:*** Physiological Integrity/Physiological Adaptation/Alterations in Body Systems

12. CORRECT ANSWER: 3. **Answer 1** is incorrect because urine production is dependent on volume status and kidney function. Suction cannot be used to create more urine output. **Answer 2** is incorrect because the dressing is changed weekly unless wet, and the bag is emptied when half to two thirds full. **Answer 3 is correct because a nephrostomy tube is inserted into the ureter, directly draining the kidney. The pelvis of the kidney cannot accommodate volumes greater than 10 mL. The procedure must be sterile.** **Answer 4** is incorrect because, unless there was ureteral flow around the nephrostomy tube, it would be dangerous to clamp the tube. Urine backing up in the kidneys could cause hydronephrosis and infection.

■ **TEST-TAKING TIP:** *Think of an action that keeps a tube patent.*

Content Area: Adult Health, Renal; ***Integrated Process:*** Nursing Process, Implementation; ***Cognitive Level:*** Application; ***Client Need:*** Physiological Integrity/Physiological Adaptation/Alterations in Body Systems

13. CORRECT ANSWER: 1. Answer 1 is correct because an indwelling catheter diverts urine away from the operative site, reducing risk of wound infection. **Answer 2** is incorrect because, with a fresh postoperative wound, urine needs to be *diverted* from the area. **Answer 3** is incorrect because fluid intake should match the needs of the body. It is *not* appropriate to restrict fluids to reduce the risk of incontinence. **Answer 4** is incorrect because diuretics facilitate removal of *excess* fluid from the body. They are *not* used to *manage incontinence.*

■ **TEST-TAKING TIP:** *The question is asking for a way to prevent wound contamination by urine. Although a catheter increases the risk of urinary tract infections, it is the only option that fully* protects *the wound.*

Content Area: Adult Health, Gastrointestinal; ***Integrated Process:*** Nursing Process, Implementation; ***Cognitive Level:*** Comprehension; ***Client Need/Subneed:*** Physiological Integrity/Reduction of Risk Potential/Potential for Alterations in Body Systems

14. CORRECT ANSWER: 2. **Answer 1** is incorrect because *pain* would not be typically seen if bladder cancer was suspected. **Answer 2 is correct because pain and blood in the urine without a fever would be more consistent with a blow or trauma to the abdomen or bladder.** **Answer 3** is incorrect because glomerulonephritis would present with a *fever.* **Answer 4** is incorrect because symptoms of pyelonephritis would include a *fever.*

■ **TEST-TAKING TIP:** *Without a fever, eliminate the options with "itis." Choose an option that would* best *explain the pain.*

Content Area: Adult Health, Renal; ***Integrated Process:*** Nursing Process, Assessment; ***Cognitive Level:*** Application; ***Client Need/Subneed:*** Physiological Integrity/Reduction of Risk Potential/System Specific Assessments

15. CORRECT ANSWER: 4. **Answer 1** is incorrect because seizures can result from very low blood sugar or Na^+, but these values are *not low enough* to be associated with seizure risk. **Answer 2** is incorrect because this Na^+ level is *only mildly* low and does not require treatment with sodium. **Answer 3** is incorrect because ingestion of free water would further dilute the sodium. **Answer 4 is correct because, as blood sugar rises, serum osmolarity increases and the pituitary secretes antidiuretic hormone. This causes the kidneys to retain free water, diluting down serum sodium. Direct treatment of the hyponatremia is not needed.**

■ **TEST-TAKING TIP:** *Ask: Is there a problem or not at this time? Understand the physiologic changes when blood sugar is lowered. The low sodium is occurring because of hemodilution. Select the answer that "monitors," rather than an action (pads, salt tablets, or water).*

Content Area: Adult Health, Endocrine; ***Integrated Process:*** Nursing Process, Implementation; ***Cognitive Level:*** Application; ***Client Need/Subneed:*** Physiological Integrity/Physiological Adaptation/Fluid and Electrolyte Imbalances

16. CORRECT ANSWERS: 3, 5, 6. **Answer 1** is incorrect because the client is *not* necessarily on *prolonged bedrest.* Immobility is *not* the priority. Bedrest is indicated until hypertension is controlled. **Answer 2** is incorrect because protein needs to be *limited* due to proteinuria, which is present with the disease. Carbohydrates are the source of energy. **Answer 3 is correct because acute glomerulonephritis (AGN) decreases glomerular function. Fluid is restricted during the edematous phase. There is a risk of renal failure as a result of the inflammation ("itis").** **Answer 4** is incorrect because the problem is *not retention* but the potential for renal failure and inadequate urine proteinuria. The disease progresses from edema to diuresis. **Answer 5 is correct because the edematous phase of AGN lasts from 4 to 10 days. Daily weight is the best indicator of fluid changes. Answer 6 is correct because hypertension occurs with AGN. Headache is common. Antihypertensives will be ordered and BP needs to be recorded q4h.**

■ **TEST-TAKING TIP:** *Choose the answers that most directly relate to monitoring renal function.*

Content Area: Adult Health, Renal; ***Integrated Process:*** Nursing Process, Planning; ***Cognitive Level:*** Application; ***Client Need/Subneed:*** Physiological Integrity/Reduction of Risk Potential/Potential for Alterations in Body Systems

17. CORRECT ANSWERS: 1, 5. Answer 1 is correct because loss of half of the visual field (hemianopsia) will be on the same side as the paralyzed side. The left visual field will be intact. **Answer 2** is incorrect because the right side will be *weak* or paralyzed. The left side will be stronger. **Answer 3** is incorrect because the client likely has right *visual field blindness.* **Answer 4** is incorrect because there is *no* expectation of deafness. Food should be placed on the *left* side. **Answer 5 is correct because the right side will be weakened or paralyzed. The client should be taught to put weight on the stronger left side when transferring from bed to chair and back.**

■ **TEST-TAKING TIP:** *Select the option that is different from others. Note that three options relate to the right. Only two options relate to the left side.*

Content Area: Adult Health, Cardiovascular; ***Integrated Process:*** Nursing Process, Implementation; ***Cognitive Level:*** Application; ***Client Need/Subneed:*** Physiological Integrity/Physiological Adaptation/Alterations in Body Systems

18. CORRECT ANSWER: 2. **Answer 1** is incorrect because a *delay* in treatment could result in *irreversible* damage. **Answer 2 is correct because a medical or surgical intervention is needed for an apparent increase in intracranial pressure.** **Answer 3** is incorrect because a change in level of consciousness is an early sign of increased intracranial pressure that requires an intervention. **Answer 4** is incorrect because this is *not* the RN's role.

■ **TEST-TAKING TIP:** *A change in level of consciousness requires immediate notification of the physician.*

Content Area: Adult Health, Neurological; *Integrated Process:* Nursing Process, Implementation; *Cognitive Level:* Analysis; *Client Need/Subneed:* Physiological Integrity/Physiological Adaptation/Medical Emergencies

19. CORRECT ANSWER: 1. Answer 1 is correct because intermittent claudication occurs with peripheral vascular disease and inadequate blood flow to the tissues. As the disease progresses, the pain will occur sooner. **Answer 2** is incorrect because pedal edema is swelling from *venous stasis—not* pain associated with *activity.* **Answer 3** is incorrect because peripheral vascular disease will affect peripheral pulses, but the question is looking for the development of *pain.* **Answer 4** is incorrect because inadequate arterial blood flow will affect the color and temperature, but the more rapid development of pain with walking is the accurate response.

■ **TEST-TAKING TIP:** *The term "intermittent" is a hint that the problem starts and stops—start walking, pain develops, stop walking.*

Content Area: Adult Health, Vascular; *Integrated Process:* Nursing Process, Analysis; *Cognitive Level:* Application; *Client Need/Subneed:* Physiological Integrity/Physiological Adaptation/Pathophysiology

20. CORRECT ANSWERS: 4, 5, 6. **Answer 1** is incorrect because hallucinations do occur but *not initially.* **Answer 2** is incorrect because the vital signs are initially *elevated.* **Answer 3** is incorrect because the client is *agitated.* **Answer 4 is correct because the client will experience autonomic overactivity causing tachycardia, dilated pupils, and profuse perspiration. Answer 5 is correct because the autonomic overactivity will cause tachycardia. Answer 6 is correct because the pupils will be dilated from the autonomic overactivity.**

■ **TEST-TAKING TIP:** *Look for an early autonomic response.*

Content Area: Adult Health, Cardiovascular; *Integrated Process:* Nursing Process, Analysis; *Cognitive Level:* Application; *Client Need/Subneed:* Physiological Integrity/Physiological Adaptation/Alterations in Body Systems

21. CORRECT ANSWER: 3. **Answer 1** is incorrect because the best protection is to receive both seasonal and novel H1N1 vaccines. The pneumonia vaccine should be given once to adults 65 years or older. If given at 60 years of age or earlier a booster may be required 5 to 10 years later. Children older than 2 years with chronic respiratory or cardiac conditions may receive the pneumonia vaccine. **Answer 2** is incorrect because healthy adults over 65 were *not as susceptible* to the novel H1N1 (swine flu) as originally feared. **Answer 3 is correct because the older adult, while less susceptible to the swine flu than younger clients, should receive both vaccines particularly if they also have pre-existing chronic conditions. The vaccines can be taken the same day.** **Answer 4** is incorrect because the vaccines can be given *the same day* in *two different syringes.* Only the *nasal* forms of the vaccine need to be given a month apart and the H1N1 nasal vaccine is reserved for ages 2 to 49 years.

■ **TEST-TAKING TIP:** *Choose the answer that focuses on* **both** *vaccines and the "same day."*

Content Area: Adult Health, Infectious Disease; *Integrated Process:* Teaching and Learning; *Cognitive Level:* Application; *Client Need/Subneed:* Safe, Effective Care Environment/Safety and Infection Control, Preventive Measures

22. CORRECT ANSWERS: 1, 5, 6. Answer 1 is correct because sweating decreases as heat exhaustion progresses to heat stroke. **Answer 2** is incorrect because the body temperature is usually *above* 104°F. **Answer 3** is incorrect because the skin may first be damp if the client has been active, then *no* perspiration. **Answer 4** is incorrect because blood pressure *decreases,* and there is tachycardia and rapid respiratory rate—the symptoms of shock. **Answer 5 is correct because the client is experiencing severe dehydration and will present with symptoms of shock. Answer 6 is correct because the client has lost the normal cooling mechanism of perspiration. The skin will be flushed and dry from the high internal body temperature.**

■ **TEST-TAKING TIP:** *Think heat stroke—a failure of the body's regulatory mechanism.*

Content Area: Adult Health, Thermoregulatory; *Integrated Process:* Nursing Process, Assessment; *Cognitive Level:* Application; *Client Need/Subneed:* Physiological Integrity/Physiological Adaptation/Medical Emergencies

23. CORRECT ANSWERS: 2, 4, 3, 1. Supplemental oxygen is the *first* action to prevent any cardiac damage from hypoxia. The oxygen can be started while continuing the client assessment and applying the ECG electrodes. The ECG leads should be applied *second,* to assess for any life-threatening arrhythmias. NTG is often given with an antacid for unexplained chest pain. It would be the *third* action after determining the cardiac rhythm. NTG can change the ECG pattern. Morphine may eventually be given if the pain is not relieved by the antacid or NTG. This would be the *fourth* action.

■ **TEST-TAKING TIP:** *When all of the options are correct, think of the priorities—prevent damage from hypoxia, gather data, and treat.*

Content Area: Adult Health, Cardiovascular; *Integrated Process:* Nursing Process, Implementation; *Cognitive Level:* Analysis; *Client Need/Subneed:* Physiological Integrity/Physiological Adaptation/Alterations in Body Systems

24. CORRECT ANSWERS: 3, 5. Answer 1 is incorrect because the problem in DVT causes phlebitis, which is characterized by *warmth, redness,* and *pain.* **Answer 2** is incorrect because the problem in DVT is circulatory, *not neurological.* **Answer 3 is correct because a clot in a leg vein will affect venous return and cause swelling and edema. Answer 4** is incorrect because the problem in DVT is in the leg, *not* the eyes. **Answer 5 is correct because pain with dorsiflexion (positive Homans' sign) may be present with DVT but should not be the only indicator of DVT.**

■ **TEST-TAKING TIP:** ***Visualize the effect a clot in the leg will have on venous circulation.***

Content Area: Adult Health, Vascular; ***Integrated Process:*** Nursing Process, Analysis; ***Cognitive Level:*** Application; ***Client Need/Subneed:*** Physiological Integrity/Physiological Adaptation/Pathophysiology

25. CORRECT ANSWER: 4. Answer 1 is incorrect because this is dangerously high potassium. It requires *immediate* treatment to avoid a lethal arrhythmia. **Answer 2** is incorrect because restricting intake or using an ion exchange agent would reduce potassium level *too slowly.* **Answer 3** is incorrect because fluid restriction does *not* reduce potassium. **Answer 4 is correct because this is dangerously high potassium. Glucose, insulin, and bicarbonate help move the potassium intracellularly. Calcium helps protect the heart from hyperkalemia-induced arrhythmias.**

■ **TEST-TAKING TIP:** ***Know the normal ranges for common electrolytes. Recognize the dangerously high level and look for an option that will produce a change rapidly—STAT. Look at the action words: "no change required," "restrict," and "give." Choose "give."***

Content Area: Adult Health, Fluid and Electrolyte Imbalances; ***Integrated Process:*** Nursing Process, Implementation; ***Cognitive Level:*** Application; ***Client Need/Subneed:*** Physiological Integrity/Physiological Adaptation/Medical Emergencies

26. CORRECT ANSWER: 3. Answer 1 is incorrect because generally clients with renal failure have trouble excreting potassium. In the days before the next dialysis treatment, the potassium will be *increasing.* It is *not* appropriate to give potassium to this client. **Answer 2** is incorrect because this client's potassium is *already too high.* More potassium is *not* needed. **Answer 3 is correct because clients with cardiac disease are vulnerable to arrhythmia when serum potassium is low. Furosemide will cause potassium loss. It is important to replace potassium before the furosemide is given. Answer 4** is incorrect because clients with cardiac disease are vulnerable to arrhythmia when serum potassium is low. Spironolactone is a potassium-sparing diuretic that would *not* be expected to drop the potassium level *as much* as furosemide would.

■ **TEST-TAKING TIP:** ***Focus on cardiac disease and the drug, if given, that will further affect the K^+ level (i.e., cause loss of K^+), so the client will need K^+ replacement.***

Content Area: Adult Health, Fluid and Electrolyte Imbalances; ***Integrated Process:*** Nursing Process, Analysis; ***Cognitive Level:*** Analysis; ***Client Need/Subneed:*** Physiological Integrity/Reduction of Risk Potential/Laboratory Values

27. CORRECT ANSWER: 3. Answer 1 is incorrect because all of the topical therapies must be effective against gram-negative organisms. The agent does not sterilize the burn but *reduces the number* of bacteria so that the body's defense mechanisms are able to overcome the infection. **Answer 2** is incorrect because the form of the topical agent is *not* important. Treatment may alternate between a liquid and a cream. **Answer 3 is correct because, since eschar is devitalized tissue, the topical agent must be able to penetrate eschar and not be systemically toxic. Answer 4** is incorrect because burn injuries are not uniform. *Variations* in burn depth and the presence of eschar affect the absorption of a topical agent.

■ **TEST-TAKING TIP:** ***Look for an option that would inhibit the absorption ability of the topical agent (e.g., eschar), and therefore render the antimicrobial less effective.***

Content Area: Adult Health, Integumentary; ***Integrated Process:*** Nursing Process, Analysis; ***Cognitive Level:*** Application; ***Client Need/Subneed:*** Physiological Integrity/Pharmacological and Parenteral Therapies/Expected Effects/Outcomes

28. CORRECT ANSWER: 1. Answer 1 is correct because TB is a bacterial infectious disease that is communicable to others and is associated with significant mortality and morbidity. Answer 2 is incorrect because scabies is a skin infection associated with an infestation of an itch mite. The mites can be transferred to family members and *close contacts,* but it is *not* an infectious disease. **Answer 3** is incorrect because Lyme disease is the result of a tick bite and is *not* infectious. **Answer 4** is incorrect because ringworm, while contagious, is a *fungal* infection.

■ **TEST-TAKING TIP:** ***Determine the potential for a community outbreak from each option.***

Content Area: Adult Health, Communicable Diseases; ***Integrated Process:*** Nursing Process, Implementation; ***Cognitive Level:*** Application; ***Client Need/Subneed:*** Safe and Effective Care Environment/Safety and Infection Control/Standard/Transmission-based/Other Precautions

29. CORRECT ANSWER: 2. Answer 1 is incorrect because the stability of the client's blood sugar is a *concern.* Also the client needs *observation* as insulin is being regulated. **Answer 2 is correct because the older adult client has a chronic problem and would be supervised in the long-term care facility. Answer 3** is incorrect because a client who is post-MI is *at risk* for possible arrhythmias and requires *continuous* monitoring. **Answer 4** is incorrect because the client's laboratory values are *abnormal,* and the client may be experiencing fatigue and weakness from the anemia.

■ **TEST-TAKING TIP:** ***Choose the client who is more stable and does not require acute care.***

Content Area: Adult Health, Triage; *Integrated Process:* Nursing Process, Analysis; *Cognitive Level:* Analysis; *Client Need/Subneed:* Safe and Effective Care Environment/ Management of Care/Establishing Priorities

30. CORRECT ANSWER: 3. **Answer 1** is incorrect because tachycardia would be the *next* concern after the blood pressure was stabilized or controlled. **Answer 2** is incorrect because blood pressure is the first concern. Hyperglycemia may be present, and insulin may be required. **Answer 3 is correct because treatment initially is directed at reducing the marked elevation of blood pressure quickly.** **Answer 4** is incorrect because dysrhythmias occur *as a result* of the elevated blood pressure. Controlling the blood pressure will reduce the likelihood that the client will develop ECG changes.

■ TEST-TAKING TIP: *Choose an option that, if treated, will likely correct other findings—that is, lower the BP, and the pulse and ECG will likely stabilize.*

Content Area: Adult Health, Hematological; *Integrated Process:* Nursing Process, Assessment; *Cognitive Level:* Analysis; *Client Need/Subneed:* Physiological Integrity/ Reduction of Risk Potential/System Specific Assessments

31. CORRECT ANSWER: 1. **Answer 1 is correct because neuropathies reduce the sensation (pain) in the client's feet. Consequently, the client is unaware of injuries or trauma to the feet that could lead to ulceration and cellulitis, which are more difficult to treat in the person who has diabetes.** **Answer 2** is incorrect because *inspection* of the feet with mirrors is most important. Foot care is important; however, any breakdown would be noted using a mirror. **Answer 3** is incorrect because *inspection* is most important. Proper foot care will prevent cracks, which would be noted by using a mirror. **Answer 4** is incorrect because, although this technique is correct and should prevent foot complications, inspection of feet is most important.

■ TEST-TAKING TIP: *All options are correct. Choose the one that has the* greatest *potential for preventing a serious problem.*

Content Area: Adult Health, Endocrine; *Integrated Process:* Nursing Process, Implementation; *Cognitive Level:* Analysis; *Client Need/Subneed:* Physiological Integrity/Basic Care and Comfort/Personal Hygiene

32. CORRECT ANSWER: 2. **Answer 1** is incorrect because treatment *will* include as much as 6 to 10 L of normal saline for 2 to 3 hours. The infusion rate will be slowed to prevent hypervolemia. **Answer 2 is correct because rehydration and the administration of insulin will cause the potassium to move back into the cells, resulting in a potentially even lower K^+ level. Potassium replacement begins when the K^+ level drops to normal to prevent hypokalemia.** **Answer 3** is incorrect because *normal saline* is the solution of choice during rehydration. **Answer 4** is incorrect because the most immediate risk is the rapid drop of *potassium* as the electrolyte moves back into the cell as a result of rehydration and the insulin drip.

■ TEST-TAKING TIP: *The question asks for the "greatest risk." Hypoglycemia is too obvious. Think about the effects of insulin on K^+.*

Content Area: Adult Health, Endocrine; *Integrated Process:* Nursing Process, Analysis; *Cognitive Level:* Analysis; *Client Need/Subneed:* Physiological Integrity/Physiological Adaptation/Fluid and Electrolyte Imbalances

33. CORRECT ANSWER: 2. **Answer 1** is incorrect because inflammation of the gallbladder interferes with the normal color of feces, and the stool color is characteristically *grayish,* like putty. Black stools would signal old blood consistent with GI bleeding. **Answer 2 is correct because biliary colic is common in cholecystitis and is associated with nausea and vomiting several hours after a heavy, high-fat meal.** **Answer 3** is incorrect because this is a dangerously high temperature for an adult, and *not a common sign.* A temperature may be present, but one this high might result from gangrene of the gallbladder and rupture, which is not common. **Answer 4** is incorrect because the pain from an acute inflammation of the gallbladder would be in the upper *right* abdomen, with radiation possible to the midsternal or right shoulder area.

■ TEST-TAKING TIP: *Think of food-related problems. Know where the gallbladder is located and a likely symptom. Often the initial warning of a gallbladder problem comes with eating.*

Content Area: Adult Health, Gastrointestinal; *Integrated Process:* Nursing Process, Assessment; *Cognitive Level:* Application; *Client Need/Subneed:* Physiological Integrity/ Physiological Adaptation/Pathophysiology

34. CORRECT ANSWER: 4. **Answer 1** is incorrect because all four quadrants should be assessed and normal bowel sounds may not occur more often than every 20 seconds, requiring a minimum of 1 minute and 20 seconds. **Answer 2** is incorrect because all four quadrants should be assessed and normal bowel sounds may not occur more often than every 20 seconds requiring, a minimum of 1 minute and 20 seconds. **Answer 3** is incorrect because, to determine if bowel sounds are absent, the nurse must listen for a minimum of 3 minutes and for as long as 5 minutes. **Answer 4 is correct because, to determine if bowel sounds are absent, the nurse must listen for a minimum of 3 minutes and for as long as 5 minutes.**

■ TEST-TAKING TIP: *Is it "seconds" or "minutes"? An accurate assessment takes time.*

Content Area: Adult Health, Gastrointestinal; *Integrated Process:* Nursing Process, Assessment; *Cognitive Level:* Comprehension; *Client Need/Subneed:* Physiological Integrity/ Reduction of Risk Potential/System Specific Assessments

35. CORRECT ANSWER: 3. **Answer 1** is incorrect because placement should be determined by instilling air rapidly, *not liquid.* Once placement is confirmed, irrigation may be done. **Answer 2** is incorrect because the concern is the placement of the *tube* first. Then, the position of the client may need to be assessed to determine if the position caused the tube to be dislodged. **Answer 3 is correct because the lack of drainage may mean the tube is no longer in the correct location.** **Answer 4** is incorrect because placement should be determined *before* removal. Reinsertion may be distressful to the client.

■ **TEST-TAKING TIP:** *This is a priority question. More than one answer may be correct, but what does the nurse do* first? *Ask yourself, where is the tube tip?*

Content Area: Adult Health, Gastrointestinal; *Integrated Process:* Nursing Process, Implementation; *Cognitive Level:* Comprehension; *Client Need/Subneed:* Physiological Integrity/Reduction of Risk Potential/System Specific Assessments

36. CORRECT ANSWERS: 2, 3, 4. **Answer 1** is incorrect because peristalsis is *diminished* and paralytic ileus may develop. **Answer 2 is correct because the pain is often diffuse initially and then localized.** **Answer 3 is correct because the abdominal muscles are rigid and the abdomen is tender and distended.** **Answer 4 is correct because, with the abdominal tenderness and distention, the client will not breathe as deeply.** **Answer 5** is incorrect because the temperature is usually 100° to 101°F.

■ **TEST-TAKING TIP:** *Think about how inflammation affects the body system as each option is considered. Think "pain," as in Answers 2, 3, and 4.*

Content Area: Adult Health, Gastrointestinal; *Integrated Process:* Nursing Process, Assessment; *Cognitive Level:* Analysis; *Client Need/Subneed:* Physiological Integrity/Reduction of Risk Potential/Potential for Complications from Surgical Procedures and Health Alterations

37. CORRECT ANSWER: 4. **Answer 1** is incorrect because nausea and vomiting are *not specific to CRF.* A client with CRF may have nausea and vomiting along with anorexia and hiccups. **Answer 2** is incorrect because these signs are consistent with *hepatic* failure. **Answer 3** is incorrect because these signs would occur during *acute* renal failure or with any developing *metabolic acidosis.* **Answer 4 is correct because the irritating toxins are accumulating and result in skin irritation. Anemia results from the inadequate erythropoietin production.**

■ **TEST-TAKING TIP:** *Look for an option that would develop over time—weeks to months (i.e., chronic)—and would occur if the* kidneys *have failed.*

Content Area: Adult Health, Renal; *Integrated Process:* Nursing Process, Assessment; *Cognitive Level:* Application; *Client Need/Subneed:* Physiological Integrity/Physiological Adaptation/Pathophysiology

38. CORRECT ANSWERS: 2, 4, 5. **Answer 1** is incorrect because this would *impair* blood flow through the fistula and potentially damage the fistula. **Answer 2 is correct because exercise increases the vessel size to better accommodate the large-bore needles used in hemodialysis.** **Answer 3** is incorrect because the fistula does *not* mature sufficiently to use for at least 14 days. **Answer 4 is correct because the arm should be reserved only for dialysis. Measuring BP or drawing blood may lead to fistula damage.** **Answer 5 is correct because tight or constricting clothing will impair blood flow through the fistula and cause loss of patency.**

■ **TEST-TAKING TIP:** *Since **Answer 5** is correct, then **Answer 1** is incorrect, because it is important to select an option that prevents constriction of the fistula and promotes development of the site.*

Content Area: Adult Health, Vascular; *Integrated Process:* Nursing Process, Planning; *Cognitive Level:* Application; *Client Need/Subneed:* Physiological Integrity/Reduction of Risk Potential/Potential for Complications from Surgical Procedures and Health Alterations

39. CORRECT ANSWER: 3. **Answer 1** is incorrect because paralytic ileus is a *surgical* complication that the client *cannot prevent.* **Answer 2** is incorrect because urinary calculi are *not* a surgical complication. A client can prevent calculi through dietary and fluid management. **Answer 3 is correct because an ileal conduit is a urinary diversion that allows direct access of organisms to the kidneys. Proper management of the appliance, good skin care, proper hand hygiene, and adequate fluids will reduce the chance of developing an infection.** **Answer 4** is incorrect because mucus in the urine is *normal* since a segment of the GI tract was used to create the diversion.

■ **TEST-TAKING TIP:** *Choose an option that can be controlled by the client directly—preventing infection (e.g., an "itis").*

Content Area: Adult Health, Renal; *Integrated Process:* Teaching and Learning; *Cognitive Level:* Application; *Client Need/Subneed:* Physiological Integrity/Reduction of Risk Potential/Potential for Complications from Surgical Procedures and Health Alterations

40. CORRECT ANSWER: 2. **Answer 1** is incorrect because the risk of infection with a Kock pouch would be related to renal deterioration from *reflux* or *fecal contamination,* not from others with URI. **Answer 2 is correct because adequate fluids will maintain the urine output and optimal renal function.** **Answer 3** is incorrect because a Kock pouch is a continent urinary diversion, and urine is drained by inserting a catheter into the stoma. There is *no appliance* to change. **Answer 4** is incorrect because irrigation is *not done* with urinary diversion. The Kock pouch collects urine, and a catheter is inserted into the stoma to remove the urine.

■ TEST-TAKING TIP: *Keep It Simple (K.I.S.) and look for the best approach to prevent a urinary tract infection for* any *client—adequate fluid intake.*
Content Area: Adult Health, Renal; *Integrated Process:* Teaching and Learning; *Cognitive Level:* Application; *Client Need/Subneed:* Physiological Integrity/Reduction of Risk Potential/Potential for Alterations in Body Systems

41. CORRECT ANSWER: 2. **Answer 1** is incorrect because the desired outcome is to reduce intraocular pressure. Upright and possibly face down would be preferred. **Answer 2 is correct because detachments or tears are toward the back of the eye. A gas bubble is frequently used to flatten the retina (pneumatic retinopexy), and the client must be positioned to make the bubble float into position.** **Answer 3** is incorrect because the desired outcome is to reduce intraocular pressure. Upright and possible face down would be preferred. **Answer 4** is incorrect because the client's head should be *higher* than the heart. Upright and face down would be desired.
■ TEST-TAKING TIP: *Visualize each position and how it would contribute to reattaching the retina to the back of the eye.*
Content Area: Adult Health, Sensory; *Integrated Process:* Nursing Process, Implementation; *Cognitive Level:* Application; *Client Need/Subneed:* Physiological Integrity/Reduction of Risk Potential/Therapeutic Procedures

42. CORRECT ANSWER: 4. **Answer 1** is incorrect because older adults appeared to have *some immunity* to the virus from previous exposure to a similar strain in the 1970s. Chronic conditions increased the risk. **Answer 2** is incorrect because the child was presumed to be *healthy.* The chronic asthma increased the risk for the 13-year-old. **Answer 3** is incorrect because the spouse was *healthy* and did not suffer from a chronic condition which would increase the risk. **Answer 4 is correct because the risk increases in a young person with a chronic condition. Ages 6 months to 24 years were effected more often than healthy older adults.**
■ TEST-TAKING TIP: *Chronic condition is more of a risk factor. Select the one answer that is different from the other three ("asthma").*
Content Area: Adult Health, Infectious Disease; *Integrated Process:* Nursing Process, Analysis; *Cognitive Level:* Analysis; *Client Need/Subneed:* Safe, Effective Care Environment/Safety and Infection Control, Prevention and Early Detection

43. CORRECT ANSWER: 2. **Answer 1** is incorrect because nasal flaring and retractions would be seen with *pulmonary edema* and *left-sided heart failure.* **Answer 2 is correct because increased intracranial pressure (ICP) presses on the structures of the brain, causing irregularities such as Cheyne-Stokes respirations.** **Answer 3** is incorrect because slow, irregular breathing is more common. Hyperventilation may occur with pressure in the *midbrain.* **Answer 4** is incorrect because paradoxical chest movements are characteristic of flail chest from *chest trauma.*
■ TEST-TAKING TIP: *Eliminate Answer 3 as it is the opposite of what occurs (Answer 2). Eliminate Answers 1 and 4, because the conditions are* not *characteristic of increased ICP, but of pulmonary edema and chest trauma. Remember that the pressure in the brain will interfere with the regulatory center. Respiratory response will be irregular.*
Content Area: Adult Health, Neurological; *Integrated Process:* Nursing Process, Assessment; *Cognitive Level:* Application; *Client Need/Subneed:* Physiological Integrity/ Physiological Adaptation/Pathophysiology

44. CORRECT ANSWER: 3. **Answer 1** is incorrect because spinal fluid does not affect the concentration of the urine. *Head trauma* may cause a disorder of the posterior pituitary, but the urine specific gravity would *be low.* **Answer 2** is incorrect because an excessive output would be more likely to result from *trauma to the posterior pituitary,* not from a cerebrospinal fluid (CSF) leak. **Answer 3 is correct because spinal fluid contains glucose. The RN should also look for the "halo" sign of blood drainage with a yellow ring of spinal fluid. In addition, nose and ears should be kept clean to reduce the chance of infection.** **Answer 4** is incorrect because the concern is leakage of CSF as a result of a *tear* that would allow fluid to leak from the nose or ears, *not* a result of a *lumbar puncture.*
■ TEST-TAKING TIP: *Remember: cerebrospinal fluid is high in glucose.*
Content Area: Adult Health, Neurological; *Integrated Process:* Nursing Process, Assessment; *Cognitive Level:* Application; *Client Need/Subneed:* Physiological Integrity/Reduction of Risk Potential/Potential for Complications from Surgical Procedures and Health Alterations

45. CORRECT ANSWERS: 1, 2, 3, 4. **Answer 1 is correct because pronator drift reflects ischemic consequences of a stroke. Answer 2 is correct because facial droop reflects ischemic consequences of a stroke. Answer 3 is correct because slurred or garbled speech reflects ischemic consequences of a stroke. Answer 4 is correct because extremity weakness on one side reflects ischemic consequences of a stroke.** **Answer 5** is incorrect because crackles in the lungs would indicate *CHF* or *pneumonia.* **Answer 6** is incorrect because decreased urine output would result from *hypotension* or impaired kidney function.
■ TEST-TAKING TIP: *Select choices that are directly influenced by the sensorimotor system, not respiratory (Answer 5) or renal (Answer 6).*
Content Area: Adult Health, Cardiovascular; *Integrated Process:* Nursing Process, Assessment; *Cognitive Level:* Comprehension; *Client Need/Subneed:* Physiological Integrity/Physiological Adaptation/Pathophysiology

46. CORRECT ANSWER: 1. Answer 1 is correct because immediate treatment is directed toward reversing circulatory shock of addisonian crisis. Replacement of sodium and the missing steroid hormones is critical. **Answer 2** is incorrect because the client needs *sodium and an increased volume.* **Answer 3** is incorrect because initial treatment is normal saline. D_5NS may be given with the glucocorticoids; however, a *vasopressor* such as dopamine would *not* be the *first* line of treatment. **Answer 4** is incorrect because the primary problem is *circulatory shock.*

■ **TEST-TAKING TIP:** *Addison's disease is a deficiency of glucocorticoids—note that the correct answer has the word "glucocorticoid."*

Content Area: Adult Health, Endocrine; ***Integrated Process:*** Nursing Process, Implementation; ***Cognitive Level:*** Application; ***Client Need/Subneed:*** Physiological Integrity/Physiological Adaptation/Fluid and Electrolyte Imbalances

47. CORRECT ANSWER: 4. **Answer 1** is incorrect because night sweats would *not* be a symptom of bone marrow depression. **Answer 2** is incorrect because these signs are consistent with *dehydration,* which may result from vomiting or diarrhea from chemotherapy if untreated. **Answer 3** is incorrect because this would indicate *nephrotoxicity* and *renal dysfunction* as a result of chemotherapy. **Answer 4 is correct because myelosuppression decreases WBCs, RBCs, and platelets. The anemia reduces oxygen-carrying capacity, leading to fatigue and weakness. The reduced platelets increases bruising and bleeding tendencies.**

■ **TEST-TAKING TIP:** *Think: blood-related symptoms. Review the role of the bone marrow in the production of red blood cells.*

Content Area: Adult Health, Oncological; ***Integrated Process:*** Nursing Process, Assessment; ***Cognitive Level:*** Comprehension; ***Client Need/Subneed:*** Physiological Integrity/Pharmacological and Parenteral Therapies/Adverse Effects/Contraindications/Interactions

48. CORRECT ANSWER: 4. **Answer 1** is incorrect because the stem says that this is a terminal admission. Dealing with the diagnosis would not be the most common fear. **Answer 2** is incorrect because a terminal admission generally means that the care will be *palliative,* not curative. **Answer 3** is incorrect because the needs of the client at the time of a terminal admission are for palliation, not continuation of a normal lifestyle. **Answer 4 is correct because the client who is terminally ill most often wishes to be pain-free and to know that someone will be there in the end.**

■ **TEST-TAKING TIP:** *Only one option relates to dying, which is the outcome of a terminal admission.*

Content Area: Adult Health, End-of-Life; ***Integrated Process:*** Nursing Process, Analysis; ***Cognitive Level:*** Comprehension; ***Client Need/Subneed:*** Psychosocial Integrity/End of Life Care

49. CORRECT ANSWER: 2. **Answer 1** is incorrect because Buck's is *skin* traction, *not* skeletal traction, which uses pins. **Answer 2 is correct because Buck's is skin traction to the lower leg. Circulatory disturbances and skin abrasions are the most important nursing concerns.** **Answer 3** is incorrect because Buck's is skin traction using an elastic bandage. The fracture site would *not* be *visible.* **Answer 4** is incorrect because Buck's uses a foam boot to *support* the foot of the affected extremity in a dorsiflexed position. This position is, therefore, *not* a complication.

■ **TEST-TAKING TIP:** *Choose the option that describes a problem from traction that is applied externally. If too tight, a limb becomes dusky, not flushed.*

Content Area: Adult Health, Musculoskeletal; ***Integrated Process:*** Nursing Process, Assessment; ***Cognitive Level:*** Application; ***Client Need/Subneed:*** Physiological Integrity/Basic Care and Comfort/Mobility/Immobility

50. CORRECT ANSWER: 1. Answer 1 is correct because there is always a risk of osteomyelitis (bone infection) with orthopedic surgery. **Answer 2** is incorrect because phlebitis, an inflammation of a vein, is *not as serious* as an infection in the bone. **Answer 3** is incorrect because urinary retention can result following hip surgery because it is difficult to relax the sphincter muscles when in pain. Retention is *not* usually life-threatening. **Answer 4** is incorrect because effective pain management following implant surgery does *not normally lead* to addiction.

■ **TEST-TAKING TIP:** *With any orthopedic surgery, the greatest risk is infection.*

Content Area: Adult Health, Musculoskeletal; ***Integrated Process:*** Nursing Process, Assessment; ***Cognitive Level:*** Application; ***Client Need/Subneed:*** Physiological Integrity/Reduction of Risk Potential/Potential for Complications from Surgical Procedures and Health Alterations

51. CORRECT ANSWER: 4. **Answer 1** is incorrect because the pulse rate and moist respirations may be *due to* the rapid IV rate. **Answer 2** is incorrect because the nurse needs to do something *immediately.* **Answer 3** is incorrect because *only the physician* can provide orders to correct the possible volume overload. **Answer 4 is correct because the assessment may indicate volume overload. Slowing the IV rate keeps the IV access open while waiting for further orders.**

■ **TEST-TAKING TIP:** *Think about what happens when the heart cannot handle the circulating volume overload, requiring ↓ IV rate and calling the physician.*

Content Area: Adult Health, Fluid and Electrolyte Imbalances; ***Integrated Process:*** Nursing Process, Implementation; ***Cognitive Level:*** Application; ***Client Need/Subneed:*** Physiological Integrity/Physiological Adaptation/Medical Emergencies

52. CORRECT ANSWER: 2. **Answer 1** is incorrect because, during the early postoperative period, pressure would *not* be the *first* concern. If edema develops, breakdown will be

ANSWERS

more likely. Answer 2 is correct because reducing edema will promote healing and prevent complications. **Answer 3** is incorrect because the wound will *not* be cleansed within the first 24 hours. The stump is wrapped securely after surgery, and the dressing would be reinforced if needed. **Answer 4** is incorrect because a prosthesis will not be indicated *until* there has been sufficient healing.

■ TEST-TAKING TIP: *With any "trauma" such as surgery, prevent swelling—in this situation look for elevation.*

Content Area: Adult Health, Musculoskeletal; ***Integrated Process:*** Nursing Process, Implementation; ***Cognitive Level:*** Application; ***Client Need/Subneed:*** Physiological Integrity/Basic Care and Comfort/Mobility/Immobility

53. CORRECT ANSWER: 3. **Answer 1** is incorrect because this choice *does not immobilize* the client's neck. **Answer 2** is incorrect because, after immobilizing the spine, *determining responsiveness* would be the *next* priority. Answer 3 is correct because, before assessing the CABs (compression, airway, and breathing) in this client, it is important to prevent further injury to the spinal cord. **Answer 4** is incorrect because this choice does *not stabilize* the spine.

■ TEST-TAKING TIP: *Whenever there is a possibility of neck injury, stabilize the neck before checking the ABCs.*

Content Area: Adult Health, Neurological; ***Integrated Process:*** Nursing Process, Implementation; ***Cognitive Level:*** Application; ***Client Need/Subneed:*** Physiological Integrity/Physiological Adaptation/Medical Emergencies

54. CORRECT ANSWER: 3. **Answer 1** is incorrect because pupillary changes related to cerebral hypoxia and increased ICP are *very* late signs. **Answer 2** is incorrect because the body would try to compensate for the drop in BP *before* a change in LOC. Answer 3 is correct because an increase in pulse would be an attempt by the body to increase the BP. **Answer 4** is incorrect because the client would be more likely to become weak (i.e., flaccid extremities) if hypotension occurs.

■ TEST-TAKING TIP: *Think how the body would respond to maintain adequate blood flow.*

Content Area: Adult Health, Cardiovascular; ***Integrated Process:*** Nursing Process, Analysis; ***Cognitive Level:*** Application; ***Client Need/Subneed:*** Physiological Integrity/Physiological Adaptation/Pathophysiology

55. CORRECT ANSWER: 2. **Answer 1** is incorrect because menopause does *not* change the risk. (Women who engage in high-risk sexual activities are at risk at *any age.*) Answer 2 is correct because older men tend to not use condoms and do not consider themselves to be at risk for HIV. **Answer 3** is incorrect because the risk is *less* (but not risk-free). **Answer 4** is incorrect because, *if* the mother with HIV uses safe sex practices, HIV can be *prevented.* The risk to the child of a mother with HIV is at birth or if being breastfed.

■ TEST-TAKING TIP: *The best answer is the least obvious one here: older-age men.*

Content Area: Adult Health, Communicable Diseases; ***Integrated Process:*** Nursing Process, Analysis; ***Cognitive Level:*** Comprehension; ***Client Need/Subneed:*** Health Promotion and Maintenance/High Risk Behaviors

56. CORRECT ANSWER: 1. Answer 1 is correct because this client will likely survive the injury with pain medication and fluids. **Answer 2** is incorrect because this client is not a priority as the injuries are *not* life-threatening. **Answer 3** is incorrect because this victim has a *normal* coma scale score, and should be seen after the victim with burns. **Answer 4** is incorrect because this client in a triage situation is not considered to be a priority.

■ TEST-TAKING TIP: *The priority in a disaster is the* most critical *with the* greatest potential *for survival if treated.*

Content Area: Adult Health, Triage; ***Integrated Process:*** Nursing Process, Assessment; ***Cognitive Level:*** Application; ***Client Need/Subneed:*** Safe and Effective Care Environment/Management of Care/Establishing Priorities

57. CORRECT ANSWER: 2. **Answer 1** is incorrect because this *delays* reestablishing the airway. Answer 2 is correct because keeping the airway open is most important. Concern for contamination of the tube can be addressed after a patent airway is established. **Answer 3** is incorrect because keeping the *airway open* is most important. **Answer 4** is incorrect because reinserting the tracheostomy tube is a *more effective* way to ventilate the client.

■ TEST-TAKING TIP: *See Answer 2 with the word "open" in the stem. Look for a nursing action that will best keep the airway open and ensure adequate ventilation.*

Content Area: Adult Health, Respiratory; ***Integrated Process:*** Nursing Process, Implementation; ***Cognitive Level:*** Application; ***Client Need/Subneed:*** Physiological Integrity/Physiological Adaptation/Medical Emergencies

58. CORRECT ANSWER: 2. **Answer 1** is incorrect because the ABGs support hypoventilation and atelectasis. Suctioning will *not reexpand* the alveoli as effectively as coughing and deep breathing. Answer 2 is correct because atelectasis is likely as a result of general anesthesia. The client also appears to be hypoventilating most likely because of abdominal pain. The client should be medicated for pain before coughing and deep breathing. **Answer 3** is incorrect because the pH is within *normal* limits, indicating compensation. **Answer 4** is incorrect because coughing and deep breathing, not just a position change, is needed. *Any degree* of head elevation will improve deep breathing.

■ TEST-TAKING TIP: *With general anesthesia and abdominal surgery, hypoventilation is likely. An independent nursing action is encouraging coughing and deep breathing.*

Content Area: Adult Health, Respiratory; ***Integrated Process:*** Nursing Process, Implementation; ***Cognitive Level:*** Analysis; ***Client Need/Subneed:*** Physiological Integrity/Reduction of Risk Potential/Laboratory Values

59. CORRECT ANSWER: 2. Answer 1 is incorrect because the heart is not beating independently, so the pulse rate would *decrease.* **Answer 2 is correct because ventricular function would be affected, causing signs of heart failure and inadequate perfusion. Answer 3** is incorrect because a pacemaker is *not* correcting atrial fibrillation but a *conduction* defect to the ventricles. **Answer 4** is incorrect because initially the client would experience symptoms consistent with *heart failure* from inadequate cardiac pumping.

■ **TEST-TAKING TIP:** *Choose the option that is different from the others. Only one describes the effects of poor perfusion.*
Content Area: Adult Health, Cardiology; ***Integrated Process:*** Nursing Process, Assessment; ***Cognitive Level:*** Application; ***Client Need/Subneed:*** Physiological Integrity/Physiological Adaptation/Pathophysiology

60. CORRECT ANSWERS: 1, 2, 4, 5. Answer 1 is correct because the heart is unable to handle the venous return, and it will back up into the venous system, causing the ankle edema. Answer 2 is correct because the heart is unable to adequately pump the blood through the right side of the heart, so there is a back-pressure and JVD. Answer 3 is incorrect because crackles would indicate *left*-sided heart failure. **Answer 4 is correct because organ enlargement will occur from the back-pressure with the failing heart. Answer 5 is correct because the right side of the heart cannot handle the venous return, and the pressure will cause systemic edema.**

■ **TEST-TAKING TIP:** *Visualize: if the* **right** *side of the heart cannot pump the blood, where would the effects of the back-pressure be noted?*
Content Area: Adult Health, Cardiology; ***Integrated Process:*** Nursing Process, Assessment; ***Cognitive Level:*** Comprehension; ***Client Need/Subneed:*** Physiological Integrity/Physiological Adaptation/Pathophysiology

61. CORRECT ANSWER: 2. Answer 1 is incorrect because cool, clammy skin occurs with *hypovolemia* and *decreased perfusion.* **Answer 2 is correct because there is an increase in the body temperature, and vasodilation would occur. Answer 3** is incorrect because a drop in the systolic pressure occurs with *hypovolemic shock,* not septic shock. **Answer 4** is incorrect because DIC is a hypercoagulable condition that would be a *late* complication of poor perfusion.

■ **TEST-TAKING TIP:** *Know the classic difference with septic shock: fever—therefore, the client is warm and flushed.*
Content Area: Adult Health, Cardiovascular; ***Integrated Process:*** Nursing Process, Assessment; ***Cognitive Level:*** Application; ***Client Need/Subneed:*** Physiological Integrity/Physiological Adaptation/Pathophysiology

62. CORRECT ANSWER: 4. Answer 1 is incorrect because a change in LOC from hypovolemia would have occurred *earlier.* **Answer 2** is incorrect because this may have been an *early* indication of a GI problem. **Answer 3** is incorrect because the respiratory change may occur as a result of metabolic acidosis. **Answer 4 is correct because the heart would attempt to increase cardiac output by increasing the pulse rate as the volume continued to decrease.**

■ **TEST-TAKING TIP:** *The key word is "worsening." Choose the option that best describes the ongoing cardiovascular response to a decrease in circulating volume.*
Content Area: Adult Health, Cardiovascular; ***Integrated Process:*** Nursing Process, Analysis; ***Cognitive Level:*** Application; ***Client Need/Subneed:*** Physiological Integrity/Physiological Adaptation/Pathophysiology

63. CORRECT ANSWERS: 1, 2, 3, 5. Answer 1 is correct because there is frequently a worsening of a cough that may have appeared to be improving. Answer 2 is correct because shortness of breath is an emergency warning sign and requires urgent care. Answer 3 is correct because swine flu may present with vomiting not typically seen with the seasonal flu. Answer 4 is incorrect because the client with swine flu does *not have a high fever* and may have a normal temperature. **Answer 5 is correct because clients with swine flu may present with diarrhea, non common in adults with seasonal flu, although diarrhea is seen in children with seasonal flu.**

■ **TEST-TAKING TIP:** *Recognize the one symptom (high fever) that is not typical.*
Content Area: Adult Health, Infectious Disease; ***Integrated Process:*** Nursing Process, Assessment; ***Cognitive Level:*** Application; ***Client Need/Subneed:*** Safe, Effective Care Environment/Safety and Infection Control

64. CORRECT ANSWER: 2. Answer 1 is incorrect because the overriding parasympathetic stimulation causes bradycardia, *not* tachycardia (pulse = 120 here). **Answer 2 is correct because the hypotension and tachycardia are classic signs of hypovolemic shock. Answer 3** is incorrect because the temperature would be *higher* in septic shock, usually greater than 38°C. **Answer 4** is incorrect because in cardiogenic shock the pulse would *not* be increased because the contractility of the heart is ineffective.

■ **TEST-TAKING TIP:** *Each type of shock has a unique characteristic. Know the clinical indications.*
Content Area: Adult Health, Cardiovascular; ***Integrated Process:*** Nursing Process, Analysis; ***Cognitive Level:*** Analysis; ***Client Need/Subneed:*** Physiological Integrity/Reduction of Risk Potential/Vital Signs Changes/Abnormalities

65. CORRECT ANSWER: 3. Answer 1 is incorrect because these findings would be consistent with *hypocalcemia* (low calcium). **Answer 2** is incorrect because these findings would be consistent with *dehydration* and metabolic acidosis. **Answer 3 is correct because potassium affects normal muscle function. Answer 4** is incorrect because these findings would be consistent with *hypoxia* and poor perfusion possibly related to cardiac failure.

■ **TEST-TAKING TIP:** *Look for the effects of low potassium on* **muscles,** *including the* **heart.**

Content Area: Adult Health, Fluid and Electrolyte Imbalances; ***Integrated Process:*** Nursing Process, Analysis; ***Cognitive Level:*** Application; ***Client Need/Subneed:*** Physiological Integrity/Physiological Adaptation/Fluid and Electrolyte Imbalances

66. CORRECT ANSWER: 1. Answer 1 is correct because the respiratory rate would increase as respiratory function improved. Respiratory acidosis occurs from slow and inadequate ventilation. Answer 2 is incorrect because an increase in creatinine and poor renal function would lead to *metabolic acidosis.* **Answer 3** is incorrect because a slow respiratory rate causes CO_2 to be retained, which will lead to respiratory acidosis. **Answer 4** is incorrect because bicarbonate *increases with respiratory acidosis.*

■ **TEST-TAKING TIP:** *Recall that a compensatory response to a metabolic problem is a change in respiratory rate. The rate should slow as CO_2 returns to normal.*

Content Area: Adult Health, Fluid and Electrolyte Imbalances; ***Integrated Process:*** Nursing Process, Analysis; ***Cognitive Level:*** Application; ***Client Need/Subneed:*** Physiological Integrity/Physiological Adaptation/Pathophysiology

67. CORRECT ANSWERS: 1, 2, 4. Answer 1 is correct because ammonia is a by-product of protein breakdown by the intestinal flora. Blood is a source of protein. Answer 2 is correct because ammonia is a by-product of protein breakdown. Reducing dietary protein will decrease the ammonia level. Answer 3 is incorrect because diarrhea actually *decreases* ammonia and may be a *desired* therapeutic effect. **Answer 4 is correct because protein is broken down to form ammonia by intestinal bacteria. Sterilizing the bowel with an antibiotic will decrease the ammonia level. Answer 5** is incorrect because the ammonia is produced in the GI system by the breakdown of protein. Ascites is in the peritoneum, *not* in the intestine.

■ **TEST-TAKING TIP:** *Review how ammonia forms in the presence of blood and bacteria.*

Content Area: Adult Health, Gastrointestinal; ***Integrated Process:*** Nursing Process, Implementation; ***Cognitive Level:*** Application; ***Client Need/Subneed:*** Physiological Integrity/Physiological Adaptation/Illness Management

68. CORRECT ANSWER: 1. Answer 1 is correct because initially peristalsis will increase in the ascending colon (right lower quadrant [RLQ]) in an attempt to clear the blockage. There will be no peristalsis distal to the obstruction. Answer 2 is incorrect because peristalsis will *increase* proximal (RLQ) to the obstruction. **Answer 3** is incorrect because initially peristalsis will *increase* proximal (RLQ) to the obstruction. **Answer 4** is incorrect because peristalsis *will be present initially* proximal (left lower quadrant [LLQ]) to the obstruction.

■ **TEST-TAKING TIP:** *Visualize the colon. Initially bowel sounds increase proximal to an obstruction and are absent distal to the obstruction.*

Content Area: Adult Health, Gastrointestinal; ***Integrated Process:*** Nursing Process, Assessment; ***Cognitive Level:*** Application; ***Client Need/Subneed:*** Health Promotion and Maintenance/Techniques of Physical Assessment

69. CORRECT ANSWERS: 2, 3, 4, 5. Answer 1 is incorrect because gatching the bed in the area of the knees *reduces* venous return. **Answer 2 is correct because these exercises prevent venous pooling. Answer 3 is correct because use of such devices prevents venous pooling. Answer 4 is correct because dehydration increases RBC concentration, resulting in sluggish circulation. Answer 5 is correct because this will increase venous return and reduce venous stasis from dependent positioning. Answer 6** is incorrect because heat will cause *vasodilation* and *venous pooling.*

■ **TEST-TAKING TIP:** *Look for strategies to prevent venous stasis and improve venous return.*

Content Area: Adult Health, Vascular; ***Integrated Process:*** Nursing Process, Implementation; ***Cognitive Level:*** Application; ***Client Need/Subneed:*** Physiological Integrity/Reduction of Risk Potential/Therapeutic Procedures

70. CORRECT ANSWERS: 1, 3, 5. Answer 1 is correct because a local anesthetic will be used to minimize pain to the puncture site. Answer 2 is incorrect because the reason for the thoracentesis is fluid in the pleural space, *not* in the *lung.* **Answer 3 is correct because this position drops the diaphragm and allows for easier access to the pleural space. Answer 4** is incorrect because upright and leaning forward is the optimal position. **Answer 5 is correct because the client needs to have been informed of the risks before the procedure is started. Answer 6** is incorrect because there is some discomfort, although use of the local anesthetic reduces the pain.

■ **TEST-TAKING TIP:** *Think client safety before, during, and after the procedure.*

Content Area: Adult Health; ***Integrated Process:*** Nursing Process, Implementation; ***Cognitive Level:*** Application; ***Client Need/Subneed:*** Physiological Integrity/Reduction of Risk Potential/Therapeutic Procedures

71. CORRECT ANSWER: 1. Answer 1 is correct because the PT is the specific test to determine the effectiveness of Coumadin therapy. Answer 2 is incorrect because the Lee-White clotting time monitors *heparin* therapy, but has been *replaced* by other tests. **Answer 3** is incorrect because the PTT is the appropriate test to determine the effectiveness of *heparin* therapy. **Answer 4** is incorrect because FCT is a measure of *thrombin* activity, and heparin prolongs the time.

■ **TEST-TAKING TIP:** *Know the differences between coumadin and heparin with regard to indications of effectiveness and monitoring of therapeutic level.*

Content Area: Adult Health, Vascular; ***Integrated Process:*** Nursing Process, Analysis; ***Cognitive Level:*** Application; ***Client Need/Subneed:*** Physiological Integrity/Reduction of Risk Potential/Laboratory Values

72. CORRECT ANSWER: 2. **Answer 1** is incorrect because a possible cause, such as dehydration or *influenza,* while potentially a concern, is not as serious as the potential of heart failure. **Answer 2 is correct because these are signs and symptoms associated with heart failure.** **Answer 3** is incorrect because a productive cough alone *without* a high fever is *not* the first priority. **Answer 4** is incorrect because palpitations *without* chest pain would *not* be a priority.

■ **TEST-TAKING TIP:** *Think* ABCs *as priority and select* "B"—*breathing. Look for the client who is most unstable, or the clinical indications that signal a potentially urgent need.*

Content Area: Adult Health, Triage; *Integrated Process:* Nursing Process, Analysis; *Cognitive Level:* Analysis; *Client Need/Subneed:* Safe and Effective Care Environment/Management of Care/Establishing Priorities

73. CORRECT ANSWER: 3. **Answer 1** is incorrect because keeping the airway open is more important than *listening* to breath sounds. **Answer 2** is incorrect because keeping the airway open is the priority, not giving oxygen. **Answer 3 is correct because, until fully awake, the tongue may obstruct the airway. Keeping the airway in place until the client pushes it out prevents obstruction.** **Answer 4** is incorrect because keeping the airway open is the priority. Side-lying may prevent aspiration in the client who may vomit, but it may not be possible, depending on type of surgery.

■ **TEST-TAKING TIP:** *Think: "ABCs" and select "airway" as the action that is most important. The best choice will increase the effectiveness of the other options.*

Content Area: Adult Health, Respiratory; *Integrated Process:* Nursing Process, Implementation; *Cognitive Level:* Application; *Client Need/Subneed:* Physiological Integrity/Reduction of Risk Potential/Potential for Complications from Surgical Procedures and Health Alterations

74. CORRECT ANSWER: 1. **Answer 1 is correct because bilateral adventitious sounds are heard early in left-sided failure. The ejection fraction is below the normal for a health heart (60% to 70%).** **Answer 2** is incorrect because the low O_2 saturation is related to *pulmonary congestion and heart failure.* A flat position may aggravate the client's condition. **Answer 3** is incorrect because crackles due to heart failure would *not clear* with deep breathing and coughing. **Answer 4** is incorrect because the ejection fraction is on the low side of normal (60% to 70% for a healthy heart). *Fatigue* would be *more common.* This degree of activity intolerance would increase as heart failure progressed.

■ **TEST-TAKING TIP:** *Know the average ejection fraction (60% to 70%). Select a finding that would be consistent with mild heart failure.*

Content Area: Adult Health, Cardiology; *Integrated Process:* Nursing Process, Analysis; *Cognitive Level:* Analysis; *Client Need/Subneed:* Physiological Integrity/Physiological Adaptation/Pathophysiology

75. CORRECT ANSWER: 1. **Answer 1 is correct because severe dehydration is often seen in DKA. This can decrease renal perfusion and cause buildup of BUN and creatinine. First, the client needs rehydration to correct prerenal failure. Then, an assessment can be made of renal function (which can be decreased in diabetes).** **Answer 2** is incorrect because fluid restriction would *exacerbate* the dehydration. **Answer 3** is incorrect because dialysis is *not* required for creatinine levels of 2.7. **Answer 4** is incorrect because a bladder catheter would not help manage the problem, only help assess the level of dehydration and the response to treatment with hourly urine output measurements.

■ **TEST-TAKING TIP:** *Remember that the client with DKA is severely dehydrated—flushed and warm. When two options are contradictory (Answers 1 and 2), often* one *of them is correct.*

Content Area: Adult Health, Endocrine; *Integrated Process:* Nursing Process, Planning; *Cognitive Level:* Application; *Client Need/Subneed:* Physiological Integrity/Physiological Adaptation/Illness Management

76. CORRECT ANSWER: 1. **Answer 1 is correct because total bilirubin comes from normal turnover of RBCs in the body. Excess destruction or inability of the liver to process waste products may cause an increase in bilirubin, which may turn the client's skin yellow. This is a normal total bilirubin.** **Answer 2** is incorrect because this is a *normal* bilirubin level, *unrelated* to presence of blood in the urine. **Answer 3** is incorrect because this is a *normal* bilirubin level, *unrelated* to blood in the *stool.* **Answer 4** is incorrect because *high* bilirubin levels may cause a yellow coloration to the skin, correctly seen in the sclera of the eye. This total bilirubin is *normal.*

■ **TEST-TAKING TIP:** *Three of the options imply that the bilirubin level is* **not** *normal. Select the one option that states it* **is** *a normal value. Memorize the ranges of common diagnostic laboratory tests.*

Content Area: Adult Health, Hematological; *Integrated Process:* Nursing Process, Implementation; *Cognitive Level:* Application; *Client Need/Subneed:* Physiological Integrity/Reduction of Risk Potential/Laboratory Values

77. CORRECT ANSWER: 2. **Answer 1** is incorrect because clients on insulin drips often require supplemental potassium to replace that carried into the cells by insulin. A K^+ of 4.4 is on the *high* end of the normal and would *not need* to be replaced. **Answer 2 is correct because this client is still acidotic, which means the cells are burning fats and releasing ketones. (Anion gap is 130 – 100 – 15 = 15, which is high; bicarbonate is low at 15). Insulin is still required. With blood sugar at 100, you will also need to give sugar.** **Answer 3** is incorrect because sodium level needs to correct *slowly* as blood sugar is lowered from the high admission level. At 130, a correction has almost occurred. Giving sodium tablets to increase sodium too quickly will pull fluid out of the cells, further dehydrating the cells. Salt may be given to correct hypertension, but is not required in this client. **Answer 4** is incorrect because clients with DKA need fluids, *not fluid restriction.* The

ANSWERS

high blood sugar creates an osmotic loss of intracellular fluids, and when sugar is spilled into the urine, there is osmotic fluid *loss* from the body.

■ **TEST-TAKING TIP:** ***Know the effects of high blood sugar levels on fluid and electrolyte levels, as well as the shifts that occur with the administration of insulin.***

Content Area: Adult Health, Endocrine; ***Integrated Process:*** Nursing Process, Implementation; ***Cognitive Level:*** Analysis; ***Client Need/Subneed:*** Physiological Integrity/Reduction of Risk Potential/Laboratory Values

78. CORRECT ANSWER: 3. Answer 1 is incorrect because clients with diabetes should manage blood sugar at a level that would result in an A_{1c} of less than 7%. An intervention is *required* to help this client better manage diabetes. **Answer 2** is incorrect because the A_{1c} would *not change acutely* with resolution of DKA. **Answer 3 is correct because the A_{1c} gives a number that reflects the average blood sugar over the last 3 months. Clients with diabetes are told to try to keep the A_{1c} less than 7% (sometimes less than 6.5%). This high level, which is getting worse, means that the client needs better management of the diabetes. Client teaching is the correct way to help a client manage this chronic disease. Answer 4** is incorrect because this client's diabetes is out of control. First, an assessment must be done to determine why the blood sugars have been chronically high. Longer-acting insulin *may or may not* be part of a reasonable intervention for this client.

■ **TEST-TAKING TIP:** ***Know that the $HgbA_{1c}$ level is too high, needing teaching.***

Content Area: Adult Health, Endocrine; ***Integrated Process:*** Nursing Process, Analysis; ***Cognitive Level:*** Analysis; ***Client Need/Subneed:*** Physiological Integrity/Reduction of Risk Potential/Laboratory Values

79. CORRECT ANSWER: 1. Answer 1 is correct because hyponatremia can precipitate seizures. Answer 2 is incorrect because the moderately high blood sugar associated with an A_{1c} of 8% would *not cause* seizures. **Answer 3** is incorrect because anion gaps less than 12 are *normal.* **Answer 4** is incorrect because neuropathies of peripheral neurons would *not* precipitate seizures.

■ **TEST-TAKING TIP:** ***Look for the most abnormal condition—a low serum sodium.***

Content Area: Adult Health, Neurological; ***Integrated Process:*** Nursing Process, Analysis; ***Cognitive Level:*** Analysis; ***Client Need/Subneed:*** Physiological Integrity/Reduction of Risk Potential/Laboratory Values

80. CORRECT ANSWERS: 4, 6. Answer 1 is incorrect because the client is *not deaf.* Speak normally. **Answer 2** is incorrect because these words *are* appropriate. **Answer 3** is incorrect because, although senses of a client with visual impairment may be extrasensitive, no voice adjustment is needed. Speak *normally.* **Answer 4 is correct because the client hears better when spoken to directly. Answer 5** is incorrect because touching a client before speaking to the client will be startling. **Answer 6 is correct because the client has no idea where "over there" is. Describe the location.**

■ **TEST-TAKING TIP:** ***Choose options that optimize the reliance on other senses of the client who is visually impaired, such as auditory (Answer 4), and avoid using vague phrases about locations that describe what the client cannot see (Answer 6).***

Content Area: Adult Health, Sensory; ***Integrated Process:*** Communication and Documentation; ***Cognitive Level:*** Application; ***Client Need:*** Psychosocial Integrity/Sensory/Perceptual Alterations

81. CORRECT ANSWER: 1. Answer 1 is correct because exercise in the absence of weight reduction is a significant factor in reducing blood pressure. Answer 2 is incorrect because support groups may *not* be beneficial to *all* clients. **Answer 3** is incorrect because avoiding tobacco doesn't reduce blood pressure but reduces the *risk of a cardiac event.* **Answer 4** is incorrect because increasing fruits and vegetables *alone* will *not* control blood pressure.

■ **TEST-TAKING TIP:** ***Look for an option that is known to manage weight and stress—exercise.***

Content Area: Adult Health, Cardiovascular; ***Integrated Process:*** Teaching and Learning; ***Cognitive Level:*** Application; ***Client Need/Subneed:*** Health Promotion and Maintenance/Health Promotion Programs

82. CORRECT ANSWER: 4. Answer 1 is incorrect because this tests the corneal reflex (*blink*). **Answer 2** is incorrect because this action tests extraocular *movements* (cranial nerve [CN] IV). **Answer 3** is incorrect because this action tests the *optic nerve* (CN II). **Answer 4 is correct because the normal response of the pupil to light is constriction, if CN III is normal.**

■ **TEST-TAKING TIP:** ***Review the correct assessment technique for each cranial nerve. Assessing CN III is part of routine neurological checks.***

Content Area: Adult Health, Sensory; ***Integrated Process:*** Nursing Process, Implementation; ***Cognitive Level:*** Application; ***Client Need/Subneed:*** Health Promotion and Maintenance/Techniques of Physical Assessment

83. CORRECT ANSWER: 3. Answer 1 is incorrect because this is seen with *tetany* (*hypo*calcemia). **Answer 2** is incorrect because this occurs from ischemia-induced *carpal spasm* from *hypocalcemia.* **Answer 3 is correct because hypercalcemia reduces neuromuscular excitability, resulting in muscle weakness and hyporeflexia. Answer 4** is incorrect because the Babinski reflex is a test of *upper motor neuron* function.

■ **TEST-TAKING TIP:** ***Eliminate the options that are clinical manifestations of*** **hypo*calcemia (Answers 1 and 2) and the option that is*** **not** ***manifested by the electrolyte imbalance (Answer 4) noted in the stem of this question.***

Content Area: Adult Health, Fluid and Electrolyte Imbalances; ***Integrated Process:*** Nursing Process, Assessment; ***Cognitive Level:*** Comprehension; ***Client Need/Subneed:*** Physiological Integrity/Physiological Adaptation/Fluid and Electrolyte Imbalances

84. CORRECT ANSWER: 4. **Answer 1** is incorrect because loss of appetite may occur in children *without* severe illness. **Answer 2** is incorrect because swine flu may present without a fever. Children also frequently have fevers *without* any underlying pathology. **Answer 3** is incorrect because vomiting would need to *be persistent* and lead to dehydration to be a concern. **Answer 4 is correct because a change in alertness or responsiveness is an emergency warning sign in children and needs urgent attention.**

■ **TEST-TAKING TIP:** *Choose a* **neurological** *sign, rather than gastrointestinal (Answers 1 and 3).*

Content Area: Child Health, Infectious Disease; ***Integrated Process:*** Teaching and Learning; ***Cognitive Level:*** Analysis; ***Client Need/Subneed:*** Safe, Effective Care Environment/ Safety and Infection Control

85. CORRECT ANSWER: 4. **Answer 1** is incorrect because the *first* priority is maintaining *circulation,* not a quiet environment. **Answer 2** is incorrect because the *first* priority is maintaining adequate perfusion, not avoiding exertion. **Answer 3** is incorrect because the inadequate perfusion must be corrected first. **Answer 4 is correct because the client is at risk for shock.**

■ **TEST-TAKING TIP:** *When all options are correct, look for the choice that responds to a "crisis" and will produce* **an immediate** *response—fluid.*

Content Area: Adult Health, Endocrine; ***Integrated Process:*** Nursing Process, Implementation; ***Cognitive Level:*** Analysis; ***Client Need/Subneed:*** Physiological Integrity/Physiological Adaptation/Alterations in Body Systems

86. CORRECT ANSWER: 4. **Answer 1** is incorrect because cerebral perfusion is determined by the *pressure* of the blood flowing into the brain and the *resistance* to inflow created by intracerebral pressure. **Answer 2** is incorrect because cerebral vasodilation is largely determined by $Paco_2$. It is important to ensure good ventilation in clients who have had trauma, but this is *unrelated to serum sodium.* **Answer 3** is incorrect because lowering the seizure threshold would make the client *more at risk* for seizures, which is never desirable. Low serum sodium levels can increase seizure risk. **Answer 4 is correct because osmolarity is largely determined by serum sodium. If the sodium level is low, water will move from the bloodstream into the cells. The client is already at risk for cerebral edema because of the injury. The swelling could result in a dangerous increase in intracerebral pressure.**

■ **TEST-TAKING TIP:** *Remember: H_2O follows sodium. The desired clinical outcome is to reduce or prevent cerebral edema.*

Content Area: Adult Health, Fluid and Electrolyte Imbalances; ***Integrated Process:*** Nursing Process, Analysis; ***Cognitive Level:*** Application; ***Client Need/Subneed:*** Physiological Integrity/ Reduction of Risk Potential/Laboratory Values

87. CORRECT ANSWER: 2. **Answer 1** is incorrect because the acidosis will correct with insulin once glucose is available to the cell so that it does not need to burn fats. Giving bicarbonate might *temporarily* fix pH, but it does not fix the problem of dehydration. **Answer 2 is correct because clients who are admitted with high blood sugar levels are very dehydrated and need IV normal saline. High blood sugar levels dehydrate cells, spilling sugar in the kidneys and causing obligate water loss.** **Answer 3** is incorrect because IV albumin is an expensive and unnecessary way to correct dehydration. This client needs sodium and water. Normal saline IV is the correct action. **Answer 4** is incorrect because, although the client needs insulin, it is *inappropriate* to give it subcutaneously. Clients who are dehydrated have poor absorption from this tissue. These clients need a *continuous* intravenous drip of insulin.

■ **TEST-TAKING TIP:** *This is a priority question. To decide between two options (fluids or bicarbonate), remember that correcting dehydration (with fluids) will improve acidosis.*

Content Area: Adult Health, Endocrine; ***Integrated Process:*** Nursing Process, Analysis; ***Cognitive Level:*** Analysis; ***Client Need/Subneed:*** Physiological Integrity/Pharmacological and Parenteral Therapies/Medication Administration

88. CORRECT ANSWER: 2. **Answer 1** is incorrect because the sodium will rise another 1 or 2 points as the blood sugar returns to normal. This will *not* require aggressive treatment; 3% NaC1 at 200 mL/hr would raise sodium levels very rapidly, and could cause seizures. **Answer 2 is correct because the anion gap is closed and the glucose is close to normal. The client can be switched to subcutaneous insulin and the insulin drip discontinued. An anion gap occurs in metabolic acidosis when there is an excessive accumulation of fixed acid. Anion gap is determined by the balance between the anions (Na^+ and K^+) and the cations (Cl^- and HCO_3^-).** **Answer 3** is incorrect because the potassium level might be treated if the client were to remain on an insulin drip. The blood sugar of 170 *without* an elevated anion gap indicates that the insulin drip can be *discontinued.* **Answer 4** is incorrect because, when the dextrose is metabolized, 5% dextrose in one-quarter normal saline (D_5 ¼NS) becomes just ¼NS. This hypotonic solution will further dilute the sodium.

■ **TEST-TAKING TIP:** *First ask: Are the values within normal limits? Then, look at the impact of each option on the laboratory values. Select the option that is different from the three others ("discontinue" versus three "gives").*

Content Area: Adult Health, Endocrine; ***Integrated Process:*** Nursing Process, Implementation; ***Cognitive Level:*** Analysis; ***Client Need/Subneed:*** Physiological Integrity/Reduction of Risk Potential/Laboratory Values

89. CORRECT ANSWER: 3. **Answer 1** is incorrect because glucocorticoids facilitate calcium *excretion.* **Answer 2** is incorrect because ketones in the urine indicate *fat* is being burned. This is *not related to calcium* level. **Answer 3 is correct because most calcium is bound to plasma proteins such as albumin. As long as the physiologically important**

portion (the ionized, nonbound calcium) is normal, low total calcium does not need to be treated. **Answer 4** is incorrect because calcium levels would *fall* with administration of phosphate.

■ **TEST-TAKING TIP:** *Total serum calcium alone does not provide sufficient data. Look for an option ("check") that collects more data before treatment. Eliminate the option with "check" that is not related to calcium (Answer 2).*

Content Area: Adult Health, Fluid and Electrolyte Imbalances; ***Integrated Process:*** Nursing Process, Implementation; ***Cognitive Level:*** Application; ***Client Need/Subneed:*** Physiological Integrity/Physiological Adaptation/Fluid and Electrolyte Imbalances

90. CORRECT ANSWER: 2. **Answer 1** is incorrect because the parathyroid is responsible for calcium absorption. High calcium levels raise BP, but a postoperative complication is *hypo*calcemia. **Answer 2 is correct because the parathyroid is responsible for calcium absorption. Numbness around the mouth is an early sign of hypocalcemia.** **Answer 3** is incorrect because the parathyroid is responsible for calcium absorption. Alteration in urine output is *not* characteristic of this disorder. **Answer 4** is incorrect because the parathyroid is responsible for calcium absorption. Muscle spasms, stiffness, and tetany are signs of hypocalcemia, *not* muscle weakness.

■ **TEST-TAKING TIP:** *Know the effect of the parathyroid on calcium—***hypo***calcemia.*

Content Area: Adult Health, Endocrine; ***Integrated Process:*** Nursing Process, Assessment; ***Cognitive Level:*** Application; ***Client Need/Subneed:*** Physiological Integrity/Reduction of Risk Potential/Potential for Complications from Surgical Procedures and Health Alterations

91. CORRECT ANSWER: 2. **Answer 1** is incorrect because 5% dextrose in water (D_5W) is not an appropriate fluid for volume resuscitation. When the sugar is metabolized, all that remains is water and almost two thirds of the infused volume will transfer into cells, which will not increase circulating volume. **Answer 2 is correct because this client is in shock and requires rapid volume infusion with IV normal saline (NS).** **Answer 3** is incorrect because, while it may be useful to have a second large-bore IV, it does not take priority over *starting* IV fluids with normal saline. **Answer 4** is incorrect because, *regardless* of the anion gap, the client will need normal saline to *raise the BP.*

■ **TEST-TAKING TIP:** *This is a priority question. The client shows signs of shock. Without additional data, choose an isotonic solution.*

Content Area: Adult Health, Cardiovascular; ***Integrated Process:*** Nursing Process, Implementation; ***Cognitive Level:*** Analysis; ***Client Need/Subneed:*** Physiological Integrity/Physiological Adaptation/Medical Emergencies

92. CORRECT ANSWER: 1. Answer 1 is correct because generally low serum sodium results from excessive water intake or retention. This client has adequate fluid levels. Fluid restriction will help treat the hyponatremia. **Answer 2** is incorrect because generally low serum sodium results from excessive water intake or retention. It is correctly treated with *water restriction.* **Answer 3** is incorrect because this client does *not need fluids.* **Answer 4** is incorrect because generally low serum sodium results indicate excessive water intake or retention. It is correctly treated with water *restriction,* not fluids by IV.

■ **TEST-TAKING TIP:** *Interpret the data. Recognize the signs of fluid excess. Three of the options add sodium; only one limits fluid.*

Content Area: Adult Health, Fluid and Electrolyte Imbalances; ***Integrated Process:*** Nursing Process, Implementation; ***Cognitive Level:*** Analysis; ***Client Need/Subneed:*** Physiological Integrity/Physiological Adaptation/Fluid and Electrolyte Imbalances

93. CORRECT ANSWER: 1. Answer 1 is correct because early ambulation is the most effective way to reduce the risk of DVT. **Answer 2** is incorrect because heparin reduces the risk of DVT in clients who will be on *bedrest* after surgery. There is *no* need for this client to be on bedrest. **Answer 3** is incorrect because alternating compression leg wraps reduce the risk of DVT in clients who will be on *bedrest* after surgery. There is *no* need for this client to be on bedrest. **Answer 4** is incorrect because DVTs generally form in the *legs* of the client who is immobilized, and would *not* be affected by *wrist* surgery. In addition, the wrist will need to be *immobilized* for a period of time after this surgery, not exercised.

■ **TEST-TAKING TIP:** *K.I.S.—Keep It Simple—if the client is not on bedrest, ambulation is the best action.*

Content Area: Adult Health, Vascular; ***Integrated Process:*** Nursing Process, Planning; ***Cognitive Level:*** Application; ***Client Need/Subneed:*** Physiological Integrity/Reduction of Risk Potential

94. CORRECT ANSWER: 3. **Answer 1** is incorrect because, although the oxygen saturation is 100%, shivering does increase oxygen consumption and *supplemental* O_2 will be needed, not removed. **Answer 2** is incorrect because warm blankets need to be applied to treat the complaints and shivering *regardless* of the client's temperature. **Answer 3 is correct because shivering increases oxygen consumption. Hypothermia associated with the perioperative period may cause arrhythmia, clotting problems, and impaired wound healing.** **Answer 4** is incorrect because the pain level is *low* at 2/10 and does *not* require treatment.

■ **TEST-TAKING TIP:** *Think patient comfort. Care for the client first, and then check the temperature.*

Content Area: Geriatrics, Musculoskeletal; ***Integrated Process:*** Nursing Process, Implementation; ***Cognitive Level:*** Application; ***Client Need/Subneed:*** Physiological Integrity/Reduction of Risk Potential/Potential for Complications from Surgical Procedures and Health Alterations

95. CORRECT ANSWER: 4. **Answer 1** is incorrect because rapid heart rate is more commonly associated with *dehydration* or *hypovolemia, not* fluid overload. **Answer 2** is incorrect because pulmonary crackles that clear with deep breathing are an indication of *atelectasis, not* heart failure from volume overload. **Answer 3** is incorrect because concentrated urine is more often seen in *dehydration* as the body tries to conserve fluid, *not* in fluid overload. **Answer 4 is correct because excess fluid in the lung is decreasing oxygen transfer into the tissues.**

■ **TEST-TAKING TIP:** *Look for an option that occurs when the heart is unable to effectively pump the circulating volume.*

Content Area: Adult Health, Fluid and Electrolyte Imbalances; ***Integrated Process:*** Nursing Process, Analysis; ***Cognitive Level:*** Application; ***Client Need/Subneed:*** Physiological Integrity/Physiological Adaptation/ Fluid and Electrolyte Imbalances

96. CORRECT ANSWER: 1. Answer 1 is correct because padding is very important before surgery begins. During surgery, the client will be immobilized on a hard surface. **Answer 2** is incorrect because turning is an excellent preventative strategy in the unit, but *not* during the surgery. **Answer 3** is incorrect because range of motion prevents *contractures, not* pressure sores. In addition, ROM is not done during surgery. **Answer 4** is incorrect because an alternating pressure mattress makes the client's body move. This is not reasonable during surgery.

■ **TEST-TAKING TIP:** *Choose the one option that is different than the others (*before *surgery). Three of the options will move the client* during *surgery, which is not feasible.*

Content Area: Adult Health, Integumentary; ***Integrated Process:*** Nursing Process, Implementation; ***Cognitive Level:*** Application; ***Client Need/Subneed:*** Physiological Integrity/Reduction of Risk Potential/Potential for Complications from Surgical Procedures and Health Alterations

97. CORRECT ANSWER: 1. Answer 1 is correct because an elevated blood sugar (over 200) is associated with an increased risk of infection and poor wound healing. **Answer 2** is incorrect because clients are not placed in contact isolation to prevent infection; it is done to prevent *transmission* of a *known* infection to *other* clients. **Answer 3** is incorrect because, to minimize the risk of bacteria developing resistance to antibiotics, *preoperative* doses are given no more than 2 hours before surgery. **Answer 4** is incorrect because glucocorticoids *increase* the risk of infection by masking symptoms.

■ **TEST-TAKING TIP:** *Prevention is the goal. Choose the answer that "monitors" a key serum level. "Diabetes" in the stem goes with "blood sugar" in the correct option. Look for an option that reduces the susceptibility of the client to an infection.*

Content Area: Adult Health, Integumentary; ***Integrated Process:*** Nursing Process, Implementation; ***Cognitive Level:*** Application; ***Client Need/Subneed:*** Physiological Integrity/Reduction of Risk Potential/Potential for Complications from Surgical Procedures and Health Alterations

98. CORRECT ANSWER: 4. **Answer 1** is incorrect because blood and mucus in the stools are *not* characteristic of gallstones. **Answer 2** is incorrect because gallstones can cause pain that is usually located in the epigastrum or the *RUQ.* It may be *precipitated* by eating, not relieved by eating. **Answer 3** is incorrect because low hemoglobin is *not* a typical feature of gallstones. **Answer 4 is correct because gallstones are asymptomatic in over 80% of clients.**

■ **TEST-TAKING TIP:** *Look for a hint in the stem. The stem says "uncomplicated." Three of the options are complications.*

Content Area: Adult Health, Gastrointestinal; ***Integrated Process:*** Teaching and Learning; ***Cognitive Level:*** Application; ***Client Need/Subneed:*** Physiological Integrity/Physiological Adaptation/Pathophysiology

99. CORRECT ANSWER: 2. **Answer 1** is incorrect because any infection growing from surgery would *not* be showing up on postoperative *day 1.* This fever is from atelectasis. **Answer 2 is correct because low-grade fever on postoperative day 1 is almost always an indication of atelectasis. This low O_2 saturation supports this. Have the client take deep breaths on the incentive spirometer to open up the alveoli.** **Answer 3** is incorrect because the fever and low O_2 Sat are most likely from atelectasis, *not* dehydration. Dehydration might be reflected in the rapid heart rate, but it would be accompanied by a *lower BP.* **Answer 4** is incorrect because, when the pain level is 2/10, medications are not indicated.

■ **TEST-TAKING TIP:** *Look for the abnormal findings. The first action to take with a lower than normal O_2 saturation is deep breathing and coughing.*

Content Area: Adult Health, Respiratory; ***Integrated Process:*** Nursing Process, Implementation; ***Cognitive Level:*** Analysis; ***Client Need/Subneed:*** Physiological Integrity/Reduction of Risk Potential/Potential for Complications from Surgical Procedures and Health Alterations

100. CORRECT ANSWER: 2. **Answer 1** is incorrect because the absence of bowel sounds *is* expected on the first postoperative day. *No action* is required. **Answer 2 is correct because paralytic ileus is expected after major abdominal surgery. The absence should be recorded in the medical record.** **Answer 3** is incorrect because the absence of bowel sounds *is* expected. It does *not* indicate *impaction.* **Answer 4** is incorrect because the absence of bowels sounds *is* expected. Massage is *not* indicated.

■ **TEST-TAKING TIP:** *The key word is "expected." Select an option that is realistic 24 hours after having been NPO (no stool will have formed in this short time period) for abdominal surgery (and massage would be painful).*

Content Area: Adult Health, Gastrointestinal; ***Integrated Process:*** Nursing Process, Implementation; ***Cognitive Level:*** Application; ***Client Need/Subneed:*** Physiological Integrity/Physiological Adaptation/Alterations in Body Systems

101. **CORRECT ANSWER: 3. Answer 1** is incorrect because African Americans have a *lower* risk of gallstones than do whites or Hispanics. **Answer 2** is incorrect because *women* are two to three times more likely to develop gallstones than men. **Answer 3 is correct because rapid weight loss is a risk factor for gallstones due to bile that becomes supersaturated with cholesterol. Also, frequent changes in weight increases the risk. Answer 4** is incorrect because coffee consumption has been associated with a *lower* risk of gallstones.

■ **TEST-TAKING TIP:** *Remember the "4 Fs" of increased risk for gallbladder disease—female, fair, fat, and forty.*

Content Area: Adult Health, Gastrointestinal; ***Integrated Process:*** Teaching and Learning; ***Cognitive Level:*** Analysis; ***Client Need/Subneed:*** Physiological Integrity/Physiological Adaptation/Pathophysiology

102. **CORRECT ANSWER: 2. Answer 1** is incorrect because a stroke in the right brain would cause paralysis or weakness on the *left* side. It is not necessary to perform range of motion on the unaffected extremity. **Answer 2 is correct because a stroke in the right brain would cause paralysis or weakness on the left side. Getting out of bed is easiest on the strong side. Answer 3** is incorrect because the client should be mobile as soon as possible. It is likely that only the left leg will be paralyzed or weak, and this may be a permanent condition. A client will need to learn mobility techniques despite the weakness. **Answer 4** is incorrect because it is important to *maintain* range of motion for the joints on the affected side, rather than immobilize the left side.

■ **TEST-TAKING TIP:** *Right brain attack leads to left-sided weakness/paralysis. Nursing actions should focus on preventing problems of immobility.*

Content Area: Adult Health, Cardiovascular; ***Integrated Process:*** Nursing Process, Planning; ***Cognitive Level:*** Application; ***Client Need/Subneed:*** Physiological Integrity/Basic Care and Comfort/Mobility/Immobility

103. **CORRECT ANSWER: 4. Answer 1** is incorrect because dysphagia refers to difficulty swallowing. *Dysphasia* (impaired speech) *may* be helped by eliminating distractions when giving directions, *not* dysphag*ia.* **Answer 2** is incorrect because dysphagia refers to difficulty swallowing. Keeping the head *elevated* might help reduce risk of aspiration. **Answer 3** is incorrect because thin liquids are *more difficult* to swallow than thick liquids and pureed foods. **Answer 4 is correct because dysphagia refers to difficulty swallowing. Nutrition may need to be provided through a feeding tube to prevent aspiration.**

■ **TEST-TAKING TIP:** *Think of the Latin meaning of the problem—"dys" means "difficulty" and "phagia" means "to eat" → feed through tube.*

Content Area: Adult Health, Cardiovascular; ***Integrated Process:*** Nursing Process, Implementation; ***Cognitive Level:*** Application; ***Client Need/Subneed:*** Physiological Integrity/Physiological Adaptation/Alterations in Body Systems

104. **CORRECT ANSWER: 1. Answer 1 is correct because, in aphasia, clients have difficulty understanding and/or using language. Nonverbal communication strategies may help this. Answer 2** is incorrect because, in aphasia, clients have *difficulty* understanding and/or using language. Making the communication *more complex* with additional words is unlikely to help. **Answer 3** is incorrect because, in aphasia, clients have difficulty understanding and/or using language. They are *not hard* of *hearing.* **Answer 4** is incorrect because *dysphagia* refers to difficulty swallowing. *Dysphasia* refers to difficulty speaking. Aphasia is absence or impairment of ability to communicate through speech, writing or signs.

■ **TEST-TAKING TIP:** *Define the word—not speaking. The question asks for a way to facilitate communication for the client. Select the answers with "communication."*

Content Area: Adult Health, Sensory; ***Integrated Process:*** Nursing Process, Implementation; ***Cognitive Level:*** Comprehension; ***Client Need/Subneed:*** Physiological Integrity/Physiological Adaptation/Alterations in Body Systems

105. **CORRECT ANSWER: 3. Answer 1** is incorrect because *neither* standard nor droplet precautions require regular use of the N95 respirator. **Answer 2** is incorrect because the N95, if used, is *not shared* and is recommended for single use. **Answer 3 is correct because the N95 is recommended when treatment may produce the potential of sputum spray, such as intubation or suctioning. Only a medical-surgical mask is necessary when entering the client room. Some hospitals may provide all direct-care providers with facemasks or respirators. Answer 4** is incorrect because the N95 is intended for use when there is a *potential* for an aerosol spray of sputum.

■ **TEST-TAKING TIP:** *Key point: "potential for aerosol spray of sputum."*

Content Area: Adult Health, Infectious Disease; ***Integrated Process:*** Teaching and Learning; ***Cognitive Level:*** Application; ***Client Need/Subneed:*** Safe, Effective Care Environment/Management of Care, Supervision

CHAPTER 7

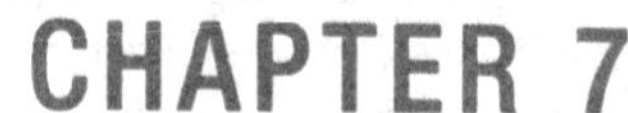

Physiological Integrity

Nursing Care of the Geriatric Client

Robyn Marchal Nelson

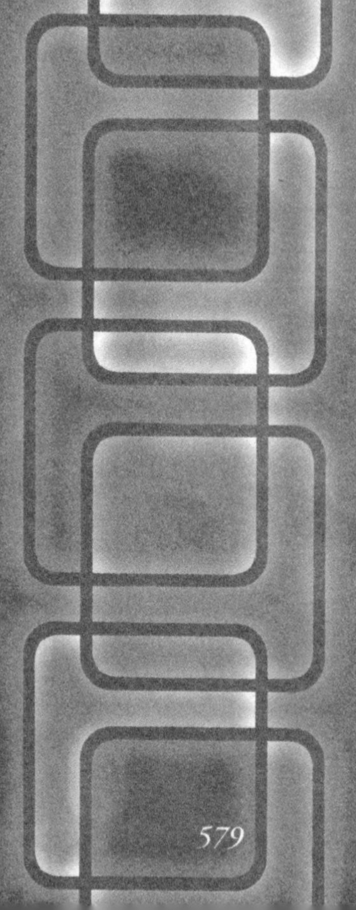

Introduction

This chapter is unique in that the primary objective is to present **practical,** concise information of **clinical** relevance for the beginning practitioner that is not covered elsewhere. The focus is on 12 significant problems and concerns associated with the older adult: *falls, use of restraints, thermoregulation, sleep disturbance, skin breakdown, polypharmacy,* specific types of *hearing changes,* age-related *macular degeneration, incontinence, sexual neglect, caregiver burden,* warning signs of *poor nutrition.*

The chapter begins with health assessment of the older adult, system by system, highlighting the most common changes associated with the aging process; it ends with several functional rating scales to assist in management of care in the home or community.

Covered elsewhere in this book are other age-relevant problems and test questions. Refer to **Chapter 10** for mental health conditions common in the older adult (e.g., *dementia, Alzheimer's disease, depression*). **Chapter 6** covers common age-relevant problems related to *immobility, bladder and bowel dysfunction, hip fracture,* use of *assistive devices,* cardiovascular conditions (*stroke, hypertension*), *cataracts,* and *glaucoma.* Also covered in **Chapter 6** are health problems that have more serious consequences in the older adult, such as *pneumonia* and *osteoporosis. Nutritional needs* of the elderly are included in **Chapter 9.**

I. HEALTH ASSESSMENT OF THE GERIATRIC CLIENT (see also **Chapter 6**)

A. *Skin:*
1. Decrease in elasticity → wrinkles and lines, dryness.
2. Loss of fullness → sagging.
3. Generalized loss of adipose and muscle tissue → wasting appearance.
4. Decrease of adipose tissue on extremities, redistributed to hips and abdomen in middle age.
5. Bony prominences become visible.
6. Excessive pigmentation → age spots.
7. Dry skin and deterioration of nerve fibers and sensory endings → pruritus.
8. Decreased blood flow → pallor and blotchiness.
9. Overgrowth of epidermal tissue → lesions (some benign, some premalignant, some malignant).

B. *Nails:*
1. Dry, brittle, peeling, ridges.
2. Increased susceptibility to fungal infections.
3. Decreased growth rate.
4. Toenails thick, difficult to cut, ingrown.

C. *Hair:*
1. Loss of pigment → graying, white.
2. Decreased density of hair follicles → thinning of hair.
3. Decreased blood flow to skin and decreased estrogen production → baldness.
   a. Hair distribution: thin on scalp, axilla, pubic area, upper and lower extremities.
   b. Decreased facial hair in *men.*
4. Decreased estrogen production → increased facial (chin, upper lip) hair in *women.*

D. *Eyes:*
1. Loss of soluble protein with loss of lens transparency → development of *cataracts.*
2. Decrease in pupil size limits amount of light entering the eye → elderly need more light to see.
3. Decreased pupil reactivity → decrease in rate of light changes to which a person can readily adapt.
4. Decreased accommodation to darkness and dim light → diminished night vision.
5. Loss of orbital fat → sunken appearance.
6. Blink reflex—slowed.
7. Eyelids—loose.
8. Visual acuity—diminished.
9. Peripheral vision—diminished.
10. Visual fields—diminished (e.g., macular degeneration).
11. Lens accommodation—decreased; requires corrective lenses.
12. *Presbyopia*—lens may lose ability to become convex enough to accommodate to nearby objects; starts at age 40 (*farsightedness*).
13. Color of iris—fades.
14. Conjunctiva—thins, looks yellow.
15. Increased intraocular pressure → *glaucoma.*
16. Previous corrective surgery.

E. *Ears:*
1. Changes in cochlea → decrease in average pitch of sound.
2. Hearing loss—greater in left ear than right; greater in *higher* frequencies than in lower.
3. Tympanic membrane—atrophied, thickened → hearing loss.
4. *Presbycusis*—progressive loss of hearing in old age.
5. Use of hearing devices.
6. Predisposed to wax buildup (cerumen).

F. *Mouth/dental health:*
1. Dental caries.
2. Poor-fitting dentures; no dentures.
3. Cancer of the mouth—increased risk.
4. Decrease in taste buds → inability to taste sweet/salty foods.
5. Olfactory bulb atrophies → decreased ability to smell due to blockage or disease of olfactory receptors in the upper sinus → decreased awareness of body odor, smoke, fumes, spoiled food.
6. Coating of tongue.

G. *Cardiovascular:*

1. Lack of elasticity of vessels → increased resistance to blood flow; decreased diameter of arteries → *increased blood pressure.*
2. Atherosclerotic and calcium plaques → *thrombosis.*
3. Valves become sclerotic, less pliable → reduced filling and emptying.
4. Diastolic murmurs heard at base of heart.
5. Loss of elasticity, decreased contractility → decreased cardiac output.
6. Changes in the coronary arteries → pooling of blood in systemic veins and shortness of breath → reduced pumping action of the heart.
7. Disturbance of the autonomic nervous system → *dysrhythmias.*
8. Extremities—arteriosclerotic changes → weaker pedal pulses, colder extremities, mottled color; pain with ambulation.

H. *Respiratory:*

1. Efficiency reduced with age.
2. Greater residual air in lungs after expiration.
3. Decreased vital capacity.
4. Weaker expiratory muscles → decreased capacity to cough → infections of lower respiratory tract.
5. Decreased ciliary activity → stasis of secretions → susceptibility to infections.
6. Oxygen debt in the muscles → dyspnea on exertion (DOE), sleep apnea due to ↓ O_2 to the brain.
7. Reduced chest wall compliance → decreased expiratory excursion, affecting inspiratory and expiratory volumes.

I. *Breasts:*

1. Atrophy.
2. Cancer risk—increased with age.

J. *Gastrointestinal:*

1. Lack of intrinsic factor → *pernicious anemia.*
2. Gastric motility—decreased → poorer, slower digestion.
3. Esophageal peristalsis—decreased.
4. Hiatal hernia—increased incidence.
5. Digestive enzymes—gradual decrease of ptyalin (which converts *starch*), pepsin and trypsin (which digest *protein*), lipase (*fat*-splitting enzyme).
6. Absorption—decreased.
7. Improper diet → constipation.
8. Decreased thirst sensation → risk for dehydration.
9. Decreased saliva → dysphagia.

K. *Endocrine:*

1. Basal metabolism rate lowered → decreased temperature.
2. Cold intolerance.
3. Women: decreased ovarian function → increased gonadotropins.
4. Decreased renal sensitivity to antidiuretic hormone (ADH) → unable to concentrate urine as effectively as younger persons.
5. Decreased clearance of blood glucose after meals → elevated postprandial blood glucose.
6. Risk of *diabetes mellitus* increases with age.

L. *Urinary:*

1. Renal function—impaired due to poor perfusion.
2. Filtration—impaired due to reduction in number of functioning nephrons → decrease in urine concentration.
3. Urgency and frequency: *men*—often due to prostatic hyperplasia; *women*—due to perineal muscle weakness.
4. Nocturia—*both* men and women.
5. Urinary tract infection (e.g., cystitis)—increased incidence.
6. Incontinence—especially with dementia; stress/exercise induced.
7. Retention—due to incomplete bladder emptying.

M. *Musculoskeletal:*

1. Muscle mass—decreased. Loss of lower limb strength.
2. Bony prominences—increased.
3. Demineralization of bone.
4. Narrowing of intervertebral space → shortening of trunk → loss of height.
5. Posture—normal; some kyphosis.
6. Range of motion—limited.
7. *Osteoarthritis*—related to extensive physical activities and joint use.
8. Gait—altered; use of cane or walker.
9. *Osteoporosis* related to menopause, immobilization, elevated levels of cortisone → increase in fractures.
10. Calcium, phosphorus, and vitamin D decreased.

N. *Neurological:*

1. Voluntary, automatic reflexes—slowed.
2. Sleep pattern—changes.
3. Mental acuity—changes.
4. Sensory interpretation and movement—changes.
5. Pain perception—diminished.
6. Dexterity and agility—lessened.
7. Reaction time—slowed.
8. Memory—past more vivid than recent memory due to loss of neurons from CNS.
9. *Depression.*
10. *Alzheimer's* disease.

O. *Sexuality:*

1. *Women:*
   a. Estrogen production—decreased with menopause.
   b. Breasts—atrophy.
   c. Vaginal secretions—reduced lubricants.
   d. Sexuality—drive continues; sexual activity declines.
2. *Men:*
   a. Testosterone production—decreased.
   b. Testes—decrease in size; decreased sperm count.
   c. Libido and sexual satisfaction—no changes.

P. *Mental status:* the **"3 Ds":**

1. *Delirium:* confusion/agitation with time and place disorientation, illusions and/or hallucinations.
2. *Dementia:* cognitive deficits (memory, reasoning, judgment).
3. *Depression:* decreased interest/pleasure in activities.

Q. *Immune system:*

1. Immune response: decreased → decreased T-cell activity and decrease in cell-mediated immunity.
2. Increased risk of nosocomial infections (e.g., *Pseudomonas,* staphylococci, enterococci, and fungi), pneumonia, cancer, reactivation of varicella-zoster virus and tuberculosis (TB).
3. Atypical inflammatory response; no elevated temperatures or white blood cell counts.

II. GENERAL NURSING DIAGNOSES IN THE GERIATRIC CLIENT

A. *Risk for loneliness* related to isolation and loss of many friends, family members, and pets due to separation and death.

B. *Self-care deficit* related to inability to complete activities of daily living.

C. *Impaired verbal communication* related to hearing loss.

D. *Fluid volume deficit* related to low fluid intake.

E. *Impaired skin integrity* related to prolonged back-lying position and inability to turn self.

F. *Body image disturbance* related to physical changes associated with the aging process.

G. *Sleep pattern disturbance* related to concern about outcomes of pending diagnostic tests.

III. PROBLEMS ASSOCIATED WITH THE GERIATRIC CLIENT*

A. *Falls:*

1. **Assessment.** *Risk factors:*
   a. Gait changes—prone to trip and stumble; do not pick feet up as high.
   b. Postural instability—tendency to lose balance; older adults take steps to correct balance and increase possibility of falling.
   c. Impaired muscular control—inability to recover from trip or unexpected step; weaker muscle cushioning and slowed righting reflexes.
   d. Deterioration of vision and hearing—impaired ability to avoid obstacles.
   e. Loss of short-term memory—prone to trip over forgotten objects.
   f. Environmental:
      (1) *Home:* unstable furniture and appliances; stairs with poor rails; throw rugs and frayed carpets; poor lighting; low beds and toilets; pets; objects on floor; medications.
      (2) *Institutions:* recent admission or transfer; furniture; slick, hard floors; unsupervised activities; mealtimes; absence of handrails; inadequate lighting, long hallways.
2. **Nursing goal/implementation:** reduce risk of falling in the older adult with *fall prevention measures.*
   a. Treat underlying condition (e.g., osteoporosis, muscle weakness, imbalance, pain).
   b. Reduce risk factors (e.g., visual problems, orthostasis).
   c. Reduce environmental hazards (e.g., provide adequate lighting and night lamps, *avoid* cluttered areas, *no* throw rugs, provide bath and shower support bars).
   d. Increase leg range-of-motion (ROM) exercises.
   e. Develop an individualized exercise plan.
   f. Support adequate nutrition (e.g., calcium intake).

B. *Use of restraints:*

1. *Definition*—any device, material, or equipment attached to the client that cannot be easily removed by the client; restricts free movement; includes leg restraints, arm restraints, hand mitts, soft ties or vests, wheelchair safety bars, "geri-chairs."
2. **Assessment** of problems resulting from use of restraints:
   a. Increased agitation, confusion.
   b. Falls.
   c. Pressure sores.
   d. Bone density loss (demineralization).
   e. Immobility hazard.
   f. Death from strangulation.
3. **Nursing goal/implementation:** provide *restraint-free care* with alternatives to restraints.
   a. *Physical:* recliners; medications for pain relief; seating adaptations (physical therapy/occupational therapy); chairs with deep seats.

**Source:* Cheryl Osborne, EdD, RN, Professor of Nursing, Director of Gerontology, California State University, Sacramento.

b. *Psychosocial:* encourage expression of feelings, giving time for client response; encourage positive self-concept; offer hope; active listening; increased or decreased sensory stimulation; increased visiting; reality orientation; clocks; animals.
c. *Activity:* structured daily routines; wandering/pacing permitted; physical exercise; nighttime activities.
d. *Environmental:* door buzzers; limb bracelet alarms; signs, call bells.
e. *Structural:* exit alarms; increased lighting; enclosed courtyards.
f. *Supervision:* family, nursing; volunteer; security.
g. Sedation.

C. *Thermoregulation*—normal oral temperature for greater than 75 years of age: oral, 96.9° to 98.3°F; rectal, 98° to 99°F. Decreased or absence of increased temperature in infection or dehydration.

1. **Assessment** of causes:
   a. Factors affecting the *hypothalmus:* decreased—muscle activity, metabolic rate, food and fluid intake, subcutaneous fat; changes in peripheral blood flow; diseases; medications.
   b. *External factors:* environmental temperature; humidity; airflow; type and amount of clothing.
2. **Nursing goal/implementation:** *prevent hypothermia and hyperthermia.*
   a. Ensure and monitor adequate fluid and food intake.
   b. Maintain constancy in environmental temperature: *avoid* drafts, overheating, prolonged exposure to cold.
   c. Monitor ventilation: provide airflow (air conditioners, fans; safe sources of heat).
   d. Use layered clothing (remove when warm; add when cold).

D. *Sleep disturbances.*

1. **Nursing goal/implementation:** promote restful sleep and *prevent sleep deprivation* with sleep care strategies.
   a. Maintain normal sleep pattern: arrange medications and therapies to minimize sleep interruptions.
   b. Encourage daytime activity; discourage daytime naps.
   c. Support bedtime routines/rituals: bedtime reading, listening to music, quiet television.
   d. Promote comfort: mattress, pillows, wrinkle-free linens, loose bed covering.
   e. Promote relaxation: warm milk or soup if not contraindicated, back rub.
   f. *Avoid*/minimize stimulation before bedtime: *no* caffeine after dinner, reduce fluid intake before sleep, refrain from smoking.

   g. *Avoid*/minimize drugs that negatively influence sleep, such as ranitidine, diltiazem, atenolol, nifedipine.
   h. Create a restful environment: turn off lights, reduce or eliminate noise, minimize disruptions for therapy or monitoring.

E. *Skin breakdown.*

1. **Assessment:**
   a. *Age-related changes:* slower rate of epidermal proliferation; thinner dermis; *decreased*—dermal blood supply, melanocytes (gray hair), moisture, sweat and sebaceous glands.
   b. Predisposing *risk factors:* exposure to ultraviolet (UV) rays (sunlight, excessive tanning); adverse medication effects; personal hygiene habits (too frequent bathing); limited activity, heredity.
   c. *Functional consequences:* dry skin; skin wrinkles; delayed wound healing; *increased*—susceptibility to burns, injury, infection, altered thermoregulation, skin cancer, cracking nails.
2. **Nursing goal/implementation:** treatment for *pressure sores.*

   Stage I—reddened broken skin: *cover* and *protect* (use sprays, gels, transparent films, transparent occlusive wafers).

   Stage II—blister or partial-thickness skin loss: *cover, protect, hydrate, insulate,* and *absorb* exudate (use transparent films, occlusive wafer dressings, calcium alginate for absorbing exudate; polyurethane foam, moistened gauze dressing).

   Stage III—full-thickness skin loss: *cover, protect, hydrate, insulate, absorb, cleanse, prevent infection,* and *promote granulation* (use occlusive wafer dressings, absorption dressing, calcium alginate, and moistened gauze dressings).

   Stage IV—full-thickness skin loss involving muscle, tendon, and bone: same as stage III except before *promoting granulation, dead eschar (tissue) is removed* (use absorption dressing, calcium alginate, and moistened gauze dressings).

F. *Polypharmacy*—concurrent use of several drugs increasing the potential for adverse reactions, drug interactions, and self-medication errors **(Table 7.1).**

1. Reasons for polypharmacy:
   a. Lack of communication among multiple health-care providers.
   b. Lack of information about over-the-counter drug use.
   c. Lack of information about client noncompliance.

Table 7.1

Medications That Should *Not* Be Used by Geriatric Clients

Medication Category	Contraindicated Medications
Antidepressants	Elavil Triavil
Cardiovascular	Aldomet Catapres Cyclospasmol Pavabid Serpasil Trental
Pain and arthritis medications	Bufferin Darvocet Darvon Feldene Talwin
Gastrointestinal	Colace Dialose-Plus Donnatal Doxidan Mylanta Surfak Tigan
Tranquilizers and hypnotics	Ativan Dalmane Halcion Librium Nembutal Restoril Valium Xanax
Neurological	Artane Cogentin

Source: Cheryl Osborne, EdD, RN, Professor of Nursing, Director of Gerontology, California State University, Sacramento.

d. Use of complementary (alternative, folk medicine) therapies and fear of telling health-care provider.
e. Assumption that, once medication is started, it should be continued indefinitely and not changed.
f. Assumption that, if there are no early side effects, there will not be any later.
g. Changes in daily habits (smoking, activity, diet/fluid intake).
h. Changes in mental-emotional status that may affect consumption patterns.
i. Changes in health status.
j. Financial limitations (drug substitution).

2. **Nursing goal/implementation:** assist the older adult to use medications safely and try **nonpharmacological interventions** for common health problems.
   a. *Constipation:* exercise, relaxation, biofeedback; increase fluid and fiber intake.
   b. *Stress incontinence:* pelvic muscle exercises, biofeedback.
   c. *Anxiety, depression:* counseling, exercise, meditation, relaxation techniques; touch, music, and pet therapy.
   d. *Arthritis:* acupuncture, heat therapy, therapeutic exercise, postural or alignment aids; touch, music, and pet therapy.
   e. *Chronic neuromuscular problems:* massage, body work, touch and music therapy.
   f. *Sleep problem* (see **D.** *Sleep disturbances*).

G. *Hearing changes*—external auditory canal atrophies, resulting in thinner walls and increased cerumen buildup; degenerative changes in ossicular joints leading to slower/stiffer movements; loss of hair cells and cochlear neurons in inner ear.

1. Types:
   a. *Presbycusis*—bilateral loss of **high-pitched** tones; slightly less severe in women than in men.
   b. *Impaired pitch discrimination*—after age 55, makes localizing and understanding sounds difficult; impaired ability to understand consonants.
   c. *Decline in speech discrimination*—after age 60, speech intelligibility declines; slowing of memory and slowing of mental processes with advancing age may also affect speech, hearing, and understanding.
   d. *Diminished vestibular function*—deficits in equilibrium and greater fall risk.
2. **Nursing goal/implementation:** *improve communication* for person who is hearing impaired.
   a. *Compensate with other senses*—face listener; make eye contact if culturally acceptable; get person's attention before talking; use touch if culturally appropriate; help with hearing aid; *avoid* walking around room while talking; write down key words if person can read.
   b. *Alter stimulus and behavior*—speak in normal volume of voice or slightly lower, *avoid* shouting; use short sentences; separate important words with pauses; allow more time for communication; have person repeat to show understanding; repeat; teach person to be more assertive about impairment.
   c. *Modify environment*—eliminate or reduce background noise (turn off running water, close doors, lower TV or radio); select areas with sound-absorbing abilities (carpets, drapes) for conversations; amplify telephone; allow for adequate light on speaker's face.

H. *Visual impairment.*

1. *Age-related macular degeneration* (AMD)—leading cause of irreversible and legal blindness for those over 65 years; blurred far and near vision; loss of central vision; difficulty going up and down steps and stairs; parts of words and letters disappear when reading; straight lines appear to be wavy. Acuity: 20/200 or less.
   a. **Assessment.** *Risk factors:* increased age, women, Caucasian, smoking, UV light exposure, diabetes, diet (low in leafy green vegetables and antioxidants).
   b. *Prevention:* UV light filters, aspirin, vitamins A and B, beta-carotene, zinc.
   c. *Prognosis:* no treatment or cure; laser may prevent spread of AMD in some clients.
   d. **Nursing goal:** assist client to maintain independent functioning.
2. See **Chapter 6** for other causes of visual problems in the older adult, such as stroke, **pp. 382–383;** glaucoma, **pp. 388–389;** cataracts, **pp. 389–390;** and diabetes, **pp. 467–470.**

I. *Loss of urinary control*—neurological mechanism controlling bladder emptying does not work effectively and results in incontinence; a symptom, *not* a diagnosis.

1. **Assessment.** *Risk factors:*
   a. Immobility.
   b. Cognitive and functional impairments—Parkinson's disease, Alzheimer's disease, multiple sclerosis, alcoholism, stroke, vitamin B deficiency, inability to walk and transfer to toilet.
   c. Medications.
   d. Institutionalization.
   e. Pathological conditions—*men:* hyperplasia leading to infection, incomplete emptying, urgency, and frequency; *women:* weakening of pelvic floor postmenopause, leading to residual urine and infection; atrophy of vaginal and trigonal tissue, leading to frequency, urgency, and incontinence.
   f. Childbirth.
2. Incontinence—possible symptom of urinary tract infection (UTI), impaction, chronic constipation, dementia, inability to walk and transfer by self to toilet, dehydration.
3. **Nursing goal/implementation:** *minimize incontinence episodes* and *reduce urinary tract infections.*
   a. Regular toileting schedule—every 2 hours, with some exceptions at night; or personalize regimen based on assessment.
   b. Modify environment—location of toilet, good lighting, prompt response to calls for assistance, use of Velcro closures on clothing, raised toilet seats with safety bars.
   c. Monitor fluid intake; adequate hydration—1 to 2 L during day; *avoid* alcohol and caffeine and restrict fluids at bedtime.
   d. *Avoid* medications contributing to incontinence.
   e. *Avoid* use of indwelling catheters if possible.
   f. Use usual undergarments; be positive about continence; use absorbent pads to improve perineal hygiene if other measures fail.
   g. Treat constipation.
   h. Observe for signs of UTI.

J. *Sexual neglect*—many myths exist about sexuality and aging.

1. *Facts* about sexuality in the older adult:
   a. Sexual desire can and does exist in advanced age.
   b. If in good health, a satisfying sex life can extend into the 80s and beyond; if sexually active in youth and middle age, vigor and interest will be retained into old age.
   c. Sexual attractiveness has little to do with age and the appearance of partner.
   d. Less than 1% of sudden coronary deaths occur during sexual intercourse; greater anxiety and tension exists if sex is restricted.
   e. Vaginal lubrication is decreased because of menopause, but sexual pleasure still exists.
   f. Sex may actually be better in later years; partners have an appreciation of intimate sharing and caring.
   g. Sexual activity is a good form of exercise and helps maintain flexibility and stamina.
   h. Older adults have a strong interest in sexual activity and physical and mental well-being; older adults should be encouraged to continue sexual interests without guilt.
   i. Male erections can continue into the 80s and beyond.
2. **Nursing goal:** assist the client to *reduce barriers* to a satisfying sexual experience.
   a. *Barriers* to a satisfying sexual experience:
      (1) Loss of sexual responsiveness—*causes:* monotony of a "same old" sexual relationship; mental or physical fatigue; overindulgence in food or drink; preoccupation with career or economic pursuits; physical or mental infirmities of either partner; performance anxiety; lack of privacy.
      (2) *Changes with aging*—hormonal; decreased muscle tone and elasticity; prostate hyperplasia; sclerosing arteries and veins; increased time needed for

arousal and rearousal; medications (e.g., antihypertensives); surgery (e.g., prostatectomy); response to menopause; availability of a partner.

K. *Caregiver burden*—80% to 90% of the care given to adults who are dependent is given by family and friends, especially middle-aged women.

1. *Negative* consequences of caregiving:
   a. Infringement on privacy.
   b. Decreased social contact.
   c. Loss of income and assets.
   d. Increased family conflict and distress.
   e. Little or no time for personal or recreational activities.
   f. Increased use of alcohol and psychotropic drugs.
   g. Changes in living arrangements (sharing households).
   h. Likelihood of decreasing or giving up job responsibilities.
   i. Increased risk of clinical depression.
   j. Feelings of anger, guilt, anxiety, grief, depression, helplessness, chronic fatigue, emotional exhaustion.
   k. Poor health and increased stress-related illness and injuries.
2. *Positive* consequences of caregiving:
   a. Family becomes closer.
   b. Making a difference in the quality of care.
   c. Companionship for adult who is dependent and caregiver.
   d. Better understanding of the needs of the adult who is dependent.
   e. Feeling useful and worthwhile.
   f. Improved relationship between caregiver and adult who is dependent.
3. Impact of hospitalization of older adult on caregiver:
   a. Frustration with delays in older adult being admitted.
   b. Perception of poor care; complaints about rudeness; upset that call lights and questions are not answered in a timely manner.
   c. Lack of involvement in decision making.
   d. Lack of preparation for discharge; too much information given too quickly; problems coordinating services (e.g., home visits, needed equipment).
   e. Fatigue/stress from going back and forth to hospital.
4. **Nursing goal/implementation:** assist the caregiver in achieving control and a sense of satisfaction.
   a. Strategies to minimize caregiver burden:
      (1) Develop and maintain a routine.
      (2) Concentrate on the present.
      (3) Talk about the reasons for being a caregiver.
      (4) Use respite care as needed.

L. *Poor nutrition.*

1. **Assessment** of warning signs:
   a. Disease, illness, or chronic condition that changes eating habits/pattern; also emotional problems: confusion, depression, or sadness.
   b. Eating too little or too much, skipping meals, drinking more than 1 to 2 alcoholic beverages daily.
   c. Missing, loose, or rotten teeth, or ill-fitting dentures.
   d. Spending less than 25 to 30 dollars per week on food.
   e. Living alone.
   f. Taking multiple medications with increased chance for side effects (change in taste, constipation, weakness, drowsiness, diarrhea, nausea).
   g. Unplanned weight loss or gain.
   h. Problems with self-care (walking, shopping, buying and preparing food).
   i. Age greater than 80 (frail elderly).
2. **Nursing goal/implementation:** promote optimal nutritional health for the older adult (see **Chapter 9** for additional information on nutrition in the older adult).
   a. Encourage fluids during meals.
   b. 5 to 6 small meals per day.
   c. Advise *not* to lie down for 1 hour after a meal.
   d. *Avoid* overuse of salt and sweets.
   e. Use alternate seasonings: herbs, garlic, lemon.

M. See **Chapter 10** for discussion of *depression, elder abuse,* and causes of *impaired cognition,* such as dementia, Alzheimer's disease, and delirium.

N. See **Chapter 6** for discussion of *osteoarthritis* and *Parkinson's disease.*

IV. SUMMARY OF MOST FREQUENT ISSUES IN THE CARE OF THE OLDER GERIATRIC CLIENT **(Table 7.2)**

V. Use the *functional rating scale for the geriatric client* **(Table 7.3)** to rate social resources, economic resources, mental health, physical health, and activities of daily living.

VI. Use the *functional screening examination* **(Table 7.4)** to help determine dependent/independent status for planning home care.

Table 7.2

Most Frequent Issues in the Care of the Geriatric Client

Complication	Cause
Loss of functional independence	Immobility, lack of time to perform task, lack of expectations by staff or family
Falling	Postural hypotension, dizziness, medication effects, unfamiliar surroundings
Confusion	Drug effects, unfamiliar environment, sensory deficits
Skin breakdown	Immobility, skin changes with aging, inadequate turning
Incontinence	Cognitive changes, inability to access toilet, need for assistance, loss of sphincter muscle control
Constipation	Drug effects, inactivity, dietary changes, changes in GI motility
Heatstroke	Altered thermoregulation response
Hypothermia	Loss of subcutaneous tissue → decreased insulation
Self-injury	Reduced tactile sensation

Source: Cheryl Osborne, EdD, RN, Professor of Nursing, Director of Gerontology, California State University, Sacramento.

Table 7.3

Functional Rating Scale for the Geriatric Client

Social Resources Rating Scale

Rate the current social resources of the person being evaluated along the six-point scale presented below. Circle the *one* number that best describes the person's present circumstances.

1. **Excellent social resources.** Social relationships are *very* satisfying and extensive; at least one person would take care of him or her indefinitely.
2. **Good social resources.** Social relationships are *fairly* satisfying and adequate, and at least one person would take care of him or her indefinitely; *or* social relationships are *very satisfying* and *extensive,* and only short-term help is available.
3. **Mildly socially impaired.** Social relationships are *unsatisfactory,* of poor quality, few, but at least one person would take care of him or her indefinitely; *or* social relationships are *fairly* satisfactory, adequate, and only short-term help is available.
4. **Moderately socially impaired.** Social relationships are *unsatisfactory,* of poor quality; few, and only short-term care is available; *or* social relationships are at least adequate or satisfactory; but help would only be available now and then.
5. **Severely socially impaired.** Social relationships are of *poor* quality, few; and help would only be available *now* and *then; or* social relationships are at least satisfactory or adequate; but help is *not* even available now and then.
6. **Totally socially impaired.** Social relationships are *unsatisfactory,* of poor quality, few, and help is *not* even available now and then.

Economic Resources Rating Scale

Rate the current economic resources of the person being evaluated along the six-point scale presented below. Circle the *one* number that best describes the person's present circumstances.

1. **Economic resources are excellent.** Income is *ample* and person has reserves.
2. **Economic resources are satisfactory.** Income is ample but person has *no* reserves; *or* income is adequate and person has reserves.
3. **Economic resources are mildly impaired.** Income is adequate but person has *no* reserves; *or* income is somewhat *inadequate* but person has reserves.
4. **Economic resources are moderately impaired.** Income is *somewhat* inadequate and person has *no* reserves.
5. **Economic resources are severely impaired.** Income is *totally* inadequate and person *may* **or** *may not* have reserves.
6. **Economic resources are completely impaired.** Person is *destitute,* completely *without* income or reserves.

Mental Health Rating Scale

Rate the current mental functioning of the person being evaluated along the six-point scale presented below. Circle the *one* number that best describes the person's present functioning.

1. **Outstanding mental health.** Intellectually alert and clearly *enjoying* life. Manages routine and major problems with *ease* and is free from any psychiatric symptoms.
2. **Good mental health.** Handles both routine and major problems *satisfactorily* and is intellectually intact and free of psychiatric symptoms.
3. **Mildly mentally impaired.** Has *mild* psychiatric symptoms and/or mild intellectual impairment. Continues to handle routine, though **not major,** problems satisfactorily.
4. **Moderately mentally impaired.** Has *definite* psychiatric symptoms and/or *moderate* intellectual impairment. Able to make routine commonsense decisions, but **unable** to handle major problems.

Continued

Table 7.3

Functional Rating Scale for the Geriatric Client—cont'd

5. **Severely mentally impaired.** Has *severe* psychiatric symptoms and/or severe intellectual impairment that *interferes* with routine judgments and decision making in everyday life.
6. **Completely mentally impaired.** *Grossly* psychotic or *completely* impaired intellectually. Requires either intermittent or constant *supervision* because of clearly abnormal or potentially harmful behavior.

Physical Health Rating Scale

Rate the current physical functioning of the person being evaluated along the six-point scale presented below. Circle the *one* number that best describes the person's present functioning.

1. **In excellent physical health.** Engages in *vigorous* physical activity, either *regularly* or at least from time to time.
2. **In good physical health.** *No* significant illnesses or disabilities. Only *routine* medical care such as annual checkups required.
3. **Mildly physically impaired.** Has only *minor* illnesses and/or disabilities that might benefit from medical treatment or corrective measures.
4. **Moderately physically impaired.** Has *one or more* diseases or disabilities that are either *painful* or require *substantial medical treatment.*
5. **Severely physically impaired.** Has one or more illnesses or disabilities that are either *severely painful* or *life-threatening* or require *extensive* medical treatment.
6. **Totally physically impaired.** Confined to *bed* and requires *full-time* medical assistance or nursing care to maintain vital bodily functions.

Performance Rating Scale For Activities of Daily Living (ADL)

Rate the current performance of the person being evaluated on the six-point scale presented below. Circle the *one* number that best describes the person's present performance.

1. **Excellent ADL capacity.** Can perform all ADL without assistance and with *ease.*
2. **Good ADL capacity.** Can perform all ADL *without assistance.*
3. **Mildly impaired ADL capacity.** Can perform *all but one to three* ADL. *Some* help is required with one to three, but not necessarily every day. Can get through any single day without help. Is able to prepare own meals.
4. **Moderately impaired ADL capacity.** *Regularly* requires assistance with *at least four ADL* but is able to get through any single day without help; *or regularly* requires help with meal preparation.
5. **Severely impaired ADL capacity.** Requires help *each day* but not necessarily throughout the day or night with *many* ADL.
6. **Completely impaired ADL capacity.** Requires help *throughout* the day and/or night to carry out ADL.

Summary of Ratings:		Projected Outcome
Social resources	______	>15— Requires help
Economic resources	______	12–15—Intermediate supports
Mental health	______	<11— Independent living
Physical health	______	
Activities of daily living	______	
Cumulative impairment score (sum of the five ratings)	______	

Source: Adapted from University of California Davis Medical Center, Alzheimer's Center, Sacramento, California.

Table 7.4

Functional Screening Examination

Test Request	Function Tested	Able, Normal	Limited but Able	Unable
Put both hands together, behind your head	Shoulder external rotation, flexion, abduction; elbow flexion; wrist extension; gross strength (managing clothing, hair combing, washing back)	☐	☐	☐
Put both hands together, behind your back	Shoulder internal rotation, adduction; elbow flexion; gross strength (managing clothing, washing lower back)	☐	☐	☐
Sitting, touch great toe with opposite hand	Back, hip, knee flexion, gross strength, balance (lower extremity dressing and hygiene)	☐	☐	☐
Squeeze my two fingers, each hand	Grasp; approximately 20-lb grasp needed for functional activities (e.g., holding a pan)	☐	☐	☐

Table 7.4

Functional Screening Examination—cont'd

Test Request	Function Tested	Able, Normal	Limited but Able	Unable
Hold paper between thumb and lateral side of index finger (while examiner tries to pull it out)	Pinch; approximately 3-lb grip needed for functional activities (e.g., turning a key)	☐	☐	☐
Show me your medicines	Cognition; knowledge; visual acuity, hand function; compliance; polypharmacy; effective management of health problems; access to health care; support system; finances; polyproviders	☐	☐	☐
Get up from the chair without using your hands, walk 10 ft down hall, turn around, stand with your eyes closed (examiner nudges to determine balance), sit down without using hands	Hip strength; gait, symmetry in posture velocity, step height; balance, ability to withstand sudden changes in position; fall risk; cardiovascular and pulmonary status; transfer ability; motion; fear of falls; judgment and cognition; environmental awareness; need for assistance/equipment; flexibility; endurance; ability to walk and function at home	☐	☐	☐
Take off your shoes and socks	Balance; fine motor skills; dexterity; hearing and receptive language; visual acuity; judgment; registration and attention span; low back flexibility and mobility; weight shifting; safety and adequacy of footware; social support if nails are cut by someone else; pain and comfort on movement	☐	☐	☐
Observe a meal being prepared/eaten	Nutritional intake; intactness of reflexes; use of utensils; hand/oral motor function; sequencing skills, visual acuity; use of utensils and equipment; ability to get needed help; ability to handle food and liquid; ability to compensate for limitations	☐	☐	☐

Summary and conclusions:

Source: Dr. Cheryl Osborne, EdD, RN, Professor of Nursing, Director of Gerontology, California State University, Sacramento.

NOTE: *Totally independent*—total score of 9 in **Able** or **Limited** columns; *dependent* > 1 in **Unable** column.

Questions

Select the one answer that is best for each question, unless otherwise directed.

1. The nurse should ensure that a healthy 89-year-old client admitted to a skilled nursing facility has received which vaccinations? *Select all that apply.*
   1. Pneumococcal.
   2. Hepatitis B (series of 3).
   3. Tetanus.
   4. Influenza.
   5. Meningococcal.
   6. Zoster.
   7. Diphtheria.

2. An elderly client has a noncemented total hip joint placed. Postoperative activity for this client should include:
   1. Bedrest for 6 weeks with continuous passive motion.
   2. Touch-down weight-bearing starting first postoperative day.
   3. Head of bed flat for 48 hours.
   4. Hip immobilization for 3 to 4 weeks with no weight-bearing.

3. A client with Alzheimer's disease has superficial skin breakdown related to functional incontinence. The correct nursing intervention includes:
   1. Inserting a continuous indwelling catheter per order.
   2. Assisting to the toilet and protecting bed with pads.
   3. Limiting oral fluid intake to 250 mL/day.
   4. Administering a loop diuretic, such as furosemide, as ordered.

4. An elderly client, who has had a stroke, is receiving full-strength tube feedings of 75 mL/hr, and an IV of D_5 ½NS at 50 mL/hr. The Na^+ level is 150. Which action should be taken by a nurse?
   1. The IV should be changed to a higher Na^+ content such as D_5NS.
   2. The rate of the IV should be slowed.
   3. Tap water should be given through the feeding tube.
   4. A diuretic should be given.

5. An elderly client with kidney disease is admitted with dementia. The laboratory values are: Ca^{++} at 7 mg/dL, PO_4 at 7 mg/dL, albumin at 2 gm, creatinine at 8 mg/dL. The laboratory findings indicate:
   1. Elevated phosphates from kidney failure.
   2. High risk for seizures from low Ca^{++}. Treatment is a priority.
   3. Need for dialysis to raise phosphate level.
   4. Need for a diet high in dairy to increase albumin.

6. An elderly client continues to have fecal incontinence with 6 to 7 small brown liquid stools each day. The client eats a soft diet and does not receive any stool softeners or laxatives. The client's primary form of activity is sitting in the wheelchair for 2 hours twice a day. What is the correct explanation for the frequent diarrhea stools?
   1. Inadequate roughage in the diet.
   2. Inactivity from sedentary lifestyle.
   3. Gastrointestinal virus.
   4. Fecal impaction.

7. An elderly client has a suspected medical diagnosis of cataracts. Which symptom is consistent with this finding?
   1. Objects are distorted and blurry.
   2. Vision is improved in bright lights.
   3. Objects have a halo around them.
   4. Single objects seem to be doubled.

8. What is the most appropriate footwear that a nurse should recommend to a client with Parkinson's disease?
   1. Open-toed sandals.
   2. Double-knotted leather wing tips.
   3. High-top sneakers.
   4. Slip-on rubber soles.

9. What are normal changes associated with aging? *Select all that apply.*
   1. Decreased salivation.
   2. Decreased ability to hear low-frequency sounds.
   3. Impaired healing of tissues.
   4. Multiple nighttime voiding.
   5. Increased sensitivity to pain.
   6. Higher than normal baseline body temperature.

10. An RN makes a home visit to a client who is 62 years old, and finds that the client is not responding to verbal stimuli and has no pulse or respirations, and the skin is cool to touch. The nurse's *first* action should be to:
    1. Do mouth-to-mouth resuscitation, 2 breaths.
    2. Do chest compression.
    3. Call emergency response (911).
    4. Call the family first.

11. In reviewing the laboratory and x-ray reports of an elderly client, which findings should a nurse identify as being consistent with a diagnosis of emphysema?
    1. Increased Pco_2, hypoinflated alveoli, and decreased Po_2.
    2. Decreased Pco_2, decreased Po_2, and decreased hematocrit.
    3. Increased Pco_2, hyperinflated alveoli, and decreased hematocrit.
    4. Increased Pco_2, increased hematocrit, and hyperinflated alveoli.

12. When a nurse shines a penlight into an elderly client's eyes to check pupil reaction, the nurse notes that one of the eyes is very cloudy and the pupil does not react. The nurse should:
    1. Check vision in the cloudy eye.
    2. Notify the MD for CT evaluation.
    3. Keep the room lights dim.
    4. Restrict dietary protein.

QUESTIONS

13. An elderly client with a history of congestive heart failure (CHF) and hypertension (HTN) had a hip prosthesis inserted. Blood pressure is 80/50 mm Hg; heart rate is 80; urine output is 15 mL during the last hour. The most appropriate nursing action would be to:
   1. Document these findings and continue to monitor vital signs.
   2. Give NS 250 mL over 15 minutes, check vital signs (VS) and lung sounds.
   3. Check Na^+ and K^+ levels before selecting IV fluids.
   4. Give 1 L lactated Ringer's as fast as possible, then check VS, neck circumference, and lab reports.

14. Following general anesthesia for a hip replacement, an elderly client's vital signs are: P: 80, R: 14, BP 110/78 mm Hg; O_2 saturation is 100% on 40% mask; and pain is 2/10. The client is shivering and complains of being cold. The *first* nursing priority should be to:
   1. Remove the oxygen.
   2. Check the temperature.
   3. Apply warm blankets.
   4. Give pain medication.

15. A 78-year-old client with CHF is being discharged home where his wife, who has chronic obstructive pulmonary disease (COPD), plans to care for him. The wife indicates that the family will help. The correct action by a nurse would be to:
   1. Recommend a nursing home placement for the couple.
   2. Contact a health-care practitioner to determine if the wife is able to provide care.
   3. Determine if the family members will help.
   4. Offer to make referrals for community resources to assist the couple.

16. A client with age-related hearing loss is complaining to a nurse about being frustrated with hearing difficulties. Which sound is most difficult for the client to hear?
   1. Recording of a march played softly.
   2. Young children talking.
   3. Motorcycle on the street.
   4. A man's voice in an elevator.

17. Which conditions increase the risk of the older adult client developing a decubitus ulcer? *Select all that apply.*
   1. Osteoarthritis.
   2. Impaired circulation.
   3. Incontinence.
   4. Malnutrition.
   5. Excessive sun exposure.

18. An older client complains of colored rings around the lightbulbs in the room. The correct response by a nurse would be:
   1. "Is there a history of cataracts in your family?"
   2. "I don't see any colored rings in the lightbulbs."
   3. "Have you had your eyes checked for glaucoma?"
   4. "Have you fallen recently and hit your head?"

19. Which condition is most likely to cause chronic pain in an older adult?
   1. Osteoarthritis.
   2. An old fracture.
   3. Sinus headaches.
   4. Peripheral neuropathy.

20. The care plan for an older adult with asthma, chronic obstructive pulmonary disease (COPD), and chronic anxiety should include:
   Select all that apply.
   1. Inhalation therapy and instruction about methods of conserving energy.
   2. An exercise program to increase the vital capacity of the lungs.
   3. Respiratory exercises with emphasis on forced inhalation.
   4. Oxygen therapy at 4 L/min as needed, and deep breathing for relaxation.
   5. Teaching the use of the diaphragm to improve breathing.

21. Which sign/symptom in an older adult is most indicative of a urinary tract infection?
   1. Confusion.
   2. Painful urination.
   3. Fever above 102°F.
   4. Urinary frequency.

22. A nurse should include the risk of developing vaginitis when teaching an older adult woman about:
   1. Anticoagulation therapy.
   2. Resuming sexual activity.
   3. Effects of poor nutrition.
   4. Prolonged antibiotic therapy.

23. An elderly client, who underwent a total hip replacement 3 days ago, asks why "crossing my legs" is prohibited. The correct response by a nurse is based on the knowledge that:
   1. Abduction can cause dislocation of the prosthesis.
   2. Adduction can cause dislocation of the prosthesis.
   3. Pressure on arteries in the legs can cause blood clots.
   4. Avoiding acute flexion of the hip prevents contractures.

24. An older adult with osteoarthritis reports pain, stiffness, and deformities of the fingers. Which nursing actions would be appropriate? *Select all that apply.*
   1. Application of cold packs.
   2. Teaching hand exercises.
   3. Scheduling meditation therapy.
   4. Giving prescribed vitamin therapy.
   5. Limiting use of affected hand to minimize pain.

25. Which older adult client is at greatest risk of developing hypothermia?
   1. A client with a sedentary lifestyle.
   2. A client who is shivering.
   3. A client who complains of being cold.
   4. A client with increased body fat.

26. A nurse is teaching an elderly client with right hemiplegia and severe speech impairment how to dress. An appropriate *first step* in the teaching would be to:
1. Ask the client to put on a shirt.
2. Demonstrate the correct way to put on a shirt.
3. Explain the difficulties in putting on a shirt.
4. Give verbal instructions on dressing techniques.

27. To prevent injury, a nurse should advise an older adult who is taking tricyclic antidepressants to:
1. Eat a diet high in roughage.
2. Get an additional night-light.
3. Provide lubrication for the oral mucosa.
4. Stand up slowly from sitting or lying positions.

28. A nurse should monitor an older adult more closely for adverse reactions to medications if the client history includes:
1. CHF and COPD.
2. Colitis and polycythemia vera.
3. Hepatitis and glomerulonephritis.
4. Diabetes and cholecystitis.

29. After reviewing an older adult client's history, a nurse should include teaching about fall prevention if the client has been taking:
1. Diphenhydramine (Benadryl).
2. Ferrous sulfate.
3. Guaifenesin (Robitussin)
4. Loratidine (Claritin)

30. While waiting to be seen in an emergency department (ED) for possible CHF, an elderly client with moderate dementia jumps up and says, "I have to go feed my chickens now." A triage nurse's most appropriate response is:
1. "All right, you may leave."
2. "Please tell us about your chickens."
3. "That noise was the TV, not chickens."
4. "You are not on the farm anymore."

31. To improve an older adult's sense of security, a nurse should:
1. Focus on increasing socialization skills in the client.
2. Connect the past with the future through pictures.
3. Provide praise and recognition for past accomplishments.
4. Review comforting memories using reminiscence.

32. A healthy, older adult client complains of dry, itchy skin. The correct response by the nurse is:
1. "Avoid scratching the skin to minimize the risk of infection."
2. "Drink fluids and shower instead of taking a bath."
3. "Take fewer baths, use soap sparingly, and apply lotion afterward."
4. "Wear cotton clothing and use a hypoallergenic soap."

33. A 90-year-old client's condition is one of lethargy, poor capillary perfusion, and urinary incontinence. These findings should indicate to a nurse that this client is at greatest risk for:
1. Aspiration.
2. Contractures.
3. Dehydration.
4. Skin breakdown.

34. An 80-year-old client complains of sleeping less and awakens several times during the night. The client takes acetaminophen at bedtime and does not drink caffeine. Which response by a nurse is most appropriate?
1. Tell the client to eliminate fluids after 6:00 p.m.
2. Recommend that the client go to bed 1 hour earlier.
3. Recommend a sleep study to diagnose sleep apnea.
4. Tell the client that the sleeping pattern is a normal age-related change.

35. Assessment of an older adult with pneumonia will often reveal:
Select all that apply.
1. Anorexia and changes in behavior.
2. Headache and difficulty breathing.
3. Muscle aches and fever.
4. Nonproductive cough and chest pain.
5. Afebrile and productive cough.

36. A 73-year-old client is admitted for rehabilitation after a mild stroke. The client complains of not feeling rested, begins to nap during the day, and sleeps only 4 to 5 hours nightly. The most appropriate nursing action is to:
1. Assess the client's sleep-wake cycle to determine necessary interventions.
2. Do nothing as the sleep pattern is associated with normal aging.
3. Determine if the client takes a medication for sleep at bedtime and request an order.
4. Relocate the client to a different room that is quieter.

37. An 87-year-old man, who has been living independently, is entering a nursing home. To help him adjust, the most effective action is to:
1. Involve him in as many activities as possible so he can meet other residents.
2. Move him as quickly as possible so that he does not have time to think.
3. Restrict family visits for the first 2 weeks to give him time to adjust.
4. Suggest that he bring his favorite things from home to make his room seem familiar.

38. When preparing to perform discharge teaching with an older adult client, which nursing actions will facilitate learning? *Select all that apply.*
1. Involving family members in the teaching sessions.
2. Keeping the pace slow, presenting a small amount of material at a time.

3. Using repetition as well as providing reinforcement, such as written material.
4. Providing ample opportunity for repeated practice sessions.
5. Scheduling a group session with other clients.

39. In preparing a health education presentation for older adults, a nurse should keep in mind that:
  1. Older adults generally prefer group teaching.
  2. Older adult learners need more than a single teaching session.
  3. Presentations should use more written materials than lectures.
  4. Videotapes and pamphlets ensure teaching effectiveness.

40. Which statement by the family caregiver of an older woman with incontinence requires teaching by a nurse?
  1. "It is too bad incontinence occurs with aging."
  2. "Incontinence has been so embarrassing for my mother."
  3. "Mother says her incontinence is related to the number of children she had."
  4. "I am relieved to know Mother's incontinence may be reversible."

41. A 63-year-old client is returning home after being hospitalized for injuries received during a home invasion and robbery. Although neighborhood robberies are rampant, the client has lived in the same house for 50 years and does not want to move. The client receives a monthly social security check in the mail. The most appropriate action by a home health nurse would be to:
Select all that apply.
  1. Advise the client to arrange for someone to visit regularly or move into the home.
  2. Advise the client to have the social security check deposited directly to the bank.
  3. Suggest the client get a dog.
  4. Advise the client to get a locking mail box to prevent mail theft.
  5. Take no action since the client has a right to autonomy.

42. A nurse in a senior adult day care program observes that the participants have long toenails, corns, calluses, and other problems indicating a need for foot care. What is a nurse's correct action?
  1. Schedule podiatry services at the site after a class on foot care.
  2. Establish a regular foot care plan whereby the participants' toenails would be cut and corns and calluses removed.
  3. Instruct family members in the proper methods of cutting toenails and using commercial foot care products.
  4. Recommend that the participants soak their feet for 10 minutes before cutting their toenails, using safe toenail clippers.

43. The incidence of tuberculosis in the older adult is significantly increased among individuals who:
  1. Are physically inactive.
  2. Are cigarette smokers.
  3. Have received the bacille Calmette-Guérin (BCG) vaccine.
  4. Reside in institutions.

44. The daughter of a client with Alzheimer's disease becomes frustrated when talking to her father. What should a nurse suggest to improve communication?
  1. Answer his questions simply even if the question is asked repeatedly.
  2. Finish his sentences before he becomes agitated.
  3. Focus the conversation on future events.
  4. Play word games to stimulate his mind and slow progression of the disease.

45. Which suggestion would be most accurate for a nurse to make to the family of a client who has Alzheimer's disease?
  1. Be sure to correct the client if the client is experiencing delusions.
  2. Avoid getting upset in front of the client.
  3. Repeat requests to the client in order to increase compliance.
  4. Activities should be done quickly to reduce client anxiety.

46. A family member asks a nurse about possible treatments for Stage III Alzheimer's disease (AD). Which statement by the nurse is correct?
  1. High doses of vitamin E may slow disease progression.
  2. The benefits of NSAIDs have been proven.
  3. The risks of herbals, such as ginkgo biloba, are greater than any benefit.
  4. Recent research has shown hormone replacement improves cognition.

47. Which assessment findings are consistent with a diagnosis of Alzheimer's disease (AD)? *Select all that apply.*
  1. Remote and recent memory impairment.
  2. No memory impairment but the client is unable to recognize familiar persons.
  3. Cognitive decline has been rapid.
  4. B_{12} deficiency or thyroid disease is often present.
  5. Impaired recall of words.
  6. Loss of ability to recognize objects.

48. A 76-year-old client with hypertension, type 2 diabetes, and a known allergy to seafood is scheduled for a cardiac catheterization. Which orders should a nurse recognize as appropriate for this client? *Select all that apply.*
  1. Administration of methylprednisolone (Solu-Medrol).
  2. Draw blood for a liver panel.
  3. Draw blood for a renal panel.
  4. Start NS IV at 125 mL/hr.
  5. Hold metformin (Glucophage).

49. A home health nurse is visiting an older client. The client asks the nurse about splitting the simvastatin tablet that has been ordered. Which response should client teaching include?

1. All medications can be split safely.
2. Let the pharmacy split an extended-release tablet.
3. Wash and dry the tablet-splitting device after each use.
4. If the drug is enteric-coated, splitting changes the therapeutic response.

50. A home health nurse is making a follow-up visit to an older adult following discharge from a hospital. Which action by the nurse is *most important* regarding medication administration in the home setting?

1. Give the ordered medication during the visit.
2. Provide comprehensive teaching.
3. Count the number of pills remaining.
4. Prepare a list of medications for client.

Answers/Rationales/Tips

1. CORRECT ANSWERS: 1, 3, 4, 6. **Answer 1 is correct because *pneumococcus* is an important cause of pneumonia in the elderly. Clients who were vaccinated more than 5 years previously or who were under 65 years old when they received the vaccination should receive a booster.** **Answer 2** is incorrect because, unless there are clients with developmental disabilities residing at the skilled nursing facility, vaccination of residents is not necessary. **Answer 3 is correct because fewer than 100 people per year become infected with tetanus in the United States, thanks to the efficiency of this vaccine. The wounds that become infected are often "inconsequential," such as pricking your finger on a rosebush thorn. Boosters are required every 10 years. Answer 4 is correct because influenza virus is an important cause of morbidity and mortality in the elderly. Although the vaccine does not always prevent disease, it lessens the severity of disease that does occur. Frequent mutation of the virus necessitates a new vaccination each year preceding or during the flu season.** **Answer 5** is incorrect because a skilled nursing facility is not considered a high-risk setting for contracting meningococcal infections. **Answer 6 is correct because varicella vaccination should be administered once, to reduce the incidence of shingles.** **Answer 7** is incorrect because, although a skilled nursing facility in the United States is an unlikely place to contract diphtheria, the product most often used to provide tetanus contains different vaccines as well (Td—tetanus/diphtheria).

■ **TEST-TAKING TIP:** *Know the high-risk groups for each virus and the effect of aging.*

Content Area: Geriatrics, Immunological; ***Integrated Process:*** Nursing Process, Analysis; ***Cognitive Level:*** Application; ***Client Need/Subneed:*** Health Promotion and Maintenance/ Immunizations

2. CORRECT ANSWER: 2. **Answer 1** is incorrect because, as long as bones and joints are stabilized, ambulation with weight-bearing improves healing. Prolonged bedrest is associated with many damaging complications, including deep vein thrombosis, pressure ulcers, and pneumonia. Continuous passive motion maintains range of motion, but does not protect from other complications of immobility. **Answer 2 is correct because early mobilization improves healing and reduces complications resulting from immobility. Because the joint is not cemented, surgeons often request less than full weight-bearing for initial mobilization.** **Answer 3** is incorrect because modern surgical procedures for hip replacement minimize damage to surrounding soft tissues; therefore, the head of the bed *can be elevated* with all surgical approaches. **Answer 4** is incorrect because immobilization of the hip is not necessary and would result in complications of immobility. Weight-bearing, as long as the joint is stable, improves healing.

■ **TEST-TAKING TIP:** *The question asks for an "activity." Only one option describes a mobility activity.*

Content Area: Geriatrics, Musculoskeletal; ***Integrated Process:*** Nursing Process, Planning; ***Cognitive Level:*** Application; ***Client Need/Subneed:*** Physiological Integrity/Basic Care and Comfort/Mobility/Immobility

3. CORRECT ANSWER: 2. **Answer 1** is incorrect because indwelling catheters are associated with a risk for infection, and should not be used as a nursing convenience. **Answer 2 is correct because, in functional incontinence, as in Alzheimer's disease, the client is usually unable to perform self-care because of alteration in mental status. Assisting the client to use a toilet and cleaning after any incontinence are appropriate.** **Answer 3** is incorrect because this severe fluid restriction would dehydrate the client and is inappropriate. **Answer 4** is incorrect because diuretics are appropriate for clients whose cardiorenal function is compromised. There is no evidence here to support use of this drug.

■ **TEST-TAKING TIP:** *Choose the option that supports normal functioning (toileting). Three of the choices alter intake or normal output.*

Content Area: Geriatrics, Integumentary; ***Integrated Process:*** Nursing Process, Implementation; ***Cognitive Level:*** Comprehension; ***Client Need/Subneed:*** Physiological Integrity/Basic Care and Comfort/Elimination

4. CORRECT ANSWER: 3. **Answer 1** is incorrect because the serum sodium is high. The client needs relatively more water and *less sodium*. **Answer 2** is incorrect because slowing the IV rate would contribute to *dehydration* and raise the serum sodium *further*. **Answer 3 is correct because hypernatremia can result from the solute load in tube feedings. Additionally, the IV contains normal saline, which could be removed. The client needs free water to dilute**

ANSWERS

the sodium level down. The enteral route is appropriate for this delivery. Answer 4 is incorrect because a diuretic would contribute to *dehydration* and raise the serum sodium *further.*

■ TEST-TAKING TIP: *Eliminate the two answers that focus on the IV (Answers 1 and 2). Recognize the* effects of tube feedings *on fluid and electrolyte levels.*

Content Area: Geriatrics, Fluid and Electrolyte Imbalances; *Integrated Process:* Nursing Process, Implementation; *Cognitive Level:* Application; *Client Need/Subneed:* Physiological Integrity/Pharmacological and Parenteral Therapies/Parenteral/Intravenous Therapies

5. CORRECT ANSWER: 1. **Answer 1 is correct because the kidneys normally excrete phosphate, which is usually maintained at a level of 2.5 to 4.5 mg/dL in adults (up to 6 mg/dL in infants and children). A low total calcium in the presence of low albumin is expected in kidney failure. Physiologically important nonbound calcium is likely to be normal so that seizure risk is not elevated.** Answer 2 is incorrect because the significance of low total serum calcium must be interpreted with consideration of the low albumin that is seen with kidney failure. Less than 50% of the plasma calcium is bound to serum protein, primarily albumin. Risk for seizures is *not increased.* Answer 3 is incorrect because the phosphate level *is already elevated.* Dialysis might be used to *bring it down.* Answer 4 is incorrect because a diet high in dairy products contains *too much* phosphate to be consumed by clients with kidney disease.

■ TEST-TAKING TIP: *Focus on the elevated phosphate level. Know the normal ranges of laboratory tests in order to recognize levels that place the client at risk.*

Content Area: Geriatrics, Renal; *Integrated Process:* Nursing Process, Analysis; *Cognitive Level:* Analysis; *Client Need/Subneed:* Physiological Integrity/Physiological Adaptation/Fluid and Electrolyte Imbalances

6. CORRECT ANSWER: 4. Answer 1 is incorrect because inadequate roughage would *not cause* diarrhea. Fecal impaction is likely causing the diarrhea. Fiber can be added to a soft diet to prevent constipation. Answer 2 is incorrect because the inactivity *contributes* to the potential for constipation and fecal impaction, but the *impaction is causing* the liquid stools. Answer 3 is incorrect because this client is more at risk to develop constipation and fecal impaction, not a GI virus. **Answer 4 is correct because the client is at risk to develop fecal impaction secondary to constipation. Pressure on the colonic mucosa causes seepage of liquid stool around the area of impaction.**

■ TEST-TAKING TIP: *Without a fever or positive stool culture, impaction should be ruled out.*

Content Area: Geriatrics, Gastrointestinal; *Integrated Process:* Nursing Process, Analysis; *Cognitive Level:* Application; *Client Need/Subneed:* Physiological Integrity/Basic Care and Comfort/Elimination

7. CORRECT ANSWER: 1. **Answer 1 is correct because the opacity and cloudiness of the lens cause blurry and dimmer vision.** Answer 2 is incorrect because in bright lights the pupil constricts and the client with cataracts *has more* difficulty seeing. Answer 3 is incorrect because the presence of a halo is characteristic of *glaucoma.* Answer 4 is incorrect because double vision is *not* a symptom of cataracts.

■ TEST-TAKING TIP: *Only one option describes impaired vision related to* cataracts.

Content Area: Geriatrics, Sensory; *Integrated Process:* Nursing Process, Assessment; *Cognitive Level:* Comprehension; *Client Need/Subneed:* Physiological Integrity/Physiological Adaptation/Pathophysiology

8. CORRECT ANSWER: 4. Answer 1 is incorrect because the client characteristically has a shuffling gait, and the foot would be prone to *injury* with an open-toed shoe. Answer 2 is incorrect because the shoes should be easy to put on so that the client could maintain some degree of independence, which would be difficult to do with double-knotted shoes. Answer 3 is incorrect because the shoes should be easy to put on so that the client could maintain some degree of independence, which would be difficult to do with high-top sneakers. **Answer 4 is correct because the client will be able to maintain a level of independence with a slip-on shoe. The rubber soles will lessen the risk of falls.**

■ TEST-TAKING TIP: *Visualize a shuffling gait and tremor. Which shoe could the client put on independently and which would not contribute to falls?*

Content Area: Adult Health, Neuromuscular; *Integrated Process:* Nursing Process, Implementation; *Cognitive Level:* Application; *Client Need/Subneed:* Health Promotion and Maintenance/Self-care

9. CORRECT ANSWERS: 1, 3, 4. **Answer 1 is correct because medications and some diseases common in the older adult affect salivation in 30% of clients.** Answer 2 is incorrect because the older adult has difficulty with *high-pitched* sounds. **Answer 3 is correct because the skin becomes more susceptible to infection and injury. Answer 4 is correct because men often have prostate enlargement, which leads to the need to urinate several times during the night.** Answer 5 is incorrect because pain sensitivity may be *decreased* because nerve cells are altered. Answer 6 is incorrect because the temperature of the older adult is often *subnormal.*

■ TEST-TAKING TIP: *Ask if each option will occur in most clients with aging.*

Content Area: Geriatrics; *Integrated Process:* Nursing Process, Assessment; *Cognitive Level:* Analysis; *Client Need/Subneed:* Health Promotion and Maintenance/Aging Process

10. CORRECT ANSWER: 3. **Answer 1** is incorrect because activating the *emergency medical services (EMS) is first,* followed by the CAB sequence (compression, airway, breathing) of cardiopulmonary resuscitation (CPR). **Answer 2** is incorrect because activating the *EMS is first,* then the CAB sequence of CPR. **Answer 3 is correct because the emergency response system needs to be activated before beginning CPR so that support services can arrive as quickly as possible.** **Answer 4** is incorrect because resuscitation of the client is a *priority.* Calling the family would delay starting CPR.

■ TEST-TAKING TIP: ***All answers are actions that need to be taken. Know the steps to take when a client is discovered who is unresponsive.***

Content Area: Geriatrics, Cardiopulmonary; ***Integrated Process:*** Nursing Process, Implementation; ***Cognitive Level:*** Analysis; ***Client Need/Subneed:*** Physiological Integrity/Physiological Adaptation/Medical Emergencies

11. CORRECT ANSWER: 4. **Answer 1** is incorrect because alveoli are *hyper*-inflated, trapping air. **Answer 2** is incorrect because CO_2 *increases.* Hypoxemia causes the body to increase red blood cell (RBC) production and hematocrit (Hct) *increases.* **Answer 3** is incorrect because hematocrit will be *increased* in response to hypoxemia. **Answer 4 is correct because emphysema is an obstructive pulmonary disease that traps air in the alveoli. The gas exchange is impaired as CO_2 increases. The body attempts to improve oxygenation by producing more red blood cells. There are immature RBCs that result in a more sluggish circulation.**

■ TEST-TAKING TIP: ***Review the physiological changes with emphysema—trapped air, poor gas exchange, production of immature RBCs to carry O_2.***

Content Area: Geriatrics, Respiratory; ***Integrated Process:*** Nursing Process, Analysis; ***Cognitive Level:*** Analysis; ***Client Need/Subneed:*** Physiological Integrity/Physiological Adaptation/Pathophysiology

12. CORRECT ANSWER: 1. **Answer 1 is correct because these are signs of cataracts, which can affect the client's vision.** **Answer 2** is incorrect because these are signs of cataracts. A CT scan is *not* needed. **Answer 3** is incorrect because these are signs of cataracts. *Increased* lighting is generally needed to assist with vision, not decreased lighting. **Answer 4** is incorrect because these are signs of cataracts. Management *is not* related to *dietary* protein.

■ TEST-TAKING TIP: ***The stem and correct option include the same world—"cloudy."***

Content Area: Geriatrics, Sensory; ***Integrated Process:*** Nursing Process, Assessment; ***Cognitive Level:*** Analysis; ***Client Need/Subneed:*** Physiological Integrity/Reduction of Risk Potential/System Specific Assessments

13. CORRECT ANSWER: 2. **Answer 1** is incorrect because the findings for BP and urine output are *not normal.* They indicate a client who has volume depletion, and an intervention is needed. **Answer 2 is correct because the low blood pressure and low urine output suggest fluid volume deficit, which should be treated with normal saline. Although it is usual to expect tachycardia in clients with hypotension, it is likely that the CHF and HTN are being managed with a beta blocker, which prevents the reflex tachycardia. Due to the client's age and heart problems, a small dose of normal saline should be given and evaluated.** **Answer 3** is incorrect because, while it is good to know these laboratory values, it is *not* necessary *before* starting some normal saline to correct the hypotension. **Answer 4** is incorrect because the nurse needs to use *caution* when administering *rapid* rates of IV fluids to *elderly* clients with CHF.

■ TEST-TAKING TIP: ***Analysis of the data is consistent with shock. Choose an action that is safest for the older adult.***

Content Area: Geriatrics, Cardiovascular; ***Integrated Process:*** Nursing Process, Analysis; ***Cognitive Level:*** Analysis; ***Client Need/Subneed:*** Physiological Integrity/Physiological Adaptation/Fluid and Electrolyte Imbalances

14. CORRECT ANSWER: 3. **Answer 1** is incorrect because, although the oxygen saturation is 100%, shivering does increase oxygen consumption and *supplemental* O_2 will be needed, not O_2 removed. **Answer 2** is incorrect because warm blankets need to be applied to treat the complaints and shivering *regardless* of the client's temperature. **Answer 3 is correct because shivering increases oxygen consumption. Hypothermia associated with the perioperative period may cause arrhythmia, clotting problems, and impaired wound healing.** **Answer 4** is incorrect because the pain level is *low* at 2/10 and does *not* require treatment.

■ TEST-TAKING TIP: ***Think client comfort. Care for the client first, and then check the temperature.***

Content Area: Geriatrics, Musculoskeletal; ***Integrated Process:*** Nursing Process, Implementation; ***Cognitive Level:*** Application; ***Client Need/Subneed:*** Physiological Integrity/Reduction of Risk Potential/Potential for Complications from Surgical Procedures and Health Alterations

15. CORRECT ANSWER: 4. **Answer 1** is incorrect because remaining in the *home* with support is a better option. **Answer 2** is incorrect because this is a decision for the client and spouse to make. **Answer 3** is incorrect because this casts doubt on wife's statement. **Answer 4 is correct because this action supports the client and wife in this decision.**

■ TEST-TAKING TIP: ***Choose the option that supports the independence of the client and family in decisions about care.***

Content Area: Geriatrics, Cardiovascular; ***Integrated Process:*** Nursing Process, Implementation; ***Cognitive Level:*** Application; ***Client Need/Subneed:*** Safe and Effective Care Environment/Management of Care/Referrals

16. CORRECT ANSWER: 2. **Answer 1** is incorrect because *volume* is *not* as much of a problem as pitch. **Answer 2 is**

ANSWERS

correct because higher pitched sounds typically made by children are more difficult to hear. **Answer 3** is incorrect because a motorcycle would likely be a *loud, low*-pitched sound. **Answer 4** is incorrect because a man's voice tends to be a *lower* pitch.

■ **TEST-TAKING TIP:** *Three of the options are low pitched. Only one choice is typically high pitched.*

Content Area: Geriatrics, Sensory; *Integrated Process:* Nursing Process, Analysis; *Cognitive Level:* Application; *Client Need/Subneed:* Health Promotion and Maintenance/ Aging Process

17. CORRECT ANSWERS: 2, 3, 4. **Answer 1** is incorrect because osteoarthritis does not predispose a client to decubitus ulcer or skin breakdown. The client would need to be immobilized by the arthritis. **Answer 2 is correct because impaired circulation *will* lead to skin breakdown and a decubitus ulcer. Answer 3 is correct because incontinence *will* cause skin breakdown and a decubitus ulcer. Answer 4 is correct because malnutrition *will* impair skin integrity leading to breakdown and decubiti.** **Answer 5** is incorrect because years of sun exposure causes the appearance of the skin to age, but the integrity of the skin is affected by circulation, moisture, and malnutrition.

■ **TEST-TAKING TIP:** *Choose the options that* directly *affect skin integrity.*

Content Area: Geriatrics, Integumentary; *Integrated Process:* Nursing Process, Analysis; *Cognitive Level:* Application; *Client Need/Subneed:* Physiological Integrity/Reduction of Risk Potential/Potential for Alterations in Body Systems

18. CORRECT ANSWER: 3. **Answer 1** is incorrect because cataracts would appear as an *opaque cloudiness* in the eye. **Answer 2** is incorrect because the response does *not address the cause.* **Answer 3 is correct because colored rings or halos are characteristic of glaucoma.** **Answer 4** is incorrect because colored rings or halos would *not* be consistent with *head injury.*

■ **TEST-TAKING TIP:** *Consider which condition would most likely cause these symptoms in the eye: cataracts or glaucoma?*

Content Area: Geriatrics, Sensory; *Integrated Process:* Communication and Documentation; *Cognitive Level:* Analysis; *Client Need/Subneed:* Physiological Integrity/Physiological Adaptation/Alterations in Body Systems

19. CORRECT ANSWER: 1. Answer 1 is correct because osteoarthritis is a common cause of chronic pain related to the aging process. **Answer 2** is incorrect because an old fracture *may or may not* be a source of chronic pain. **Answer 3** is incorrect because this condition is *not due to aging.* **Answer 4** is incorrect because this condition is related to *diabetes* or *liver* disease, not aging.

■ **TEST-TAKING TIP:** *Choose the option that can occur in any client from normal aging*—not *from* injury or illness.

Content Area: Geriatrics, Musculoskeletal; *Integrated Process:* Nursing Process, Analysis; *Cognitive Level:* Application; *Client Need/Subneed:* Health Promotion and Maintenance/ Aging Process

20. CORRECT ANSWERS: 1, 5. Answer 1 is correct because the actions are appropriate for the older adult and will improve ventilation. **Answer 2** is incorrect because lung capacity *diminishes* with age and this is not reversible. **Answer 3** is incorrect because COPD traps air, so the client should learn *pursed-lip breathing,* not forced inhalation. **Answer 4** is incorrect because the oxygen level is higher than recommended for COPD. The stimulus to breathe is hypoxia. **Answer 5 is correct because the diaphragm should be used to facilitate inspiration and expiration rather than the accessory muscles of breathing.**

■ **TEST-TAKING TIP:** *Think about the pathophysiology involved and the impact of aging.*

Content Area: Geriatrics, Respiratory; *Integrated Process:* Nursing Process, Planning; *Cognitive Level:* Application; *Client Need/Subneed:* Physiological Integrity/Physiological Adaptation/Alterations in Body Systems

21. CORRECT ANSWER: 1. Answer 1 is correct because, by the time a UTI is diagnosed, the older adult may begin to show signs of urosepsis, with altered mental status. **Answer 2** is incorrect because the older adult may be *asymptomatic.* **Answer 3** is incorrect because aging alters the thermoregulatory response, and the older adult may not have fever with a lower urinary tract infection. **Answer 4** is incorrect because the older adult may *already* have a problem with frequency, as part of the aging process.

■ **TEST-TAKING TIP:** *Choose the option that is different from the others (not urine or fever), and unique to the older adult.*

Content Area: Geriatric, Urological; *Integrated Process:* Nursing Process, Assessment; *Cognitive Level:* Analysis; *Client Need/Subneed:* Physiological Integrity/Reduction of Risk Potential/System Specific Assessments

22. CORRECT ANSWER: 4. **Answer 1** is incorrect because vaginitis is *not* associated with anticoagulation. **Answer 2** is incorrect because vaginitis is associated with increased sexual activity or multiple partners, *not just resuming* sex. **Answer 3** is incorrect because vaginitis occurs because of a yeast, fungal, or bacterial *infection.* Poor nutrition *may* lead to *decreased* resistance. **Answer 4 is correct because antibiotic therapy alters the normal protective organisms and allows fungal or yeast infections to develop.**

■ **TEST-TAKING TIP:** *More than one option may increase the risk for vaginitis, but select the one that is designed to "destr organisms—even the protective ones.*

Content Area: Geriatrics, Genitourinary; *Integrated Process:* Teaching and Learning; *Cognitive Level:* Application; *Client Need/Subneed:* Physiological Integrity/Reduction of Risk Potential/Potential for Alterations in Body Systems

23. CORRECT ANSWER: 2. Answer 1 is incorrect because abduction *prevents* dislocation. **Answer 2 is correct because crossing the legs, or bringing the legs together, exerts pressure on the hip and increases the risk of dislocation. Answer 3** is incorrect because blood clots develop in the *veins,* not arteries. **Answer 4** is incorrect because acute flexion (greater than 90 degrees) *increases* the risk of dislocation.

■ **TEST-TAKING TIP:** *Visualize the position of the client after surgery with the "abductor" pillow to prevent dislocation. Think: the opposite of abduction—adduction.*

Content Area: Adult Health, Musculoskeletal; ***Integrated Process:*** Teaching and Learning; ***Cognitive Level:*** Application; ***Client Need/Subneed:*** Physiological Integrity/Reduction of Risk Potential/Potential for Complications from Surgical Procedures and Health Alterations

24. CORRECT ANSWERS: 1, 2, 3. Answer 1 is correct because cold or heat will help the pain, but *not* flexibility. Answer 2 is correct because range of motion maintains flexibility and functional ability. Answer 3 is correct because meditation may help with chronic *pain.* Answer 4 is incorrect because vitamins or herbal therapies do *not* produce *consistent* results. Anti-inflammatory drugs may help, but exercises will be needed to maintain function. **Answer 5** is incorrect because exercise is important to prevent contractures of the hand.

■ **TEST-TAKING TIP:** *Look for actions that will manage pain and increase flexibility.*

Content Area: Geriatrics, Musculoskeletal; ***Integrated Process:*** Nursing Process, Implementation; ***Cognitive Level:*** Application; ***Client Need/Subneed:*** Physiological Integrity/Basic Care and Comfort/Non-pharmacological Comfort Interventions

25. CORRECT ANSWER: 1. Answer 1 is correct because the older client who is inactive is likely to have poor circulation and loss of subcutaneous fat. Answer 2 is incorrect because shivering *increases* body heat. **Answer 3** is incorrect because this client is *aware* of the cold, is likely to do something about it, and therefore is less likely to develop a problem. **Answer 4** is incorrect because fat acts as *insulation.*

■ **TEST-TAKING TIP:** *Three options protect from hypothermia. Select the one option that would not protect the client from hypothermia.*

Content Area: Geriatrics, Thermoregulatory; ***Integrated Process:*** Nursing Process, Analysis; ***Cognitive Level:*** Application; ***Client Need/Subneed:*** Health Promotion and Maintenance/ Health Screening

26. CORRECT ANSWER: 2. Answer 1 is incorrect because the client needs *to see* how to manage the right-sided hemiplegia. **Answer 2 is correct because demonstration is the best approach to teaching this client. Answer 3** is incorrect because the client *does not need to know* the difficulties but rather the best approach. **Answer 4** is incorrect because there may be some *processing problems* following a stroke; verbal instructions may not be clear to the client.

■ **TEST-TAKING TIP:** *Choose the option that is different from the others. Three options involve "talk"; only one "shows" how to put on the shirt.*

Content Area: Geriatrics, Cardiovascular; ***Integrated Process:*** Nursing Process, Implementation; ***Cognitive Level:*** Application; ***Client Need/Subneed:*** Health Promotion and Maintenance/ Self-care

27. CORRECT ANSWER: 4. Answer 1 is incorrect because constipation is a side effect but *not* an *imminent* cause for injury. **Answer 2** is incorrect because blurred vision is a side effect; however, the improved lighting is *not* the best answer. **Answer 3** is incorrect because dry mouth is a side effect but *not* a *cause* of injury. **Answer 4 is correct because tricyclic antidepressants cause orthostatic hypotension.**

■ **TEST-TAKING TIP:** *Select the option that provides the greatest client safety.*

Content Area: Geriatrics, Vascular; ***Integrated Process:*** Nursing Process, Implementation; ***Cognitive Level:*** Application; ***Client Need/Subneed:*** Physiological Integrity/Pharmacological and Parenteral Therapies/Adverse Effects/Contraindications/ Interactions

28. CORRECT ANSWER: 3. Answer 1 is incorrect because clients with cardiac and respiratory problems would be more prone to side effects, but kidney and liver problems will cause *toxic responses.* **Answer 2** is incorrect because *neither* condition will interfere with the detoxification or breakdown of drugs. **Answer 3 is correct because drugs are detoxified by the liver or the kidney. The client would be at risk for adverse drug effects when the function of the liver or kidneys is impaired. Answer 4** is incorrect because a client who has diabetes and gallbladder problems would *not* pose the greatest concern for reaction to medications detoxified by the liver or kidneys.

■ **TEST-TAKING TIP:** *Think about the role each condition has in drug metabolism and detoxification.*

Content Area: Geriatrics, Pharmacology; ***Integrated Process:*** Nursing Process, Analysis; ***Cognitive Level:*** Application; ***Client Need/Subneed:*** Physiological Integrity/Pharmacological and Parenteral Therapies/Adverse Effects/Contraindications/ Interactions

29. CORRECT ANSWER: 1. Answer 1 is correct because Benadryl causes drowsiness. Answer 2 is incorrect because there is *no effect* from *iron* that would interfere with balance. **Answer 3** is incorrect because there is *no effect* from Robitussin that would affect the client's balance. **Answer 4** is incorrect because Claritin is a *nondrowsy* allergy formula.

■ **TEST-TAKING TIP:** *Look for a drug that would interfere with balance.*

Content Area: Geriatrics, Pharmacology; **Integrated Process:** Teaching and Learning; **Cognitive Level:** Application; **Client Need/Subneed:** Safe and Effective Care Environment/Safety and Infection Control/Accident Prevention and Injury Prevention

30. CORRECT ANSWER: 2. **Answer 1** is incorrect because the client *needs* to be seen in the ED. Engage the client in conversation, which will hopefully have a calming effect. **Answer 2 is correct because, unlike techniques used with the client who is mentally ill, the nurse would not attempt to orient the client with moderate or severe dementia to person, place, or thing.** **Answer 3** is incorrect because the client with moderate dementia usually cannot be oriented to person, place, or thing. **Answer 4** is incorrect because the client with moderate dementia usually cannot be oriented to person, place, or thing.

■ **TEST-TAKING TIP:** *Select an option that engages the client without attempting to orient the client with dementia.*

Content Area: Geriatrics, Neurological; **Integrated Process:** Communication and Documentation; **Cognitive Level:** Analysis; **Client Need/Subneed:** Psychosocial Integrity/Therapeutic Communications

31. CORRECT ANSWER: 4. **Answer 1** is incorrect because effects of aging may be interfering with increasing the social skills of the client; focusing on this area could cause more difficulties in maintaining self-esteem. **Answer 2** is incorrect because the older adult may be feeling that the future is *hopeless.* **Answer 3** is incorrect because the older adult does not need praise for past accomplishments as much as a focus on remembering happy events for self-esteem. **Answer 4 is correct because focusing on long-term memory helps maintain self-worth and self-esteem in the client.**

■ **TEST-TAKING TIP:** *Talking about the* past *is a source of comfort for the older adult, not talking about the future (Answers 1 and 2).*

Content Area: Geriatrics, Mental Health; **Integrated Process:** Nursing Process, Implementation; **Cognitive Level:** Application; **Client Need/Subneed:** Psychosocial Integrity/Mental Health Concepts

32. CORRECT ANSWER: 3. **Answer 1** is incorrect because this response does *not* provide *relief.* **Answer 2** is incorrect because this response would help with dryness, but offers *no relief.* **Answer 3 is correct because this response will lessen the dryness and relieve the itching.** **Answer 4** is incorrect because this response does *not* provide *relief.*

■ **TEST-TAKING TIP:** *Look for actions that do not contribute to the dryness* and *provide relief.*

Content Area: Geriatrics, Integumentary; **Integrated Process:** Nursing Process, Implementation; **Cognitive Level:** Application; **Client Need/Subneed:** Physiological Integrity/Physiological Adaptation/Alterations in Body Systems

33. CORRECT ANSWER: 4. **Answer 1** is incorrect because these conditions do *not* cause *aspiration,* for which risk factors would come from secretions, food, or fluid. **Answer 2** is incorrect because these conditions do *not* cause *contractures.* **Answer 3** is incorrect because these conditions do *not* cause *dehydration.* **Answer 4 is correct because all of the conditions are risk factors for skin breakdown—inactivity, poor circulation, and skin wet from urine.**

■ **TEST-TAKING TIP:** *Ask what the three presenting conditions will cause. Eliminate the options where the client's condition is not a risk factor: tracheobronchial disorders (Answer 1), musculoskeletal problems (Answer 2), and fluid and electrolyte imbalances (Answer 3).*

Content Area: Geriatrics, Integumentary; **Integrated Process:** Nursing Process, Analysis; **Cognitive Level:** Application; **Client Need/Subneed:** Physiological Integrity/Reduction of Risk Potential/Potential for Alterations in Body Systems

34. CORRECT ANSWER: 4. **Answer 1** is incorrect because the problem is *not* due to *urinary frequency.* **Answer 2** is incorrect because the action will *not promote* sleep. **Answer 3** is incorrect because the complaint of waking up at night is *not* indicative of sleep apnea. The client with sleep apnea doesn't usually wake up at night. **Answer 4 is correct because the older adult does experience changes in sleeping. It is important to rule out any pathological patterns.**

■ **TEST-TAKING TIP:** *Recognize the normal changes of aging affecting the sleep-wake cycle.*

Content Area: Geriatrics; **Integrated Process:** Nursing Process, Implementation; **Cognitive Level:** Application; **Client Need/Subneed:** Health Promotion and Maintenance/Aging Process

35. CORRECT ANSWERS: 1, 5. **Answer 1 is correct because the signs of pneumonia are more subtle and subjective and are related to developing sepsis.** **Answer 2** is incorrect because headache is *not* common; respiratory rate increases. **Answer 3** is incorrect because the older adult typically has *no fever* with pneumonia. **Answer 4** is incorrect because the client may have *increased* sputum and *no chest* (pleuritic) pain. **Answer 5 is correct because sputum will be increased, causing a productive cough. The older adult often has a subnormal temperature, so that the temperature with an infection is often not elevated.**

■ **TEST-TAKING TIP:** *The* typical *sign of pneumonia is often* not *present in the older adult (high fever). Look for less specific symptoms (Answer 1) and a choice consistent with the altered thermoregulatory system in the older adult.*

Content Area: Geriatrics, Respiratory; **Integrated Process:** Nursing Process, Assessment; **Cognitive Level:** Application; **Client Need/Subneed:** Physiological Integrity/Physiological Adaptation/Alterations in Body Systems

36. CORRECT ANSWER: 1. Answer 1 is correct because these are strategies to promote better sleep. **Answer 2** is incorrect because *more information* is needed to ensure there is not a pathological cause. **Answer 3** is incorrect because *more information* is needed *before* an intervention is selected. **Answer 4** is incorrect because this may be a solution but *more information* is needed.

■ **TEST-TAKING TIP:** *First priority—Assess.*

Content Area: Geriatrics; ***Integrated Process:*** Nursing Process, Implementation; ***Cognitive Level:*** Application; ***Client Need/Subneed:*** Physiological Integrity/Basic Care and Comfort/Rest and Sleep

37. CORRECT ANSWER: 4. **Answer 1** is incorrect because this strategy will be important but *not* the *most* effective. **Answer 2** is incorrect because the speed of the move is *irrelevant.* The client will still think about the change. **Answer 3** is incorrect because family will be *important* in making this transition. **Answer 4 is correct because it is important to create a familiar environment.**

■ **TEST-TAKING TIP:** *Eliminate the options with the words "many" (Answer 1), "quickly" (Answer 2), and "restrict" (Answer 3). The most effective approach is to make the environment* familiar.

Content Area: Geriatrics, Mental Health; ***Integrated Process:*** Nursing Process, Implementation; ***Cognitive Level:*** Application; ***Client Need/Subneed:*** Psychosocial Integrity/Mental Health Concepts

38. CORRECT ANSWERS: 1, 2, 3, 4. Answer 1 is correct because family members provide a source for reinforcement as well as valuable assessment information about the client's living situation and learning needs. Answer 2 is correct because a slower pace and more frequent sessions with smaller amounts of information will contribute to better understanding. Answer 3 is correct because reinforcement of the content in writing is an appropriate action when teaching an older adult. Answer 4 is correct because learning improves with the opportunity to practice. **Answer 5** is incorrect because visual problems may require special lighting, and difficulty hearing compounded by background noises make a group session a less effective teaching approach.

■ **TEST-TAKING TIP:** *When all of the options are accepted teaching strategies, look for the options that accommodate the sensory and possible cognitive limitations seen with aging.*

Content Area: Geriatrics; ***Integrated Process:*** Teaching and Learning; ***Cognitive Level:*** Application; ***Client Need/Subneed:*** Health Promotion and Maintenance/Principles of Teaching and Learning

39. CORRECT ANSWER: 2. **Answer 1** is incorrect because *not everyone* relates to or learns well in groups. If group teaching is used, follow-up is essential to ensure that an individual client has attained sufficient knowledge. **Answer 2 is correct because a single teaching strategy is rarely adequate. Learning takes time. Follow-up sessions are important to building confidence in the client and to assess the effectiveness of prior teaching.** **Answer 3** is incorrect because the teaching techniques *vary* with older adults. The nurse needs to assess *each* client. A combination of lecture, visual aids, and discussion is commonly used. **Answer 4** is incorrect because there is no substitute for *human interaction.* Teaching aids are invaluable, but there must be discussion following use of such aids.

■ **TEST-TAKING TIP:** *Eliminate the options that imply a "one size fits all" approach to teaching older adults.*

Content Area: Geriatrics; ***Integrated Process:*** Teaching and Learning; ***Cognitive Level:*** Application; ***Client Need/Subneed:*** Health Promotion and Maintenance/Principles of Teaching and Learning

40. CORRECT ANSWER: 1. Answer 1 is correct because incontinence is *not* a normal consequence of aging. Age-related changes in the urinary tract predispose the older client to incontinence, but incontinence is a symptom of *many* possible disorders—not just aging. **Answer 2** is incorrect because incontinence *is* embarrassing. Many clients conceal the problem and fail to seek help that may reverse the problem. **Answer 3** is incorrect because the number of vaginal births *does* increase the incidence of incontinence in women—young and old. **Answer 4** is incorrect because collaboration with the family, the client, and the health-care team *may reverse* incontinence.

■ **TEST-TAKING TIP:** *The stem asks for what is not correct information and needs further teaching by the nurse. Incontinence* is not a fact *of aging. Look for an option* that implies *it is an expected consequence of aging and therefore is an incorrect statement that requires teaching.*

Content Area: Geriatrics, Renal; ***Integrated Process:*** Nursing Process, Evaluation; ***Cognitive Level:*** Analysis; ***Client Need/Subneed:*** Physiological Integrity/Basic Care and Comfort/Elimination

41. CORRECT ANSWERS: 2, 3. **Answer 1** is incorrect because this will *not* necessarily stop the robbery attempts, which are targeting people who are vulnerable and may have money. **Answer 2 is correct because removing the target (the Social Security check) reduces the risk. Answer 3 is correct because a dog will likely deter a robber.** **Answer 4** is incorrect because the Social Security check would *still* be delivered to the home. **Answer 5** is incorrect because the client is *at risk* for a repeat home invasion. The nurse needs to address strategies to reduce or eliminate the risk.

■ **TEST-TAKING TIP:** *Think safety; reduce the risk of being targeted and offer a deterrent—a dog.*

Content Area: Geriatrics, Safety; ***Integrated Process:*** Caring; ***Cognitive Level:*** Application; ***Client Need/Subneed:*** Safe and Effective Care Environment/Safety and Infection Control/Home Safety

42. **CORRECT ANSWER: 1. Answer 1 is correct because ideally foot care should be provided by podiatric care providers. The service is covered by insurance.** **Answer 2** is incorrect because the calluses should only be removed by a podiatric specialist. This option does not indicate who is doing the foot care. **Answer 3** is incorrect because this choice does not include the importance of being seen by a podiatric specialist. **Answer 4** is incorrect because the older adult should not cut his or her own toenails. Care should be provided by an expert.

■ **TEST-TAKING TIP:** *Only one option includes the importance of being seen by an expert in foot care.*

Content Area: Geriatrics, Integumentary; ***Integrated Process:*** Nursing Process, Implementation; ***Cognitive Level:*** Application; ***Client Need/Subneed:*** Physiological Integrity/Basic Care and Comfort/Personal Hygiene

43. **CORRECT ANSWER: 4.** **Answer 1** is incorrect because inactivity does *not* increase susceptibility. The client needs to be in *close contact* with someone who *has* the disease. **Answer 2** is incorrect because smoking does *not* increase susceptibility, *but* the *potential* for lung damage may be greater. **Answer 3** is incorrect because recipients of BCG should be *less* likely to contract the infection. **Answer 4 is correct because the spread of the infection increases in crowded, close living conditions since TB is spread from person to person by airborne transmission—droplets from talking, coughing, sneezing, laughing, or singing.**

■ **TEST-TAKING TIP:** *Think about how tuberculosis is spread—airborne from person to person.*

Content Area: Geriatrics, Infectious Disease; ***Integrated Process:*** Nursing Process, Analysis; ***Cognitive Level:*** Comprehension; ***Client Need/Subneed:*** Safe and Effective Care Environment/Safety and Infection Control/Standard/Transmission-based/Other Precautions

44. **CORRECT ANSWER: 1. Answer 1 is correct because the client with Alzheimer's disease typically has lost short-term memory. Understanding of the father's disease will decrease the daughter's frustration.** **Answer 2** is incorrect because this inappropriate action does *not* address daughter's frustration nor does it improve communication. **Answer 3** is incorrect because the client will *not recall* the conversation. **Answer 4** is incorrect because the cognitive problem is *not reversible.* Word games, such as crossword puzzles, *may delay* development of the disease.

■ **TEST-TAKING TIP:** *Only one option gives the family member a strategy to address the frustration.*

Content Area: Geriatric, Neurological; ***Integrated Process:*** Nursing Process, Implementation; ***Cognitive Level:*** Application; ***Client Need/Subneed:*** Psychosocial Integrity/Therapeutic Communications

45. **CORRECT ANSWER: 2.** **Answer 1** is incorrect because correcting the client will not increase the client's compliance, and may increase agitation. Attempting to orient the client to person, place, or time increases agitation in the client with dementia. **Answer 2 is correct because, if the family becomes upset and angry, the client's agitation and anxiety will likely increase.** **Answer 3** is incorrect because repetition will not improve the client's condition. **Answer 4** is incorrect because this will *increase* client anxiety. The client with dementia *cannot* process rapid stimuli.

■ **TEST-TAKING TIP:** *Think of the effect that each option will have on the client.*

Content Area: Geriatrics, Neurological; ***Integrated Process:*** Teaching and Learning; ***Cognitive Level:*** Application; ***Client Need/Subneed:*** Psychosocial Integrity/Sensory/Perceptual Alterations

46. **CORRECT ANSWER: 3.** **Answer 1** is incorrect because only drugs that are reversible inhibitors of cholinesterase have benefitted in slowing disease progression in *mild to moderate* Alzheimer's disease. Stage III is a late stage with severe dementia. **Answer 2** is incorrect because only drugs that are reversible inhibitors of cholinesterase have benefitted *mild to moderate* Alzheimer's disease, not Stage III. **Answer 3 is correct because families are often desperate to find a treatment, and there may be serious side effects. They need to discuss alternative therapies with the physician.** **Answer 4** is incorrect because only drugs that are reversible inhibitors of cholinesterase have benefitted cognition in *mild to moderate* Alzheimer's disease, not Stage III.

■ **TEST-TAKING TIP:** *Look for an option that is different from the others—only one option raises the potential risks of a drug. Drug therapy does not work consistently in all AD clients.*

Content Area: Geriatrics, Neurological; ***Integrated Process:*** Teaching and Learning; ***Cognitive Level:*** Application; ***Client Need/Subneed:*** Physiological Integrity/Physiological Adaptation/Alterations in Body Systems

47. **CORRECT ANSWERS: 1, 5, 6. Answer 1 is correct because there is recent and remote memory impairment, as well as anomia, agnosia, and aphasia.** **Answer 2** is incorrect because the client *loses* short-term memory and may *not* remember younger family members, like grandchildren. **Answer 3** is incorrect because the cognitive decline is *slow* and *gradual.* **Answer 4** is incorrect because these causes of cognitive impairment would have been *ruled out before* a diagnosis of AD was made. **Answer 5 is correct because it describes anomia, which occurs with AD. Answer 6 is correct because it describes agnosia, which is consistent with AD.**

■ **TEST-TAKING TIP:** *AD is the leading cause of dementia—memory impairment as well as language disorders.*

Content Area: Geriatrics, Neurological; ***Integrated Process:*** Nursing Process, Analysis; ***Cognitive Level:*** Application; ***Client Need/Subneed:*** Physiological Integrity/Physiological Adaptation/Pathophysiology

48. CORRECT ANSWERS: 1, 3, 4, 5. **Answer 1** is correct because antihistamines (Solu-Medrol) may be ordered before the procedure because of the known allergy to seafood. **Answer 2** is incorrect because the contrast dye in this procedure will have the greatest effect on the kidneys, not the liver. **Answer 3** is correct because the client's age and history of diabetes combined with the nephrotoxic effects of the contrast dye may lead to acute renal failure. **Answer 4** is correct because IV hydration is a key to preventing acute renal failure secondary to the contrast dye used during catheterization. **Answer 5** is correct because metformin is excreted in the kidneys. If the client develops renal failure secondary to the contrast media, the drug will accumulate and the client may develop fatal lactic acidosis.

■ **TEST-TAKING TIP:** *Think safety first. Protect the kidneys.*

Content Area: Geriatric, Endocrine; ***Integrated Process:*** Nursing Process, Analysis; ***Cognitive Level:*** Analysis; ***Client Need/Subneed:*** Physiological Integrity/Reduction of Risk Potential/Therapeutic Procedures

49. CORRECT ANSWER: 3. **Answer 1** is incorrect because this is an incorrect statement. **Answer 2** is incorrect because extended-release tablets should *never* be split. **Answer 3** is correct because, if splitting can be done, an approved device should be used. Clean between usages. **Answer 4** is incorrect because, while splitting enteric-coated tablets defeats the protective function of the enteric coating, it does not change the drug effect. Enteric-coated tablets should *never* be split; gastric irritation would be likely.

■ **TEST-TAKING TIP:** *Review the rules for safely splitting tablets.*

Content Area: Geriatrics, Pharmacology; ***Integrated Process:*** Teaching and Learning; ***Cognitive Level:*** Application; ***Client Need/Subneed:*** Physiological Integrity/Pharmacological and Parenteral Therapies/Medication Administration

50. CORRECT ANSWER: 2. **Answer 1** is incorrect because giving the medication *without* ensuring that the client understands the orders after the nurse leaves would not be the best action. **Answer 2** is correct because effectiveness of the discharge orders will depend on the client understanding the regimen. **Answer 3** is incorrect because this may indicate a problem that teaching will correct. **Answer 4** is incorrect because this will most likely have been part of the predischarge teaching.

■ **TEST-TAKING TIP:** *"Teaching" is an umbrella answer that encompasses the other options.*

Content Area: Geriatrics, Pharmacology; ***Integrated Process:*** Nursing Process, Implementation; ***Cognitive Level:*** Application; ***Client Need/Subneed:*** Physiological Integrity/Pharmacological and Parenteral Therapies/Medication Administration

CHAPTER 8

Physiological Integrity

Pharmacological and Parenteral Therapies

Sally Lambert Lagerquist • Janice Lloyd McMillin • Robyn Marchal Nelson • Kathleen E. Snider

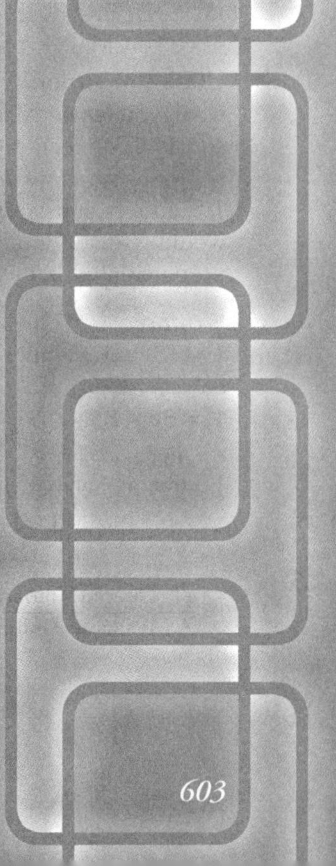

CONVERSIONS AND CALCULATIONS IN MEDICATION ADMINISTRATION

I. COMMON METRIC CONVERSION

A. *Weight:*
1 gram (gm) = 1,000,000 micrograms (mcg)
1 milligram (mg) = 1,000 micrograms (mcg)
1,000 milligrams (mg) = 1 gram (gm)
1 kilogram (kg) = 1,000 grams (gm)

B. *Volume:*
1 liter (L) = 1,000 milliliters (mL)
1 kiloliter (kL) = 1,000 liters (L)
1 milliliter (mL) = 1 cubic centimeter (cc)

II. APOTHECARY SYSTEM (*Note:* metric is preferred for medication administration.)

A. *Weight:*
60 grains (gr) = 1 dram (dr)
8 drams (dr) = 1 ounce (oz)

B. *Liquid:*
60 minims = 1 fluidram (fl dr)
8 fluidrams (fl dr) = 1 fluidounce (fl oz)
16 fluidounces (fl oz) = 1 pint (pt)
2 pints (pt) = 1 quart (qt)
4 quarts (qt) = 1 gallon (gal)

III. EQUIVALENT HOUSEHOLD CONVERSIONS

20 drops (gtt) = 1 milliliter (mL)
1 teaspoon (tsp) = 5 milliliters (mL)
1 ounce (oz) = 30 milliliters (mL)
1 cup (C) = 240 milliliters (mL)
1 liter (L) = 1,000 milliliters (mL)

IV. DETERMINING EQUIVALENCY FROM ONE SYSTEM TO ANOTHER

Use a proportion. On the left side of the proportion is what you *know* to be an equivalent (e.g., 30 milliliters equals 1 ounce). On the right side of the proportion is what you *need to determine* (e.g., you want to give 1.5 ounces and your medicine cup is in milliliters—you would write "x" milliliters equals 1.5 ounces). Rewrite the proportion without using the symbols.

Example:
1 oz : 30 mL :: x mL : 1.5 oz
Solve for x:
$1x = 30 \times 1.5$
$x = 45$
1.5 ounces equals 45 milliliters (mL)

V. ALTERNATE FORMULA FOR CALCULATION WITH LIKE UNITS

$$\frac{\text{D (Desired Amount)}}{\text{A (Available Amount)}} \times \text{Q (Quantity Available)} = x$$

Example: the order is for 50 mg of phenobarbital, which comes in 20 mg per 5 mL.

$$\frac{\text{50 mg (Desired)}}{\text{20 mg (Available)}} \times \frac{\text{5 mL (Quantity)}}{1} = x$$

Solve for x:

$$x = \frac{50}{\overset{}{\cancel{20}}_{4}} \times \frac{\overset{1}{\cancel{5}}}{1}$$

$$x = \frac{50 \times 1}{4 \times 1}$$

$$x = \frac{50}{4}$$

$x = 12.5$ mL

VI. DIMENSIONAL ANALYSIS FOR CONVERSION AND CALCULATION

Another format for dosage calculation that uses only one equation even when conversion to like units is needed.

Example with *like* units: penicillin 500 mg comes in 250-mg capsules. You would give _______ capsules.
On the left side of the equation is the drug form you are solving for:
x capsules =
On the right side, place the known information in a common fraction with the numerator matching the x quantity (capsules). The amount in each capsule that is known is the denominator (250 mg):

$$x \text{ capsules} = \frac{1 \text{ capsule}}{250 \text{ mg}}$$

Next set up a proportion with the information that matches the denominator (500 mg):

$$x \text{ capsules} = \frac{1 \text{ capsule}}{250 \text{ mg}} \times \frac{500 \text{ mg}}{1}$$

$$x = 1 \times \frac{500}{250}$$

$x = 2$ capsules

Example with *different* units: Keflin 400 mg IM q10h. The drug is available in 0.5 gm per 2 mL.

$$x \text{ mL} = \frac{2 \text{ mL}}{0.5 \text{ g}}$$

Because the available drug is in grams (gm), an additional fraction is added for the conversion from grams to milliliters. Remember: the numerator of each fraction must match the denominator of the fraction before.

$$x \text{ mL} = \frac{2 \text{ mL}}{0.5 \text{ g}} \times \frac{1 \text{ g}}{1{,}000 \text{ mg}}$$

$$x \text{ mL} = \frac{2 \text{ mL}}{0.5 \text{ g}} \times \frac{1 \text{ g}}{1{,}000 \text{ mg}} \times \frac{400 \text{ mg}}{1}$$

(amount of drug ordered)

Cancel out the like abbreviations on the right side of the equation. If the equation is correct, the only abbreviation remaining on the right side will match the abbreviation on the left side (mL):

$$x \text{ mL} = \frac{2 \text{ mL}}{0.5 \not{g}} \times \frac{1 \not{g}}{1{,}000 \not{mg}} \times \frac{400 \not{mg}}{1}$$

Solve for x:

$$x = \frac{2 \times 400}{0.5 \times 1000}$$

$$x = \frac{800}{500}$$

$$x = 1.6 \text{ mL}$$

VII. DETERMINING FLOW RATES FOR PARENTERAL INFUSION (see **Intravenous Therapy, II. B, p. 606).**

MEDICATION ADMINISTRATION: INFANTS AND CHILDREN

I. DEVELOPMENTAL CONSIDERATIONS

A. Be honest. Do *not* bribe or threaten child to obtain cooperation.

B. When administering medication, do so in the least traumatic manner possible.

C. Describe any sensations child may expect to experience (e.g., "pinch" of needle during IM).

D. Explain how child can "help" nurse (e.g., "Lie as still as you can").

E. Tell child that it is OK to cry; provide privacy.

F. Offer support, praise, and encouragement during and after giving medication.

G. Allow child opportunity for age-appropriate therapeutic play to work through feelings and experiences, to clarify any misconceptions, and to teach child more effective coping strategies.

II. SAFETY CONSIDERATIONS

A. Be absolutely sure dose you are giving is both safe (check recommended mg/kg) and accurate (have another nurse check your calculations). Remember: dose should generally be smaller than adult dose.

B. Check identification band or ask parent or another nurse for child's first and last name.

C. Restrain child to avoid injury while giving medication; a second person is often required to help hold child.

III. ORAL MEDICATIONS

A. Use syringe without needle to draw up medication.

B. *Position:* upright or semireclining.

C. Place tip of syringe along the side of infant's tongue, and give medication slowly, in small amounts, allowing infant to swallow. Medicine cups can be used for older infants and children. ***Never*** pinch infant or child's nostrils to force the child to open mouth.

D. When giving tablets or capsules (that are *not* enteric coated), crush and mix into smallest possible amount of food or liquid to ensure that child takes entire dose. Do *not* mix with essential food or liquid (e.g., milk); select an "optional" food, such as applesauce.

IV. OPHTHALMIC INSTILLATIONS

A. *Position:* supine or sitting with head extended.

B. For eye*drops:* hold dropper 1 to 2 cm above middle of conjunctival sac.

C. For eye *ointment:* squeeze 2 cm of ointment from tube onto conjunctival sac.

D. After giving drops or ointment, encourage child to keep eyes closed briefly, to maximize contact with eyes. Child should be asked to look in all directions (with eyes closed) to enhance even distribution of medication.

E. Whenever possible, administer eye ointments at nap time or bedtime, due to possible blurred vision. Administer eyedrops *prior* to ointment (if both are ordered for the same time). Eyedrops may "roll off" the slick surface of the eye ointment.

V. OTIC INSTILLATIONS

A. *Position:* head to side so that affected ear is uppermost.

B. For child ***under*** 3 years of age: pull pinna gently ***down*** and back.

C. For child 3 years of age and ***over:*** pull pinna gently ***up*** and back.

D. After administering eardrops, encourage child to remain with head to side with affected ear uppermost, to maximize contact with entire external canal to reach eardrum. Gentle massage of area in front of ear will facilitate entry of eardrops into canal.

E. If eardrops are kept in refrigerator, allow to warm to room temperature before instilling.

VI. DERMATOLOGICAL INSTILLATIONS

A. Remember: young child's skin is more permeable; therefore, there is increased risk for medication absorption and resultant systemic effects. Monitor for systemic effects.

B. Apply thin layer of cream or ointment, and confine it to portions of skin where it is essential.

VII. RECTAL MEDICATIONS

A. Prepare child emotionally and physically; rectal route is invasive and embarrassing, particularly for children.

B. *Position:* side-lying with upper leg flexed.

C. Lubricate rounded end of suppository and insert past anal sphincter with gloved fingertip (wear double *gloves* when inserting rectal medication).

D. Remove fingertip but hold child's buttocks gently together until child no longer strains or indicates urge to expel medication.

VIII. INTRAMUSCULAR MEDICATIONS

A. Because the infant or child is much smaller physically than an adult, the nurse should select a shorter needle, generally *5/8 inch* (infant) to 1 inch (child).

B. Preferred injection sites in infants and young children include the vastus lateralis and ventrogluteal muscles. The deltoid muscle, though small, provides easy access and can be used in children over 12 months of age with adequate muscle mass.

C. Usually *1 mL* is the maximum volume that should be administered in a single site to infants and children.

D. Because of vast differences in size, muscle mass, and subcutaneous tissue, it is especially important to note bony prominences as landmarks for intramuscular injections.

E. Have a second adult present to help restrain the child.

F. Once the nurse has told the child he or she is to receive an injection, the procedure should be carried out as quickly and skillfully as possible.

INTRAVENOUS THERAPY/BLOOD ADMINISTRATION

I. INFUSION SYSTEMS

A. Plastic bag:
1. Contains no vacuum—needs no air to replace fluid as it flows from container.
2. Medication can be added with syringe through a resealable latex port.
   a. During infusion, administration set should be completely clamped before medications are added.
   b. Prevents undiluted, and perhaps toxic, dose from entering administration set.

B. Closed system:
1. Requires partial vacuum—however, only filtered air enters container.
2. Medication may be added during infusion through air vent in administration set.

C. Administration sets:
1. *Standard sets*—deliver 10 to 15 drops (gtt)/mL.
2. *Pediatric or minidrop sets*—deliver 60 drops (gtt)/mL.
3. *Controlled-volume sets*—permit accurate infusion of measured volumes of fluids.
   a. Particularly valuable when piggybacked into primary infusion.
   b. Solutions containing drugs can then be administered intermittently.
4. *Y-type administration sets*—allow for simultaneous or alternate infusion of two fluids.
   a. May contain filter and pressure unit for blood transfusions.
   b. *Air embolism* significant hazard with this type of administration set.
5. *Positive-pressure sets*—designed for rapid infusion of replacement fluids.
   a. In emergency, built-in pressure chamber increases rate of blood administration.
   b. Pump chamber *must* be filled at all times to avoid air embolism.
   c. Application of positive pressure to infusion fluids is responsibility of *physician.*
6. *Infusion pumps*—used to deliver small volumes of fluid or doses of high-potency drugs.
   a. Used primarily in neonatal, pediatric, and adult intensive care units.
   b. Have increased the safety of parenteral therapy and reduced nursing time.

D. Long-term delivery systems—centrally placed venous access catheters and ports for the administration of drugs (e.g., chemotherapy), blood and blood products, antibiotics, analgesics, antiemetics, and total parenteral nutrition (TPN). Types: Hickman/Broviac, Groshong, venous access port (VAP).
1. Inserted under strict aseptic conditions using local or general anesthesia.
2. Major concern: prevention of infection.

II. FLUID ADMINISTRATION

A. Factors influencing rate:
1. Client's size.
2. Client's physical condition.
3. Age of client.
4. Type of fluid.
5. Client's tolerance to fluid.
6. Client's position.

B. *Flow rates for parenteral infusions* can be computed using the following formula:

$$\frac{\text{gtt/mL of given set}}{\text{60 min/hr}} \times \text{total volume/hr} = \text{gtt/min}$$

Example: if 1,000 mL is to be infused in an 8-hr period (125 mL/hr) and the administration set delivers 15 gtt/mL, the rate is 31.2 gtt/min:

$$\frac{15}{60} \times 125 = \frac{1}{4} \times 125 = 31.2 \text{ gtt/min}$$

IV THERAPY

C. Generally the type of fluid administration set determines its rate of flow.
1. *Fluid* administration sets—approximately 15 gtt/min.
2. *Blood* administration sets—approximately 10 gtt/min.
3. *Pediatric* administration sets—approximately 60 gtt/min.
4. Always check information on the administration set box to determine the number of gtt/mL before calculating; varies with manufacturer.

D. Factors influencing flow rates:
1. *Gravity*—a change in the height of the infusion bottle will increase or decrease the rate of flow; for example, raising the bottle *higher* will *increase* the rate of flow, and vice versa.
2. *Blood clot* in needle—stopping the infusion for any reason or an increase in venous pressure may result in partial or total obstruction of needle by clot due to:
   a. *Delay* in changing infusion bottle.
   b. Blood pressure cuff on, or restraints *on* or *above* infusion needle.
   c. Client *lying on arm* in which infusion is being made.
3. Change in *needle position*—against or away from vein wall.
4. *Venous spasm*—due to cold blood or irritating solution.
5. *Plugged vent*—causes infusion to stop.

III. FLUID AND ELECTROLYTE THERAPY

A. Types of therapy:
1. *Maintenance therapy*—provides water, electrolytes, glucose, vitamins, and in some instances protein to meet daily requirements.
2. *Restoration of deficits*—in addition to maintenance therapy, fluid and electrolytes are added to replace *previous* losses.
3. *Replacement therapy*—infusions to replace *current* losses in fluid and electrolytes.

B. Types of intravenous fluids **(Table 8.1):**
1. *Isotonic solutions*—fluids that approximate the osmolarity (280 to 300 mOsm/L) of normal blood plasma.
   a. Sodium chloride (0.9%)—normal saline.
      (1) *Indications:*
         (a) Extracellular fluid replacement when Cl^- loss is equal to or greater than Na^+ loss.
         (b) Treatment of metabolic alkalosis.
         (c) Na^+ depletion.
         (d) Initiating and terminating blood transfusions.
      (2) Possible *side effects:*
         (a) Hypernatremia.
         (b) Acidosis.
         (c) Hypokalemia.
         (d) Circulatory overload.
   b. Five percent dextrose in water (D_5W).
      (1) *Provides calories* for energy, *sparing body protein* and *preventing* ketosis resulting from fat breakdown.
         (a) 3.75 calories are provided per gram of glucose.
         (b) United States Pharmacopeia (USP) standards require use of monohydrated glucose, so only 91% is actually glucose.
         (c) D_5W yields 170.6 calories; D_5W means 5 grams glucose/100 mL water.
         $50 \times 3.75 = 187.5$ calories/L
         $0.91 \times 187.5 = 170.6$ calories/L
      (2) *Indications:*
         (a) Dehydration.
         (b) Hypernatremia.
         (c) Drug administration.

Table 8.1

Commonly Used Intravenous Fluids

IV Solution	Na^+ (mEq/L)	K^+ (mEq/L)	Ca^{++} (mEq/L)	Cl^- (mEq/L)	Lactate (mEq/L)	Calories/L
0.9% NaCl (NS)	154	0	0	154	0	0
5% Dextrose (D_5W)	0	0	0	0	0	170
5% Dextrose + 0.9% NaCl (D_5NS)	154	0	0	154	0	170
5% Dextrose + 0.45% NaCl (D_5 1/2NS)	77	0	0	77	0	170
Lactated Ringer's solution	130	4	3	109	28	9
3% NaCl	462	0	0	462	0	0
5% NaCl	770	0	0	770	0	0
0.45% NaCl	69.3	0	0	69.3	0	0
10% Dextrose ($D_{10}W$)	0	0	0	0	0	340

(3) Possible *side effects:*
(a) Hypokalemia.
(b) Osmotic diuresis—dehydration.
(c) Transient hyperinsulinism.
(d) Water intoxication.

c. Five percent dextrose in normal saline (D_5NS).
(1) *Prevents* ketone formation and *loss* of potassium and intracellular water.
(2) *Indications:*
(a) Hypovolemic shock—temporary measure.
(b) Burns.
(c) Acute adrenocortical insufficiency.
(3) Same *side effects* as normal saline.

d. Isotonic multiple-electrolyte fluids—*used for* replacement therapy; ionic composition approximates blood plasma.
(1) Types—Plasmanate, Polysol, and lactated Ringer's.
(2) *Indicated in:* vomiting, diarrhea, excessive diuresis, and burns.
(3) Possible *side effect*—circulatory overload.
(4) Lactated Ringer's is *contraindicated* in severe metabolic acidosis and/or alkalosis and liver disease.
(5) Same *side effects* as normal saline.

2. *Hypertonic solutions*—fluids with an osmolarity much higher than 310 mOsm (+50 mOsm); increase osmotic pressure of blood plasma, thereby drawing fluid from the cells.
a. Ten percent dextrose in normal saline ($D_{10}NS$).
(1) Administered in large vein to dilute and prevent venous trauma.
(2) *Used for:* nutrition and to replenish Na^+ and Cl^-.
(3) Possible *side effects:*
(a) Hypernatremia (excess Na^+).
(b) Acidosis (excess Cl^-).
(c) Circulatory overload.
b. Sodium chloride solutions, 3% and 5%.
(1) Slow administration essential to prevent overload (100 mL/hr).
(2) *Indicated in* water intoxication and severe sodium depletion.

3. *Hypotonic solutions*—fluids whose osmolarity is significantly less than that of blood plasma (–50 mOsm); these fluids lower plasma osmotic pressures, causing fluid to enter cells.
a. 0.45% sodium chloride—used for replacement when requirement for Na^+ use is questionable.
b. 2.5% dextrose (D) in 0.45% saline, also 5% D in 0.2% NaCl—common rehydrating solution.
(1) *Indications:*
(a) Fluid replacement when some Na^+ replacement is also necessary.
(b) Encourage diuresis in clients who are dehydrated.
(c) Evaluate kidney status before instituting electrolyte infusions.
(2) Possible *side effects:*
(a) Hypernatremia.
(b) Circulatory overload.
(c) Use with *caution* in clients who are edematous with cardiac, renal, or hepatic disease.
(d) After adequate renal function is established, appropriate electrolytes should be given to *avoid hypokalemia.*

4. *Alkalizing agents*—fluids used in the treatment of *metabolic acidosis:*
a. Ringer's:
(1) Administration—rate usually not more than 300 mL/hr.
(2) *Side effects*—observe carefully for signs of *alkalosis.*
b. Sodium bicarbonate:
(1) *Indications:*
(a) Replace excessive loss of bicarbonate ion.
(b) Emergency treatment of life-threatening acidosis.
(2) Administration:
(a) Depends on client's weight, condition, and carbon dioxide level.
(b) Usual dose is 500 mL of a 1.5% solution (89 mEq).
(3) *Side effects:*
(a) Alkalosis.
(b) Hypocalcemic tetany.
(c) Rapid infusion may induce cellular acidity and death.

5. *Acidifying solutions*—fluids used in treatment of *metabolic alkalosis.*
a. Types:
(1) Normal saline (see **B.1.** Isotonic solutions, **pp. 607–608**).
(2) Ammonium chloride.
b. Administration—dosage depends on client's condition and serum laboratory values.
c. *Side effects:*
(1) Hepatic encephalopathy in presence of decreased liver function because ammonia is metabolized by liver.
(2) Toxic effects: irregular respirations, twitching, and bradycardia.
(3) *Contraindicated* with renal failure.

6. *Blood and blood products* **(Table 8.2).**
a. *Indications:*
(1) Maintenance of blood volume.
(2) Supply red blood cells to maintain oxygen-carrying capacity.

Table 8.2

Transfusion with Blood or Blood Products

Blood or Blood Product	Indications	Assessment: Side Effects	Nursing Care Plan/ Implementation
Whole blood	1. Acute hemorrhage 2. Hypovolemic shock	1. Hemolytic reaction 2. Fluid overload 3. Febrile reaction 4. Pyrogenic reaction 5. Allergic reaction	1. See **Chapter 6, Table 6.9 (p. 374)**, for complete discussion of nursing responsibilities 2. Protocol for checking blood before transfusion is begun varies with each institution; however, at least *two* RNs must verify that the unit of blood has been crossmatched for a specific client
Red blood cells, packed	1. Acute anemia with hypoxia 2. Aplastic anemia 3. Bone marrow failure due to malignancy 4. Clients who need red blood cells but not volume	*See* Whole blood	*See* Whole blood
Red blood cells, frozen	1. *See* Red blood cells, packed 2. Clients sensitized by previous transfusions	1. Less likely to cause antigen reaction 2. Decreased possibility of transmitting hepatitis	*See* Whole blood
White blood cells (leukocytes)	Currently being used in severe leukopenia with infection (research still being done)	1. Elevated temperature 2. Graft-versus-host disease	1. Careful monitoring of temperature 2. *Must* be given as soon as collected
Platelet concentrate	1. Severe deficiency 2. Clients who have thrombocytopenia and are bleeding, with platelet counts *below* 10,000/mm^3	1. Fever, chills 2. Hives 3. Development of antibodies that will destroy platelets in future transfusions *Contraindications:* 1. Idiopathic thrombocytopenic purpura 2. Disseminated intravascular coagulation (DIC)	Monitor temperature
Single-donor fresh plasma	1. Clotting deficiency or concentrates not available or deficiency not fully diagnosed 2. Shock	1. Side effects rare 2. Heart failure 3. Possible hepatitis	Use sterile, pyrogen-free filters
Plasma removed from whole blood (up to 5 days after expiration date, which is 21 days)	1. Shock due to loss of plasma 2. Burns 3. Peritoneal injury 4. Hemorrhage 5. While awaiting blood crossmatch results	*See* Single-donor fresh plasma	*See* Single-donor fresh plasma
Freeze-dried plasma	*See* Plasma removed from whole blood	*See* Single-donor fresh plasma	Must be reconstituted with sterile water before use
Single-donor fresh frozen plasma	1. *See* Single-donor fresh plasma 2. Inherited or acquired disorders of coagulation 3. Preoperatively for hemophilia	*See* Single-donor fresh plasma	1. Notify blood bank to thaw about 30 min before administration 2. Give *immediately*

Continued

Table 8.2

Transfusion with Blood or Blood Products—cont'd

Blood or Blood Product	Indications	Assessment: Side Effects	Nursing Care Plan/ Implementation
Cryoprecipitate concentrate (factor VIII—antihemophilic factor)	For hemophilia: 1. Prevention 2. Preoperatively 3. During bleeding episodes	Rare	0.55 mL of cryoprecipitate concentrate has same effect on serum level as 1,600 mL of fresh frozen plasma
Factors II, VII, IX, and X compiled	Specific deficiencies	Hepatitis	Commercially prepared
Fibrinogen (factor I)	Fibrinogen deficiency	Increased risk of hepatitis because the hepatitis virus combines with fibrinogen during fractionation	1. Reconstitute with sterile water 2. Do *not* warm fibrinogen or use hot water to reconstitute 3. Do *not* shake 4. Must be given with a filter
Albumin or salt-poor albumin	1. Shock due to hemorrhage, trauma, infection, surgery, or burns 2. Treatment of cerebral edema 3. Low serum protein levels	None; these are heat-treated products	Commercially prepared

(3) Supply clotting factors to maintain coagulation properties.

(4) Exchange transfusion.

IV. INTRAVENOUS CANCER CHEMOTHERAPY

A. Usual sites: forearm, dorsum of hand, wrist, antecubital fossa.

B. Procedure:

1. Normal saline infusion usually started first, to verify vein patency, position of needle. Chemotherapy "piggybacked" into IV line that is running.
2. Rate: usually 1 mL/min. Running slowly decreases nausea, vomiting, and the degree of vein damage.
3. Check vein patency every 3 to 5 minutes.
4. If more than one drug is to be infused, normal saline should be infused between drugs.
5. **Never** infuse against resistance.
6. **Stop** treatment if client reports pain at needle site. Extravasation (infiltration of toxic drugs into tissue surrounding vessel) may be present
7. If extravasation present, begin protocol appropriate to drug administered (e.g., flushing of line with saline, applying ice or heat, local injection of site with antidote drugs, topical application of steroid creams).
8. Once treatment is completed, remove needle, apply Band-Aid, exert pressure to prevent hematoma formation.

V. COMPLICATIONS OF IV THERAPY **(Table 8.3).**

VI. TOTAL PARENTERAL NUTRITION (TPN): nutrition through a central venous line to clients who are in a catabolic state; are malnourished and cannot tolerate food by mouth or enteral nutrition; are in negative nitrogen balance; or have conditions that interfere with protein ingestion, digestion, and absorption (e.g., Crohn's disease, major burns, and side effects of radiation therapy of abdomen). Least desirable route for nutrition.

A. Types of solutions:

1. Hydrolyzed proteins (Hyprotein, Amigen).
2. Synthetic amino acids (Freamine).
3. Usual components:
   a. 3% to 8% amino acid.
   b. 10% to 25% glucose.
   c. Multivitamins.
   d. Electrolytes.
4. Supplements that can be added:
   a. Fructose.
   b. Alcohol.
   c. Minerals: iron, copper, calcium.
   d. Trace elements: iodine, zinc, magnesium.
   e. Vitamins: A, B, C.
   f. Androgen hormone therapy.
   g. Insulin.
   h. Heparin.
   i. Fats (lipid or fat emulsions) with prolonged use. Lipid emulsions are *contraindicated* if client has allergy to eggs or is on ↑ lipid-containing medications such as propofol (Diprivan).

(text continues on page 612)

Table 8.3

Complications of IV Therapy

Complication	Assessment: Subjective Data	Assessment: Objective Data	Nursing Care Plan/Implementation
Infiltration—fluid infusing into surrounding tissue rather than into vessel	Pain around needle insertion	1. Infusion rate slow 2. Swelling, hardness, coolness, blanching of tissue at site of needle 3. Blood does not return into tubing when bag/bottle lowered 4. Puffiness under surface of arm	1. Stop IV 2. Apply warm towel to area 3. Restart at another site 4. Record
Thrombophlebitis—inflammatory changes in vessel; *thromboemboli*—the development of venous clots within the inflamed vessel	Pain along the vein	Redness, swelling around affected area (red line)	1. Stop IV 2. Notify physician 3. Cold compresses or warm towel, as ordered 4. Restart in another site 5. *Rest affected limb; do not rub* 6. *See* nursing care of thrombophlebitis, **Chapter 6, p. 434**
Pyrogenic reaction—contaminated equipment/solution	1. Headache 2. Backache 3. Nausea 4. Anxiety	1. ↑ Temperature 2. Chills 3. Face flushed 4. Vomiting 5. ↓ BP 6. Cyanosis	1. Discontinue IV 2. Vital signs 3. Send equipment for culture/analysis 4. Antibiotic ointment, as ordered, at injection site 5. *Prevention:* change tubing q24–48h; meticulous sterile technique; check for precipitation, expiration dates, damage to containers, tubings, etc.; refrigerate hyperalimentation fluids; discard hyperalimentation fluids that have been at room temperature for 8–12 hr and use new bag regardless of amount left in first bag (change, to prevent infection—excellent medium for bacterial growth)
Fluid overload—excessive amount of fluid infused; infants/elderly at risk	1. Headache 2. Shortness of breath 3. Syncope 4. Dyspnea	1. ↑ Pulse, venous pressure 2. Venous distention 3. Flushed skin 4. Coughing 5. ↑ Respirations 6. Cyanosis, pulmonary edema 7. Shock	1. Stop IV 2. Semi-Fowler's *position* 3. Notify physician 4. Be prepared for diuretic therapy 5. *Preventive measures:* monitor flow rate and client's response to IV therapy (see **Chapter 6,** Fluid volume excess, **p. 358,** for subjective and objective data)
Air emboli—air in circulatory system	Loss of consciousness	1. Hypotension, cyanosis 2. Tachycardia 3. ↑ Venous pressure 4. Tachypnea	1. Turn on *left* side, with head *down* 2. Administer oxygen therapy 3. **Medical emergency—call physician**
Nerve damage—improper position of limb during infusion or *tying* limb down too tight during infusion → damage to nerve	Numbness: fingers, hands	Unusual position for limb	1. Untie 2. Passive ROM exercises 3. Monitor closely for return of function 4. Record limb status
Pulmonary embolism—blood clot enters pulmonary circulation and obstructs pulmonary artery	Dyspnea	1. Orthopnea 2. Signs of circulatory and cardiac collapse	1. Slow IV to keep vein open (rate: 5–6 drops/min) 2. Notify physician 3. **Medical emergency** 4. Be prepared for lifesaving measures and *anticoagulation* therapy

B. Administration:

1. Dosage varies with clinical condition; 1 to 2 L over 24 hours at a constant IV drip rate. If TPN is discontinued, the rate *must be tapered over 4 to 8 hours* to avoid fluid, electrolyte abnormalities.
2. Solution prepared under laminar flow hood (usually in pharmacy); solution must be *refrigerated;* when refrigerated, expires in *24* hours; once removed from refrigerator, expires in *12* hours.
3. Incompatible with most medications; check with pharmacy. Give in a dedicated TPN line. Do **not** inject IV push medications into TPN line.
4. Route: *Must* be given via central line catheter—double- or triple-lumen catheter or infusion port of pulmonary artery (PA) catheter inserted by physician into internal jugular or subclavian vein. More commonly given via peripherally inserted central catheter (PICC line), inserted by specially trained IV nurses into brachial or cephalic veins. Placement *must* be confirmed by x-ray before beginning infusion. Catheter tip in superior vena cava or right atrium.
5. Management of PICC line:
   a. Always wash hands before handling.
   b. Do **not** take BP in PICC arm.
   c. **No** needle sticks near or above PICC. If possible draw blood from opposite arm.
   d. **Avoid** excessive shoulder use; if sent home with PICC, cautious use of backpacks, playing basketball, shoveling, weight lifting.
   e. Cover PICC arm before bathing/showering.
   f. If dressing becomes wet, soiled, or loose, change as soon as possible.
   g. If catheter breaks, secure with tape and call care provider.
   h. If sudden chest pain, shortness of breath (SOB), or gurgling sensation heard near ear with catheter breakage, clamp or pinch catheter, have client lie on left side with head down. **Call physician.**
6. *Side effects:*
   a. Hyperosmolar coma.
   b. Hyperglycemia greater than 130 mg/dL.
   c. Septicemia.
   d. Thrombosis/sclerosis of vein.
   e. Air embolus.
   f. Pneumothorax.

C. Analysis/nursing diagnosis:

1. *Fluid volume excess, potential,* related to inability to tolerate amount and consistency of solution.
2. *Fluid volume deficit* related to state of malnutrition.
3. *Risk for injury* related to possible complications.
4. *Altered nutrition, more or less than body requirements,* related to ability to tolerate parenteral nutrition.

D. Nursing care plan/implementation:

1. Goal: *prevent infection.*
   a. Dressing change:
      (1) Strict *aseptic* technique.
      (2) Nurse and client wear mask during dressing change.
      (3) Cleanse skin with solution as ordered:
         (a) Acetone to defat the skin, destroy the bacterial wall.
         (b) Iodine 1% solution as *antiseptic* agent.
      (4) Dressing changed q48–72h; transparent polyurethane dressings may be changed weekly.
      (5) Mark with nurse's initials, date and time of change.
      (6) Air-occlusive dressing.
   b. Attach final filter on tubing setup, to prevent air embolism.
   c. Solution: change q24h to prevent infection.
   d. Culture wound and catheter tip if signs of infection appear.
   e. Monitor temperature q4h.
   f. Use lumen line for feeding *only* (not for CVP or medications).
2. Goal: *prevent fluid and electrolyte imbalance.*
   a. Daily weights.
   b. I&O.
   c. Blood glucose q6h for 24 hours using glucometer; may need insulin coverage. If normal range, change to daily.
   d. Monitor Chem 20 electrolytes biweekly initially.
   e. Infusion pump to maintain constant infusion rate.
3. Goal: *prevent complications.*
   a. Warm TPN solution to room temperature to prevent chills.
   b. Monitor for signs of complications **(Table 8.4).**
      (1) Infiltration.
      (2) Thrombophlebitis.
      (3) Fever.
      (4) Hyperglycemia.
      (5) Fluid and electrolyte imbalance.
   c. Have client perform *Valsalva maneuver* or apply a plastic-coated clamp when changing tubing to prevent air embolism.
   d. Tape tubings together to prevent accidental separation.

E. Evaluation/outcome criteria:

1. No signs of infection.
2. Blood sugar less than 130 mg/dL.

Table 8.4

Complications Associated with Total Parenteral Nutrition

Problem	Nursing Interventions
Infection	
Local infection (pain, redness, edema) Generalized, systemic infection (elevated temperature, WBC count)	Sterile dressings; administer *antibiotics* as ordered; general comfort measures
Arterial Puncture	
Artery is punctured instead of vein Physician aspirates bright-red blood that is pulsating strongly	Needle is withdrawn and pressure is applied
Air Embolus	
Air enters venous system during catheter insertion or tubing changes; or catheter/tubing pull apart Chest pain, dizziness, cyanosis, confusion	STAT arterial blood gases (ABGs), chest x-ray, ECG Connect catheter to sterile syringes, and aspirate air Clean catheter tip, connect to new tubing 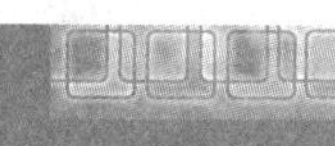 *Place client on left side with head lowered* (left Trendelenburg prevents air from going into pulmonary artery) *Prevention: have client perform Valsalva maneuver or use plastic-coated clamp on catheter at insertion or tubing changes*
Catheter Embolus	
Catheter must be checked for placement by x-ray and observed when removed to be sure it is intact	Careful observation of catheter Monitor for signs of distress
Pneumothorax	
If needle punctures pleura, client reports dyspnea, chest pain	May seal off or may need chest tubes

3. Electrolytes within normal limits.
4. Wounds begin to heal.
5. Weight: no further loss, begins to gain.

PSYCHOTROPIC MEDICATIONS

I. ANTIPSYCHOTICS (also called *neuroleptics, major tranquilizers*)

A. Typical antipsychotics:

1. **Phenothiazines** (prochlorperazine [Compazine], promazine HCl [Sparine], chlorpromazine HCl [Thorazine], thioridazine [Mellaril], trifluoperazine HCl [Stelazine], perphenazine [Trilafon], triflupromazine HCl [Vesprin], fluphenazine enanthate [Prolixin]).
2. **Butyrophenones** (haloperidol [Haldol, Serenace], droperidol fentanyl citrate [Innovar]).
3. **Thiothixenes** (chlorprothixene [Taractan], thiothixene [Navane])—chemically related to phenothiazines, with similar therapeutic effects.
4. **Dibenzoxazepines**—loxapine succinate [Loxitane])

B. Atypical antipsychotics:

1. Risperidone (Risperdal), olanzapine (Zyprexa), quetiapine (Seroquel), ziprasidone (Geodon).
   a. ***Use***—incremental increases for first 3 days to manage psychotic symptoms. Effective for *both positive and negative symptoms* of schizophrenia. Risperidone also available as long-acting injection (Risperdal Consta): IM q 2 wk in alternate gluteal muscle site; delayed onset of action. *Benefit:* lower incidence of extrapyramidal symptoms.
   b. **Assessment**—*side effects:* same as for typical antipsychotics but with higher incidence of weight gain.
2. Clozapine (Clozaril).
   a. ***Use***—those who do not respond to other neuroleptic antipsychotic drugs; offers relief from schizophrenic symptoms: hallucinations, delusions, flat affect, apathy.
   b. **Assessment**—*side effects:*
      (1) Most serious is *agranulocytosis* (potentially fatal; reversible if diagnosed within 1 to 2 weeks of onset).
         (a) *Symptoms* of agranulocytosis: infection, high fever, chills, sore throat, malaise, ulceration of mucous membranes.
         (b) Laboratory value: Discontinue drug with white blood cell (WBC) count less than 2,000 mcg/L or granulocyte count less than 1,000 mcg/L.
      (2) Other side effects: seizures, tachycardia, orthostatic hypotension.

(3) *Caution:* must have weekly blood tests for WBC count; do **not** resume clozapine once it is discontinued, due to side effects.

C. General use of antipsychotic medications—acute and chronic psychoses; most useful in cases of disorganization of thought or behavior; to decrease panic, fear, hostility, restlessness, aggression, and withdrawal.

D. General assessment—*side effects:*

1. *Hypersensitivity* effects:
   a. *Blood dyscrasia*—agranulocytosis, leukopenia, granulocytopenia.
   b. *Skin reactions*—solar sensitivity, allergic dermatitis, flushing, blue-gray skin.
   c. *Obstructive jaundice.*
2. *Extrapyramidal symptoms (EPS)* affecting voluntary movement and skeletal muscles
   a. *Parkinsonism* (also called pseudoparkinsonism)—tremors, cogwheel rigidity, shuffling gait, pill-rolling, masklike facies, salivation, and difficulty starting muscular movement (dyskinesia).
   b. *Dystonia*—limb and neck spasms (torticollis), extensive rigidity of back muscles (opisthotonos), oculogyric crisis, speech and swallowing difficulties, and protrusion of tongue.
   c. *Akathisia*—motor restlessness, pacing, foot tapping, inner tremulousness, and agitation.
   d. ***Tardive dyskinesia (TD)***—excessive blinking; vermiform tongue movement; stereotyped, abnormal, involuntary sucking, chewing, licking, and pursing movements of tongue and mouth; grimacing, frowning, rocking.
      (1) *Cause*—long-term use of high doses of antipsychotic drugs.
      (2) *Predisposing factors*—age, women, organic brain syndrome (OBS); history of electroconvulsive therapy (ECT) or use of tricyclic antidepressants or anti-Parkinson drugs.
3. *Potentiates* central nervous system depressants.
4. *Orthostatic hypotension* (less with butyrophenones).
5. *Anticholinergic effects* (atropine-like)—dry mouth, stuffy nose, blurred vision, urinary retention, and constipation.
6. Pigmentary retinopathy—ocular changes (lens and corneal opacity).
7. Photosensitivity.
8. Weight gain (especially true of the atypical antipsychotic medications).
9. ***Neuroleptic malignant syndrome (NMS):***
   a. *Description:* a rare complication of antipsychotic drugs, with a rapid progression (1 to 3 days) and a 20% mortality rate. It is a **serious medical emergency** for which early recognition of symptoms is critical. *Onset:* at start, after change, or dose increase, when used with combination of medications.
   b. **Assessment:**
      (1) ↑**Vital signs: extreme** temperature of 107°F (leading to seizures, diaphoresis, confusion, → stupor, coma), fluctuating BP, *pulse:* irregular, tachycardia.
      (2) Laboratory values: *increased* creatine phosphokinase (CPK), *increased* potassium, leukocytosis (↑ WBC).
      (3) Renal failure.
      (4) Muscular: parkinsonian rigidity (lead-pipe skeletal muscle rigidity) that leads to dyspnea and dysphagia, tremors, dyskinesia.
      (5) *At risk:* clients with organic brain disorders and severe dehydration.
   c. *Medical treatment:*
      (1) Discontinue all drugs *STAT.*
      (2) Institute supportive care.
      (3) Administer bromocriptine (Parlodel) or dantrolene (Dantrium), dopamine function–enhancing substances (e.g., levodopa, carbidopa, bromocriptine, amantadine).

   d. *Health teaching: avoid* overheating or dehydration; diet: ↑ fluids, ↑ fiber, hard candy.

E. Antipsychotic agents—comparison of side effects (Table 8.5).

F. General nursing care plan/implementation:

1. Goal: *anticipate and check for side effects.*
   a. Protect the person's skin from *sunburn* when outside.
   b. For *hypotension:* take BP and have person lie down for 30 minutes, especially after an injection.
   c. Watch for signs of *blood dyscrasia:* sore throat, fever, malaise.
   d. Observe for symptoms of *hypothermic* or *hyperthermic* reaction due to effect on heat-regulating mechanism.
   e. Observe for, withhold drug for, and report early symptoms of: *jaundice* and bile tract obstruction; high fever; upper abdominal pain, nausea, diarrhea; rash; monitor *liver function.*
   f. Relieve excessive *mouth dryness:* mouth rinse, *increase* fluid intake, gum or hard candy.
   g. Relieve gastric irritation, *constipation:* take with and *increase fluids* and *roughage* in diet.
   h. Observe for and report changes in carbohydrate metabolism (glycosuria, weight gain, polyphagia); change diet.
   i. Check blood sugar levels periodically.

Table 8.5

Antipsychotic Agents—Comparison of Side Effects

Classification	Name Generic	Trade	Extrapyramidal Symptoms (EPS)*	Sedation*	Anticholinergic*	Orthostatic Hypotension*
Typical antipsychotics						
Phenothiazine	Chlorpromazine	Thorazine	3	4	3	4
	Fluphenazine	Prolixin	5	2	2	2
	Perphenazine	Trilafon	4	2	2	2
	Prochlorperazine	Compazine	4	3	2	2
	Promazine	Sparine	3	3	4	3
	Thioridazine	Mellaril	2	4	4	4
	Triflupromazine	Vesprin	3	4	4	3
Butyrophenone	Haloperidol	Haldol	5	1	1	1
Thioxanthene	Thiothixene	Navane	4	2	2	2
Dibenzoxazepine	Loxapine	Loxitane	4	3	2	3
Atypical antipsychotics	Clozapine	Clozaril	1	5	5	4
	Olanzapine	Zyprexa	1	3	2	1
	Quetiapine	Seroquel	1	3	2	1
	Risperidone	Risperdal	1	1	1	3
	Ziprasidone	Geodon	1	2	1	1

*Key: 1 = very low; 2 = low; 3 = moderate; 4 = high; 5 = very high.

2. Goal: *health teaching.*
   a. Dangers of drug potentiation with alcohol or sleeping pills.
   b. Advise about driving or occupations where blurred vision may be a problem.
   c. Caution against abrupt cessation at high doses.
   d. Warn regarding dark urine (sign of jaundice, urinary retention).
   e. Have client with respiratory disorder breathe deeply and cough (drug is a cough depressant).
   f. Need for continuous use of drug and follow-up care.
   g. Prompt reporting of hypersensitivity symptoms: fever, laryngeal edema; abdominal distention (constipation, urinary retention); jaundice; blood dyscrasia.

G. General evaluation/outcome criteria:
1. Behavior is less agitated.
2. Knows side effects to observe for, lessen, and/or prevent.
3. Continues to use drug.

II. ANTIDEPRESSANTS

A. Tricyclic antidepressants (TCAs) (imipramine HCl [Tofranil], desipramine HCl [Norpramine, Pertofrane], nortriptyline HCl [Pamelor, Aventyl], trimipramine [Surmontil], clomipramine [Anafranil], amitriptyline HCl [Elavil, Endep], amitriptyline HCl/perphenazine [Triavil], protriptyline HCl [Vivactil], doxepin HCl [Sinequan, Adapin]), bupropion (Wellbutrin), trazodone (Desyrel), amoxapine (Asendin)—effective in 2 to 4 weeks.

1. **Use**—elevate mood in depression, increase physical activity and mental alertness; may bring relief of symptoms of depression so that client can attend individual or group therapy; bipolar disorder, depressed; dysthymic disorder; sleep disturbance; agitation.
2. **Assessment**—*side effects:*
   a. *Behavioral*—activation of latent schizophrenia (hallucinations); hypomania; suicide attempts; mental *confusion.* Withhold drug if observed.
   b. *Central nervous system* (CNS)—*tremors, seizures,* ataxia, jitteriness, irritability.
   c. *Autonomic nervous system* (ANS)—*dry mouth,* nasal congestion, aggravation of glaucoma (blurred vision), constipation, urinary retention, edema, paralysis, *ECG* changes (flattened T waves; **arrhythmia** severe in overdose).
3. **Nursing care plan/implementation:**
   a. Goal: *assess risk of suicide during initial improvement*—careful, close observation.
   b. Goal: *prevent risk of tachycardia and cardiac arrhythmias and orthostatic hypotension*—use caution with client with cardiovascular disease, hyperthyroidism, having ECT or surgery (gradually discontinue 2 to 3 days *before* surgery). Monitor BP, pulse twice a day; ECGs, 2 to 3/wk until dose adjusted.
      (1) *Avoid* long hot showers or baths.

c. Goal: *observe for signs of urinary retention, constipation:* monitor I&O and *weight gain* (encourage exercise).
   (1) Fiber diet.
   (2) Reduced calories.

d. Goal: *cautious drug use with glaucoma or history of seizures.* Observe seizure precautions due to lowered seizure threshold.

e. Goal: *health teaching.*
   (1) Advise against driving car or participating in activities requiring mental alertness, due to *sedative* effects.
   (2) Encourage increased fluid intake and frequent mouth rinsing to combat dry mouth; use candy, ice; take with food.
   (3) *Avoid* smoking, which decreases drug effects.
   (4) *Avoid* use of alcohol and other drugs, due to adverse interactions, especially over-the-counter (OTC) drugs (e.g., antihistamines).
   (5) Advise of *delay* in desired effect (2 to 4 weeks).
   (6) Instruct *gradual* discontinuance to *avoid* withdrawal symptoms.

4. **Evaluation/outcome criteria:** diminished symptoms of agitated depression and anxiety.

B. Monoamine oxidase inhibitors (MAOIs) (phenelzine sulfate [Nardil], isocarboxazid [Marplan], tranylcypromine sulfate [Parnate], iproniazid [Marsilid], pargiline HCl [Eutonyl], nialamide [Niamid]).

1. **Assessment**—*side effects:*
   a. *Behavioral*—may activate latent schizophrenia, mania, excitement.
   b. *CNS*—tremors; **hypertensive crisis** (*avoid:* cheese, colas, caffeine, red wine, beer, yeast, chocolate, chicken liver, and other substances high in *tyramine or pressor amines* [e.g., amphetamines and cold and hay fever medication]); *intracerebral hemorrhage; hyperpyrexia.*
   c. *ANS—dry mouth,* aggravation of glaucoma, bowel and bladder control problems; edema, paralysis, ECG changes (severe arrhythmia in overdose).
   d. *Allergic* hepatocellular jaundice.

2. **Nursing care plan/implementation:**
   a. Goal: *reduce risk of hypertensive crisis*—diet restrictions of foods high in *tyramine* content.
   b. Goal: *observe for urinary retention*—measure I&O.
   c. Goal: *health teaching.*
      (1) Therapeutic response takes 2 to 3 weeks.
      (2) *Food and alcohol restrictions:* avocados, bananas, raisins, licorice, chocolate, aged cheese, yogurt, sour cream, papaya, figs, overripe fruit, sausages, salami, bologna, liver, herring, soy sauce, meat tenderizers, red wine, beer, caffeine, cola, yeast, chocolate.
      (3) Change position gradually to prevent postural hypotension.
      (4) Report any stiff neck, palpitations, chest pain, headaches because of possible hypertensive crises (can be fatal).
      (5) Take *no nonprescribed* drugs.

3. **Evaluation/outcome criteria:**
   a. Improvement in sleep, appetite, activity, interest in self and surroundings.
   b. Lessening of anxiety and complaints.

C. Selective serotonin reuptake inhibitors (SSRIs) (fluoxetine [Prozac], paroxetine [Paxil], sertraline [Zoloft], fluvoxamine [Luvox], citalopram hydrobromide [Celexa])—SSRIs are generally the first-line choice because they have fewer side effects, do not require blood monitoring, and are safe in overdose.

1. **Assessment**—*side effects: CNS stimulation*—insomnia, agitation, headache (especially with Prozac); weight loss; sexual dysfunction (men: impotence; women: loss of orgasm, decreased libido). Other side effects are similar to TCAs (dry mouth, sedation, nausea).

2. **Nursing care plan/implementation:**
   a. Goal: *reduce insomnia, agitation*—take early in day; *avoid* alcohol, caffeine; teach relaxation before sleep time.
   b. Goal: *reduce headaches*—give analgesics.
   c. Goal: *prevent weight loss*—weigh every day or every other day, same time and scale; do *not* use with clients who are anorexic.

3. **Evaluation/outcome criteria:**
   a. Improvement in mood and hygiene, thought and communication patterns.
   b. Has not harmed self.
   c. No significant anticholinergic and cardiovascular side effects.

III. ANTIANXIETY AGENTS (also called anxiolytics, minor tranquilizers) **(Table 8.6)**

A. Benzodiazepines, beta-adrenergic blockers, buspirone HCl, diphenylmethane antihistamines

1. **Use**—acute alcohol withdrawal, tension, and irrational fears; anxiety disorders, preoperative sedation; have muscle relaxant and anticonvulsant properties.

2. **Assessment**—*side effects:* hypotension, drowsiness, motor uncoordination, confusion, skin eruptions, edema, menstrual irregularities, constipation, extrapyramidal symptoms, blurred vision, lethargy; increased or decreased libido.

Table 8.6

Antianxiety Agents: Comparison

Drug	Use	Side Effects/Cautions
Benzodiazepines *Ativan* (lorazepam)	For specific stress: Medium acting	Drowsiness, ↓ mental alertness, ↓ BP, headache Lethal overdose with alcohol
Klonopin (clonazepam) *Librium* (chlordiazepoxide)	Long acting Long acting	High risk for dependency with long-term use; taper gradually over 2–6 wk
Serax (oxazepam) *Valium* (diazepam)	 Short acting	Symptoms with abrupt withdrawal: irritability, dizziness
Tranxene (clorazepate) *Xanax* (alprazolam)	 Short acting	Do *not* use in pregnancy Paradoxical reactions (euphoria, excitement)
Beta-adrenergic blocker *Inderal* (propranolol hydrochloride)	Stage fright Relief of physical signs of anxiety (tachycardia)	Hypotension Bradycardia No risk of dependence or abuse
Buspirone hydrochloride *BuSpar*	Long-term use	Less sedation; no risk of dependence *Delayed* effect (3 wk); no CNS depression
Diphenylmethane antihistamines *Atarax* (hydroxyzine hydrochloride) *Vistaril* (hydroxyzine pamoate)	Safe for long-term use	No risk of physical dependency or abuse; minimal toxicity May cause drowsiness

Adapted from ©Lagerquist S: *Nurse Notes: Psychiatric-Mental Health*. Philadelphia, Lippincott.

3. **Nursing care plan/implementation:**
   a. Goal: *administer cautiously, because drug may:*
      (1) Be habituating (causing withdrawal convulsions; therefore, *gradual withdrawal* necessary).
      (2) Potentiate CNS depressants.
      (3) Have adverse effect on pregnancy.
      (4) Be dangerous for those: with suicidal tendencies or severe psychoses, narrow-angle glaucoma, elderly or debilitated.

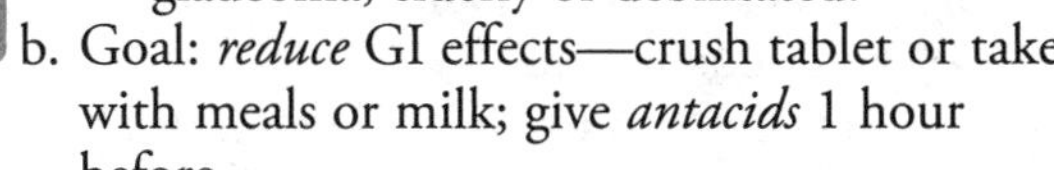

   b. Goal: *reduce* GI effects—crush tablet or take with meals or milk; give *antacids* 1 hour before.
   c. Goal: *monitor effects on liver function:* Periodic liver function tests and blood counts, especially with upper respiratory infection, hepatic or renal dysfunction.
   d. Goal: *reduce* risk of—hypotension, respiratory depression, phlebitis, venous thrombosis.
   e. Goal: *health teaching.*
      (1) Advise against suddenly stopping drug (withdrawal symptoms begin in 5 to 7 days).
      (2) Talk with physician if plans to be or is pregnant or lactating.
      (3) Urge to drink fluids.
      (4) *Avoid:* alcohol, OTC drugs (due to potentiation of other CNS depressants), and heavy smoking and caffeine.
      (5) Problem with habituation.
4. **Evaluation/outcome criteria:** decreased alcohol withdrawal symptoms or preoperative anxiety; no seizures or confusion; relief of tension, anxiety, skeletal muscle spasm.

IV. ANTIMANIC AGENTS

A. Lithium (Eskalith, Lithane, Lithobid)—effect occurs 1 to 3 weeks after first dose.

1. **Use**—acute manic attack and prevention of recurrence of cyclic manic-depressive episodes of bipolar disorders.
2. **Assessment:**
   a. *Side effects*—levels from 1.6 to 2.0 mEq/L may cause: blurred vision, tinnitus, tremors, nausea and vomiting, severe diarrhea, polyuria, polydipsia; ataxia. Levels greater than 2 mEq/L may cause: motor weakness, headache, edema, and lethargy. Levels greater than 2.5 mEq/L *may exhibit signs of severe toxicity:* arrhythmias, myocardial infarction (MI), cardiovascular collapse, oliguria/anuria; *neurological* (twitching, marked drowsiness, slurred speech, dysarthria, athetotic movements, convulsions, delirium, stupor, coma).
   b. *Precautions*—cautious use with clients on *diuretics;* with abnormal *electrolytes* (sweating, dehydrated, and clients who are postoperative); with *thyroid* problems, on *low-salt diets;* with *heart failure;* with *impaired renal function;* with *pregnancy and lactation;* risk of suicide.
   c. *Dosage*—**therapeutic** level 0.8 to 1.6 mEq/L; dose for maintenance 300 to 1,200 mg/day; *toxic* level greater than 2.0 mEq/L; blood sample drawn in acute phase 10 to 14 hours after last dose, taken three times a day.

3. **Nursing care plan/implementation:**
   a. Goal: *anticipate and check for signs and symptoms of toxicity.*
      (1) Reduce GI symptoms: take *with meals.*
      (2) Check for edema: daily weight, I&O.
      (3) Monitor blood levels greater than 2.0 mEq/L for side effects and signs of *toxicity:* nausea, vomiting, diarrhea, anorexia, ataxia, weakness, drowsiness, fine tremor or muscle twitching, slurred speech.
      (4) Monitor results from repeat thyroid and kidney function tests.
      (5) Withhold drug and notify physician when 1.5 mEq/L is reached.
      (6) Monitor vital signs 2 to 3 times/day (pulse irregularities, hypotension, arrhythmias).
   b. Goal: *report fever, diarrhea, prolonged vomiting immediately.*
   c. Goal: *monitor effect* (therapeutic and toxic) through blood samples taken:
      (1) 10 to 14 hours after last dose.
      (2) Every 2 to 3 days until 1.6 mEq/L is reached.
      (3) Once a week while in hospital.
      (4) Every 2 to 3 months to maintain blood levels less than 2 mEq/L.
   d. Goal: *health teaching.*
      (1) Advise client of 1- to 3-week lag time for effect.
      (2) Urge to drink adequate *liquids* (2 to 3 L/day), ice; strict oral hygiene.
      (3) Report: *polyuria* and polydipsia.
      (4) *Diet: avoid* caffeine, crash diets, diet pills, self-prescribed low-salt diet, alcohol, antacids, high-sodium foods (which increase lithium excretion and reduce drug effect); take *with meals.* Use sugarless candy.
      (5) Caution against driving, operating machinery that requires mental alertness until drug is effective.
      (6) Warn *not* to change or omit dose.
4. **Evaluation/outcome criteria:**
   a. Changed facial affect.
   b. Improved posture, ability to concentrate, sleep patterns; mood is stabilized.
   c. Assumption of self-care.
   d. No signs of lithium toxicity.

PSYCHOTROPIC

V. ANTIPARKINSONIAN AGENTS

A. Trihexyphenidyl HCl (Artane) and benztropine mesylate (Cogentin).

1. **Use**—counteract drug-induced extrapyramidal reactions.
2. **Assessment:**
   a. Trihexyphenidyl HCl:
      (1) *Side effects*—anticholinergic: *dry mouth, blurred vision,* dizziness, nausea, *constipation,* drowsiness, *urinary hesitancy* or *retention;* pupil dilation; headache; weakness; *tachycardia.*
      (2) *Precautions*—cautious use with: cardiac, liver, or kidney disease or obstructive gastrointestinal-genitourinary disease, benign prostatic hyperplasia (BPH), or myasthenia gravis. Do *not* give if glaucoma present.
   b. Benztropine mesylate—*side effects:* same as for trihexyphenidyl HCl *plus:*
      (1) Effect on *body temperature* (hyperpyrexia) may result in life-threatening state (heatstroke).
      (2) *GI distress.*
      (3) Inability to concentrate, memory difficulties, and mild confusion (often mistaken for senility); *drowsiness.*
      (4) May lead to toxic *psychotic* reactions.
      (5) *Subjective sensations*—light or heavy feelings in legs, numbness and tingling of extremities, *light-headedness* or tightness of head, and giddiness.
3. **Nursing care plan/implementation:**
   a. Goal: *relieve GI distress* by giving *after* or *with* meals or at bedtime.
   b. Goal: *monitor adverse effects.*
      (1) Hypotension, tachycardia: check pulse, blood pressure; increased temperature; decreased sweating.
      (2) Constipation and fecal impaction: add roughage to *diet.*
      (3) Dry mouth: increase *fluid* intake; encourage frequent mouth rinsing; offer sugarless candy or gum, ice.
      (4) Blurred vision: suggest reading glasses.
      (5) Dizziness: assist with ambulation; use side rails.
      (6) Urinary retention: maintain I&O.
   c. *Health teaching:*
      (1) *Avoid* driving, and limit activities requiring alertness.
      (2) Delayed drug effect (2 to 3 days).
      (3) Potential abuse due to hallucinogenic effects.
      (4) *Avoid* alcohol and other CNS depressants; *avoid* hot weather.
      (5) Take with food.
      (6) Do *not* stop drug abruptly.
4. **Evaluation/outcome criteria:**
   a. Less rigidity, drooling, and oculogyric crisis.
   b. Improved gait, balance, posture.
   c. Has not experienced symptoms of hyperthermia.

MIND-ALTERING SUBSTANCES

Major substances used by the public to alter mental states are compared in **Table 8.7.**

Table 8.7

Major Substances Used for Mind Alteration

Official Name	Slang Name	Usual Single Adult Dose/Duration	Legitimate Medical Uses—Present and Projected	Short-Term Effects	Long-Term Effects
Alcohol—whisky, gin, beer, wine	Booze, hooch, suds, moonshine, firewater, nightcap	1½ oz gin or whiskey, 12 oz beer/2–4 hr	Rare: sometimes used as a sedative (for tension)	CNS depressant; relaxation (sedation); euphoria; drowsiness; impaired: judgment, reaction time, coordination, and emotional control; frequent aggressive behavior and driving accidents; loss of inhibitions; slurred speech	Diversion of energy and money from more creative and productive pursuits; habituation; possible obesity with chronic excessive use; irreversible damage to brain and liver; addiction with severe withdrawal illness (delirium tremens [DTs]) with heavy use; many deaths
Caffeine—coffee, tea, cola, No-Doz, APC	Java, mud, brew	1–2 cups, 1 bottle, 5 mg/2–4 hr	Mild stimulant; treatment of some forms of coma	CNS stimulant; increased alertness; reduction of fatigue	Sometimes insomnia, restlessness, or gastric irritation; habituation
Nicotine (and coal tar)—cigarettes, cigars, pipe tobacco, snuff	Fags, nails, weeds, butts, chaw, cancer sticks	1–2 cigarettes/1–2 hr	None (used as an insecticide)	CNS stimulant; relaxation or distraction	Lung (and other) cancer, heart and blood vessel disease, cough, etc.; higher infant mortality rate; many deaths; habituation; diversion of energy and money; air pollution; fire
SEDATIVES	Downers				
Alcohol—see above					
Barbiturates—amobarbital (Amytal, Tuinal), pentobarbital (Nembutal), secobarbital (Seconal), phenobarbital	Barbs, blue, angel, blue devils, yellow jackets, yellow birds, dolls, red devils, red birds, phennies, goofers, jelly beans, tooies	50–100 mg	Treatment of insomnia and tension Induction of anesthesia As an anticonvulsant	CNS depressants; sleep induction; relaxation (sedation); sometimes euphoria; drowsiness; impaired: judgment, reaction time, coordination, and emotional control; relief of anxiety/tension; muscle relaxation	Irritability, weight loss, addiction with severe withdrawal illness (like DTs); diversion of energy and money; habituation, addiction
Glutethimide (Doriden)	Gorilla pills, CBs, D	500 mg			
Chloral hydrate (Noctec)	Peter, Mickey	500 mg			
Meprobamate (Miltown, Equanil)	Dolls, dollies	400 mg/4 hr*			

Continued

Table 8.7

Major Substances Used for Mind Alteration—cont'd

Official Name	Slang Name	Usual Single Adult Dose/Duration	Legitimate Medical Uses—Present and Projected	Short-Term Effects	Long-Term Effects
STIMULANTS	Uppers				
Caffeine—see above					
Nicotine—see above					
Amphetamines Methamphetamine (Methedrine, Pesoxyn)	Pep pills, wake-ups, Bennies, splash, peaches Water crystal, speed, meth	2.5–15.0 mg	Treatment of: obesity, narcolepsy, fatigue, depression, hyperkinesia	CNS stimulants; increased alertness; reduction of fatigue; loss of appetite; insomnia; often euphoria, agitation	Restlessness, weight loss, toxic psychosis (mainly paranoid); diversion of energy and money; habituation; extreme irritability, toxic psychosis
Dextroamphetamine (Dexedrine)	Dexies, uppers Diet pills	25 mg		*Symptoms of overdose:* hallucinations, convulsions; cardiac, respiratory failure; coma; pulmonary edema	
Phenmetrazine HCl (Preludin) Cocaine	Coke, snow, blow, happy gold dust, toot, lady, flake, crack, cecil, girl, C	Variable/4 hr*	Anesthesia of the eyes and throat		
TRANQUILIZERS					
Chlordiazepoxide (Librium) Phenothiazines: Chlorpromazine HCl (Thorazine) Perchlorperazine (Compazine) Trifluoperazine HCl (Stelazine) Reserpine (rauwolfia)	Green and whites, roaches	5–25 mg 10–50 mg 5–10 mg 2–5 mg 0.10–0.25 mg/4–6 hr*	Treatment of: anxiety, tension, alcoholism, neurosis, psychosis, psychosomatic disorders, and vomiting	Selective CNS depressants; relaxation, relief of anxiety/tension; suppression of hallucinations or delusions, improved functioning	Sometimes drowsiness, dryness of mouth, blurring of vision, skin rash, tremor; occasionally jaundice, agranulocytosis, or death
Marijuana or cannabis	Pot, grass, Texas tea, weed, stuff, joint, reefers, Mary Jane, MJ, hay, locoweed	Variable—1 cigarette or pipe, or 1 drink or cake (India)/4 hr*	Treatment of: depression, tension, loss of appetitie, high blood pressure, nausea and vomiting from chemotherapy	Relaxation, euphoria, increased appetite; some alteration of time perception; possible impairment of judgment and coordination; mixed CNS depressant-stimulant; lowered inhibitions	Memory impairment; possible diversion of energy and money; habituation; occasional acute panic reactions (with paranoia, delusions, hallucinations)
Hashish†	Hash, rope, Sweet Lucy				

ANTIDEPRESSANTS					
Dibenzazepine (imipramine [Tofranil], amitriptyline HCl [Elavil])		25 mg, 10 mg	Treatment of moderate to severe depression	Relief of depression (elevation of mood), stimulation	Basically the same as tranquilizers above
MAO inhibitors (phenelzine sulfate [Nardil], tranylcypromine sulfate [Parnate])		10 mg, 15 mg/4–6 hr*			
NARCOTICS (OPIATES, ANALGESICS)					
Opium	Op, black, poppy, tar, Big O	10–12 "pipes" (Asia)/4 hr*	Treatment of severe pain, diarrhea, and cough	CNS depressants; sedation, euphoria, relief of pain, impaired intellectual functioning and coordination	Constipation, loss of appetite and weight, temporary impotency or sterility; habituation, addiction with unpleasant and painful withdrawal illness
Heroin	Horse, H, smack, shit, junk, brown, pcag, TNT	Variable—bag or paper with 5%–10% heroin			
Morphine (Astramorph)	M, white stuff, Miss Emma	10–15 mg			
Codeine	Terp, robo, romo, syrup	15–30 mg	Topical anesthetic		
Aspirin/oxycodone HCl (Percodan)	Perks, Perkies	1 tablet			
Meperidine HCl (Demerol)	Doctors	50–100 mg			
Methadone (Dolophine)	Dollies, done	2.5–40.0 mg			
Cough syrups (Cheracol, Hycodan, Romilar, etc.)		2–4 oz (for euphoria)/ 4–6 hr*			
Dilaudid	DLs, 4s, lords, little D				
HALLUCINOGENS					
LSD (Lysergic acid diethylamide)	Acid, sugar cube, trip, big D	150 mcg/10–12 hr	Experimental study of mind and brain function; enhancement of creativity and problem-solving; treatment of alcoholism, mental illness, and reduction of intractable pain in the person who is dying; chemical warfare	Production of visual imagery, increased sensory awareness, anxiety, nausea, impaired coordination; sometimes consciousness expansion	Usually none; sometimes precipitates or intensifies an already existing psychosis (hallucinations); more commonly can produce a panic reaction (extreme hyperactivity)
Psilocybin	Magic mushrooms, God's flesh, 'rooms	25 mg			
STP	Serenity, tranquility, peace	6 mg			
DMT	Businessman's Trip				

Continued

Table 8.7

Major Substances Used for Mind Alteration—cont'd

Official Name	Slang Name	Usual Single Adult Dose/Duration	Legitimate Medical Uses—Present and Projected	Short-Term Effects	Long-Term Effects
Mescaline (peyote)	Cactus, mesc, mescal, half moon, big chief, bad seed	350 mg/12–14 hr			
PCP (Phencyclidine)	Angel dust, hog, rocket fuel				
MDMA	Ecstasy, XTC, Adam				
MISCELLANEOUS					
Glue, gasoline, and solvents		Variable	None except for antihistamines used for allergy and amyl nirite for fainting	When used for mind alteration generally produces a "high" (euphoria) with impaired coordination and judgment	Variable—some of the substances can seriously damage the liver or kidney, and some produce hallucinations
Amyl nitrite	Pearls, poppers	1–2 ampules			
Antihistamines		25–50 mg			
Nutmeg		Variable/2 hr			
Nonprescription "sedatives" (Compoze)					
Catnip					
Nitrous oxide					

*Time given pertains to all drugs listed.

†Hashish or charas is a more concentrated form of the active ingredient THC (tetrahydrocannabinol) and is consumed in smaller doses, analogous to vodka-beer ratios.

ABSORPTION RATES BY DIFFERENT ROUTES

Table 8.8 lists the rates of absorption in a healthy person with normal perfusion by various routes.

Table 8.8

Rates of Absorption by Different Routes

Route of Administration	Time Until Drug Takes Effect*
Topical	Hours to days
Oral	30–90 min
Rectal	5–30 min (unpredictable)
Subcutaneous injection	15–30 min
Intramuscular injection	10–20 min
Sublingual tablet	3–5 min
Inhalation	3 min
Endotracheal	3 min
Intravenous	30–60 sec
Intracardiac	15 sec

*In a healthy person with normal perfusion.

REGIONAL ANALGESIA-ANESTHESIA IN LABOR AND BIRTH

The characteristics and nursing implications for regional analgesia-anesthesia in labor and delivery are detailed in **Table 8.9.**

Table 8.9

Regional Analgesia-Anesthesia for Labor and Birth

Types	Characteristics	Nursing Implications
Common Agents in 0.5%–1.0% Solution		
Lidocaine (Xylocaine) Bupivacaine HCl (Marcaine) Tetracaine HCl (Pontocaine) Mepivacaine HCl (Carbocaine) Chloroprocaine HCl (Nesacaine) Ropivacaine (Norapin)	Used with epinephrine (or other vasoconstrictor drug) to delay absorption, prolong anesthetic effect, and decrease chance of hypotension	*Note any history of allergy;* note response: allergic reaction, hypotension, and lack of wearing off of anesthetic effect; observe for hypertensive crisis if agent combined with epinephrine and oxytocin is also being given
Peripheral Nerve Block		
Pudendal (5–10 mL each side) anesthetizes lower two thirds of vagina and perineum	Perineal anesthesia of short duration (30 min); local anesthesia; simple and safe; does not depress neonate; may inhibit bearing-down reflex	To get cooperation, give explanation during procedure
Paracervical (uterosacral) block (5–10 mL given into each side) anesthetizes cervix and upper two thirds of vagina; *note:* used more for gynecological surgery than for labor	When the cervix is dilated, may be given between 3 and 8 cm by physician when woman is having at least 3 contractions in 10 min; lasts 45–90 min; can be repeated; can be followed by local, epidural, or other; may cause temporary fetal bradycardia	Explain: especially length and type of needle; take maternal vital signs and fetal heart rate (FHR); have her void; help position; monitor FHR continuously; monitor contractions; and watch for return of pain
Local infiltration	Useful for perineal repairs	No special nursing care
Epidural lumbar block	Useful during first and second stages; can be given "one shot" or continuously; T10 to S5 for vaginal birth; T8 to S1 for abdominal birth; complete anesthesia for labor and birth	*Hypotension* (with resultant fetal bradycardia): (a) turn from supine to lateral, or *elevate* legs, (b) administer humidified oxygen by mask at 8–10 L/min, (c) increase rate of IV fluids (use infusate *without* oxytocin); will need coaching to push, and low forceps or vacuum may be required

Continued

Table 8.9

Regional Analgesia-Anesthesia for Labor and Birth—cont'd

Types	Characteristics	Nursing Implications
Peripheral Nerve Block		
Subarachnoid spinal		
Continuous	Useful during first or second stage of labor, or for abdominal surgery	Instruct when to bear down
Low spinal ("saddle," "one shot") block	Same as continuous	Same as continuous
Intrathecal (spinal): morphine, fentanyl, sufentanil	0.5 mg produces marked analgesia for 12–24 hr; onset in 20–30 min Fentanyl and sufentanil produce short-acting analgesia (1½–3½ hr)	*Side effects:* respiratory depression, pruritus, nausea, vomiting, sleepiness, urinary retention; keep *naloxone* 0.4 mg at bedside and respiratory support equipment readily available

FOOD/FLUID-MEDICATION INTERACTIONS

Food and fluid considerations with various drugs are detailed in **Table 8.10.**

Table 8.10

Food and Fluid Considerations with Drugs

Key:

1. Take with food or milk
2. Take on empty stomach (1 hr ac or 2 hr pc)
3. Don't drink milk or eat dairy products
4. Take with full glass of water
5. Take ½ hr before meals
6. Take with or without food

A

Albuterol 1
Allopurinol 1
Aminophylline 1
Amiodarone 1
Amlodipine 6
Amoxicillin 6
Ampicillin 2
Aspirin 1
Augmentin 6
Azo Gantrisin 4, 6

B

Baclofen 1
Bactrim 4, 6
Belladonna 5
Benemid 1, 4
Bisacodyl 3

C

Captopril 2
Cefaclor 6
Cefuroxime axetil 6
Cephalexin 6
Chlorothiazide 1
Cholestyramine 5
Cimetidine 1
Ciprofloxacin 4, 6
Clonazepam 1
Clopidogrel 6
Cloxacillin 2
Co-trimoxazole 4, 6
Cyclosporine 1

D

Demeclocycline 2, 3
Diltiazem 1
Diuril 1
Donnatal 5
Dopar 1
Doxycycline hyclate 3, 6
Dulcolax 3

E

Ecotrin 3
Enalapril 6
Erythromycin stearate 2
Ethosuximide 1
Etodolac 2

F

Famotidine 6
Feldene 1
Ferrous sulfate 3
Flecainide 6
Fluoxetine 6

G

Gantrisin 4, 6
Gemfibrozil 5
Glycopyrrolate 5

H

Hismanal 2
Hydrocodone/acetaminophen 1
Hydromorphone 1

I

Ibuprofen 1, 2
Ilosone 6
Indinavir 2, 4
Indomethacin 1
Isoniazid 2

K

Keflex 6
Ketoconazole 1
Ketoprofen 1
K-Lor 1

L

Levodopa 1
Librium 1
Lisinopril 6
Lovastatin 1

M

Macrodantin 1
Marax 1
Metronidazole 1
Mexiletine 1
Mycophenolate 2

N

Nafcillin 2
Naproxen 4
Neostigmine 5
Niacin 1
Nicardipine 5
Nitrofurantoin 1

P

Parlodel 1
Penicillamine 2
Penicillin G 2
Penicillin V 2
Persantine 2
Phenylbutazone 1
Phenytoin 1

Table 8.10

Food and Fluid Considerations with Drugs—cont'd

Key:

Prednisone 1
Pro-Banthine 5
Probenecid 4

Q

Quinidine 1

R

Ranitidine 6
Rifampin 2
Robinul 5

S

Simvastatin 6
Sinemet 1
Slow-K 1
Sucralfate 2
Sulfisoxazole 4, 6

T

Tedral 1
Tetracycline 2, 3
Theophylline 1, 4
Ticlopidine 1
Trimethoprim 2

V

Vasotec 6

Z

Zestril 6

ANTINEOPLASTIC DRUG CLASSIFICATIONS

Table 8.11 provides a classification of the antineoplastic drugs.

Table 8.11

Antineoplastic Drug Classifications

I. Alkylating agents
- **A.** Alkyl sulfonates
  1. Busulfan (*Myleran*)
- **B.** Ethylenimines
  1. Thiotepa
- **C.** Nitrogen mustards
  1. Chlorambucil (*Leukeran*)
  2. Cyclophosphamide (*Cytoxan*)
  3. Ifosfamide (*Ifex*)
  4. Mechlorethamine hydrochloride (*Mustargen*, HN_2, nitrogen mustard)
  5. Melphalan (*Alkeran, L-PAM,* L-phenylalanine mustard)
- **D.** Nitrosoureas
  1. Carmustine (BCNU, *BiCNU*)
  2. Lomustine (CCNU, *CeeNu*)
  3. Semustine (methyl-CCNU)
  4. Streptozocin (*Zanosar*, streptozotocin)
- **E.** Triazenes
  1. Dacarbazine (*DTIC-Dome*)

II. Antibiotics
- **A.** Anthracyclines
  1. Daunorubicin (daunomycin, *Cerubidine*)
  2. Doxorubicin hydrochloride (*Adriamycin*)
  3. Idarubicin (*Idamycin*)
- **B.** Bleomycins
  1. Bleomycin sulfate (*Blenoxane*)
- **C.** Dactinomycin (actinomycin D, *Cosmegen*)
- **D.** Mitomycin (mitomycin C, *Mutamycin*)
- **E.** Plicamycin (*Mithracin*)

III. Antimetabolites
- **A.** Folate antagonist
  1. Methotrexate (*Folex, Mexate*)
- **B.** Purine analogues
  1. Cladribine (2-chlorodeoxyadenosine, *Leustatin*)
  2. Fludarabine (*Fludara*)
  3. Mercaptopurine (6-MP, *Purinethol*)
  4. Pentostatin (deoxycoformycin, *Nipent*)
  5. Thioguanine (6-TG, 6-thioguanine)
- **C.** Pyrimidine analogues
  1. Cytarabine (cytosine arabinoside, *Cytosar-U*, ara-C)
  2. Fluorouracil (5-FU, 5-fluorouracil)

IV. Cellular growth factors
- **A.** Filgrastim (*Neupogen*)
- **B.** Sargramostim (*Leukine, Prokine*)

V. Enzymes
- **A.** L-Asparaginase (*Elspar*)

VI. Hormonal agents
- **A.** Androgens/antiandrogens
  1. Flutamide (*Eulexin*)
- **B.** Estrogens/antiestrogens
  1. Estramustine phosphate sodium (*Emcyt*)
  2. Tamoxifen citrate (*Nolvadex*)
- **C.** Glucocorticoids
- **D.** Luteinizing hormone–releasing hormone (LH-RH) antagonists
  1. Buserelin (*Suprefact*)
  2. Leuprolide (*Lupron*)
- **E.** Octreotide acetate (*Sandostatin*)

VII. Immunomodulating agents
- **A.** Interferons
  1. Interferon alfa-2a (*Roferon-A*)
  2. Interferon alfa-2b (*Intron A*)
- **B.** Interleukins: aldesleukin (interleukin-2, IL-2, *Proleukin*)
- **C.** Levamisole (*Ergamisol*)

VIII. Miscellaneous agents
- **A.** Carboplatin (*Paraplatin*)
- **B.** Cisplatin (*cis*-platinum II, *Platinol*)
- **C.** Hexamethylmelamine (HMM)
- **D.** Hydroxyurea (*Hydrea*)
- **E.** Mitotane (o,p′-DDD, *Lysodren*)
- **F.** Mitoxantrone (*Novantrone*)
- **G.** Procarbazine (*N*-methylhydrazine, *Matulane, Natulan*)

IX. Monoclonal antibodies

X. Plant-derived products
- **A.** Epipodophyllotoxins
  1. Etoposide (*VePesid*)
  2. Teniposide (*Vumon*)
- **B.** Taxanes: paclitaxel (*Taxol*)
- **C.** Vinca alkaloids
  1. Vinblastine (*Velban*)
  2. Vincristine (*Oncovin*)

COMMON SIDE EFFECTS OF CHEMOTHERAPEUTIC AGENTS

The common side effects of various chemotherapeutic agents are detailed in **Table 8.12.**

Table 8.12

Common Side Effects of Chemotherapeutic Agents*

	Nausea and Vomiting	Mucositis	Diarrhea	Skin Reactions	Lung	Neurological
Alkylating Agents						
Busulfan	0	+	0	Hyperpigmentation	0	0
Carboplatin	+	0	0	0	0	0
Chlorambucil	0	0	0	0	+	0
Cisplatin	+	0	0	Alopecia	0	+
Cyclophosphamide	+	0	0	0	+	0
DTIC	+	0	0	0	0	0
Ifosfamide	+	0	0	Alopecia	0	Encephalopathy
Mechlorethamine	+	+	+	Alopecia, rash	0	0
Melphalan	0	0	0	0	0	0
Antimetabolites						
2-Chlorodeoxyadenosine	+	0	0	0	0	0
Cytosine arabinoside	0	0	+	0	+	0
2-Deoxycoformycin	+	0	0	Erythema	0	Lethargy, coma
Fludarabine	+	0	0	0	0	0
5-Fluorouracil	0	+	+	Phlebitis	0	Cerebellar
Hydroxyurea	0	0	0	Skin atrophy	0	0
6-Mercaptopurine	+	0	0	Rash	0	0
Methotrexate	+	+	+	Dermatitis	+	0
with leucovorin	+	+	+	Dermatitis	+	0
Thioguanine	+	+	0	0	0	0
Antitumor Antibiotics						
Bleomycin	0	0	0	Erythema	+	0
Dactinomycin	+	+	0	Alopecia, rash	0	0
Daunorubicin	+	+	+	Alopecia, vesicant	0	0
Doxorubicin	+	+	+	Alopecia, vesicant	0	0
Idarubicin	+	+	+	Alopecia, vesicant	0	0
Mitomycin C	+	+	0	Vesicant	+	0
Mitoxantrone	+	+	+	Alopecia, vesicant	0	0
Nitrosoureas						
Carmustine (BCNU)	+	0	0	0	+	0
Lomustine (CCNU)	+	0	0	0	0	0
Streptozocin	+	0	0	0	0	0
Thiotepa	+	+	+	Alopecia, rash	0	0
Plant Alkaloids						
Etoposide (VP-16)	0	0	0	0	0	0
Taxol	+	0	0	Alopecia	0	Neuropathy
Vinblastine	+	+	0	Alopecia, vesicant	0	+
Vincristine	0	0	0	Vesicant	0	+ Neuropathy

*Key: +, present; 0, absent.

Adapted from Ewald G, McKenzie C: *Manual of Medical Therapeutics.* Little, Brown, Boston (out of print).

CHEMOTHERAPY

PROPERTIES OF SELECTED ANALGESIC AGENTS

Table 8.13 lists the properties of some nonopioid and nonsteroidal analgesic agents.

Table 8.13

Properties of Selected Analgesic Agents

Specific Group	Analgesic	Antipyretic	Anti-inflammatory
Nonopioid			
Acetaminophen	*	*	0
Fenoprofen	*	*	*
Flurbiprofen	*	*	*
Ibuprofen	*	*	*
Ketoprofen	*	*	*
Naproxen	*	*	*
Nonsteroidal			
Aspirin	*	*	*
Diclofenac	*	*	*
Diflunisal	*	0	*
Etodolac	*	0	*
Indomethacin	*	*	*
Meclofenamate	*	0	*
Nabumetone	*	*	*
Piroxicam	*	*	*
Sulindac	*	0	*
Tolmetin	*	*	*

* = possesses the property assigned; 0 = lacks the property assigned.

EQUIANALGESIC DOSING FOR OPIOID ANALGESICS

Table 8.14 provides information on equianalgesic dosing for the opioid analgesics.

Table 8.14

Equianalgesic Dosing for Opioid Analgesics

Drug	Approximate Equianalgesic Dose		Recommended Starting Dose (adults >50 kg body weight)		Recommended Starting Dose (children and adults >50 kg body weight)*	
	Oral	*Parenteral*	*Oral*	*Parenteral*	*Oral*	*Parenteral*
Opioid Agonist						
Morphine†	30 mg q3–4h (around-the-clock dosing) 60 mg q3–4h (single dose or intermittent dosing)	10 mg q3–4h	30 mg q3–4h	10 mg q3–4h	0.3 mg/kg q3–4h	0.1 mg/kg q3–4h
Codeine‡	180–200 mg q3–4h	130 mg q3–4h	60 mg q3–4h	60 mg q2h (intramuscular/ subcutaneous)	1 mg/kg q3–4h§	Not recommended
Hydrocodone (in Lorcet, Lortab, Vicodin, others)	30 mg q3–4h	Not available	10 mg q3–4h	Not available	0.2 mg/kg q3–4h§	Not available

Continued

ANALGESICS

Table 8.14

Equianalgesic Dosing for Opioid Analgesics—cont'd

Drug	Approximate Equianalgesic Dose		Recommended Starting Dose (adults >50 kg body weight)		Recommended Starting Dose (children and adults >50 kg body weight)*	
	Oral	*Parenteral*	*Oral*	*Parenteral*	*Oral*	*Parenteral*
Opioid Agonist						
Hydromorphone† (Dilaudid)	7.5 mg q3–4h	1.5 mg q3–4h	6 mg q3–4h	1.5 mg q3–4h	0.06 mg/kg q3–4h	0.015 mg/kg q3–4h
Levorphanol (Levo-Dromoran)	4 mg q6–8h	2 mg q6–8h	4 mg q6–8h	2 mg q6–8h	0.04 mg/kg q6–8h	0.02 mg/kg q6–8h
Meperidine (Demerol)	300 mg q2–3h	100 mg q3h	Not recommended	100 mg q3h	Not recommended	0.75 mg/kg q2–3h
Methadone (Dolophine, others)	20 mg q6–8h	10 mg q6–8h	20 mg q6–8h	10 mg q6–8h	0.2 mg/kg q6–8h	0.1 mg/kg q6–8h
Oxycodone (Roxicodone, also in Percocet, Percodan, Tylox, others)	30 mg q3–4h	Not available	10 mg q3–4h	Not available	0.2 mg/kg q3–4h§	Not available
Oxymorphone† (Numorphan)	Not available	1 mg q3–4h	Not available	1 mg q3–4h	Not recommended	Not recommended
Opioid Agonist-Antagonist and Partial Agonist						
Buprenorphine (Buprenex)	Not available	0.3–0.4 mg q6–8h	Not available	0.4 mg q6–8h	Not available	0.004 mg/kg q6–8h
Butorphanol (Stadol)	Not available	2 mg q3–4h	Not available	2 mg q3–4h	Not available	Not recommended
Dezocine (Dalgan)	Not available	10 mg q3–4h	Not available	10 mg q3–4h	Not available	Not recommended
Nalbuphine (Nubain)	Not available	10 mg q3–4h	Not available	10 mg q3–4h	Not available	0.1 mg/kg q3–4h
Pentazocine (Talwin, others)	150 mg q3–4h	60 mg q3–4h	50 mg q4–6h	Not recommended	Not recommended	Not recommended

Note: Published tables vary in the suggested doses that are equianalgesic to morphine. Clinical response is the criterion that must be applied for each client; titration to clinical response is necessary. Because there is not complete cross-tolerance among these drugs, it is usually necessary to use a lower-than-equianalgesic dose when changing drugs and to retitrate to response.

Caution: Recommended doses do not apply to clients with renal or hepatic insufficiency or other conditions affecting drug metabolism and kinetics.

***Caution:** Doses listed for clients with body weight less than 50 kg cannot be used as initial starting doses in babies less than 6 mo of age.

†For morphine, hydromorphone, and oxymorphone, *rectal* administration is an alternate route for clients *unable* to take oral medications, but equianalgesic doses may differ from oral and parenteral doses because of pharmacokinetic differences.

‡**Caution:** Codeine doses *above 65 mg often are not appropriate* because of diminishing incremental analgesia with increasing doses but continually *increasing constipation* and other side effects. Oral doses refer to *combination* with aspirin or acetaminophen.

§**Caution:** Doses of aspirin and acetaminophen in combination opioid/NSAID preparations must also be adjusted to the client's body weight.

Adapted from Acute Pain Management Guideline Panel: *Acute Pain Management in Adults: Operative Procedures. Quick Reference Guide for Clinicians.* Agency for Health Care Policy and Research, Department of Health and Human Services, Rockville, MD. AHCPR Publication No. 92–0019.

DIETARY SUPPLEMENTS AND HERBS

Information on dietary supplements and herbal products used for psychiatric conditions is provided in **Table 8.15, and Table 8.16** lists the potential dangers of various herbs.

Table 8.15

Dietary Supplements and Herbal Products Used for Psychiatric Conditions

Herb	Action/Use	Caution	Drug Interactions
DHEA (dehydroepiandrosterone)	• Depression • ↓ Fatigue	• Hx of prostatic or breast carcinoma • Hepatic dysfunction • Diabetes	• Antidiabetic agents • Estrogen • Corticosteroids
Ginkgo biloba	• ↑ Mental function (e.g., Alzheimer's disease) • Antiplatelet agent • CNS stimulant	*Contraindication:* • Discontinue 2 wk before surgery • Blood clotting disorder • Renal failure • Acute infection • ↑ or ↓ BP	• Blood-thinning medications (e.g., Coumadin, heparin, NSAIDs, ASA) • Hormonal • Monoamine oxidase (MAO) inhibitors • Antihypertensives • Caffeine • Decongestants
Ginseng	• ↓ Fatigue, stress • ↑ Mental alertness • ↑ Physical endurance • ↑ Appetite • Antidepressant • ↑ Immune response	*Contraindicated* with: • Peptic ulcer • Intracranial bleeding • Elderly with cardiovascular disease • Diabetes	• MAO inhibitors • Antihypertensives • Barbiturates • Anticoagulants • Insulin and oral hypoglycemics • Digoxin

Kava	• ↓ Anxiety
	• ↓ Stress
	• ↓ Restlessness
	• ↑ Sleep (↓ insomnia)
	• ↑ Relaxation
		• Discontinue after 3 mo (yellow hair, skin, nails)
		• Reaction:
		  • Euphoria
		  • Depression
		  • Somnolence
		  • Eye accommodation disturbance
		  • Muscle weakness
			• Alcohol/CNS depressants
			• Barbiturates
			• Antipsychotics (e.g., Haldol)
			• Antianxiety drugs (Valium, Xanax, Ativan)
			• ↓ Effects of levodopa (Parkinson's disease)
			• Statins (liver injury)

SAMe (S-adenosylmethionine)	• Depression (not bipolar)	• Bleeding	• Other antidepressants (MAO inhibitors, tricyclic antidepressants [TCAs], selective serotonin reuptake inhibitors [SSRIs]) • Potentiates St. John's wort

St. John's wort	• ↓ Mild depression	• ↑ Panic, agitation, confusion
		• ↑ Skin sensitivity in sun (if also on sulfa, Feldane, Prilosec, Prevacid)
			• ↑ Serotonin level if on antidepressants (e.g., MAO inhibitors, SSRIs, TCAs)
			• Reduces effect of:
			  • Digoxin
			  • Immunosuppressants
			  • Protease inhibitors (HIV)
			  • Oral contraceptives
			  • Coumadin
			  • Theophylline (asthma)
			  • Antipsychotics (e.g., clozapine)
			  • Chemotherapy

Valerian	• Minor tranquilizer • Anxiety, panic attacks • Sleep disorders (insomnia)	• Light-headedness • Restless • Fatigue • Nausea • Tremor • Blurred vision	• Potentiates other CNS depressants (e.g., alcohol) • Benzodiazepines (e.g., Xanax, Valium) • Anticonvulsants (e.g., Dilantin, phenobarbital) • Antidepressants (e.g., Elavil, Tofranil, Prozac) • *Avoid* taking with substances that cause drowsiness

Table 8.16

Herbs and Potential Dangers

Herb	Use	Adverse Effects/Drug Interactions/Cautions
Aloe	**External:** • Heal burns, wounds • Anti-infective • Moisturizer **Internal:** • Laxative • General healing	**Adverse effect:** • Contact dermatitis **Adverse effect:** • Hypokalemia **Caution:** • *Avoid* oral use in GI conditions (e.g., inflammation, ulcers, pain of unknown origin)
Arnica	**External:** • Inflammation caused by insect bites • After muscular and joint injuries (e.g., bruises)	**Adverse effect:** • Toxic skin reaction • *Avoid* use on broken skin
Black cohosh	• Premenstrual syndrome (PMS) • Menopause	**Interaction with:** • Oral contraceptives • Anticoagulants (e.g., Coumadin) • Hormone replacement therapy (HRT) **Caution with:** • Estrogen-sensitive cancers (breast, ovarian) • Salicylate allergies • History of thromboembolic disease
Burdock leaf and root	• Severe skin problems • Arthritis	**Adverse effect:** • Contaminated with belladonna
Chamomile	**External:** • Topical anti-inflammatory agent (for eczema, hemorrhoids, mastitis, leg ulcers) **Internal:** • Indigestion • Antispasmodic (irritable bowel syndrome)	**Caution with:** • Asthma
Echinacea	• Immune system stimulant at onset of cold • Anti-infective • Antipyretic	**Interaction with:** • Immunosuppressants (e.g., cyclosporine, anabolic steroids) **Caution with:** • Lupus • Multiple sclerosis
Evening primrose oil	• Asthma • Diabetic neuropathy • Eczema • Hyperglycemia • Irritable bowel syndrome • Menopause • Multiple sclerosis • Rheumatoid arthritis	**Interaction with:** • Phenothiazines • ASA • NSAIDs • Anticoagulants • Antiplatelet agents • Anticonvulsants **Caution with:** • Peptic ulcer • Intracranial bleeding • Epilepsy • Schizophrenia
Feverfew (see also **Appendix E**)	• Migraines	**Adverse effect:** • Increase bleeding • Spontaneous abortion in early pregnancy **Interaction with:** • Anticoagulants • Antiplatelets • NSAIDs **Caution:** • Do *not* use before or after surgery

Table 8.16

Herbs and Potential Dangers—cont'd

Herb	Use	Adverse Effects/Drug Interactions/Cautions
Ginger	• Antiemetic • Colds, flu • Headaches	**Interaction with:** • Anticoagulants • Antiplatelets • Cardiac glycosides • Hypoglycemic agents **Caution with:** • Diabetes • Gallstones
Goldenseal	Topical treatment of: • Sores • Inflamed mucous membranes	**Interaction with:** • Tretinoins (Retin-A) • Anticoagulants **Adverse effect:** • Causes uterine contractions **Caution with:** • Women who are pregnant • Lactation
Hawthorne	• Dementia • Congestive heart failure (CHF) • Angina	**Interaction with:** • Angiotensin-converting enzyme (ACE) inhibitors • Anticoagulants • Coronary vasodilators **Caution with:** • Lactation
Melaleuca oil®	• Topical use for burns • Bactericidal • Fungicidal	**Adverse effect:** • CNS depression • Allergic dermatitis
Milk thistle	• Liver: hepatitis and cirrhosis • Gallstones • Psoriasis	**Interaction with:** • Oral contraceptives **Adverse effect:** • Laxative effect
Nettle leaf	• Kidney, bladder stones • UTI	**Caution with:** • Pregnancy • Lactation
Pennyroyal	**External:** • Skin disease **Internal:** • Digestive disorders • Liver and gallbladder disorders • Gout	***Use not recommended because of hepatotoxicity***
Sassafras oil	• Lice • Insect bites	**Adverse effect:** • ***Carcinogenesis*** (e.g., hepatic tumors)
Saw palmetto	• Antiandrogen therapy • Benign prostatic hyperplasia (BPH)	**Interaction with:** • HRT • Proscar
Senna	• Catharsis • Laxative	**Adverse effect:** • Electrolyte imbalance (decreased K^+) **Caution with:** • Acute intestinal inflammation (e.g., Crohn's disease, ulcerative colitis, appendicitis)

HERBS

COMMON MEDICATIONS

Dosages, uses, mechanism of action, and assessment of side effects of common medications are detailed in **Table 8.17.**

Table 8.17

Common Medications

Drug and Dosage	Use	Action	Assessment: Side Effects
Adrenergics			
Alpha and Beta Agonists			
Epinephrine (Adrenalin)—Subcu or IM 0.1–1 mg in 1:1000 solution; IV—intracardiac 1:10,000 solution; ophthalmic 1:1000–1:50,000 solution	Asystole, bronchospasm, anaphylaxis, glaucoma	Stimulates pacemaker cells; inhibits histamine and mediates bronchial relaxation; ↓ intraocular pressure	Ventricular arrhythmias, fear, anxiety, anginal pain, decreased renal blood flow, burning of eyes, headache
NURSING IMPLICATIONS: Use TB syringe for greater accuracy; massaging injection site hastens action; repeated injections may cause tissue necrosis; *avoid* injection in buttocks because bacteria in area may lead to gas gangrene; may make mucous plugs in lungs more difficult to dislodge			
Norepinephrine (Levophed)—IV 8–12 mcg/min titrated to desired response	Acute hypotension, cardiogenic shock	Increases rate and strength of heartbeat; increases vasoconstriction	Palpitations, pallor, headache, hypertension; anxiety, insomnia; dilated pupils, nausea, vomiting; glycosuria, tissue sloughing
NURSING IMPLICATIONS: Observe vital signs, mentation, skin temperature, and color (earlobes, lips, nailbeds); tissue necrosis occurs with infiltration; *antidote* is phentolamine 5–10 mg in 10–15 mL normal saline			
Beta Agonists			
Dobutamine (Dobutrex)—IV 1.5–10 mcg/kg/min	Acute heart failure	Stimulates cardiac contractile force (positive inotropy); fewer changes in heart rate than dopamine or isoproterenol	Tachycardia, arrhythmias
NURSING IMPLICATIONS: Mix with 5% dextrose; do *not* dilute until ready to use; protect from light; administer with infusion pump; check vital signs constantly; extravasation can produce tissue necrosis; see Norepinephrine			
Dopamine (Inotropin)—IV 1–5 mcg/kg/min titrated to desired response; gradually increase in 1- to 4-mcg/kg/min increments at 10- to 30-min intervals; must maintain at 20 mcg/kg/min or less	Acute heart failure	↑ Cardiac contractility; ↑ renal blood flow	Ectopic beats; nausea, vomiting; tachycardia, anginal pain, dyspnea, hypotension
NURSING IMPLICATIONS: Monitor vital signs, urine output, and signs of peripheral ischemia; will cause tissue sloughing if infiltration occurs			
Isoproterenol (Isuprel)—sublingual 10–15 mg; IV 0.5–5.0 mcg/min in solution	Cardiogenic shock, heart block, bronchospasm—asthma, emphysema	↑ Cardiac contractility; facilitates atrioventricular (AV) conduction and pacemaker automaticity	Tachyarrhythmias, hypotension, headache, flushing of skin; nausea; tremor; dizziness
NURSING IMPLICATIONS: Monitor vital signs, ECG; oral inhalation solutions must *not* be injected			
Analgesics (see Table 8.14 for Equianalgesic Dosing)			
Acetaminophen (Tylenol, Datril, Panadol)—PO 325–650 mg q4h	Simple fever or pain	Analgesic and antipyretic actions; no anti-inflammatory or anticoagulant effects	No remarkable side effects when taken for a short period
NURSING IMPLICATIONS: Consult with physician if no relief after 4 days of therapy			
Aspirin (acetylsalicylic acid)—PO or rectal 0.3–0.6 gm Ecotrin (enteric-coated aspirin)—PO 81–325 mg	Minor aches and pains; fever from colds and influenza; rheumatoid arthritis; anticoagulant therapy	Selectively depresses subcortical levels of CNS	Erosive gastritis with bleeding; coryza, urticaria; nausea, vomiting; tinnitus, impaired hearing, and respiratory alkalosis

Table 8.17

Common Medications—cont'd

Drug and Dosage	Use	Action	Assessment: Side Effects
NURSING IMPLICATIONS: Administer *with food or after meals;* observe for nasal, oral, or subcutaneous bleeding; push fluids; check *hematocrit (Hct), hemoglobin (Hgb), prothrombin times* frequently; *avoid* use in children with flu; do *not* take ecotrin with milk or dairy			
Butorphanol (Stadol)—IM 1–2 mg; IV 0.5–2 mg	**Obstetric use:** Control pain, especially during labor. Avoid in clients who are opioid addicted.	30–40 times more potent than meperidine; onset: 2–15 min; duration; 0.5–2 hr	No excessive sedation. Neonatal respiratory depression less than with meperidine. Pseudo-sinusoidal FHR pattern after administration.
NURSING IMPLICATIONS: Care must be taken that drug is *not* given with meperidine, as it may potentiate effects of meperidine; *avoid* in clients who are opioid addicted			
Celecoxib (Celebrex)—PO 100–200 mg twice daily or 200 mg daily	Arthritis; acute pain; dysmenorrhea	NSAID, anti-inflammatory, analgesic, antipyretic; inhibits prostaglandin synthesis	Back pain; peripheral edema; diarrhea; dizziness; rash, rhinitis
NURSING IMPLICATIONS: Monitor for signs of fluid retention and edema; report *promptly* unexplained weight gain, rash			
Codeine—PO, IM, Subcu 15–60 mg (gr ¼ to 1)	Control pain; may be used during the puerperium	Nonsynthetic narcotic analgesic	Of little use during labor; allergic response; constipation; GI upset
NURSING IMPLICATIONS: Note response to the medication; less respiratory depression; preferred for client with head injury			
Etodolac (Lodine)—PO 400–1,200 mg/day, 300–400 q6–8h	Management of osteoarthritis; mild to moderate pain	Inhibits prostaglandin synthesis; suppression of inflammation and pain (NSAID)	Dyspepsia; asthma; drowsiness, dizziness; rash, tinnitus, anaphylaxis
NURSING IMPLICATIONS: Give 30 min *before or* 2 hr *after* meals for rapid effect; may be taken with food to decrease GI irritation			
Fentanyl transdermal (Duragesic)—25–100 mcg/hr	Chronic pain; not recommended for postoperative pain **Obstetric use:** Short-acting pain control during labor	Binds to opiate receptors in the CNS to alter response to and perception of pain	Drowsiness, confusion, weakness; constipation, dry mouth, nausea, vomiting, anorexia; sweating
NURSING IMPLICATIONS: Apply to upper torso, flat, nonirritated surface; when applying, hold firmly with palm of hand 10–20 sec			
Hydrocodone/Acetaminophen (Vicodin)—PO 5–10 mg q4–6h	Moderate to severe pain **Obstetric use:** in postpartum to control pain	Bind to opiate receptors in CNS; alter perception of and response to painful stimuli	Confusion, sedation, hypotension, constipation
NURSING IMPLICATIONS: Assess: type, location, and intensity of pain before and 1 hr (peak) after giving; prolonged use may lead to physical and psychological dependence; give with *food or milk* to reduce GI irritation			
Hydromorphone (Dilaudid)—PO 2–4 mg q3–6h; IM 1–2 mg q3–6h up to 2–4 mg q4–6h; IV 0.5–1.0 mg q3h	Moderate to severe pain; antitussive	Binds to opiate receptors in the CNS; alters perception and response to pain	Sedation, confusion, hypotension, constipation
NURSING IMPLICATIONS: Give PO with *food or milk*; give IV 2 mg over 3–5 min; *fluids, bulk,* and laxatives to minimize constipation			
Ibuprofen (Motrin)—PO 300–800 mg 3–4 times/day (not to exceed 3,200 mg/day)	Nonsteroid anti-inflammatory, antirheumatic used in chronic arthritis pain **Obstetric use:** uterine cramping postpartum (not used during pregnancy)	Inhibition of prostaglandin synthesis or release	GI upset, leukopenia; sodium/water retention

Continued

Table 8.17

Common Medications—cont'd

Drug and Dosage	Use	Action	Assessment: Side Effects
NURSING IMPLICATIONS: Give on *empty stomach* for best result; may mix with food if GI upset severe; teach caution when using other medications			
Indomethacin (Indocin)—PO 25 mg 3–4 times/day; increase to max. 200 mg daily in divided doses	Rheumatoid arthritis; bursitis; gouty arthritis Closure of patent ductus arteriosus (PDA) in premature infants and some newborn	Antipyretic/anti-inflammatory action; inhibits prostaglandin biosynthesis	GI distress, bleeding; rash; headache; blood dyscrasias; corneal changes
NURSING IMPLICATIONS: Monitor GI side effects; administer *after* meals for best effect or *with* food, milk, or antacids if GI symptoms severe			
Ketorolac (Toradol)—PO, IV 10 mg q4–6h; IM 30–60 mg initially, then 15–30 mg q6h; ophthalmic 1 gtt 4 times daily for 1 wk	Short-term management of pain; ocular itching due to allergies (NSAID)	Inhibits prostaglandin synthesis, producing peripherally mediated analgesia; antipyretic/anti-inflammatory	Drowsiness, dizziness, dyspnea; prolonged bleeding time; dyspepsia
NURSING IMPLICATIONS: May be given routinely or prn; *advise* dentist or physician before any procedure			
Meperidine HCl (Demerol)—PO, IM 50–100 mg q3–4h	Pain due to trauma or surgery; allay apprehension before surgery	Acts on CNS to produce analgesia, sedation, euphoria, and respiratory depression	Palpitations, bradycardia, hypotension; nausea, vomiting; syncope, sweating, tremors, convulsions
NURSING IMPLICATIONS: Check *respiratory rate* and depth before giving drug; give IM, because subcutaneous administration is painful and can cause local irritation			
	Obstetric use: maternal relaxation may either slow labor or speed up labor	Acts as a uterine irritant; depresses CNS, maternal and fetal; allays apprehension; PO peak action 1–2 hr; IM peak action first hour	Maternal side effects same as above; also can depress fetus
NURSING IMPLICATIONS: Monitor maternal vital signs, contractions, progress of labor, and response to drug; fetal heart rate; if delivery occurs during peak action, prepare to give *narcotic antagonist* to mother or neonate or both			
Morphine SO_4—PO 10–30 mg (Roxanol, MS Contin); Subcu 8–15 mg; IV 4–10 mg; rectal 10–20 mg	Control pain and relieve fear, apprehension, restlessness, as in pulmonary edema	Depresses CNS reception of pain and ability to interpret stimuli; depresses respiratory center in medulla	Nausea, vomiting; flushing; confusion; urticaria; depressed rate and depth of respirations, decreased blood pressure
NURSING IMPLICATIONS: Check rate and depth of *respirations* before administering drug; observe for gas pains and *abdominal distention;* smaller doses for aged; monitor vital signs; observe for postural hypotension			
	Obstetric use: preeclampsia, eclampsia; uterine dysfunction; pain relief	Increases cerebral blood flow; provides antihypertensive action; CNS depressant	Respiratory and circulatory depression in mother and neonate; may depress contractions
NURSING IMPLICATIONS: Observe for level of sedation, respirations, arousability, and deep tendon reflex; give *narcotic antagonist* as necessary; check I&O (*urinary retention* possible)			
Nalbuphine (Nubain)—IV 1 mg at 6- to 10-min intervals	**Obstetric use:** pain relief during labor. *Avoid* in clients who are opioid addicted.	Onset: 2–15 min; duration 1–4 hr	Increased sedation and limited ceiling effect; ceiling effect for neonatal respiratory depression
NURSING IMPLICATIONS: Less nausea and vomiting and sedation if given with patient-controlled analgesia (PCA). Prophylactic nalbuphine seems unable to prevent pruritus			
Naproxen (Naprosyn)—PO 250–500 mg twice daily	Mild to moderate pain; dysmenorrhea; rheumatoid arthritis; osteoarthritis (NSAID)	Inhibits prostaglandin synthesis; suppression of inflammation	Headache, drowsiness, dizziness, nausea, dyspepsia, constipation, bleeding

Table 8.17

Common Medications—cont'd

Drug and Dosage	Use	Action	Assessment: Side Effects
NURSING IMPLICATIONS: Take with a full glass of *water; avoid* exposure to sun			
Oxycodone HCl (OxyContin)—PO 3–20 mg; Subcu 5 mg	**Postpartum use:** control pain; may be used during puerperium; 5–6 times more potent than codeine	Less potent and addicting than morphine; for moderate pain—episiotomy and "afterpains"; peak action 1 hr	See Morphine SO_4
NURSING IMPLICATIONS: Administer per order and observe for effect			
Pentazocine (Talwin)—PO 50–100 mg; IM 30–60 mg q3–4h	Relief of moderate to severe pain	Narcotic antagonist, opioid antagonist properties, equivalent to codeine	Respiratory depression, nausea, vomiting, dizziness, light-headedness, seizures
NURSING IMPLICATIONS: Monitor *respirations,* BP; *caution* with client with myocardial infarction (MI), head injuries, chronic obstructive pulmonary disease (COPD)			
Antacids (see Antiulcer Agents)			
Antiadrenal Agent			
Aminoglutethimide (Cytadren)—PO 250 mg q6h	Cushing's syndrome	Inhibits enzymatic conversion of cholesterol to pregnenolone, thus reducing synthesis of adrenal glucocorticoids/mineralocorticoids	Cortical hypofunction, hypotension, hypothyroidism
NURSING IMPLICATIONS: Monitor: vital signs, laboratory values, disease signs and symptoms; observe frequently during periods of stress			
Antianemic Agents			
Ferrous sulfate (Feosol, Fer-In-Sol)—adults, PO 300 mg–1.2 gm daily; children under 6 yr, PO 75–225 mg daily; 6–12 yr, PO 120–600 mg daily	Iron-deficiency anemia; prophylactically during infancy, childhood, pregnancy	Corrects nutritional iron-deficiency anemia	Nausea, vomiting, anorexia, constipation, diarrhea; yellow-brown discoloration of eyes, teeth
NURSING IMPLICATIONS: To minimize GI distress, give *with* meals; do *not* give with antacids or tea; liquid form should be taken through straw to prevent *staining* of teeth; causes dark-green/black stool			
Filgrastim (Neupogen)—Subcu, IV 5-mcg/kg/day increments	Neutropenia from cancer, chemotherapy, bone marrow transplantation	Stimulates white blood cell production, specifically neutrophil count; a biologic response modifier	Bone pain, fever
NURSING IMPLICATIONS: Monitor WBC count as indication of effectiveness			
Lenalidomide (Revlimid)—PO 5–25 mg daily for 21 days	Slow progression of multiple myeloma; transfusion-dependent anemia	Works in bone marrow to slow growth of cancerous myeloma cells	Deep vein thrombosis, neutropenia, thrombocytopenia, birth defects
NURSING IMPLICATIONS: Clients with multiple myeloma take the drug with dexamethasone			
Pegfilgrastim (Neulasta)—Subcu 6 mg per chemotherapy cycle	Neutropenia from chemotherapy	Stimulates bone marrow and promotes neutrophils (WBCs)	Infection, skin rash, splenic rupture, acute respiratory distress syndrome (ARDS)
NURSING IMPLICATIONS: Do not give 14 days before or 24 hours after chemotherapy. Instruct client to **report immediately sudden, severe pain in left upper stomach spreading to shoulder**			
Antianginals			
Atenolol (Tenormin)—PO 50–150 mg daily; IV 5 mg initially, wait 10 min, then another 5 mg	Hypertension: angina; arrhythmias	Blocks (cardiac) beta-adrenergic receptors	Fatigue, weakness, bradycardia, heart failure, pulmonary edema
NURSING IMPLICATIONS: Give 1 mg/min IV; check vital signs; assess for signs of fluid *overload*			

Continued

Table 8.17

Common Medications—cont'd

Drug and Dosage	Use	Action	Assessment: Side Effects
Isosorbide dinitrate (Isordil, Isorbid)—sublingual 2.5–10.0 mg q5–10 min for 3 doses; PO 5–10 mg initially, 10–40 mg q6h	Acute angina: long-term prophylaxis for angina; heart failure	Produces vasodilation, decreases preload	Headache, dizziness, hypotension, tachycardia
NURSING IMPLICATIONS: *Avoid* eating, drinking, or smoking until sublingual tablets are dissolved; change positions *slowly;* aspirin or acetaminophen for headache. Determine if client is taking drugs for erectile dysfunction—serious drug interaction!			
Nitroglycerin—sublingual 0.25–0.6 mg prn; transdermal (patch) 2.5–15.0 mg/day; topical 2–3 inches q8h; IV 10–20 mcg/min	Angina pectoris; adjunctive treatment in MI, heart failure, hypertension (IV form)	Directly relaxes smooth muscle, dilating blood vessels; lowers peripheral vascular resistance; increases blood flow	Faintness, throbbing headache; vomiting; flushing, hypotension; visual disturbances
NURSING IMPLICATIONS: Instruct client to sit or lie down when taking drug, to reduce *hypotensive* effect; onset 1–3 min; may take 1–3 doses at 5-min intervals to relieve pain; up to *10/day* may be allowed; if headache occurs, tell client to expel tablet as soon as pain relief occurs; keep drug at bedside or on person; watch *expiration* dates—tablets lose potency with exposure to air and humidity; *alcohol* ingestion soon after taking may produce shocklike syndrome from drop in BP; *smoking* causes vasoconstricting effect; causes burning under tongue; may crush between teeth to ↑ absorption			
Antiarrhythmics (also see Calcium Channel Blockers)			
Amiodarone hydrochloride (Cordarone)—PO 800–1,600 mg/day loading dose; 400–600 mg/day maintenance	Life-threatening ventricular arrhythmias; supraventricular arrhythmias (e.g., atrial fibrillation)	Class III antiarrhythmic; antianginal, antiadrenergic	Muscle weakness, fatigue, dizziness, hypotension with IV; corneal microdeposits; anorexia, nausea, vomiting; photosensitivity
NURSING IMPLICATIONS: Monitor vital signs (VS). Expect possible CNS symptoms 1 wk after beginning drug. Instruct client to protect eyes and skin from sun			
Bretylium (Bretylol)—IV 0.5–10 mg/kg q6h; IM 5–10 mg/kg (max. 250 mg in one site)	Ventricular fibrillation; ventricular tachycardia	Inhibits norepinephrine release from sympathetic nerve endings; increased fibrillation threshold	Worsening of arrhythmia; tachycardia and increased BP initially; nausea, vomiting; hypotension later
NURSING IMPLICATIONS: Monitor BP and cardiac status closely; *rotate* IM injection sites; no more than 5 mL/site			
Diphenylhydantoin (Dilantin)—PO 100–200 mg 3–4 times daily; IV loading dose 10–15 mg/kg (not to exceed 50 mg/min), 50–100 mg over 5–10 min	Digitalis toxicity; ventricular ectopy	Depresses pacemaker activity in sinoatrial (SA) node and Purkinje tissue without slowing conduction velocity	Severe pain if administered in small vein; ataxia, vertigo, nystagmus, seizures, confusion; skin eruptions, hypotension if administered too fast
NURSING IMPLICATIONS: With IV use, monitor vital signs; observe for CNS side effects; have O_2 on hand; seizure precautions (padded side rails, nonmetal airway; suction, mouth gag); also see Anticonvulsants			
Lidocaine HCl—IV 50–100 mg, bolus; 1–4 mg/kg/min, IV drip	Ventricular tachycardia; premature ventricular contractions (PVCs)	Depresses myocardial response to abnormally generated impulses	Drowsiness, dizziness, nervousness, confusion, paresthesias
NURSING IMPLICATIONS: Monitor vital signs; observe for signs of CNS toxicity; monitor ECG for *prolonged P-R* interval			
Metoprolol tartrate (Lopressor)—PO 25 mg/day; range 25–300 mg/day	Hypertension; angina; MI	Beta-adrenergic blocker; ↓ cardiac output (CO), ↓ heart rate (HR)	Dizziness, fatigue, insomnia; bradycardia, shortness of breath (SOB)
NURSING IMPLICATIONS: Monitor: vital signs carefully; I&O, daily weight; check for *rales.* Give with or without food—be consistent			
Procainamide HCl (Pronestyl)—PO, IM 500–1,000 mg 4–6 times daily; IV 1 gm	Atrial and ventricular arrhythmias; PVCs; overdose of digitalis; general anesthesia	Depresses myocardium; lengthens conduction time between atria and ventricles	Polyarthralgia; fever, chills, urticaria; nausea, vomiting; psychoses; rapid decrease in BP
NURSING IMPLICATIONS: Check pulse rate *before* giving; monitor heart action during IV administration			

Table 8.17

Common Medications—cont'd

Drug and Dosage	Use	Action	Assessment: Side Effects
Propranolol HCl (Inderal)—IV push 0.5–3.0 mg (up to 3 mg); PO 20–60 mg 3–4 times daily	Ventricular ectopy; angina unresponsive to nitrites, paroxysmal atrial tachycardia (PAT); hypertension	Beta-adrenergic blocker, ↓ cardiac contractility, ↓ heart rate, ↓ myocardial oxygen requirements	Bradycardia, hypotension, vertigo, paresthesia of hands
NURSING IMPLICATIONS: Instruct client to take pulse *before* each dose; do *not* give to clients with history of asthma or chronic obstructive pulmonary disease; no smoking, because hypertension may occur			
Quinidine SO_4—PO 0.2–0.6 gm q2h loading dose; maintenance: 400–1,000 mg 3–4 times daily; IV 5–10 mg/kg over 30–60 min	Atrial fibrillation; PAT; ventricular tachycardia; PVCs	Lengthens conduction time in atria and ventricles; blocks vagal stimulation of heart	Nausea, vomiting, diarrhea; vertigo, tremor, headache; abdominal cramps; AV block, cardiac arrest
NURSING IMPLICATIONS: *Count pulse before* giving; report changes in rate, quality, or rhythm; give drug *with food;* monitor BP daily			
Antiasthmatic			
Cromolyn sodium—inhalation 1 capsule 4 times daily	Perennial bronchial asthma (*not acute* asthma or status asthmaticus)	Inhibits release of bronchoconstrictors—histamine and slow-reacting substance of anaphylaxis (SRS-A); suppresses allergic response	Cough, hoarseness, wheezing; dry mouth, bitter aftertaste, urticaria; urinary frequency
NURSING IMPLICATIONS: Instruct on use of inhaler—exhale; tilt head back; inhale rapidly, deeply, steadily; remove inhaler, exhale—repeat until dose is taken; gargle or drink water after treatment			
Anticholelithic			
Ursodeoxycholic (Actigall)—PO 300–600 mg	Gallstones	Dissolves gallstones	Diarrhea; *avoid* concurrent use with bile acid sequestrants
NURSING IMPLICATIONS: *Monitor* for pain, GI distress			
Anticholinergics (Antimuscarinics)			
Atropine SO_4—PO, Subcu, IM, IV 0.3–1.2 mg; ophthalmic 0.5%–1.0% up to 6 times daily	Peptic ulcer; spasms of GI tract, Stokes-Adams syndrome; control excessive secretions during surgery	Blocks parasympathomimetic effects of acetylcholine on effector organs	Dry mouth, tachycardia, blurred vision, drowsiness, skin flushing; urinary retention; *contraindications:* glaucoma and paralytic ileus
NURSING IMPLICATIONS: Observe for postural *hypotension* in clients who are ambulating; administer cautiously in aged; and monitor vital signs for pulse and respiratory rate changes			
Dicyclomine (Bentyl)—PO 10–20 mg 3–4 times/day	Diverticulosis	Antispasmodic	Blurred vision; constipation; dry eyes, dry mouth
NURSING IMPLICATIONS: Report symptoms listed under side effects, abdominal pain			
Glycopyrrolate (Robinul)—PO 1–2 mg 2–3 times per day; IM, IV 4.4 mcg/kg (preop); 100–200 mcg 4 times a day (ulcer)	Inhibit salivation and respiratory secretions; peptic ulcer disease	Inhibits action of acetylcholine (antimuscarinic action)	Tachycardia; dry mouth; urinary hesitancy
NURSING IMPLICATIONS: Give 30–60 min *before* meals; do *not* give within 1 hr of antacids; IM or IV may be given undiluted			
Hyoscyamine (Levsinex)—PO 0.125–0.5 mg 3–4 times/day; or PO 0.375 mg twice a day in extended-released tablets	Diverticulosis	Manages spasms of irritable bowel syndrome	Constipation; dry mouth, blurred vision
NURSING IMPLICATIONS: *Monitor* for: pain, bleeding, constipation, drug reaction			

Continued

Table 8.17

Common Medications—cont'd

Drug and Dosage	Use	Action	Assessment: Side Effects
Propantheline bromide (Pro-Banthine)—PO 15 mg 4 times daily; IM, IV 30 mg	Decreases hypertonicity and hypersecretion of GI tract; ulcerative colitis; peptic ulcer	Blocks neural transmission at ganglia of autonomic nervous system and at parasympathetic effector organs	Nausea, gastric fullness, constipation; mydriasis
NURSING IMPLICATIONS: Give *before* meals; observe urinary output to *avoid retention,* particularly in elderly; mouth care to relieve dryness; *contraindicated* with glaucoma			
Tincture of belladonna—PO 0.3–0.6 mL 3 times daily	Hypermotility of stomach; bowel, biliary, and renal colic; prostatitis	Blocks parasympathomimetic effects of acetylcholine	Dry mouth, thirst; dilated pupils; skin flushing; elevated temperature; delirium
NURSING IMPLICATIONS: Administer 30–60 min *before* meals; observe for side effects; *physostigmine salicylate* is antidote			
Tolterodine tartrate (Detrol LA)—PO 2 mg twice daily; 4 mg sustained release (SR) daily	Overactive bladder	Selective muscarinic urinary bladder receptor antagonist	Dry mouth; back pain; fatigue, weight gain
NURSING IMPLICATIONS: Report eye pain *promptly.* Blurred vision, sensitivity to light, and dry mouth should be reported if bothersome			
Anticoagulants			
Enoxaparin (Lovenox)—Subcu 30–40 mg twice daily, 7–10 days; or 1 mg/kg q12h	Deep vein thrombosis; prophylaxis before knee and abdominal surgery	Potentiates inhibitory effect of antithrombin	Bleeding, anemia, thrombocytopenia
NURSING IMPLICATIONS: Observe injection sites for hematomas, ecchymosis, or inflammation; *ice cube massage* at site prior to injection may lessen bruising			
Heparin—initial dose: IV bolus of 5,000 units, followed by infusion of 20,000–40,000 units over 24 hr	Acute thromboembolic emergencies	Prevents thrombin formation	Hematuria, bleeding gums, ecchymosis
NURSING IMPLICATIONS: Observe clotting times—should be 20–30 min; antagonist is *protamine sulfate*			
Warfarin sodium (Coumadin)—initial dose: PO 10–15 mg; maintenance dose: PO 2–10 mg daily	Venous thrombosis; atrial fibrillation with embolization; pulmonary emboli; myocardial infarction	Depresses liver synthesis of prothrombin and factors VII, IX, and X	Minor or major hemorrhage; alopecia; fever; nausea, diarrhea; dermatitis
NURSING IMPLICATIONS: Drug effects last 3–4 days; antagonist is vitamin K; *avoid* foods high in vitamin K; *no* aspirin			
Anticoagulant Antidotes			
Protamine sulfate 1%—IV 10 mg/mL slowly; 1 mg/100 units heparin	Overdose of heparin	Positive electrostatic charge inactivates negatively charged heparin molecules	Excessive coagulation; hypotension, bradycardia, dyspnea
NURSING IMPLICATIONS: Slow IV; no more than 50 mg in 10-min period; monitor VS continuously; check *activated partial thromboplastin time (aPTT)* for effectiveness			
Vitamin K (Aquamephyton, Konakion)—PO, IM, Subcu 2.5–25.0 mg; 0.5–1.0 mg in newborns	Warfarin (Coumadin) hypoprothrombinemia; hemorrhagic disease in newborns	Counteracts the inhibitory effects of oral anticoagulants on hepatic synthesis of vitamin K–dependent clotting factors	Flushing, hypotension, allergic reactions; reappearance of clotting problems (high doses)
NURSING IMPLICATIONS: Give IV only if absolutely necessary; dilute with preservative-free 0.9% NaCl, D_5W, or 5% dextrose in NaCl; protect solution *from light;* repeat injection may cause redness and pain; check *prothrombin time (PT)* for drug effect			
Anticonvulsants			
Carbamazepine (Tegretol)—PO 200 mg twice/day (range: 600–1,200/day in divided doses)	Multiple sclerosis	Decreases synaptic transmission in CNS by affecting sodium channels in neurons	Contraindicated in hypersensitivity, bone marrow depression; drowsiness, ataxia, agranulocytosis, aplastic anemia
NURSING IMPLICATIONS: *Monitor:* complete blood count (CBC), liver function, electrocardiogram (ECG). Therapeutic levels should be 6–12 mcg/mL; take medication as directed around the clock; use sunscreen due to photosensitivity			

Table 8.17

Common Medications—cont'd

Drug and Dosage	Use	Action	Assessment: Side Effects
Clonazepam (Klonopin)—PO 1.5 mg in 3 doses initially, 0.5–1.0 mg every third day	Absence seizures (petit mal seizures, myoclonic seizures)	Produces anticonvulsant and sedative effects in the CNS; mechanism unknown	Drowsiness, ataxia, behavioral changes
NURSING IMPLICATIONS: Give *with* food; evaluate *liver enzymes, CBC,* and *platelets; avoid* abrupt withdrawal—may cause status epilepticus			
Diazepam (Valium)—PO 2–10 mg 2–4 times daily; IM, IV 5–10 mg	All types of seizures **Obstetric use:** eclampsia	Induces calming effect on limbic system, thalamus, and hypothalamus	Drowsiness, ataxia, paradoxical increase in CNS excitability
NURSING IMPLICATIONS: IV may cause phlebitis; give IV injection *slowly,* because respiratory arrest can occur; inject IM *deeply* into tissue			
Ethosuximide (Zarontin)—PO 500 mg/day, increase by 250 mg/day until effective	Absence seizures	Depresses motor cortex and reduces CNS sensitivity to convulsive nerve stimuli	GI distress: nausea, vomiting, cramps, diarrhea, anorexia; blood dyscrasias
NURSING IMPLICATIONS: Administer *with* meals; regular *CBC;* precautions to avoid injury from drowsiness			
Magnesium salts—IV infusion 4–5 gm	Cirrhosis	Osmotically active in GI tract	Use caution in renal failure; *contraindicated* in: hypermagnesemia, anuria, heart block
NURSING IMPLICATIONS: *Monitor:* vital signs, seizure precautions, I&O; *respiratory rate must be 16* before administration			
Magnesium sulfate—IM or IV 1- to 4-gm loading dose, followed by continuous infusion (2–3 gm/hr)	Control seizures in pregnancy, epilepsy; relief of acute constipation; reduces edema, inflammation, and itching of skin; may inhibit preterm contractions	Depresses CNS and smooth, cardiac, and skeletal muscle; promotes osmotic retention of fluid	Flushing, sweating, extreme thirst; complete heart block; dehydration; depressed or absent reflexes, ↓ respirations
NURSING IMPLICATIONS: If given IV, monitor vital signs continuously; I&O; use with caution in clients with *impaired renal* functions; observe mother and newborn for signs of toxicity if given near birth; *antidote:* calcium gluconate			
Phenytoin or diphenylhydantoin (Dilantin) SO_4—PO 30–100 mg 3–4 times daily; IM 100–200 mg 3–4 times daily; IV 150–250 mg	Psychomotor epilepsy, convulsive seizures; ventricular arrhythmias	Depresses motor cortex by preventing spread of abnormal electrical impulses	Nervousness, ataxia; gastric distress; nystagmus; slurred speech; hallucinations; gingival hyperplasia
NURSING IMPLICATIONS: Give *with* meals *or* after meals (pc); frequent and diligent mouth care; advise client that urine may turn *pink to red-brown;* teach client signs of adverse reactions; mix IV with normal saline (precipitates with D_5W)			
Primidone (Mysoline)—PO 100–250 mg, increase over 10 days (not to exceed 2 gm/day)	Tonic-clonic, focal, or local seizures	Inhibits abnormal brain electrical activity; dose-dependent CNS depression	Excessive sedation or ataxia, vertigo
NURSING IMPLICATIONS: Careful neurological, cardiovascular, and respiratory assessment; have resuscitation equipment available			
Valproic acid (Depakene)—PO 15 mg/kg/day, increase up to 60 mg/kg/day	Absence, tonic-clonic, myoclonic, focal, or local seizures	Inhibits spread of abnormal discharges through brain	Nausea, vomiting, diarrhea (disappear over time); drowsiness or sedation if taken in combination with other anticonvulsants
NURSING IMPLICATIONS: Assess responses; monitor blood levels; precautions against excessive sedation; *discourage alcohol* use			
Antidiarrheals			
Diphenoxylate HCl with atropine sulfate (Lomotil)—PO 5–10 mg 3–4 times daily	Diarrhea	Increases intestinal tone and decreases propulsive peristalsis	Rash; drowsiness, dizziness; depression; abdominal distention; headache, blurred vision; nausea
NURSING IMPLICATIONS: May *potentiate* action of barbiturates, opiates, and other depressants; closely observe clients receiving these drugs, and administer *narcotic antagonists* such as levallorphan tartrate (Lorfan), naloxone HCl (Narcan), and nalorphine HCl (Naline) as ordered; administer cautiously to clients with hepatic dysfunction—may precipitate *hepatic coma*			

Continued

Table 8.17

Common Medications—cont'd

Drug and Dosage	Use	Action	Assessment: Side Effects
Kaolin with pectin (Kaopectate)—adults, PO 60–120 mL after each bowel movement (BM); children over 12, PO 60 mL; 6–12 yr, PO 30–60 mL; 3–6 yr, PO 15–30 mL after each BM	Diarrhea	Reported to absorb irritants and soothe	Granuloma of the stomach
NURSING IMPLICATIONS: Do *not* administer for more than 2 days, in presence of fever, or to children younger than 3 yr			
Paregoric or camphorated opium tincture—PO 5–10 mL q2h, not more than 4 times daily	Diarrhea	Acts directly on intestinal smooth muscle to increase tone and decrease propulsive peristalsis	Occasional nausea; prolonged use may produce dependence
NURSING IMPLICATIONS: Contains approximately 1.6 mg morphine or 16 mg opium and is subject to federal narcotic regulations; administer with partial glass of water to facilitate passage into stomach; observe number and consistency of stools—discontinue drug as soon as diarrhea is controlled; keep in tight *light-resistant* bottles			
Antiemetics			
Chlorpromazine (Thorazine)—preop IM 12.5–25.0 gm 1–2 hr before; IV 25–50 mg; PO 10–25 mg q4–6h; IM 25–50 mg q3–4h; suppository 50–100 mg q6–8h	Nausea, vomiting, hiccups, preoperative sedation, psychoses	Alters the effects of dopamine in the CNS; anticholinergic, alpha-adrenergic blocking	Sedation, extrapyramidal reactions; dry eyes, blurred vision; hypotension; constipation, dry mouth; photosensitivity
NURSING IMPLICATIONS: Keep *flat* 30 min after IM; change positions slowly; frequent mouth care; may turn urine *pink* to *red-brown*			
Prochlorperazine dimaleate (Compazine)—PO, IM, rectal 5–30 mg 4 times daily	Nausea, vomiting, and retching	See Trimethobenzamide HCl	Drowsiness, orthostatic hypotension, palpitations, blurred vision, diplopia, headache
NURSING IMPLICATIONS: Use *cautiously* in children, women who are pregnant, and clients with liver disease			
Trimethobenzamide HCl (Tigan)—PO, IM, rectal 250 mg 4 times daily	Nausea; vomiting	Suppresses chemoreceptors in the trigger zone located in the medulla oblongata	Drowsiness, vertigo; diarrhea, headache, hypotension; jaundice; blurred vision; rigid muscles
NURSING IMPLICATIONS: Give *deep* IM to prevent escape of solution; can cause edema, pain, and burning			
Antifungals			
Amphotericin B (Fungizone)—IV 5 mg/250 mL dextrose over 4–6 hr (to 1 mg/kg body weight)	Severe fungal infections; histoplasmosis	Fungistatic or fungicidal; binds to sterols in fungal cell membrane, altering cell permeability	Febrile reactions; chills, nausea, vomiting; muscle/joint pain; renal damage; hypotension, tachycardia, arrhythmias; hypokalemia
NURSING IMPLICATIONS: Monitor for side effects, thrombophlebitis at IV site; blood urea nitrogen (BUN) >40; creatinine >3; stop drug because of *nephrotoxicity*			
Ketoconazole (Nizoral)—PO 200–400 mg daily	Histoplasmosis, systemic fungal infections	Antifungal	Headache, fatigue, dizziness; nausea, vomiting; decreased libido, impotence; gynecomastia, especially in men
NURSING IMPLICATIONS: Administer *with* food; *avoid* concomitant use of antacids, histamine$_2$ (H_2) blockers; advise to report side effects			
Nystatin (Nilstat, Mycostatin)—PO, rectal, vaginal 100,000–1,000,000 units 3–4 times daily	Skin, mucous membrane infections (*Candida albicans*); oral thrush, vaginitis; intestinal candidiasis	Fungistatic and fungicidal; binds to sterols in fungal cell membrane	Nausea, vomiting, GI distress, diarrhea

Table 8.17

Common Medications—cont'd

Drug and Dosage	Use	Action	Assessment: Side Effects
NURSING IMPLICATIONS: *Oral* use—clear mouth of food; keep medication in mouth several minutes before swallowing; *vaginal*—usually requires 2 wk therapy; continue use during menses; consult physician before using anti-infective douches; determine predisposing factors to infection (diabetes, pregnancy, antibiotics, tight-fitting nylon pantyhose)			
Antigout Agents			
Allopurinol (Lopurin, Zyloprim)—PO 100 mg initially, 300 mg daily with meals or pc	Primary hyperuricemia, secondary hyperuricemia with cancer therapy	Lowers plasma and urinary uric acid levels; no analgesic, anti-inflammatory, or uricosuric actions	Rash, itching; nausea, vomiting; anemia, drowsiness
NURSING IMPLICATIONS: Report side effects, particularly *rash,* because drug *must be stopped; avoid* driving or other complex tasks until drug effects known; give at least *3,000 mL* fluid daily; minimum urine output of *2,000 mL/day;* keep urine neutral or *alkaline* with sodium bicarbonate or potassium citrate; use *cautiously* with: liver disease, impaired renal function, history of peptic ulcers, lower GI disease, or bone marrow depression			
Colchicine—PO 1.0–1.2 mg acute phase; 0.5–2.0 mg nightly with milk or food; IV 1–2 mg initially	Gouty arthritis, acute gout	Inhibits leukocyte migration and phagocytosis in gouty joints; nonanalgesic, nonuricosuric	Nausea, vomiting, diarrhea, abdominal pain; peripheral neuritis; bone marrow depression (sore throat, bleeding gums, sore mouth); tissue and nerve necrosis with IV use
NURSING IMPLICATIONS: Do *not* dilute IV form with normal saline or 5% dextrose—use sterile water to prevent precipitation; infuse over 3–5 min IV; potentiate drug action with *alkali-ash foods* (milk, most fruits and vegetables)			
Probenecid (Benemid)—PO 0.25–0.50 gm twice daily pc	Chronic gouty arthritis (no value in acute); adjuvant therapy with penicillin to increase plasma levels	Inhibits renal tubular resorption of uric acid; no analgesic or anti-inflammatory activity; competitively inhibits renal tubular secretion of penicillin and many weak organic acids	Headache; nausea, vomiting, anorexia, sore gums; urinary frequency, flushing
NURSING IMPLICATIONS: Give *with* food, milk, or prescribed antacid; 3,000 mL/day fluids; *avoid* alcohol, which increases serum urates; do *not* take with aspirin—inhibits action of drug; renal function and hematology should be evaluated frequently; during acute gout, give with colchicine			
Antihistamines			
Astemizole (Hismanal)—PO 10 mg/day	Relief of allergic symptoms (rhinitis, urticaria); less sedating	Blocks the effects of histamine	Drowsiness, headache, fatigue; stimulation; dry mouth; rash; increased appetite (none of these are frequent)
NURSING IMPLICATIONS: Take *1 hr before* or *2 hr after* eating; good oral hygiene; may need to reduce calories			
Cetirizine (Zyrtec)—PO 5–10 mg/day; 10 mg daily or twice daily for urticaria	Seasonal and perennial allergic rhinitis; chronic urticaria	Potent histamine$_1$ (H_1) receptor antagonist	Drowsiness, sedation, headache
NURSING IMPLICATIONS: Sedation more common in older adult. Do **not** take with OTC antihistamines			
Chlorpheniramine maleate (Chlor-Trimeton)—PO 2–4 mg 3 or 4 times daily; Subcu, IM, IV 10–20 mg	Asthma; hay fever; serum reactions; anaphylaxis	Inhibits action of histamine	Nausea, gastritis, diarrhea; headache; dryness of mouth and nose; nervousness, irritability
NURSING IMPLICATIONS: IV may drop BP; give slowly; caution client about drowsiness			
Diphenhydramine HCl (Benadryl)—PO 25–50 mg 3 or 4 times daily; IM, IV 10–20 mg	Allergic and pyrogenic reactions; motion sickness; radiation sickness; hay fever; Parkinson's disease	Inhibits action of histamine on receptor cells; decreases action of acetylcholine	Sedation, dizziness, inability to concentrate; headache; anorexia; dermatitis; nausea; diplopia, insomnia

Continued

Table 8.17

Common Medications—cont'd

Drug and Dosage	Use	Action	Assessment: Side Effects
NURSING IMPLICATIONS: *Avoid* use in newborn or preterm infants and clients with glaucoma; supervise ambulation; *caution* against driving or operating mechanical devices; excitation or hallucinations may occur in *children*			
Fexofenadine (Allegra)—PO 50 mg twice daily	Seasonal allergic rhinitis; chronic urticaria	Antagonizes histamine at the H_1 receptor site	Headache, drowsiness, fatigue; dyspepsia; throat irritation
NURSING IMPLICATIONS: Monitor effectiveness; well tolerated; consult physician *if breastfeeding*			
Loratidine (Claritin)—PO 10 mg daily on empty stomach	Seasonal allergic rhinitis; idiopathic chronic urticaria	Selective peripheral H_1 receptor sites, blocking histamine release	Dizziness; dry mouth, thirst; fatigue; headache
NURSING IMPLICATIONS: Causes significant drowsiness in *older* adult			
Nedocromil (Tilade)—inhalation 2 sprays	Asthma	Prevents the release of histamine from sensitized mast cells	Hypersensitivity, acute asthma attacks; does not relieve (may accelerate) bronchospasm
NURSING IMPLICATIONS: Monitor pulmonary function; use only as prescribed; if symptoms increase, notify health-care professional; teach proper use of metered-dose inhaler			
Antihyperglycemics			
Alpha-Glucosidase Inhibitor			
Acarbose (Precose)—PO 25 mg 3 times daily; may be increased q4–8 wk (range: 50–100 mg 3 times daily)	Type 2 diabetes	Alpha-glucosidase inhibitors/ oral hypoglycemic	*Overdose signs:* flatulence, diarrhea, abdominal discomfort
NURSING IMPLICATIONS: Observe for side effects of hypoglycemia; take same time each day; do *not* double dose; therapy is long term			
Biguanide			
Metformin (Glucophage)—PO 500 mg twice daily; may increase by 500 mg to 2,000 mg/day	Type 2 diabetes **Obstetric Use:** Also used for infertility when the client has polycystic ovary syndrome and gestational diabetes after first trimester.	Decreases hepatic production of glucose; decreases intestinal absorption of glucose	Lactic acidosis; nausea, vomiting, diarrhea, abdominal bloating
NURSING IMPLICATIONS: Monitor glucose levels; take medication as directed; dietary compliance; metallic taste resolves spontaneously			
Sulfonylureas			
Acetohexamide (Dymelor)—PO 200–1,500 mg daily; 1–2 doses/day; duration 12–24 hr	Oral hypoglycemic; antidiabetic **Obstetric Use:** May be used after first trimester of pregnancy for controlling blood sugar in gestational diabetes	Lowers blood glucose by stimulating insulin release from beta cells; effective only if pancreas has ability to produce insulin	Hypoglycemia (profuse sweating, hunger, headache, nausea, confusion, ataxia, coma; skin rashes; bone marrow depression, liver toxicity
NURSING IMPLICATIONS: Drug therapy must be combined with diet therapy, weight control, and planned, graded exercise; alcohol intolerance may occur (disulfiram reaction—flushing, pounding headache, sweating, nausea, vomiting); should *not* be taken at bedtime unless specifically ordered (nocturnal hypoglycemia more likely); take at *same time* each day; *contraindicated* in liver disease, renal disease, pregnancy			
Chlorpropamide (Diabinese)—PO 100–500 mg maintenance; not to exceed 750 mg/day; duration 30–60 hr	See Acetohexamide	See Acetohexamide	See Acetohexamide

Table 8.17

Common Medications—cont'd

Drug and Dosage	Use	Action	Assessment: Side Effects
NURSING IMPLICATIONS: See Acetohexamide			
Glimepiride (Amaryl), glipizide (Glucotrol)—PO 1–2 mg once daily; increase slowly up to 8 mg in one dose; 15 mg/day in divided dose	Type 2 diabetes mellitus	Stimulate release of insulin from pancreas	Photosensitivity; hypoglycemia; ingestion of alcohol may induce reaction
NURSING IMPLICATIONS: Observe for signs of hypoglycemia; long-term therapy; *avoid* aspirin, alcohol; follow prescribed diet/exercise program			
Glyburide (Micronase)—PO 2.5–5 mg initially; 1.25–20 mg/day	See Acetohexmide	See Acetohexamide	See Acetohexamide
NURSING IMPLICATIONS: See Acetohexamide			
Tolazamide (Tolinase)—PO 100–500 mg; once/day; duration 10–14 hr	See Acetohexamide	See Acetohexamide	See Acetohexamide
NURSING IMPLICATIONS: See Acetohexamide			
Tolbutamide (Orinase)—PO 500–3,000 mg; 2–3 doses/day; duration 6–12 hr	See Acetohexamide	See Acetohexamide	See Acetohexamide
NURSING IMPLICATIONS: See Acetohexamide			
Insulin—Rapid Acting			
Crystalline zinc insulin (regular) (Humulin R) (clear)—onset 0.5–1.0 hr; peak 2–4 hr; duration 6–8 hr	Poorly controlled diabetes; trauma; surgery, coma	Enhances transmembrane passage of glucose into cells; promotes carbohydrate, fat, and protein metabolism	Hypoglycemia (profuse sweating, nausea, hunger, headache, confusion, ataxia, coma); allergic reaction at injection site
Insulin analogue: lispro (Humalog), aspart (Novolog)		More rapid absorption and shorter duration	
NURSING IMPLICATIONS: Monitor blood and urine for glucose and acetone levels; insulin currently being used can be kept at *room temperature for 1 mo;* refrigerate stock insulin only; rotate injection sites; cold insulin leads to lipodystrophy, reduced absorption, and local reaction; *only* form of insulin that is given IV; need to eat *within 15 min* of insulin analogue injection			
Insulin—Intermediate Acting Basal			
NPH insulin (isophane insulin suspension) (cloudy)—onset 1–2 hr; peak 5–8 hr; duration 10–20 hr	Clients who can be controlled by one dose per day	See Crystalline zinc insulin (regular)	See Crystalline zinc insulin (regular)
NURSING IMPLICATIONS: Gently rotate vial between palms, invert several times to mix; do *not* shake; see Crystalline zinc insulin (regular)			
Insulin zinc suspension (lente insulin) (cloudy)—onset 1–3 hr; peak 6–12 hr; duration 18–24 hr	Clients allergic to NPH	See Crystalline zinc insulin (regular)	See Crystalline zinc insulin (regular)
NURSING IMPLICATIONS: See Crystalline zinc insulin (regular)			
Insulin—Slow Acting			
Extended insulin zinc suspension (ultralente) (Humulin U)—onset 4–8 hr; peak 12–24 hr; duration 36 hr	Often mixed with semilente for 24-hr curve	See Crystalline zinc insulin (regular)	See Crystalline zinc insulin (regular)
NURSING IMPLICATIONS: See Crystalline zinc insulin (regular)			

Continued

Table 8.17

Common Medications—cont'd

Drug and Dosage	Use	Action	Assessment: Side Effects
Insulin—Long Acting Basal			
Insulin glargine (Lantus) (clear)—onset 1–2 hr; duration 24 hr		Closely imitates pancreas's basal insulin release	Absorbs equally over 24-hr period
NURSING IMPLICATIONS: See Crystalline zinc insulin (regular); glargine may cause mild pain at injection site and *cannot be mixed* with other insulins			
Antihypertensives			
Captopril (Capoten)—PO 50 mg 3 times daily	Hypertension, heart failure	Prevents production of angiotensin II; vasodilation	Hypotension; loss of taste perception; proteinuria; rashes
NURSING IMPLICATIONS: Monitor VS and weight; take 1 hr *before* or 2 hr *after* meals; change positions *slowly; avoid* salt and salt substitutes			
Clonidine (Catapres)—PO 200–600 mcg/day; transdermal 100–300 mcg applied every 7 days	Mild to moderate hypertension; also used for epidural pain management	Stimulates alpha-adrenergic receptors in CNS	Drowsiness; dry mouth; postural hypotension
NURSING IMPLICATIONS: Instruct client to take same time each day; *avoid* sudden position changes; *report:* mental depression, swelling of feet, paleness or cold feeling in fingertips or toes, vivid dreams or nightmares			
Guanadrel (Hylorel)—PO 5 mg twice daily (range: 20–75 mg/day)	Moderate to severe hypertension	Prevents release of norepinephrine in response to sympathetic stimulation	Confusion; fainting; fatigue; diarrhea; orthostatic hypotension; dizziness
NURSING IMPLICATIONS: Give with *diuretics* to minimize tolerance and fluid retention; *weigh* twice weekly; fewer side effects after 8 wk of therapy			
Guanethidine SO_4 (Ismelin)—PO 10–50 mg daily in divided doses	Severe to moderately severe hypertension	Blocks norepinephrine at postganglionic synapses	Orthostatic hypotension; diarrhea; inhibition of ejaculation
NURSING IMPLICATIONS: *Postural hypotension* is marked in the morning, *accentuated* by hot weather, alcohol, and exercise; teach to rise slowly, with assistance			
Guanfacine hydrochloride (Tenex)—PO 1 mg daily to maximum dose of 3 mg/day	Hypertension, in combination with thiazide-like diuretics	Centrally acting alpha-adrenergic receptor agonist	Drowsiness; weakness; dizziness; dry mouth; constipation; impotence
NURSING IMPLICATIONS: Warn client *not* to drive or perform activities requiring alertness; take at *bedtime* to minimize sedation; monitor BP and pulse			
Hydralazine HCl (Apresoline)—PO 10–50 mg 4 times daily	Moderate hypertension	Dilates peripheral blood vessels, increases renal blood flow	Palpitations, tachycardia, angina pectoris, tremors; depression
NURSING IMPLICATIONS: Encourage moderation in exercise and identification of stressful stimuli			
	Obstetric use: preeclampsia, eclampsia	Relaxes peripheral blood vessels (opens vascular bed—physiological dehydration)	Headache, heart palpitation; gastric irritation; coronary insufficiency; edema; chills, fever; severe depression
NURSING IMPLICATIONS: Side rails up; must *not* stand without assistance; may be given with diuretics; observe carefully; IM route *only;* monitor BP; IV for severe hypertension and preeclampsia; in pregnancy, must *not* decrease arterial pressure too much or too rapidly; otherwise, will jeopardize uteroplacental perfusion			
Lisinopril (Prinivil)—PO 10 mg/day, up to 20–40 mg daily or twice daily	Hypertension; heart failure; post-MI	Inhibits angiotensin-converting enzyme; alters hemodynamics without reflex tachycardia	Headache, fatigue, hypotension; cough, rash; ↑ BUN and creatinine
NURSING IMPLICATIONS: *Notify physician* if sudden drop in BP with supine positioning 1–5 hr after initial drug dose. Check BP before dose to determine 24-hr control			
Methyldopa (Aldomet)—PO 500 mg–2 gm in divided doses	Severe to moderately severe hypertension	Inhibits formation of dopamine, a precursor of norepinephrine	Initial drowsiness, depression with feelings of unreality, edema, jaundice, dry mouth

Table 8.17

Common Medications—cont'd

Drug and Dosage	Use	Action	Assessment: Side Effects
NURSING IMPLICATIONS: *Contraindicated* in acute and chronic liver disease; encourage not to drive car if drowsy			
Minoxidil (Loniten)—PO 5 mg/day (range: 10–40 mg/day)	Severe hypertension; end-stage organ failure	Relaxes vascular smooth muscle	ECG changes; tachycardia; Na^+, water retention; hypertrichosis
NURSING IMPLICATIONS: Depilatory cream may minimize increased hair growth; report resting pulse *increase more than 20 beats/min;* caution client to change positions *slowly*			
Phentolamine hydrochloride (Regitine)—PO 50 mg 4–6 doses daily; IV, IM, local 5–10 mg, diluted in minimum 10 mL normal saline	Prevents dermal necrosis; hypertensive crisis; pheochromocytoma	Blocks alpha-adrenergic receptors	Weakness, dizziness, orthostatic hypotension; nausea, vomiting, abdominal pain
NURSING IMPLICATIONS: When giving parenterally, client should be *supine;* monitor for overdosage (precipitous drop in BP); do *not* give with epinephrine			
Prazosin (Minipress)—PO 6–15 mg 2 or 3 times daily	Mild to moderate hypertension	Dilates arteries and veins by blocking postsynaptic $alpha_1$-adrenergic receptors	Dizziness, headache, weakness, palpitations; orthostatic hypotension with first dose
NURSING IMPLICATIONS: Monitor: I&O, VS, and *weight* at beginning of therapy; teach client/family to check BP at least weekly; need to comply with other interventions (weight reduction, diet, smoking cessation, exercise)			
Reserpine (Serpasil)— PO 0.25 mg daily	Mild to moderate hypertension	Depletes catecholamines and decreases peripheral vasoconstriction, heart rate, and BP	Depression; nasal stuffiness; increased gastric secretions; rash, pruritus
NURSING IMPLICATIONS: Watch for signs of *mental depression;* closely monitor pulse rates of clients *also receiving digitalis; avoid* alcohol			
	Obstetric use: Preeclampsia-eclampsia	CNS-depressant tranquilizer; sedation is major effect; decreases neural transmission to nerves; decreases tone in blood vessels	Low level of toxicity; weight gain; diarrhea; allergic reactions—dry mouth, itching, skin eruptions
NURSING IMPLICATIONS: Side rails up; must *not* stand up without assistance; observe carefully; monitor *BP*			
Timolol (Timoptic)—PO 20–40 mg/day; ophthalmic 1 gtt 1–2 times/day	Hypertension, migraine, glaucoma	Blocks stimulation of myocardial ($beta_1$) and pulmonary/vascular ($beta_2$) receptors	Fatigue, weakness; depression; insomnia; peripheral vasoconstriction; diarrhea, nausea, vomiting
NURSING IMPLICATIONS: Check VS and evidence of heart failure; do *not* take if pulse <50; *avoid* OTC cold remedies, coffee, tea, and cola			
Antihypotensives			
Metaraminol (Aramine)—IM 2–10 mg, or IV 15–100 mg in 500 mL NaCl	Adrenalectomy	Elevated systolic and diastolic BP by vasoconstriction	Hypertension, cardiac arrhythmias; may cause hypertensive crisis, if on MAO inhibitors or antidepressants
NURSING IMPLICATIONS: *Monitor* VS frequently (q3–5 min); observe for side effects; have *phentolamine available as antidote*			
Anti-infectives			
Amoxicillin (Amoxil)—PO 250–500 mg q8h; sexually transmitted infection (STI): 3-gm single dose with probenecid	Ear, nose, and throat (ENT) infections; soft tissue infections (cellulitis); gonorrhea	Broad spectrum; bactericidal	Rash, diarrhea; anaphylaxis
NURSING IMPLICATIONS: Determine allergies to penicillin, cephalosporins. Instruct client to take drug around the clock, and to complete therapy			

Continued

Table 8.17

Common Medications—cont'd

Drug and Dosage	Use	Action	Assessment: Side Effects
Cefazolin (Ancef, Kefzol)—IM, IV 250 mg–1.5 gm q6–12h	*Staphylococcus aureus; Escherichia coli; Klebsiella;* group A and B *Streptococcus; Pneumococcus*	Bactericidal	Allergic reaction; urticaria, rash; abnormal bleeding
NURSING IMPLICATIONS: See Penicillin; may cause *false-positive* laboratory tests (Coombs', urine glucose); oral probenecid may be taken concurrently to prolong effects of drug			
Cephalexin (Keflex)—PO 1–4 gm daily in 2–4 equally divided doses	Infections caused by gram-positive cocci; infections: respiratory, biliary, urinary, bone, septicemia, abdominal; surgical prophylaxis	Bactericidal effects on susceptible organisms, inhibition of bacterial cell wall synthesis	Nausea, vomiting; urticaria; toxic paranoid reactions; dizziness; increased alkaline phosphatase; nephrotoxicity; bone marrow suppression
NURSING IMPLICATIONS: Peak blood levels delayed when given with food; *report:* nausea, flushing, tachycardia, headache; monitor for *nephrotoxicity* and for bleeding			
Cephalothin (Keflin, Seffin)—IM, IV 2–12 gm/day in 4–6 equally divided doses	Same as cephalexin, except not recommended for biliary tract infections	See Cephalexin	See Cephalexin
NURSING IMPLICATIONS: See Cephalexin; pain at site of IM injection; given in large muscle; rotate sites			
Ciprofloxacin (Cipro)—PO 250–750 mg q12h; IV 200–400 mg q12h; ophthalmic 1–2 gtt q15–30 min, then 4–6 times daily	Lower respiratory tract infections; skin, bone, and joint infections; urinary tract infection (UTI)	Inhibits bacterial DNA synthesis	Restlessness; nausea, diarrhea, vomiting, abdominal pain
NURSING IMPLICATIONS: Give PO on an *empty stomach* unless GI irritation occurs, then take with food; *do not* take with milk or yogurt; IV over 60 min			
Clarithromycin (Biaxin)—PO 7.5 mg/kg q12h; usual 500 mg q12h	Peptic ulcer	Inhibits protein synthesis of bacterial ribosome	Hypersensitivity to other antibiotics; use with caution in *liver/renal* impairment
NURSING IMPLICATIONS: Take medication around the clock; report signs of superinfection, diarrhea; do *not* take during pregnancy			
Cloxacillin (Tegopen)—PO 250–500 mg q6h	Penicillinase-producing staphylococci infections: respiratory, sinus, and skin	Binds to bacterial cell wall, leading to cell death	Nausea, vomiting, diarrhea; rashes, allergic reactions; seizures (high doses)
NURSING IMPLICATIONS: *Give around the clock* on an *empty* stomach; observe for signs of *superinfection* (black, furry tongue, vaginal itching, loose stools)			
Co-trimoxazole (Bactrim, Septra)—PO 160 mg twice daily or 20 mg/kg/day for *P. jiroveci* pneumonia	Acute otitis media; urinary tract infection; shigellosis; *P. jiroveci* pneumonia; prostatitis	Bacteriostatic; anti-infective; antagonizes folic acid production; combination of sulfamethoxazole and trimethoprim	Hypersensitivity; see Sulfisoxazole
NURSING IMPLICATIONS: IV administration can cause phlebitis and *tissue damage* with extravasation			
Doxycycline (Vibramycin)—PO 100 mg q12h on day 1; then 100 mg/day × 7 days; IV 200 mg in 1–2 infusions on day 1; then 100–200 mg/day	Chlamydia, other STIs; Lyme disease	Inhibits bacterial protein of the 30S bacterial ribosome	Urticaria, diarrhea; nausea, vomiting; photosensitivity
NURSING IMPLICATIONS: Take prescribed medications as ordered; use sunscreen or protective clothing due to photosensitivity; report signs of superinfection, if original symptoms not improved			
Erythromycin—adults, PO 250 mg q6h; children, PO 30–50 mg/kg daily	Pneumonia; pelvic inflammatory disease; intestinal amebiasis; ocular infections; used if allergic to penicillin	Inhibits protein synthesis of microorganism; more effective against gram-positive organisms	Abdominal cramping, distention, diarrhea

Table 8.17

Common Medications—cont'd

Drug and Dosage	Use	Action	Assessment: Side Effects
NURSING IMPLICATIONS: Be sure culture and sensitivity done *before* treatment; give on *empty* stomach 1 hr before or 3 hr after meals; do *not* crush or chew tablets; do *not* give with fruit juice			
Gentamicin (Garamycin)—IM, IV 3–5 mg/kg/day in 3–4 divided doses; topical; skin, eye	Serious gram-negative infections; possible *S. aureus,* uncomplicated urinary tract infections	Bactericidal effects on susceptible gram-positive and gram-negative organisms and mycobacteria	Serious toxic effects: kidneys, ear; causes muscle weakness/paralysis
NURSING IMPLICATIONS: Monitor *plasma* levels (peak is 4–10 mcg/mL); clients with burns, cystic fibrosis may need higher doses			
Metronidazole (Flagyl)—PO 7.5 mg/kg q6h (not to exceed 4 gm/day)	Diverticulosis	Disrupts DNA and protein synthesis in susceptible organisms	Cimetidine may decrease metabolism; seizures, dizziness, abdominal pain
NURSING IMPLICATIONS: Administer with *food or milk* to decrease GI symptoms; *avoid* alcohol; has unpleasant metallic taste; *avoid* OTC medication while on this drug			
Penicillin: penicillin G, penicillin G potassium, penicillin G procaine, ampicillin—IM 400,000–1.2 million units q8h × 10 days, or single dose of 2.4 million units	*Streptococcus; Staphylococcus; Pneumococcus; Gonococcus; Treponema pallidum*	Primarily bactericidal	Dermatitis and delayed or immediate anaphylaxis
	Obstetric use: group B β-hemolytic streptococcus—prophylaxis	Prophylaxis	
NURSING IMPLICATIONS: Outpatients should be observed for *20 min after injection;* hospitalized clients should be observed at frequent intervals for 20 min after injection			
Pentamidine (Pentam)—IV 4 mg/kg once daily; inhalation 300 mg via nebulizer	Prevention or treatment of *P. jiroveci* pneumonia	Appears to disrupt DNA or RNA synthesis to protozoa	Anxiety, headache; bronchospasm, cough; hypotension, arrhythmias; nephrotoxicity; hypoglycemia; leukopenia, thrombocytopenia, anemia, chills
NURSING IMPLICATIONS: Assess for infection and respiratory status; unpleasant metallic taste may occur (not significant)			
Sulfisoxazole (Gantrisin), sulfamethizole (Thiosulfil), and sulfisomidine (Elkosin)—PO 2.4-gm loading dose, then 1–2 gm 4 times daily × 7–10 days	Acute, chronic, and recurrent urinary tract infections	Bacteriostatic and bactericidal	Nausea, vomiting; oliguria, anuria; anemia, leukopenia; dizziness; jaundice, skin rashes, and photosensitivity
NURSING IMPLICATIONS: Maintenance of blood levels is important; encourage *fluids* to prevent crystal formation in kidney tubules—push up to 3,000 mL/day; *avoid* in later stage of pregnancy and first month of life for newborn (may cause kernicterus)			
Tetracyclines: doxycycline hyclate (Vibramycin), oxytetracycline (Terramycin), tetracycline HCl (Sumycin)—PO 250–500 mg q6h; IM 250 mg/day; IV 250–500 mg q8–12h	Broad-spectrum antibiotic	Primarily bacteriostatic	GI upsets such as diarrhea, nausea, vomiting; sore throat; black, hairy tongue; glossitis; inflammatory lesions in anogenital region
 **NURSING IMPLICATIONS:** *Phototoxic* reactions have been reported; clients should be advised to stay out of direct sunlight; medication should *not* be given with milk or snacks, because food interferes with absorption of tetracyclines; do *not* give to women who are pregnant and children under 8 yr			
Trimethoprim (TMP)/sulfamethoxazole (SMZ) (Bactrim)—PO 160 mg TMP or 800 mg SMZ q12h for 14–21 days; IV 8–10 mg/kg (TMP 40–50 mg/kg) q6–12h	Bronchitis, *Shigella* enteritis, otitis media, *P. jiroveci* pneumonia, UTI, traveler's diarrhea	Combination inhibits the metabolism of folic acid in bacteria; bactericidal	Nausea, vomiting; rashes; phlebitis at IV site; aplastic anemia; hepatic necrosis

Continued

Table 8.17

Common Medications—cont'd

Drug and Dosage	Use	Action	Assessment: Side Effects
NURSING IMPLICATIONS: Check IV site frequently; do *not* give IM; give PO on *empty stomach;* take *around the clock; avoid* exposure to sun			
Anti-inflammatory Agents			
Gastrointestinal			
Infliximab (Remicade)—IV 3 mg/kg up to 10 mg/kg	Autoimmune disorders (e.g., Crohn's disease, ulcerative colitis, psoriatic arthritis)	Blocks the action of tumor necrosis factor-alpha, which attacks normal healthy parts of the body	Allergic reactions, bleeding problems
NURSING IMPLICATIONS: Infuse over 2 hr; use in-line filter. Medication to treat hypersensitivity should be available			
Mesalamine (Asacol, Pentusa, Rowasa)—PO 800 mg 3 times/day for 6 wk	Ulcerative colitis	Local-acting anti-inflammatory in GI tract	*Contraindicated* if client has allergy to sulfonamides or salicylates; acceleration of symptoms; abdominal pain
NURSING IMPLICATIONS: *Monitor* for: abdominal pain, diarrhea, blood in stools, superinfection; if no improvement notify health-care professional; may need diagnostic studies			
Olsalazine (Dipentum)—PO 1 gm/day in 2 divided doses	See Mesalamine	See Mesalamine	See Mesalamine
NURSING IMPLICATIONS: See Mesalamine			
Sulfasalazine (Azulfidine)—PO 3–4 gm/day in divided doses	See Mesalamine	See Mesalamine	See Mesalamine
NURSING IMPLICATIONS: See Mesalamine			
Inhalants			
Beclomethasone (Beclovent, Vanceril)—42–50 mcg/spray; 2 metered sprays 3–4 times/day	Emphysema	Glucocorticoid (inhalation)	Headache, hypersensitivity to fluorocarbon propellant; used with *caution* in diabetes or glaucoma
NURSING IMPLICATIONS: Do *not* exceed 1 mg/day			
Flunisolide (AeroBid)—42–50 mcg/spray; 2 metered sprays 2–4 times/day	Emphysema	Potent locally acting anti-inflammatory and immune modifier	Headache, dysphonia; fungal infections; adrenal suppression with long-term use
NURSING IMPLICATIONS: *Monitor* respiratory status and lung sounds; *assess* clients changing from systemic to inhaled glucocorticoids for signs of *adrenal insufficiency* (anorexia, nausea, weakness, hypotension, hypoglycemia)			
Triaminolone (Azmacort)—See Beclomethasone	Asthma	See Beclomethasone	See Beclomethasone
NURSING IMPLICATIONS: See Beclomethasone			
Systemics			
Cortisone acetate—PO, IM 20–100 mg daily in single or divided doses	Adrenocorticotropic hormone (ACTH) insufficiency; rheumatoid arthritis; allergies; ulcerative colitis; nephrosis	Anti-inflammatory effect of unknown action	Moon facies, hirsutism, thinning of skin, striae; hypertension; menstrual irregularities, delayed healing; psychoses
NURSING IMPLICATIONS: Give oral form pc, with snack at bedtime; give deep IM (*never* deltoid); monitor vital signs; observe for behavior changes; skin care and activity to tolerance; *diet*—salt *restricted, high* protein, KCl supplement; protect from injury			
Desoxycorticosterone acetate (hydrocortisone)—IM, IV 100–500 mg q2–6h; PO 3–5 mg 2–4 times daily	Addison's disease; burns; surgical shock; adrenal surgery	Promotes reabsorption of sodium; restores plasma volume, BP, and electrolyte balance	Edema, hypertension, pulmonary congestion, hypokalemia

Table 8.17

Common Medications—cont'd

Drug and Dosage	Use	Action	Assessment: Side Effects
NURSING IMPLICATIONS: Salt restriction according to BP readings; *monitor* vital signs; weigh daily			
Dexamethasone (Decadron)—PO 0.5–5.0 mg daily; IM, IV 4–20 mg daily	Addison's disease; allergic reactions; leukemia; Hodgkin's disease; iritis; dermatitis; rheumatoid arthritis **Obstetric use:** stimulate surfactant production in client with premature labor	Anti-inflammatory effect	See Cortisone acetate
NURSING IMPLICATIONS: *Contraindicated* in tuberculosis; see Cortisone acetate for nursing care			
Methylprednisolone sodium (Solu-Medrol)—IV, IM 10–40 mg, slowly	Glucocorticoid, corticosteroid	See Dexamethasone	See Dexamethasone
NURSING IMPLICATIONS: See Dexamethasone			
Prednisolone (Deltsone)—PO 5–60 mg/day single or divided doses	Multiple sclerosis	Suppress inflammation and normal immune response	Depression, euphoria; peptic ulceration; thromboembolism
NURSING IMPLICATIONS: *Monitor* for: *Homans' sign,* abdominal pain, vomiting, tarry stools, mental status or mood changes			
Prednisone—PO 2.5–15.0 mg daily	Rheumatoid arthritis; cancer therapy	Anti-inflammatory effect of unknown action	Insomnia and gastric distress
NURSING IMPLICATIONS: See Cortisone acetate			
Rituximab (Rituxan)—IV 1,000-mg doses separated by 2 wk	Non-Hodgkin's lymphoma; rheumatoid arthritis	Monoclonal antibody that interferes with growth and spread of certain B cells	Infusion reaction; tumor lysis syndrome, skin reaction, fever, headache, chills, sneezing
NURSING IMPLICATIONS: Give *slowly* IV. *Avoid* vaccines during treatment			
Antilipemics			
Atorvastatin calcium (Lipitor)—PO 10 mg daily up to 80 mg/day	Reduce: low-density lipoprotein (LDL), cholesterol, triglycerides	Increases number of hepatic LDL receptors	Back pain, myalgia; constipation, diarrhea; ↑ liver function tests
NURSING IMPLICATIONS: Assess for: muscle pain, tenderness, or weakness—check creatine phosphokinase (CPK) level. Use *cautiously* with: antifungals, niacin, erythromycin			
Cholestyramine (Questran)—PO 4 gm 1–4 times/day	Hypercholesterolemia; pruritus from increased bile	Binds bile acids in GI tract, increased clearance of cholesterol	Nausea, constipation, abdominal discomfort
NURSING IMPLICATIONS: Take *before* meals; do *not* take with other medications; give others 1 hr before or 4–6 hr after			
Gemfibrozil (Lopid)—PO 1,200 mg/day	Hypercholesterolemia	May inhibit peripheral lipolysis and reduce triglyceride synthesis in liver	GI upset (abdominal pain, epigastric pain, diarrhea, nausea, vomiting); rash; headache, dizziness, blurred vision
NURSING IMPLICATIONS: Use *caution* when driving or doing tasks requiring alertness; take *before* meals			
Niacin (vitamin B_3, nicotinic acid)—PO 1.5–6.0 gm	Hypercholesterolemia	Decreases liver's production of LDLs and synthesis of triglycerides	GI upset, flushing; pruritus, hyperuricemia, hyperglycemia

Continued

Table 8.17

Common Medications—cont'd

Drug and Dosage	Use	Action	Assessment: Side Effects
NURSING IMPLICATIONS: Take the drug *with* meals; prevent flushing by taking an *aspirin 30 min before*; monitor closely during first year of therapy			
Simvastatin (Zocor)—PO 10–20 mg daily	Lipid-lowering	Inhibits enzyme responsible for increased synthesis of cholesterol	Abdominal cramps, constipation, diarrhea, flatus; heartburn; elevation of liver enzymes, pancreatitis
NURSING IMPLICATIONS: Give once in the *evening* with or without food			
Antineoplastics			
6-Mercaptopurine (Purinethol)—PO 2.5 mg/kg/day; may increase to 5 mg/kg after 4 wk; maintenance 1.5–2.5 mg/kg/day	Leukemia (ulcerative)	Antineoplastic	Bone marrow depression, severe hepatotoxicity
NURSING IMPLICATIONS: *Monitor:* bleeding, infection, *liver* function tests, skin care, nausea and vomiting			
Methotrexate (Rheumatrex)—PO, IM 15–30 mg/day for 5 days; repeat after 1 wk for 3–5 courses	Leukemia Breast, lung cancer	Interferes with folic acid metabolism, resulting in inhibition of DNA synthesis and cell reproduction	Pulmonary fibrosis; hepatotoxicity; stomatitis, signs and symptoms of chemotherapy side effects
NURSING IMPLICATIONS: Monitor: *liver* function; *assess* respiratory status; see nursing care of clients receiving chemotherapy, **pp. 526–527**			
Mitotane (Lysodren)—PO 9–10 gm/day in 3–4 divided doses initially; decrease for maintenance	Adrenocortical carcinoma	Affects pituitary disorders	GI complaints; lethargy, somnolence
NURSING IMPLICATIONS: *Monitor:* signs of disease progression, GI abnormalities, abdominal pain			
Anti-Parkinson Agents			
Benztropine (Cogentin)—PO 1–2 mg/day (range: 0.5–6 mg/day)	Parkinson's disease	Blocks cholinergic activity in CNS	Blurred vision, dry eyes; constipation; *caution* with antihistamines, phenothiazines
NURSING IMPLICATIONS: Take as directed for best results; monitor for drowsiness, dizziness, orthostatic hypotension; good mouth care; use *caution* with OTC drugs, overheating (drug causes a decrease in perspiration)			
Biperiden (Akineton)—PO 2 mg 3–4 times/day; *not to exceed* 16 mg/day	Parkinson's disease	Restores natural balance of neurotransmitters in CNS	Same as Benztropine
NURSING IMPLICATIONS: See Benztropine			
Carbidopa/levodopa (Sinemet)—PO (10/100, 25/100 carbidopa/levodopa ratio) 1 tablet 3 times/day up to 8 tablets daily	Parkinson's disease	Levodopa is converted to dopamine in CNS, where it serves as a neurotransmitter	Use with MAO inhibitors may result in hypertensive crisis; some drugs can reverse effects (e.g., phenothiazines, reserpine)
NURSING IMPLICATIONS: Rate of dosage increase determined by client response; make accurate observations. May experience "on-off" phenomenon—loss of drug effects and sudden return. Prevent falling from postural hypotension, "leg freezing," instability			
Trihexyphenidyl (Artane)— PO 1–2 mg daily; usual maintenance dose: 5–15 mg/day in divided dose	Parkinson's disease	Inhibits action of acetylcholine	Dizziness, nervousness, blurred vision, mydriasis
NURSING IMPLICATIONS: Monitor symptoms; *avoid* orthostatic hypotension; mouth care			
Antiplatelet Agents			
Clopidogrel (Plavix)—PO 75 mg daily	Reduce risk of atherosclerotic event (MI, stroke)	Inhibits platelet aggregation	Bleeding; neutropenia; reactions similar to aspirin
NURSING IMPLICATIONS: Give once daily without regard to food; *avoid* aspirin, NSAIDs; observe for symptoms of: stroke, peripheral vascular disease, MI			

Table 8.17

Common Medications—cont'd

Drug and Dosage	Use	Action	Assessment: Side Effects
Dipyridamole (Persantine)—PO 70–100 mg 4 times/day; IV 570 mcg/kg	Prevent thromboembolism; surgical graft patency; *diagnostic* agent in myocardial perfusion studies	Decreases platelet aggregation; coronary vasodilator	Headache, dizziness, hypotension; nausea; MI, arrhythmias with IV
NURSING IMPLICATIONS: Take at *evenly* spaced intervals; *avoid* use of alcohol; if no GI irritation, take 1 hr before or 2 hr after meals			
Eptifibatide (Integrilin)—IV 180-mcg/kg bolus; 2 mcg/kg/min until discharge or up to 72 hr	Severe chest pain; small heart attacks; unstable angina; before balloon angioplasty	Binds to glycoprotein receptor sites of platelets	Bleeding
NURSING IMPLICATIONS: Minimize any vascular trauma during treatment. Monitor laboratory tests for indications of bleeding or clotting disorders; **stop drug immediately** if bleeding occurs			
Ticlopidine (Ticlid)—PO 250 mg twice daily	Stroke prevention; prevent early restenosis of coronary stents	Inhibits platelet aggregation; prolongs bleeding time	Diarrhea, rashes, bleeding, intracerebral bleeding
NURSING IMPLICATIONS: Give *with* food or immediately *after* eating			
Antituberculosis Agents*			
First-Line Drugs			
Ethambutol—PO 15–25 mg/kg	See Isoniazid	See Isoniazid	Optic neuritis (reversible with discontinuation of drug; very rare at 15 mg/kg); skin rash
NURSING IMPLICATIONS: Use with *caution* with renal disease or when eye testing is not feasible; used *in combination with* other drug			
Isoniazid—PO, IM 5–10 mg/kg up to 300 mg	Tuberculosis	Suppresses or interferes with biosynthesis; bacteriostatic	Peripheral neuritis; hepatitis; hypersensitivity
NURSING IMPLICATIONS: Give pyridoxine (vitamin B_6) 10 mg as prophylaxis for neuritis; 50–100 mg as treatment			
Pyrazinamide—PO 15–30 mg/kg up to 3 gm	Tuberculosis	Bactericidal	Hyperuricemia, hepatotoxicity
NURSING IMPLICATIONS: Loss of glycemic control in those with diabetes			
Rifampin—PO 10–20 mg/kg; IV 600 mg Rifamate combination (isoniazid with rifampin) Rifater combination (isoniazid and pyrazinamide with rifampin)—see Rifampin	Tuberculosis, meningitis, *Haemophilus influenzae*	Impairs RNA synthesis; bactericidal	Hepatitis, febrile reaction, purpura (rare)
NURSING IMPLICATIONS: *Orange* urine color; *negates* effect of birth control pills			
Streptomycin—IM 15–20 mg/kg up to 1 gm	Tuberculosis, endocarditis, tularemia	Inhibits protein synthesis; bactericidal	*Eighth cranial* nerve damage, *nephrotoxicity*
NURSING IMPLICATIONS: Use with caution in *older* clients or those with *renal* disease			
Antiulcer Agents			
Aluminum hydroxide gel (Amphojel)—PO 5–10 mL q2–4h or 1 hr pc	Gastric acidity; peptic ulcer; phosphatic urinary calculi; ↓ phosphorus level in chronic renal failure	Buffers HCl in gastric juices without interfering with electrolyte balance	Constipation and fecal impaction
NURSING IMPLICATIONS: *Shake well* before administering; encourage *fluids* to prevent impaction and milk-alkali syndrome			
Calcium carbonate (Titralac)—PO 1–2 gm taken with H_2O after meals and at bedtime	Peptic ulcer and chronic gastritis	Reduces hyperacidity	Constipation or laxative effect

*To minimize resistant strains, combination therapy is used long-term.

Continued

Table 8.17

Common Medications—cont'd

Drug and Dosage	Use	Action	Assessment: Side Effects
NURSING IMPLICATIONS: See Aluminum hydroxide gel			
Cimetidine (Tagamet)—PO 300–600 mg q6h; IM, IV 300 mg q6h	Duodenal ulcers, gastroesophageal reflux disease (GERD), gastric hypersecretion; peptic acid gastritis, heartburn; esophagitis	Inhibits action of histamine at H_2 receptor site, inhibits gastric acid secretion; neutralizes and absorbs excess acid	Confusion, dizziness; nausea; rash; diarrhea, constipation; hypermagnesemia
NURSING IMPLICATIONS: Give *with* meals or immediately *after; avoid* smoking; *avoid* prolonged administration to clients with renal insufficiency			
Famotidine (Pepcid)—PO 40 mg/day at bedtime or 20 mg twice a day	Peptic ulcer	Inhibits gastric acid secretion by inhibiting histamine at H_2 receptor site	Use with caution: elderly, renal failure; confusion, arrhythmias, agranulocytosis, aplastic anemia
NURSING IMPLICATIONS: Assess for: epigastric pain, blood in stool, or emesis; monitor laboratory values to avoid side effects; take medication for full course of treatment; *avoid* self-medication with OTC drugs; *avoid* smoking			
Lansoprazole (Prevacid)—PO 15 mg/day; with *Helicobacter pylori:* 30 mg twice a day with amoxicillin	Peptic ulcer	Binds to an enzyme in presence of gastric acid; prevents final transport of hydrogen ions into gastric lumen	Hypersensitivity; use with caution in elderly; dosage change needed with hepatic impairment
NURSING IMPLICATIONS: *Avoid* alcohol; *report* signs of: GI bleeding, cramping, abdominal pain, vomiting			
Magnesium and aluminum hydroxides (Maalox suspension)—PO 5–30 mL q1–3h pc and at bedtime	Gastric hyperacidity; peptic ulcer; heartburn; reflux esophagitis	Neutralizes and binds gastric acids, heals ulcers	Constipation from aluminum hydroxide; diarrhea from magnesium hydroxide
NURSING IMPLICATIONS: Encourage fluid intake; *contraindicated* for clients who are debilitated or those with renal insufficiency			
Misoprostol (Cytotec)—PO 200 mcg 4 times/day; rectal 800 mcg; vaginal 25–50 mcg	Peptic ulcer **Obstetric use:** labor induction, to control postpartum hemorrhage	Prostaglandin analogue	Hypersensitivity to prostaglandins; diarrhea; *avoid* during pregnancy
NURSING IMPLICATIONS: Monitor effectiveness of the drug; report increase in abdominal pain, bleeding			
Nizatidine (Axid) see Cimetidine	See Cimetidine	See Cimetidine	See Cimetidine
NURSING IMPLICATIONS: See Cimetidine			
Omeprazole (Prilosec)—PO 20 mg once daily	Peptic ulcer GERD	Gastric acid–pump inhibitor	Abdominal pain; *contraindicated:* hypersensitivity
NURSING IMPLICATIONS: May cause drowsiness, dizziness; *avoid:* alcohol, aspirin, NSAIDs, foods that cause GI irritation			
Ranitidine (Zantac)—PO 150 mg twice daily; IM 50 mg q6–8h; IV 50 mg q6–8h	Duodenal ulcer, gastric ulcer, GERD, gastric hypersecretion	Inhibits action of histamine at H_2 receptor site, inhibits gastric acid secretion	Headache, malaise; nausea, constipation, diarrhea
NURSING IMPLICATIONS: Food does *not* affect absorption; give 1 hr *apart* from antacids; *smoking* interferes with action			
Sucralfate (Carafate)—PO 1 gm 4 times daily	Prevention and treatment of duodenal ulcer	Reacts with gastric acid to form a thick paste that adheres to the ulcer surface	Constipation
NURSING IMPLICATIONS: Give 1 hr *before meals* and *at bedtime; do not* crush or chew tablets; take *antacids* 30 min before or 1 hr after sucralfate; increase *fluids and dietary* bulk			
Antivirals			
Acyclovir (Zovirax)—PO 200 mg 3–5 times/day; IV 5 mg/kg q8h over 1 hr; topical 6 times daily for 1 wk	Herpes simplex (types 1, 2)	Converts to an active cytotoxic metabolite that inhibits viral DNA replication	Headache, nausea, vomiting, diarrhea; *increased* serum BUN and creatinine

Table 8.17

Common Medications—cont'd

Drug and Dosage	Use	Action	Assessment: Side Effects
NURSING IMPLICATIONS: Measure I&O q8h; ensure adequate *hydration;* assess for common side effects; apply topical with *finger cot* or rubber glove; refer for counseling			
Indinavir (Crixivan)—PO 800 mg q8h	HIV; possible prevention in combination therapy	Inhibits action of HIV protease and cleavage of viral polyproteins	Ketoacidosis; kidney stones; hyperglycemia; altered taste; acid regurgitation
NURSING IMPLICATIONS: Give with *water or other liquids* (skim milk, coffee, tea, juice) *1 hr before* or *2 hr after* meal; *avoid* high-fat, high-protein meal within 2 hr; with concurrent therapy, may need to take drugs 1 hr apart; capsules are sensitive to moisture—keep desiccant in bottle			
Nevirapine (Viramune)—PO 200 mg daily for 2 wk, then twice daily	HIV; delays disease progression	Binds to the enzyme reverse transcriptase; disrupts DNA synthesis	Rash; *Stevens-Johnson syndrome* (severe erythema multiforme)
NURSING IMPLICATIONS: Give with or without food; drug does not cure AIDS—decreases opportunistic infections			
Zidovudine (AZT, Retrovir)—PO 200 mg q4h	AIDS and related disorders	Inhibits HIV replication	Blood disorders, especially anemia and granulocytopenia; headache; nausea; insomnia; myalgia
NURSING IMPLICATIONS: Monitor for signs of opportunistic infection and adverse drug effects; drug must be taken *around the clock;* regular blood tests (q2 wk)			
Blood Viscosity–Reducing Agent			
Pentoxifylline (Trental)—PO 400 mg 3 times daily	Peripheral vascular disease (intermittent claudication)	Increases flexibility of red blood cells (RBCs); inhibits platelet aggregation	Nausea, vomiting, GI upset; drowsiness; dizziness; headache
NURSING IMPLICATIONS: Give *with* meals to minimize GI irritation; take tablets whole; report persistent GI or CNS side effects			
Bronchodilators			
Albuterol (Ventolin)—PO 2–6 mg 3–4 times/day; inhalation q4–6h or 2 puffs 15 min before exercise	Bronchodilator	Results in accumulation of cyclic adenosine monophosphate (cAMP) at beta-adrenergic receptors	Nervousness, restlessness, tremor, hypertension, nausea
NURSING IMPLICATIONS: Give *with* meals; allow 1 min *between* inhalations; rinse mouth with water *after* inhalation			
Aminophylline—PO 250 mg 2–4 times daily; rectal 250–500 mg; IV 250–500 mg over 10–20 min	Rapid relief of bronchospasm; asthma; pulmonary edema	Relaxes smooth muscles and increases cardiac contractility; interferes with reabsorption of Na^+ and Cl^- in proximal tubules	Nausea, vomiting; cardiac arrhythmias; intestinal bleeding; insomnia, restlessness; rectal irritation from suppository
NURSING IMPLICATIONS: Give oral *with* or *after meals;* monitor *vital signs* for changes in BP and pulse; weigh daily; IM injections are painful			
Ephedrine SO_4—PO, Subcu, IM 25 mg 3 or 4 times daily	Asthma: allergies; bradycardia; nasal decongestant	Relaxes hypertonic muscles in bronchioles and GI tract	Wakefulness, nervousness, dizziness, palpitations, hypertension
NURSING IMPLICATIONS: Monitor vital signs; *avoid* giving dose near bedtime; *check urine* output in older adults			
Ipratropium (Atrovent)—1–4 inhalations	Emphysema	Inhibits cholinergic receptors in bronchial smooth muscle	Nasal dryness, epistaxis; fluorocarbon toxicity when used with other inhalants
NURSING IMPLICATIONS: Instruct in proper use of inhaler; do *not* use more than 12 metered doses in 12 hr; if severe bronchospasm occurs, consult physician/nurse practitioner			
Isoproterenol HCl (Isuprel)—inhalation of 1:100 or 1:200 solution	Mild to moderately severe asthma attack; bronchitis; pulmonary emphysema	Relaxes hypertonic bronchioles	Nervousness, tachycardia; hypertension; insomnia
NURSING IMPLICATIONS: Monitor vital signs *before and after* treatment; teach client how to use nebulizer			

Continued

Table 8.17

Common Medications—cont'd

Drug and Dosage	Use	Action	Assessment: Side Effects
Metaproterenol (Alupent)—PO 20 mg 3–4 times/day; inhalation 2–3 metered-dose inhalations	Asthma	Bronchodilation	Nervousness, restlessness, tremor, paradoxical bronchospasm
NURSING IMPLICATIONS: Assess lung sounds, observe for wheezing (paradoxical bronchospasm); observe clients' respiratory signs and symptoms; refer to health-care professional if symptoms persist or shortness of breath continues			
Salmeterol (Serevent)—inhalation 50 mcg twice a day (2 inhalations)	Asthma	Produces accumulation of cAMP at beta-adrenergic receptors	Headache, palpitations, abdominal pain; *avoid* use when on beta-adrenergic agents (decreases effectiveness)
NURSING IMPLICATIONS: Assess lung sounds; *monitor* pulmonary function; do *not* use for acute symptoms			
Terbutaline (Brethine)—PO 2.5–5.0 mg q6h (*not* to exceed 20 mg/24 hr); Subcu 0.25 mg, repeat 15–30 min (*not* to exceed 0.5 mg/hr); inhalation 2 puffs (0.2 mg each) q4–6h	Bronchospasm **Obstetric use:** may be used for premature labor; not Food and Drug Administration (FDA) approved for use as tocolytic agent, but widely used	See Isoproterenol	See Isoproterenol If used in pregnancy: maternal and fetal tachycardia
NURSING IMPLICATIONS: See Isoproterenol			
Theophylline—PO 400 mg/day in divided doses; max. adult dose: 900-mg divided dose	Treatment/prevention of emphysema, asthma (bronchoconstriction); chronic bronchitis	Bronchodilation	Restlessness; increased respiration, heart rate; palpitations, arrhythmias; nausea, vomiting; increased urine output → dehydration
NURSING IMPLICATIONS: Monitor theophylline levels: 10–20 mcg/mL; monitor signs of toxicity; take with 8 oz water or *with* meals to decrease GI symptoms			
Zafirlukast (Accolate)—PO 20 mg twice daily	Asthma	Antagonizes the effects of leukotrienes	Headache, fever, infection, pain
NURSING IMPLICATIONS: *Monitor* lung sounds, respiratory function			
Zileuton (Zyflo)—PO 600 mg 4 times daily	Asthma	Enzyme inhibitor	Headache, dizziness; chest pain; increases blood level of theophylline, propranolol, warfarin
NURSING IMPLICATIONS: Assess lung sounds; do *not* discontinue or reduce dosage without consulting health-care professional; not used to treat acute attack			
Calcium Channel Blockers			
Amlodipine (Norvasc)—PO 5–10 mg daily	Hypertension, angina pectoris, vasospastic (Prinzmetal's) angina, muscle cells	Inhibits the transport of calcium into myocardial and vascular smooth muscle	Arrhythmias, peripheral edema, heart failure; photosensitivity; gingival hyperplasia
NURSING IMPLICATIONS: Instruct client to: monitor pulse, report rate <50 beats/min, take with or without food			
Diltiazem (Cardizem)—PO 30–120 mg 3–4 times/day; IV 5–15 mg/hr	Angina, hypertension, atrial arrhythmias	Inhibits excitation-contraction coupling; decreased SA, AV node conduction	Headache, fatigue, arrhythmias, edema, hypotension; constipation; rash
NURSING IMPLICATIONS: May take *with* meals; take pulse; do *not* give drug if pulse <50 beats/min; change positions slowly; may take nitroglycerin sublingually concurrently			
Metoprolol (Lopressor)—PO 100 mg/day up to 450 mg/day	Hypertension	Blocks stimulation of myocardial adrenergic receptors ($beta_1$)	*Contraindicated* in: congestive heart failure (CHF), pulmonary edema; *caution* with renal impairment

Table 8.17

Common Medications—cont'd

Drug and Dosage	Use	Action	Assessment: Side Effects
NURSING IMPLICATIONS: Monitor vital signs, especially BP; prevent *orthostatic hypotension; avoid* self-medication with OTC; may cause drowsiness; medication may increase *sensitivity to cold*			
Nicardipine (Cardene)—PO 20–40 mg 3 times daily	Angina, hypertension	Inhibits excitation-contraction coupling	Dizziness, light-headedness, headache; peripheral edema; flushing
NURSING IMPLICATIONS: Give on an *empty* stomach; chest pain may occur 30 min after dose (temporary, from *reflex tachycardia*)			
Nifedipine (Procardia)—PO 10–30 mg 3 times daily (*not* to exceed 180 mg/day); sublingual 10 mg repeated in 15 min	Angina, hypertension **Obstetric use:** may be used for premature labor; not FDA approved for use as tocolytic agent, but widely used	Vasodilation	Dizziness, light-headedness, giddiness, headache, nervousness; nasal congestion; sore throat, dyspnea, cough, wheezing; nausea; flushing, warmth
NURSING IMPLICATIONS: May take *with* meals; make position changes *slowly;* angina may occur 30 min after dose (temporary)			
Verapamil (Calan, Isopten)—PO 240–480 mg, 3–4 times/day; IV 75–150 mcg/kg over 2 min	Angina; supraventricular arrhythmias; essential hypertension	Inhibits calcium movement into smooth-muscle cells; lowers pressure by reducing cardiac contractility	Constipation, AV block, hepatotoxicity
NURSING IMPLICATIONS: Monitor VS and ECG for *bradycardia* and *arrhythmias;* observe for *jaundice, abdominal pain;* encourage *fluids* and *bulk-forming* foods			
Cardiac Glycosides			
Digitoxin—digitalizing dose: PO 200 mcg twice/day; IM, IV 200–400 mcg; maintenance dose: PO 50–300 mcg daily	Heart failure: atrial fibrillation and flutter; supraventricular tachycardia	Increases force of cardiac contractility, slows heart rate, decreases right atrial pressures, promotes diuresis	Arrhythmias; nausea, vomiting; anorexia, malaise; color vision, yellow or blue
NURSING IMPLICATIONS: Hold medication if pulse rate less than *50* or over *120;* encourage foods high in *potassium* (e.g., bananas, orange juice); observe for signs of electrolyte depletion, apathy, disorientation, and anorexia			
Digoxin (Lanoxin)—digitalizing dose: PO 10–15 mcg/kg; IV 0.6–1 mg/kg; maintenance dose: PO 0.125–0.375 mg daily	See Digitoxin	See Digitoxin	See Digitoxin
NURSING IMPLICATIONS: See Digitoxin			
Central Nervous System Stimulants			
Amphetamine SO_4—PO 5–60 mg daily in divided doses	Mild depressive states; narcolepsy; postencephalitic parkinsonism; obesity control; minimal brain dysfunction in children (attention deficit disorder)	Raises BP, decreases sense of fatigue, elevates mood	Restlessness, dizziness, tremors, insomnia; increased libido; suicidal and homicidal tendencies; palpitations; anginal pain
NURSING IMPLICATIONS: Give *before* 4 p.m. to avoid sleep disturbance; dependence on drug may develop; *contraindicated* with: MAO inhibitors, hyperthyroidism, and psychotic states			
Methylphenidate hydrochloride (Ritalin)—PO 0.3 mg/kg/day or adults 20–60 mg in divided doses	Childhood hyperactivity; narcolepsy; attention deficit disorder in children	Mild CNS and respiratory stimulation	Anorexia; dizziness, drowsiness, insomnia, nervousness; BP and pulse changes
NURSING IMPLICATIONS: To avoid insomnia, take last dose 4–5 hr before bedtime; monitor vital signs; check weight 2–3 times weekly and report weight losses			

Continued

Table 8.17

Common Medications—cont'd

Drug and Dosage	Use	Action	Assessment: Side Effects
Chemotherapy and Antineoplastics (see Table 8.11 and Table 8.12)			
Cholinergics			
Bethanechol chloride (Urecholine)—PO 5–30 mg; Subcu 2.5–5.0 mg	Postoperative abdominal atony and distention; bladder atony with retention; postsurgical or postpartum urinary retention; myasthenia gravis	Increases GI and bladder tone; decreases sphincter tone	Belching, abdominal cramps, diarrhea, nausea, vomiting; incontinence; profuse sweating, salivation; respiratory depression
NURSING IMPLICATIONS: Check *respirations;* have urinal or bedpan close at hand and answer calls quickly; atropine SO_4 is the *antidote* for cholinergic drugs			
Edrophonium (Tensilon)—IV 2 mg; IM 10 mg	Diagnosis of myasthenia gravis; reversal of neuromuscular blockers	Inhibits breakdown of acetylcholine; anticholinesterase	Excess secretions; bronchospasm; bradycardia; abdominal cramps, vomiting, diarrhea; excess salivation; sweating
NURSING IMPLICATIONS: Effects last up to 30 min; give IV *undiluted* with *TB* syringe			
Neostigmine (Prostigmin)—PO 15–30 mg q3–4h; Subcu, IM 0.25–1 mg	Myasthenia gravis, postoperative bladder distention, urinary retention, reversal of neuromuscular blockers	Inhibits breakdown of acetylcholine	Excess secretions; bronchospasm; bradycardia; abdominal cramps, nausea, vomiting, diarrhea; excess salivation; sweating
NURSING IMPLICATIONS: Take oral form *with* food or milk; with chewing difficulty, take 30 min before eating			
Physostigmine salicylate (Eserine)—ophthalmic 0.1 mL of 0.25%–10% solution: not more than 1 drop 4 times daily; IM, IV 0.5–3 mg	Glaucoma; reverse effects of: tricyclic antidepressants, overdose, toxic effects of atropine and diazepam	Increases concentration of acetylcholine	Sweating; marked miosis, lacrimation; nausea, diarrhea
NURSING IMPLICATIONS: If *brown eyed,* may require stronger solution or more frequent dose			
Pilocarpine HCl—ophthalmic 1–2 gtt 1%–2% solution up to 6 times/day	Chronic open-angle and acute closed-angle glaucoma	Contraction of the sphincter muscle of iris, resulting in miosis	Brow ache, headache, ocular pain, blurring and dimness of vision, allergic conjunctivitis; nausea, vomiting, profuse sweating; bronchoconstriction in clients with bronchial asthma
NURSING IMPLICATIONS: Initially the medication may be irritating; teach proper sterile technique for instilling drops—wipe excess solution to prevent systemic symptoms; discard cloudy solutions			
Pyridostigmine (Mestinon)—PO 60 mg/day × 3 days; IM, IV 2 mg q2–3h; maintenance: 60–150 mg/day	Myasthenia gravis; reversal of neuromuscular blockers	Inhibits breakdown of acetylcholine and prolongs its effects	See Neostigmine
NURSING IMPLICATIONS: See Neostigmine			
Decongestants			
Phenylephrine (Neo-Synephrine, Sinex)—Subcu, IM 2–5 mg q10–15 min, *not to exceed* 5 mg; IV 40–60 mcg/min; nasal 2–3 gtt or 1–2 sprays q3–4h; ophthalmic 3 gtt/day	Shock, hypotension, decongestant, adjunct to spinal anesthesia, mydriatic	Constricts blood vessels by stimulating alpha-adrenergic receptors	Dizziness, restlessness, dyspnea, tachycardia, arrhythmias; ophthalmological: burning, photophobia, tearing
NURSING IMPLICATIONS: Check for correct concentration; protect eyes from *light sensitivity;* blow nose before using; *rebound congestion* will occur with prolonged use			
Pseudoephedrine (Sudafed)—PO 60 mg q4–6h	Nasal congestion, allergies, chronic ear infections	Produces vasoconstriction in respiratory tract and possibly bronchodilation	Nervousness, anxiety, palpitations, anorexia

Table 8.17

Common Medications—cont'd

Drug and Dosage	Use	Action	Assessment: Side Effects
NURSING IMPLICATIONS: Give at least 2 hr before bedtime to minimize *insomnia*			
Electrolyte and Water Balance Agents			
Acetazolamide (Diamox)—PO 250–1,000 mg/day; IV 500 mg	Glaucoma; heart failure; convulsive disorders	Weak diuretic; produces acidosis; self-limiting effect; increases bicarbonate excretion	Electrolyte depletion symptomatology—lassitude, apathy, decreased urinary output, mental confusion
NURSING IMPLICATIONS: Weigh daily, I&O; assess edema; give *early* in day to allow sleep at night; observe for side effects; replace electrolytes as ordered			
Ethacrynic acid (Edecrin)—PO 50–200 mg daily in divided doses	Pulmonary edema; ascites; edema of heart failure	Inhibits the reabsorption of Na^+ in the ascending loop of Henle	Nausea, vomiting, diarrhea; hypokalemia; hypotension; gout; dehydration; deafness; metabolic acidosis
NURSING IMPLICATIONS: Assess for dehydration—skin turgor, neck veins; hypotension; *KCl* supplement			
Furosemide (Lasix)—PO 40–80 mg daily in divided doses	Edema and associated heart failure; cirrhosis; renal disease; nephrotic syndrome: hypertension	Inhibits Na^+ and Cl^- reabsorption in the loop of Henle	Dermatitis, pruritus; paresthesia; blurring of vision; postural hypotension; nausea, vomiting, diarrhea, dehydration, electrolyte depletion; hearing loss (usually reversible)
NURSING IMPLICATIONS: Assess for weakness, lethargy, leg cramps, anorexia; peak action in 1–2 hr; duration 6–8 hr; do *not* give at bedtime; supplemental *KCl* indicated; may induce *digitalis toxicity*			
Hydrochlorothiazide (HydroDIURIL, Esidrix, Microzide)—PO 25–100 mg 3 times daily Chlorothiazide (Diuril)—PO 500–1,000 mg daily oral suspension	Edema; heart failure; Na^+ retention in steroid therapy; hypertension	Inhibits NaCl and water reabsorption in the distal ascending loop and the distal convoluted tubule of the kidneys	Hypokalemia, nausea, vomiting, diarrhea; dizziness; paresthesias; may exacerbate diabetes
NURSING IMPLICATIONS: Watch for muscle weakness; give well-diluted potassium chloride supplement; *monitor* urine for changes in sugar and acetone			
Mannitol (Osmitrol)—IV 50–100 mg/24 hr as 15%–20% solution	Cerebral edema, oliguria, acute renal failure, drug intoxication	Hypertonic solution that kidney tubules cannot reabsorb, thereby causing obligatory water loss	Diarrhea; water intoxication, thirst, headache
NURSING IMPLICATIONS: Usually Foley catheter required; monitor *cardiac and respiratory* status; a rate of infusion to elicit 30–50 mL urine/hr			
Sevelamer hydrochloride (Renagel)—PO 2 capsules or tablets 3 times daily	Reduction of serum phosphorus level	Polymer binds intestinal phosphate	Headache; infection; pain; diarrhea, constipation; cough
NURSING IMPLICATIONS: Important to take multivitamin supplement approved by physician. Do **not** take after printed expiration date			
Spironolactone (Aldactone)—PO 25 mg 2–4 times daily	Cirrhosis of liver; when other diuretics are ineffective	Inhibits effects of aldosterone in distal tubules of kidney	Headache; lethargy; diarrhea; ataxia; skin rash; gynecomastia
NURSING IMPLICATIONS: Potassium-sparing drug; do *not* give supplemental KCl; monitor for signs of electrolyte imbalance			
Emetic			
Ipecac syrup—*Adults, elderly adults, children >12 yr:* PO 15–30 mL followed by 3–4 glasses of water. *Children 1–12 yr:* PO 15 mL followed by 1–2 glasses of water. *Infants 6 mo–1 yr:* PO 5–10 mL followed by 1 glass of water	Emergency emetic for poison ingestion	NH_4 ions cause gastric irritation	Violent emesis, tachycardia, decreased BP, dyspnea

EMETIC

Continued

Table 8.17

Common Medications—cont'd

Drug and Dosage	Use	Action	Assessment: Side Effects
NURSING IMPLICATIONS: *Contraindicated* in liver and renal disease; if given for emesis, follow dose with as much *water* as client will drink. Should **not** be used in the home. Dosage and usage are *controversial,* as is repetition of dose if vomiting has not occurred in 20–30 min after giving first dose.			
Enzyme			
Pancrelipase (Viokase)—adults, PO 325 mg–1 gm daily, during meals; children, PO 300–600 mg 3 times daily	Chronic pancreatitis; cystic fibrosis; gastrectomy; pancreatectomy; sprue	Assists in digestion of starch, protein, and fats; decreases nitrogen and fat content of stool	Anorexia, nausea, vomiting, diarrhea; buccal/anal soreness (infants); sneezing; skin rashes; diabetes
NURSING IMPLICATIONS: May be taken with antacid or cimetidine; do *not* crush or chew tablets; *monitor* I&O, weight; be alert for signs of diabetes; children may use sprinkles			
Erectile Dysfunction			
Sildenafil citrate (Viagra)—PO 50 mg 0.5–4 hr before sexual activity	Erectile dysfunction	Vasodilation of nitric oxide in the corpus cavernosum of penis	Headache; cardiac arrest with *sudden death;* exfoliative dermatitis
NURSING IMPLICATIONS: High-fat meal delays drug action. Report to physician: headaches, flushing, chest pain, indigestion, blurred vision, changes in color vision; safety issue if taking nitrates			
Expectorants			
Guaifenesin (Robitussin)—PO 100–400 mg q4h	Respiratory congestion	Increases expectoration by causing irritation of gastric mucosa; reduces adhesiveness/surface tension of respiratory tract fluid	Low incidence of GI upset; drowsiness
NURSING IMPLICATIONS: Encourage to stop smoking; increase fluid intake; respiratory hygiene			
Terpin hydrate—PO 5–10 mL q3–4h	Bronchitis; emphysema	Liquefies bronchial secretions	Nausea, vomiting, gastric irritation
NURSING IMPLICATIONS: Give undiluted; *push* fluids			
Fibrinolytic Agents			
Alteplase, recombinant (Activase, tPA)—IV bolus 100 mg over 90 min: 15-mg bolus given over 1–2 min; then 50 mg over 30 min; then 35 mg over 60 min	Acute MI; under investigation for pulmonary emboli, deep vein thrombosis, and peripheral artery thrombosis	Promotes conversion of plasminogen to plasmin, which is fibrinolytic	Internal or local bleeding; urticaria; dysrhythmias related to reperfusion; hypotension; nausea, vomiting
NURSING IMPLICATIONS: Assess for signs of reperfusion (relief of chest pain, no ST-segment elevation); observe for *bleeding; avoid* IM injection; do *not* mix other medications in line			
Streptokinase (Stretase)—IV 1.5 million units initially diluted; infused over 60 min	Lysis of pulmonary or systemic emboli or thrombi; acute MI	Reacts with plasminogen, dissolves fibrin clots	Prolonged coagulation; allergic reactions; mild fever
NURSING IMPLICATIONS: Monitor for signs of *excessive bleeding,* particularly at injection sites; *avoid* nonessential handling of client			
Urokinase—IV 4,400 IU/kg over 10 min; 1.0–1.8 mL of 5,000 IU/mL into catheter	Massive pulmonary emboli, coronary artery thrombi, occluded IV catheter	Directly activates plasminogen	Bleeding, anaphylaxis, rash
NURSING IMPLICATIONS: Vital signs; check *q15 min* for bleeding during first hr; q15–30 min for 8 hr; have *epinephrine* ready			
Fibrinolytic Antidote			
Aminocaproic acid (Amicar)—PO, IV 5-gm loading dose; 1 gm/hr to 30 gm in 24 hr	Management of streptokinase or urokinase overdose	Inhibits plasminogen activator and antagonizes plasmin	Hypotension, bradycardia, cardiac arrhythmias
NURSING IMPLICATIONS: Give slowly IV to prevent side effects; not recommended for disseminated intravascular coagulation (DIC)			

Table 8.17

Common Medications—cont'd

Drug and Dosage	Use	Action	Assessment: Side Effects
Hematopoietic Agents			
Darbepoetin alfa (Aranesp)—IV, Subcu 25–500 mcg/kg once weekly	Treatment of anemia with chronic renal failure, chemotherapy	Erythropoiesis-stimulating protein	Peripheral edema; infection; headache, hypertension, hypotension; arrhythmias; nausea, vomiting, diarrhea; myalgia, respiratory infection
NURSING IMPLICATIONS: See Epoetin			
Epoetin alfa (Epogen, Procrit)—Subcu, IV 3–500 units/kg/dose 3 times/wk	Anemia secondary to chronic kidney failure, chemotherapy, HIV treatment	Glycoprotein that stimulates RBC production	Headache, hypertension; iron deficiency, clotting of AV fistula
NURSING IMPLICATIONS: Monitor BP closely. Headache is common; report severe or persistent problem			
Hormones			
Chlorotrianisene (TACE), estrogen—PO 12–50 mg	Prostatic cancer; menopause	Nonsteroidal synthetic estrogen	Rare after one course of treatment; thromboembolism; impotence and gynecomastia in men
NURSING IMPLICATIONS: Supply client with package insert; *contraindicated* in blood coagulation disorders			
Diethylstilbestrol (DES)—PO, IM 0.2–5.0 mg daily; vaginal suppository 0.1–0.5 mg at bedtime	Prostate carcinoma; menopausal symptoms; osteoporosis; pain; mammary carcinoma; atrophic vaginitis	Synthetic nonsteroidal compound with estrogenic effects on pituitary, ovaries, myometrium, endometrium, and other tissues	Anorexia, nausea, vomiting, headache, diarrhea, dizziness, fainting—many side effects with long-term use
NURSING IMPLICATIONS: *Never* give if woman is pregnant—predisposes to vaginal cancer in female offspring at puberty			
Estradiol—PO 1–2 mg for replacement therapy; up to 10 mg for cancer daily and up to 3 times daily; cyclic (on 3 wk, off 1 wk)	Menopausal symptoms; osteoporosis; hypogenitalism; sexual infantilism; breast and prostatic carcinoma	Inhibits release of pituitary gonadotropins; promotes growth of female genital tissues	Anorexia, nausea, vomiting, diarrhea, fluid retention; mental depression; headache, thromboembolism; feminization in men
NURSING IMPLICATIONS: Baseline VS; weigh daily; encourage frequent physical checkups to check serum lipids; teach breast self-examination			
Medroxyprogesterone (Provera)—PO 2.5–10.0 mg; IM 400–1,000 mg weekly	Amenorrhea; functional uterine bleeding; threatened abortion; dysmenorrhea; adjunctive and palliative with renal cancer and endometriosis; premenstrual syndrome (PMS)	Similar to progesterone, but can be taken orally; thickens uterine decidua	Drowsiness; cyclic menstrual withdrawal bleeding; GI upset; headache; edema; breast congestion
NURSING IMPLICATIONS: Teach client regarding self-administration; breast self-examination for possible breast changes			
Menotropins (Pergonal)—IM 1 ampule (FSH + LH)/day for 9–12 days (followed by 5,000–10,000 units human chorionic gonadotropin (HCG); if ovulation does not occur, repeat with 2 ampules)	**Infertility use:** treatment of secondary anovulation; stimulation of spermatogenesis	Human gonadotropic responses; induces ovulation; sperm stimulation	Abortions occur in 25%; failure rate 55%–80% of clients: possible multiple births; ovarian enlargement; gynecomastia in men
NURSING IMPLICATIONS: Assist in collection of urine to assess estrogen levels; counsel regarding couple's need to have daily intercourse from day of HCG injection until ovulation			
Progesterone—Subcu, IM 5–10 mg daily; sublingual 5–10 mg	Amenorrhea; dysmenorrhea; endometriosis; habitual abortion	Converts endometrium into secreting structure; prevents ovulation; stimulates growth of mammary tissue	Nausea, vomiting; dizziness, edema, headache; protein metabolism

Continued

Table 8.17

Common Medications—cont'd

Drug and Dosage	Use	Action	Assessment: Side Effects
NURSING IMPLICATIONS: Give *deep* IM and rotate sites; weigh daily to ascertain fluid retention			
Testosterone—PO 5–10 mg daily; IM 25–50 mg 2–3 times/wk; 200–400 mg IM q2–4 wk for breast cancer	Hypogonadism; eunuchism; impotence, advanced cancer of breast	Growth of sex organs and appearance of secondary male sex characteristics; counteracts excessive amounts of estrogen	Nausea, dyspepsia; masculinization; hypercalcemia; menstrual irregularities; renal calculi; Na^+, K^+, and H_2O retention
NURSING IMPLICATIONS: Observe for edema; weigh daily; I&O; *push fluids* for clients who are bedridden, to prevent renal calculi			
Vasopressin (Pitressin)—IM, Subcu 5–10 mcg 2–4 times daily; IM, Subcu 2.5–5 mcg 2–3 times daily for chronic therapy	Diabetes insipidus	Antidiuretic	Nausea, flatus; tremor; pounding in head; water intoxication
NURSING IMPLICATIONS: *Monitor* fluid balance, vital signs			
Immune Modifiers			
Glatiramer acetate (Copaxone)—Subcu 20 mg/day	Multiple sclerosis (MS)	Management of relapsing-remitting MS	Allergic reactions; anxiety; chest pain; weight gain; cough
NURSING IMPLICATIONS: Monitor for side effects; new drug to attempt to control signs and symptoms of progressing multiple sclerosis			
Interferon beta-1b (Betaseron)—Subcu 30 mcg once a week	Multiple sclerosis	Reduce incidence of relapse	Seizures; GI symptoms; flu-like symptoms; neutropenia, injection site reactions
NURSING IMPLICATIONS: Monitor progress of multiple sclerosis; determine if drug is effective in reducing incidence of relapse; provide information about multiple side effects			
Immunosuppressant Agents			
Azathioprine (Imuran)—PO, IV 3–5 mg/kg/day initially; maintenance: 1–3 mg/kg/day	Prevent renal transplant rejection Ulcerative colitis Rheumatoid arthritis	Antagonizes purine metabolism/inhibition of DNA/RNA synthesis	Hypersensitivity; additive myelosuppression with antineoplastics; hepatotoxicity, leukopenia
NURSING IMPLICATIONS: Assess for infection; monitor I&O and *daily weight*			
Cyclosporine (Sandimmune)—PO 5–10 mg/kg several hours before surgery; daily for 2 wk; reduce dosage by 2.5 mg/kg/wk to 5–10 mg/kg/day; IV 5–6 mg/kg several hours before surgery; switch to PO form as soon as possible	Prevent organ rejection Ulcerative colitis; Rheumatoid arthritis	Inhibits interleukin-2, which is necessary for initiation of T-cell activity	Hypersensitivity; *caution* with alcohol, renal impairment
NURSING IMPLICATIONS: *Monitor:* I&O, daily weight, blood pressure; take as directed (time of day and with food); observe for *nephrotoxicity,* gingival hyperplasia; *avoid* self-administration of OTC drugs			
Muromonab-CD 3 (Orthoclone OKT3)—IV 5 mg/day, 10–14 days	Renal, liver, or cardiac transplant rejection	Immunosuppression of T-cell function	Tremor; dyspnea, shortness of breath, wheezing; chest pain; diarrhea, nausea, vomiting; chills, fever
NURSING IMPLICATIONS: Draw solution into filter; give IV push over <1 min; do *not* give as IV infusion; do *not* mix with other medications			
Mycophenolate (CellCept)—PO 1 gm twice daily	Prevent renal transplant rejection	Inhibits purine synthesis; suppresses T and B lymphocytes	Diarrhea; vomiting; leukopenia; sepsis
NURSING IMPLICATIONS: Give initial dose *within* 72 hr of transplant surgery; give on *empty* stomach 1 hr before or 2 hr after meals; do *not* open, crush, or chew capsules; do *not* give with *magnesium or aluminum* antacids			
Tacrolimus—PO 0.075–0.15 mg/kg q12h; IV 0.05–0.1 mg/kg/day	Prevent rejection of liver transplant	Inhibits T-lymphocyte activation	Headache, insomnia, tremor; ascites; hypertension; peripheral edema; abdominal pain; rash; hyperglycemia, anemia

Table 8.17

Common Medications—cont'd

Drug and Dosage	Use	Action	Assessment: Side Effects
NURSING IMPLICATIONS: Give *6 hr after* transplant surgery; oral therapy is preferred because of anaphylaxis with IV; therapy is lifelong			
Mineralocorticoid Agent			
Fludrocortisone (Florinef)—PO 0.1–0.2 mg daily	Addison's disease	Causes sodium reabsorption, hydrogen and potassium excretion, and water retention	Heart failure; adrenal suppression, hypertension
NURSING IMPLICATIONS: Do *not* miss dose; therapy is lifelong; high potassium; *report:* weight gain, muscle weakness, cramps, nausea, anorexia, dizziness			
Mucolytic Agent			
Acetylcysteine (Mucomyst)—inhalation 1–5 mL of 20% solution or 1–10 mL of 10% solution per nebulizer 3 times daily	Emphysema; pneumonia; tracheostomy care; atelectasis; cystic fibrosis Antidote to acetaminophen overdose, to protect against hepatotoxicity	Lowers viscosity of respiratory secretions by opening disulfide linkages in mucus	Stomatitis, nausea; rhinorrhea; bronchospasm
NURSING IMPLICATIONS: Observe *respiratory rate;* maintain open airway with suctioning as necessary; observe clients with asthma carefully for *increased bronchospasm*; discontinue treatment **immediately** if this occurs; odor disagreeable initially			
Muscle Relaxants			
Baclofen (Lioresal)—PO 5 mg 3 times daily up to 10–20 mg 4 times/day maintenance dose	Relief of spasticity of multiple sclerosis, spinal cord injury	Centrally acting skeletal muscle relaxant; depresses polysynaptic afferent reflex activity at spinal cord level	Pruritis, tinnitus; nausea, vomiting; diarrhea or constipation; drowsiness
NURSING IMPLICATIONS: Administer *with* food if GI symptoms; monitor for safety when ambulating; do *not* discontinue abruptly			
Dantrolene sodium (Dantrium)—PO 25 mg/day–25 mg 2–3 times daily to 100 mg 4 times daily max.	See Baclofen	See Baclofen	See Baclofen
NURSING IMPLICATIONS: See Baclofen			
Narcotic Antagonist			
Naloxone HCl (Narcan)—IV 0.1–0.2 mg repeated q2–3 min prn up to 0.4–2 mg for narcotic-induced respiratory depression	Reverses respiratory depression due to narcotics	Reverses respiratory depression of morphine SO_4, meperidine HCl, and methadone HCl; does not itself cause respiratory depression, sedation, or analgesia	No common side effects; tachycardia, hypertension; nausea and vomiting with high doses
NURSING IMPLICATIONS: Note time, type of narcotic, dosage received; not useful with CNS depression from other drugs; respiratory depression *may return;* monitor closely			
Sedatives and Hypnotics			
Chloral hydrate—PO 250 mg 3 times daily; hypnotic: PO 0.5–1.0 gm; rectal suppository 0.3–0.9 gm	Sedation for elderly; delirium tremens; pruritus; mania; barbiturate and alcohol withdrawal	Depresses sensorimotor areas of cerebral cortex	Nausea, vomiting, gastritis; pinpoint pupils; delirium; rash; decreased BP, pulse, respirations, temperature; hepatic damage
NURSING IMPLICATIONS: *Caution:* should not be taken in combination with alcohol; dependency is possible			
Chlordiazepoxide HCl (Librium)—PO 5–10 mg; IM, IV 50–100 mg	Psychoneuroses; preoperative apprehension; chronic alcoholism; anxiety	CNS depressant resulting in mild sedation; appetite stimulant; anticonvulsant	Ataxia, fatigue; blurred vision, diplopia; lethargy; nightmares; confusion
NURSING IMPLICATIONS: Ensure anxiety relief by allowing client to verbalize feelings; advise client to *avoid* driving and alcoholic beverages			

Continued

Table 8.17

Common Medications—cont'd

Drug and Dosage	Use	Action	Assessment: Side Effects
Diazepam (Valium)—PO 2–10 mg 3–4 times daily; IM, IV 2–10 mg q3–4h	Anxiety disorders; alcohol withdrawal; adjunctive therapy in seizure disorders; status epilepticus; eclamptic seizures; tetanus, preoperative or preprocedural sedation (also see Midazolam)	Induces calming effect on limbic system, thalamus, and hypothalamus	CNS depression—sedation or ataxia (dose related); dry mouth; blurred vision; mydriasis; constipation; urinary retention
NURSING IMPLICATIONS: Do *not* mix with other drugs; IM injection painful; observe for *phlebitis;* monitor response; measures to ensure client safety (e.g., falls); high potential for abuse; *contraindicated* in acute closed-angle glaucoma and porphyria			
Flurazepam (Dalmane)—PO >15 yr, 30 mg at bedtime; elderly or debilitated, 15 mg at bedtime	Hypnotic	Fastest acting; see Diazepam	See Diazepam
NURSING IMPLICATIONS: See Diazepam			
Hydroxyzine pamoate (Vistaril)—PO 25–100 mg 4 times daily	See Chlordiazepoxide (Librium); antiemetic in postoperative conditions; adjunctive therapy	CNS relaxant with sedative effect on limbic system and thalamus	Drowsiness; headache; itching; dry mouth; tremor
	Obstetric use: prodromal labor	Allows relaxation	
NURSING IMPLICATIONS: Give *deep* IM only; *potentiates* action of: warfarin (Coumadin), narcotics, and barbiturates			
Lorazepam (Ativan)—PO 1–2 mg 2–3 times daily (up to 10 mg); 2–4 mg at bedtime; IM 4 mg max.; IV 2 mg max.	Anxiety disorders; insomnia; alternative to diazepam for status epilepticus; preanesthesia	See Diazepam	See Diazepam
NURSING IMPLICATIONS: See Diazepam			
Meprobamate (Equanil, Miltown)—PO 400 mg 3–4 times daily	Anxiety; stress; absence seizures	See Hydroxyzine pamoate (Vistaril)	Voracious appetite; dryness of mouth; ataxia
NURSING IMPLICATIONS: Older clients prone to drowsiness and hypotension; observe for *jaundice*			
Midazolam (Versed)—IM 0.05–0.08 mg/kg; IV 0.1–0.15 mg/kg	Preanesthesia; prediagnostic procedures; induction of general anesthesia	Penetrates blood-brain barrier to produce sedation and amnesia	Respiratory depression, apnea; disorientation, behavioral excitement
NURSING IMPLICATIONS: Monitor ventilatory status and oxygenation; prevent injuries from CNS depression; nonirritating to vein			
Phenobarbital—sedative, PO 20–30 mg 3 times daily; hypnotic, PO 50–100 mg; IV, IM 100–300 mg; also butabarbital (Butisol), pentobarbital (Nembutal), secobarbital (Seconal)	Preoperative sedation; emergency control of convulsions; absence seizures	Depresses CNS, promoting drowsiness	Cough, hiccups; restlessness; pain; hangover; CNS and circulatory depression
NURSING IMPLICATIONS: Observe for hypotension during IV administration; put up side rails on bed of older clients; observe for increased tolerance			
Promethazine (Phenergan)—IV, IM, PO 25–50 mg	Preoperative sedation; postoperative sedation	Antihistaminic; sedative, antiemetic, anti–motion sickness	Drowsiness; coma; hypotension; hypertension; leukopenia; photosensitivity; irregular respirations; blurred vision; urinary retention; dry mouth, nose, throat
NURSING IMPLICATIONS: Administer PO *with* food, milk; IM *deep* into large muscles, rotate sites; verify compatibility with other drugs; safety concerns due to sedative effect			

Table 8.17

Common Medications—cont'd

Drug and Dosage	Use	Action	Assessment: Side Effects
Zolpidem (Ambien)—PO 5–10 mg at bedtime, limited to 7–10 days	Short-term treatment of insomnia	Nonbenzodiazepine hypnotic; preserves deep sleep (stages 3 and 4)	Headache on awakening; drowsiness, fatigue; confusion and falls in elderly; myalgia
NURSING IMPLICATIONS: Monitor for: compromised respiratory status, increased depression, cognitive impairment. Onset more rapid on empty stomach. Do **not** breastfeed while taking this medication			
Serum			
Immune globulin—IM 0.02 mL/kg	Hepatitis	Provides passive immunity	Do *not* use if client is hypersensitive
NURSING IMPLICATIONS: Should be administered within *2 wk* of exposure			
Thyroid Hormone Inhibitors			
Propylthiouracil—PO 300–400 mg/day, divided initial dose; 100–150 mg/day maintenance dose; methimazole (Tapazole) 15–60 mg/day initial dose; 5–15 mg/day maintenance dose	Hyperthyroidism; return client to euthyroid state; also used preoperatively	Inhibits functional thyroid hormone synthesis by blocking reactions; responsible for iodide conversion to iodine; inhibition of thyroxine (T_4) conversion to triiodothyronine (T_3)	Blood dyscrasias, hepatotoxicity, hypothyroidism
NURSING IMPLICATIONS: Teach importance of compliance with medication protocol; *avoid* iodine-rich foods (seafood, iodized salt); caution when using other drugs			
Saturated potassium iodide (SSKI)—PO 300 mg 3 or 4 times daily	To reduce size, vascularity of thyroid before thyroid surgery; emergency treatment of thyroid storm; or control of hyperthyroid symptoms after radioiodine (^{131}I) therapy	Inhibits thyroid hormone secretion, synthesis	GI distress; stained teeth; increased respiratory secretions; rashes; acne
NURSING IMPLICATIONS: *Dilute in juice,* give through *straw*; bloody diarrhea/vomiting indicates acute poisoning			
Thyroid Hormone Replacement			
Levothyroxine (Levothroid, Synthroid)—PO 0.05–0.10 mg/day; IV 200–500 mcg	Hypothyroidism Myxedema coma	Replacement therapy to alleviate symptoms Emergency replacement therapy	Symptoms of hyperthyroidism
NURSING IMPLICATIONS: Teach signs and symptoms of hyperthyroidism, hypothyroidism; monitor bowel activity; teach diet to combat constipation; keep medication in tight light-proof container; *avoid foods* that inhibit thyroid secretion (turnips, cabbage, carrots, peaches, peas, strawberries, spinach, radishes)			
Liothyronine (Cytomel)—PO 25 mcg/day to maintenance dose 25–75 mcg	Mild hypothyroidism in adults	Replacement therapy	See Levothyroxine
NURSING IMPLICATIONS: See Levothyroxine			
Uterine Contractants			
Ergonovine maleate (Ergotrate)—PO, IM, IV 0.2 mg (gr 1/320)	Postabortal or postpartum hemorrhage; promotes involution after delivery of placenta	Stimulates uterine contractions for 3 hr or more	Nausea, vomiting; occasional transient hypertension, especially if given IV; cramping
NURSING IMPLICATIONS: Store in *cool* place; monitor maternal BP and pulse; *do not use in labor*			
Methylergonovine maleate (Methergine)—PO 0.2 mg; IM, IV 0.2 mg (gr 1/320)	Postpartum hemorrhage, after delivery of placenta	Stimulates stronger and longer contractions than ergonovine maleate (Ergotrate)	Nausea, vomiting; transient hypertension, dizziness, tachycardia; cramping
NURSING IMPLICATIONS: Do *not* give if mother is hypertensive; do *not* use if solution is discolored; *do not use in labor*			

Continued

Table 8.17

Common Medications—cont'd

Drug and Dosage	Use	Action	Assessment: Side Effects
Oxytocin (Pitocin, Syntocinon)—IV 2 mL (15 units) in 250-mL solution; 1 mL IM after delivery	Stimulates rhythmic contractions of uterus	Induces labor; augments contractions; prevents or controls postpartum atony; antidiuretic effect	Tetanic contractions, uterine rupture; cardiac arrhythmias, FHR deceleration
NURSING IMPLICATIONS: *Contraindicated* if cervix is unripe, in cephalopelvic disproportion (CPD), abruptio placentae, and cardiovascular disease; *monitor:* FHR, contractions, maternal BP, pulse, I&O; watch for signs of water intoxication with prolonged IV use; drug of choice in presence of hypertension; *never* use undiluted; discontinue if tetanic contractions occur; *antidote:* propranolol			
Volume Expander			
Albumin 5%, 25%—IV 500 mL as needed	Cirrhosis Nephrotic syndrome	Provides colloidal oncotic pressure, which mobilizes fluid from extracellular back into intravascular space	Hypersensitivity, CHF, hepatic failure
NURSING IMPLICATIONS: Monitor progress of disease; monitor for signs of shock; if fever, tachycardia, or hypotension occur, *stop* treatment and call physician			

Questions

Select the one answer that is best for each question, unless otherwise directed.

1. A nursing *priority* when administering a blood transfusion is to:
1. Check the fibrinogen level before infusing.
2. Infuse blood slowly the first 20 minutes.
3. Warm the blood prior to administration.
4. Infuse the blood over 1 to 2 hours.

2. Blood sugar management for a client who has type 2 diabetes with nausea and decreased appetite should include:
1. Continuing insulin even if the client is vomiting.
2. Continuing insulin if blood sugar is less than 80 mg/dL.
3. Stopping insulin if urine is positive for ketones.
4. Stopping insulin until the client is able to tolerate food.

3. Which finding indicates that epoetin alfa (Epogen) has been effective?
1. Negative Homans' sign, aPTT of 35 to 55.
2. Guaiac-negative gastric secretions and stool.
3. Hematocrit of 33%.
4. Creatinine of 1.4.

4. A nurse should locate and remove a client's clonidine patch if:
1. The client complains of numbness and tingling down the arm that is nearest to the patch.
2. The blood pressure is 80/50 mm Hg.
3. The client tells the nurse about being allergic to sulfa products.
4. The potassium level is 3.0 mg/dL.

5. Managing a sodium level of 120 in a client with diabetic ketoacidosis is correctly accomplished with:
1. Oral salt tablets.
2. Intravenous 3% sodium chloride solution.
3. Fluid restriction.
4. Insulin and 0.9% sodium chloride.

6. The correct time for a nurse to administer pancrelipase (Pancrease) is:
1. One hour after meals.
2. With meals.
3. At bedtime.
4. With insulin.

7. Before administering furosemide (Lasix), a nurse should verify that:
1. The blood pressure is under 180/90 mm Hg.
2. The potassium is over 4 mg/dL.
3. There are no crackles in the lungs.
4. The client has an indwelling catheter in place.

8. One hour after starting the insulin drip at 10 units/hr, the client's blood sugar has fallen from 899 to 750. Which action should a nurse take?
1. Increase the insulin drip rate to 20 units/hr.
2. Decrease the insulin drip rate to 7 units/hr.
3. Give a bolus of 10 units of regular insulin and increase the drip rate to 8 units/hr.
4. Keep the rate the same and do not bolus.

9. Which IV fluid order is most appropriate for a client on dialysis?
1. D_5 ½NS at 20 mL/hr.
2. NS at 150 mL/hr.
3. ¼NS with 20 mEq KCl at 75 mL/hr.
4. $D_{10}W$ with 40 mEq KCl at 50 mL/hr.

10. Teaching for a client starting on spironolactone (Aldactone) should include:
   1. The importance of removing the patch at bedtime.
   2. Food sources to replace lost potassium.
   3. The purpose of this drug is to prevent fibrosis in the heart.
   4. Taking the medication just before bed.

11. A nurse should hold administration of a nitrate if:
   1. Pulse rate is under 60.
   2. Client is allergic to sulfa.
   3. Blood pressure is less than 90/50 mm Hg.
   4. Drug therapy has exceeded 2 weeks.

12. A client has a blood pressure of 145/83 mm Hg and an ejection fraction of 50%. Before discharge from the hospital, the client will need instructions on taking which drug(s)?
   1. A thiazide diuretic.
   2. Digoxin and furosemide.
   3. A beta blocker and an ACE inhibitor.
   4. An anticoagulant.

13. A client with a sexually transmitted infection (STI) is to receive azithromycin. Before the medication is given, which nursing assessment is a *priority?*
   1. Obtain a CBC.
   2. Ask the client about allergies.
   3. Check the blood pressure.
   4. Ask the client about sexual contact.

14. Which intervention would most likely prevent nausea in a client receiving cisplatin chemotherapy?
   1. Administering trimethobenzamide prn nausea.
   2. Administering dexamethasone and ondansetron prior to chemotherapy.
   3. Serving all food warm or hot.
   4. Keeping client NPO 24 hours before chemotherapy.

15. The most important nursing assessment to make before a client is started on indomethacin is:
   1. Asking if there is a history of sulfa allergies.
   2. Asking if there is a history of gastric bleeding.
   3. Checking blood pressure.
   4. Checking blood sugar.

16. A client, who is postoperative, has the anesthetic bupivacaine infusing into an epidural catheter for pain control. On assessment, a nurse notes the client has decreased sensation and numbness in the lower abdomen. The pain level is 3/10. The nurse should:
   1. Record this expected finding.
   2. Increase the epidural infusion rate.
   3. Turn the epidural infusion off and raise the head of bed.
   4. Turn the epidural infusion off and lower the head of bed.

17. A client who is postoperative needs to walk, but even turning in bed is very painful. A patient-controlled analgesia (PCA) pump is set with a lock-out of 6 minutes. A nurse notes 45 attempts to get medication and 2 injections received in the last 2 hours. The correct nursing action is to:
   1. Get client out of bed now while pain level is low.
   2. Teach client how and why to use the pump more effectively.
   3. Record client's refusal to get out of bed.
   4. Push pain button before getting client out of bed.

18. A client is due to receive Novolog insulin. When should it be administered?
   1. 60 minutes before the meal.
   2. 15 minutes before the meal.
   3. As soon as the meal is finished.
   4. Without regard to meals.

19. A client with a duodenal ulcer has been taking sucralfate (Carafate). Which statement by the client would be a *priority* for a nurse to address?
   1. "I don't like the taste, so I mix it in pudding."
   2. "I wish I could take Carafate at the same time as my other pills."
   3. "I have found that stewed prunes help prevent constipation from the drug."
   4. "Taking Carafate with H_2O has helped my fluid intake."

20. A client in diabetic ketoacidosis (DKA) has an order for an insulin drip at 4 units/hr. The pharmacy prepared a solution of 10 units of insulin in 100 mL normal saline. The nurse correctly sets the infusion pump at _______ mL/hr. *Fill in the blank.*

21. A nurse is concerned that a client may be at risk for oversedation from opioid therapy using a patient-controlled analgesia pump. The most reliable assessment for possible oversedation would be to check:
   1. Changes in the level of pain reported by the client.
   2. The oxygen saturation level recorded by pulse oximetry.
   3. How easily the client can be roused from sleeping.
   4. The level of carbon dioxide in the blood using capnography.

22. For optimal effects from thrombolytic therapy given for a brain attack (cerebrovascular accident [CVA]), treatment should be given:
   1. Within 3 hours of the onset of symptoms.
   2. When signs of increased intracranial pressure occur.
   3. As pulse pressure begins to increase.
   4. No later than 24 hours after the onset of symptoms.

23. What observation should indicate to a nurse that the therapeutic effect of calcium gluconate has been achieved?
  1. Thyroid gland shrinks.
  2. Blood loss is curtailed during surgery.
  3. Trousseau's sign is absent.
  4. Chvostek's sign is positive.

24. Which common systemic side effect of chemotherapy will a nurse note in an oncology client?
  1. Ascites.
  2. Septicemia.
  3. Polycythemia.
  4. Leukopenia.

25. Which order by a physician should a nurse question?
  1. A client with COPD who is prescribed metoprolol (Lopressor).
  2. A client with chronic renal failure receiving an aluminum hydroxide gel (Amphogel).
  3. A client with an abdominal aortic aneurysm (AAA) taking diltiazem (Cardizem).
  4. A client on long-term hemodialysis receiving epoetin alfa (Epogen).

26. Which prescribed drugs would a nurse most likely give the client for respiratory stridor, with wheezing, and hypotension after a bee sting? *Select all that apply.*
  1. Epinephrine.
  2. Diphenhydramine (Benadryl).
  3. Corticosteroid (Solu-Medrol).
  4. Furosemide (Lasix).
  5. Acetaminophen (Tylenol).
  6. Ranitidine (Zantac).

27. During cardiopulmonary resuscitation (CPR) for ventricular fibrillation, which drug would an RN most likely prepare *first?*
  1. Atropine sulfate.
  2. Epinephrine.
  3. Furosemide (Lasix).
  4. Lidocaine.

28. A nurse should teach a client with angina about the common side effects of nitroglycerin, including: *Select all that apply.*
  1. Headache.
  2. Hypotension.
  3. Shock.
  4. Flushing.
  5. Dizziness.
  6. Shortness of breath.
  7. Abdominal cramps.

29. The cardiac glycosides are essential in the therapy of a client with a myocardial infarction (MI). What should indicate to a nurse that a therapeutic response to this medication has been achieved?
  1. A 15% increase in apical pulse rate.
  2. A rise in CVP from 12 to 15 cm.
  3. Urine output 30 mL/hr (previously 40 to 50 mL/hr).
  4. Diminished crackles in the lungs.

30. To prevent a common adverse effect of prolonged use of phenytoin sodium (Dilantin), a client should be instructed to:
  1. Obtain an annual influenza vaccination.
  2. Drink at least 8 to 10 glasses of water daily.
  3. Eat a diet low in sodium and high in potassium.
  4. Report gum swelling or bleeding to the physician.

31. A client is being discharged and instructed to take furosemide (Lasix) every morning. A nurse tells the client to notify the health provider in the event of:
  1. Increased appetite.
  2. Disruption in sleep patterns.
  3. Increased urinary frequency.
  4. Leg cramps.

32. A client is planning a cruise and wants to use the scopolamine patch. Which frequent side effect should a nurse tell the client to expect?
  1. Irregular pulse.
  2. Dry mouth.
  3. Drop in blood pressure.
  4. Slurred speech.

33. A nurse instructs a client about taking an angiotensin-converting enzyme (ACE). The client should be warned to continue therapy even when which common side effect occurs?
  1. A dry, persistent cough.
  2. Exacerbation of heart failure.
  3. Sedation.
  4. Urinary incontinence.

34. Which solution will a client most likely receive for fluid replacement in the first 24 hours after a burn injury that covers a large area?
  1. D_5W.
  2. Lactated Ringer's.
  3. Dextran.
  4. Normal saline with added K^+.

35. A client is to receive oxycodone for acute pain. Adverse effects of opioid analgesics include: *Select all that apply.*
  1. Agitation.
  2. Constipation.
  3. Diarrhea.
  4. Vomiting
  5. Pruritus
  6. Sedation.

36. The treatment for a client suffering from hypovolemic shock following extensive burns will focus on controlling fluid loss and replacing fluid volume. A nurse should expect the client with burns to receive solutions that expand volume. To pull fluid from the interstitial spaces,

which solutions should the nurse prepare? *Select all that apply.*
1. A unit of whole blood.
2. Hespan (hetastarch).
3. Albumin.
4. Lactated Ringer's.
5. Packed red blood cells.

37. During a blood transfusion, a client reports a throbbing headache, chills, and nausea. What ordered drugs should a nurse prepare for administration? *Select all that apply.*
1. Epinephrine.
2. Sodium bicarbonate.
3. Theophylline.
4. Solu-Cortef.
5. Dopamine.

38. Upon discharge from a hospital, teaching for a client with osteoporosis about proper administration of calcium supplements should include:
1. Taking calcium with vitamin D to increase absorption.
2. Taking calcium citrate at meal time.
3. Taking a calcium carbonate on an empty stomach.
4. Taking calcium once a day.

39. A common symptom for Sjögren's syndrome, an autoimmune disorder in women, is dry eyes. A client asks a nurse what she can do for relief. Which suggestion given by the nurse would be correct for *initial* treatment?
1. Use artificial tears 3 to 4 times a day.
2. Use cyclosporine A (Restasis) ophthalmic drops.
3. Schedule punctal occlusion.
4. Use pilocarpine drops 3 times a day.

40. A nurse is to administer nitroprusside (Nipride) 4 mcg/kg/min intravenously to a client with severe hypertension who weighs 75 kg .The pharmacy prepares a solution of 50 mg nitroprusside in 500 mL D_5W. The nurse correctly calculates that _______ mL/hr of this medication should be administered to the client. *Fill in the blank.*

41. Epidural analgesia has been started for a client who is experiencing chronic pain that is unrelieved by other methods. Proper positioning of the client should include: *Select all that apply.*
1. Side-lying, semi-Fowler's.
2. Supine, head of bed flat, thin pillow.
3. Side-lying, head of bed flat.
4. High Fowler's, supine.
5. Prone.

42. Cefotetan disodium (Cefotan) 2 grams IV over 30 minutes is to be administered to a client 1 hour before surgery. The available IV solution contains 2 grams Cefotan in 100 mL of normal saline. A nurse calculates that the client should receive _______ mL/hr of this medication. *Fill in the blank.*

43. The correct nursing actions when administering a vesicant chemotherapeutic agent are to: *Select all that apply.*
1. Assess the site for swelling, redness, or presence of vesicles.
2. Administer the drug by IV push.
3. Give the drug slowly to minimize cardiac toxicity.
4. Apply ice to the site if infiltration occurs.
5. Apply heat to the site if extravasation occurs.

44. A client with diabetic ketoacidosis is to receive regular insulin IV at 5 units/hr. The solution received from the pharmacy includes 100 units of regular insulin in 500 mL of NS. A nurse carefully calculates that the insulin dip should infuse at a rate of _______ mL/hr. *Fill in the blank.*

45. A nurse is to give metoclopramide (Reglan) 10 mg IV over 15 minutes. The dose on hand is 10 mg metoclopramide in 50 mL D_5W. The nurse should infuse this medication at a rate of _______ mL/hr. *Fill in the blank.*

46. A nurse is to give 0.01 mcg/kg/min of nesiritide (Natrecor) to a client weighing 110 pounds. The premixed solution contains 1.5 mg of the drug in 250 mL of D_5W. The nurse correctly calculates that the client should receive _______ mL/hr of this medication. *Fill in the blank.*

47. A client with hyperglycemia is to receive an insulin drip at 12 units/hr. The premixed bag contains 50 units of regular insulin in 100 mL of normal saline. The nurse should set the infusion pump to administer the drip at a rate of _______ mL/hr. *Fill in the blank.*

48. A client's blood pressure drops to 70/40 mm Hg. Albumin 500 mL is to be given IV over 30 minutes. Using a macrodrip system (10 gtt/min), the IV rate should be _______ gtt/min. *Fill in the blank.*

49. A client reports unexplained weight loss and palpitations. Assessment findings include: exophthalmos, tachycardia, decreased thyroid-stimulating hormone (TSH), and increased triiodothyronine (T_3) and thyroxine (T_4). Which treatments would be most appropriate for this client? *Select all that apply.*
1. Levothyroxine (Synthroid).
2. Radioactive iodine.
3. Propylthiouracil (PTU).
4. Methimazole (Tapazole).
5. Liothyronine (Cytomel).

50. A client with diabetes is admitted with symptoms of diabetic ketoacidosis. Which type of insulin IV should a nurse expect to administer?
1. NPH.
2. Regular.
3. Lantus.
4. Intermediate- and short-acting mix.

51. Which combination of insulins, if ordered, should a nurse question?
   1. Regular and NPH.
   2. Regular and Humulin-N.
   3. Lantus and Lispro.
   4. Humulin-R and Lente.

52. When drawing up two different insulins in one syringe, which insulin should a nurse draw up *first?*
   1. Lispro.
   2. NPH.
   3. Lantus.
   4. Novolin 70/30.

53. When administering nitroglycerin to a client for chest pain, a nurse knows that a second dose can be safely given in:
   1. 5 minutes.
   2. 10 minutes.
   3. 15 minutes.
   4. 20 minutes.

54. A client is to start on an enteral tube feeding. What should a nurse do to make this as comfortable as possible for the client?
   1. Keep the head of the bed flat.
   2. Give the feeding as quickly as possible.
   3. Chill the feeding to improve the taste.
   4. Start the tube feeding slowly.

55. A physician orders furosemide (Lasix) for a client. What should a nurse tell the client to expect if the medication is having the desired effect?
   1. Elevated blood pressure.
   2. Elevated heart rate.
   3. More frequent urination.
   4. Nighttime urination will decrease.

56. When administering a beta blocker, a nurse should *first:*
   1. Take the client's temperature and heart rate.
   2. Place the client in an upright position before the client swallows the drug.
   3. Take the client's blood pressure and heart rate.
   4. Ask the client if there have been any adverse effects.

57. Maintaining the infusion rate of total parenteral nutrition (TPN) is a nursing responsibility. If the infusion rate is too rapid, which side effects would the nurse observe?
   1. Serum sodium and potassium excess.
   2. Increased blood pressure and hyperglycemia.
   3. Hypoglycemia and low blood pressure.
   4. Potassium excess and congestive heart failure.

58. An older client complains that, in the past, some analgesics have caused urinary retention and constipation. Which analgesic should a nurse tell the client would *not* cause those problems?
   1. Lomotil.
   2. Morphine.
   3. Meperidine.
   4. Fentanyl.

59. A client weighing 70 kg has received 10 mg of morphine sulfate (MS) IM for pain rated at 5/10 postappendectomy. Which outcome should a nurse expect?
   1. Blood pressure and pulse will increase.
   2. Moderate pain will be relieved for 4 hours.
   3. Dose is insufficient for the client's size.
   4. Another dose will be needed in 2 hours.

60. A nursing student asks an RN why clients who have had myocardial infarctions (MIs) should receive medications intravenously rather than intramuscularly. The best response by the RN would be:
   1. "A larger dose of medication would be required to bring relief from chest pain."
   2. "The trauma from more frequent needle sticks would cause stress and increase the serum enzymes."
   3. "Tissue perfusion is poor and venous return is diminished following an MI, which affects results."
   4. "Intramuscular injections should be avoided if the client is also receiving an anticoagulant drug post-MI."

61. A client with a history of alcohol abuse returns to a postanesthesia care unit (PACU) following abdominal surgery. A nurse knows pain management may be more difficult because of:
   1. Potential diminished drug effects related to impaired liver blood flow.
   2. Possible drug tolerance requiring higher dosages to produce desired effects.
   3. The need for higher dosages of medications because of accelerated liver detoxification.
   4. Increased sensitivity to the anesthetic agents used, requiring higher dosages than normal.

62. A client, who is gravida 6, para 4, has blood drawn for routine prenatal first-trimester laboratory work. Upon reviewing the client's laboratory results, which result should a nurse consider within normal limits for this stage of pregnancy?
   1. Hemoglobin of 11 gm/dL.
   2. Hemoglobin of 18 gm/dL.
   3. Fasting serum glucose of 110 mg/dL.
   4. White blood cell count of 18,000/mL.

63. A client, who is gravida 1, para 0, is admitted with a diagnosis of severe preeclampsia. A nurse starts the client on intravenous magnesium sulfate. For which expected side effect should the nurse closely observe the client?
   1. Decreased urinary output.
   2. Hypersomnolence.
   3. Absence of knee jerk reflex.
   4. Decreased respiratory rate.

64. A client, who is gravida 5, para 3, requests epidural anesthesia to relieve the discomfort of labor. After placement

of her epidural and a loading dose of medication, which assessment should be a nurse's *priority?*
1. Checking for cervical dilation.
2. Placing the client in a supine position.
3. Obtaining a fetal heart rate.
4. Checking the client's blood pressure.

65. A client, who is gravida 2, para 1, is at 42 weeks' gestation with gestational diabetes that is controlled with diet. A physician orders an intravenous infusion of oxytocin for the induction of labor due to postdates pregnancy. When caring for the client who is receiving intravenous oxytocin, the nurse should monitor for:
1. Maternal hypoglycemia.
2. Fetal movement.
3. Maternal hyperreflexia.
4. Fetal bradycardia.

66. A client, who is gravida 2, para 1 at 14 weeks gestation, has a routine ultrasound that shows no fetal cardiac motion. Which medication should a nurse anticipate being ordered for this client?
1. Magnesium sulfate.
2. Clomiphene citrate (Clomid).
3. Calcium gluconate.
4. Misoprostol (Cytotec).

67. A client, who is gravida 1, para 0 with severe preeclampsia, has been on a magnesium sulfate infusion at 2 gm/hr for the past 6 hours. Her recent assessment reveals a blood pressure 150/88 mm Hg, pulse 88, respirations 16, 1+ deep tendon reflexes, with 80 mL of urinary output during the past hour. Which action should a nurse take?
1. Decrease the infusion rate to 1 gm/hr and turn the client on her left side.
2. Continue the infusion of magnesium sulfate and monitor the client's blood pressure.
3. Stop the infusion of magnesium sulfate and notify the physician.
4. Administer calcium gluconate IV push and notify the physician.

68. A client is having severe pain in the lower back and left leg. The client has sensation in all extremities, but is not moving the left leg. While waiting for a diagnostic x-ray, the client asks for pain medication. The correct response by the nurse would be to:
1. Tell the client nothing can be given until a diagnosis is made.
2. Give half of the usual dose of analgesic to minimize pain.
3. Request order for an opioid to achieve maximum relief.
4. Offer two acetaminophen tablets.

69. A 35-year-old man has been experiencing low back pain for 2 days with no relief from ibuprofen 400 mg 4 times daily. His pain is 7 on a scale of 1 to 10. An opioid is prescribed by a physician for pain. A nurse should know that the most important barrier to the use of opioids for pain is:
1. Clients fear becoming addicted.
2. Physicians' concern about drug abuse.
3. Possible side effects of the drug.
4. Lack of accurate pain screening tools.

70. A client with intractable chest pain is to receive nitroglycerin 50 mg/250 mL and the rate is to be titrated until chest pain is relieved. The IV is infusing at 27 mL/hr and the client is pain-free. A nurse determines that the client is receiving nitroglycerin at a rate of _______ mcg/min. *Fill in the blank.*

71. A nurse enters a client's room to administer an IV medication and finds that the IV site is swollen, cool, and pale. The client reports discomfort at the insertion site. The nurse recognizes that this may be:
1. Infiltration.
2. Phlebitis.
3. Sepsis.
4. An allergic reaction.

72. Medications are absorbed differently with aging. A nurse should expect the dosage for an older adult to be:
1. Doubled to achieve the same effectiveness.
2. Reduced to prevent excessive systemic levels.
3. Increased slightly to make up for diminished liver function.
4. Monitored for reduced clinical effectiveness.

73. A client is scheduled for an inguinal herniorrhaphy in the morning and wants to know when to take the blood pressure pill before surgery. The best response by a nurse would be:
1. "No medications are taken by mouth the morning of surgery."
2. "Since you will not be taking anything by mouth after midnight, your drug won't be absorbed as well in the stomach."
3. "You will probably take your medicine with a small amount of water in the morning as usual."
4. "Your medication will be given to you intravenously just before surgery."

74. A client, who is newly diagnosed with tuberculosis, is being seen in a clinic. Current treatment includes isoniazid (INH) and rifampin (Rifadia). During the assessment, the client states that there has been blood in the urine since starting treatment. The best response by a nurse would be:
1. "One of your medications changes the color of body fluids."
2. "This is expected. There is nothing to worry about."
3. "I will send a urine specimen to the lab for analysis."
4. "Have you had any pain on urination or more frequent urination?"

75. A child is hospitalized for moderate respiratory distress caused by asthma. A physician orders a corticosteroid. A nurse knows that the main rationale for this medication is to:
1. Improve circulation.
2. Cause bronchodilation.
3. Reduce inflammation.
4. Thin respiratory secretions.

76. A child with gastroenteritis is admitted to a pediatric unit. The child is severely dehydrated and anuric. After the child receives a fluid bolus, a physician orders continuous IV fluids. Which IV fluid order should a nurse question?
1. 0.45% NaCl with KCl 20 mmol/L.
2. 0.45% NaCl with 5% glucose.
3. 0.9% NaCl.
4. 0.9% NaCl with 5% glucose.

77. A pediatric nurse prepares to infuse a fluid bolus of 300 mL NS over 1 hour. A nurse plans to use microdrip IV tubing. The nurse calculates that the drip rate for this infusion should be _______ gtt/min. *Fill in the blank.*

78. A nurse admits a preschooler with sickle cell anemia. Which medications should the nurse expect that the child has been receiving at home? *Select all that apply.*
1. Fer-In-Sol.
2. Penicillin.
3. Ibuprofen.
4. Folic acid.
5. Desferal.

79. A child recovering from abdominal surgery is receiving morphine for pain via PCA at a concentration of 1 mg/mL. The child receives a basal rate of 1 mg/hr and is able to self-administer up to four 1-mg boluses each hour. A nurse hangs a 50-mL syringe at the start of the shift and reviews the child's PCA record 4 hours later to find that the child self-administered a total of 7 boluses during that time. The nurse calculates that _______ mL of morphine should be left in the syringe. *Fill in the blank.*

80. A 44-pound child is to receive a 20-mL/kg bolus of IV fluid over 2 hours. A nurse correctly sets the infusion pump at a rate of _______ mL/hr. *Fill in the blank.*

81. A client, who is gravida 4, para 3 at 28 weeks' gestation, is dilated 2 cm. A physician has prescribed nifedipine to treat her preterm labor. For which common maternal side effect of the medication should a nurse assess?
1. Decreased deep tendon reflexes.
2. Bradycardia.
3. Hypotension.
4. Tachycardia.

82. A client, who is gravida 2, para 0 at 31 weeks' gestation, has been hospitalized for 5 days on oral terbutaline. A physician discharges the client with a prescription for terbutaline 5 mg PO q4h. When giving discharge instructions, which instruction should a nurse include?
1. "Call your physician if your heart rate is higher than 120 before you take your terbutaline."
2. "You can double your dose of terbutaline if you are having more than 2 contractions per hour."
3. "Call your physician if your fetus moves more than 10 times per hour."
4. "You can increase your activity each day if you are not fatigued."

83. A client, who is gravida 1, para 0, is at 39 weeks' gestation. She has an uncomplicated prenatal history. Her recent cervical examination reveals that she is 4 to 5 cm dilated, 100% effaced, and at a +1 station. She is asking for an epidural for labor pain control. Which order should a nurse anticipate to prevent hypotension in this client?
1. Administer a 500- to 2,000-mL bolus of IV fluid.
2. Administer oxygen at 12 L/min via face mask.
3. Place the client in high Fowler's position.
4. Administer epinephrine to raise her blood pressure.

84. A client, who is a 17-year-old gravida 1, para 0, is at 35 weeks' gestation with a blood pressure of 164/116 mm Hg on her left side, 4+ deep tendon reflexes, and 3+ proteinuria. Her physician orders a 4-gram loading dose of magnesium sulfate over 30 minutes, followed by 2 gm/hr. After administration of the bolus, the client complains of chest heaviness. A nurse assesses the client's deep tendon reflexes, which are now absent. The nurse should anticipate that the physician will most likely order:
1. Butorphanol tartrate.
2. Furosemide.
3. Diazepam.
4. Calcium gluconate.

85. A client, who is a 44-year-old gravida 2, para 1, is at 18 weeks' gestation with consistent blood pressures ranging from 130 to 140/80 to 90 mm Hg during her last two prenatal visits. She has no proteinuria or hyperreflexia. Which medication should a nurse anticipate being prescribed for this client?
1. Vasotec.
2. Aldomet.
3. Diazepam.
4. Magnesium sulfate.

86. A client, who is gravida 6, para 5 and in the fourth stage of labor, receives an injection of carboprost (Hemabate) 250 mcg IM. The nurse knows that the expected outcomes of this medication are:
Select all that apply.
1. Increased uterine atony.
2. Delayed uterine involution.

3. Increased myometrial contractions.
4. Decreased blood pressure.
5. Increased contractility of gastrointestinal smooth muscle.

87. A physician orders oxytocin IV for the augmentation of labor. The premixed IV has 20 units of oxytocin in 1,000 mL of lactated Ringer's solution. The oxytocin is ordered to begin at 6 milliunits/min. To administer the correct dose, a nurse should begin the infusion at _______ mL/hr via infusion pump. *Fill in the blank.*

88. A client, who is gravida 3, para 1, is being induced for pregnancy-induced hypertension using IV oxytocin. Under which circumstances should a nurse discontinue infusion of oxytocin? *Select all that apply.*
1. Three contractions in a 10-minute window of time.
2. Contractions every 3 minutes, lasting 90 seconds each.
3. Decrease in fetal heart rate after the peak of the contraction during each of the last three contractions.
4. Five contractions in the past 8 minutes.
5. Client is completely dilated.

89. The nursing instructor questions a nursing student about an analgesic that may be ordered for a child with otitis media who is complaining of mild ear pain. Which medication should the nursing student correctly expect to be ordered?
1. Ibuprofen.
2. Acetaminophen.
3. Codeine.
4. Dilaudid.

90. An adolescent who has attention deficit-hyperactivity disorder (ADHD) complies with taking the prescribed once-a-day medication. The adolescent's academic classes (e.g., math, science, etc.) should be scheduled by the school nurse for the:
1. Morning.
2. Midday.
3. Afternoon.
4. Intermingled with high-interest classroom activities.

91. A client is to receive 5 mcg/min of isoproterenol hydrochloride (Isuprel). The pharmacy prepares 1 mg of Isuprel in 500 mL of D_5W. A nurse should regulate the infusion rate to _______ mL/hr. *Fill in the blank.*

92. A client, who is an 18-year-old primigravida with gestational diabetes, is admitted to a labor and delivery unit at 34 weeks' gestation in preterm labor. Which physician's order for this client should a nurse question?
1. Magnesium sulfate 4 gm IV bolus over 30 minutes.
2. Brethine 10 mcg IV.
3. Stadol 1 mg IV push every 4 hours as needed for pain.
4. Ancef 2 gm IVPB every 6 hours.

93. A client, who is gravida 1, para 0, delivers an infant at 39 weeks' gestation. The client's blood type is O negative and the baby is O positive. A physician orders an injection of $Rh_o(D)$ immune globulin. To provide adequate postpartum prophylaxis, when should a nurse administer $Rh_o(D)$ immune globulin?
1. Within 72 hours of delivery.
2. Within 1 week of delivery.
3. Before 12 hours after delivery.
4. Within 2 weeks of delivery.

Answers/Rationales/Tips

1. **CORRECT ANSWER: 2. Answer 1** is incorrect because there is no risk to the client from fibrinogen, which is a protein that is converted into fibrin to form a thrombus or clot. **Answer 2 is correct because a hemolytic reaction will most likely occur during the first 20 minutes. Answer 3** is incorrect because warming is *not* required, but may be more comfortable for the client. **Answer 4** is incorrect because the rate of infusion could be up to *4* hours.

■ **TEST-TAKING TIP:** ***This is a priority question; therefore, other options could be correct. Look for the action that protects the client from injury—think safety.***

Content Area: Adult Health, Hematological; ***Integrated Process:*** Nursing Process, Analysis; ***Cognitive Level:*** Application; ***Client Need/Subneed:*** Physiological Integrity/Pharmacological and Parenteral Therapies/Blood and Blood Products

2. **CORRECT ANSWER: 1. Answer 1 is correct because during illness the cells still need insulin. Failure to give it will likely put the client into a hyperosmolar, if nonketotic state (type 1 diabetes is more likely to cause ketoacidosis). Since the client will not be eating very much, the insulin dose may be reduced, and it is hard to predict by how much. Clients with diabetes need to prepare a "sick day strategy," which will include checking blood sugar, and possibly ketone level, more frequently. Answer 2** is incorrect because insulin should *not* be administered if the blood glucose is low. **Answer 3** is incorrect because ketone-positive urine indicates that there is inadequate insulin carrying glucose into the cells. Insulin *is* needed. **Answer 4** is incorrect because, when unable to ingest food, the liver breaks down glycogen, which provides glucose for the body. Insulin is *still* required to take this glucose into the cell.

■ **TEST-TAKING TIP:** ***Totally stopping insulin is not advised as a general management strategy; therefore, eliminate Answers 3 and 4.***

Content Area: Adult Health, Endocrine; ***Integrated Process:*** Nursing Process, Planning; ***Cognitive Level:*** Application; ***Client Need/Subneed:*** Physiological Integrity/Pharmacological and Parenteral Therapies/Expected Effects/Outcomes

3. CORRECT ANSWER: 3. Answer 1 is incorrect because Epogen is given to treat *anemia.* Negative Homans' sign and elevated activated partial thromboplastin time (aPTT) are used to monitor *thromboembolism.* **Answer 2** is incorrect because Epogen is given to treat anemia. Guaiac-negative gastric secretions might indicate effectiveness of *stress ulcer* prevention. **Answer 3 is correct because epoetin alfa (Epogen) stimulates the development of red blood cells (RBCs). It is given to anemic clients to increase hematocrit (Hct). Answer 4** is incorrect because Epogen is given to treat anemia. It is *not measured by creatinine.*

■ **TEST-TAKING TIP:** *Think: Epogen = erythropoietin =* erythro *(red) → increased RBCs → increased Hct.*

Content Area: Adult Health, Hematological; ***Integrated Process:*** Nursing Process, Analysis; ***Cognitive Level:*** Application; ***Client Need/Subneed:*** Physiological Integrity/Pharmacological and Parenteral Therapies/Expected Effects/Outcomes

4. CORRECT ANSWER: 2. Answer 1 is incorrect because clonidine patches are used to manage pain or hypertension. Numbness or tingling down the arm is *not related* to the patch. **Answer 2 is correct because clonidine is an alpha-2 receptor stimulator, working at the presynaptic receptor of the sympathetic nervous system. Thus, it reduces the output of norepinephrine and is used to treat hypertension. If the BP is too low, antihypertensive medications should not be given. It is important for the nurse to remember that drugs in patches are in a constant state of "being given," and the patch would need to be removed. Answer 3** is incorrect because clonidine patches are *not sulfa-based.* **Answer 4** is incorrect because clonidine patches *do not affect* serum potassium.

■ **TEST-TAKING TIP:** *If the drug is an antihypertensive, select the answer that relates to blood pressure, not neurology (Answer 1) or allergy (Answer 3).*

Content Area: Adult Health, Cardiovascular; ***Integrated Process:*** Nursing Process, Analysis; ***Cognitive Level:*** Application; ***Client Need/Subneed:*** Physiological Integrity/Pharmacological and Parenteral Therapies/Adverse Effects/Contraindications/Interactions

5. CORRECT ANSWER: 4. Answer 1 is incorrect because clients in diabetic ketoacidosis are dehydrated. They need salt and *fluids,* which are generally given *intravenously.* **Answer 2** is incorrect because hypertonic saline solutions are not appropriate. Fluids must run fast in these clients who are dehydrated, and this would change sodium levels *too quickly.* Rapid changes in serum sodium can precipitate a dangerous fluid shift. **Answer 3** is incorrect because clients with diabetic ketoacidosis are *dehydrated.* Fluid restriction is *inappropriate.* **Answer 4 is correct because high blood sugar increases the osmolarity of the blood and stimulates the body to secrete antidiuretic hormone (ADH) to help the kidneys to retain free water, which dilutes the sodium. Obligate diuresis from the osmotic action of sugar in the tubules of the kidneys forces water and sodium loss even though the client is dehydrated. Clients in diabetic ketoacidosis need fluid replacement with normal saline and insulin to return the blood sugar to a normal level.**

■ **TEST-TAKING TIP:** *Select the option with* **insulin.** *Think about the fluid and electrolyte imbalances that occur from a* **high blood glucose:** *Blood glucose is elevated (>200 mg/dL) in diabetic ketoacidosis. Knowing why the low sodium (<135) has occurred is important for selecting the correct action.*

Content Area: Adult Health, Endocrine; ***Integrated Process:*** Nursing Process, Implementation; ***Cognitive Level:*** Analysis; ***Client Need/Subneed:*** Physiological Integrity/Pharmacological and Parenteral Therapies/Expected Effects/Outcomes

6. CORRECT ANSWER: 2. Answer 1 is incorrect because taking this medication 1 hour *after* a meal does *not* replace enzymes that would be released by the pancreas in response to food intake. Taking it with meals stimulates the normal pancreas activity. **Answer 2 is correct because this medication is replacing enzymes that would be released by the pancreas in response to food intake. Taking it with meals stimulates the normal pancreatic activity and helps with the digestion of proteins, starches, and fats. Answer 3** is incorrect because taking this medication at bedtime does *not replace* enzymes that would be released by the pancreas in response to food intake. Taking it with meals stimulates the normal pancreatic activity. **Answer 4** is incorrect because clients with deficiencies in pancreatic enzymes do *not* necessarily have any *deficit* in insulin secretion. Pancrease should be administered with the meal; insulin (*if* administered) would need to be given *before* the meal to allow for absorption.

■ **TEST-TAKING TIP:** *Knowing the importance of pancreatic enzymes in facilitating digestion makes the choice easier*—**with** *meals,* **not** *before or after.*

Content Area: Adult Health, Gastrointestinal; ***Integrated Process:*** Nursing Process, Implementation; ***Cognitive Level:*** Application; ***Client Need/Subneed:*** Physiological Integrity/Pharmacological and Parenteral Therapies/Medication Administration

7. CORRECT ANSWER: 2. Answer 1 is incorrect because *high blood pressure* (e.g., 180/90) is treated with diuretics and does *not* need to be verified (although furosemide is not usually the first choice). **Answer 2 is correct because this diuretic will cause potassium to be lost in the urine. Clients receiving furosemide often need K^+ replacement. Answer 3** is incorrect because crackles that are present with *pulmonary edema may be* treated with furosemide. **Answer 4** is incorrect because, although the urine volume will be increased, there is *no need* for a bladder catheter if the client can void.

■ **TEST-TAKING TIP:** *Only one of the options relates to the importance of the potassium level. The other options relate to assessing and managing the impact of fluid in the client.*

Content Area: Adult Health, Fluid and Electrolyte Imbalances; ***Integrated Process:*** Nursing Process, Assessment; ***Cognitive Level:*** Application; ***Client Need/Subneed:*** Physiological

Integrity/Pharmacological and Parenteral Therapies/ Medication Administration

8. CORRECT ANSWER: 2. Answer 1 is incorrect because rapid reduction in blood glucose reduces serum osmolarity and may shift fluids into cells, *causing cerebral edema.* The blood glucose level should not fall by more than 15% an hour. The insulin infusion rate should be *reduced,* not increased. **Answer 2 is correct because rapid reduction in blood glucose reduces serum osmolarity and may shift fluids into cells, causing cerebral edema. The blood glucose should not fall by more than 15% an hour. Slow the insulin infusion rate. Answer 3** is incorrect because rapid reduction in blood glucose reduces serum osmolarity and may shift fluids into cells, *causing cerebral edema.* The blood glucose level has fallen by more than 15% an hour. The insulin infusion rate is too fast and *no bolus* is needed. **Answer 4** is incorrect because blood glucose level has dropped by more than 15% in 1 hour. This reduces serum osmolarity and may shift fluids into cells, causing cerebral edema. The insulin infusion rate should be *reduced.*

■ **TEST-TAKING TIP:** *Recognize a* therapeutic *drop in blood glucose versus a change that will potentially cause a* problem.
Content Area: Adult Health, Endocrine; ***Integrated Process:*** Nursing Process, Implementation; ***Cognitive Level:*** Analysis; ***Client Need/Subneed:*** Physiological Integrity/Pharmacological and Parenteral Therapies/Adverse Effects/Contraindications/ Interactions

9. CORRECT ANSWER: 1. Answer 1 is correct because clients on dialysis should receive minimal fluids and *no* potassium, since these agents cannot be removed until the next dialysis treatment. Answer 2 is incorrect because this IV rate is *too fast* for a client who is unable to excrete fluids via the kidney. **Answer 3** is incorrect because potassium is *rarely* given to clients requiring dialysis since they are unable to secrete any excess. **Answer 4** is incorrect because potassium is *rarely* given to clients requiring dialysis since they are unable to secrete any excess.

■ **TEST-TAKING TIP:** *First, eliminate the two options with potassium (Answers 3 and 4). Then, select the option with the* slowest *rate. Look for the option that best addresses the fluid and sodium restrictions usually required for the client with chronic renal failure.*
Content Area: Adult Health, Renal; ***Integrated Process:*** Nursing Process, Analysis; ***Cognitive Level:*** Analysis; ***Client Need/Subneed:*** Physiological Integrity/Pharmacological and Parenteral Therapies/ Parenteral/Intravenous Therapies

10. CORRECT ANSWER: 3. Answer 1 is incorrect because this diuretic is taken in *pill* form. **Answer 2** is incorrect because spironolactone is a potassium-sparing diuretic. Supplemental potassium is *not* advised. **Answer 3 is correct because spironolactone has antiproliferative effects and prevents fibrotic remodeling of heart tissue. It is the only diuretic that reduces mortality in heart failure. Answer 4** is incorrect because generally diuretics are taken in the *morning* to prevent having to wake up from sleep to urinate.

■ **TEST-TAKING TIP:** *Three of the options focus on administration and adverse effects of the medication. Only one option states a* desired *outcome. Choose the option that is different. Review the common classifications of diuretics—thiazides, loop, and potassium-sparing—and know examples for each type.*
Content Area: Adult Health, Cardiology; ***Integrated Process:*** Teaching and Learning; ***Cognitive Level:*** Application; ***Client Need/Subneed:*** Physiological Integrity/Pharmacological and Parenteral Therapies/Medication Administration

11. CORRECT ANSWER: 3. Answer 1 is incorrect because nitrates vasodilate veins but do *not decrease* heart rate. This would not be a reason to hold the drug. **Answer 2** is incorrect because nitrates are *not sulfa* drugs. **Answer 3 is correct because nitrates are potent vasodilators. This reduces the venous return, cardiac output, and BP. The drug should be held if the BP is too low. Answer 4** is incorrect because, with prolonged therapy, the client may develop tolerance to nitrates. Efficacy can be retained by providing a "nitrate-free" interval each day to allow the receptor to regain sensitivity. Therefore, therapy *can* proceed over weeks and years.

■ **TEST-TAKING TIP:** *An example of a nitrate is nitroglycerin. Note the similarity to the drug classification—nitrate and "nitro-." Nitroglycerin is a vasodilator, leading to ↓ BP.*
Content Area: Adult Health, Cardiovascular; ***Integrated Process:*** Nursing Process, Implementation; ***Cognitive Level:*** Application; ***Client Need/Subneed:*** Physiological Integrity/Pharmacological and Parenteral Therapies/Medication Administration

12. CORRECT ANSWER: 3. Answer 1 is incorrect because, although thiazide diuretics are often first-line therapy for hypertension, the heart failure is correctly managed with beta blockers and angiotensin-converting enzyme (ACE) inhibitors. Diuretics would be added *only* if there was *insufficient* clinical response to the other drugs. **Answer 2** is incorrect because digoxin and furosemide, long considered the treatment of choice in heart failure, were found *not* to reduce mortality. Heart failure should be treated with beta blockers and/or ACE inhibitors. **Answer 3 is correct because the ejection fraction is low, indicating a problem with cardiac output. The ejection fraction of a healthy heart is 60% to 70%. Beta blockers and ACE inhibitors reduce morbidity and mortality in heart failure. Answer 4** is incorrect because, although heart failure can increase the risk of thromboembolism, the usefulness of anticoagulation in clients without atrial fibrillation or a history of blood clots is *not well established.*

■ **TEST-TAKING TIP:** *The problem is with the pumping effectiveness of the heart. Select the option with the greatest effect on improving cardiac output and client survival.*
Content Area: Adult Health, Cardiovascular; ***Integrated Process:*** Nursing Process, Analysis; ***Cognitive Level:*** Analysis; ***Client Need/Subneed:*** Physiological Integrity/Pharmacological and Parenteral Therapies/Medication Administration

13. CORRECT ANSWER: 2. **Answer 1** is incorrect because data from a complete blood count (CBC) are *rarely* required in the assessments of clients with STIs, and would *not* be a priority. **Answer 2 is correct because clients should always be questioned about allergies before medications are administered.** **Answer 3** is incorrect because *none* of the adverse effects, contradictions, or cautions associated with azithromycin involves blood pressure. **Answer 4** is incorrect because, although it is important to get information about sexual contacts, this information does not alter the decision to treat the current client, and thus is not a priority before giving azithromycin.

■ TEST-TAKING TIP: *With priority questions, look for the option that provides the client with the greatest safety.*
Content Area: Adult Health, Communicable Disease; *Integrated Process:* Nursing Process, Assessment; *Cognitive Level:* Application; *Client Need/Subneed:* Physiological Integrity/Pharmacological and Parenteral Therapies/Medication Administration

14. CORRECT ANSWER: 2. **Answer 1** is incorrect because nausea is prevented by giving the antidote *before* chemotherapy. Anticholinergics, such as trimethobenzamide, have limited usefulness in chemotherapy-induced nausea. **Answer 2 is correct because there is often specific matching of nausea treatments and chemotherapeutic agents. Nausea is better prevented than treated by giving the antiemetic before the chemotherapy.** **Answer 3** is incorrect because heat increases the odor of foods, which may *worsen* nausea. **Answer 4** is incorrect because there is no reason to have a client NPO for 24 hours before chemotherapy. This would promote dehydration and malnutrition *unnecessarily.*

■ TEST-TAKING TIP: *Look for an action prior to chemotherapy.*
Content Area: Adult Health, Oncology; *Integrated Process:* Nursing Process, Implementation; *Cognitive Level:* Application; *Client Need/Subneed:* Physiological Integrity/Pharmacological and Parenteral Therapies/Expected Effects/Outcomes

15. CORRECT ANSWER: 2. **Answer 1** is incorrect because indomethacin is *not* a sulfa-based drug and may be used safely in clients with sulfa allergies. **Answer 2 is correct because a side effect of indomethacin is gastrointestinal bleeding. This risk is greater in clients with history of GI bleeding.** **Answer 3** is incorrect because, even though indomethacin can worsen hypertension, a greater risk is hemorrhage. **Answer 4** is incorrect because indomethacin does *not* affect blood sugar.

■ TEST-TAKING TIP: *Only one option addresses a side effect of the drug.*
Content Area: Adult Health, Pharmacology; *Integrated Process:* Nursing Process, Assessment; *Cognitive Level:* Application; *Client Need/Subneed:* Physiological Integrity/Pharmacological and Parenteral Therapies/Medication Administration

16. CORRECT ANSWER: 1. **Answer 1 is correct because bupivacaine blocks neuron transmission, numbing tissue and reducing pain. This is the desired effect and the data should be recorded.** **Answer 2** is incorrect because pain levels of 3/10 *rarely* require additional medication. **Answer 3** is incorrect because the medication is working well and the client is *not* showing adverse effects. Raising the head of the bed may be helpful when too much medication has been administered, as gravity would help keep the medicine from anesthetizing nerves involved in breathing. **Answer 4** is incorrect because the medication is working well and the client is *not* showing adverse effects. There is *no* reason to turn the infusion off. Lowering the head would facilitate movement of the medication to a higher spinal level. This is *not needed* for this client with good pain control.

■ TEST-TAKING TIP: *Know the normal level of numbness with an epidural. Select the only option that does* not *reequire an active intervention (e.g., "increase," "raise," "lower").*
Content Area: Adult Health, Pain Control; *Integrated Process:* Nursing Process, Implementation; *Cognitive Level:* Application; *Client Need/Subneed:* Physiological Integrity/Pharmacological and Parenteral Therapies/Expected Effects/Outcomes

17. CORRECT ANSWER: 2. **Answer 1** is incorrect because, if the pain level is too high for the client to turn in bed, the client will not do well with walking. **Answer 2 is correct because, with lock-out of 6 minutes, the client could have received 20 injections over the last 2 hours, yet only received 2. The high pain level will prevent the client from engaging in health promoting activities: 45 attempts indicates that the client wants more medicine. Teaching is required to help the client spread out the attempts.** **Answer 3** is incorrect because the nurse might record it if the client refuses ambulation, but it would be better to help the client control the pain to make ambulation possible. **Answer 4** is incorrect because *only the client* should push the PCA button. This helps prevent overdoses.

■ TEST-TAKING TIP: *Look for the option that is different from the others. Three of the options refer to "getting out of bed."*
Content Area: Adult Health, Pain Control; *Integrated Process:* Nursing Process, Implementation; *Cognitive Level:* Application; *Client Need/Subneed:* Physiological Integrity/Pharmacological and Parenteral Therapies/Pharmacological Pain Management

18. CORRECT ANSWER: 2. **Answer 1** is incorrect because, if given 60 minutes before a meal, this rapidly absorbing insulin could cause *hypoglycemia* before the client begins to eat. **Answer 2 is correct because the "log" ending indicates this drug is one of the insulin analogues. Very small changes in the amino acid sequence facilitate rapid absorption of this drug.** **Answer 3** is incorrect because regular and rapid-acting insulin should be given *before meals* so that they are active in the blood as sugars are being absorbed from the intestine. **Answer 4** is incorrect because regular and rapid-acting insulin should be given *before* meals so that they are active in the blood as sugars are being absorbed from the intestine.

■ TEST-TAKING TIP: *The goal is to* prevent *hyperglycemia—give* before *eating. Choose between short (15 minutes) and*

long (60 minutes) interval. Know the peak effect time for rapid-*acting insulin. Choose the* shortest *time period.*
Content Area: Adult Health, Endocrine; ***Integrated Process:*** Nursing Process, Implementation; ***Cognitive Level:*** Application; ***Client Need/Subneed:*** Physiological Integrity/Pharmacological and Parenteral Therapies/Medication Administration

19. CORRECT ANSWER: 1. Answer 1 is correct because Carafate should be given *alone* 30 to 60 minutes before mealtime. It is activated by stomach acid and coats a stomach ulcer. **Answer 2** is incorrect because the drug *may be taken* with other drugs. Only digoxin and tetracycline should be taken at different times. **Answer 3** is incorrect because constipation is *not* a side effect. Diarrhea would be more common. **Answer 4** is incorrect because the drug should *not be diluted* to obtain maximum effect; water does not coat the stomach.
■ **TEST-TAKING TIP:** *Look for the option that would maximize the therapeutic* coating *effect of Carafate.*
Content Area: Adult Health, Gastrointestinal; ***Integrated Process:*** Nursing Process, Evaluation; ***Cognitive Level:*** Application; ***Client Need/Subneed:*** Physiological Integrity/Pharmacological and Parenteral Therapies/Medication Administration

20. CORRECT ANSWER: 40. Calculate the rate using the following formula:

$$\frac{10 \text{ units}}{100 \text{ mL}} \times \frac{4 \text{ units}}{x \text{ mL}}$$

■ **TEST-TAKING TIP:** *Memorize the formulas for calculating infusion rates.*
Content Area: Adult Health, Endocrine; ***Integrated Process:*** Nursing Process, Implementation; ***Cognitive Level:*** Analysis; ***Client Need/Subneed:*** Physiological Integrity/Pharmacological and Parenteral Therapies/Dosage Calculation

21. CORRECT ANSWER: 4. **Answer 1** is incorrect because there may be improvement in the client's perception of pain; however, the concern is about oversedation by the drug. There are sedation scales available that do help the nurse identify the onset of sedation in a client. **Answer 2** is incorrect because the client may be receiving supplemental oxygen. **Answer 3** is incorrect because a client who is oversedated can be awakened and will respond to questions appropriately. **Answer 4 is correct because opioids will depress ventilation, causing a buildup of carbon dioxide in the blood. If hypoventilation is present, measuring the level of carbon dioxide is the most reliable indication of possible respiratory depression. Capnography measures breath by breath the level of CO_2 and is most often used during anesthesia, in critical care, and in emergency medicine to prevent respiratory depression. If capnography is not available with the client who is on PCA, monitoring the client's respiratory rate and depth and assessing sedation levels is essential.**
■ **TEST-TAKING TIP:** *This question is asking for the "most reliable" indication. If a client is oversedated, ventilation will be affected. Hypoventilation affects CO_2.*
Content Area: Adult Health, Pain Control; ***Integrated Process:*** Nursing Process, Assessment; ***Cognitive Level:*** Application; ***Client Need/Subneed:*** Physiological Integrity/Pharmacological and Parenteral Therapies/Pharmacological Pain Management

22. CORRECT ANSWER: 1. Answer 1 is correct because administration of therapy within 3 hours decreases the size of the stroke and improves client outcome. **Answer 2** is incorrect because the typical signs of a stroke occur *earlier.* By the time the signs of increased intracranial pressure (ICP) are present, there has been distortion of brain centers. **Answer 3** is incorrect because this is a sign of *increased intracranial pressure* and the Cushing response. Numbness, trouble speaking, or loss of balance would be *earlier* signs of brain attack. **Answer 4** is incorrect because clinical research has shown that therapy is most effective when given *within 3 hours* after the onset of symptoms.
■ **TEST-TAKING TIP:** *Think "the sooner the better."*
Content Area: Adult Health, Cardiovascular; ***Integrated Process:*** Nursing Process, Implementation; ***Cognitive Level:*** Application; ***Client Need/Subneed:*** Physiological Integrity/Pharmacological and Parenteral Therapies/Medication Administration

23. CORRECT ANSWER: 3. **Answer 1** is incorrect because calcium therapy is indicated for hypocalcemia, *not* hyperthyroidism. **Answer 2** is incorrect because calcium gluconate is used to treat hypocalcemia, *not* blood loss. **Answer 3 is correct because Trousseau's sign is present with hypocalcemia. The carpal spasm will not occur if treatment has been effective.** **Answer 4** is incorrect because Chvostek's sign, the twitching of facial muscles when tapped, indicates *hypocalcemia.*
■ **TEST-TAKING TIP:** *Know why calcium gluconate is given—for low calcium, which causes tetany as evidenced by Trousseau's sign.*
Content Area: Adult Health, Fluid and Electrolyte Imbalances; ***Integrated Process:*** Nursing Process, Evaluation; ***Cognitive Level:*** Application; ***Client Need/Subneed:*** Physiological Integrity/Pharmacological and Parenteral Therapies/Expected Effects/Outcomes

24. CORRECT ANSWER: 4. **Answer 1** is incorrect because ascites is the accumulation of fluid in the peritoneal space. This may occur as the result of a *disease process,* such as liver failure, *not* from chemotherapy. **Answer 2** is incorrect because septicemia is the presence of an infection in the blood. Chemotherapy can increase the client's risk of infection because of the decreased WBCs, which if not treated could result in septicemia. **Answer 3** is incorrect because polycythemia is an increase in immature RBCs. Chemotherapy *suppresses* RBC production in the bone marrow. **Answer 4 is correct because chemotherapy causes myelosuppression (depression of bone marrow function). WBCs, RBCs and platelets are decreased.**
■ **TEST-TAKING TIP:** *Think of a common side effect—one that all clients who are on chemotherapy usually experience.*
Content Area: Adult Health, Oncological; ***Integrated Process:*** Nursing Process, Assessment; ***Cognitive Level:*** Application; ***Client Need/Subneed:*** Physiological Integrity/Pharmacological and Parenteral Therapies/Adverse Effects/Contraindications/Interactions

25. CORRECT ANSWER: 1. Answer 1 is correct because beta blockers (metoprolol) cause bronchoconstriction. Note that the client already has a respiratory problem. **Answer 2** is incorrect because an aluminum hydroxide gel *is used* to *reduce the elevated phosphate level,* which results in renal failure. **Answer 3** is incorrect because calcium channel blockers (diltiazem) *are used* to *control blood pressure* in the client with an AAA. **Answer 4** is incorrect because clients on *hemodialysis* are often *anemic.* Epoetin stimulates RBC production.

■ TEST-TAKING TIP: *Three of the answers produce the* desired *effect for the* condition; *one does not. Think about the drug action and the potential for an adverse effect as the result of the drug's normal action.*

Content Area: Adult Health, Respiratory; ***Integrated Process:*** Nursing Process, Analysis; ***Cognitive Level:*** Analysis; ***Client Need/Subneed:*** Physiological Integrity/ Pharmacological and Parenteral Therapies/Adverse Effects/Contraindications/Interactions

26. CORRECT ANSWERS: 1, 2, 3. Answer 1 is correct because subcutaneous epinephrine is the first line of treatment. Clients with bee sting allergies should carry an EpiPen. Answer 2 is correct because Benadryl is a standard treatment for an allergic reaction. The client should chew the tablets. Answer 3 is correct because Solu-Medrol is a standard anti-inflammatory drug for anaphylaxis or an allergic reaction. **Answer 4** is incorrect because the diuretic effects of Lasix will *not* help anaphylaxis. **Answer 5** is incorrect because the analgesic or antipyretic effects of Tylenol will *not* help anaphylaxis. **Answer 6** is incorrect because a histamine$_2$ (H_2) blocker such as Zantac is *not a first* line of defense, although the drug may be given.

■ TEST-TAKING TIP: *Anaphylaxis is the concern here. Know the first-line drugs for* anaphylaxis. *Eliminate the drugs used for diuretic and antipyretic effects.*

Content Area: Adult Health, Respiratory; ***Integrated Process:*** Nursing Process, Analysis; ***Cognitive Level:*** Application; ***Client Need/Subneed:*** Physiological Integrity/Pharmacological and Parenteral Therapies/Expected Effects/Outcomes

27. CORRECT ANSWER: 2. **Answer 1** is incorrect because atropine is used for *bradycardia* or *first-degree atrioventricular (AV) blocks.* Answer 2 is correct because epinephrine (adrenalin) is a first-line drug used during CPR to stimulate cardiac activity. **Answer 3** is incorrect because Lasix is a *diuretic,* not an antiarrhythmic. **Answer 4** is incorrect because lidocaine is indicated for ventricular arrhythmias, specifically *premature ventricular contractions (PVCs).*

■ TEST-TAKING TIP: *Consider the cardiac effects of each drug and the nature of the arrhythmia. The best choice is a drug that will stimulate normal cardiac activity.*

Content Area: Adult Health, Cardiology; ***Integrated Process:*** Nursing Process, Implementation; ***Cognitive Level:*** Application; ***Client Need/Subneed:*** Physiological Integrity/Pharmacological and Parenteral Therapies/Expected Effects/Outcomes

28. CORRECT ANSWERS: 1, 2, 4, 5. Answer 1 is correct because the vasodilating effect of the drug causes increased cerebral blood flow and headache. Answer 2 is correct because the drug causes vasodilation, which decreases venous return, cardiac output, and BP. **Answer 3** is incorrect because the effects reduce the O_2 demand on the heart, but there is *no change* in volume or pumping effectiveness. Answer 4 is correct because the vasodilating effect causes flushing. Answer 5 is correct because vasodilation and the drop in BP could cause dizziness and light-headedness. **Answer 6** is incorrect because the drug should decrease the O_2 demand, and workload to cardiac function would be improved. Shortness of breath indicates *heart failure.* **Answer 7** is incorrect because the drug does *not* interfere with gastric or intestinal functions.

■ TEST-TAKING TIP: *Focus on the vasodilation effect of nitroglycerin on blood vessels. Consider if vasodilation will produce each of the signs or symptoms.*

Content Area: Adult Health, Cardiology; ***Integrated Process:*** Nursing Process, Assessment; ***Cognitive Level:*** Application; ***Client Need/Subneed:*** Physiological Integrity/Pharmacological and Parenteral Therapies/Expected Effects/Outcomes

29. CORRECT ANSWER: 4. **Answer 1** is incorrect because an increase in rate would not be desired post-MI. **Answer 2** is incorrect because an increase in central venous pressure (CVP) would signal *increasing* demand on the heart. **Answer 3** is incorrect because this would indicate a *decrease in renal* perfusion. Answer 4 is correct because improved cardiac contractions will increase cardiac output. Crackles would be heard if *heart failure* were present.

■ TEST-TAKING TIP: *Only one of the options indicates an improvement in cardiac function.*

Content Area: Adult Health, Cardiology; ***Integrated Process:*** Nursing Process, Evaluation; ***Cognitive Level:*** Application; ***Client Need/Subneed:*** Physiological Integrity/Pharmacological and Parenteral Therapies/Expected Effects/Outcomes

30. CORRECT ANSWER: 4. **Answer 1** is incorrect because there is *no* increased incidence of viral infections while taking the drug. A need for an annual influenza vaccination is not related to taking this drug. **Answer 2** is incorrect because the drug does *not affect renal* function or fluid balance. **Answer 3** is incorrect because the drug does *not affect electrolyte* levels. Answer 4 is correct because gingival hyperplasia is a noninflammatory enlargement of the gingiva from an increase in normal cells. Good dental hygiene may reduce the swelling.

■ TEST-TAKING TIP: *The question asks for a common side effect. Choose the option that is different from the others—only one has the* client report *an adverse effect.*

Content Area: Adult Health, Neurological; ***Integrated Process:*** Teaching and Learning; ***Cognitive Level:*** Application; ***Client Need/Subneed:*** Physiological Integrity/ Pharmacological and Parenteral Therapies/Adverse Effects/Contraindications/Interactions

31. CORRECT ANSWER: 4. **Answer 1** is incorrect because this loop diuretic does *not* affect appetite. **Answer 2** is incorrect because taking the diuretic in the *morning* should *not* increase nighttime urination, with sleep disturbances. **Answer 3** is incorrect because this is a *desired* outcome of the drug, not an adverse effect. **Answer 4 is correct because leg cramps could indicate excessive loss of potassium.**

■ TEST-TAKING TIP: ***Choose an option that has potentially the greatest risk if not corrected. Eliminate options that involve the GI (Answer 1) and urinary (Answer 3) systems because, in this case, they do not cause at-risk effects.***

Content Area: Adult Health, Fluid and Electrolyte Imbalances; ***Integrated Process:*** Nursing Process, Implementation; ***Cognitive Level:*** Application; ***Client Need/Subneed:*** Physiological Integrity/Pharmacological and Parenteral Therapies/Adverse Effects/Contraindications/Interactions

32. CORRECT ANSWER: 2. **Answer 1** is incorrect because the drug *increases* heart rate. Irregularity is *not* expected. **Answer 2 is correct because scopolamine has the same effects as atropine, which is used to dry secretions preoperatively.** **Answer 3** is incorrect because the drug *increases* the heart rate, so hypotension is *not* expected. **Answer 4** is incorrect because the drug affects salivation, *not speech.*

■ TEST-TAKING TIP: ***Look for a side effect that would be annoying but not have a severe consequence.***

Content Area: Adult Health, Gastrointestinal; ***Integrated Process:*** Nursing Process, Implementation; ***Cognitive Level:*** Application; ***Client Need/Subneed:*** Physiological Integrity/Pharmacological and Parenteral Therapies/Adverse Effects/Contraindications/Interactions

33. CORRECT ANSWER: 1. **Answer 1 is correct because a dry cough might be annoying, but would not place the client at increased risk for injury or debilitation.** **Answer 2** is incorrect because progression of heart failure would *not* be an *acceptable* side effect. **Answer 3** is incorrect because sedation would be an *unsafe* consequence of the drug. **Answer 4** is incorrect because incontinence would not be an acceptable side effect for an adult.

■ TEST-TAKING TIP: ***The question focuses on what is an "OK" side effect so that the drug doesn't have to be stopped. Three of the choices have the potential to incapacitate the client.***

Content Area: Adult Health, Cardiovascular; ***Integrated Process:*** Teaching and Learning; ***Cognitive Level:*** Application; ***Client Need/Subneed:*** Physiological Integrity/Pharmacological and Parenteral Therapies/Adverse Effects/Contraindications/Interactions

34. CORRECT ANSWER: 2. **Answer 1** is incorrect because dextrose can cause a *pseudodiabetes* during the first 24 hours after a burn. **Answer 2 is correct because a crystalloid, such as lactated Ringer's, will correct the volume deficit, sodium loss, and metabolic acidosis that is present in the client with burns.** **Answer 3** is incorrect because colloids, such as Dextran or albumin, are *not* used for *primary* fluid replacement. **Answer 4** is incorrect because this client would be hyperkalemic and should *not* receive additional K^+. NS *without* K^+ would be appropriate for fluid replacement.

■ TEST-TAKING TIP: ***Look for a solution that will not contribute to any shift of fluids or electrolytes in the first 24 hours.***

Content Area: Adult Health, Fluid and Electrolyte Imbalances; ***Integrated Process:*** Nursing Process, Analysis; ***Cognitive Level:*** Application; ***Client Need/Subneed:*** Physiological Integrity/Pharmacological and Parenteral Therapies/Parenteral/Intravenous Therapies

35. CORRECT ANSWERS: 2, 4, 5, 6. **Answer 1** is incorrect because opioids act on the brain to decrease pain—agitation would *not* be expected. **Answer 2 is correct because opioids do affect the GI tract. Constipation will persist even with long-term use of opioids.** **Answer 3** is incorrect because opioids are *constipating.* **Answer 4 is correct because nausea and vomiting are common, and may subside in a few days. Fluids and an antiemetic may help.** **Answer 5 is correct because itching *does* occur. However, it is not considered an "allergy" to the drug. Antihistamines are given.** **Answer 6 is correct because the drug acts directly on the brain and produces sedation. However, the client will quickly develop *tolerance* to sedation.**

■ TEST-TAKING TIP: ***When two options are contradictory (e.g., Answers 1 and 6, and Answers 2 and 3), one of them is incorrect.***

Content Area: Adult Health, Pain Control; ***Integrated Process:*** Nursing Process, Assessment; ***Cognitive Level/Subneed:*** Analysis; ***Client Need:*** Physiological Integrity/Pharmacological and Parenteral Therapies/Adverse Effects/Contraindications/Interactions

36. CORRECT ANSWERS: 2, 3. **Answer 1** is incorrect because *volume* will increase, but fluid will *not be pulled* from the tissue. **Answer 2 is correct because this solution is classified as a hypertonic volume expander, pulling fluids from the tissues.** **Answer 3 is correct because albumin is a hypertonic solution and will increase the osmotic pressure, pulling fluid into the vascular space.** **Answer 4** is incorrect because lactated Ringer's is considered to be isotonic, not causing any shift of fluids. Volume will increase, but fluid will *remain* in the tissues. **Answer 5** is incorrect because packed red blood cells improve oxygen-carrying capacity, but *not* volume.

■ TEST-TAKING TIP: ***Look for a solution that will increase osmotic (pull) pressure in the intravascular (venous) system.***

Content Area: Adult Health, Fluid and Electrolyte Imbalances; ***Integrated Process:*** Nursing Process, Analysis; ***Cognitive Level:*** Application; ***Client Need/Subneed:*** Physiological Integrity/Pharmacological and Parenteral Therapies/Expected Effects/Outcomes

37. CORRECT ANSWERS: 2, 4, 5. **Answer 1** is incorrect because epinephrine is the first line of treatment for an *allergic* reaction. This client is experiencing a *hemolytic* reaction. Epinephrine blocks the effects of the histamine released during an allergic reaction. **Answer 2 is correct because the client is experiencing hemolytic shock and sodium bicarbonate will be needed to reverse metabolic acidosis.** **Answer 3** is incorrect because theophylline is a bronchodilator, and would improve wheezing, but it would *not reverse* the antibody effects and the potential for shock, which is causing the signs and symptoms. **Answer 4 is correct because hydrocortisone will be given to control the effects of the antigen-antibody reaction that has occurred from apparent ABO incompatibility. Answer 5 is correct because this client is experiencing a hemolytic reaction that can progress to septic shock. A vasopressor will be needed to maintain the blood pressure.**

■ **TEST-TAKING TIP:** *Recognize the difference between a hemolytic reaction (ABO incompatibility) and an allergic reaction to the donor protein (likely a hereditary component to this reaction).*

Content Area: Adult Health, Pharmacology; *Integrated Process:* Nursing Process, Implementation; *Cognitive Level:* Application; *Client Need/Subneed:* Physiological Integrity/ Pharmacological and Parenteral Therapies/Blood and Blood Products

38. CORRECT ANSWER: 1. Answer 1 is correct because 400 to 800 IU of vitamin D is needed a day for proper absorption and metabolism of calcium. **Answer 2** is incorrect because calcium citrate can be taken *anytime.* **Answer 3** is incorrect because calcium carbonate should be taken with *food.* **Answer 4** is incorrect because calcium is frequently taken in *divided* doses.

■ **TEST-TAKING TIP:** *Choose the answer that is different from the others. Three options deal with the time that calcium is taken.*

Content Area: Adult Health, Musculoskeletal; *Integrated Process:* Teaching and Learning; *Cognitive Level:* Application; *Client Need/Subneed:* Physiological Integrity/Pharmacological and Parenteral Therapies/Medication Administration

39. CORRECT ANSWER: 1. Answer 1 is correct because over-the-counter artificial tears are effective for dry eyes initially. **Answer 2** is incorrect because conservative treatment, such as artificial tears, is indicated before use of a prescriptive treatment to increase tear production and reduce inflammation. **Answer 3** is incorrect because this would slow the rate of tear drainage and more tears would stay on the eyes. **Answer 4** is incorrect because pilocarpine drops are ordered to treat dry *mouth, not* dry eyes.

■ **TEST-TAKING TIP:** *Think conservative treatment initially.*

Content Area: Adult Health, Sensory; *Integrated Process:* Nursing Process, Implementation; *Cognitive Level:* Application; *Client Need/Subneed:* Physiological Integrity/Pharmacological and Parenteral Therapies/Expected Effects/Outcomes

40. CORRECT ANSWER: 180. This is a three-step problem. First, calculate the ordered dose. Second, convert milligrams to micrograms. Third, calculate the flow rate.

1. **4 mcg/min × 75 kg = 300 mcg/min**
2. **50 mg × 1,000 mcg = 50,000 mcg**
3. **50,000 mcg divided by 500 mL = 100 mcg/mL; then**

$$\frac{300 \text{ mcg/min}}{100 \text{ mcg/mL}} = 3 \text{ mL/min} \times 60 \text{ min} = 180 \text{ mL/hr}$$

■ **TEST-TAKING TIP:** *Don't forget to convert mg to mcg.*

Content Area: Adult Health, Pharmacology; *Integrated Process:* Nursing Process, Implementation; *Cognitive Level:* Analysis; *Client Need/Subneed:* Physiological Integrity/Pharmacological and Parenteral Therapies/Dosage Calculation

41. CORRECT ANSWERS: 1, 4. Answer 1 is correct because the client's head is elevated, which prevents the analgesia from affecting the respiratory muscles. **Answer 2** is incorrect because the client's head needs to be elevated, *not* flat, to prevent the drug from affecting the respiratory muscles. **Answer 3** is incorrect because the client's head needs to be elevated, *not* flat, to prevent the drug from affecting the respiratory muscles. **Answer 4 is correct because head elevation prevents migration of the drug toward the respiratory muscles.** **Answer 5** is incorrect because the client's head needs to be *elevated* and *not* face down, to prevent the drug from affecting the respiratory muscles.

■ **TEST-TAKING TIP:** *Eliminate the two answers with "flat." Picture "prone" and eliminate Answer 5. Choose the two answers that maximize analgesia without affecting the respiratory muscles.*

Content Area: Adult Health, Pain Control; *Integrated Process:* Nursing Process, Implementation; *Cognitive Level:* Application; *Client Need/Subneed:* Physiological Integrity/Pharmacological and Parenteral Therapies/Pharmacological Pain Management

42. CORRECT ANSWER: 200. The solution contains the prescribed dose. Infuse the 100 mL at a rate of 200 mL/hr and the drug will be received in 30 minutes as ordered.

■ **TEST-TAKING TIP:** *To calculate the flow rate, double the volume in order to infuse in half the time.*

Content Area: Adult Health, Pharmacology; *Integrated Process:* Nursing Process, Analysis; *Cognitive Level:* Application; *Client Need/Subneed:* Physiological Integrity/Pharmacological and Parenteral Therapies/Dosage Calculation

43. CORRECT ANSWERS: 1, 5. Answer 1 is correct because these are local signs of tissue damage from infiltration of a vesicant, which causes blistering or necrosis with infiltration. **Answer 2** is incorrect because IV push *increases* the chance of infiltration. Nonvesicants, which may cause little to no irritation if infiltration occurs, are given safely by IV push. **Answer 3** is incorrect because *not all* vesicants are cardiotoxic. **Answer 4** is incorrect because ice or a cold pack should *not* be used with vinca alkaloids. **Answer 5 is correct because heat is specifically recommended to prevent ulceration with vincristine or vinblastine if extravasation of the drug occurs.**

■ TEST-TAKING TIP: *"Assess" and "heat" are the best answers.*

Content Area: Adult Health, Oncological; *Integrated Process:* Nursing Process, Assessment; *Cognitive Level:* Application; *Client Need/Subneed:* Physiological Integrity/Pharmacological and Parenteral Therapies/Medication Administration

44. CORRECT ANSWER: 25. Calculate the rate using the following formula:

$$\frac{\text{Desired amount}}{\text{Available amount}} \times \text{Quantity available} = x$$

$$\frac{5 \text{ units}}{100 \text{ units}} \times \frac{500 \text{ mL}}{1} = \frac{2500x}{100} = 25$$

■ TEST-TAKING TIP: *Memorize the formula to solve for mL/hr.*

Content Area: Adult Health, Pharmacology; *Integrated Process:* Nursing Process, Analysis; *Cognitive Level:* Application; *Client Need/Subneed:* Physiological Integrity/Pharmacological and Parenteral Therapies/Dosage Calculation

45. CORRECT ANSWER: 200. The solution contains the prescribed dose. Simply calculate the infusion rate. Since 15 minutes is one fourth of an hour, multiply the volume times 4.

■ TEST-TAKING TIP: *No formula is needed. Don't make this question more difficult.*

Content Area: Adult Health, Pharmacology; *Integrated Process:* Nursing Process, Analysis; *Cognitive Level:* Application; *Client Need/Subneed:* Physiological Integrity/Pharmacological and Parenteral Therapies/Dosage Calculation

46. CORRECT ANSWER: 5.

Step 1: Convert the lb to kg: 110 lb × 1 kg/2.2 lb = 50 kg

Step 2: Calculate drug delivery rate for this client, who weighs 50 kg:

0.01 mcg/kg/min × 50 kg = 0.5 mcg/min

Step 3: Calculate volume delivery:

$$\frac{x \text{ mL}}{\text{hr}} = \frac{250 \text{ mL}}{1.5 \text{ mg}} \times \frac{1 \text{ mg}}{1000 \text{ mcg}} \times \frac{0.5 \text{ mcg}}{\text{min}} = \frac{60 \text{ min}}{1 \text{ hr}} = 5 \text{ mL/hr}$$

■ TEST-TAKING TIP: *Use dimensional analysis to solve for* x.

Content Area: Adult Health, Pharmacology; *Integrated Process:* Nursing Process, Analysis; *Cognitive Level:* Analysis; *Client Need/Subneed:* Physiological Integrity/Pharmacological and Parenteral Therapies/Dosage Calculation

47. CORRECT ANSWER: 24. Calculate the rate using the following formula:

$$\frac{\text{mL}}{\text{hr}} = \frac{100 \text{ mL}}{50 \text{ units}} \times \frac{12 \text{ units}}{1 \text{ hour}} \times 24 \text{ mL/hr}$$

■ TEST-TAKING TIP: *Use the correct formula to compute the rate.*

Content Area: Adult Health, Pharmacology; *Integrated Process:* Nursing Process, Analysis; *Cognitive Level:* Analysis; *Client Need/Subneed:* Physiological Integrity/Pharmacological and Parenteral Therapies/Dosage Calculation

48. CORRECT ANSWER: 167. Calculate the rate using the following formula:

$$\frac{\text{gtt}}{\text{min}} = \frac{10 \text{ gtt}}{\text{mL}} \times \frac{500 \text{ mL}}{30 \text{ min}} = \frac{5000 \text{ gtt}}{30 \text{ min}} = 166.6 \text{ or } 167 \text{ gtt/min}$$

■ TEST-TAKING TIP: *Use a ratio formula when calculating.*

Content Area: Adult Health, Pharmacology; *Integrated Process:* Nursing Process, Analysis; *Cognitive Level:* Analysis; *Client Need/Subneed:* Physiological Integrity/Pharmacological and Parenteral Therapies/Dosage Calculation

49. CORRECT ANSWER: 2, 3, 4. Answer 1 is incorrect because Synthroid would be ordered for *hypo*thyroidism. **Answer 2 is correct because radioactive iodine is an appropriate drug treatment for hyperthyroidism. Answer 3 is correct because PTU is used in the treatment of hyperthyroidism. Answer 4 is correct because Tapazole is an appropriate drug for the treatment of hyperthyroidism.** Answer 5 is incorrect because Cytomel is used in the treatment of *hypo*thyroidism.

■ TEST-TAKING TIP: *The symptoms are for* hyper*thyroidism. Therefore, eliminate the drugs that appear to include a thyroid* replacement*—"thyro" in the name.*

Content Area: Adult Health, Endocrine; *Integrated Process:* Nursing Process, Analysis; *Cognitive Level:* Analysis; *Client Need/Subneed:* Physiological Integrity/Pharmacological and Parenteral Therapies/Expected Effects/Outcomes

50. CORRECT ANSWER: 2. Answer 1 is incorrect because NPH is an intermediate-acting insulin given *subcutaneously.* **Answer 2 is correct because regular insulin is the only form of insulin that can be given IV.** Answer 3 is incorrect because Lantus is a long-acting insulin. It should be used to maintain a normal blood sugar, and is given *subcutaneously.* Answer 4 is incorrect because Lispro, a rapid-acting insulin, *cannot* be given IV.

■ TEST-TAKING TIP: *The stem asks for IV administration.* ***Only regular insulin can be given both IV and subcutaneously.***

Content Area: Adult Health, Endocrine; *Integrated Process:* Nursing Process, Implementation; *Cognitive Level:* Application; *Client Need/Subneed:* Physiological Integrity/Pharmacological and Parenteral Therapies/Expected Effects/Outcomes

51. CORRECT ANSWER: 3. Answer 1 is incorrect because regular insulin *is* safe to mix with NPH. Answer 2 is incorrect because NPH *is* safe to mix with Humulin-N, another name for NPH or Lente insulin. **Answer 3 is correct because, when Lantus is mixed with other insulins, it is rendered useless. Lantus is a long-acting insulin with no peak.** Answer 4 is incorrect because Humulin-R *is* safe to mix with Lente (or NPH).

■ TEST-TAKING TIP: *Select the option that includes Lantus, which is not in any other option.*

Content Area: Adult Health, Endocrine; *Integrated Process:* Nursing Process, Analysis; *Cognitive Level:* Application; *Client Need/Subneed:* Physiological Integrity/Pharmacological and Parenteral Therapies/Adverse Effects/Contraindications/Interactions

52. CORRECT ANSWER: 1. **Answer 1 is correct because Lispro is a rapid-acting insulin and should always be drawn up first, to avoid contaminating the bottle of the fast-acting insulin with intermediate- or slow-acting insulin.** **Answer 2** is incorrect because NPH could contaminate the Lispro. **Answer 3** is incorrect because Lantus should *never* be mixed. It is rendered useless when mixed. **Answer 4** is incorrect because Novolin 70/30 is a mixture of long lasting (70 units) with rapid (30 units); therefore, further mixings should be questioned.

■ TEST-TAKING TIP: ***It is more important to remember to draw the rapid-acting insulin first, rather than remembering "clear to cloudy."***

Content Area: Adult Health, Endocrine; ***Integrated Process:*** Nursing Process, Implementation; ***Cognitive Level:*** Application; ***Client Need/Subneed:*** Physiological Integrity/Pharmacological and Parenteral Therapies/Medication Administration

53. CORRECT ANSWER: 1. **Answer 1 is correct because, following the first dose, a second or third dose can be given in 5-minute intervals.** **Answer 2** is incorrect because, if the pain is due to angina, the greatest effect occurs with 5-minute intervals. **Answer 3** is incorrect because waiting *too long* may result in *ischemic damage.* **Answer 4** is incorrect because *repeated* doses in a *shorter* period of time are needed to determine the cause of the chest pain.

■ TEST-TAKING TIP: ***Remember: the maximum effect of nitroglycerin is achieved in 5 minutes . . . "take five."***

Content Area: Adult Health, Cardiovascular; ***Integrated Process:*** Nursing Process, Planning; ***Cognitive Level:*** Comprehension; ***Client Need/Subneed:*** Physiological Integrity/Pharmacological and Parenteral Therapies/Medication Administration

54. CORRECT ANSWER: 4. **Answer 1** is incorrect because the head of the bed should be *elevated,* not flat, to prevent aspiration. **Answer 2** is incorrect because the feeding should be given *slowly* to prevent diarrhea and vomiting. **Answer 3** is incorrect because the feeding should be warm. Also, clients cannot "taste" the feedings; improving taste is not a concern. **Answer 4 is correct because giving the feeding too fast could upset the client's stomach and cause diarrhea.**

■ TEST-TAKING TIP: ***Choose an option that minimizes vomiting and aspiration.***

Content Area: Adult Health, Gastrointestinal; ***Integrated Process:*** Nursing Process, Implementation; ***Cognitive Level:*** Application; ***Client Need/Subneed:*** Physiological Integrity/Pharmacological and Parenteral Therapies/Total Parenteral Nutrition

55. CORRECT ANSWER: 3. **Answer 1** is incorrect because furosemide *lowers* blood pressure, not elevates. **Answer 2** is incorrect because furosemide does *not usually* cause tachycardia; however, the heart rate might increase if too much fluid is removed. **Answer 3 is correct because the drug is a diuretic and there should be an increase in frequency and volume of urine if furosemide is working.** **Answer 4** is incorrect because the client needs to be told that, if the drug is taken near bedtime, the increased need to urinate will disrupt sleep.

■ TEST-TAKING TIP: ***The question is asking for the* desired *effect of a diuretic—look for a description that shows fluid is being removed (i.e., excreted).***

Content Area: Adult Health, Renal; ***Integrated Process:*** Nursing Process, Implementation; ***Cognitive Level:*** Application; ***Client Need/Subneed:*** Physiological Integrity/Pharmacological and Parenteral Therapies/Expected Effects/Outcomes

56. CORRECT ANSWER: 3. **Answer 1** is incorrect because a client's temperature has *nothing* to do with giving a beta blocker. **Answer 2** is incorrect because there are *no required* positions for ingestion. The client chooses a position that facilitates swallowing. **Answer 3 is correct because a beta blocker can decrease blood pressure and heart rate to unsafe levels.** **Answer 4** is incorrect because the client may *not be aware* of the effects of the drug on heart rate and blood pressure. Also, the nurse needs *objective* data to assess the response, not subjective data.

■ TEST-TAKING TIP: ***Ask yourself: Which vital sign is most relevant to the drug's antihypertensive effect, BP or temperature?***

Content Area: Adult Health, Cardiovascular; ***Integrated Process:*** Nursing Process, Implementation; ***Cognitive Level:*** Application; ***Client Need/Subneed:*** Physiological Integrity/Pharmacological and Parenteral Therapies/Medication Administration

57. CORRECT ANSWER: 2. **Answer 1** is incorrect because the increase in vascular volume might result in hemo*dilution* of sodium, not excess. **Answer 2 is correct because TPN is a high-glucose and hyperosmolar solution that would result in increased vascular volume.** **Answer 3** is incorrect because the blood glucose level and blood pressure would *increase* with rapid infusion, not decrease. **Answer 4** is incorrect because an increase in blood pressure and hyperglycemia would occur *before* hyperkalemia and heart failure.

■ TEST-TAKING TIP: ***Focus on two contradictory options: ↑ BP and hyperglycemia vs. ↓ BP and hypoglycemia. Think "too fast" → "too high."***

Content Area: Adult Health, Total Parenteral Nutrition; ***Integrated Process:*** Nursing Process, Analysis; ***Cognitive Level:*** Application; ***Client Need/Subneed:*** Physiological Integrity/Pharmacological and Parenteral Therapies/Total Parenteral Nutrition

58. CORRECT ANSWER: 3. **Answer 1** is incorrect because Lomotil, an opioid, is used to *control diarrhea.* **Answer 2** is incorrect because constipation and urinary retention *are* common with morphine. **Answer 3 is correct because meperidine produces *less* constipation. However, all opioids used in the management of pain can cause constipation.** **Answer 4** is incorrect because fentanyl *does* cause constipation. This drug is usually reserved for anesthesia or cancer-related pain.

■ TEST-TAKING TIP: ***Look at the two frequently used opioid analgesics (morphine and meperidine). Select the option that has fewer GI problems.***

Content Area: Geriatrics, Pain Control; ***Integrated Process:*** Nursing Process, Implementation; ***Cognitive Level:*** Application; ***Client Need/Subneed:*** Physiological Integrity/Pharmacological and Parenteral Therapies/Adverse Effects/Contraindications/ Interactions

59. CORRECT ANSWER: 2. **Answer 1** is incorrect because blood pressure and pulse should *decrease* since MS is a vasodilator. **Answer 2 is correct because, without any further client information, this is an appropriate dosage for relief of moderate pain.** **Answer 3** is incorrect because the dose *is* sufficient for a client whose weight is 154 lb. **Answer 4** is incorrect because the pain relief should be near *4* hours.

■ TEST-TAKING TIP: *Focus on two options with a time frame. Select the option with the longer lasting effect when the pain is moderate.*

Content Area: Adult Health, Pain Control; ***Integrated Process:*** Nursing Process, Analysis; ***Cognitive Level:*** Application; ***Client Need/Subneed:*** Physiological Integrity/Pharmacological and Parenteral Therapies/Expected Effects/Outcomes

60. CORRECT ANSWER: 3. **Answer 1** is incorrect because increasing the dosage to compensate for the poor perfusion would be *unsafe.* There would be an increased risk of side effects with a larger dose. **Answer 2** is incorrect because these are enzymes that are *cardiac specific* and that do not increase from other causes of muscle trauma such as injections. **Answer 3 is correct because drug effectiveness would be less predictable with the change in perfusion.** **Answer 4** is incorrect because anticoagulant therapy does *not prevent* the use of IM injections.

■ TEST-TAKING TIP: *Look for the answer that refers to tissue perfusion after an MI. Remember: tissue perfusion is* needed *for drug absorption with the IM route.*

Content Area: Adult Health, Cardiovascular; ***Integrated Process:*** Teaching and Learning; ***Cognitive Level:*** Application; ***Client Need/Subneed:*** Physiological Integrity/Pharmacological and Parenteral Therapies/Medication Administration

61. CORRECT ANSWER: 2. **Answer 1** is incorrect because effects of the drug may *increase* with liver damage because the liver is responsible for detoxification of drugs. **Answer 2 is correct because the client will likely need a higher dose because alcohol is a CNS depressant. The client will have developed a drug tolerance to a standard does of pain medication.** **Answer 3** is incorrect because the dosage should be *lowered* if there is liver damage, where there would be *impaired* ability of the liver to detoxify medications. **Answer 4** is incorrect because the client will likely have a *decreased* sensitivity that requires a higher dosage.

■ TEST-TAKING TIP: *Eliminate the two answers that focus on the liver (Answers 1 and 3). The reason for a higher dose is because alcohol depresses the normal nervous system response to pain.*

Content Area: Adult Health, Pain Control; ***Integrated Process:*** Nursing Process, Analysis; ***Cognitive Level:*** Application; ***Client Need/Subneed:*** Physiological Integrity/Pharmacological and Parenteral Therapies/Pharmacological Pain Management

62. CORRECT ANSWER: 1. **Answer 1 is correct because blood volume increases by 30% to 50% in pregnancy. This causes hemodilution of RBCs and physiological anemia. Normal hemoglobin levels in pregnancy range from 11 to 12 gm/dL.** **Answer 2** is incorrect because plethora (hemoglobin >15.5 gm/dL for women) is *not a normal* finding in pregnancy. **Answer 3** is incorrect because normal fasting serum glucose in pregnancy is *less* than 95 mg/dL. **Answer 4** is incorrect because a normal WBC for first trimester pregnancy is 6,600 to 14,100/mL.

■ TEST-TAKING TIP: *This question asks to identify the normal value for the first trimester of pregnancy. Know that laboratory values change during pregnancy.*

Content Area: Maternity, Antepartum; ***Integrated Process:*** Nursing Process, Analysis; ***Cognitive Level:*** Application; ***Client Need/Subneed:*** Physiological Integrity/Reduction of Risk Potential/Laboratory Values

63. CORRECT ANSWER: 2. **Answer 1** is incorrect because decreased urinary output is *not* an *expected* side effect of magnesium sulfate; it is an indicator of *worsening* preeclampsia. **Answer 2 is correct because hypersomnolence (excessive sleepiness) is an expected side effect not associated with magnesium toxicity, an unexpected side effect related to a high serum level.** **Answer 3** is incorrect because the absence of knee jerk reflex is a symptom of magnesium *toxicity.* **Answer 4** is incorrect because decreased respiratory rate is a symptom of magnesium *toxicity.*

■ TEST-TAKING TIP: *This question is asking for the* expected *side effect of magnesium sulfate administration. Eliminate the answers that are indicative of magnesium* toxicity.

Content Area: Maternity, Intrapartum; ***Integrated Process:*** Nursing Process, Assessment; ***Cognitive Level:*** Application; ***Client Need/Subneed:*** Physiological Integrity/Pharmacological and Parenteral Therapies/Expected Effects/Outcomes

64. CORRECT ANSWER: 4. **Answer 1** is incorrect because the side effect from epidural anesthesia that the nurse needs to monitor is *hypotension.* Cervical dilation is an assessment that is *common to all* clients in labor. **Answer 2** is incorrect because placing the client in a supine position will *worsen* the hypotension. **Answer 3** is incorrect because obtaining a fetal heart rate is a *common* assessment to all clients in labor, and does not address the *specific* side effect of epidural anesthesia. **Answer 4 is correct because checking the client's blood pressure is most important with epidural anesthesia.**

■ TEST-TAKING TIP: *This question is asking about a side effect that is common in epidural anesthesia. Regular assessments of cervical dilation and fetal heart rate are common to* all clients *in labor and do not address the* specific *condition in the question.*

Content Area: Maternity, Intrapartum; ***Integrated Process:*** Nursing Process, Assessment; ***Cognitive Level:*** Application; ***Client Need/Subneed:*** Physiological Integrity/Pharmacological and Parenteral Therapies/Pharmacological Pain Management

65. CORRECT ANSWER: 4. Answer 1 is incorrect because maternal hypoglycemia is *unrelated* to the administration of oxytocin, either for induction of labor or for use after delivery. **Answer 2** is incorrect because fetal movement is a *general* assessment for *all clients* in labor; it is not specific to the administration of oxytocin. **Answer 3** is incorrect because maternal hyperreflexia is an assessment specifically for a client with *preeclampsia, not* Pitocin induction. **Answer 4 is correct because oxytocin administration can be associated with tetanic contractions and inadequate resting period between contractions, resulting in fetal bradycardia.**

■ **TEST-TAKING TIP:** *Look for an assessment specific to the side effects of oxytocin induction, not general assessments or assessment of a condition that the client does not have. The effect on the fetus (Answer 4) is most significant for the nurse to monitor.*

Content Area: Maternity, Intrapartum; ***Integrated Process:*** Nursing Process, Assessment; ***Cognitive Level:*** Application; ***Client Need/Subneed:*** Physiological Integrity/Pharmacological and Parenteral Therapies/Adverse Effects/Contraindications/Interactions

66. CORRECT ANSWER: 4. Answer 1 is incorrect because magnesium sulfate is a treatment for *preterm* labor and *preeclampsia;* it is *not* a treatment to induce labor. **Answer 2** is incorrect because Clomid is a treatment to induce *ovulation, not delivery.* **Answer 3** is incorrect because calcium gluconate is an *antidote* for *magnesium toxicity, not* a treatment for inducing labor. **Answer 4 is correct because this client has a fetus that has died. Cytotec is an appropriate treatment for inducing delivery of a fetal demise.**

■ **TEST-TAKING TIP:** *The question is asking how to induce delivery in a client with a fetal demise or a missed abortion. Eliminate the drugs that do not induce labor.*

Content Area: Maternity, Intrapartum; ***Integrated Process:*** Nursing Process, Planning; ***Cognitive Level:*** Application; ***Client Need/Subneed:*** Physiological Integrity/Pharmacological and Parenteral Therapies/Expected Effects/Outcomes

67. CORRECT ANSWER: 2. Answer 1 is incorrect because the assessment is *normal* for this client; there is no reason to decrease the infusion. Decreasing the magnesium level may put the client at risk for eclampsia. **Answer 2 is correct because the assessment findings are *normal* for this client; continuing the infusion *is* the *appropriate* action for the nurse. Answer 3** is incorrect because the assessment is *normal* for this client; there is no reason to stop the infusion. Decreasing the magnesium level may put the client at risk for eclampsia. **Answer 4** is incorrect because the assessment is *normal* for this client; there is no reason to administer an antidote to the client. Decreasing the magnesium level may put the client at risk for eclampsia.

■ **TEST-TAKING TIP:** *This question is asking if the client is having symptoms consistent with magnesium toxicity. Since the client has a normal assessment, there is no need for intervention.*

Content Area: Maternity, Antepartum; ***Integrated Process:*** Nursing Process, Implementation; ***Cognitive Level:*** Application; ***Client Need/Subneed:*** Physiological Integrity/Pharmacological and Parenteral Therapies/Expected Effects/Outcomes

68. CORRECT ANSWER: 3. Answer 1 is incorrect because treatment of pain *is* a *priority* and will not interfere with the ability to diagnose a fracture of back or limb. **Answer 2** is incorrect because the pain needs to be relieved, *not* minimized. **Answer 3 is correct because pain needs to be treated immediately and maximally, to avoid potential complications such as shock. Answer 4** is incorrect because this analgesic choice will *not* relieve *severe* pain.

■ **TEST-TAKING TIP:** *Relief of pain is a priority. Unrelieved pain can cause shock.*

Content Area: Adult Health, Pain Control; ***Integrated Process:*** Nursing Process, Implementation; ***Cognitive Level:*** Application; ***Client Need/Subneed:*** Physiological Integrity/Pharmacological and Parenteral Therapies/Pharmacological Pain Management

69. CORRECT ANSWER: 2. Answer 1 is incorrect because, while a specific client may have concerns about becoming addicted to opioids, it is more often physicians who are concerned about abuse. **Answer 2 is correct because physicians often undermedicate clients because of fear that the client is abusing a narcotic opioid. Answer 3** is incorrect because the *side effects can be managed* if they occur. **Answer 4** is incorrect because there *are* accurate assessment tools.

■ **TEST-TAKING TIP:** *Choose the option that is the greatest barrier . . . staff's concern.*

Content Area: Adult Health, Pain Control; ***Integrated Process:*** Nursing Process, Analysis; ***Cognitive Level:*** Application; ***Client Need/Subneed:*** Physiological Integrity/Pharmacological and Parenteral Therapies/Pharmacological Pain Management

70. CORRECT ANSWER: 90. Calculate the delivery rate using the following formula:

$$\frac{1000\ \text{mcg}}{1\ \text{mg}} \times \frac{50\ \text{mg}}{250\ \text{mL}} \times \frac{27\ \text{mL}}{1\ \text{hr}} \times \frac{1\ \text{hour}}{60\ \text{min}} = 90\ \text{mcg/min}$$

■ **TEST-TAKING TIP:** *First, convert mg to mcg, then use the formula.*

Content Area: Adult Health, Pharmacology; ***Integrated Process:*** Nursing Process, Analysis; ***Cognitive Level:*** Analysis; ***Client Need/Subneed:*** Physiological Integrity/Pharmacological and Parenteral Therapies/Dosage Calculation

71. CORRECT ANSWER: 1. Answer 1 is correct because it is the only one that fits all four symptoms. Answer 2 is incorrect because with phlebitis the skin would be *warm* and *red.* **Answer 3** is incorrect because sepsis is a *systemic* problem, *not* a *localized* complication. **Answer 4** is incorrect because an allergic response is *usually* systemic, or if localized, it would produce *redness.*

■ TEST-TAKING TIP: *What would be the expected* **color** *and* **skin temperature** *for each option? Only one of the options would be cool and pale.*

Content Area: Adult Health, Integumentary; *Integrated Process:* Nursing Process, Analysis; *Cognitive Level:* Application; *Client Need/Subneed:* Physiological Integrity/Pharmacological and Parenteral Therapies/Adverse Effects/Contraindications/Interactions

72. CORRECT ANSWER: 2. **Answer 1** is incorrect because older adults usually require *lower* dosages. **Answer 2 is correct because changes in kidney and/or liver function will affect excretion of drugs. The chance of toxicity increases.** **Answer 3** is incorrect because liver impairment would result in a *greater risk* of toxicity from too high of a dosage. **Answer 4** is incorrect because the monitoring should be for *clinical effectiveness, not* for *reduced* effectiveness.

■ TEST-TAKING TIP: *Remember: older adults are more sensitive to drug effects; therefore, eliminate Answers 1 and 3.*

Content Area: Geriatrics, Aging Process; *Integrated Process:* Nursing Process, Analysis; *Cognitive Level:* Application; *Client Need/Subneed:* Physiological Integrity/Pharmacological and Parenteral Therapies/Medication Administration

73. CORRECT ANSWER: 3. **Answer 1** is incorrect because *oral* medications may be taken because of the *type* of anesthesia used for the surgery. **Answer 2** is incorrect because this is not an accurate statement. Nothing has affected absorption yet. **Answer 3 is correct because antihypertensive medications may still be given because the procedure is usually done by using local, spinal, or epidural anesthesia.** **Answer 4** is incorrect because IV drugs would *only* be given for an *emergency.*

■ TEST-TAKING TIP: *Consider the type of surgery (GI) and the anesthesia (not general). Eliminate the two options with "no medications . . . by mouth" and "not . . . anything by mouth."*

Content Area: Adult Health, Gastrointestinal; *Integrated Process:* Nursing Process, Implementation; *Cognitive Level:* Application; *Client Need/Subneed:* Physiological Integrity/Pharmacological and Parenteral Therapies/Medication Administration

74. CORRECT ANSWER: 1. **Answer 1 is correct because rifampin changes tears, sweat, saliva, and urine to an *orange-red color.* This is an expected effect.** **Answer 2** is incorrect because this response does *not explain* the cause *or address* the client's worry. **Answer 3** is incorrect because this color change is *normal.* **Answer 4** is incorrect because this change does *not* indicate a urinary tract *infection.*

■ TEST-TAKING TIP: *Eliminate the trite reassurance response (Answer 2), and the other two answers that relate to possible problems (Answers 3 and 4). Select the answer about an expected effect.*

Content Area: Adult Health, Infectious Disease; *Integrated Process:* Teaching and Learning; *Cognitive Level:* Application; *Client Need/Subneed:* Physiological Integrity/Pharmacological and Parenteral Therapies/Expected Effects/Outcomes

75. CORRECT ANSWER: 3. **Answer 1** is incorrect because a corticosteroid is *not* given to improve circulation. **Answer 2** is incorrect because albuterol, *not* a corticosteroid, is administered to cause bronchodilation during asthma attacks. **Answer 3 is correct because corticosteroids are used in the treatment of acute asthma exacerbation to reduce inflammation of the airways.** **Answer 4** is incorrect because a corticosteroid is given to reduce inflammation, *not* thin secretions.

■ TEST-TAKING TIP: *Corticosteroids are used in the treatment of many diseases; do not let the diagnosis of asthma fool you into choosing the answer option that is specific to the lungs. Two of the answer options are specific to respiration and can be eliminated; only one option has a general action—"reduce inflammation"—which is the best response.*

Content Area: Child Health, Respiratory; *Integrated Process:* Nursing Process, Planning; *Cognitive Level:* Analysis; *Client Need/Subneed:* Physiological Integrity/Pharmacological and Parenteral Therapies/Expected Effects/Outcomes

76. CORRECT ANSWER: 1. **Answer 1 is correct because the nurse should question an order to administer an IV solution containing potassium to a child who is anuric. Potassium should not be added to a child's IV until kidney function is established by the return of urine output.** **Answer 2** is incorrect because this would be an *acceptable* order for continuous IV fluids. **Answer 3** is incorrect because this would be an *acceptable* order for continuous IV fluids. **Answer 4** is incorrect because this would be an *acceptable* order for continuous IV fluids.

■ TEST-TAKING TIP: *Look for the answer that is different from the group. Answer 1 is the only one containing potassium.*

Content Area: Child Health, Gastrointestinal; *Integrated Process:* Nursing Process, Analysis; *Cognitive Level:* Analysis; *Client Need/Subneed:* Physiological Integrity/Pharmacological and Parenteral Therapies/Parenteral/Intravenous Therapies

77. CORRECT ANSWER: 300. **To arrive at the correct answer, first recall that microdrip tubing has a drip rate of 60 mL/min. Next, multiply the volume to be infused by the drop factor (300 × 60) to arrive at 18,000. Then, divide this answer by the infusion time (18,000/60) to arrive at the correct response of 300 drops per minute.**

■ TEST-TAKING TIP: *Determine the infusion time in* **minute** *rather than* **hour** *increments to arrive at the correct response.*

Content Area: Child Health, Pharmacology; *Integrated Process:* Nursing Process, Implementation; *Cognitive Level:* Analysis; *Client Need/Subneed:* Physiological Integrity/Pharmacological and Parenteral Therapies/Dosage Calculation

78. CORRECT ANSWERS: 2, 3, 4, 5. **Answer 1** is incorrect because iron supplementation is typically not prescribed for children with sickle cell anemia, because there already is a risk of excess iron in the blood. **Answer 2 is correct because children with sickle cell anemia frequently take prophylactic antibiotics because of an increased risk for infection. Answer 3 is correct because these children may take NSAIDs for pain relief. Answer 4 is correct because folic acid is commonly prescribed to assist in the production of healthy red blood cells. Answer 5 is correct because these children are at risk for iron overload and are commonly prescribed chelation agents such as Desferal.**

■ TEST-TAKING TIP: *Recall that children who are likely to receive multiple blood transfusions (as in sickle cell anemia) are at risk for hemosiderosis, or iron overload. Select the options that will not worsen this condition.*

Content Area: Child Health, Hematological; *Integrated Process:* Nursing Process, Analysis; *Cognitive Level:* Analysis; *Client Need/Subneed:* Physiological Integrity/Pharmacological and Parenteral Therapies/Medication Administration

79. CORRECT ANSWER: 39. **To solve this calculation, first determine how many mL of morphine has been administered over the past 4 hours. The child has self-administered 7 boluses of 1 mg each. If the syringe has a concentration of 1 mg/1 mL, the child has received 7 mL. The basal rate is 1 mg/hr; 4 hours at this rate is equal to 4 mL. Add the self-administered doses to the basal rate to get a total of 11 mL administered in 4 hours. Finally, subtract 11 mL from the 50-mL syringe starting volume to arrive at the correct response of 39 mL left in the syringe after 4 hours.**

■ TEST-TAKING TIP: *Do not be confused by extra information in pharmacology questions. For this item, the information states the child can only self-administer up to 4 boluses per hour. This information is not to be considered; no information is given regarding the number of boluses the child administered in a single hour—only the total amount for a 4-hour period.*

Content Area: Child Health, Pharmacology; *Integrated Process:* Nursing Process, Analysis; *Cognitive Level:* Analysis; *Client Need/Subneed:* Physiological Integrity/Pharmacological and Parenteral Therapies/Dosage Calculation

80. CORRECT ANSWER: 200. **First, determine the child's weight in kilograms by taking 44 and dividing by 2.2 to arrive at a weight of 20 kilograms. Then, determine the total amount of fluid to be administered by multiplying 20 kg by 20 mL/kg to arrive at 400 mL. If the 400 mL is to be delivered over 2 hours, divide 400 mL by 2 to arrive at a rate of 200 mL/hr.**

■ TEST-TAKING TIP: *Always perform medication calculations twice, especially when caring for children.*

Content Area: Child Health, Pharmacology; *Integrated Process:* Nursing Process, Implementation; *Cognitive Level:* Analysis; *Client Need/Subneed:* Physiological Integrity/Pharmacological and Parenteral Therapies/Dosage Calculation

81. CORRECT ANSWER: 3. **Answer 1** is incorrect because decreased deep tendon reflexes are a side effect of *magnesium sulfate* therapy. **Answer 2** is incorrect because bradycardia is *not* a common side effect of a calcium channel blocker, such as nifedipine. **Answer 3 is correct because nifedipine is a calcium channel blocker, more commonly used to treat high blood pressure and heart disease. Nifedipine blocks the passage of calcium into certain tissues, relaxing the uterine muscles and smooth muscles of blood vessels throughout the body. Use of nifedipine for the treatment of preterm labor is an unlabeled use of the drug. Hypotension is a side effect of nifedipine.** **Answer 4** is incorrect because tachycardia is a side effect of *beta-sympatholytic* medications, such as terbutaline.

■ TEST-TAKING TIP: *All tocolytics are smooth muscle relaxers and act on the smooth muscles throughout the body. None of the tocolytics cause bradycardia; therefore, eliminate Answer 2. Eliminate also two other options that relate to* other *medications: magnesium sulfate (Answer 1) and a beta sympatholytic (Answer 4).*

Content Area: Maternity, Intrapartum; *Integrated Process:* Nursing Process, Assessment; *Cognitive Level:* Application; *Client Need/Subneed:* Physiological Integrity/Pharmacological and Parenteral Therapies/Expected Effects/Outcomes

82. CORRECT ANSWER: 1. **Answer 1 is correct because terbutaline is considered to be working at a therapeutic level when a woman's resting heart rate is between 90 and 105 beats per minute. If the heart rate is higher than 120, the physician should be notified before taking the terbutaline.** **Answer 2** is incorrect because a client should *not be doubling* the dose of terbutaline *without consulting* her physician. Also, the client can have up to 5 contractions per hour; more than 6 contractions per hour is a reason to notify the physician. **Answer 3** is incorrect because *normal* fetal movement is 10 or more movements per hour. There is *no need* to call the physician for normal fetal movement. **Answer 4** is incorrect because clients with preterm labor should be *resting* as much as possible. It is *not appropriate* to instruct a client to increase her activity.

■ TEST-TAKING TIP: *Focus on a side effect of the drug: heart rate.*

Content Area: Maternity, Antepartum; *Integrated Process:* Nursing Process, Implementation; *Cognitive Level:* Application; *Client Need/Subneed:* Physiological Integrity/Pharmacological and Parenteral Therapies/Expected Effects/Outcomes

83. CORRECT ANSWER: 1. **Answer 1 is correct because administering a fluid bolus before beginning the epidural can prevent hypotension that is associated with anesthesia administration.** **Answer 2** is incorrect because administering oxygen can assist in providing additional oxygen to the fetus, but does *not prevent hypotension.* **Answer 3** is incorrect because placing the client in high Fowler's position will *not* prevent hypotension, and may actually decrease the effectiveness of the epidural anesthesia by *decreasing the dermatome level.* **Answer 4** is incorrect because administering epinephrine is not an appropriate prevention measure. It is used to *treat, not prevent,* hypotension.

■ **TEST-TAKING TIP:** *The key word in this question is "prevent." Preventing a side effect is different than treating the condition. An IV fluid bolus prevents hypotension; epinephrine* treats *hypotension after it has developed.*

Content Area: Maternity, Intrapartum; ***Integrated Process:*** Nursing Process, Planning; ***Cognitive Level:*** Application; ***Client Need/Subneed:*** Physiological Integrity/Pharmacological and Parenteral Therapies/Expected Effects/Outcomes

84. CORRECT ANSWER: 4. Answer 1 is incorrect because butorphanol tartrate is a pain medication, and does *not* treat the client's condition of magnesium toxicity. **Answer 2** is incorrect because furosemide works by blocking the absorption of salt and fluid in the kidney tubules, causing a profound increase in urine output (diuresis). The diuretic effect of furosemide can cause body water and electrolyte depletion and is *not* used to treat pregnancy-induced hypertension, and does *not* treat magnesium toxicity. **Answer 3** is incorrect because diazepam is used to treat seizures related to eclampsia. Diazepam is *not* used to *reverse* magnesium toxicity. **Answer 4 is correct because this client most likely is experiencing magnesium toxicity. Calcium gluconate is the *antidote* for magnesium overdose.**

■ **TEST-TAKING TIP:** *The key is to recognize that the client is experiencing magnesium toxicity. Do not get distracted by other possible drugs used in treating preeclampsia. Remember that the antidote for magnesium is another electrolyte, calcium.*

Content Area: Maternity, Intrapartum; ***Integrated Process:*** Nursing Process, Analysis; ***Cognitive Level:*** Application; ***Client Need/Subneed:*** Physiological Integrity/Pharmacological and Parenteral Therapies/Medication Administration

85. CORRECT ANSWER: 2. Answer 1 is incorrect because Vasotec is an angiotensin-converting enzyme (ACE) inhibitor. ACE inhibitors are *not* used in pregnancy due to the potential for certain *fetal defects.* **Answer 2 is correct because this client is in the second trimester of pregnancy and has a history of high blood pressure during the pregnancy, an indicator of chronic hypertension. Aldomet is an antihypertensive drug that is safe during pregnancy, and is commonly used for chronic hypertension during pregnancy. Answer 3** is incorrect because diazepam is used to treat *seizures* in eclampsia. This client has chronic *hypertension, not* preeclampsia. **Answer 4** is incorrect because magnesium sulfate is used to *prevent seizures* in eclampsia. This client has chronic *hypertension, not* preeclampsia, and magnesium is *not* an *antihypertensive* agent.

■ **TEST-TAKING TIP:** *This key to this question is that the client has chronic hypertension and is in the second trimester. Preeclampsia generally begins in the* third *trimester with proteinuria and hyperreflexia; this client has* no *proteinuria* or *hyperreflexia.*

Content Area: Maternity, Antepartum, At-risk; ***Integrated Process:*** Nursing Process, Planning; ***Cognitive Level:*** Application; ***Client Need/Subneed:*** Physiological Integrity/Pharmacological and Parenteral Therapies/Expected Effects/Outcomes

86. CORRECT ANSWERS: 3, 5. Answer 1 is incorrect because Hemabate *decreases* uterine atony, by increasing smooth muscle contractions. **Answer 2** is incorrect because Hemabate *increases* uterine contractions, *not* decreases uterine contractions (the process of involution). **Answer 3 is correct because the major action of Hemabate is to increase uterine (myometrial) contractions and decrease uterine bleeding. Answer 4** is incorrect because Hemabate increases smooth muscle contractions, including vascular smooth muscles. Hemabate usually results in an *increase* in blood pressure, *not* a decrease in blood pressure. **Answer 5 is correct because Hemabate causes increased smooth muscle contractions, including gastrointestinal smooth muscle, which can lead to diarrhea.**

■ **TEST-TAKING TIP:** *A memory tip: the name of the medication is "heme" "abate"; "heme" means blood and "abate" means to decrease or reduce. This medication is used to reduce bleeding after delivery.*

Content Area: Maternity, Intrapartum; ***Integrated Process:*** Nursing Process, Analysis; ***Cognitive Level:*** Analysis; ***Client Need/Subneed:*** Physiological Integrity/Pharmacological and Parenteral Therapies/Expected Effects/Outcomes

87. CORRECT ANSWER: 18 mL/hr. The answer is calculated as follows:

20 units/1,000 mL = 0.02 units/mL. This is the concentration of the drug.

A pump rate of 1 mL/hr = 0.02 units/hr.

Pitocin is most commonly expressed as milliunits/minute. Convert 6 milliunits/min to units/min by dividing by 1,000 mL (volume of infusion). The result is 0.006 unit/min. Multiply by 60 minutes = 0.36 units/hr × 0.02 units/hr (amount delivered in 1 mL/hr). Pump would be set to a rate of 18 mL/hr.

■ **TEST-TAKING TIP:** *The initial concentration of oxytocin is in units/mL, which needs to be converted to milliunits/min. Pay attention to the complex conversion from units/mL to milliunits per minute.*

Content Area: Maternity, Intrapartum; ***Integrated Process:*** Nursing Process, Implementation; ***Cognitive Level:*** Application; ***Client Need/Subneed:*** Physiological Integrity/Pharmacological and Parenteral Therapies/Dosage Calculation

88. **CORRECT ANSWERS: 2, 3, 4.** **Answer 1** is incorrect because 3 contractions in a 10-minute window is a *normal* pattern for contractions, and *not* a reason to discontinue the oxytocin infusion. **Answer 2 is correct because contractions that occur every 3 minutes, lasting 90 seconds, do not allow adequate resting time for the uterus, and the oxytocin should be discontinued. Answer 3 is correct because this pattern describes late decelerations, which are a sign of fetal distress, and the oxytocin should be discontinued. Answer 4 is correct because more than 5 contractions in a 10-minute window is hyperstimulation, and the oxytocin should be discontinued.** **Answer 5** is incorrect because being completely dilated is *not* a reason to discontinue the oxytocin infusion. Contractions are still needed for the second stage of labor. Discontinuing the oxytocin may decrease the number of contractions and increase the length of the second stage.

■ **TEST-TAKING TIP:** *Draw out the pattern of contractions described to see if the contractions are too frequent or too long as reasons for stopping the oxytocin.*

Content Area: Maternity, Intrapartum; ***Integrated Process:*** Nursing Process, Evaluation; ***Cognitive Level:*** Analysis; ***Client Need/Subneed:*** Physiological Integrity/Pharmacological and Parenteral Therapies/Adverse Effects/Contraindications/Interactions

89. **CORRECT ANSWER: 1.** **Answer 1 is correct because ibuprofen has a longer duration of action (about 6 hours) than acetaminophen (about 4 hours), which is a distinct advantage for nighttime comfort or when a child is resistant to taking medication. Selecting ibuprofen would require giving fewer doses to the child.** **Answer 2** is incorrect because acetaminophen has a *shorter* duration of action (about 4 hours) than ibuprofen (about 6 hours). This is a distinct disadvantage for nighttime comfort or when a child is resistant to taking medication because acetaminophen would result in giving more doses to the child. **Answer 3** is incorrect because, while codeine is recommended as an analgesic in the treatment of otitis media, it is reserved for *severe* pain rather than the mild pain about which the child is complaining. **Answer 4** is incorrect because, while Dilaudid is used in the pediatric population, it is reserved for the severe pain associated with *cancer* or *major* surgeries.

■ **TEST-TAKING TIP:** ↑ *duration* = ↓ *doses.*

Content Area: Pediatrics, Pharmacology; ***Integrated Process:*** Nursing Process, Implementation; ***Cognitive Level:*** Analysis; ***Client Need/Subneed:*** Physiological Integrity/Pharmacological and Parenteral Therapies/Expected Effects/Outcomes

90. **CORRECT ANSWER: 1.** **Answer 1 is correct because the adolescent's schedule should be arranged so that academic subjects (e.g., math, science, etc.) are taught in the morning when the adolescent is experiencing the effect of the morning dose of medication. This will allow the adolescent to focus more readily on difficult content, and to avoid sleep disturbances.** **Answer 2** is incorrect because the adolescent's schedule should be arranged so that academic subjects (e.g., math, science, etc.) are taught in the *morning,* when the adolescent is experiencing the effect of the morning dose of medication, not midday. This will allow the adolescent to focus more readily on difficult content. **Answer 3** is incorrect because the adolescent's schedule should be arranged so that academic subjects (e.g., math, science, etc.) are taught in the *morning,* when the adolescent is experiencing the effect of the morning dose of medication, not in the afternoon. This will allow the adolescent to focus more readily on difficult content, and to avoid sleep disturbances. **Answer 4** is incorrect because, while intermingling high-interest classroom activities with the adolescent's academic classes (e.g., math, science, etc.) will assist in maintaining the adolescent's attention and interest in learning, it does not take into account the timing of the effectiveness of the morning dose of medication. This would not allow the adolescent to more readily focus on difficult content.

■ **TEST-TAKING TIP:** *Once-a-day medication typically means morning.*

Content Area: Pediatrics, Pharmacology; ***Integrated Process:*** Nursing Process, Planning; ***Cognitive Level:*** Application; ***Client Need/Subneed:*** Physiological Integrity/Pharmacological and Parenteral Therapies/Medication Administration

91. **CORRECT ANSWER: 150. First, convert milligrams to micrograms. Second, calculate micrograms per mL, and third, calculate the flow rate.**

■ **TEST-TAKING TIP:** *Be sure to convert the order into the same unit of measure as the available solution.*

Content Area: Adult Health, Pharmacology; ***Integrated Process:*** Nursing Process, Analysis; ***Cognitive Level:*** Analysis; ***Client Need/Subneed:*** Physiological Integrity/Pharmacological and Parenteral Therapies/Dosage Calculation

92. **CORRECT ANSWER: 2.** **Answer 1** is incorrect because magnesium sulfate 4 gm IV bolus over 30 minutes *is* an appropriate order for this client for preterm labor. **Answer 2 is correct because the correct dosage and route for Brethine is *0.25 mg SQ.* Both the dosage and route are wrong for this drug.** **Answer 3** is incorrect because Stadol 1 mg IV push every 4 hours as needed for pain *is* an appropriate order. **Answer 4** is incorrect because Ancef 2 gm intravenous piggyback (IVPB) every 6 hours *is* an appropriate order.

■ **TEST-TAKING TIP:** *This question is asking for the order that is wrong or inappropriate for this client. Look for the order that is incorrect.*

Content Area: Maternity, Intrapartum; ***Integrated Process:*** Nursing Process, Analysis; ***Cognitive Level:*** Application; ***Client Need/Subneed:*** Physiological Integrity/Pharmacological and Parenteral Therapies

93. CORRECT ANSWER: 1. Answer 1 is correct because Rh_0(D) immune globulin needs to be administered before 72 hours after delivery to be effective. **Answer 2** is incorrect because 1 week is *too long* after delivery for adequate prophylaxis. **Answer 3** is incorrect because Rh_0(D) immune globulin *does not need* to be administered by 12 hours of age. Adequate prophylaxis is obtained if administration is *within 72* hours after delivery. **Answer 4** is incorrect because 2 weeks is *too long* after delivery for adequate prophylaxis.

■ **TEST-TAKING TIP:** *Since Rh_0(D) immune globulin is administered* in *the hospital, eliminate the time frames that would be longer than the average hospital stay for delivery. Is it hours or weeks? 72 hours is a reasonable length of time.*

Content Area: Maternity, Postpartum; ***Integrated Process:*** Nursing Process, Implementation; ***Cognitive Level:*** Application; ***Client Need/Subneed:*** Physiological Integrity/Pharmacological and Parenteral Therapies/Medication Administration

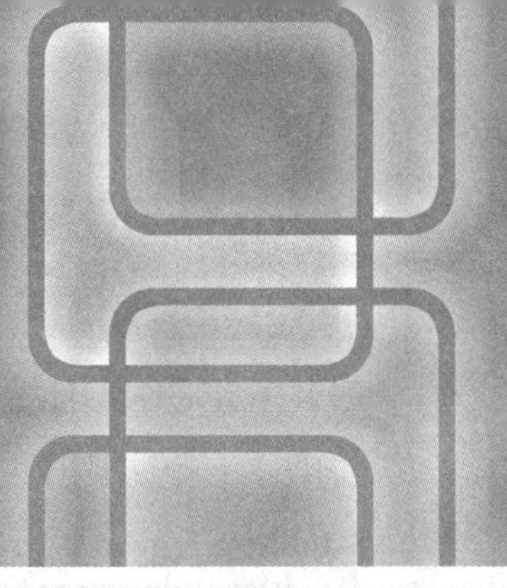

CHAPTER 9

Physiological Integrity:

Basic Care and Comfort—Nutrition

Sally Lambert Lagerquist • Janice Lloyd McMillin • Robyn Marchal Nelson • Denise Wall Parilo • Kathleen E. Snider

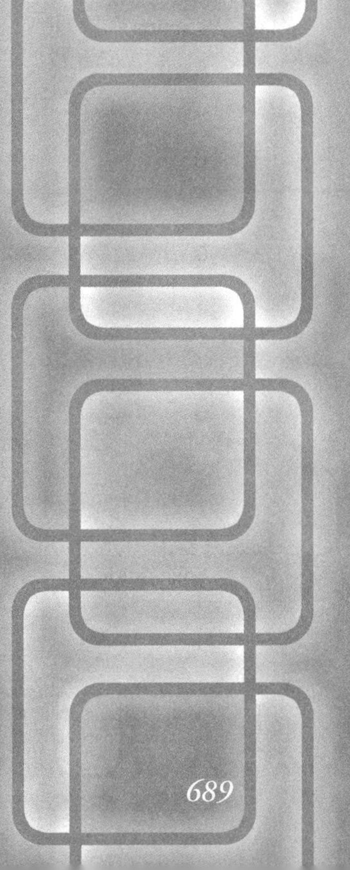

POPULATION-SPECIFIC NUTRITIONAL NEEDS

Nutrition During Pregnancy and Lactation

Table 9.1 gives a summary of nutrient needs (maternal and fetal) during pregnancy.

I. MILK GROUP—**important for calcium, protein of high biological value, and other vitamins and minerals.**
  A. *Pregnancy*—three to four servings (four to five for adolescents).
  B. *Lactation*—four to five servings.
  C. *Count as one serving*—1 cup milk; ½ cup undiluted evaporated milk; ¼ cup dry milk; 1¼ cups cottage cheese; 2 cups low-fat cottage cheese; 1½ oz cheddar or Swiss cheese; or 1½ cups ice cream.

II. MEAT, POULTRY, FISH, DRY BEANS, NUTS, AND EGGS GROUP—**important for protein, iron, and many B vitamins.**
  A. *Pregnancy*—three servings.
  B. *Lactation*—three servings.
  C. *Count as one serving*—½ cup cooked dry beans, 1 egg, or 1½ tbsp peanut butter is equivalent to 1 oz meat; use peanut butter or nuts rarely to *avoid*

Table 9.1

Nutrient Needs During Pregnancy

Nutrient	Maternal Need	Fetal Need	Food Source
Protein—75 gm/day	Maternal tissue growth: uterus, breasts, blood volume, storage	Rapid fetal growth	Milk and milk products; animal meats—muscle, organs; grains, legumes; eggs
Calories—2,500/day	Increased basal metabolic rate (BMR)	Primary energy source for growth of fetus	Carbohydrates: 4 kcal/gm Proteins: 4 kcal/gm Fats: 9 kcal/gm
Minerals—1,200 mg/day (*calcium* and *phosphorus*)	Increase in maternal Ca^{++} metabolism	Skeleton and tooth formation	Milk and milk products, especially natural cheese*
Iron—30 mg/day	Increase in red blood cell (RBC) mass Prevent anemia Decrease infection risk	Liver storage (especially in third trimester)	Organ meats—liver, animal meat; egg yolk; whole or enriched grains; green leafy vegetables; nuts
Vitamins			
A	Tissue growth	Cell development—tissue and bone growth and tooth bud formation	Butter, cream, fortified margarine; green and yellow vegetables
B	Coenzyme in many metabolic processes	Coenzyme in many metabolic processes	Animal meats, organ meats; milk and cheese; beans, peas, nuts; enriched grains
C	Tissue formation and integrity Increase iron absorption	Tissue formation and integrity	Citrus fruits, berries, melons, papaya, kiwi, strawberries; peppers; green, leafy vegetables; broccoli, brussels sprouts, snow pea pods; potatoes
D	Absorption of Ca^{++}, phosphorus	Mineralization of bone tissue and tooth buds	Fortified milk and margarine
E	Tissue growth; cell wall integrity; RBC integrity	Tissue growth; cell integrity; RBC integrity	Widely distributed: meat, milk, eggs, grains, leafy vegetables, vegetable oils
Folic acid	Meet increased metabolic demands in pregnancy Production of blood products	Meet increased metabolic demands, including production of cell nucleus material Prevent neural tube defects	Liver; deep-green, leafy vegetables; asparagus; avocado

*Natural cheese contains less lactose; therefore, it is a good source for those with lactose intolerance.
Tofu (soybean cake) is also high in calcium and contain *no* lactose.

excessive fat intake; limit eggs to reduce cholesterol intake; trim fat from meat, and remove skin from poultry.

III. VEGETABLE AND FRUIT GROUP—**vitamins and minerals (especially vitamins A and C) and roughage.**

- **A.** *Vegetables:*
  1. *Pregnancy*—three to four servings.
  2. *Lactation*—three to five servings.
  3. *Count as one serving*—1 cup raw leafy greens, ½ cup of others.
- **B.** *Fruits:*
  1. *Pregnancy*—two to four servings.
  2. *Lactation*—two to four servings.
  3. *Count as one serving*—½ medium grapefruit; 1 medium apple, banana, or orange; ¾ cup fruit juice.
- **C.** *Good sources of vitamin C*—citrus, cantaloupe, mango, papaya, strawberries, broccoli, and green and red bell peppers.
- **D.** *Fair sources of vitamin C*—tomatoes, honeydew melon, asparagus tips, raw cabbage, collards, kale, mustard greens, potatoes (white and sweet), spinach, and turnip greens.
- **E.** *Good sources of vitamin A*—dark-green or deep-yellow vegetables and a few fruits (apricots, broccoli, pumpkin, sweet potato, spinach, cantaloupe, carrots, and winter squash).
- **F.** *Good sources of folic acid*—dark-green *foliage*-type vegetables.

IV. BREAD AND CEREAL GROUP—**good for thiamine, iron, niacin, and other vitamins and minerals.**

- **A.** *Pregnancy*—6 to 11 servings.
- **B.** *Lactation*—6 to 11 servings.
- **C.** *Count as one serving*—1 slice bread, 1 oz ready-to-eat cereal, ½ to ¾ cup cooked cereal, cornmeal, grits, macaroni, noodles, rice, or spaghetti.

V. NOTE: use dark-green leafy and deep-yellow vegetables often; eat dry beans and peas often; count ½ cup cooked dry beans or peas as a serving of vegetables or 1 oz from meat group.

Nutritional Needs of the Newborn

I. CALORIES—108 kcal/kg/day.

II. PROTEIN—2.2 gm/kg/day (1 gm protein = 1 oz milk).

III. FLUIDS—3.5 oz/kg/day.

IV. VITAMIN D—400 IU daily for infants who are bottle-fed after week 2.

V. FLUORIDE—0.25 mg daily up to 3 years old when local water supply has less than 0.3 ppm content.

Nutritional Needs of the Geriatric Client

I. CALORIES—1,500 to 2,000 kcal/day to maintain ideal weight; 12% of calories from protein sources; 50% to 60% of calories from carbohydrates; 20% to 30% of calories from fats.

II. HIGH FIBER—prevent or alleviate constipation and dependence on laxatives.

III. SODIUM—3 to 4 gm/day according to cardiac and renal status.

IV. FATS—limit to help retard the development of cancer, atherosclerosis, obesity, and other diseases.

V. FLUIDS—6 to 8 glasses/day.

VI. COMMON DEFICIENCIES: calories; calcium; folic acid; iron; thiamine; vitamins A, B_{12}, C, and D; niacin; zinc.

VII. FACTORS CONTRIBUTING TO FOOD PREFERENCES:

- **A.** Physical ability to prepare, shop for, and eat food.
- **B.** Income.
- **C.** Availability of food if dependent on others.
- **D.** Food intolerances.

VIII. COMMON EATING PROBLEMS: **Table 9.2** provides interventions for common eating problems of the geriatric client.

CULTURAL FOOD PATTERNS

Table 9.3 gives a summary of the cultural food patterns of various ethnic groups, and **Table 9.4** details the "hot" versus "cold" theory of disease treatment.

RELIGIOUS CONSIDERATIONS IN MEAL PLANNING

I. ORTHODOX JEWS:

- **A.** Kosher meat and poultry.
- **B.** *No* shellfish, eels, or pork products.
- **C.** Milk and dairy products *cannot* be consumed with meat or poultry; requires separate utensils.
- **D.** *No* eggs with a blood spot may be eaten. Eggs may be used with either meat or dairy meals.

II. CONSERVATIVE AND REFORM JEWS: dietary practices may vary from religious laws.

III. MUSLIMS: *no* pork or alcohol.

IV. HINDUS: vegetarianism (cows are sacred).

Table 9.2

Eating Problems of the Geriatric Client and Ways to Improve Nutrition

Problem	Cause	Dietary Interventions
Within the mouth	Impaired taste buds Dental caries Chewing difficulty due to: Poorly fitting dentures No dentures No saliva Paralysis Metallic taste from medications	• Referral for correction of dental problems • Mouthwash/oral care before meals • Food prepared to meet client's needs (chopped, pureed, soft)
In the upper GI tract	Swallowing difficulty Paralysis due to stroke Food causing GI distress	• Thickened and jellied liquids • Soft, chopped foods • Small, frequent meals • Presentation important (how food looks on serving plate) • *Avoid* expression such as "baby food" (negative connotation)
In the lower GI tract	Constipation Diarrhea Bloating	• Add fruits/liquids to restore bowel function (see **Table 11.12, p. 844**) • *Avoid* foods that cause diarrhea • Plan meals at appropriate times for ease of digestion • *Avoid* salt
Psychosocial	Loneliness Meals no longer social event Depression Anorexia	• Encourage attendance at meal program if available • Arrange group meals/activities when possible • Emphasize best nutrition when appetite is at peak (breakfast) • Allow time to complete meal • Interact with others whenever possible
In the environment	Inability to shop for, prepare, or cook food Impaired vision Lack of resources Difficulty in feeding self Acute or chronic illnesses present (e.g., arthritis, stroke)	• Refer to Meals-on-Wheels • Encourage family involvement; describe how food is arranged on plate • Refer to social services • Assess need for assistive devices • Assess ability to grasp utensils and guide food to mouth • Open packages and milk cartons; butter the bread; cut meat and vegetables

From Thomas, CL (ed): *Taber's Cyclopedic Medical Dictionary,* ed 18. FA Davis, Philadelphia, 1997.

Table 9.3

Cultural Food Patterns

Ethnic Group	Cultural Food Patterns	Dietary Excesses or Omissions
Mexican (native)	• Basic sources of protein—dried beans, flan, cheese, many meats, fish, eggs • Chili peppers and many deep-green and yellow vegetables • Fruits include: zapote, guava, papaya, mango, citrus • Tortillas (corn, flour); sweet bread; fideo; tacos, burritos, enchiladas	• *Limited* meats, milk, and milk products • Some are using flour tortillas more than the more nutritious corn tortillas • ***Excessive*** use of lard (manteca), sugar • Tendency to boil vegetables for long periods of time

Table 9.3

Cultural Food Patterns—cont'd

Ethnic Group	Cultural Food Patterns	Dietary Excesses or Omissions
Filipino (Spanish-Chinese influence)	Most meats, eggs, nuts, legumes Many different kinds of vegetables Large amounts of rice and cereals	• May *limit* meat, milk, and milk products (the latter may be due to **lactose intolerance**) • Tend to prewash rice • Tend to fry many foods
Chinese (mostly Cantonese)	• Cheese, soybean curd (tofu), many meats, chicken and pigeon eggs, nuts, legumes • Many different vegetables, leaves, bamboo sprouts • Rice and rice-flour products; wheat, corn, millet seed; green tea • Mixtures of fish, pork, and chicken with vegetables—bamboo shoots, broccoli, cabbage, onions, mushrooms, pea pods	• Tendency among some immigrants to use *excess* grease in cooking. • May be *low* in protein, milk, and milk products (the latter may be due to **lactose intolerance**) • Often wash rice before cooking • **Large** amounts of soy and oyster sauces, both of which are *high in salt;* monosodium glutamate (MSG)
Puerto Rican	• Milk with coffee • Pork, poultry, eggs, dried fish; beans (habichuelas) • Viandas (starchy vegetables; starchy ripe fruits) • Avocados, okra, eggplant, sweet yams • Rice, cornmeal	Use *large* amounts of lard for cooking *Limited* use of milk and milk products *Limited* amounts of pork and poultry
African American	• Milk with coffee • Pork, poultry, eggs • *Fruit:* strawberries, watermelon • *Vegetables:* turnip, collard, mustard greens; kale, okra, sweet potatoes • Cereals (including grits, hominy, cornbread, hot breads) • Molasses (dark molasses is especially good source of calcium, iron, vitamins B_1 and B_2, and niacin)	• *Limited* use of milk group **(lactose intolerance)** • Extensive use of frying, "smothering," simmering for cooking • *Large* amounts of fat: salt pork, bacon drippings, lard, gravies • May have *limited* use of citrus and enriched breads
Middle Eastern (Greek, Syrian, Armenian)	• Yogurt • Predominantly lamb, nuts, dried peas, beans, lentils • Deep-green leaves and vegetables; dried fruits • Dark breads and cracked wheat	• Tend to use *excessive* sweeteners, lamb fat, olive oil • Tend to fry meats and vegetables • *Insufficient* milk and milk products (almost no butter—use olive oil, which has no nutritive value except for calories) • *Deficiency* in fresh fruits
Middle European (Polish)	Many milk products Pork, chicken Root vegetables (potatoes), cabbage, fruits Wheat products • Sausages, smoked and cured meats, noodles, dumplings, bread, cream with coffee	• Tend to use *excessive* sweets and to overcook vegetables • *Limited* amounts of fruits (citrus), raw vegetables, and meats
Native American (American Indian—much variation)	• If "Americanized," use milk and milk products • Variety of meats: game, fowl, fish; nuts, seeds, legumes • Variety of vegetables, some wild • Variety of fruits, some wild, rose hips; roots • Variety of breads, including tortillas, cornmeal, rice	• *Nutrition-related problems:* obesity, diabetes, dental problems, iron-deficiency anemia; alcoholism • *Limited* quantities of high-protein foods depending on availability (flocks of game, fowl) and economic situation • *Excessive* use of sugar
Italian	• Staples are pasta with sauces; bread; eggs; cheese; tomatoes; and vegetables such as artichokes, eggplant, greens, and zucchini • Only small amount of meat is used	*Limited* use of whole grains *Insufficient* servings from milk group Tendency to overcook vegetables Enjoy sweets

Table 9.4

Hot-Cold Theory of Disease Treatment*

Hot Diseases or Conditions	Cold Diseases or Conditions	Hot Foods	Cold Foods	Hot Medicines and Herbs	Cold Medicines and Herbs
Constipation	Cancer	Beverages, aromatic	Barley water	Anise	Bicarbonate of soda
Diarrhea	Common cold	Cereal grains	Cod	Aspirin	Linden
Infections	Earache	Cheese	Dairy products	Castor oil	Milk of magnesia
Kidney diseases	Headache	Chili peppers	Fruits, tropical	Cinnamon	Orange flower water
Liver complaints	Joint pain	Chocolate	Honey	Cod liver oil	Sage
Skin eruptions	Malaria	Coffee	Meats (goat, fish, chicken)	Garlic	
Throat (sore)	Menstrual period	Eggs	Milk, bottled	Ginger root	
Ulcers	Paralysis	Fruits, temperate zone	Raisins	Iron preparations	
Warts	Pneumonia	Goat milk	Vegetables, fresh	Mint	
	Rheumatism	Hard liquor		Penicillin	
	Stomach cramps	Meats (beef, water fowl, mutton)		Tobacco	
	Teething	Oils		Vitamins	
	Tuberculosis	Onions			
		Peas			

*A Latin American, particularly Puerto Rican, approach to treating diseases. A "hot" disease is treated with "cold" treatments (foods, medicines) and vice versa.
Adapted from Wilson, HS, & Kneisl, CR: *Psychiatric Nursing,* ed 2. Addison-Wesley, Menlo Park, CA. (out of print)

V. SEVENTH-DAY ADVENTISTS:

A. Vegetarianism is common (lacto-ovo).
B. *No* shellfish or pork products.
C. *Avoid* stimulants (coffee, tea, other caffeine sources).
D. *No* alcohol.

VI. MORMONS (LATTER-DAY SAINTS [LDS]): *no* coffee, tea, or alcohol.

VII. CATHOLICS: some still adhere to meatless Fridays and fasting during Lent.

COMMON VITAMINS AND NUTRIENTS AND RELATED DEFICIENCIES

Table 9.5 gives a summary of the physiological functions of common vitamins and the results of deficiencies. **Table 9.6** gives a similar summary of essential nutrients.

MEDICAL CONDITIONS WITH DIETARY MANAGEMENT

The dietary management of various medical conditions is detailed in **Table 9.7.**

SPECIAL DIETS

I. LOW-CARBOHYDRATE DIET—ketogenic: low carbohydrate, high fat; *dumping syndrome:* low carbohydrate, high fat, high protein.

II. GLUTEN-FREE DIET—elimination of all foods made from oats, barley, wheat, and rye; may have corn and rice. Used for *celiac* disease.

III. HIGH-PROTEIN DIET—lean meat, cheese, and green vegetables.

A. *Nephrotic* syndrome (may also be on low-sodium diet).
B. *Acute leukemia* (combined with high-calorie and soft food diets).
C. *Neoplastic* disease.

IV. LOW-PROTEIN DIET:

A. Usually accompanied by high-carbohydrate diet and normal fats and calories.
B. *Renal* failure, uremia, anuria, acute glomerulonephritis.

V. LOW-SODIUM DIET:

A. *Heart* failure.
B. *Nephrotic* syndrome.
C. *Acute glomerulonephritis* (varies with degree of oliguria).

(text continues on page 699)

Table 9.5

Physiological Functions of Common Vitamins and Related Deficiencies

Vitamin	Chief Functions	Results of Deficiency	Characteristics	Good Sources
Vitamin A				
Retinol (animal source) Carotene Beta-carotene	• Essential for maintaining the integrity of epithelial membranes • Helps maintain resistance to infections • Necessary for the formation of rhodopsin and prevention of night blindness • Necessary for proper bone growth • Facilitates RNA formation from DNA • Thought to be cancer preventive because of antioxidant properties associated with control of free radical damage to DNA and cell membranes	***Mild:*** • Retarded growth • Increased susceptibility to infection • Abnormal function of gastrointestinal, genitourinary, and respiratory tracts due to altered epithelial membranes • Skin dries, shrivels, thickens; sometimes pustule formation • Night blindness ***Severe:*** • Xerophthalmia, a characteristic eye disease, and other local infections	• Fat soluble* • Not destroyed by ordinary cooking temperatures • Is destroyed by high temperatures when oxygen is present • Marked capacity for storage in the liver **NOTE:** Excessive intake of carotene, from which vitamin A is formed, may produce yellow discoloration of the skin (*carotenemia*); excessive vitamin A intake causes symptoms similar to those of deficiency conditions	Liver Animal fats: Butter Cheese Cream Egg yolk Whole milk Fish liver oil Liver Vegetables: • Green leafy, especially escarole, kale, parsley • Yellow, especially carrots *Artificial:* • Concentrates in several forms • Irradiated fish oils
Vitamin B_6				
Pyridoxine Pyridoxal Pyridoxamine	• Used in hemoglobin synthesis • Essential for metabolism of tryptophan to niacin • Needed for utilization of certain other amino acids	• Anemias • Depressed immunity • Dermatitis around eyes and mouth • Neuritis • Anorexia, nausea, and vomiting	• Soluble in water and alcohol • Rapidly inactivated in presence of heat, sunlight, or air	Meats Cereal grains Some fruits Nuts
Vitamin B_{12}				
Cyanocobalamin Hydroxycobalamin	• Necessary for myelin synthesis • Essential for normal development of red blood cells • Associated with folate metabolism	• Pernicious anemia • Neurological disorders	• Soluble in water or alcohol • Unstable in hot alkaline or acid solutions	• Found only in animal products (e.g., meats, eggs, dairy products) • Most of vitamin B_{12} required by humans is synthesized by intestinal bacteria; can also be recycled
Vitamin C				
Ascorbic acid	• Essential to formation of intracellular cement substances in a variety of tissues, including skin, dentin, cartilage, and bone matrix • Important in healing of wounds and bone fractures • Prevents scurvy • Facilitates absorption of iron • Protects folate • Antioxidant • Promotes capillary permeability	***Mild:*** • Lowered resistance to infections • Joint tenderness • Susceptibility to dental caries, pyorrhea, and bleeding gums • Delayed wound healing • Bruising ***Severe:*** • Hemorrhage • Anemia • Scurvy **NOTE:** Many drugs affect availability	• Soluble in water • Easily destroyed by oxidation; heat hastens the process • Lost in cooking, particularly if water in which food was cooked is discarded; loss is greater if cooked in iron or copper utensils • Quick-frozen foods lose little of their vitamin C • Stored in the body to a limited extent	• Abundant in most fresh fruits and vegetables, especially citrus fruit and juices, tomato and orange • *Artificial:* Ascorbic acid Cevitamic acid

Continued

VITAMINS

Table 9.5

Physiological Functions of Common Vitamins and Related Deficiencies—cont'd

Vitamin	Chief Functions	Results of Deficiency	Characteristics	Good Sources
Vitamin D				
Calciferol Ergocalciferol Cholecalciferol Calcitriol Antirachitic factor	Hormone-like regulation of calcium and phosphorus metabolism by promotion of: Gastrointestinal absorption Bone and tooth mineralization Renal reabsorption Skeletal reserves Antirachitic	***Mild:*** Interferes with utilization of calcium and phosphorus in bone and tooth formation Irritability Weakness ***Severe:*** Rickets in young children Osteomalacia in adults	Soluble in fats and organic solvents* Relatively stable under refrigeration Stored in liver Often associated with vitamin A	• Formed in the skin by exposure to sunlight • Fortified milk and dairy products Egg yolk Fish liver oils • Fish having fat distributed through the flesh, salmon, tuna, herring sardines Liver Oysters • Artifically prepared forms
Vitamin E				
Alpha-tocopherol Beta-tocopherol Gamma-tocopherol	Important antioxidant that: • Prevents red blood cell hemolysis • Protects vitamin A and unsaturated fatty acids from oxidation • Promotes cell membrane integrity • Improves immune response • May protect against cancer	• Red blood cell resistance to rupture is decreased, but deficiency seldom occurs except in *premature* infants and people with *chronic fat malabsorption*	Soluble in fat* Stable to heat in absence of oxygen and ultraviolet light Unstable under freezing and processing	Vegetable oils Margarine Whole-grain or fortified cereals Wheat germ Green leafy vegetables
Folate				
Folacin Folic acid	• Essential for normal functioning of hematopoietic system Important coenzyme for RNA and DNA synthesis Important in fetal development • Functions interrelated with those of vitamin B_{12}	Anemia **NOTE:** Neural tube defects (e.g., *spina bifida*) are associated with maternal deficiency; alcohol and contraceptives interfere with absorption	Slightly soluble in water Easily destroyed by heat in presence of acid Decreases when food is stored at room temperature **NOTE:** A large dose may prevent appearance of anemia in a case of pernicious anemia but still permit neurological symptoms to develop	Liver Eggs Fish Green leafy vegetables Asparagus Peas, beans, legumes Nuts, seeds, wheat germ Avocado Some fruits
Vitamin K				
Menadione Phylloquinone Menaquinone	Promotes synthesis of clotting factors	• Prolonged clotting time, resulting in bleeding **NOTE:** Seldom occurs in the absence of anticoagulant drugs; in addition to food sources, intestinal bacteria manufacture approximately half the body's requirement • Fat malabsorption can cause deficiency • Synthetic form (menadione) does not depend on fat absorption	Soluble in fat* Stable to heat	Green leafy vegetables Meats Dairy products Intestinal bacteria

Table 9.5

Physiological Functions of Common Vitamins and Related Deficiencies—cont'd

Vitamin	Chief Functions	Results of Deficiency	Characteristics	Good Sources
Niacin				
Nicotinic acid Nicotinamide Antipellagra vitamin	As the component of two important enzymes, it is important in glycolysis, tissue respiration, fat synthesis, and cellular energy production Nicotinic acid, but not nicotinamide, causes vasodilation and flushing Prevents pellagra	Pellagra Gastrointestinal disturbances Mental disturbances **NOTE:** Associated with alcoholism	Soluble in hot water and alcohol Not destroyed by heat, light, air, or alkali Not destroyed in ordinary cooking	Milk Eggs Meats Legumes Enriched foods Whole-grain cereals Nuts **NOTE:** Also formed in the body from dietary tryptophan (amino acid)
Riboflavin				
Vitamin B_2	Important as coenzyme in cellular oxidation Essential to normal growth Participates in light adaptation Vital to protein metabolism Associated with niacin and vitamin B_6 functions	Impaired growth Lassitude and weakness Cheilosis Glossitis Dermatitis Anemia Photophobia Cataracts	Water soluble Alcohol soluble Not destroyed by heat in cooking unless with alkali Unstable in light, especially in presence of alkali	Milk and milk products Enriched foods Whole-grain breads and cereals Liver Meats Eggs
Thiamine				
Vitamin B_1	Important role in carbohydrate metabolism Essential for maintenance of normal appetite Essential for normal functioning of nervous tissue Coenzyme for cellular energy production	***Mild:*** Loss of appetite Impaired metabolism of starches and sugars Emaciation Irritability ***Severe:*** Various nervous disorders Loss of coordinating power of muscles Beriberi Paralysis in humans	Soluble in water Not readily destroyed by ordinary cooking temperatures Destroyed by exposure to heat, alkali, or sulfites Not stored in body **NOTE:** Deficiency is often associated with alcoholism	Widely distributed in plant and animal tissues but seldom occurs in high concentration, except in brewer's yeast Enriched or whole-grain cereals Pork Peas, beans Nuts *Artificial:* Concentrates from yeast Rice polishings Wheat germ

*Vitamins A, D, E, and K are available in water-soluble forms and are used in children with cystic fibrosis and celiac disease.
Adapted from Venes, D (ed): *Taber's Cyclopedic Medical Dictionary,* ed 20. FA Davis, Philadelphia, 2005.

Table 9.6

Essential Nutrients and Potential Deficiencies

Nutrient	Function	Deficiency Leads to
Calcium	Aids in formation and maintenance of bones and teeth; permits healthy nerve functioning and normal blood clotting	↑ Neuromuscular irritability Impaired blood clotting
Phosphorus	Bone building	Rickets

Continued

Table 9.6

Essential Nutrients and Potential Deficiencies—cont'd

Nutrient	Function	Deficiency Leads to
Magnesium	Cellular metabolism of carbohydrates and protein	↓ Cellular metabolism of carbohydrates and protein Tetany
Sodium	Fluid and electrolyte balance; acid-base balance; electrochemical impulses of nerves and muscles	Fluid and electrolyte imbalance ↓ Muscle contraction
Potassium	Osmotic pressure and water balance	Fluid and electrolyte imbalance ↓ Cardiac and skeletal muscular contractility
Chloride	Fluid and electrolyte balance; acid-base balance Digestion	Fluid imbalances; alkalosis
Iron	Hemoglobin formation Cellular oxidation	Anemia; ↑ risk of infection
Iodine	Synthesis of thyroid hormone; overall body metabolism	Goiter
Zinc	Constituent of cell enzyme system; CO_2 carrier in RBCs	↓ Metabolism of protein and carbohydrates Delayed wound healing; ↑ risk of infection
Vitamin A	Collagen synthesis	Poor healing; scaly skin
Vitamin C	Capillary integrity	Poor healing; bruising
Vitamin K	Coagulation	Bruising and hemorrhage
Pyridoxine and thiamine	Antibody, RBC, and WBC formation	↑ Risk of infection Anemia
Protein	Wound repair; clotting WBC production Phagocytosis	Poor healing; edema
Fats	Cellular energy Cell membrane integrity	Impaired tissue repair
Carbohydrates	Cellular energy; spare protein	Interference with healing

Table 9.7

Medical Conditions with Dietary Management

Condition	Recommended Diet
Celiac sprue	*Avoid* glutens (wheat, buckwheat, rye, oats, barley)
Cholelithiasis	*Avoid* fatty food
Cirrhosis	↓ Sodium; limit protein
Diverticulosis	Low residue
Esophagitis	Thick liquids; *avoid* alcohol
Gastroesophageal reflux disease (GERD)	*Avoid:* late meals, chocolate, caffeine, mints
Gout	↓ Alcohol, ↓ purine (organ meats, anchovies, sardines, consommé, gravies, fish roes, herring); ↑ fluid
Hyperhomocysteinemia	↑ Vitamin B_{12}; ↑ folates
Hypertension	DASH (**D**ietary **A**pproaches to **S**top **H**ypertension) diet: ↓ saturated fats and cholesterol; ↓ total fats and dairy fats; ↑ fruits, vegetables, whole grains, fish, poultry, and nuts
Iron-deficiency anemia	Vitamin C with iron supplements
Irritable bowel syndrome (IBS)	↑ Fiber, ↓ dairy products
Nephrotic syndrome	↓ Sodium
Osteoporosis	↓ Alcohol; supplement calcium and vitamin D
Pernicious anemia	Vitamin B_{12} supplements
Renal failure	↓ Sodium, potassium, protein, fluids

VI. HIGH-PHOSPHORUS DIET:

A. Use when serum phosphorus level is less than 2.7 mg/dL due to:
1. *Insufficient* intake (e.g., malnutrition, starvation).
2. *Increased* phosphorus excretion due to:
   a. Renal failure.
   b. Hyperparathyroidism.
   c. Malignancy.
   d. Antacids that are aluminum hydroxide–based or magnesium-based.

B. Sources of phosphorus: beef, chicken, fish, organ meats, pork, nuts, legumes, whole-grain breads and cereals, milk, egg, cheese, ice cream, carbonated beverages.

COMMON THERAPEUTIC DIETS

I. CLEAR LIQUID DIET

A. *Purpose:* relieve thirst and help maintain fluid balance.

B. *Use:* postsurgically and following acute vomiting or diarrhea.

C. *Foods allowed:* carbonated beverages; coffee (caffeinated and decaffeinated); tea; fruit-flavored drinks; strained fruit juices; clear, flavored gelatins; broth, consommé; sugar; popsicles; commercially prepared clear liquids; and hard candy.

D. *Foods avoided:* milk and milk products, fruit juices with pulp, and fruit.

II. FULL LIQUID DIET

A. *Purpose:* provide an adequately nutritious diet for clients who cannot chew or who are too ill to do so.

B. *Use:* acute infection with fever, gastrointestinal upsets, after surgery as a progression from *clear liquids.*

C. *Foods allowed:* clear liquids, milk drinks, cooked cereals, custards, ice cream, sherbets, eggnog, all strained fruit juices, vegetable juices, creamed vegetable soups, puddings, mashed potatoes, instant breakfast drinks, yogurt, mild cheese sauce or pureed meat, and seasonings.

D. *Foods avoided:* nuts, seeds, coconut, fruit, jam, and marmalade.

III. SOFT DIET

A. *Purpose:* provide adequate nutrition for those who have trouble chewing.

B. *Use:* clients with no teeth or ill-fitting dentures; transition from full liquid to general diet; and for those who cannot tolerate highly seasoned, fried, or raw foods following acute infections or gastrointestinal disturbances, such as gastric ulcer or cholelithiasis.

C. *Foods allowed:* very tender minced, ground, baked, broiled, roasted, stewed, or creamed beef, lamb, veal, liver, poultry, or fish; crisp bacon or sweetbreads; cooked vegetables; pasta; all fruit juices; soft raw fruits; soft breads and cereals; all desserts that are soft; and cheeses.

D. *Foods avoided:* coarse whole-grain cereals and breads; nuts; raisins; coconut; fruits with small seeds; fried foods; high-fat gravies or sauces; spicy salad dressings; pickled meat, fish, or poultry; strong cheeses; brown or wild rice; raw vegetables, as well as lima beans and corn; spices such as horseradish, mustard, and catsup; and popcorn.

IV. SODIUM-RESTRICTED DIET

A. *Purpose:* reduce sodium content in the tissues and promote excretion of water.

B. *Use:* heart failure, hypertension, renal disease, cirrhosis, toxemia of pregnancy, and cortisone therapy.

C. *Modifications:* mildly restrictive 2-gm sodium diet to extremely restricted 200-mg sodium diet.

D. *Foods avoided:* table salt; all commercial soups, including bouillon; gravy, catsup, mustard, meat sauces, and soy sauce; buttermilk, ice cream, and sherbet; sodas; beet greens, carrots, celery, chard, sauerkraut, and spinach; *all canned* vegetables; frozen peas; all baked products containing salt, baking powder, or baking soda; potato chips and popcorn; fresh or canned shellfish; all cheeses; smoked or commercially prepared meats; salted butter or margarine; bacon; olives; and commercially prepared salad dressings.

V. RENAL DIET

A. *Purpose:* control protein, potassium, sodium, and fluid levels in body.

B. *Use:* acute and chronic renal failure, hemodialysis.

C. *Foods allowed:* high-biological proteins such as meat, fowl, fish, cheese, and dairy products—range between 20 and 60 mg/day. Potassium is usually limited to 1,500 mg/day. Vegetables such as cabbage, cucumber, and peas are lowest in potassium. Sodium is restricted to 500 mg/day. Fluid intake is restricted to the daily urine volume plus 500 mL, which represents insensible water loss. Fluid intake measures water in fruit, vegetables, milk, and meat.

D. *Foods avoided:* cereals, bread, macaroni, noodles, spaghetti, avocados, kidney beans, potato chips, raw fruit, yams, soybeans, nuts, gingerbread, apricots, bananas, figs, grapefruit, oranges, percolated coffee, Coca-Cola, Orange Crush, sport drinks, and breakfast drinks such as Tang or Awake.

VI. HIGH-PROTEIN, HIGH-CARBOHYDRATE DIET

A. *Purpose:* corrects large protein losses and raises the level of blood albumin. May be modified to include low-fat, low-sodium, and low-cholesterol diets.

B. *Use:* burns, hepatitis, cirrhosis, pregnancy, hyperthyroidism, mononucleosis, protein deficiency due to poor eating habits, geriatric clients with poor food intake, nephritis, nephrosis, and liver and gallbladder disorders.

C. *Foods allowed:* general diet with added protein. In adults, high-protein diets usually contain 135 to 150 gm protein.

D. *Foods avoided:* restrictions depend on modifications added to the diet. These modifications are determined by the client's condition.

VII. PURINE-RESTRICTED DIET

A. *Purpose:* designed to reduce intake of uric acid–producing foods.

B. *Use:* high uric acid retention, uric acid renal stones, and gout.

C. *Foods allowed:* general diet plus 2 to 3 quarts of liquid daily.

D. *Foods avoided:* cheese containing spices or nuts, fried eggs, meat, liver, seafood, lentils, dried peas and beans, broth, bouillon, gravies, oatmeal and whole wheats, pasta, noodles, and alcoholic beverages. *Limited* quantities of meat, fish, and seafood allowed.

VIII. BLAND DIET

A. *Purpose:* provision of a diet low in fiber, roughage, mechanical irritants, and chemical stimulants.

B. *Use:* gastritis, hyperchlorhydria, functional GI disorders, gastric atony, diarrhea, spastic constipation, biliary indigestion, and hiatus hernia.

C. *Foods allowed:* varied to meet individual needs and food tolerances.

D. *Foods avoided:* fried foods, including eggs, meat, fish, and seafood; cheese with added nuts or spices; commercially prepared luncheon meats; cured meats such as ham; gravies and sauces; raw vegetables; potato skins; fruit juices with pulp; figs; raisins; fresh fruits; whole wheats; rye bread; bran cereals; rich pastries; pies; chocolate; jams with seeds; nuts; seasoned dressings; caffeinated coffee; strong tea; cocoa; alcoholic and carbonated beverages; and pepper.

IX. LOW-FAT, CHOLESTEROL-RESTRICTED DIET

A. *Purpose:* reduce hyperlipidemia, provide dietary treatment for malabsorption syndromes and clients having acute intolerance for fats.

B. *Use:* hyperlipidemia, atherosclerosis, pancreatitis, cystic fibrosis, sprue, gastrectomy, massive resection of the small intestine, and cholecystitis.

C. *Foods allowed:* nonfat milk; low-carbohydrate, low-fat vegetables; most fruits; breads; pastas; cornmeal; lean meats; unsaturated fats such as corn oil; desserts made without whole milk; and unsweetened carbonated beverages.

D. *Foods avoided:* **remember to avoid the "5 Cs" of cholesterol—cookies, cream, cake, coconut, chocolate;** whole milk and whole-milk or *cream* products, avocados, olives, commercially prepared *baked* goods such as donuts and muffins, poultry skin, highly marbled meats, shellfish, fish canned in oil, nuts, *coconut,* commercially prepared meats, butter, ordinary margarines, olive oil, lard, pudding made with whole milk, *ice cream,* candies with *chocolate, cream,* sauces, gravies, and commercially fried foods.

X. DIABETIC DIET

A. *Purpose:* maintain blood glucose as near normal as possible; prevent or delay onset of diabetic complications.

B. *Use:* diabetes mellitus.

C. *Foods allowed:* choose foods with low *glycemic index;* composed of 45% to 55% carbohydrates, 30% to 35% fats, and 10% to 25% protein. Foods are divided into groups from which exchanges can be made. Coffee, tea, broth, bouillon, spices, and flavorings can be used as desired. Exchange groups include: *milk, vegetables, fruit, starch/bread* (includes starchy vegetables), *meat* (divided into lean, medium fat, and high fat), and *fat* exchanges. The number of exchanges allowed from each group is dependent on the total number of calories allowed. Nonnutritive sweeteners (aspartame) if desired. Nutritive sweeteners (sorbitol) in moderation for those who have controlled diabetes and have normal weight.

D. *Foods avoided:* concentrated sweets or regular soft drinks.

XI. ACID-ASH AND ALKALI-ASH DIETS

A. *Purpose:* furnish a well-balanced diet in which the total acid ash is greater than the total alkali ash each day.

B. *Use:* retard the formation of renal calculi. The type of diet chosen depends on laboratory analysis of the stones.

C. *Acid-ash and alkali-ash food groups:*

1. *Acid ash:* meat, whole grains, eggs, cheese, cranberries, prunes, plums.
2. *Alkali ash:* milk, vegetables, fruit (except cranberries, prunes, and plums).
3. *Neutral:* sugars, fats, beverages (coffee and tea).

D. *Foods allowed:* all the client wants of the following:

1. Breads: any, preferably whole grain; crackers; rolls.
2. Cereals: any, preferably whole grain.
3. Desserts: angel food or sunshine cake; cookies made without baking powder or soda; cornstarch pudding, cranberry desserts, custards, gelatin desserts, ice cream, sherbet, plum or prune desserts; rice or tapioca pudding.
4. Fats: any, such as butter, margarine, salad dressings, Crisco, Spry, lard, salad oils, olive oil, etc.

5. Fruits: cranberries, plums, prunes.
6. Meat, eggs, cheese: any meat, fish, or fowl, two servings daily; at least one egg daily.
7. Potato substitutes: corn, hominy, lentils, macaroni, noodles, rice, spaghetti, vermicelli.
8. Soup: broth as desired; other soups from foods allowed.
9. Sweets: cranberry or plum jelly; sugar; plain sugar candy.
10. Miscellaneous: cream sauce, gravy, peanut butter, peanuts, popcorn, salt, spices, vinegar, walnuts.

E. *Restricted foods:* no more than the amount allowed each day.

1. Milk: 1 pint daily (may be used in other ways than as beverage).
2. Cream: ⅓ cup or less daily.
3. Fruits: one serving of fruit daily (in addition to the prunes, plums, and cranberries); certain fruits listed under *Foods avoided* (following) are *not allowed at any time.*
4. Vegetables, including potatoes: two servings daily; certain vegetables listed under *Foods avoided* (following) are *not allowed at any time.*

F. *Foods avoided:*

1. Carbonated beverages, such as ginger ale, cola, root beer.
2. Cakes or cookies made with baking powder or soda.
3. Fruits: dried apricots, bananas, dates, figs, raisins, rhubarb.
4. Vegetables: dried beans, beet greens, dandelion greens, carrots, chard, lima beans.
5. Sweets; chocolate or candies other than those listed under *Foods allowed* (preceding); syrups.
6. Miscellaneous: other nuts, olives, pickles.

XII. HIGH-FIBER DIET

A. *Purpose:* soften stool; exercise digestive tract muscles; speed passage of food through digestive tract to prevent exposure to cancer-causing agents in food; lower blood lipids; prevent sharp rise in blood glucose after eating.

B. *Use:* diabetes, hyperlipidemia, constipation, diverticulosis, anticarcinogenic (colon).

C. *Foods allowed:* recommended intake about 6 gm crude fiber daily: all bran cereals; watermelon, prunes, dried peaches, apple with skin; parsnips, peas, brussel sprouts; sunflower seeds.

XIII. LOW-RESIDUE (LOW-FIBER) DIET

A. *Purpose:* reduce stool bulk and slow transit time.

B. *Use:* bowel inflammation during acute diverticulitis or ulcerative colitis, preparation for bowel surgery, esophageal and intestinal stenosis.

C. *Foods allowed:* eggs; ground or well-cooked tender meat, fish, poultry; milk; mild cheeses; strained fruit juice (except prune); cooked or canned apples, apricots, peaches, pears; ripe bananas; strained vegetable juice; canned, cooked, or strained asparagus, beets, green beans, pumpkin, acorn squash, spinach; white bread; refined cereals (Cream of Wheat).

XIV. LACTOSE-FREE DIET

A. *Purpose:* decrease symptoms that occur after having milk products: diarrhea, cramps, abdominal pain, increased flatus.

B. *Use:* in lactose intolerance, where there is an inability to tolerate lactose because of absence or deficiency of lactase, an enzyme found in the secretions of the small intestine required for digestion of lactose.

C. *Foods avoided:* milk products.

D. *Foods allowed:* soy-based milk foods; hard cheese, cottage cheese, yogurt (contains inactive lactose enzyme).

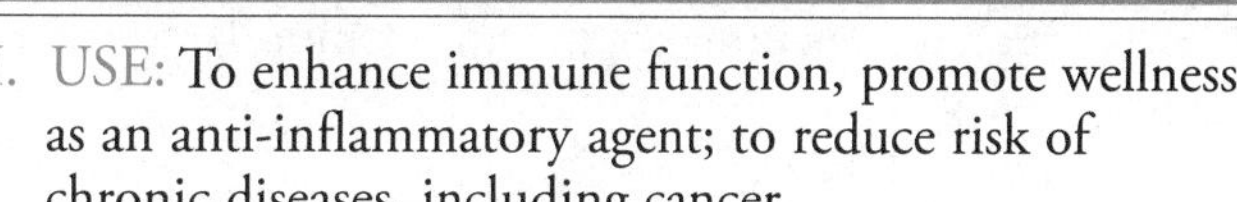

ANTICANCER NUTRIENTS AND NONNUTRITIVE COMPOUNDS

I. USE: To enhance immune function, promote wellness as an anti-inflammatory agent; to reduce risk of chronic diseases, including cancer.

II. SOURCE FOODS:

A. *Berries.*

1. Rich in: vitamin C, fiber, potassium, phytochemicals (flavonoids).
2. *Effect:*
   a. Antioxidants: protect against cell damage.
   b. Anti-inflammatory.
   c. Antiulcerative.
   d. Antiviral.
   e. May help to inhibit tumor formation in: liver, colon, esophageal, and oral cancer.
3. Servings: daily.

B. *Citrus fruits.*

1. Rich in: vitamin C, folic acid, phytochemicals (e.g., beta-carotene, limonoids, monoterpenes, phenols).
2. *Effect:*
   a. Inhibit activation of cancer cells; detoxify cancer promoters.
   b. Aid protective enzymes.
   c. Stimulate cancer-killing immune cells.
   d. May reduce risk of: breast, skin, colon cancers.
3. Servings: daily.

C. *Cruciferous vegetable family.*

1. Rich in: antioxidants (e.g., beta-carotene and vitamin C); also isothiocyanates; including sulforaphane.
2. Group includes: broccoli, kale, cauliflower, cabbage, bok choy, brussels sprouts.

3. *Effect:*
   a. Isothiocyanates: interfere with tumor growth.
   b. Neutralize cancer-causing chemicals.
   c. Stimulate enzymes (e.g., glutathione *S*-transferase) that inactivate carcinogens.
   d. May help reduce risk of hormone-related cancers (e.g., breast, prostate, and thyroid).
   e. May help reduce risk of: lung, GI, oral, pharyngeal, and esophageal cancers.
4. Servings: 3 servings/week.

D. *Fatty fish* (salmon, trout, herring, bluefish, sardines).
1. Rich in: omega-3 fatty acids, iron, B vitamins, selenium, vitamin D.
2. *Effect:*
   a. Inhibit growth of cancer cells.
   b. Stimulate the immune system.
   c. Help prevent or reduce muscle wasting.
   d. May reduce the risk of cancers of: breast, prostate, endometrium, colon.
3. Servings: twice/week or more often.

E. *Flaxseed.*
1. Rich in: omega-3 fatty acids, lignans, fiber, protein, calcium, potassium, vitamin B, iron.
2. *Effect:*
   a. Block tumor growth.
   b. Inhibit angiogenesis.
   c. Enhance immune system.
   d. Anti-inflammatory.
3. **Caution:** Not to be used by clients with hormone-sensitive breast cancer and/or if using tamoxifen or other antiestrogenic drugs.

F. *Garlic and onions.*
1. *Effect:*
   a. Increase detoxification of enzymes.
   b. Stimulate cancer-fighting immune cells.
   c. May decrease risk of: prostate, breast, gastric, and colon cancer.
   d. May also have antiasthma and cardioprotective effects.
2. Servings: use in any recipe.

G. *Green tea.*
1. Rich in: polyphenols (antioxidants that prevent DNA damage).
2. *Effect:*
   a. Catechins (a type of polyphenol) may help to rid body of carcinogens.
   b. May neutralize cell-damaging free radicals.
   c. Stimulates immune response.
   d. May suppress the growth of cancer cells.
   e. May reduce the risk of: colorectal, prostate, breast, bladder, gastric, esophageal, liver, lung, skin, and head and neck cancers.
3. Servings: 2 to 4 cups daily.

H. *Herbs and spices.*
1. *Rosemary:* rich in carnosol and ursolic acid with strong antioxidant activity.
2. *Turmeric* and *cumin:* rich in curcumin that may reduce risk of leukemia, skin, and liver cancers.
3. *Chili peppers:* rich in capsaicin that helps to prevent formation of nitrosamines; may reduce risk of colon, gastric and rectal cancers.

I. *Legumes/beans.*
1. Rich in: low-fat source of protein and dietary fiber, iron, folic acid, calcium, zinc, phytochemicals (e.g., phytosterols, saponins, phytic acid, isoflavones).
2. *Effect:* prevent DNA damage → provide anticancer activity.
3. Servings: 3 to 4/week.

J. *Nuts.*
1. Rich in: dietary fiber, vitamin E, healthy fats.
   a. Brazil nuts: high amount of selenium.
   b. Walnuts: high in omega-3 fatty acids.
2. *Effect:* encourage "suicide" (apoptosis) of cancer cells.
3. Servings: 2 Brazil nuts daily; 2 tbsp of walnuts daily.

K. *Olive oil* (extra virgin).
1. Rich in: monounsaturated fats, polyphenols.
2. *Effect:*
   a. Inhibit oxidative stress.
   b. Arrest cell proliferation.
   c. Induce cell death (apoptosis).
3. May reduce risk of: breast, prostate, and colorectal cancers.

L. *Vegetables/fruits*—**orange-colored** (carrots, sweet potatoes, winter squash, mangoes, papayas).
1. Rich in: vitamin C, folic acid, other B vitamins, fiber and beta-carotene.
2. *Effect:* carotenoids strengthen immune system.
3. May reduce risk of: lung, colorectal, uterine, prostate, and breast cancers.
4. Servings: daily servings of dark-orange and green foods.

M. *Soy foods.*
1. Rich in: protein, fiber, calcium, variety of vitamins and minerals; phytoestrogens (e.g., isoflavones, lignans).
2. Dietary sources: soybeans (edamame), tofu, tempeh, miso, soy nuts, soy milk.
3. **Caution:** Those with breast cancer are advised to limit soy consumption to 3 to 4 servings/week.
4. May reduce risk of cancers: breast, prostate, thyroid, and colon.
5. Servings: 1 to 2 daily soy servings (10 to 30 gm soy protein and 30 to 90 mg isoflavones). **Avoid excesses** of more than 200 mg isoflavones daily.

N. *Tomatoes.*
1. Rich in: lycopene, vitamin C, beta-carotene, potassium.

2. *Effect:*
   a. Antioxidants that scavenge free radicals.
   b. Reduce tissue damage.
   c. Protect cell membranes.
   d. Prevent formation of nitrosamines.
3. Have been shown to inhibit growth of: prostate, colon, bladder, cervical, stomach, esophageal, and lung cancers.
4. Servings: 4 or more daily.

O. *Whole grains.*
1. Rich in: fiber, vitamins, trace minerals, antioxidants, plant sterols, phytoestrogens, phytases, tocotrienols, lignans, ellagic acid, saponins.
2. Dietary sources: oats, barley, mullet, brown rice, bulgur.
3. *Effect:* may reduce risk of various cancers, as well as hypertension, heart disease, obesity, and diabetes.
4. Servings: 3 times daily.

P. *Yogurt* with live, active cultures.
1. Rich in: protein, calcium, and probiotics.
2. *Effect:*
   a. Boost immunity.
   b. Inhibit cell proliferation.
   c. Induce cell death.
3. May protect against colorectal cancer.

FOOD LIST FOR MENU PLANNING

I. HIGH-CHOLESTEROL FOODS—over 50 mg/100-gm portion: beef, butter, cheese, egg yolks, shellfish, kidney, liver, pork, veal.

II. HIGH-SODIUM FOODS—over 500 mg/100-gm portion: bacon (cured, Canadian); beef (corned, cooked, canned, dried, creamed); biscuits, baking powder; bouillon cubes; bran, added sugar and malt; bran flakes with thiamine; breads (wheat, French, rye, white, whole wheat); butter, cheese (cheddar, Parmesan, Swiss, pasteurized American); cocoa; cookies, gingersnaps; cornflakes; cornbread; crackers (graham, saltines); margarine; milk (dry, skim); mustard; oat products; olives (green, ripe); peanut butter; pickles, dill; popcorn with oil and salt; raisins; salad dressing (blue cheese, Roquefort, French, Thousand Island); sausages (bologna, frankfurters); soy sauce; tomato catsup; tuna in oil.

III. HIGH-POTASSIUM FOODS—more than 400 mg/100-gm portion: almonds; bacon, Canadian; baking powder, low sodium; beans (white, lima); beef, hamburger; bran with sugar and malt; cake (fruitcake, gingerbread); cashew nuts; chicken, light meat; cocoa; coffee, instant; cookies, gingersnaps; dates; fruits, fruit juices; garlic; milk (skim, powdered); peanuts, roasted; peanut butter; peas; pecans; potatoes, boiled in skin; scallops; tea, instant; tomato puree; turkey, light meat; veal; walnuts, black; yeast, brewer's.

IV. FOODS HIGH IN B VITAMINS

A. *Thiamine:* pork, dried beans, dried peas, liver, lamb, veal, nuts, peas.

B. *Riboflavin:* liver, poultry, milk, yogurt, whole-grain cereals, beef, oysters, tongue, fish, cottage cheese, veal.

C. *Niacin:* liver, fish, poultry, peanut butter, whole grains and enriched breads, lamb, veal, beef, pork.

V. FOODS HIGH IN VITAMIN C: oranges, strawberries, dark-green leafy vegetables, potatoes, grapefruit, tomato, cabbage, broccoli, melon, liver.

VI. FOODS HIGH IN IRON, CALCIUM, AND RESIDUE

A. *Iron:* breads (brown, corn, ginger); fish (tuna); poultry; organ meats; whole-grain cereals; shellfish; egg yolk; fruits (apples, berries); dried fruits (dates, prunes, apricots, peaches, raisins); vegetables (dark-green leafy, potatoes, tomatoes, rhubarb, squash); molasses; dried beans and peas; peanut butter; brown sugar; noodles; rice.

B. *Calcium:* milk (dry, skim, whole, evaporated, buttermilk); cheese (American, Swiss, hard); dark green leafy vegetables (kale, turnip greens, mustard greens, collards); black-eyed peas; tofu; canned fish with bones; figs.

C. *Residue:* whole-grain cereals (oatmeal, bran, shredded wheat); breads (whole wheat, cracked wheat, rye, bran muffins); vegetables (lettuce, spinach, Swiss chard, raw carrots, raw celery, corn, cauliflower, eggplant, sauerkraut, cabbage); fruits (bananas, figs, apricots, oranges).

VII. FOODS TO BE USED IN LOW-PROTEIN AND LOW-CARBOHYDRATE DIETS

A. *Low protein* (these proteins are allowed in various amounts in controlled-protein diets for *renal decompensation*): milk (buttermilk, reconstituted evaporated, low sodium, skim, powdered); meat (chicken, lamb, turkey, beef [lean], veal); fish (sole, flounder, haddock, perch); cheese (cheddar, American, Swiss, cottage); eggs; fruits (apples, grapes, pears, pineapple); vegetables (cabbage, cucumbers, lettuce, tomatoes); cereals (cornflakes, puffed rice, puffed wheat, farina, rolled oats).

B. *Low carbohydrate:* all meats; cheese (hard, soft, cottage); eggs; shellfish (oysters, shrimp); fats (bacon, butter, French dressing, salad oil, mayonnaise, margarine); vegetables (asparagus, green beans, beet greens, broccoli, brussels sprouts, cabbage, celery, cauliflower, cucumber, lettuce, green pepper, spinach, squash, tomatoes); fruits (avocados, strawberries, cantaloupe, lemons, rhubarb).

VIII. DIETARY GUIDE—MyPlate has replaced the Food Pyramid as a guide to daily food selection **(Fig. 9.1)**

A. Balance calories:
1. Enjoy food, but eat less.
2. Avoid oversized portions.

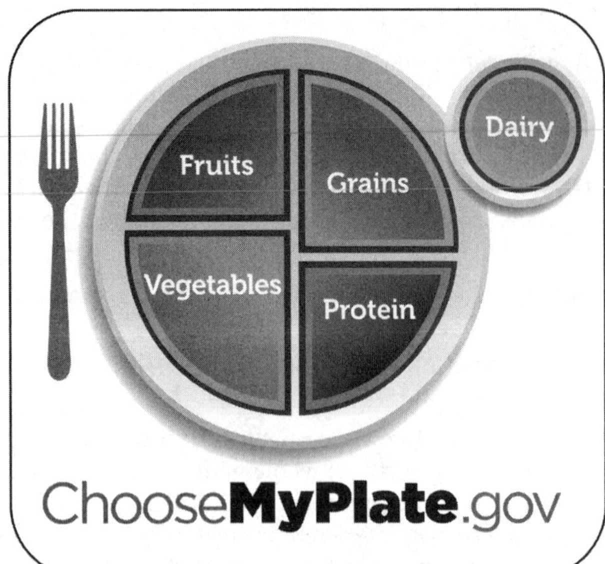

Figure 9.1 MyPlate—guide to daily food choices.
(www.choosemyplate.gov.)

B. Increase the following foods:
   1. Half the plate should be fruits and vegetables.
   2. Grains should be whole grains (e.g., whole wheat, oatmeal, brown rice).
   3. Switch to fat-free or low-fat milk.

C. Reduce the following foods:
   1. Sodium—read the label.
   2. Soda—drink water instead of sugary drinks.

Questions

Select the one answer that is best for each question, unless otherwise directed.

1. A client is discharged on a 2-gm sodium-restricted diet. Which menu choice would indicate the client understands the restriction?
1. Chow mein, egg roll, hot tea.
2. Onion soup, unsalted crackers, 1 oz cheddar cheese.
3. Corned beef sandwich, dill pickle, ginger ale.
4. Turkey breast Divan, rice pilaf, iced tea.

2. A client with Parkinson's disease will likely have the greatest difficulty swallowing:
1. Apple juice.
2. Cottage cheese.
3. Milk shake.
4. Ground beef.

3. Which statement by a client with hypokalemia indicates a need for further teaching by a nurse?
1. "I will eat more bananas and cantaloupes."
2. "I will eat more bran."
3. "I will take my K-Lor on a full stomach."
4. "I will call my provider for weakness, confusion, abdominal cramping, or anxiety."

4. A nurse should determine that a client understands the dietary restrictions with a low-cholesterol diet if the client selects a larger portion of:
1. Cottage cheese.
2. Cheese.
3. Beef.
4. Brown rice.

5. A nurse instructs a client to eat a low-iodine diet before a thyroid study. A client should be told to avoid:
1. Shellfish.
2. Coffee and chocolate.
3. Dark-green leafy vegetables.
4. Tap water unless it is run through a filter.

6. A client would demonstrate awareness of dietary influences in the prevention of dumping syndrome if the intake were adjusted by:
Select all that apply.
1. Increasing fats as tolerated.
2. Eating more dry items than liquid.
3. Consuming fluids before or after mealtimes.
4. Avoiding concentrated carbohydrates.
5. Increasing simple carbohydrates.

7. In preparation for surgery, a client is placed on a low-residue diet. In discussing the kinds of foods that will be allowed, a nurse should list:
1. Ground lean beef, soft-boiled eggs.
2. Lettuce, spinach, corn.
3. Prunes, grapes, apples.
4. Bran cereal, whole-wheat toast, milk.

8. In Ménière's disease, the diet is modified as a part of the treatment plan. Which diet is most appropriate?
1. Low sodium.
2. High protein.
3. Low carbohydrate.
4. Low fat.

9. The results of a client's complete blood count are: RBC 3.2 million/mm^3, Hgb 10 gm/dL, Hct 29%, and mean corpuscular hemoglobin (MCH) 25 pg/cell. Which foods should the nurse recommend to the client? *Select all that apply.*
1. Peas.
2. Cauliflower.
3. Milk.
4. Eggs.
5. Raisins.

10. A client is admitted with a diagnosis of brain attack (stroke). A physician orders a diet as tolerated. Before feeding the client, a nurse should *first:*
1. Wait for a specific diet order.
2. Elevate the head of the bed 30 degrees.
3. Evaluate the client's swallow reflex.
4. Delegate feeding to the nursing assistant.

11. A client is admitted to a hospital for pneumonia and it is discovered that the client also has a stage II pressure ulcer. When planning a diet for this client, what foods should a nurse encourage the client to eat?
   1. Fruits and vegetables.
   2. Whole grains.
   3. Milk, yogurt, and cheese.
   4. Lean meats and low-fat milk.

12. A 16-year-old client, who is gravida 1, para 0, is attending a class on pregnancy and nutrition. Which menu selection should a nurse recommend that would best meet the nutritional needs of the client who is pregnant?
   1. Hamburger patty, green beans, French fries, and iced tea.
   2. Roast beef sandwich, potato chips, baked beans, and cola.
   3. Baked chicken, fruit cup, potato salad, coleslaw, yogurt, and herbal tea.
   4. Fish sandwich, gelatin with fruit, and coffee.

13. A client, who is 23 years old, gravida 3, para 1, has a hemoglobin of 9 gm/dL. She has been prescribed an exogenous iron supplement, but tells a nurse that she cannot take pills. Which food should the nurse recommend that is high in iron?
   1. Dried apricots.
   2. Lima beans.
   3. Tofu.
   4. Milk.

14. A neonatal nurse is caring for a newborn who is breastfeeding. How many kilocalories are present in an ounce of maternal breast milk?
   1. 10 kcal/ounce.
   2. 20 kcal/ounce.
   3. 30 kcal/ounce.
   4. 40 kcal/ounce.

15. A child is diagnosed with cystic fibrosis. Which food(s) should the child avoid? *Select all that apply.*
   1. Low-fat yogurt.
   2. Nuts.
   3. Ham.
   4. Hot dogs.
   5. Sugar-free Jello.
   6. Low-salt crackers.

16. What would be allowed in the diet of a client with peptic ulcer disease (PUD)?
   1. Milk.
   2. Caffeinated coffee.
   3. Alcohol.
   4. Tomato juice.

17. Sodium intake is recommended to be no more than 2,400 mg each day. Which client is most at risk for stroke and heart attack with a higher than recommended Na^+ intake?
   1. A woman.
   2. A client who is overweight.
   3. A man.
   4. A client who is Hispanic.

18. Which food would be restricted in a low-sodium diet?
   1. Whole milk.
   2. Ginger ale.
   3. Orange juice.
   4. Black coffee.

19. A client is attending an informational session for in-vitro fertilization. The client asks a nurse, "What foods can I eat to increase my intake of folic acid?" The nurse suggests that the best source of folic acid is:
   1. Green vegetables and liver.
   2. Yellow vegetables and red meat.
   3. Carrots and onions.
   4. Milk and eggs.

20. A 40-year-old client at 9 weeks' gestation presents to an obstetric clinic complaining of nausea and vomiting every morning when she awakens. Which intervention should a nurse recommend for this client?
   1. Eat a handful of peanuts before getting out of bed.
   2. Increase her intake of high-fat foods.
   3. Drink a carbonated beverage before bedtime.
   4. Eat dry, unsalted crackers before getting out of bed.

21. A nurse prepares to give maternal breast milk to an infant via a bottle. Which steps should the nurse take when preparing and administering breast milk? *Select all that apply and place in priority order.*
   1. Review the diet orders.
   2. Compare the infant's identification band against the label on the milk.
   3. Discard thawed milk after 1 hour.
   4. Thaw frozen milk slowly in the microwave.
   5. Put on gloves.

22. A client, who has not been eating or drinking, is admitted to a hospital. Which sign of dehydration should a nurse expect?
   1. Tachycardia.
   2. Hypertension.
   3. Shortness of breath.
   4. Crackles in the lungs.

23. A client, who is 24 years old and has gestational diabetes, is getting instructions about her diet. A nurse knows that her teaching has been successful when the client correctly identifies that she should avoid: *Select all that apply.*
   1. White rice.
   2. Fruit juice.
   3. Cold cereal.
   4. Hot cereal.
   5. Milk.

24. A client, who is a 17-year-old gravida 2, para 1, practices a strict vegetarian diet. She has been prescribed an iron supplement during her second trimester of pregnancy. To promote better absorption, a nurse should instruct the client to take the iron supplement with which beverage?
1. Milk.
2. Iced tea.
3. Soy milk.
4. Orange juice.

25. A client is attending a class on prenatal nutrition. The client asks why vitamin C is important during pregnancy. A nurse's best response would be:
1. Vitamin C is needed to promote collagen formation.
2. Eating foods high in vitamin C helps metabolize fats and carbohydrates.
3. Supplemental vitamin C in large doses can prevent neural tube defects.
4. Studies have shown that vitamin C deficiency leads to pregnancy-induced hypertension.

Answers/Rationales/Tips

1. CORRECT ANSWER: 4. **Answer 1** is incorrect because ethnic foods, such as Chinese, are high in sodium. **Answer 2** is incorrect because the broth used in onion soup, and cheeses, are both high in sodium. **Answer 3** is incorrect because the brining processes for corned beef, as well as the sodium contained in ginger and dill pickle, all make this a poor choice for the diet. **Answer 4 is correct because turkey and rice are lowest in sodium. The sauce used on the turkey Divan can be made with a low-sodium soup.**

■ TEST-TAKING TIP: *Eliminate the choices that are known to be high in sodium—ethnic foods, canned or processed foods, or those prepared with large amounts of salt.*

Content Area: Adult Health, Nutrition; *Integrated Process:* Nursing Process, Evaluation; *Cognitive Level:* Application; *Client Need/Subneed:* Physiological Integrity/Basic Care and Comfort/Nutrition and Oral Hydration

2. CORRECT ANSWER: 1. **Answer 1 is correct because any thin liquid or food increases the chance of aspiration.** **Answer 2** is incorrect because thicker foods *will reduce the risk* of aspiration. **Answer 3** is incorrect because thick liquids *are* less likely to be aspirated. **Answer 4** is incorrect because ground beef is soft, does not required chewing, and the risk of aspiration is *minimized.*

■ TEST-TAKING TIP: *Look for the option that is different from the others—one is a thin consistency, and like saliva, is more likely to cause aspiration.*

Content Area: Adult Health, Neuromuscular; *Integrated Process:* Nursing Process, Analysis; *Cognitive Level:* Application; *Client Need/Subneed:* Physiological Integrity/Basic Care and Comfort/Nutrition and Oral Hydration

3. CORRECT ANSWER: 2. **Answer 1** is incorrect because bananas and cantaloupes *are* good sources of potassium. **Answer 2 is correct because bran has fiber but little potassium for a client with low potassium.** **Answer 3** is incorrect because potassium is irritating and *is* correctly taken with food or plenty of liquids. **Answer 4** is incorrect because these *are* signs of hypokalemia.

■ TEST-TAKING TIP: *The question calls for selecting the wrong statement as the best answer. Review good sources of potassium and signs/symptoms of low potassium.*

Content Area: Adult Health, Fluid and Electrolyte Imbalances; *Integrated Process:* Nursing Process, Evaluation; *Cognitive Level:* Application; *Client Need/Subneed:* Physiological Integrity/Basic Care and Comfort/Nutrition and Oral Hydration

4. CORRECT ANSWER: 4. **Answer 1** is incorrect because cottage cheese is a source of protein (which comprises only 15% of calories) and contains more cholesterol. **Answer 2** is incorrect because cheese, a source of protein, should be limited because of fat and calories. **Answer 3** is incorrect because beef, higher in fat than fish or chicken, should be limited. **Answer 4 is correct because 50% to 60% of the calories should come from a carbohydrate source such as brown rice.**

■ TEST-TAKING TIP: *Only brown rice is a low-carbohydrate and low-fat choice. The other three options are sources of protein.*

Content Area: Adult Health, Nutrition; *Integrated Process:* Nursing Process, Evaluation; *Cognitive Level:* Application; *Client Need/Subneed:* Physiological Integrity/Basic Care and Comfort/Nutrition and Oral Hydration

5. CORRECT ANSWER: 1. **Answer 1 is correct because shellfish are high in iodine. Also, some brands of table salt should be avoided.** **Answer 2** is incorrect because coffee and chocolate are *not* rich in iodine. **Answer 3** is incorrect because dark-green leafy vegetables are *not* rich in iodine. **Answer 4** is incorrect because water is *not* rich in iodine.

■ TEST-TAKING TIP: *Eliminate caffeine and water as sources of iodine (Answers 2 and 4). Shellfish are the most obvious source of iodine.*

Content Area: Adult Health, Endocrine; *Integrated Process:* Nursing Process, Implementation; *Cognitive Level:* Comprehension; *Client Need/Subneed:* Physiological Integrity/Basic Care and Comfort/Nutrition and Oral Hydration

6. CORRECT ANSWERS: 1, 2, 3, 4. **Answer 1 is correct because dietary fat does not contribute to dumping syndrome like carbohydrates do. Answer 2 is correct because fluid with meals or near mealtime (less than 1 hour before or 1 hour after) contributes to dumping syndrome. Answer 3 is correct because fluid should not be consumed with meals. Fluids, 1 hour before or 1 hour after a meal, reduce the potential for dumping syndrome. Answer 4 is correct because carbohydrates increase the chance of dumping syndrome because they speed up gastric emptying.** **Answer 5** is incorrect because the diet should keep carbohydrate intake *low.*

■ **TEST-TAKING TIP:** *Ask how each option will affect gastric emptying. Will it speed or slow the "dumping" of gastric contents?*
Content Area: Adult Health, Gastrointestinal; *Integrated Process:* Nursing Process, Evaluation; *Cognitive Level:* Analysis; *Client Need/Subneed:* Physiological Integrity/Basic Care and Comfort/Nutrition and Oral Hydration

7. CORRECT ANSWER: 1. Answer 1 is correct because residue is produced by high-fiber foods. Lean beef, well cooked, and eggs are not good sources of fiber. Low residue reduces the amount of stool in the large bowel. **Answer 2** is incorrect because leafy greens (particularly in the cruciferous family) are high in roughage and fiber. **Answer 3** is incorrect because only grapes would be allowed on a low-residue diet. Generally fruit juices (except prune) are permitted. **Answer 4** is incorrect because grains such as bran and whole wheat are high fiber sources. Dairy may be permitted. In a low-residue diet, refined, plain foods are permitted.
■ **TEST-TAKING TIP:** *Know that high-fiber foods influence stool production. The goal before surgery is to reduce the amount of stool. Eliminate most vegetables (Answer 2), fruits (Answer 3), and bran and whole wheat (Answer 4).*
Content Area: Adult Health, Gastrointestinal; *Integrated Process:* Nursing Process, Implementation; *Cognitive Level:* Comprehension; *Client Need/Subneed:* Physiological Integrity/Basic Care and Comfort/Nutrition and Oral Hydration

8. CORRECT ANSWER: 1. Answer 1 is correct because fluid retention is thought to aggravate the symptoms of Ménière's disease. Foods high in sodium contribute to fluid retention. **Answer 2** is incorrect because foods high in protein do *not* contribute to fluid retention, which is the concern. **Answer 3** is incorrect because reducing the carbohydrate content of the diet will *not* decrease fluid retention, which is the concern. **Answer 4** is incorrect because reducing the fat intake in the diet will *not* decrease fluid retention, which is the concern.
■ **TEST-TAKING TIP:** *Consider which option could have a direct effect on the ear—sodium would increase fluid retention.*
Content Area: Adult Health, Sensory; *Integrated Process:* Nursing Process, Planning; *Cognitive Level:* Application; *Client Need/Subneed:* Physiological Integrity/Basic Care and Comfort/Nutrition and Oral Hydration

9. CORRECT ANSWERS: 1, 4, 5. Answer 1 is correct because the client's red blood cell (RBC), hemoglobin (Hgb), and hematocrit (Hct) levels are low and indicate iron-deficiency anemia, and legumes are a good source of iron. **Answer 2** is incorrect because the *green* vegetables (particularly *leafy*) are iron-rich food sources. **Answer 3** is incorrect because milk is *not* an iron-rich food source. **Answer 4 is correct because the laboratory results reflect iron-deficiency anemia, and animal protein is an excellent source of iron. Answer 5 is correct because the RBC count indicates iron-deficiency anemia, and dried fruits are a rich source of iron.**
■ **TEST-TAKING TIP:** *Choose common food sources of iron.*
Content Area: Adult Health, Hematological; *Integrated Process:* Teaching and Learning; *Cognitive Level:* Application; *Client Need/Subneed:* Physiological Integrity/Basic Care and Comfort/Nutrition and Oral Hydration

10. CORRECT ANSWER: 3. **Answer 1** is incorrect because the RN can offer the client *any* preferred foods. **Answer 2** is incorrect because this would *not* be the *first* nursing action. **Answer 3 is correct because the client may be at risk for aspiration if the ability to swallow has been affected.** **Answer 4** is incorrect because the RN must *assess* the client and determine ability to swallow *before* delegating care.
■ **TEST-TAKING TIP:** *Focus on a step of the nursing process: "evaluate" before any action (wait, elevate, delegate). Think client safety.*
Content Area: Adult Health, Cardiovascular; *Integrated Process:* Nursing Process, Planning; *Cognitive Level:* Application; *Client Need/Subneed:* Physiological Integrity/Basic Care and Comfort/Nutrition and Oral Hydration

11. CORRECT ANSWER: 4. **Answer 1** is incorrect because fruits and vegetables are mostly carbohydrates. **Answer 2** is incorrect because whole grains are not complete proteins. **Answer 3** is incorrect because this choice has a lot of fats as well as carbohydrates. **Answer 4 is correct because proteins help to repair and build cells.**
■ **TEST-TAKING TIP:** *The client is likely in a catabolic state and cells are being destroyed. Look for the option with the most amount of protein.*
Content Area: Adult Health, Integumentary; *Integrated Process:* Nursing Process, Implementation; *Cognitive Level:* Application; *Client Need/Subneed:* Physiological Integrity/Basic Care and Comfort/Nutrition and Oral Hydration

12. CORRECT ANSWER: 3. **Answer 1** is incorrect because the hamburger patty and French fries are choices that are *high* in *fat* and have *fewer nutrients. Caffeine*-containing beverages such as iced tea should be avoided in pregnancy. **Answer 2** is incorrect because this option has *no fresh vegetable or fruit* choices, and cola with *caffeine* should be avoided in pregnancy. **Answer 3 is correct because this menu has a variety of lean protein, carbohydrates, fruits, vegetables, and dairy. While the choices within the categories are not ideal, it is the most balanced of the options.** **Answer 4** is incorrect because this option has *no fresh vegetable or fruit* choices, and *coffee* with caffeine should be avoided in pregnancy.
■ **TEST-TAKING TIP:** *Three of the options have beverages with caffeine, which should be avoided in pregnancy.*
Content Area: Maternity, Antepartum; *Integrated Process:* Nursing Process, Implementation; *Cognitive Level:* Analysis; *Client Need/Subneed:* Physiological Integrity/Basic Care and Comfort/Nutrition and Oral Hydration

13. CORRECT ANSWER: 1. **Answer 1 is correct because dried apricots are a good source of iron, require no cooking, and are palatable for a young mother.** **Answer 2** is incorrect because, even though lima beans are a good source of iron, they require preparation and are not usually a primary choice for *a younger client.* **Answer 3** is incorrect because, even though tofu is a good source of iron, it requires preparation and is not usually a primary choice for *a younger client.* **Answer 4** is incorrect because milk is *not* a good source of iron; it is a good source of *calcium.* You also need to consider if the client has lactose intolerance.

■ **TEST-TAKING TIP:** ***The key to this question is the client's age. Iron-rich foods can be less palatable. Even if a food is a good source of iron, the young adult may not eat it or take time to prepare anything. Choose the best food for this young busy mother.***

Content Area: Maternity, Antepartum; ***Integrated Process:*** Nursing Process, Implementation; ***Cognitive Level:*** Application; ***Client Need/Subneed:*** Physiological Integrity/Basic Care and Comfort/Nutrition and Oral Hydration

14. CORRECT ANSWER: 2. **Answer 1** is incorrect because it is too few kilocalories. **Answer 2 is correct because maternal breast milk contains 20 kilocalories per ounce.** **Answer 3** is incorrect because it is too many kilocalories. **Answer 4** is incorrect because it is too many kilocalories.

■ **TEST-TAKING TIP:** ***Recall that maternal breast milk contains the same number of kilocalories per ounce as regular infant formula.***

Content Area: Child Health, Newborn; ***Integrated Process:*** Nursing Process, Analysis; ***Cognitive Level:*** Comprehension; ***Client Need/Subneed:*** Physiological Integrity/Basic Care and Comfort/Nutrition and Oral Hydration

15. CORRECT ANSWERS: 1, 5, 6. **Answer 1 is correct because the child with cystic fibrosis *should avoid* low-fat foods and eat foods that are high in calories instead, such as *full-fat* yogurt.** **Answer 2** is incorrect because children with cystic fibrosis *should* eat foods high in calories, such as nuts. **Answer 3** is incorrect because children with cystic fibrosis *should* eat meats, such as ham. **Answer 4** is incorrect because children with cystic fibrosis *should* eat foods *high in calories,* such as hot dogs. **Answer 5 is correct because children with cystic fibrosis *should* eat foods *high in calories,* such as puddings.** **Answer 6 is correct because children with cystic fibrosis *should* eat foods that contain *salt,* as they tend to lose salt.**

■ **TEST-TAKING TIP:** ***Note the key word in the stem: "avoid." These children need high-calorie diets to maintain body weight because children with cystic fibrosis are likely to have failure to thrive and require nighttime gastrostomy feedings.***

Content Area: Child Health, Respiratory; ***Integrated Process:*** Nursing Process, Analysis; ***Cognitive Level:*** Application; ***Client Need/Subneed:*** Physiological Integrity/Basic Care and Comfort/Nutrition and Oral Hydration

16. CORRECT ANSWER: 4. **Answer 1** is incorrect because milk is known to *increase* acid production and is restricted in a PUD diet. **Answer 2** is incorrect because coffee is known to *increase* acid production and is restricted in a PUD diet. **Answer 3** is incorrect because alcohol is known to *increase* acid production and is restricted in a PUD diet. **Answer 4 is correct because, although tomato juice may be acidic, it does *not* increase acid production. The guideline for the diet with PUD is to avoid foods that increase symptoms, and these vary from client to client.**

■ **TEST-TAKING TIP:** ***The key concept is avoiding food/fluid that increases acid production.***

Content Area: Adult Health, Gastrointestinal; ***Integrated Process:*** Nursing Process, Planning; ***Cognitive Level:*** Application; ***Client Need/Subneed:*** Physiological Integrity/Basic Care and Comfort/Nutrition and Oral Hydration

17. CORRECT ANSWER: 2. **Answer 1** is incorrect because, based on current research, the only population having an association between salt intake and hypertension are clients who are *obese.* **Answer 2 is correct because high sodium intake increases the risk of cardiovascular disease and death in clients who are obese.** **Answer 3** is incorrect because, based on current research, the only population having an association between salt intake and hypertension are clients who are *obese.* **Answer 4** is incorrect because, based on current research, the only population having an association between salt intake and hypertension are clients who are *obese.*

■ **TEST-TAKING TIP:** ***Eliminate gender and ethnic factors. Choose the client who will be most affected by fluid retention associated with an increase in sodium intake.***

Content Area: Adult Health, Cardiovascular; ***Integrated Process:*** Nursing Process, Analysis; ***Cognitive Level:*** Comprehension; ***Client Need/Subneed:*** Physiological Integrity/Basic Care and Comfort/Nutrition and Oral Hydration

18. CORRECT ANSWER: 1. **Answer 1 is correct because whole milk has 120 mg of sodium per 8 oz.** **Answer 2** is incorrect because 8 oz of ginger ale has *only* 6 mg of sodium. **Answer 3** is incorrect because the sodium content of orange juice is *so low* it is not even listed in the nutrition books. **Answer 4** is incorrect because 8 oz of coffee has *only* 1 mg of sodium.

■ **TEST-TAKING TIP:** ***Recall that dairy products are high in sodium. Review therapeutic diets for restricted foods.***

Content Area: Adult Health, Cardiovascular; ***Integrated Process:*** Nursing Process, Analysis; ***Cognitive Level:*** Application; ***Client Need/Subneed:*** Physiological Integrity/Basic Care and Comfort/Nutrition and Oral Hydration

19. CORRECT ANSWER: 1. **Answer 1 is correct because green vegetables and liver are rich sources of folic acid, an essential nutrient to prevent neural tube defects in the developing fetus.** **Answer 2** is incorrect because *green* vegetables are the *best* source of folic acid. Yellow vegetables *are* a source of folic acid, but *red meat* is *not* a good source of folic acid. **Answer 3** is incorrect because carrots are a good source of *vitamin A,* but *not* folic acid, and onions are *not* a particularly rich source of folic acid. **Answer 4** is incorrect because milk and eggs are *not* the best source of folic acid.

■ **TEST-TAKING TIP:** *Folic acid is highest in leafy green vegetables. Even though many foods have some folic acid, the option with the green vegetables is the best choice.*
Content Area: Maternity, Antepartum; *Integrated Process:* Teaching and Learning; *Cognitive Level:* Application; *Client Need/Subneed:* Physiological Integrity/Basic Care and Comfort/Nutrition and Oral Hydration

20. CORRECT ANSWER: 4. Answer 1 is incorrect because eating peanuts before getting out of bed avoids having an empty stomach, but the peanuts are high in fat and slowly digested, which can add to the hyperemesis symptoms. **Answer 2** is incorrect because a client with hyperemesis should eat foods that are easy to digest, such as: toast, crackers, bagels, pretzels, cereal, rice, pasta, and potatoes. A high-carbohydrate, *low-fat* diet is best *tolerated* by clients with hyperemesis. **Answer 3** is incorrect because drinking carbonated beverages can assist in preventing the dehydration associated with hyperemesis, but it will *not help* with nausea and vomiting that the client experiences *upon waking*. She should be drinking throughout the day to avoid dehydration. Suggestions include: tea, juices, water and carbonated beverages. **Answer 4 is correct because eating a small amount of easily digested carbohydrate can help decrease nausea and vomiting. To avoid having an empty stomach, the crackers should be eaten before getting out of bed.**
■ **TEST-TAKING TIP:** *The key to this question is assisting the client to manage her symptoms that occur upon waking. Choose the option that best treats the client's major concern (nausea and vomiting).*
Content Area: Maternity, Antepartum; *Integrated Process:* Nursing Process, Implementation; *Cognitive Level:* Application; *Client Need/Subneed:* Physiological Integrity/Basic Care and Comfort/Nutrition and Oral Hydration

21. CORRECT ANSWERS: 1, 2, 5, 3. Answer 1 is correct because the *first* step is to confirm the diet order. Answer 2 is correct because the *second* step should be to verify that the correct client is receiving the breast milk. Answer 3 is correct because the *final* step is to discard thawed breast milk after 1 hour. **Answer 4** is incorrect because breast milk should *never* be warmed in the microwave; this destroys the immune properties and creates hot spots in the bottle, which could burn the infant. **Answer 5 is correct because the *third* step is to put on gloves, since breast milk is a body fluid and may be a route of exposure to infectious organisms. Universal precautions (applying protective barriers such as gloves, gowns, and mask) should be applied when handling blood or body fluids.**
■ **TEST-TAKING TIP:** *Breast milk is a body fluid that has the potential for transmitting infectious disease. A nurse should take similar steps as when administering blood products, including confirming the "five rights," and following standard precautions.*
Content Area: Child Health, Nutrition; *Integrated Process:* Nursing Process, Implementation; *Cognitive Level:* Application; *Client Need/Subneed:* Physiological Integrity/Basic Care and Comfort/Nutrition and Oral Hydration

22. CORRECT ANSWER: 1. Answer 1 is correct because the body is trying to compensate for the fluid loss by stimulating the heart rate to increase cardiac output and perfusion. **Answer 2** is incorrect because *hypo*tension would be more common with dehydration or hypovolemia. **Answer 3** is incorrect because shortness of breath would be more likely with volume *overload*. **Answer 4** is incorrect because crackles in the lungs are a sign of increased fluid in the *lungs, not* dehydration.
■ **TEST-TAKING TIP:** *Look for the option that would be the compensatory response to the hypovolemia resulting from dehydration. Three of the options are seen with hypervolemia or volume overload, not dehydration.*
Content Area: Adult Health, Fluid and Electrolyte Imbalances; *Integrated Process:* Nursing Process, Assessment; *Cognitive Level:* Application; *Client Need/Subneed:* Physiological Integrity/Basic Care and Comfort/Nutrition and Oral Hydration

23. CORRECT ANSWERS: 1, 2, 3. Answer 1 is correct because white rice has a *high glycemic index* and results in a rapid increase in the client's blood sugar, and it should be avoided. Answer 2 is correct because fruit juice has a *high glycemic index* and results in a rapid increase in the client's blood sugar, and it should be avoided. Answer 3 is correct because cold cereal has a *high glycemic index* and results in a rapid increase in the client's blood sugar, and it should be avoided. **Answer 4** is incorrect because hot cereal does *not* have a high glycemic index, does *not* result in a rapid increase in the client's blood sugar, and *can* be part of the diet in gestational diabetes. **Answer 5** is incorrect because milk does *not* have a high glycemic index, does not result in a rapid increase in the client's blood sugar, and *can* be part of the diet in gestational diabetes.
■ **TEST-TAKING TIP:** *Clients with gestational diabetes need to have blood sugar that is well controlled; foods that cause a spike in blood sugar are to be avoided.*
Content Area: Maternity, Antepartum; *Integrated Process:* Nursing Process, Evaluation; *Cognitive Level:* Application; *Client Need/Subneed:* Physiological Integrity/Basic Care and Comfort/Nutrition and Oral Hydration

24. CORRECT ANSWER: 4. Answer 1 is incorrect because cow's milk contains *little* iron and can *reduce* iron absorption. **Answer 2** is incorrect because iced tea contains *tannins,* which are known to *reduce* the absorption of iron. **Answer 3** is incorrect because studies have shown soy to have an *inhibitory* effect on iron absorption. **Answer 4 is correct because orange juice is high in vitamin C, which can increase the absorption of iron and is needed for the production of hemoglobin.**
■ **TEST-TAKING TIP:** *Remember:* acidic *beverages can assist in absorption of iron supplements. Milk, antacids, soy, and tannins decrease absorption.*
Content Area: Maternity, Antepartum; *Integrated Process:* Nursing Process, Implementation; *Cognitive Level:* Application; *Client Need/Subneed:* Physiological Integrity/Basic Care and Comfort/Nutrition and Oral Hydration

25. CORRECT ANSWER: 1. Answer 1 is correct because **vitamin C is important in the synthesis of collagen, which is the main structural component of the skin as well as many other body tissues. Vitamin C also works as a powerful antioxidant, aids in the absorption of iron, is critical in fighting off infections, helps alleviate allergic reactions, and aids in wound healing. Vitamin C helps the fetus grow and builds strong bones and teeth.** **Answer 2** is incorrect because vitamin C does *not* assist in metabolizing fats and carbohydrates. Vitamin B complex, especially thiamine, helps with metabolism of fats and carbohydrates. **Answer 3** is *incorrect* because *folic acid, not* vitamin C, prevents neural tube defects. **Answer 4** is incorrect because there are *no* studies that have shown that vitamin C deficiency leads to pregnancy-induced hypertension.

■ **TEST-TAKING TIP:** *Since the cause of pregnancy-induced hypertension has not been found, eliminate the response that correlates vitamin C deficiency and pregnancy-induced hypertension (Answer 4). Eliminate Answers 2 and 3, as they relate to vitamin B complex and folic acid.*

Content Area: Maternity, Antepartum; ***Integrated Process:*** Nursing Process, Implementation; ***Cognitive Level:*** Application; ***Client Need/Subneed:*** Physiological Integrity/Basic Care and Comfort/Nutrition and Oral Hydration

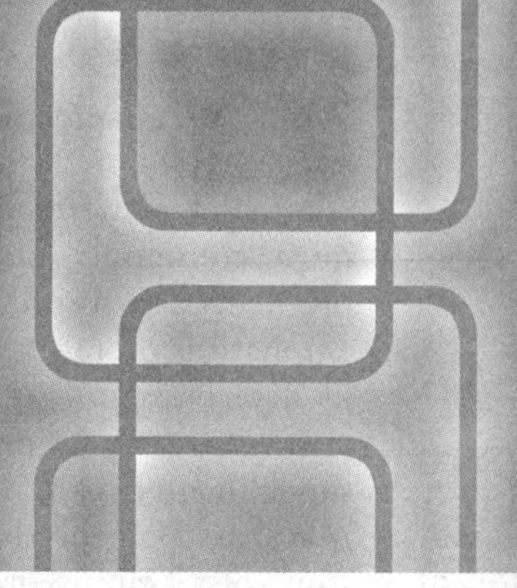

CHAPTER 10

Psychosocial Integrity

Behavioral/Mental Health Care Throughout the Life Span

Sally Lambert Lagerquist • Janis Ryan Wisherop (Reviewer and Contributor to Selected Sections)

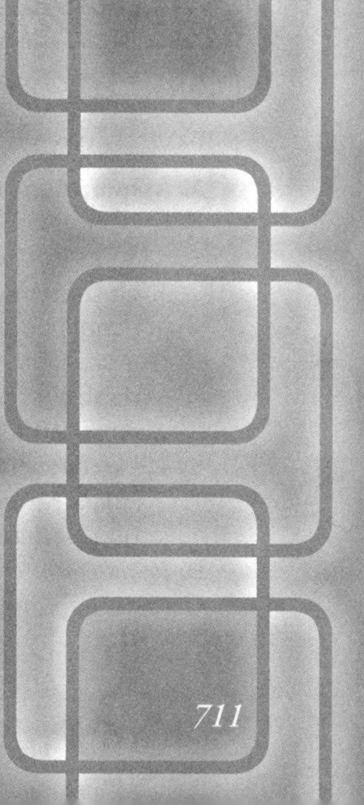

The chief *objective* of this chapter is to highlight the most commonly observed behavioral and emotional problems and disorders in the mental health field. The emphasis is on (a) main points for *assessment,* (b) *analysis* of data based on underlying *basic concepts and general principles* drawn from a psychodynamic and interpersonal theoretical framework, and (c) *nursing interventions* based on the therapeutic use of self as the cornerstone of a helping process. Nursing actions are listed in *priority* whenever possible. Hence the **nursing process framework** is followed throughout. Note that nursing interventions are divided into *planning* and *implementation* (covering long-term and short-term *goals* and stressing *priority* of actions) and *health teaching. Evaluation* of results is listed separately, although this step of the nursing process is circular and relates back to "assessment" and "goals."

The categorization of psychiatric-emotional disorders can be complex and controversial. For purposes of clarity and simplicity, an attempt has been made here to capsulize many theoretical principles and component skills of the helping process that these disorders have *in common.* That the term *client* is often used in place of *patient* reflects the interpersonal rather than medical model of psychiatric nursing. The diagnostic categorization of disorders (based on a synthesis of the North American Nursing Diagnosis Association [NANDA], Psychiatric Nursing Diagnosis [PND-I], and American Nurses Association [ANA] classification system for psychiatric nursing diagnoses) is included here to update the reader in current terminology in the mental health field.

The underlying organizational framework for this chapter is based on applicable **categories of client needs and subneeds** from the official NCLEX-RN® Test Plan.

PSYCHOSOCIAL GROWTH AND DEVELOPMENT

Major Theoretical Models

I. PSYCHODYNAMIC MODEL **(Freud)**

A. Assumptions and key ideas:

1. No human behavior is accidental; each psychic event is determined by preceding ones.
2. Unconscious mental processes occur with great frequency and significance.
3. Psychoanalysis is used to uncover childhood trauma, which may involve conflict and repressed feelings.
4. Psychoanalytic methods are used: therapeutic alliance, transference, regression, dream association, catharsis.

B. *Freud*—shifted from classification of behavior to understanding and explaining in psychological terms and changing behavior under structured conditions.

1. Structure of the mind: id, ego, superego; unconscious, preconscious, conscious.
2. Stages of psychosexual development **(Table 10.1).**
3. Defense mechanisms (see **pp. 772–774**).

II. PSYCHOSOCIAL DEVELOPMENT MODEL **(Erikson, Maslow, Piaget, Duvall)**

A. *Erik Erikson—Eight Stages of Man* (1963)

1. Psychosocial development—interplay of biology with social factors, encompassing total life span, from birth to death, in progressive developmental tasks.
2. *Stages of life cycle*—life consists of a series of developmental phases (**Table 10.2** and **Table 10.3**).
   a. Universal sequence of biological, social, psychological events.
   b. Each person experiences a series of normative conflicts and crises and thus needs to accomplish specific psychosocial tasks.
   c. Two opposing energies (positive and negative forces) coexist and must be synthesized.
   d. How each age-specific task is accomplished influences the developmental progress of the next phase and the ability to deal with life.

B. *Abraham Maslow—Hierarchy of Needs* (1962)

1. Beliefs regarding emotional health based on a comprehensive, multidisciplinary approach to human problems, involving all aspects of functioning.
   a. *Premise:* mental illness cannot be understood without prior knowledge of mental health.
   b. *Focus:* positive aspects of human behavior (e.g., contentment, joy, happiness).

(text continues on page 714)

Table 10.1

Freud's Stages of Psychosexual Development

Stage	Age	Behaviors
Oral	Birth–1 yr	Dependency and oral gratification
Anal	1–3 yr	Creativity, stinginess, cruelty, cleanliness, self-control, punctuality
Phallic or oedipal	3–6 yr	Sexual, aggressive feelings; guilt
Latency	6–12 yr	Reactivation of pregenital impulses; intellectual and social growth
Genital	12–18 yr	Displacement of pregenital impulses; learns responsibility for self; establishes identity

Table 10.2

Erikson's Stages of the Life Cycle

Age and Stage of Development	Conflict Areas Needing Resolution	Evaluation: Result of Resolution/Nonresolution
Infancy (birth–18 mo)	Trust vs. Mistrust	Shows affection, gratification, recognition; trusts self and others; begins to tolerate frustrations; develops *hope.* Uses primary caregiver as a base for exploration. Withdrawn, alienated.
Early childhood (18 mo–3 yr)	Autonomy vs. Shame and doubt	Cooperative, self-controlled, self-expressive, can delay gratification; develops *will.* Exaggerated self-restraint; defiance; compulsive; overly compliant.
Late childhood (3–5 yr)	Initiative vs. Guilt	Realistic goals; can evaluate self; explorative; imitates adult, shows imagination; tests reality; anticipates roles; develops *purpose,* self-motivation. Self-imposed restrictions relative to jealousy, guilt, and denial.
School age (5–12 yr)	Industry vs. Inferiority	Sense of duty; acquires self-confidence from social and school *competencies;* persevering in real tasks. School and social dropout; social loner; incompetent.
Adolescence (12–18 yr)	Identity vs. Role diffusion	Has ideological commitments, self-actualizing; sense of self; experiments with roles; experiences sexual polarizations; develops *fidelity.* Ambivalent, confused, indecisive; may act out (antisocial acts).
Young adulthood (18–25 yr)	Intimacy, solidarity vs. Isolation	Makes commitments to love, work relationships, a cause or creative effort; able to sustain mutual *love* relationships. Superficial, impersonal, biased.
Adulthood (25–60 yr)	Generativity vs. Self-absorption, stagnation	Productive, creative, procreative, concerned for others; develops *care.* Self-indulgent.
Late adulthood (60 yr–death)	Ego integrity vs. Despair	Appreciates past, present, and future; self-acceptance of own contribution to others, of own *self-worth,* and of changes in lifestyle and life cycle; can face "not being"; develops *wisdom.* Preoccupied with loss of hope, of purpose; contemptuous, fears death.

From ©Lagerquist, S: *Nursing Examination Review,* ed 4. Addison-Wesley, Redwood City, CA.

Table 10.3

Summary of Theories of Psychosocial Development Throughout the Life Cycle

Freud	Piaget	Sullivan	Erikson
Emphasis on:			
Pathology (intrapsychic)	*Normal* children	Pathology (interpersonal)	Both health and illness
Anxiety	*No* emphasis on ego, anxiety, identity, libido	Anxiety	
Unconscious, uncontrollable drives	Cognitive development	Unconscious, uncontrollable drives	Problems are manageable and can be solved
Ego needing defense	Tasks can be accomplished through learning process	Self-system needing defense	Need to integrate individual and society
Pathological Development Influenced by:			
Early feelings; repressed experiences in unconscious mind	Individual differences and social influences on the mind	Unconscious mind *and* interpersonal relationships (IPRs)	Ego, anxiety, identity, libido concepts *combined* with social forces

Continued

Table 10.3

Summary of Theories of Psychosocial Development Throughout the Life Cycle—cont'd

Freud	Piaget	Sullivan	Erikson
Change Possible With:			
Understanding content and meaning of unconscious	Socialization process to facilitate cognitive development	Improved IPRs and understanding basic good-bad transformations	Integration of attitudes, libido, and social roles for strong ego identity
Age Group:			
First 5 yr of life	Middle childhood years	Adolescence	Middle age, old age
Focus on:			
Emotional development	Cognitive skills	Emotional and interpersonal development; relationships with opposite sex	Emotional, interpersonal, spiritual
Psychosexual aspects	Cognitive, interactive aspects	Psychosocial aspects; developing sense of identity	Psychosocial aspects
Cause of Conflicts and Problems:			
Oral, anal, genital stage problems (especially unresolved oedipal/castration conflicts)	Faulty adaptation between individual and environment for intellectual development	Threats to self-system; disturbed communication process; 7 stages not complete	Unresolved conflicts, crises in 8 successive life cycle stages
Prognosis:			
Few changes possible after age 5	Little change in adult cognitive structure after middle adolescence	Change usually possible with improved IPRs	Change not only possible but *expected* throughout life
Sexual problems part of disturbed behavior	Sex as a variable in learning (age, IQ)	Sexual problems are only one type of faulty IPRs affecting behavior	Sexual identity as one of many problems solved by interaction of desire and social process

2. *Hierarchy of needs*—physiological, safety, love and belonging, self-esteem and self-recognition, self-actualization, aesthetic. As each stage is mastered, the next stage becomes dominant **(Fig. 10.1).**
3. *Characteristics of optimal mental health*—keep in mind that *wellness is on a continuum with cultural variations.*
   a. *Self-esteem:* entails self-confidence and self-acceptance.
   b. *Self-knowledge:* involves accurate self-perception of strengths and limitations.
   c. *Satisfying interpersonal relationships:* able to meet reciprocal emotional needs through collaboration rather than by exploitation or power struggles or jealousy; able to make full commitments in close relationships.
   d. *Environmental mastery:* can adapt, change, and solve problems effectively; can make decisions, choose from alternatives, and predict consequences. Actions are conscious, not impulsive.
   e. *Stress management:* can delay seeking gratification and relief; does not blame or dwell on past; assumes self-responsibility; either modifies own expectations, seeks substitutes, or withdraws from stressful situation when cannot reduce stress.

C. *Jean Piaget—Cognitive and Intellectual Development* (1963)

1. **Assumptions**—child development is steered by interaction of environmental and genetic influences; therefore, focus is on environmental and social forces (see **Table 10.3** for comparison with other theories).
2. **Key concepts:**
   a. *Assimilation:* process of acquiring new knowledge, skills, and insights by using what the child already knows and has.
   b. *Accommodation:* adjusts to change by solving previously unsolvable problems because of newly assimilated knowledge.

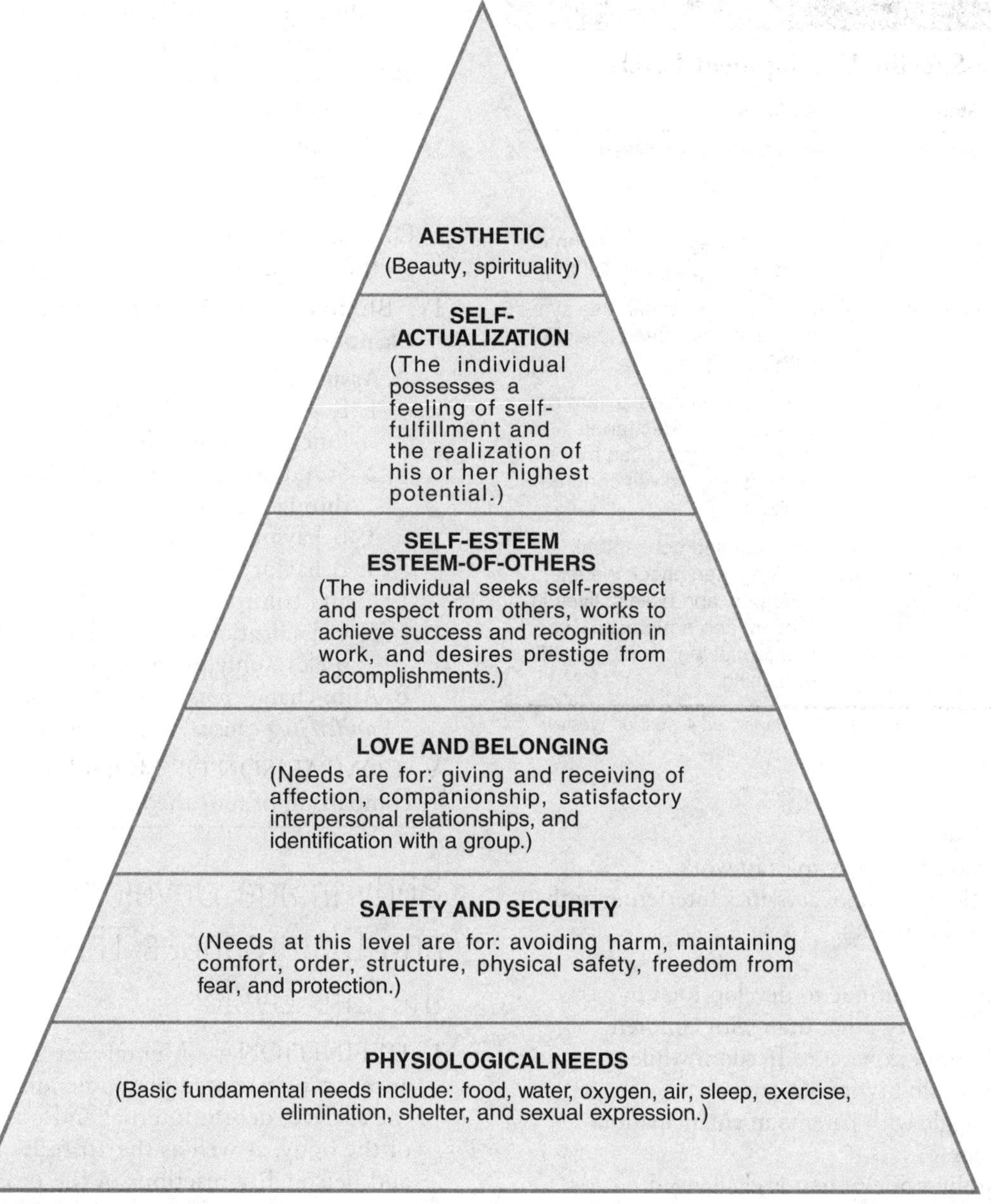

Figure 10.1 Maslow's hierarchy of needs. (Modified from Townsend M: *Essentials of Psychiatry/Mental Health Nursing.* FA Davis, Philadelphia.)

   c. *Adaptation:* coping process to handle environmental demands.
3. **Age-specific developmental levels**—sensorimotor, preconceptual, intuitive, concrete, formal operational thought **(Table 10.4).**

D. *E. M. Duvall—Family Development* (1971)—developmental tasks are family oriented, presented in eight stages throughout the life cycle.

1. *Married couple:*
   a. Establishing relationship.
   b. Defining mutual goals.
   c. Developing intimacy: issues of dependence-independence-interdependence.
   d. Establishing mutually satisfying relationship.
   e. Negotiating boundaries of couple with families.
   f. Discussing issue of childbearing.
2. *Childbearing years:*
   a. Working out authority, responsibility, and caregiver roles.
   b. Having children and forming new unit.
   c. Facilitating child's trust.
   d. Need for personal time and space while sharing with each other and child.
3. *Preschool-age years:*
   a. Experiencing changes in energy.
   b. Continuing development as couple, parents, family.
   c. Establishing own family traditions without guilt related to breaks with tradition.

Table 10.4

Piaget's Age-Specific Development Levels

Age	Stage	Abilities
Infancy–2 yr	Sensorimotor	Preverbal; uses all senses; coordinates simple motor actions
2–4 yr	Preconceptual	Can use language; egocentric; imitation in play, parallel play
4–7 yr	Intuitive	Asks questions; can use symbols and associate subjects with concepts
7–11 yr	Concrete	Sees relationships, aware of viewpoints; understands cause and effect, can make conclusions; solves concrete problems
11 yr and older	Formal operational thought	Abstract and conceptual thinking; can check ideas, thoughts, and beliefs; lives in present and nonpresent; can use formal logic and scientific reasoning

From ©Lagerquist, S: *Nursing Examination Review*, ed 4. Addison-Wesley, Redwood City, CA.

4. *School-age years:*
   a. Establishing new roles in work.
   b. Children's school activities interfering with family activities.
5. *Teenage years:*
   a. Parents continue to develop roles in community other than with children.
   b. Children experience freedom while accepting responsibility for actions.
   c. Struggle with parents in emancipation process.
   d. Family value system is challenged.
   e. Couple relationships may be strong or weak depending on responses to needs.
6. *Families as launching centers:*
   a. Young adults launched with rites of passage.
   b. Changes in couple's relationship due to empty nest and increased leisure time.
   c. Changes in relationship with children away from home.
7. *Middle-aged parents:* Dealing with issues of aging of own parents.
8. *Aging family members:*
   a. Sense of accomplishment and desire to continue to live fully.
   b. Coping with bereavement and living alone.

III. COMMUNITY MENTAL HEALTH MODEL **(Gerald Kaplan)—levels of prevention**

A. *Primary prevention*—lower the risk of mental illness and increase capacity to resist contributory influences by providing anticipatory guidance and maximizing strengths.

B. *Secondary prevention*—decrease disability by shortening its duration and reducing its severity through detection of early-warning signs and effective intervention following case-finding.

C. Crisis intervention (see **pp. 795–796**).

D. *Tertiary prevention*—avoid permanent disorder through rehabilitation.

IV. BEHAVIORAL MODEL **(Pavlov, Watson, Wolpe, Skinner)**

A. Assumptions:
1. Roots in neurophysiology (i.e., neurotransmitter functions versus effects).
2. Stimulus-response learning can be *conditioned* through *reinforcement.*
3. Behavior is what one does.
4. Behavior is observable, describable, predictable, and controllable.
5. Classification of mental disease is clinically useless, only provides legal labels.

B. Aim: change *observable* behavior. There is *no underlying* cause, *no internal* motive.

V. COMPARISON OF MODELS: see **Table 10.3** for comparison of four theories.

Body Image Development and Disturbances Throughout the Life Cycle

I. DEFINITION— "Mental picture of body's appearance; an interrelated phenomenon which includes the surface, depth, internal and postural picture of the body, as well as the attitudes, emotions, and personality reactions of the individual in relation to his body as an object in space, apart from all others."*

II. OPERATIONAL DEFINITION†

A. Body image is created by social interaction.
1. Approval given for "normal" and "proper" appearance, gestures, posture, etc.
2. Behavioral and physical deviations from normality not given approval.
3. Body image formed by the person's response to the approval and disapproval of others.
4. Person's values, attitudes, and feelings about self continually evolving and unconsciously integrated.

*Adapted from Kolb, L: Disturbances in body image. In Arieti, S (ed): *American Handbook of Psychiatry.* Basic Books, New York.

†Adapted from Norris, C: Body image. In Carlson, C, & Blackwell, B (eds): *Behavioral Concepts and Nursing Intervention,* ed 2. JB Lippincott, Philadelphia.

B. Self-image, identity, personality, sense of self, and body image are interdependent.
C. Behavior is determined by body image.

III. CONCEPTS RELATED TO PERSONS WITH PROBLEMS OF BODY IMAGE

A. Image of self changes with *changing posture* (walking, sitting, gestures).
B. *Mental picture of self* may not correspond with the actual body; subject to continual but slow revision.
C. The degree to which people like themselves (good self-concept) is directly related to how well defined they perceive their body image to be.
1. *Vague, indefinite, or distorted body image* correlates with the following personality traits:
   a. Sad, empty, hollow feelings.
   b. Mistrustful of others; poor peer relations.
   c. Low motivation.
   d. Shame, doubt, sense of inferiority, poor self-concept.
   e. Inability to tolerate stress.
2. *Integrated body image* tends to correlate positively with the following personality traits:
   a. Happy, good self-concept.
   b. Good peer relations.
   c. Sense of initiative, industry, autonomy, identity.
   d. Able to complete tasks.
   e. Assertive.
   f. Academically competent; high achievement.
   g. Able to cope with stress.

D. Child's concept of body image can indicate degree of *ego strength* and personality integration; vague, distorted self-concept may indicate *schizophrenic* processes.
E. *Successful* completion of various developmental phases determines body concept and degree of *body boundary definiteness.*
F. *Physical changes* of height, weight, and body build lead to changes in perception of body appearance and of how body is used.
G. Success in *using* one's body (motor ability) influences the value one places on self (self-evaluation).
H. *Secondary sex characteristics* are significant aspects of body image (*too much, too little, too early, too late,* in the *wrong place,* may lead to disturbed body image). Sexual differences in body image are in part related to differences in anatomical structure and body function, as well as to contrasts in lifestyles and cultural roles.
I. Different *cultures and families* value bodily traits and bodily deviations differently.
J. Different *body parts* (e.g., hair, nose, face, stature, shoulders) have varying personal significance; therefore, there is variability in degree of threat, personality integrity, and coping behavior.
K. *Attitudes* concerning the self will influence and be influenced by person's physical appearance and ability. Society has developed stereotyped ideas regarding outer body structure (body physique) and inner personalities (temperament). Current stereotypes are:
1. *Endomorph*—talkative, sympathetic, good natured, trusting, dependent, lazy, fat.
2. *Mesomorph*—adventuresome, self-reliant, strong, tall.
3. *Ectomorph*—thin, tense and nervous, suspicious, stubborn, pessimistic, quiet.

L. Person with a *firm ego boundary or body image* is more likely to be independent, striving, goal oriented, influential. Under stress, *may develop skin and muscle disease.*
M. Person with *poorly integrated body image and weak ego boundary* is more likely to be passive, less goal oriented, less influential, more prone to external pressures. Under stress, *may develop heart and GI diseases.*
N. Any situation, *illness,* or *injury* that causes a change in body image is a crisis, and the person will go through the *phases of crisis* in an attempt to reintegrate the body image **(Table 10.5).**

IV. ASSESSMENT: (Table 10.6).

V. ANALYSIS/NURSING DIAGNOSIS—*body image development disturbance may be related to:*

A. *Obvious loss* of a major body part—amputation of an extremity; hair, teeth, eye, breast.
B. Surgical procedures in which the relationship of body parts is *visibly* disturbed—colostomy, ileostomy, gastrostomy, ureteroenterostomy.
C. Surgical procedures in which the loss of body parts is *not visible* to others—hysterectomy, lung, gallbladder, stomach.
D. Repair procedures (plastic surgery) that do *not* reconstruct body image as assumed—rhinoplasty, plastic surgery to correct large ears, breasts.
E. *Changes in body size and proportion*—obesity, emaciation, acromegaly, gigantism, pregnancy, pubertal changes (*too early, too late, too big, too small, too tall, too short*).
F. Other changes in *external body* surface—hirsutism in women, mammary glands in men.
G. Skin *color* changes—chronic dermatitis, Addison's disease.
H. Skin *texture* changes—scars, thyroid disease, excoriative dermatitis, acne.
I. *Crippling* changes in bones, joints, muscles—arthritis, multiple sclerosis, Parkinson's disease.
J. Failure of a body part to *function*—quadriplegia, paraplegia, stroke (brain attack).

Table 10.5

Four Phases of Body Image Crisis

Phase	Assessment	Nursing Care Plan/Implementation
Acute shock	Anxiety, numbness, helplessness.	• Provide sustained support, be available to listen, express interest and concern. • Allow time for silence and privacy.
Denial	Retreats from reality; fantasy about the wholeness and capability of the body; euphoria; rationalization; refusal to participate in self-care.	• Accept denial without reinforcing it. *Avoid* arguing and overloading with reality. Gradually raise questions, reply with doubt to convey unrealistic ideas. • Follow client's suggestions for personal-care routine to help increase feelings of adequacy and to decrease helplessness.
Acknowledgment of reality	Grief over loss of valued body part, function, or role; depression, apathy; agitation, bitterness; physical symptoms (insomnia, anorexia, nausea, crying) serve as outlet for feeling; redefinition of body structure and function, with implications for change in lifestyle; acceptance of and cooperation with realistic goals for care and treatment; preoccupation with body functions.	• Expect and accept displacement onto nurse of anger, resentment, projection of client's inadequacy. • Examine own behavior to see if client's remarks are justified. • Simply listen if this is the only way the client can handle feelings at this time. • Offer sustained, nonjudgmental listening without being defensive or taking remarks personally. • Help dispel anger by encouraging its ventilation. • Encourage self-care activities. • Support family members as they cope with changes in client's health or body image, role changes, treatment plans.
Resolution and adaptation	Perceives crisis in new light; increased mastery leads to increased self-worth; can look at, feel, and ask questions regarding altered body part; tests others' reactions to changed body; repetitive talk on painful topic of changed self; concentration on *normal* functions in order to increase sense of control.	• Teaching and counseling by same nurse in warm, supportive relationship. • Assess level of knowledge; begin at that level. • Consider motivational state. • Provide gradual, nontechnical medical information and specific facts. • Repeat instructions frequently, patiently, consistently. • Support sense of mastery in self-care; draw on inner resources. • Do *not* discourage dependence while gradually encouraging independence. • Focus on necessary adaptations of lifestyle due to realistic limitations. • Provide follow-up care via referral to community resources after client is discharged.

From ©Lagerquist, S: *Nursing Examination Review,* ed 4. Addison-Wesley, Redwood City, CA.

Table 10.6

Body Image Development and Disturbance Throughout the Life Cycle: Assessment

Age Group	Development of Body Image	Developmental Disturbances in Body Image
Infant and toddler	• Becomes aware of body boundaries and separateness of own external body from others through sensory stimulation. • Explores external body parts; handles and controls the environment and body through play, bathing, and eating. • Experiences pain, shame, fear, and pleasure. Feels doubt or power in mastery of motor skills and strives for autonomy. Learns who one is in relation to the world.	***Infant*** • Inadequate somatosensory stimulation → impaired ego development, increased anxiety level, poor foundation for reality testing. • Continues to see external objects as extension of self → unrealistic, *distorted* perceptions of significant persons, inability to form normal attachments to others (possessive, engulfing, autistic, withdrawn). ***Toddler*** • If body fails to meet parental expectations → shameful, self-deprecating feelings. • Failure to master environment and control own body → helplessness, inadequacy, and doubt.

Table 10.6

Body Image Development and Disturbance Throughout the Life Cycle: Assessment—cont'd

Age Group	Development of Body Image	Developmental Disturbances in Body Image
Preschool and school age	• Experiences praise, blame, derogation, or criticism for body, its parts, or use (pleasure, pain, doubt, or guilt). • Explores genitals—discovers anatomical differences between sexes with joy, pride, or shame. • Begins awareness of *sexual identity.* • Differentiates self as a body and self as a mind.	***Preschool*** • Distortion of body image of genital area due to conflict over pleasure versus punishment. • If body build does not conform to sex-typed expectations and sex role identification → body image confusion.
	• Beginning of *self-concept;* of self as man or woman. • Learns mastery of the body (to *do,* to protect *self,* to protect *others*) and environment (run, skip, skate, swim); feels pleasure, competence, worth, or inadequacy.	***School age*** • Physical impairments (speech, poor vision, poor hearing) → feelings of inadequacy and inferiority. • Overly self-conscious about, and excessive focus on, body changes in puberty.
Adolescent	• Physical self is of more concern than at any other time except old age. • Forced body awareness due to physical changes (new senses, proportions, features); feelings of pleasure, power, confidence, or helplessness, pain, inadequacy, doubt, and guilt. • Adult body proportions emerge. • Anxiety over *ideal self versus emerging/emerged physical self;* body is compared competitively with same-sex peers. • Use of body (adolescents' values and attitudes) to relate with opposite sex. • Body image crucial for self-concept formation, status achievement, and adequate social relations. • Physical changes need to be integrated into evolving body image (strong, competent, powerful, or weak and helpless).	• Growth and changes may produce distorted view of self → overemphasis on defects with compensations; inflated ideas of body ability, beauty, perfection; preoccupation with body appearance or body processes, women more likely than men to see body fatter than it is; egocentrism.
Early adulthood	• Learns to accept own body without undue preoccupation with its functions or control of these functions. • Stability of body image.	• Less dependable, less likable body → regression to adolescent behavior and dress due to denial of aging, defeat, depression, self-pity, egocentrism due to fear of loss of sexual identity, withdrawal to early old age.
Middle age	• New challenges due to differential rates of aging in various body parts. • Body not functioning as well; unresolved fears, misconceptions, and experiences in relation to body image persist and become recognized.	• Women more likely to judge themselves uglier than do men or younger and older women.
Old age	• Accelerated physical decline with influence on self-concept and lifestyle. • Can accept self and personality as a whole; continued emphasis on physical self, with increased emphasis on inner, emotional self.	• Ill health → fear of invalidism, hypochondriasis. • Denial related to feelings of threatened incapacity and fear of declining functions. • Despair over loss of beauty, strength, and youthfulness, with self-disgust about body → projection of criticism onto others. • Regression. • Isolation (separation of affect and thought) leads to less intense response to death, disease, aging. • Compartmentalization (focus on one thing at a time) causes narrowing of consciousness, resistance, rigidity, repetitiveness. • Resurgence of egocentrism.

K. Distorted ideas of structure, function, and significance stemming from *symbolism* of disease seen in terms of *life and death* when heart or lungs are afflicted—heart attacks, asthmatic attacks, pneumonia.

L. *Side effects* of drug therapy—moon facies, hirsutism, striated skin, changes in body contours.

M. *Violent attacks* against the body—incest, rape, shooting, knifing, battering.

N. *Mental, emotional disorders*—schizophrenia with depersonalization, somatic delusions, and hallucinations about the body; anorexia nervosa, hypochondriasis; hysteria, malingering.

O. *Diseases requiring isolation* may convey attitude that body is undesirable, unacceptable—tuberculosis, AIDS, malodorous conditions (e.g., gangrene, cancer).

P. *Women's movement and sexual revolution*—use of body for pleasure, not just procreation, sexual freedom, wide range of normality in sex practices, legalized abortion.

Q. *Medical technology*—organ transplants, lifesaving but scar-producing burn treatment, alive but hopeless, alive but debilitated with chronic illnesses.

VI. GENERAL NURSING CARE PLAN/IMPLEMENTATION:

A. *Protect from psychological threat* related to impaired *self-attitudes.*
1. Emphasize person's *normal* aspects.
2. Encourage self-performance.

B. *Maintain warm, communicating relationship.*
1. Encourage awareness of positive responses from others.
2. Encourage expression of feelings.

C. *Increase reality perception.*
1. Provide *reliable* information about health status.
2. Provide *kinesthetic* feedback to paralyzed part (e.g., "I am raising your leg.").
3. Provide *perceptual* feedback (e.g., touch, describe, look at scar).
4. Support a realistic assessment of the situation.
5. Explore with the client his or her strengths and resources.

D. *Help achieve positive feelings about self, about adequacy.*
1. Support strengths *despite* presence of handicaps.
2. Assist client to look at self in *totality* rather than focus on limitations.

E. *Health teaching:*
1. Teach client and family about expected changes in functioning.
2. Explain importance of maintaining a positive self-attitude.
3. Advise that negative responses from others be regarded with minimum significance.

VII. EVALUATION/OUTCOME CRITERIA:

A. Able to resume function in activities of daily living rather than prolonging illness.

B. Able to accept limits imposed by physical or mental conditions and not attempt unrealistic tasks.

C. Can shift focus from reminiscence about the healthy past to present and future.

D. Less verbalized discontent with present body; diminished display of self-displeasure, despair, weeping, and irritability.

Body Image Disturbance—Selected Examples

I. DEFINITION—a body image disturbance arises when a person is unable to accept the body as is and to adapt to it; a conflict develops between the body as it actually is and the body that is pictured mentally—that is, the ideal self.

II. ANALYSIS/NURSING DIAGNOSIS: *body image disturbance* may be related to:

A. Sensation of *size change* due to obesity, pregnancy, weight loss.

B. Feelings of being *dirty*—may be imaginary due to hallucinogenic drugs, psychoses.

C. Dual change of body *structure and function* due to trauma, amputation, stroke, etc.

D. Progressive *deformities* due to chronic illness, burns, arthritis.

E. Loss of body boundaries and *depersonalization* due to sensory deprivation, such as blindness, immobility, fatigue, stress, anesthesia. May also be due to psychoses or hallucinogenic drugs.

III. ASSESSMENT: see **Table 10.6**.

Body Image Disturbance Caused by Amputation

A. Assessment:
1. Loss of self-esteem; feelings of helplessness, worthlessness, shame, and guilt.
2. Fear of abandonment may lead to appeals for sympathy by exhibiting helplessness and vulnerability.
3. Feelings of castration (loss of self) and symbolic death; loss of wholeness.
4. Existence of phantom pain (most clients).
5. Passivity, lack of responsibility for use of disabled body parts.

B. Nursing care plan/implementation:
1. *Avoid* stereotyping person as being less competent now than previously by *not* referring to client as the "amputee."

2. Foster independence; encourage self-care by assessing what client *can* do for himself or herself.
3. Help person set *realistic* short-term and long-term goals by exploring with the client his or her strengths and resources.
4. *Health teaching:*
   a. Encourage family members to work through their feelings, to accept person as he or she presents self.
   b. Teach how to set realistic goals and limitations.
   c. Explain what phantom pain is; that it is a normal experience.
   d. Explain role and function of prosthetic devices, where and how to obtain them, and how to find assistance in their use.

C. Evaluation/outcome criteria:

1. Can acknowledge the loss and move through three stages of mourning (shock and disbelief, developing awareness, and resolution).
2. Can discuss fears and concerns about loss of body part, its meaning, the problem of compensating for the loss, and reaction of persons (repulsion, rejection, and sympathy).

Body Image Disturbance in Brain Attack (Stroke)

A. Assessment:

1. Feelings of shame (personal, private, self-judgment of failure) due to loss of bowel and bladder control, speech function.
2. Body image boundaries disrupted; contact with environment is hindered by inability to ambulate or manipulate environment physically; may result in personality deterioration due to diminished number of sensory experiences. Loses orientation to body sphere; feels confused, trapped in own body.

B. Nursing care plan/implementation:

1. Reduce frustration and infantilism due to communication problems by:
   a. Rewarding all speech efforts.
   b. Listening and observing for all nonverbal cues.
   c. Restating verbalizations to see if correct meaning is understood.
   d. Speaking slowly, using two- to three-word sentences.
2. Assist *reintegration* of body parts and function; help regain awareness of paralyzed side by:
   a. Tactile stimulation.
   b. Verbal reminders of existence of affected parts.
   c. Direct visual contact via mirrors and grooming.
   d. Use of safety features (e.g., Posey belt).
3. *Health teaching:* control of bowel and bladder function; how to prevent problems of immobility.

C. Evaluation/outcome criteria: dignity is maintained while relearning to control elimination.

Body Image Disturbance in Myocardial Infarction

Emotional problems (e.g., anxiety, depression, sleep disturbance, fear of another myocardial infarction [MI]) during convalescence can seriously hamper rehabilitation. The adaptation and convalescence are influenced by the multiple symbolic meanings of the heart, for example:

1. Seat of emotions (love, pride, fear, sadness).
2. Center of the body (one-of-a-kind organ).
3. Life itself (can no longer rely on the heart; failure of the heart means failure of life).

A. Assessment:

1. *Attitude*—overly cautious and restrictive; may result in boredom, weakness, insomnia, exaggerated dependency.
2. *Acceptance* of illness—use of denial may result in noncompliance.
3. *Behavior*—self-destructive.
4. *Family conflicts*—related to activity, diet.
5. *Effects of MI on:*
   a. *Changes in lifestyle*—eating, smoking, drinking; activities, employment, sex.
   b. *Family members*—may be anxious, overprotective.
   c. *Role in family*—role reversal may result in loss of incentive for work.
   d. *Dependence-independence*—issues related to family conflicts (especially restrictive attitudes about desirable activity and dietary regimen).
   e. *Job*—social pressure to "slow down" may result in loss of job, reassignment, forced early retirement, "has-been" social status.

B. Nursing care plan/implementation:

1. Prevent "cardiac cripple" by shaping person's and family's attitude toward damaged organ.
   a. Instill optimism.
   b. Encourage *productive* living rather than inactivity.
2. Set up a physical and mental activity program with client and mate.
3. Provide anticipatory guidance regarding expected weakness, fear, uncertainty.
4. *Health teaching:* nature of coronary disease, interpretation of medical regimen, effect on sexual behavior.

C. Evaluation/outcome criteria:
1. Adheres to medical regimen.
2. Modifies lifestyle without becoming overly dependent on others.

Body Image and Obesity (see Chapter 6)

A. Definition: body weight exceeding 20% above the norm for person's age, sex, and height constitutes obesity. Body mass index (BMI) is also used. Although a faulty adaptation, obesity may serve as a protection against more severe illness; it represents an effort to function better, be powerful, stay well, or be less sick. The *problem* may *not* be difficulty in losing weight; reducing may *not* be the appropriate *cure.*

B. Assessment—characteristics:
1. Age—one out of three persons under 30 years of age is more than 10% overweight.
2. Increase risks for stroke, MI, diabetes.
3. Feelings: self-hate, self-derogation, failure, helplessness; tendency to avoid clothes shopping and mirror reflections.
4. Viewed by others as ugly, repulsive, lacking in will power, weak, unwilling to change, neurotic.
5. Discrepancy between actual body size (real self) and person's concept of it (ideal self).
6. Pattern of successful weight loss followed quickly and repetitively by failure; that is, weight gain.
7. Eating in response to outer environment (e.g., food odor, time of day, food availability, degree of stress, anger); *not inner* environment (hunger, increased gastric motility).
8. Experiences less pleasure in physical activity; less active than others.
9. All people who are obese are *not* the same.
   a. In *newborns and infants who are obese,* there is an increased *number* of adipocytes via *hyperplastic* process.
   b. In *adults who are obese,* there may be increased body fat deposits, resulting in increased *size* of adipocytes via *hypertrophic* process.
   c. When an *infant who is obese becomes an adult who is obese,* the result may be an increased *number* of cells available for fat *storage.*
10. Loss of control of own body or eating behavior.

C. Analysis/nursing diagnosis: *defensive coping* related to eating disorder. Contributing factors:
1. Genetic.
2. Thermodynamic.
3. Endocrine.
4. Neuroregulatory.
5. Biochemical factors in metabolism.
6. Ethnic and family practices.
7. *Psychological:*
   a. Compensation for feelings of helplessness and inadequacy.
   b. Maternal overprotection; overfed and force-fed, especially infants who are formula-fed.
   c. Food offered and used to relieve anxiety, frustration, anger, and rage can lead to difficulty in differentiating between hunger and other needs.
   d. As a child, food offered instead of love.
8. *Social:*
   a. Food easily available.
   b. Use of motorized transportation and labor-saving devices.
   c. Refined carbohydrates.
   d. Social aspects of eating.
   e. Restaurant meals high in salt, sugar, trans-fats, and larger portions.

D. Nursing care plan/implementation:
1. Encourage *prevention* of lifelong body image problems.
   a. Support *breastfeeding,* where infant determines quantity consumed, *not* mother; work through her feelings against breastfeeding (fear of intimacy, dependence, feelings of repulsion, concern about confinement, and inability to produce enough milk).
   b. Help mothers to *not overfeed* the infant if formula-fed: suggest water between feedings; do *not* start solids until 6 months old or 14 pounds; do *not* enrich the prescribed formula.
   c. Help mothers *differentiate* between hunger and other infant cries; help mothers to try out different responses to the expressed needs other than offering food.
2. Use *case findings* of infants who are obese, as well as young children, and adolescents.
3. Assess current eating patterns.
4. Identify need to eat, and relate need to preceding events, hopes, fears, or feelings.
5. Employ behavior modification techniques.
6. Encourage outside interests not related to food or eating.
7. Alleviate guilt, reduce stigma of being obese.
8. *Health teaching:*
   a. Promote awareness of certain *stressful* periods that can produce maladaptive responses such as obesity (e.g., puberty, postnuptial, postpartum, menopause).
   b. Assist in drawing up a meal plan for slow, steady weight loss.
   c. Advise eating five small meals a day and increase exercises.

E. Evaluation/outcome criteria: goal for desired weight is reached; weight-control plan is continued.

Human Sexuality Throughout the Life Cycle

Human sexuality refers to all the characteristics of an individual (social, personal, and emotional) that are manifest in his or her relationships with others and that reflect gender-genital orientation.

I. COMPONENTS OF SEXUAL SYSTEM

A. *Biological sexuality*—refers to chromosomes, hormones, primary and secondary sex characteristics, and anatomical structure.

B. *Sexual identity*—based on own feelings and perceptions of how well traits correspond with own feelings and concepts of maleness and femaleness; also includes gender identity.

C. *Gender identity*—a sense of masculinity and femininity shaped by biological, environmental, and intrapsychic forces, as well as cultural traditions and education.

D. *Sex role behavior*—includes components of both sexual identity and gender identity. Aim: sexual fulfillment through masturbation, heterosexual, or homosexual experiences. Selection of behavior is influenced by personal value system and sexual, gender, and biological identity. Gender identity and roles are learned and constantly reinforced by input and feedback regarding social expectations and demands (**Table 10.7**).

Table 10.7

Sexual Behavior Throughout the Life Cycle

Age	Development of Sexual Behavior
First 18 mo	Major source of pleasure from touch and oral exploration.
18 mo–3 yr	Pleasurable and sexual feelings are associated with genitals (acts of urination and defecation). Masturbation without fantasy or eroticism.
3–6 yr	Beginning resolution of Oedipus and Electra complexes; foundation for heterosexual relationships; masturbation with curiosity about genitals of opposite sex.
6–12 yr	Peer relations with same sex; onset of sex play; morality and sexual attitudes taught and learned; phase of sexual tranquility.
12–18 yr (adolescence)	Onset of puberty with biological development of secondary sex characteristics; menstruation and ejaculation occur. Frequent masturbation. Intense anxiety and guilt may occur over heterosexual or homosexual behavior (petting, coitus, masturbation, STI, pregnancy, genital size).
18–23 yr (early adulthood)	Maximum interpersonal and intrapsychic self-consciousness about sexuality. Issues: premarital coitus, sexual freedom. Anxiety about: sexual competency, genital size, impotence, fear of pregnancy, rejection.
23–30 yr	Focus on sexual activity in coupling and parenthood; mutual masturbation.
30–45 yr (middle adulthood)	For women—peak sexuality without new sexual experiences. Conflict regarding extramarital sex may increase. **Purpose of Intercourse:** Need for body contact (and procreation until age 35+). Physical expression of trust, love, and affection. Reaffirmation of self-concept, as sexually desirable and sexually competent due to worry about effects of aging. **Sexual Dysfunctions:** *Men:* erectile dysfunction, premature ejaculation, decreasing libido. *Women:* intermittent lack of orgasmic response, vaginismus, dyspareunia. *For either or both:* changes or divergences in degree of sexual interest. **Causes of Sexual Dysfunction (Men):** Overindulgence in food or drink. Preoccupation with career and economic pursuits. Mental or physical fatigue. Boredom with monotony of relationship. Drug dependency: alcohol, tobacco, certain medications. Fear of failure. Chronic illness: diabetes, alcoholism → peripheral neuropathy → impotence (smoking and drinking may result in decreased testosterone production); excessive smoking → vascular constriction → decreased libido; spinal cord injuries; prostatectomy, androgen deprivation therapy (for prostate cancer). Self-devaluation due to accumulation of role function losses, sexual self-image, and body image. Past history of lack of sexual enjoyment in younger years. **Causes of Sexual Dysfunction (Women):** Belief in myths regarding "shoulds and should nots" of frequency, variations, and enjoyment. Widowhood: inhibition and loyalty to deceased.

Continued

Table 10.7

Sexual Behavior Throughout the Life Cycle—cont'd

Age	Development of Sexual Behavior
45–65 yr (later adulthood)	Menopause occurs. Little or no fear of pregnancy; evidence of sexual activity differences in men and women: women may have increased pleasure, men take longer to reach orgasm; may prefer less strenuous mutual masturbation.
Over 65 yr (old age)	Activity depends on earlier sexual attitude. May suffer guilt and shame when engaging in sex. Can have active and enjoyable sex life with continuing sex needs. Age is not a barrier provided there is opportunity for sexual activity with a partner or for sublimated activities. Women in this age group outnumber men; single women outnumber single men by an even larger margin.

From ©Lagerquist, S: *Nursing Examination Review,* ed 4. Addison-Wesley, Redwood City, CA.

II. CONCEPTS AND PRINCIPLES OF HUMAN SEXUAL RESPONSE

A. Human sexual response involves not only the genitals but the total body.

B. Factors in early postnatal and childhood periods influence gender identity, gender role, sex typing, and sexual responses in later life.

C. Cultural and personally subjective variables influence ways of sexual expression and perception of what is satisfying.

D. Healthy sexual expressions vary widely.

E. Requirements for human sexual response:

1. Intact central and peripheral nervous system to provide *sensory* perception, *motor* reaction.
2. Intact circulatory system to produce *vasocongestive* response.
3. Desirable and interested partner, if sex outlet involves mutuality.
4. *Freedom* from guilt, anxiety, misconceptions, and interfering conditioned responses.
5. Acceptable physical *setting,* usually private.

Sexual-Health Counseling

General Issues

I. ISSUES in sexual practices with implications for counseling:

A. *Sex education*—need to provide accurate and complete information on all aspects of sexuality to all people.

B. *Sexual-health care*—should be part of total health-care planning for all.

C. *Sexual orientation*—need to avoid discrimination based on sexual orientation (such as homosexuality); the right to satisfying, nonexploitive relationships with others, regardless of gender.

D. *Sex and the law*—sex between consenting adults not a legal concern.

E. *Explicit sexual material* (pornography)—can be useful in fulfilling various needs in life, as in quadriplegia.

F. *Masturbation*—a natural behavior at all ages; can fulfill a variety of needs (see Masturbation, **p. 726**).

G. Availability of *contraception* for minors—the right of access to medical contraceptive care should be available to all ages.

H. *Abortion*—confidentiality for minors.

I. *Treatment for sexually transmitted infections (STIs)*—naming of partners as part of STI control.

J. *Sex and the elderly*—need opportunity for sexual expression; need privacy when in communal living setting.

K. *Sex and the disabled*—need to have possible means available for rewarding sexual expressions.

II. SEXUAL MYTHS*

A. *Myth:* Ignorance is bliss.

Fact: What you don't know *can* hurt you (note the high frequency of STI and abortions); *myths* can perpetuate fears and such misinformation as:

1. *Masturbation causes mental illness.*
2. *Women don't or shouldn't have orgasms.*
3. *Tampons cause STI.*
4. *Plastic wrap works better than condoms.*
5. *Coca-Cola is an effective douche.*

Fact: Lack of knowledge during initial experiences may result in fear and set precedent for future sexual reactions.

B. *Myths:* The planned sex act is not OK and is immoral for "nice" girls. If a woman gets pregnant, it is her own fault. Contraceptives are solely a woman's responsibility.

Fact: Sex and contraception are the prerogative and responsibility of both partners.

C. *Myth:* A good relationship is harmonious, free of conflict and disagreement (which are signs of rejection and incompatibility).

Fact: Conflict can induce growth in self-understanding and in understanding of others.

*Adapted from Sedgwick, R: Myths in human sexuality: a social-psychological perspective. *Nurs Clin North Am* 10(3):539–550. Philadelphia, WB Saunders.

D. *Myth:* Sexual deviance (such as homosexuality) is a sign of personality disturbance.
Fact: No single sexual behavior is the most desirable, effective, or satisfactory. Personal sexual choice is a fundamental right.

E. *Myth:* A woman's sexual needs and gratification should be secondary to her partner's; a woman's role is to satisfy others.
Fact: A woman has as much right to sexual freedom and experience as a man.

F. *Myth:* Menopause is an affliction signifying the end of sex.
Fact: Many women do not suffer through menopause, and many report renewed sexual interest.

G. *Myth:* Sexual activity past 60 years of age is not essential.
Fact: Sexual activity is therapeutic because it:

1. Affirms identity.
2. Provides communication.
3. Provides companionship.
4. Meets intimacy needs.

H. *Myth:* A woman's sex drive decreases in postmenopausal period.
Fact: The strength of the sex drive becomes greater as androgen overcomes the inhibitory action of estrogen.

I. *Myth:* Men over age 60 cannot achieve an erection.
Fact: According to Masters and Johnson, a major difference between the aging man and the younger man is the duration of each phase of the sexual cycle. The older man is slower in achieving an erection.

J. *Myth:* Regular sexual activity cannot help the aging person's loss of function.
Fact: Research is revealing that "disuse atrophy" may lead to loss of sexual capacity. Regular sexual activity helps preserve sexual function.

III. BASIC PRINCIPLES OF SEXUAL-HEALTH COUNSELING

A. There is *no* universal consensus about acceptable values in human sexuality. Each social group has very definite values regarding sex.

B. Counselors need to examine own feelings, attitudes, values, biases, knowledge base.

C. Help reduce fear, guilt, ignorance.

D. Offer guidance and education rather than indoctrination or pressure to conform.

E. Each person needs to be helped to make personal choices regarding sexual conduct.

IV. COUNSELING IN SEXUAL HEALTH

A. General considerations:

1. Create atmosphere of *trust and acceptance* for objective, nonjudgmental dialogue.
2. Use *language* related to sexual behavior that is mutually comfortable and understood between client and nurse.
   a. Use alternative terms for definitions (e.g., "being intimate" vs. "having sex").
   b. Determine exact meaning of words and phrases because sexual words and expressions have different meanings to people with different backgrounds and experiences.
3. *Desensitize* own stress reaction to the emotional component of taboo topics.
   a. Increase awareness of own sexual values, biases, prejudices, stereotypes, and fears.
   b. *Avoid* overreacting, underreacting.
4. Become sensitively aware of *interrelationships* between sexual needs, fears, and behaviors and other aspects of living.
5. Begin with *commonly* discussed areas (such as menstruation) and progress to discussion of individual sexual experiences (such as masturbation). Move from areas where there is less voluntary control (nocturnal emissions) to more responsibility and voluntary behavior (premature ejaculation).
6. Offer *educational information* to dispel fears, myths; give tacit permission to explore sensitive areas.
7. Bring into awareness possibly *repressed* feelings of guilt, anger, denial, and suppressed sexual feelings.
8. Explore possible *alternatives* of sexual expression.
9. Determine *interrelationships* among mental, social, physical, and sexual well-being.

B. Assessment parameters:

1. Self-awareness of body image, values, and attitudes toward human sexuality; comfort with own sexuality.
2. Ability to identify sex problems on basis of own satisfaction or dissatisfaction.
3. Developmental history, sex education, family relationships, cultural and ethnic values, and available support resources.
4. Type and frequency of sexual behavior.
5. Nature and quality of sex relations with others.
6. Attitude toward and satisfaction with sexual activity.
7. Expectations and goals.

C. Nursing care plan/implementation:

1. *Long-term goals:*
   a. Increase knowledge of reproductive system and types of sex behavior.
   b. Promote positive view of body and sex needs.
   c. Integrate sex needs into self-identity.
   d. Develop adaptive and satisfying patterns of sexual expression.
   e. Understand effects of physical illness on sexual performance.

2. *Primary sexual-health interventions:*
   a. Goals: minimize stress factors, strengthen sexual integrity.
   b. Provide education to uninformed or misinformed.
   c. Identify stress factors (myths, stereotypes, negative parental attitudes).
3. *Secondary sexual-health interventions:* identify sexual problems early and refer for treatment.

D. Evaluation/outcome criteria:
1. Reduced impairment or dysfunction from acute sex problem or chronic, unresolved sex problem.
2. Evaluate how client's goals were achieved in terms of *positive* thoughts, feelings, and *satisfying* sexual behaviors.

Specific Situations

I. MASTURBATION

A. Definition—act of achieving sexual arousal and orgasm through manual or mechanical stimulation of the sex organs.

B. Characteristics:
1. Can be an interpersonal as well as a solitary activity.
2. "It is a healthy and appropriate sexual activity, playing an important role in ultimate consolidation of one's sexual identity."*
3. Accompanied by fantasies that are important for:
   a. Physically disabled.
   b. Fatigued.
   c. Compensation for unreachable goals and unfulfilled wishes.
   d. Rehearsal for future sexual relations.
   e. Absence or impersonal action of partner.
4. Can help release tension harmlessly.

C. Concepts and principles related to masturbation:
1. Staff's feelings and reactions influence their responses to client and affect continuation of masturbation (i.e., negative staff actions increase client's frustration, which increases masturbation).
2. Masturbation is normal and universal, *not* physically or psychologically harmful in itself.
3. Pleasurable genital sensations are important for increasing *self-pride,* finding *gratification* in *own* body, increasing sense of *personal value* of being lovable, helping to *prepare for adult* sexual role.
4. Excessive masturbation—some needs not being met through interpersonal relations; may use behavior to *avoid* interpersonal relations.
5. Activity may be related to:
   a. Curiosity, experimentation.
   b. Tension reduction, pleasure.
   c. Enhanced interest in sexual development.
   d. Fear and avoidance of social relationships.

D. Nursing care plan:
1. *Long-term goals:*
   a. Gain insight into *preference* for masturbation.
   b. Relieve accompanying guilt, worry, self-devaluation **(Fig. 10.2).**
2. *Short-term goals:*
   a. Clarify myths regarding masturbation.
   b. Help client see masturbation as an acceptable sexual activity for individuals of all ages.
   c. Set limits on masturbation in inappropriate settings.

E. Nursing implementation:
1. Examine, control nurse's own negative feelings; show respect.
2. *Avoid:* reinforcement of guilt and self-devaluation; scorn; threats, punishment, anger, alarm reaction; use of masturbation for rebellion in power struggle between staff and client.
3. *Identify* client's unmet needs; consider purpose served by masturbation (may be useful behavior).
4. *Examine* pattern in which behavior occurs.
5. Intervene when degree of functioning in other daily life activities is *impaired.*
   a. Remain calm, accepting, but nonsanctioning.
   b. Promptly help clarify client's feelings, thoughts, at stressful time.
   c. Review precipitating events.
   d. Be a neutral "sounding board"; *avoid* evasiveness.
   e. If unable to handle situation, find someone who can.
6. For clients who masturbate at *inappropriate* times or in inappropriate places:
   a. Give special attention when they are not masturbating.
   b. Encourage new interests and activities, but *not* immediately after observing masturbation.
   c. Keep clients distracted, occupied with interesting activities.
7. *Health teaching:* explain myths and teach facts regarding cause and effects.

F. Evaluation/outcome criteria:
1. Acknowledges function of own sexual organs.
2. States sexual experience is satisfying.
3. Views sexuality as pleasurable and wholesome.
4. Views sex organs as acceptable, enjoyable, and valued part of body image.
5. Self-image as fully functioning person is restored and maintained.

II. HOMOSEXUALITY

A. Definition—alternative sexual behavior; applied to sexual relations between persons of the same sex.

---

*Marcus, IM, & Francis, JJ: *Masturbation from Infancy to Senescence.* International Universities Press, New York.

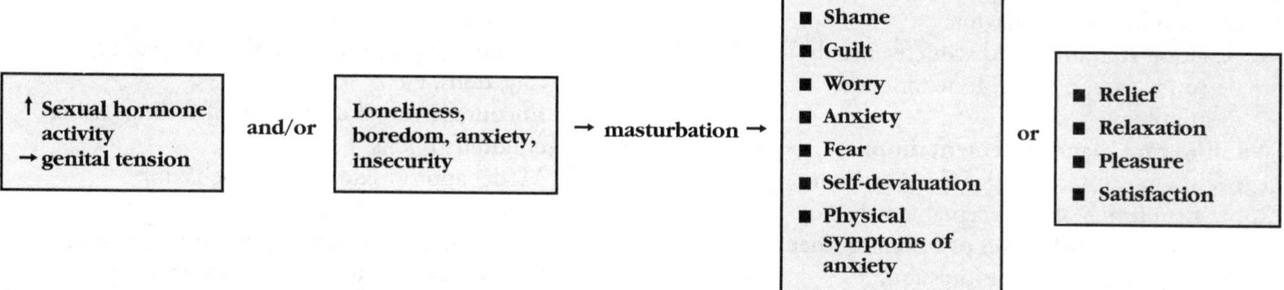

Figure 10.2 **Operationalization of the behavioral concept of masturbation.**

B. Theories regarding causes:
1. Hereditary tendencies.
2. Imbalance of sex hormones.
3. Environmental influences and conditioning factors, related to learning and psychodynamic theories.
   a. Defense against unsatisfying relationship with father.
   b. Unsatisfactory and threatening early relationships with opposite sex.
   c. Oedipal attachment to parent.
   d. Parent who is seductive (incest).
   e. Castration fear.
   f. Labeling and guilt leading to sexual acting out.
   g. Faulty sex education.
4. Preferred choice as a lifestyle.

C. Nursing care plan/implementation:
1. Nurse needs to be aware of and work through own attitudes that may interfere with providing care.
2. Accept and respect lifestyle of a client who is gay (man who is homosexual) or lesbian (woman who is homosexual).
3. Assess and treat for possible sexually transmitted infections and hepatitis.
4. *Health teaching:* assess and add to knowledge base about alternatives in sexual behavior.

D. Evaluation/outcome criteria: expresses self-confidence and positive self-image; able to sustain satisfying sexual behavior with chosen partner and avoid at-risk behaviors for STIs.

III. SEX AND THE PERSON WHO IS DISABLED

A. Assessment parameters:
1. Previous level of sex functioning and conflict.
2. Client's view of sex activity (self and mutual pleasure, tension release, procreation, control).
3. Cultural environment (influence on body image).
4. Degree of acceptance of illness.
5. Support system (partner, family, support group).
6. Body image and self-esteem.
7. Outlook on future.

B. Analysis/nursing diagnosis: *sexual dysfunction* associated with physical illness related to:
1. Disinterest in sexual activity.
2. Fear of precipitating or aggravating physical illness through sexual activity.
3. Use of illness as excuse to avoid feared or undesired sex.
4. Physical inability or discomfort during sexual activity.

C. Nursing care plan/implementation:
1. Approach with nonjudgmental attitude.
2. Elicit concerns about current physical state and perceptions of changes in sexuality.
3. Observe nonverbal clues of concern.
4. Identify genital assets.
5. Support client and partner during adjustment to current state.
6. Explore culturally acceptable sublimation activities.
7. Promote adjustment to body image change.
8. *Health teaching:*
   a. Teach self-help skills.
   b. Teach partner to care for client's physical needs.
   c. Teach alternate sex behaviors and acceptable sublimation (e.g., touching).

D. Evaluation/outcome criteria: attains satisfaction with adaptive alternatives of sexual expressions; has a positive attitude toward self, body, and sexual activity.

IV. INAPPROPRIATE SEXUAL BEHAVIOR

A. Assessment: public exhibitions of sexual behaviors that are offensive to others; making sexual advances to other clients or staff.

B. Analysis/nursing diagnosis: *conflict with social order* related to:
1. Acting out angry and hostile feelings.
2. Lack of awareness of hospital and agency rules regarding acceptable public behavior.

3. Variation in cultural interpretations of what is acceptable public behavior.
4. Reaction to unintended seductiveness by person's attire, posture, tone, or choice of terminology.

C. Nursing care plan/implementation:
1. Maintain calm, nonjudgmental attitude.
2. Set firm limits on unacceptable behavior.
3. Encourage verbalization of feelings rather than unacceptable physical expression.
4. Reinforce appropriate behavior.
5. Provide constructive diversional activity for clients.
6. *Health teaching:* explain rules regarding public behavior; teach acceptable ways to express anger.

D. Evaluation/outcome criteria: verbalizes anger rather than acting out; accepts rules regarding behavior in public.

Concept of Death Throughout the Life Cycle

I. AGES 1 TO 3

A. No concept per se, but experiences *separation anxiety and abandonment* any time significant other disappears from view over a period of time.

B. *Coping* means: fear, resentment, anger, aggression, regression, withdrawal.

C. Nursing care plan/implementation—help the family:
1. Facilitate transfer of affectional ties to another nurturing adult.
2. Decrease separation anxiety of child who is hospitalized by encouraging family visits and rooming in, reassuring child that she or he will not be alone.
3. Provide stable environment through consistent staff assignment.

II. AGES 3 TO 5

A. Least anxious about death.

B. Denial of death as inevitable and final process.

C. Death is separation, being alone.

D. Death is *sleep* and sleep is death.

E. "Death" is part of vocabulary; seen as real, gradual, *temporary,* not permanent.

F. Dead person is seen as alive, but in altered form, that is, lacks movement.

G. There are *degrees* of death.

H. Death means not being here anymore.

I. "Living" and "lifeless" are not yet distinguished.

J. Illness and death seen as *punishment* for "badness"; fear and guilt about sexual and aggressive impulses.

K. Death happens, but only to others.

L. Nursing care plan/implementation (in addition to previous):
1. Encourage play for expression of feelings; use clay, dolls, etc.
2. Encourage verbal expression of feelings using children's books.
3. Model appropriate grieving behavior.
4. Protect child from the overstimulation of hysterical adult reactions by limiting contact.
5. Clearly state what death is—death is final, no breathing, eating, awakening—and that death is *not* sleep.
6. Check child at night and provide support through holding and staying with child.
7. Allow a choice of attending the funeral and, if child decides to attend, describe what will take place.
8. If parents are grieving, have other family or friends attend to child's needs.

III. AGES 5 TO 10

A. Death is cessation of life; question of what happens after death.

B. Death seen as definitive, *universal,* inevitable, *irreversible.*

C. Death occurs to all living things, including self; may express, "It isn't fair."

D. Death is distant from self (an eventuality).

E. Believe death occurs by accident, happens only to the very *old* or very sick.

F. Death is personified (as a separate person) in fantasies and magical thinking.

G. Death anxiety handled by *nightmares, rituals,* and *superstitions* (related to fear of darkness and sleeping alone because death is an external person, such as a skeleton, who comes and takes people away at night).

H. Dissolution of bodily life seen as a perceptible result.

I. Fear of body mutilation.

J. Nursing care plan/implementation (in addition to previous):
1. Allow child to experience the loss of pets, friends, and family members.
2. Help child talk it out and experience the appropriate emotional reactions.
3. Understand need for increase in play, especially competitive play.
4. Involve child in funeral preparation and rituals.
5. Understand and accept regressive or protest behaviors.
6. Rechannel protest behaviors into constructive outlets.

IV. ADOLESCENCE

A. Death seen as inevitable, *personal,* universal, and *permanent;* corporal life stops; body decomposes.

B. Does not fear death, but concerned with how to *live now,* what death feels like, *body changes.*

C. Experiences *anger, frustration, and despair* over lack of future, lack of fulfillment of adult roles.
D. Openly asks *difficult,* honest, *direct* questions.
E. Anger at healthy peers.
F. Conflict between *developing* body versus *deteriorating* body, *independent* identity versus *dependency.*
G. **Nursing care plan/implementation** (in addition to previous):
   1. Facilitate full expression of grief by answering direct questions.
   2. Help let out feelings, especially through creative and aesthetic pursuits.
   3. Encourage participation in funeral ritual.
   4. Encourage full use of peer group support system, by providing opportunities for group talks.

V. YOUNG ADULTHOOD

A. Death seen as *unwelcome* intrusion, *interruption* of what might have been.
B. Reaction: *rage, frustration, disappointment.*
C. **Nursing care plan/implementation:** all of previous, especially *peer group support.*

VI. MIDDLE AGE

A. Concerned with *consequences* of own death and that of significant others.
B. Death seen as disruption of involvement, responsibility, and *obligations.*
C. End of plans, projects, experiences.
D. Death is *pain.*
E. **Nursing care plan/implementation** (in addition to previous): assess need for counseling when also in midlife crisis.

VII. OLD AGE

A. *Philosophical* rationalizations: death as inevitable, final process of life, when "time runs out."
B. *Religious* view: death represents only the dissolution of life and is a doorway to a new life (a preparatory stage for another life).
C. Time of rest and peace, supreme refuge from turmoil of life.
D. **Nursing care plan/implementation** (in addition to previous):
   1. Help person prepare for own death by helping with funeral prearrangements, wills, and sharing of mementos.
   2. Facilitate life review and reinforce positive aspects.
   3. Provide care and comfort.
   4. Be present at death.

End-of-Life: Death and Dying

Too often the process of death has had such frightening aspects that people have suffered alone. Today there has been a vast change in attitudes; death and dying are no longer taboo topics. There is a growing realization that we need to accept death as a natural process. Elisabeth Kübler-Ross has written extensively on the process of dying, describing the stages of *denial* ("not me"), *anger* ("why me?"), *bargaining* ("yes me—but"), *depression* ("yes, me"), and *acceptance* ("my time is close now, it's all right"), with implications for the helping person.

I. CONCEPTS AND PRINCIPLES RELATED TO DEATH AND DYING:

A. Persons may know or *suspect* they are dying and may want to talk about it; often they look for someone to share their fears and the process of dying.
B. Fear of death can be reduced by helping clients feel that they are *not alone.*
C. The dying need the opportunity to live their final experiences to the fullest, in their *own* way.
D. People who are dying remain more or less the *same* as they were during life; their approaches to death are consistent with their approaches to life.
E. Dying persons' need to review their lives may be a purposeful attempt to reconcile themselves to what "was" and what "could have been."
F. *Three ways* of facing death are (a) quiet acceptance with inner strength and peace of mind; (b) restlessness, impatience, anger, and hostility; and (c) depression, withdrawal, and fearfulness.
G. *Four tasks* facing a person who is dying are (a) reviewing life, (b) coping with physical symptoms in the end stage of life, (c) making a transition from known to unknown state, and (d) reaction to separation from loved ones.
H. Crying and tears are an important aspect of the grief process.
I. There are many *blocks* to providing a helping relationship with the dying and bereaved:
   1. Nurses' unwillingness to share the process of dying—minimizing their contacts and blocking out their own feelings.
   2. Forgetting that a person who is dying may be feeling lonely, abandoned, and afraid of dying.
   3. Reacting with irritation and hostility to the person's frequent calls.
   4. Nurses' failure to seek help and support from team members when feeling afraid, uneasy, and frustrated in caring for a person who is dying.
   5. Not allowing client to talk about death and dying.
   6. Nurses' use of technical language or social chit-chat as a defense against their own anxieties.

II. ASSESSMENT OF DEATH AND DYING:

A. *Physical:*
   1. Observable deterioration of physical and mental capacities—person is unable to fulfill physiological needs, such as eating and elimination.
   2. Circulatory collapse (blood pressure and pulse).

3. Renal or hepatic failure.
4. Respiratory decline.

B. *Psychosocial:*
1. Fear of death is signaled by agitation, restlessness, and sleep disturbances at night.
2. Anger, agitation, blaming.
3. Morbid self-pity with feelings of defeat and failure.
4. Depression and withdrawal.
5. Introspectiveness and calm acceptance of the inevitable.

III. ANALYSIS/NURSING DIAGNOSIS:

A. *Terminal illness response.*
B. *Altered feeling states* related to fear of being alone.
C. *Altered comfort patterns* related to pain.
D. *Altered meaningfulness* related to depression, hopelessness, helplessness, powerlessness.
E. *Altered social interaction* related to withdrawal.

IV. NURSING CARE PLAN/IMPLEMENTATION:

A. *Long-term goal:* foster environment where person and family can experience dying with dignity.
B. *Short-term goals:*
1. Express feelings (person and family).
2. Support person and family.
3. Minimize physical discomfort.

C. Explore own feelings about death and dying with team members; form support groups.
D. Be aware of the *normal grief* process.
1. *Allow* person and family to do the work of grieving and mourning.
2. Allow crying and mood swings, anger, demands.
3. Permit yourself to cry.

E. Allow person to *express* feelings, fears, and concerns.
1. *Avoid* pat answers to questions about "why."
2. Pick up symbolic communication.

F. Provide care and comfort with *relief from pain;* do not isolate person.
G. Stay *physically close.*
1. Use touch.
2. Be available to form a consistent relationship.

H. *Reduce isolation and abandonment* by assigning person to room in which isolation is less likely to occur and by allowing flexible visiting hours.
I. Keep activities in room as *near normal* and *constant* as possible.
J. Speak in *audible* tones, not whispers.
K. Be alert to cues when person needs to be alone (*disengagement process*).
L. Leave room for *hope.*
M. Help person die with peace of mind by lending support and providing opportunities to express anger, pain, and fears to someone who will accept her or him and not censor verbalization.
N. *Health teaching:* teach grief process to family and friends; teach methods to relieve pain.

V. EVALUATION/OUTCOME CRITERIA:

A. Remains comfortable and free of pain as long as possible.
B. Dies with dignity.

Grief/Bereavement

Grief is a typical reaction to the loss of a source of psychological gratification. It is a syndrome with somatic and psychological symptoms that diminish when grief is resolved. Grief processes have been extensively described by Erich Lindemann and George Engle.*

I. CONCEPTS AND PRINCIPLES RELATED TO GRIEF:

A. Cause of grief: reaction to loss (real or imaginary, actual or pending).
B. Healing process can be interrupted.
C. Grief is universal.
D. Uncomplicated grief is a self-limiting process.
E. Grief responses may vary in degree and kind (e.g., *absence* of grief, *delayed* grief, and *unresolved* grief).
F. People go through stages similar to stages of death described by Elisabeth Kübler-Ross.
G. Many factors influence successful outcome of grieving process:
1. The more *dependent* the person on the lost relationship, the greater the difficulty in resolving the loss.
2. A *child* has greater difficulty resolving loss.
3. A person with *few meaningful relationships* also has greater difficulty.
4. The *more losses* the person has had in the past, the more affected that person will be, because losses tend to be cumulative.
5. The more *sudden* the loss, the greater the difficulty in resolving it.
6. The more *ambivalence* (love-hate feelings, with guilt) there was toward the dead, the more difficult the resolution.
7. *Loss of a child* is harder to resolve than loss of an older person.

II. ASSESSMENT—CHARACTERISTIC STAGES OF GRIEF RESPONSES:

A. *Shock and disbelief* (initial and recurrent stage):
1. *Denial* of reality ("No, it can't be.")
2. Stunned, *numb* feeling.

*Adapted from a *classic* article by George Engel: Grief and grieving. *Am J Nurs* 9(64):93–98, 1964.

3. Feelings of loss, *helplessness,* impotence.
4. Intellectual acceptance.

B. *Developing awareness:*
1. Anguish about loss.
   a. *Somatic* distress.
   b. Feelings of emptiness.
2. *Anger* and hostility toward person or circumstances held responsible.
3. Guilt feelings—may lead to self-destructive actions.
4. Tears (inwardly, alone; or inability to cry).

C. *Restitution:*
1. Funeral *rituals* are an aid to grief resolution by emphasizing the reality of death.
2. Expression and sharing of feelings by gathered family and friends are a source of acknowledgment of grief and support for the bereaved.

D. *Resolving the loss:*
1. Increased *dependency* on others as an attempt to deal with painful void.
2. More aware of own *bodily sensations*—may be identical with symptoms of the deceased.
3. Complete *preoccupation* with thoughts and memories of the dead person.

E. *Idealization:*
1. All hostile and negative feelings about the dead are *repressed.*
2. Mourner may *assume* qualities and attributes of the dead.
3. Gradual lessening of preoccupation with the dead; *reinvesting* in others.

III. ANALYSIS: **Table 10.8** and **Figure 10.3**.

IV. NURSING CARE PLAN/IMPLEMENTATION IN GRIEF STAGES:

A. *Apply crisis theory and interventions.*

B. *Demonstrate unconditional respect* for cultural, religious, and social mourning customs.

C. *Utilize knowledge of the stages of grief* to anticipate reactions and facilitate the grief process.
1. Anticipate and permit expression of different manifestations of shock, disbelief, and denial.
   a. News of impending death is best communicated to a family group (rather than an individual) in a private setting.
   b. *Let mourners see the dead or dying,* to help them accept reality.
   c. Encourage description of circumstances and nature of loss.
2. *Accept guilt, anger, and rage* as common responses to coping with guilt and helplessness.
   a. Be aware of potential suicide by the bereaved.
   b. Permit crying; stay with the bereaved.
3. Mobilize social support system; promote hospital policy that allows gathering of friends and family in a private setting.

Table 10.8

Analysis/Nursing Diagnosis: Altered Feeling States Related to Grief

Problem Classification	Characteristics
1. Somatic distress	• Occurs in waves lasting from 20 min to 1 hr • Deep, sighing respirations most common when discussing grief • Lack of strength • Loss of appetite and sense of taste • Tightness in throat • Choking sensation accompanied by shortness of breath
2. Preoccupation with image of deceased	• Similar to daydreaming • May mistake others for deceased person • May be oblivious to surroundings • Slight sense of unreality • Fear that he or she is becoming "insane"
3. Feelings of guilt	• Accuses self of negligence • Exaggerates existence and importance of negative thoughts, feelings, and actions toward deceased • Views self as having failed deceased—"if I had only . . ."
4. Feelings of hostility	• Irritability, anger, and loss of warmth toward others • May attempt to handle feelings of hostility in formalized and stiff manner of social interaction
5. Loss of patterns of conduct	• Inability to initiate or maintain organized patterns of activity • Restlessness, with aimless movements • Loss of zest—tasks and activities are carried on as though with great effort • Activities formerly carried on in company of deceased have lost their significance • May become strongly dependent on whomever stimulates him or her to activity

4. Allow dependency on staff for initial decision making while person is attempting to resolve loss.
5. Respond to somatic complaints.
6. Permit reminiscence.
7. Encourage mourner to relate accounts connected with the lost relationship that reflect positive and negative feelings and remembrances; *place loss in perspective.*
8. Begin to encourage and reinforce new interests and social relations with others by the end of the idealization stage; loosen bonds of attachment.

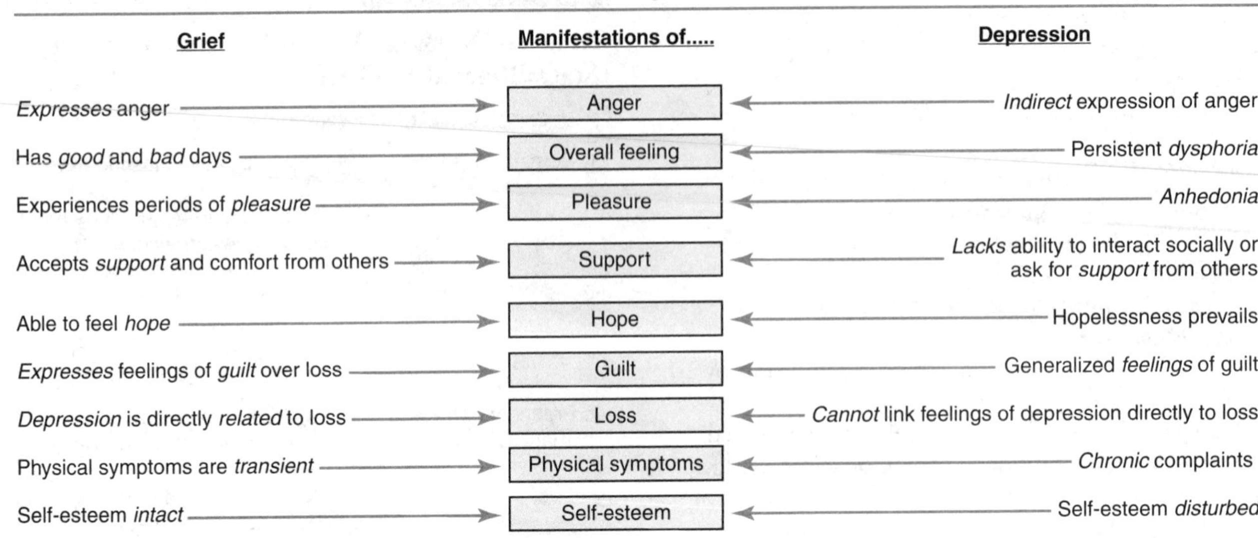

Figure 10.3 Grief versus depression.

9. Identify high-risk persons for maladaptive responses (see **I. G.** Many factors influence successful outcome of grieving process, **p. 730**).
10. *Health teaching:*
    a. Explain that emotional response is appropriate and common.
    b. Explain and offer hope that emotional pain will diminish with time.
    c. Describe normal grief stages.

V. EVALUATION/OUTCOME CRITERIA: outcome may take 1 year or more—can remember comfortably and realistically both pleasurable and disappointing aspects of the lost relationship.

A. Can express feelings of sorrow caused by loss.
B. Can describe ambivalence (love, anger) toward lost person, relationship.
C. Able to review relationship, including pleasures, regrets, etc.
D. Bonds of attachment are loosened and new object relationships are established.

Mental Status Assessment

I. COMPONENTS OF MENTAL STATUS EXAMINATION:

A. *Appearance*—appropriate dress, piercings, tattoos, hair color/texture, grooming, facial expression, eye contact, stereotyped movements, tremors, tics, gestures, gait, mannerisms, rigidity, height and weight.
B. *Behavior*—anxiety level, congruence with situation, impulse control (aggression, sexual), cooperativeness, openness, hostility, reaction to interview (guarded, defensive, apathetic), consistency.
C. *Speech characteristics*—relevance, coherence, meaning, repetitiveness, qualitative (*what* is said), quantitative (*how much* is said), abnormalities, inflections, affectations, congruence with level of education, impediments (e.g., stutter), tone quality.
D. *Mood*—appropriateness, intensity, hostility turned inward or toward others, swings, guilty, despairing, irritable, sad, depressed, anxious, fearful.
E. *Thought content*—delusions, hallucinations, obsessive ideas, suicidal, homicidal, paranoid, religiosity, magical, phobic ideas, themes, areas of concern, self-concept.
F. *Thought processes*—organization and association of ideas, coherence, ability to abstract and understand symbols.
G. *Sensorium:*
1. *Orientation* to person, time and place, situation.
2. *Memory*—immediate, rote, remote, and recent.
3. *Attention and concentration*—susceptibility to distraction.
4. *Information and intelligence*—account of general knowledge, history, and reasoning powers.
5. *Comprehension*—concrete and *abstract.*
6. *Stage of consciousness*—alert/awake, somnolent, lethargic, delirious, stuporous, comatose.

H. *Insight and judgment:*
1. Extent to which client sees self as having problems, needing treatment.
2. Client awareness of intrapsychic nature of own difficulties.
3. Soundness of judgment, problem-solving, decision making.

I. *Spiritual.*

II. INDIVIDUAL ASSESSMENT—consider the following (**Table 10.9**):

A. Physical and intellectual factors.

B. Socioeconomic factors.

Table 10.9

Individual Assessment

Physical and Intellectual
1. Presence of physical illness or disability. 2. Appearance and energy level. 3. Current and potential levels of intellectual functioning. 4. How client sees personal world, translates events around self; client's perceptual abilities. 5. Cause-and-effect reasoning, ability to focus.
Socioeconomic Factors
1. Economic factors—level of income, adequacy of subsistence; how this affects lifestyle, sense of adequacy, self-worth. 2. Employment and attitudes about it. 3. Racial, cultural, and ethnic identification; sense of identity and belonging. 4. Religious identification and link to significant value systems, norms, and practices.
Personal Values and Goals
1. Presence or absence of congruence between values and their expression in action; meaning of values to individual. 2. Congruence between individual's values and goals and the immediate systems with which client interacts. 3. Congruence between individual's values and assessor's values; meaning of this for intervention process.
Adaptive Functioning and Response to Present Involvement
1. Manner in which individual presents self to others—grooming, appearance, posture. 2. Emotional tone and change or constancy of levels. 3. Style of communication—verbal and nonverbal; ability to express appropriate emotion, follow train of thought; factors of dissonance, confusion, uncertainty. 4. Symptoms or symptomatic behavior. 5. Quality of relationship individual seeks to establish—direction, purposes, and uses of such relationships for individual. 6. Perception of self. 7. Social roles that are assumed or ascribed; competence in fulfilling these roles. 8. Relational behavior: a. Capacity for intimacy. b. Dependence-independence balance. c. Power and control conflicts. d. Exploitiveness. e. Openness.
Developmental Factors
1. Role performance equated with life stage. 2. How developmental experiences have been interpreted and used. 3. How individual has dealt with past conflicts, tasks, and problems. 4. Uniqueness of present problem in life experience.

Adapted from Wilson, HS, and Kneisl, CR: *Psychiatric Nursing*, ed. 2. Addison-Wesley, Menlo Park, CA. (out of print)

C. Personal values and goals.

D. Adaptive functioning and response to present involvement.

E. Developmental factors.

III. CULTURAL ASSESSMENT (see **Chapter 3**):

A. Knowledge of ethnic beliefs and cultural practices can assist the nurse in the planning and implementation of holistic care.

B. Consider the following:

1. *Demographic data:* is this an "ethnic neighborhood"?
2. *Socioeconomic status:* occupation, education (formal and informal), income level; who is employed?
3. *Ethnic/racial orientation:* ethnic identity, value orientation.
4. *Country of immigration:* date of immigration; where were the family members born? Where has the family lived?
5. *Languages spoken:* does family speak English? Language and dialect preferences.
6. *Family relationships:* what are the formal roles? Who makes the decisions within the family? What is the family lifestyle and living arrangements?
7. *Degree of acculturation* of family members: how are the family customs and beliefs similar to or different from the dominant culture?
8. *Communication patterns:* social customs, nonverbal behaviors.
9. *Religious preferences:* what role do beliefs, rituals, and taboos play in health and illness? Is there a significant religious person? Are there any dietary symbolisms or preferences or restrictions due to religious beliefs?
10. *Cultural practices related to health and illness:* does the family use folk medicine practices or a folk healer? Are there specific dietary practices related to health and illness?
11. *Support systems:* do extended family members provide support?
12. *Health beliefs:* response to pain and hospitalization; disease predisposition and resistance.
13. Other significant factors related to ethnic identity: what health-care facilities does the family use?
14. Communication barriers:
    a. Differences in language.
    b. Technical languages.
    c. Inappropriate place for discussion.
    d. Personality or gender of the nurse.
    e. Distrust of the nurse.
    f. Time-orientation differences.
    g. Differences in pain perception and expression.
    h. Variable attitudes toward death and dying.

Interviewing

I. DEFINITION: a goal-directed method of communicating facts, feelings, and meanings. For interviewing to be successful, interaction between two persons involved must be effective.

II. NINE PRINCIPLES OF VERBAL INTERACTION:

A. *Client's initiative* begins the discussion.
B. *Indirect approach,* moving from the periphery to the core.
C. *Open-ended* statements, using incomplete forms of statements such as "You were saying . . ." to prompt rather than close off an exchange.
D. *Minimal verbal activity* in order not to obstruct thought process and client's responses.
E. *Spontaneity,* rather than fixed interview topics, may bring out much more relevant data.
F. *Facilitate expression of feelings* to help assess events and reactions by asking, for example, "What was that like for you?"
G. *Focus on emotional areas* about which client may be in conflict, as noted by repetitive themes.
H. *Pick up cues, clues, and signals from client,* such as facial expressions and gestures, behavior, emphatic tones, and flushed face.
I. *Introduce material related to content* already brought up by client; do *not* bring in a tangential focus from "left field."

III. PURPOSE AND GOALS OF INTERVIEWING:

A. *Initiate and maintain a positive nurse-client relationship,* which can decrease symptoms, lessen demands, and move client toward optimum health when nurse demonstrates understanding and sharing of client's concerns.
B. *Determine client's view of nurse's role* in order to utilize it or change it.
C. *Collect information on emotional crisis* to plan goals and approaches in order to increase effectiveness of nursing interventions.
D. *Identify and resolve crisis;* the act of eliciting cause or antecedent event may in itself be therapeutic.
E. *Channel feelings directly* by exploring interrelated events, feelings, and behaviors in order to discourage displacement of feelings onto somatic and behavioral symptoms.
F. *Channel communication* and transfer significant information to the physician and other team members.
G. *Prepare for health teaching* in order to help the client function as effectively as possible.

General Principles of Health Teaching

One key nursing function is to promote and restore health. This involves teaching clients new psychomotor skills, general knowledge, coping attitudes, and social skills related to health and illness (e.g., proper diet, exercises, colostomy care, wound care, insulin injections, urine testing). The teaching function of the nurse is vital in assisting normal development and helping clients meet health-related needs.

I. PURPOSE OF HEALTH TEACHING:

A. *General goal:* motivate health-oriented behavior.
B. *Nursing interventions:*
1. Fill in *gaps* in information.
2. *Clarify* misinformation.
3. Teach necessary *skills.*
4. *Modify* attitudes.

II. EDUCATIONAL THEORIES on which effective health teaching is based:

A. *Motivation theory:*
1. Health-oriented behavior is determined by the degree to which person sees health problem as *threatening,* with *serious consequences, high probability of occurrence,* and *belief in availability of effective course of action.*
2. Non–health-related motives may *supersede* health-related motives.
3. Health-related motives may not always give rise to health-related behavior, and vice versa.
4. Motivation may be influenced by:
   a. *Phases of adaptation* to crisis (poor motivation in early phase).
   b. *Anxiety and awareness of need* to learn. (Mild anxiety is highly motivating.)
   c. *Mutual* versus externally imposed goal setting.
   d. Perceived *meaningfulness* of information and material. (If within client's frame of reference, both meaningfulness and motivation increase.)

B. *Theory of planned change:*
1. *Unfreeze* present level of behavior—develop awareness of problem.
2. Establish *need* for change and relationship of trust and respect.
3. *Move* toward change—examine alternatives, develop intentions into real efforts.
4. *Freeze* on a new level—generalize behavior, stabilize change.

C. Elements of *learning theory:*
1. *Drive* must be present based on experiencing uncertainty, frustration, concern, or curiosity; hierarchy of needs exists.
2. *Response* is a learned behavior that is elicited when associated stimulus is present.
3. *Reward and reinforcement* are necessary for response (behavior) to occur and remain.
4. *Extinction of response,* that is, elimination of undesirable behavior, can be attained through conditioning.

5. Memorization is the easiest level of learning, but least effective in changing behavior.
6. Understanding involves the incorporation of generalizations and specific facts.
7. After introduction of new material, there is a period of floundering when assimilation and insight occur.
8. Learning is a two-way process between learner and teacher; defensive behavior in either makes both activities difficult, if not impossible.
9. Learning flourishes when client feels respected, accepted by nurse who is enthusiastic; learning occurs best when differing value systems are accepted.
10. Feedback increases learning.
11. Successful learning leads to more successes in learning.
12. Teaching and learning should take place in the area where *targeted activity* normally occurs.
13. Priorities for learning are dependent on client's *physical and psychological status.*
14. Decreased visual and auditory perception leads to decreased readiness to learn.
15. Content, terminology, pacing, and spacing of learning must correspond to client's *capabilities, maturity level, feelings, attitudes, and experiences.*

III. ASSESSMENT OF THE CLIENT-LEARNER:

A. *Characteristics:* age, sex, race, medical diagnosis, prognosis.

B. *Sociocultural-economic:* ethnic, religious group beliefs and practices; family situation (roles, support); job (type, history, options, stress); financial situation, living situation (facilities).

C. *Psychological:* own and family's response to illness; premorbid personality; current self-image.

D. *Educational:*
1. Client's *perception* of current situation: what is wrong? Cause? How will lifestyle be affected?
2. *Past experience:* previous hospitalization and treatment; past compliance.
3. *Level of knowledge:* what has client been told? From what source? How accurate? Known others with the same illness?
4. *Goals:* what client *wants* to know.
5. *Needs:* what nurse thinks client *should* know for self-care.
6. Readiness for learning.
7. *Educational* background; ability to read and learn.

IV. ANALYSIS OF FACTORS INFLUENCING LEARNING:

A. *Internal:*
1. Physical condition.
2. Senses (sight, hearing, touch).
3. Age.
4. Anxiety.
5. Motivation.
6. Experience.
7. Values (cultural, religious, personal).
8. Comprehension.
9. Education and language deficiency.

B. *External:*
1. Physical environment (heat, light, noise, comfort).
2. Timing, duration, interval.
3. Teaching methods and aids.
4. Content, vocabulary.

V. TEACHING PLAN must be:

A. Compatible with the *three* domains of learning:
1. *Cognitive* (knowledge, concepts): use written and audiovisual materials, discussion.
2. *Psychomotor* (skills): use demonstrations, illustrations, role models.
3. *Affective* (attitudes): use discussions, maintain atmosphere conducive to change; use role models.

B. Appropriate to educational material.

C. Related to client's abilities and perceptions.

D. Related to objectives of teaching.

VI. IMPLEMENTATION—*teaching guidelines* to use with clients:

A. Select conducive *environment* and best *timing* for activity.

B. Assess the client's *needs,* interests, *perceptions,* motivations, and *readiness* for learning.

C. State purpose and *realistic goals* of planned teaching/learning activity.

D. Actually involve the client by giving him or her the opportunity to *do, react, experience,* and *ask questions.*

E. Make sure that the client views the activity as useful and worthwhile and that it is within the client's grasp.

F. Use comprehensible terminology.

G. Proceed from the *known to the unknown,* from *specific to general* information.

H. Provide opportunity for client to *see results* and progress.

I. Give *feedback* and *positive reinforcement.*

J. Provide opportunities to achieve *success.*

K. Offer repeated practice in *real-life* situations.

L. *Space and distribute* learning sessions over a period of time.

VII. EVALUATION/OUTCOME CRITERIA:

A. Client's deficit of knowledge is lessened.

B. Increased compliance with treatment.

C. Length of hospital stay is reduced.

D. Rate of readmission to hospital is reduced.

The Therapeutic Nursing Process*

A *therapeutic nursing process* involves an interaction between the nurse and client in which the nurse offers a series of planned, goal-directed activities that are useful to a particular client in relieving discomfort, promoting growth, and satisfying interpersonal relationships.

I. CHARACTERISTICS of therapeutic nursing:

A. Movement from first contact through final outcome:

1. *Eight general phases* occur in a typical unfolding of a natural process of problem-solving.
2. Stages are not always in the same sequence.
3. Not all stages are present in a relationship.

B. Phases†

1. *Beginning* the relationship. *Goal:* build trust.
2. *Formulating* and clarifying a problem and concern. *Goal:* clarify client's statements.
3. *Setting a contract* or working agreement. *Goal:* decide on terms of the relationship.
4. *Building* the relationship. *Goal:* increase depth of relationship and degree of commitment.
5. *Exploring goals* and solutions, gathering data, expressing feelings. *Goals:* (a) maintain and enhance relationship (trust and safety), (b) explore blocks to goal, (c) expand self-awareness, and (d) learn skills necessary to reach goal.
6. *Developing action plan. Goals:* (a) clarify feelings, (b) focus on and choose between alternative courses of action, and (c) practice new skills.
7. *Working through* conflicts or disturbing feelings. *Goals:* (a) channel earlier discussions into specific course of action and (b) work through unresolved feelings.
8. *Ending* the relationship. *Goals:* (a) evaluation of goal attainment; (b) pointing out assets and gains; and (c) leave-taking reactions (repression, regression, anger, withdrawal, acting out).

II. THERAPEUTIC NURSE-CLIENT INTERACTIONS:

A. Plans/goals:

1. Demonstrate unconditional *acceptance,* interest, concern, and respect.
2. Develop trust—be *consistent and congruent.*
3. Make *frequent* contacts with the client.
4. Be *honest* and *direct, authentic* and spontaneous.
5. Offer support, security, and empathy, *not* sympathy.
6. Focus comments on concerns of client (*client centered*), not self (social responses). *Refocus* when client changes subject.
7. Encourage expression of *feelings;* focus on feelings and *here-and-now* behavior.
8. Give attention to a client who complains.
9. Give information at client's level of understanding, at appropriate time and place.
10. Use open-ended questions; ask *how, what, where, who,* and *when* questions; avoid *why* questions; *avoid* questions that can be answered by *yes* or *no.*
11. Use feedback or reflective listening.
12. Maintain hope, but *avoid* false reassurances, clichés, and pat responses.
13. *Avoid* verbalizing value judgments, giving personal opinions, or moralizing.
14. Do *not* change the subject *unless* the client is redundant or focusing on physical illness.
15. Point out *reality;* help the client leave "inner world."
16. Set *limits* on behavior when client is acting out unacceptable behavior that is self-destructive or harmful to others.
17. Assist clients in arriving at their own decisions by demonstrating problem-solving or involving them in the process.
18. Do *not* talk if it is not indicated.
19. Approach, sit, or walk with clients who are agitated; stay with the person who is upset, if he or she can tolerate it.
20. Focus on nonverbal communication.
21. Remember the *psyche has a soma!* Do *not* neglect appropriate physical symptoms.

B. Examples of **therapeutic** responses as interventions:

1. Being *silent*—being able to sit in silence with a person can connote acceptance and acknowledgment that the person has the right to silence. (*Dangers:* The nurse may wrongly give the client the impression that there is a lack of interest, or the nurse may discourage verbalization if acceptance of this behavior is prolonged; it is not necessarily helpful with acutely psychotic behavior.)
2. Using *nonverbal communication*—for example, nodding head, moving closer to the client, and leaning forward; use as a way to encourage client to speak.
3. Give encouragement to continue with *open-ended leads*—nurse's responses: "Then what?" "Go on," "For instance," "Tell me more," "Talk about that."
4. *Accepting, acknowledging*—nurse's responses: "I hear your anger," or "I see that you are sitting in the corner."
5. *Commenting on nonverbal behavior* of client—nurse's responses: "I notice that you are swinging your leg," "I see that you are tapping your foot," or "I notice that you are wetting your

---

*Source: ©Lagerquist, S: *Addison-Wesley's Nursing Examination Review,* ed 4. Addison-Wesley, Redwood City, CA.

†Adapted from Brammer, LM: *The Helping Relationship; Process and Skills.* Prentice Hall, Englewood Cliffs, NJ. (out of print)

lips." Client may respond with, "So what?" If she or he does, the nurse needs to reply why the comment was made—for example, "It is distracting," "I am giving the nonverbal behavior meaning," "Swinging your leg makes it difficult for me to concentrate on what you are saying," or "I think when people tap their feet it means they are impatient. Are you impatient?"

6. Encouraging clients to *notice with their senses* what is going on—nurse's response: "What did you see (or hear)?" or "What did you notice?"
7. Encouraging *recall and description* of details of a particular experience—nurse's response: "Give me an example," "Please describe the experience further," "Tell me more," or "What did you say then?"
8. *Giving feedback by reflecting, restating, and paraphrasing* feelings and content:
   Client: I cried when he didn't come to see me.
   Nurse: You cried. You were expecting him to come and he didn't?
9. *Picking up on latent content* (what is implied)—nurse's response: "You were disappointed. I think it may have hurt when he didn't come."
10. *Focusing, pinpointing,* asking "what" questions:
    Client: They didn't come.
    Nurse: Who are "they"?
    Client: [Rambling.]
    Nurse: Tell it to me in a sentence or two. What is your main point? What would you say is your main concern?
11. *Clarifying*—nurse's response: "What do you mean by 'they'?" "What caused this?" or "I didn't understand. Please say it again."
12. *Focusing on reality* by expressing doubt on "unreal" perceptions:
    Client: Run! There are giant ants flying around after us.
    Nurse: That is unusual. I don't see giant ants flying.
13. *Focusing on feelings,* encouraging client to be aware of and describe personal feelings:
    Client: Worms are in my head.
    Nurse: That must be a frightening feeling. What did you feel at that time? Tell me about that feeling.
14. Helping client to *sort and classify impressions, make speculations, abstract* and *generalize* by making connections, seeing common elements and similarities, making comparisons, and placing events in logical sequence—nurse's responses: "What are the common elements in what you just told me?" "How is this similar to . . .?" "What happened just before?" or "What is the connection between this and . . .?"
15. *Pointing out discrepancies* between thoughts, feelings, and actions—nurse's response: "You say you were feeling sad when she yelled at you, yet you laughed. Your feelings and actions do not seem to fit together."
16. *Checking perceptions* and *seeking agreement* on how the issue is seen, *checking* with the client to see if the message sent is the same one that was received—nurse's response: "Let me restate what I heard you say," "Are you saying that . . .?" "Did I hear you correctly?" "Is this what you mean?" or "It seems that you were saying . . ."
17. *Encouraging client to consider alternatives*—nurse's response: "What else could you say?" or "Instead of hitting him, what else might you do?"
18. *Planning a course of action*—nurse's response: "Now that we have talked about your on-the-job activities and you have thought of several choices, which are you going to try out?" or "What would you do next time?"
19. *Imparting information*—give additional data as new input to help client (e.g., state facts and reality-based data that client may lack).
20. *Summing up*—nurse's response: "Today we have talked about your feelings toward your boss, how you express your anger, and about your fear of being rejected by your family."
21. *Encouraging client to appraise and evaluate* the experience or outcome—nurse's response: "How did it turn out?" "What was it like?" "What was your part in it?" "What difference did it make?" or "How will this help you later"?

C. Examples of **nontherapeutic** responses:

1. *Changing the subject, tangential response,* moving away from problem or focusing on incidental, superficial content:
   Client: I hate you.
   Nurse: Would you like to take your shower now?
   Suggested responses: use reflection: "You hate me; tell me about this," or "You hate me; what does hate mean to you?"
   Client: I want to kill myself today.
   Nurse: Isn't today the day your mother is supposed to come?
   Suggested responses: (a) give open-ended lead, (b) give feedback: "I hear you saying today that you want to kill yourself," or (c) clarifying: "Tell me more about this feeling of wanting to kill yourself."
2. *Moralizing:* saying with approval or disapproval that the person's behavior is good or bad, right or wrong; *arguing* with stated belief of person; directly opposing the person:
   Nurse: That's good. It's wrong to shoot yourself.
   Client: I have nothing to live for.

Nurse: You certainly do have a lot!
Suggested responses: similar to those in **C. 1.** previous.

3. *Agreeing with client's autistic inventions:*
Client: The eggs are flying saucers.
Nurse: Yes, I see. Go on.
Suggested response: use clarifying response first: "I don't understand," and then, depending on client's response, use either *accepting and acknowledging, focusing on reality,* or *focusing on feelings.*
4. *Agreeing with client's negative view of self:*
Client: I have made a mess of my life.
Nurse: Yes, you have.
Suggested response: use clarifying response about "mess of my life"—"Give me an example of one time where you feel you messed up in your life."
5. *Complimenting, flattering:*
Client: I have made a mess of my life.
Nurse: How could you? You are such an attractive, intelligent, generous person.
Suggested response: same as in **C. 4.**
6. *Giving opinions and advice* concerning client's life situation—examples of poor responses include: "In my opinion . . ." "I think you should . . ." or "Why not?"
Suggested responses: (a) encourage the client to consider alternatives ("What else do you think you could try?"); (b) encourage the client to appraise and evaluate for himself or herself ("What is it like for you?").
7. *Seeking agreement* from client with nurse's personal opinion—examples of poor responses include: "I think . . . don't you?" and "Isn't that right?"
Suggested responses: (a) it is best to keep personal opinion to oneself and only give information that would aid the client's orientation to reality; (b) if you give an opinion as a *model* of orienting to reality, ask client to *state his or her* opinion ("My opinion is . . . what is your opinion?").
8. *Probing* or *offering premature solutions and interpretations;* jumping to conclusions:
Client: I can't find a job.
Nurse: You could go to an employment agency.
Client: I'd rather not talk about it.
Nurse: What are you unconsciously doing when you say that? What you really mean is . . .
Client: I don't want to live alone.
Nurse: Are you afraid of starting to drink again?
Suggested responses: use responses that seek clarification and elicit more data.
9. *Changing client's words* without prior validation:
Client: I am *not feeling well* today.
Nurse: What makes you feel so *depressed?*
Suggested response: "In what way are you not feeling well?" Use the same language as the client.
10. *Following vague content* as if understood or *using vague global* pronouns, adverbs, and adjectives:
Client: People are so *unfair.*
Nurse: I know what you mean.
Suggested response: clarify vague referents such as "people" and "unfair."
Client: I feel sad.
Nurse: Everyone feels that way at one time or another.
Suggested response: "What are you sad about?"
11. *Questioning on different topics without waiting for a reply:*
Client: [Remains silent.]
Nurse: What makes you so silent? Are you angry? Would you like to be alone?
Suggested response: choose one of the above and wait for a response before asking the next question.
12. *Ignoring client's questions or comments:*
Client: Am I crazy, nurse?
Nurse: [Walking away as if he or she did not hear the client.]
Suggested responses: "I can't understand what makes you bring this up at this time," or "Tell me what makes you bring this up at this time." Ignoring questions or comments usually implies that the nurse is feeling uncomfortable. It is important not to "run away" from the client.
13. *Closing off exploration* with questions that can be answered by *yes* or *no:*
Client: I'll never get better.
Nurse: Is something making you feel that way?
Suggested response: "What makes you feel that way?" Use open-ended questions that start with *what, who, when, where,* etc.
14. *Using clichés* or stereotyped expressions:
Client: The doctor took away my weekend pass.
Nurse: The doctor is only doing what's best for you. Doctor knows best. [Comment: also an example of moralizing.]
Suggested response: "Tell me what happened when the doctor took away your weekend pass."
15. *Overloading:* giving too much information at one time:
Nurse: Hello, I'm Mr. Brown. I'm a nurse here. I'll be here today, but I'm off tomorrow. Ms. Anderson will assign you another nurse tomorrow. This unit has five RNs, three LVNs, and students from three nursing schools who will all be taking care of you at some time.

Suggested response: "Hello, I'm Mr. Brown, your nurse today." Keep your initial orienting information simple and brief.

16. *Underloading:* not giving enough information, so that meaning is not clear; withholding information:
    Client: What are visiting hours like here?
    Nurse: They are flexible and liberal.
    Suggested response: "They are flexible and liberal, from 10 a.m. to 12 noon and from 6 to 8 p.m." Use specific terms and give specific information.
17. *Saying no without saying no:*
    Client: Can we go for a walk soon?
    Nurse: We'll see. Perhaps. Maybe. Later.
    Suggested response: "I will check the schedule in the nursing office and let you know within an hour." Vague, ambiguous responses can be seen as "putting the client off." It is best to be clear, specific, and direct.
18. *Using double-bind communication:* sending conflicting messages that do not have "mutual fit," or are incongruent:
    Nurse: [Continuing to stay and talk with the client.] It's time for you to rest.
    Suggested response: "It's time for you to rest and for me to leave [proceeding to leave]."
19. *Protecting:* defending someone else while talking with client; implying client has no right to personal opinions and feelings:
    Client: This hospital is no good. No one cares here.
    Nurse: This is an excellent hospital. All the staff were chosen for their warmth and concern for people.
    Suggested response: focus on feeling tone or on clarifying information.
20. *Asking "why" questions* implies that the person has immediate conscious awareness of the reasons for his or her feelings and behaviors. Examples of this include: "Why don't you?" "Why did you do that?" or "Why do you feel this way?"
    Suggested response: ask clarifying questions using *how, what,* etc.
21. *Coercion:* using the interaction between people to force someone to do *your* will, with the implication that if he or she does not "do it for your sake," you will not love or stay with him or her:
    Client: I refuse to talk with him.
    Nurse: Do it for my sake, before it's too late.
    Suggested response: "Something keeps you from wanting to talk with him?"
22. Focusing on *negative* feelings, thoughts, actions:
    Client: I can't sleep; I can't eat; I can't think; I can't do anything.
    Nurse: How long have you not been sleeping, eating, or thinking well?
    Suggested response: "What *do* you do?"
23. *Rejecting* client's behavior or ideas:
    Client: Let's talk about incest.
    Nurse: Incest is a bad thing to talk about; I don't want to.
    Suggested response: "What do you want to say about incest?"
24. *Accusing, belittling:*
    Client: I've had to wait five minutes for you to change my dressing.
    Nurse: Don't be so demanding. Don't you see that I have several people who need me?
    Suggested response: "It must have been hard to wait for me to come when you wanted it to be right away."
25. *Evading a response* by asking a question in return:
    Client: I want to know your opinion, nurse. Am I crazy?
    Nurse: Do you think you are crazy?
    Suggested response: "I don't know. What do you mean by 'crazy'?"
26. *Circumstantiality:* communicating in such a way that the main point is reached only after many side comments, details, and additions:
    Client: Will you go out on a date with me?
    Nurse: I work every evening. On my day off I usually go out of town. I have a steady boyfriend. Besides that, I am a nurse and you are a client. Thank you for asking me, but no, I will not date you.
    Suggested response: abbreviate your response to: "Thank you for asking me, but no, I will not date you."
27. *Making assumptions* without checking them:
    Client: [Standing in the kitchen by the sink, peeling onions, with tears in the eyes.]
    Nurse: What's making you so sad?
    Client: I'm not sad. Peeling onions always makes my eyes water.
    Suggested response: use simple acknowledgment and acceptance initially, such as "I notice you have tears in your eyes."
28. *Giving false, premature reassurance:*
    Client: I'm scared.
    Nurse: Don't worry; everything will be all right. There's nothing to be afraid of.
    Suggested response: "I'd like to hear about what you're afraid of, so that together we can see what could be done to help you." Open the way for clarification and exploration, and offer yourself as a helping person—not someone with magic answers.

Common Behavioral Problems

I. ANGER

A. Definition: feelings of resentment in response to anxiety when threat is perceived; need to discharge tension of anger.

B. Assessment:

1. *Degree of anger and frequency:* scope of anger ranges on a continuum from *everyday mild annoyance* → *frustration* from interference with goal accomplishment → *assertiveness* (behavior used to deal with anger effectively) → *anger* related to helplessness and powerlessness that may interfere with functioning → *rage and fury,* when coping means are depleted or not developed.
2. *Mode of expression of anger:*
   a. *Covert, passive* expression of anger: being overly nice; body language with little or no eye contact, arms close to body, soft voice, little gesturing; sarcasm through humor; *sublimation* through art and music; projection onto others; *denying* and pushing anger out of awareness; *psychosomatic* illness in response to internalized anger (e.g., headache).
   b. *Overt,* active expression of anger: physical activity to work off excess physical energy associated with biological response (e.g., hitting a punching bag, taking a walk); *aggression,* assertiveness.
3. *Physiological behaviors*—result of secretion of epinephrine and sympathetic nervous system stimulation preparing for fight-flight.
   a. *Cardiovascular* response: increased blood pressure and pulse, increased free fatty acid in blood.
   b. *Gastrointestinal* response: increased nausea, salivation; decreased peristalsis.
   c. *Genitourinary* response: urinary frequency.
   d. *Neuromuscular* response: increased alertness, increased muscle tension and deep tendon reflexes, electrocardiographic (ECG) changes.
4. *Positive functions of anger:*
   a. Energizes behavior.
   b. Protects positive image.
   c. Provides ego defense during high anxiety.
   d. Gives greater control over situation.
   e. Alerts to need for coping.
   f. A sign of a healthy relationship.

C. Analysis/nursing diagnosis: *defensive coping* related to source of stress (stressors):

1. *Biological stressors*—instinctual drives (Lorenz, on aggressive instincts, and Freud), *endocrine imbalances,* seizures, tumors, *hunger, fatigue.*
2. *Psychological stressors*—inability to resolve frustration that leads to aggression; real or imagined threatened loss of self-esteem; conflict, lack of control; anger as a learned expression and a reinforced response. Prolonged stress; an attempt to protect self; a desire for retaliation; a normal part of grief process.
3. *Sociocultural stressors*—lack of early training in self-discipline and social skills; crowding, personal space intrusion; *role modeling of abusive behavior* by significant others and by media personalities.

D. Nursing care plan/implementation—*long-term goals:* constructive use of angry energy to accomplish tasks and motivate growth.

1. *Prevent* and *control* violence.
   a. Approach unhurriedly.
   b. Provide atmosphere of acceptance; listen attentively, refrain from arguing and criticizing.
   c. Encourage expression of feelings.
   d. Offer feedback of client's expressed feelings.
   e. Encourage mutual problem-solving.
   f. Encourage realistic perception of others and situation and respect for the rights of others.
2. *Limit setting:*
   a. Clearly state *expectations* and *consequences* of acts.
   b. Enforce consequences.
   c. Encourage client to assume responsibility for behavior.
   d. Explore reasons and meaning of negative behavior.
3. Promote *self-awareness* and *problem-solving* abilities. Encourage and assist client to:
   a. Accept self as a person with a right to experience angry feelings.
   b. Explore reasons for anger.
   c. Describe situations where anger was experienced.
   d. Discuss appropriate alternatives for expressing anger (including assertiveness training).
   e. Decide on one feasible solution.
   f. Act on solution.
   g. Evaluate effectiveness.
4. *Health teaching:*
   a. Explore other ways to express feelings, and provide activities that allow appropriate expression of anger.
   b. Recommend that behavioral limits be set (by the family).
   c. Explain how to set behavioral limits.
   d. Advise against causing defensive patterns in others.

E. Evaluation/outcome criteria:

1. Demonstrates insight (awareness of factors that precipitate anger; identifies disturbing topics, events, and inappropriate use of coping mechanisms).

2. Uses appropriate coping mechanisms.
3. Reaches out for emotional support before stress level becomes excessive.
4. Evidence of increased reality perception and problem-solving ability.

II. COMBATIVE-AGGRESSIVE BEHAVIOR

A. Definition: *acting out* feelings of frustration, anger, anxiety, etc., through *physical or verbal* behavior.

B. Assessment: recognize *precombative* behavior:
1. Demanding, fist clenching.
2. Boisterous, loud.
3. Vulgar, profane.
4. Limited attention span.
5. Sarcastic, taunting, verbal threats.
6. Restless, agitated, elated.
7. Frowning.

C. Analysis/nursing diagnosis: *risk for self-injury* and *violence directed at others* related to:
1. Frustration as response to *breakdown of self-control* coping mechanisms.
2. Acting out as customary response to anger (*defensive coping*).
3. Confusion (*sensory/perceptual alterations*).
4. Physical restraints, such as when clients are postoperative and discover wrist restraints.
5. Fear of intimacy, intrusion on emotional and physical space (*altered thought processes*).
6. Feelings of helplessness, inadequacy *(situational or chronic low self-esteem).*

D. Nursing care plan/implementation:
1. *Long-term goal:* channel aggression—help person express feelings rather than act them out.
2. *Immediate goal: prevent injury to self and others.*
   a. Calmly call for assistance; do *not* try to handle *alone.*
   b. Approach cautiously. Keep client within *eye contact,* observing client's personal space.
   c. *Protect* against self-injury and injury to others; be aware of your position in relation to the weapon, door, escape route.
   d. *Minimize* stimuli, to control the environment—clear the area, close doors, turn off TV so person can hear you.
   e. *Divert* attention from the act; engage in talk and lead away from others.
   f. Assess *triggering* cause.
   g. Identify immediate problem.
   h. Focus on *remedy for immediate* problem.
   i. Choose one individual who has a calm, quiet presence to interact with person; nonauthoritarian, nonthreatening.
   j. Maintain *verbal contact* to keep communication open; offer empathetic ear, but be firm and consistent in setting *limits* on dangerous behavior.
   k. Negotiate, but do not make false promises or argue.
   l. Restraints may be necessary as a *last* resort.
   m. Place person in quiet room so he or she can calm down.
3. *Health teaching:*
   a. Explain how to obtain relief from stress and how to rechannel emotional energy into acceptable activity.
   b. Advise against causing defensive responses in others.
   c. Explain what is justifiable aggression.
   d. Emphasize importance of how to recognize tension in self.
   e. Explain why self-control is important.
   f. Explain to family, staff, how to set behavioral limits.
   g. Explain causes of maladaptive coping related to anger.
   h. Teach how to use problem-solving method.

E. Evaluation/outcome criteria:
1. Is aware of causes of anger; can recognize the feeling of anger and use alternative methods of expressing anger.
2. Expression of anger is appropriate, congruent with the situation.
3. Replaces aggression and acting out with assertiveness.

III. CONFUSION/DISORIENTATION

A. Definition: loss of reality orientation as to person, time, place, events, ideas.

B. Assessment: note unusual behavior:
1. Picking, stroking movements in the air or on clothing and linens.
2. Frequent crying or laughing.
3. Alternating periods of confusion and lucidity (e.g., confused at night, when alone in the dark).
4. Fluctuating mood, actions, rationality (argumentative, combative, withdrawn).
5. Increasingly restless, fearful, leading to insomnia, nightmares.
6. Acts bewildered; has trouble identifying familiar people.
7. Preoccupied; irritable when interrupted.
8. Unresponsive to questions; problem with concentration and setting realistic priorities.
9. Sensitive to noise and light.
10. Has unrealistic perception of time, place, and situation.
11. Nurse no longer seen as supportive but as threatening.

C. Analysis/nursing diagnosis: *altered thought processes and sensory/perceptual alterations* related to:
1. *Physical and physiological disturbances*—metabolic (uremia, diabetes, hepatic dysfunction), fluid

MENTAL HEALTH

and electrolyte imbalances, cardiac arrhythmias, heart failure; anemia, massive blood loss with low hemoglobin; brain lesions; nutritional deficiency; pain; sleep disturbance; drugs (antidepressants, tranquilizers, sedatives, antihypertensives, diuretics, alcohol, phencyclidine [PCP], street drugs).
2. *Unfamiliar environment*—unfamiliar routine and people; procedures that threaten body image; *noisy* equipment.
3. *Loss of sensory acuity* from partial or incomplete reception of orienting stimuli or information.
4. *Disability in screening out* irrelevant and excessive sensory input.
5. *Memory impairment.*

D. Nursing care plan/implementation:
1. Check *physical signs* (e.g., vital signs, neurological status, fluid and electrolyte balance, and blood urea nitrogen [BUN]).
2. Be calm; make contact to *reorient to reality:*
   a. *Avoid* startling if person is alone, in the dark, sedated.
   b. Make sure person can *see, hear, and talk* to you—turn off TV; turn on light, put on client's glasses, hearing aids, dentures.
   c. Call by name, clearly and distinctly.
   d. Approach cautiously, close to *eye* level.
   e. Keep your *hands visible;* for example, on bed.
3. *Take care of immediate problem* (e.g., disconnected IV tube or catheter).
   a. Give instructions slowly and distinctly; *avoid* threatening tone and comments.
   b. *Stay* with person until reoriented.
   c. Put *side rails* up.
4. Use conversation to *reduce* confusion.
   a. Use *simple, concrete phrases;* language the person can understand; *repeat* as needed.
   b. *Avoid:* shouting, arguing, false promises, use of medical abbreviations (e.g., NPO).
   c. Give *more time to concentrate* on what you said.
   d. Focus on *reality-oriented* topics or objects in the environment.
5. *Prevent confusion by establishing a reality-oriented relationship.*
   a. Introduce self by name.
   b. Jointly establish routines to prevent confusion from unpredictable changes and variations. Determine client's usual routine; attempt to incorporate this to lessen disruption in lifestyle.
   c. Explain what to expect in understandable words—where client is and why, what will happen, noises and activities client will hear and see, people client will meet, tests and procedures client will have.
   d. Find out what meaning hospitalization has to client; reduce anxiety related to feelings of apprehension and helplessness.
   e. Spend as much time as possible with client.
6. *Maintain orientation by providing nonthreatening environment.*
   a. Assign to room *near nurses' station.*
   b. Surround with *familiar* objects from home (e.g., photos).
   c. Provide *clock, calendar, and radio.*
   d. Have flexible visiting hours.
   e. Open curtain for *natural light.*
   f. Keep glasses, dentures, hearing aids nearby.
   g. Check client often, especially at night.
   h. *Avoid* using intercom to answer calls.
   i. *Avoid* low-pitched conversation.
7. *Take care of other needs.*
   a. Promote sleep according to usual habits and patterns to *prevent sleep deprivation.*
   b. *Avoid sedatives,* which may lead to or increase confusion.
   c. Promote independent functions, self-help activities, to *maintain dignity.*
   d. Encourage *nutritional* adequacy; incorporate familiar foods, ethnic preferences.
   e. Maintain *routine; avoid* being late with meals, medication, or procedures.
   f. Have *realistic expectations.*
   g. *Discover hidden fears.*
      (1) Do *not* assume confused behavior is unrelated to reality.
      (2) Look for clues to meaning from client's background, occupation.
   h. *Provide support to family.*
      (1) Encourage expression of feelings; *avoid* being judgmental.
      (2) Check what worked in previous situations.
8. *Health teaching:* explain possible causes of confusion. Reassure that it is common. Teach family, friends how to react to confused behavior.

E. Evaluation/outcome criteria:
1. Less restlessness, fearfulness, mood lability.
2. More frequent periods of lucidity; oriented to time, place, and person; responds to questions.

IV. DEMANDING BEHAVIOR

A. Definition: a strong and persistent struggle to obtain satisfaction of self-oriented needs (e.g., control, self-esteem) or relief from anxiety.

B. Assessment:
1. Attention-seeking behavior.
2. Multiple requests.
3. Frequency of questions.
4. Lack of reasonableness; irrationality of request.

C. Analysis/nursing diagnosis: *defensive coping and impaired social interaction* related to:
1. Feelings of *helplessness* and *hopelessness.*
2. Feelings of *powerlessness* and *fear.*
3. A way of coping with anxiety.

D. Nursing care plan/implementation:
1. *Control* own irritation; assess reasons for own annoyance.
2. *Anticipate* and meet client's needs; set time to discuss requests.
3. *Confront* with behavior; discuss reasons for behavior.
4. *Ignore* negative attention seeking and *reinforce appropriate* requests for attention.
5. Make plans with *entire staff* to set *limits.*
6. Set up *contractual* arrangement for brief, frequent, regular, uninterrupted attention.
7. *Health teaching:* teach appropriate methods for gaining attention.

E. Evaluation/outcome criteria: fewer requests for attention; assumes more responsibility for self-care.

V. DENIAL OF ILLNESS

A. Definition: an attempt or refusal to acknowledge some anxiety-provoking aspect of oneself or external reality. Denial may be an acceptable *first phase of coping* as an attempt to allow time for adaptation.

B. Assessment:
1. Observe for *defense and coping mechanisms* such as: dissociation, repression, selective inattention, suppression, displacement of concern to another person.
2. Note behaviors that may indicate *denial* of diagnosis:
   a. Failure to follow treatment plan.
   b. Missed appointment.
   c. Refusal of medication.
   d. Inappropriate cheerfulness.
   e. Ignoring symptoms.
   f. Use of flippant humor.
   g. Use of second or third person in reference to illness.
   h. Flight into wellness, overactivity.
3. Use of earliest and most primitive defense by closing eyes, turning head away to separate from what is unpleasant and anxiety provoking.
4. Note *range* of denial: *explicit* verbal denial of obvious facts, disowning or *ignoring* aspects or *minimizing* by understatement.
5. Be aware of situations such as long-term physical disability that make people more prone to denial of illness. *Denial of illness protects the ego from overwhelming anxiety.*

C. Analysis/nursing diagnosis: *ineffective denial* related to:
1. Untenable wishes, needs, ideas, deeds, or reality factors.
2. Inability to adapt to full realization of painful experience or to accept changes in body image or role perception.
3. Intense stress and anxiety.

D. Nursing care plan/implementation:
1. *Long-term goal:* understand needs met by denial.
2. *Short-term goals: avoid* reinforcing denial patterns.
   a. Recognize behavioral cues of denial of some reality aspect; be aware of level of awareness and degree to which reality is excluded.
   b. Determine if denial interferes with treatment.
   c. Support moves toward greater reality orientation.
   d. Determine person's stress tolerance.
   e. Supportively help person discuss events leading to, and feelings about, hospitalization.
3. *Health teaching:*
   a. Explain that emotional response is appropriate and common.
   b. Explain to family and staff that emotional adjustment to painful reality is done at own pace.

E. Evaluation/outcome criteria: indicates desire to discuss painful experience.

VI. DEPENDENCE

A. Definition: reliance on other people to meet basic needs, usually for love and affection, security and protection, and support and guidance; *acceptable in early phases* of coping.

B. Assessment:
1. Excessive need for advice and answers to problems.
2. Lack of confidence in own decision-making ability and lack of confidence in self-sufficiency.
3. Clinging, too-trusting behavior.
4. Gestures, facial expressions, body posture, recurrent themes conveying "I'm helpless."

C. Analysis/nursing diagnosis:
1. *Chronic low self-esteem* related to inability to meet basic needs or role expectations.
2. *Helplessness* and *hopelessness* related to inadvertent reinforcement by staff's expectations.
3. *Powerlessness* related to holding a belief that one's own actions cannot affect life situations.

D. Nursing care plan/implementation:
1. *Long-term goal:* increase self-esteem, confidence in own abilities.
2. *Short-term goal:* provide activities that promote independence.
   a. *Limit setting*—clear, firm, consistent; acknowledge when demands are made; accept client but refuse to respond to demands.

MENTAL HEALTH

b. *Break cycle* of nurse avoids client when he or she is clinging and demanding → a client's anxiety increases → demands for attention increase → frustration and avoidance on nurse's part increase.
c. *Give attention before* demand exists.
d. Use *behavior modification* approaches:
   (1) *Reward* appropriate behavior (such as making decisions, helping others, caring for own needs) with attention and praise.
   (2) Give *no response* to attention-seeking, dependent, infantile behavior; goal is to increase incidence of mature behavior as client realizes little gratification from dependent behavior.
e. *Avoid secondary gains* of being cared for, which impede progress toward aforementioned goals.
f. Assist in developing *ability to control* panic by responding less to client's high anxiety level.
g. Help client develop ways to seek gratification other than excessive turning to others.
h. *Resist* urge to act like a parent when client becomes helpless, demanding, and attention seeking.
i. *Promote decision making* by not giving advice.
j. *Encourage accountability* for own feelings, thoughts, and behaviors.
   (1) Help identify feelings through nonverbal cues, thoughts, recurrent themes.
   (2) Convey expectations that client does have opinions and feelings to share.
   (3) Role model how to express feelings.
k. *Reinforce self-esteem* and ability to work out problems independently. (Consistently ask: "How do you feel about . . ."; "What do you think?")

3. *Health teaching:*
   a. Teach family ways of interacting to enforce less dependency.
   b. Teach problem-solving skills, assertiveness.

E. Evaluation/outcome criteria:

1. Performs self-care.
2. Asks less for approval and praise.
3. Seeks less attention, proximity, physical contact.

VII. HOSTILITY

A. Definition: a feeling of *intense* anger or an attitude of antagonism or animosity, with the *destructive* component of intent to inflict harm and pain to another or to self; may involve *hate, anger, rage, aggression, regression.*

B. Operational definition:

1. Past experience of frustration, loss of self-esteem, unmet needs for status, prestige, or love.
2. Present expectations of self and others not met.
3. Feelings of humiliation, inadequacy, emotional pain, and conflict.
4. Anxiety experienced and converted into hostility, which can be:
   a. Repressed, with result of becoming withdrawn.
   b. Disowned to the point of overreaction and extreme compliance.
   c. Overtly exhibited: verbal, nonverbal.

C. Concepts and principles:

1. Aggression and violence are two *outward* expressions of hostility.
2. Hostility is often unconscious, automatic response.
3. Hostile wishes and impulses may be underlying motives for many actions.
4. Perceptions may be *distorted* by hostile outlook.
5. Continuum: from extreme politeness to *externalization* as murderous rage or homicide or *internalization* as depression or suicide.
6. Hostility seen as a defense *against* depression, as well as a *cause* of it.
7. Hostility may be repressed, dissociated, or expressed covertly or overtly.
8. *Normal* hostility may come from justifiable fear of *real* danger; *irrational* hostility stems from *anxiety.*
9. Developmental roots of hostility:
   a. *Infants* look away, push away, physically move away from threat; give defiant look. Role modeling by parents.
   b. *Three-year-olds* replace overt hostility with protective shyness, retreat, and withdrawal. Feel weak, inadequate in face of powerful person against whom cannot openly ventilate hostility.
   c. Frustrated or unmet needs for status, prestige, or power serve as a basis for *adult* hostility.

D. Assessment:

1. Fault-finding, scapegoating, sarcasm, derision.
2. Arguing, swearing, abusiveness, verbal threatening.
3. Deceptive sweetness, joking at other's expense, gossiping.
4. Physical abusiveness, violence, murder, vindictiveness.

E. Analysis/nursing diagnosis:

1. *Causes:*
   a. *Anxiety* related to a learned means of dealing with an interpersonal threat.
   b. *Risk for violence* related to a reaction to *loss of self-esteem* and *powerlessness.*
   c. *Defensive coping* related to intense frustration, insecurity, or apprehension.
   d. *Impaired social interaction* related to low anxiety tolerance.
2. *Situations with high potential for hostility:*
   a. *Enforced illness and hospitalization* cause anxiety, which may be expressed as hostility.
   b. Dependency feelings related to acceptance of illness may result in hostility as a coping mechanism.

c. Certain illnesses or physical disabilities may be conducive to hostility:
   (1) Client who has *preoperative cancer* and is displacing hostility onto staff and family.
   (2) Postoperatively, if diagnosis is *terminal,* the family may displace hostility onto nurse.
   (3) Anger, hostility is a *stage of dying* the person may experience.
   (4) Client who had *amputation* may focus frustration on others due to dependency and jealousy.
   (5) Clients on *hemodialysis* are prone to helplessness, which may be displaced as hostility.

F. Nursing care plan/implementation:

1. *Long-term goal:* help alter response to fear, inadequacy, frustration, threat.
2. *Short-term goal:* express and explore feelings of hostility without injury to self or others.
   a. Remain calm, nonthreatening; endure verbal abuse in impartial manner, within limits; speak quietly.
   b. *Protect from self-harm,* acting out.
   c. Discourage hostile behavior while showing acceptance of client.
   d. Offer support to *express* feelings of frustration, anger, and fear *constructively, safely,* and *appropriately.*
   e. Explore hostile feelings *without* fear of retaliation, disapproval.
   f. *Avoid:* arguing, giving advice, reacting with hostility, punitiveness, finding fault.
   g. *Avoid* joking, teasing, which can be misinterpreted.
   h. *Avoid* words such as *anger, hostility;* use client's words (*upset, irritated*).
   i. Do *not* minimize problem or give client reassurance or hasty, general conclusions.
   j. *Do not stop verbal* expression of anger unless detrimental.
   k. Respond *matter-of-factly* to attention-seeking behavior, not defensively.
   l. *Avoid* physical contact; allow client to set pace in "closeness."
   m. Look for clues to antecedent events and focus *directly* on those areas; *do not evade* or ignore.
   n. Constantly focus on *here and now* and affective component of message rather than on content.
   o. Reconstruct what happened and why, discuss client's reactions; seek observations, *not* inferences.
   p. Learn how client would like to be treated.
   q. Look for ways to help client relate better without defensiveness, *when ready.*
   r. Plan to channel feelings into *motor* outlets (occupational and recreational therapy, physical activity, games, debates).
   s. Explain procedures beforehand; approach frequently.
   t. Withdraw attention, *set limits,* when acting out.
3. *Health teaching:* teach acceptable motor outlets for tension.

G. Evaluation/outcome criteria: identifies sources of threat and experiences success in dealing with threat.

VIII. MANIPULATION

A. Definition: process of playing on and using others by unfair, insidious means to serve own purpose without regard for others' needs; may take many forms; occurs consciously, unconsciously to some extent, in all interpersonal relations.

B. Operational definition (Fig. 10.4):

1. Conflicting needs, goals exist between client and other person (e.g., nurse).
2. Other person perceives need as unacceptable, unreasonable.
3. Other person refuses to accept client's need.
4. Client's tension increases, and he or she begins to relate to others as objects.
5. Client increases attempts to influence others to fulfill his or her needs.
   a. Appears unaware of others' needs.
   b. Exhibits excessive dependency, helplessness, demands.
   c. Sets others at odds (especially staff).
   d. *Rationalizes,* gives logical reasons.
   e. Uses deception, false promises, insincerity.
   f. Questions and *defies nurse's authority* and competence.
6. Nurse feels powerless and angry at having been used.

C. Assessment:

1. Acts out sexually, physically.
2. Dawdles, always last minute.
3. Uses insincere flattery; expects special favors, privileges.
4. Exploits generosity and fears of others.
5. Feels no guilt.
6. Plays one staff member against another.
7. *Tests limits.*
8. Finds weaknesses in others.
9. Makes excessive, unreasonable, unnecessary *demands* for staff time.
10. *Pretends* to be helpless, lonely, distraught, tearful.
11. Cannot distinguish between truth and falsehood.
12. *Plays on sympathy* or *guilt.*

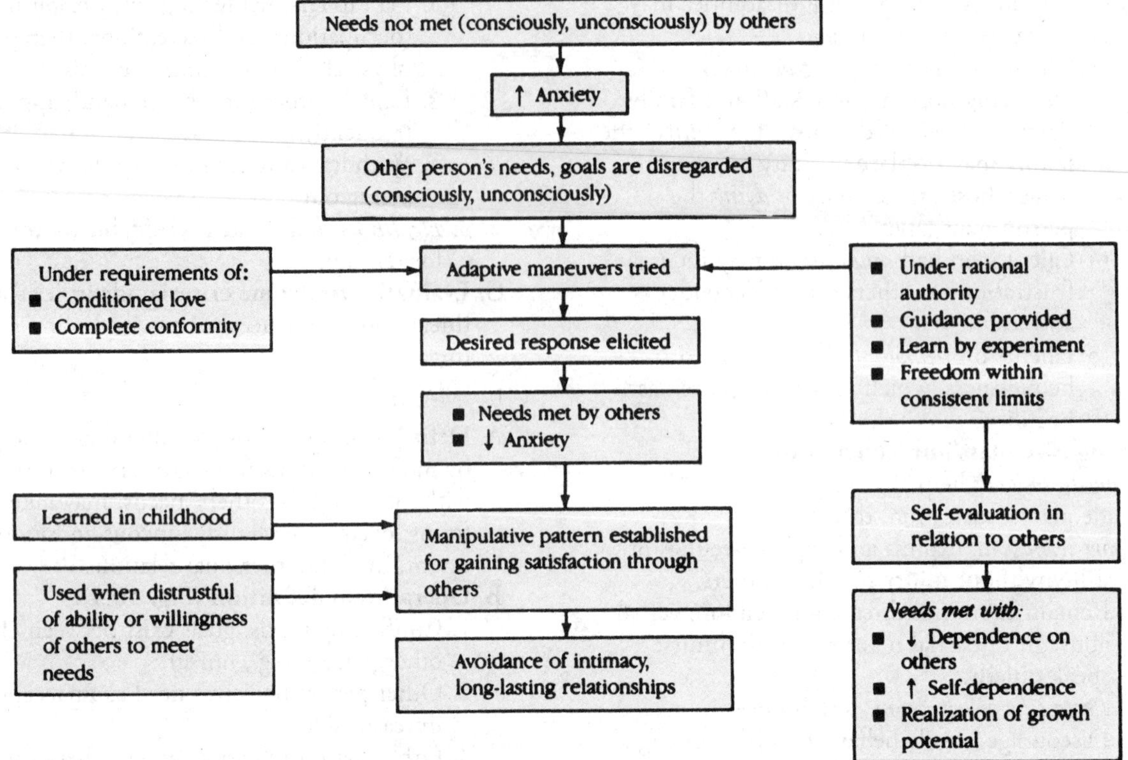

Figure 10.4 Operationalization of the behavioral concept of manipulation.

13. Offers many excuses, lacks insight.
14. Pursues unpleasant issues without genuine regard for feelings of individuals involved.
15. *Intimidates,* derogates, threatens, bargains, cajoles, violates rules to obtain reactions or privileges.
16. Betrays information.
17. Uses communication as a medium for manipulation, as verbal, nonverbal means to get others to cooperate, to behave in certain way, to get something from another for own use.
18. May be coercive, illogical, or skillfully deceptive.
19. *Unable to learn from experience* (i.e., repeats unacceptable behaviors despite negative consequences).

D. Analysis/nursing diagnosis: *ineffective individual coping and impaired adjustment* related to:

1. Mistrust and contemptuous view of others' motivations.
2. Life experience of rejection, deception.
3. Low anxiety tolerance.
4. Inability to cope with tension.
5. Unmet dependency needs.
6. Need to avoid anxiety when cannot obtain gratification.
7. Need to obtain something that is forbidden, or need for *instant gratification.*
8. Attempt to put something over on another when no real advantage exists.
9. *Intolerance of intimacy,* maneuvering effectively to keep others at a safe distance to dilute the relationship by withdrawing and frustrating others or distracting attention away from self.
10. Attempt to demand attention, approval, disapproval.

E. Nursing care plan/implementation:

1. *Long-term goal:* define relationship as a mutual experience in *learning and trust* rather than a struggle for *power and control.*
2. *Short-term goals:* increase awareness of self and others; increase self-control; learn to accept limitations.
3. Promote use of **"3 Cs"**—*cooperation, compromise, collaboration*—rather than exploitation or deception.
4. *Decrease level and extent of manipulation.*
   a. Set *firm, realistic goals,* with clear, consistent expectations and limits.
   b. *Confront* client regarding exploitation attempts; examine, discuss behavior.
   c. Give *positive reinforcement* with concrete reinforcers for nonmanipulation, to lessen need for exploitive, deceptive, and self-destructive behaviors.

d. *Ignore* "wooden-leg" behavior (feigning illness to evoke sympathy).
e. *Allow verbal* anger; do *not* be intimidated; *avoid* giving desired response to obvious attempts to irritate.
f. Set *consistent, firm, enforceable limits* on *destructive,* aggressive behavior that impinges on others' health, rights, and interests, and on excessive dependency; *give reasons* when you cannot meet requests.
g. Keep staff informed of rules and reasons; obtain staff *consensus.*
h. Enforce *direct* communication; encourage openness about *real* needs, feelings.
i. Do *not* accept gifts, favors, flattery, or other guises of manipulation.

5. Increase responsibility for *self-control* of actions.
   a. Decide who (client, nurse) is responsible for what.
   b. Provide opportunities for *success* to increase self-esteem, experience acceptance by others.
   c. Evaluate actions, *not* verbal behavior; point out the difference between talk and action.
   d. Support efforts to be responsible.
   e. Assist client to increase emotional repertoire; explore *alternative* ways of relating interpersonally.
   f. *Avoid submission* to control based on fear of punishment, retaliation, loss of affection.
6. Facilitate awareness of, and *responsibility* for, manipulative behavior and its *effects on others.*
   a. Reflect back client's behavior.
   b. Discourage distortion and misuse of information.
   c. *Increase tolerance* for differences and *delayed gratification* through behavior modification.
   d. Insist on clear, consistent staff communication.
7. *Avoid:*
   a. Labeling client as a "problem."
   b. Hostile, negative attitude.
   c. Making a public issue of client's behavior.
   d. Being excessively rigid or permissive, inconsistent or ambiguous, argumentative or accusatory.
8. *Health teaching:* act as a role model; demonstrate how to deal with mistakes, human imperfections, by admitting mistakes in nonshameful, nonvirtuous ways.

F. Evaluation/outcome criteria: accepts limits; able to compromise, cooperate rather than deceive and exploit; acts responsibly, self-dependent.

IX. NONCOMPLIANCE AND UNCOOPERATIVE BEHAVIOR

A. Definition: consistently failing to meet the requirements of the prescribed treatment regimen (e.g., refusing to adhere to dietary restrictions or take required medications).

B. Assessment:
1. Refuses to participate in routine or planned activities.
2. Refuses medication.
3. Violates rules, ignores limits, and abuses privileges; acts out anger and frustration.

C. Analysis/nursing diagnosis: *noncompliance* related to:
1. *Psychological factors:* lack of knowledge; attitudes, beliefs, and values; denial of illness; rigid, defensive personality type; anxiety level (very high or very low); cannot accept limits or dependency (rebellious counterdependency).
2. *Environmental factors:* finances, transportation, lack of support system.
3. *Health-care agent–client relationship:* client feels discounted and like an "object"; sees staff as uncaring, authoritative, controlling.
4. *Health-care regimen:* too complicated; not enough benefit from following regimen; results in social stigma or social isolation; unpleasant side effects.

D. Nursing care plan/implementation:
1. *General goal:* reduce need to act out by nonadherence.
   a. Take *preventive* action—be alert to signs of noncompliance, such as intent to leave against medical advice.
   b. *Explore* feelings and reasons for lack of cooperation.
   c. Assess and *allay fears* in client in reassuring manner.
   d. Provide *adequate* information about, and reasons for, rules and procedures.
   e. *Avoid* threats or physical restraints; maintain calm composure.
   f. Demonstrate *tact and firmness* when confronting violations.
   g. Offer *alternatives.*
   h. Firmly insist on cooperation in selected important activities but not all activities.
2. *Health teaching:* increase knowledge base regarding health-related problem, procedures, or treatments and consequences.

E. Evaluation/outcome criteria: follows prescribed regimen.

Mental and Emotional Disorders in Children and Adolescents

Children have certain developmental tasks to master in the various stages of development (e.g., learning to trust, control primary instincts, and resolve basic social roles.

MENTAL HEALTH

I. CONCEPTS AND PRINCIPLES RELATED TO MENTAL AND EMOTIONAL DISORDERS IN CHILDREN AND ADOLESCENTS:

A. Most emotional disorders of children are related to family dynamics and the place the child occupies in the family group.

B. Children must be understood and treated within the context of their *families.*

C. Many disorders are related to the phases of development through which the children are passing. (Erik Erikson's developmental tasks for children are *trust, autonomy, initiative, industry, identity,* and *intimacy.*)

D. Table 10.10 summarizes key age-related disturbances, lists main *symptoms* and *analyses* of causes, and highlights *medical interventions* and *nursing plan/implementation.*

E. Children are not miniature adults; they have special needs.

F. Play and food are important media to make contact with children and help them release emotions in

(text continues on page 754)

Table 10.10

Emotional Disturbances in Children

Stage	Disturbance	Assessment: Symptoms or Characteristics	Analysis: Behavior Related To:	Plan/Implementation
Oral (birth–1 yr)	Feeding disturbances	Refusal of food.	1. Rigid feeding schedule. 2. *Psychological* stress.	Pediatric evaluation, especially if infant is not gaining weight or is losing weight.
			3. Incompatible formula.	Rule out physiological etiology or incompatible formula.
			4. *Physiological:* pyloric stenosis.	Evaluate *feeding style* of caregiver. Is infant on-demand feeding? Is caregiver sensitive to infant's needs or communications about holding, hunger, or satiation?
		Colic. Crying is usually confined to one part of day and starts after a feeding. Commonly lasts from first to third month.	Periodic tension in infant's immature nervous system, causing gas and sharp intestinal pains.	Reassure parents and teach about condition and how to relieve it with *hot water bottle, rocking, rubbing back, pacifier,* which may soothe infant.
	Sleeping disturbances	Infant resists being put down for sleep or going to sleep.	1. Need for parental attention. 2. A pattern formed during period of colic or other illness. 3. Emotional disturbance related to *anxiety.*	If it is attention-getting strategy, suggest parental lack of response for a few nights to break pattern. If emotional disturbance is suspected, evaluate *infant-caregiver interaction* and refer for psychotherapeutic intervention.
	Failure to thrive	Infant does not grow or develop over a period of time.	1. *Psychological:* inadequate caregiving. 2. *Physiological:* heart, kidneys, central nervous system (CNS) malfunction.	*Hospitalization* is essential. Assist in evaluation of physiological functioning, especially heart, kidneys, and CNS. *Nurturing plan* for infant, using specifically assigned personnel and the caregiver parent. If the infant grows and develops with nurturing, thus confirming problems of parenting as causative factor, psychotherapeutic and child protective interventions are necessary.

Table 10.10

Emotional Disturbances in Children—cont'd

Stage	Disturbance	Assessment: Symptoms or Characteristics	Analysis: Behavior Related To:	Plan/Implementation
	Severe disturbances	**Pervasive developmental disorders:** Very early onset; lack of response to others; bizarre, repetitive behavior; normal to above-normal intelligence; failure to develop language or use communicative speech. Autism is one of the most severe and debilitating psychiatric disturbances.	1. Uncertain etiology; *regression* or *fixation* at earlier developmental stage, before child differentiates "me" from "not me." 2. A "*nature versus nurture*" controversy over the causative factors. These are variously thought to be: a. *Environment only:* Infant is tabula rasa and all disturbance is directly attributable to the environment (primarily the parenting). b. *Heredity only:* For genetic, biochemical, or other predetermined reasons, some infants will be psychotic regardless of the environment. c. *Combination of environment and heredity* plus *the interaction between them:* An infant who is *susceptible, less* than optimal parenting, and *negative* interaction between parent and infant will combine to produce disturbance.	The child who is severely disturbed requires intensive psychotherapy and often milieu therapy available in residential or day-care programs. Therapy is usually indicated for parents also. Nurses can work on a *primary level* of prevention by assessing parenting skills of prospective parents and *teaching* them these skills. On a *secondary level of prevention*, nurses can be knowledgeable about and *teach* others the early signs of childhood psychosis, making appropriate referrals. The earlier the intervention, the better the prognosis. On a *tertiary level of prevention*, nurses work with children who are severely disturbed and their families in child guidance clinics and residential and day-care settings. *Occupational therapy:* provide tactile, oral-tactile, visual, auditory, gravitational sensory input to normalize response. *Health teaching* would include play activities that foster support, acceptance, and a nonthreatening mode of communication and interaction with a significant other. *Simplify* language by avoiding abstracts and metaphors. Keep gestures clear and simple. Give one instruction at a time, not a sequence. Give time to respond.
		Symbiotic psychosis: Identified later than autistic type, usually between 2 and 5 yr of age. These children seem to be unable to function independently of the caregiving parent. A situational stress, such as hospitalization of parent or child or entry into school, may precipitate a psychotic break in the child.	The same "*nature versus nurture*" controversy with respect to the origin of symbiotic psychosis. The child progresses beyond the self-absorbed autistic stage to form an object relationship with another (usually the mother). Having progressed to this stage, the child then *fails to differentiate his or her own identity* from that of the mother.	

Continued

Table 10.10

Emotional Disturbances in Children—cont'd

Stage	Disturbance	Assessment: Symptoms or Characteristics	Analysis: Behavior Related To:	Plan/Implementation
Anal (1–3 yr)	Elimination disorders (disturbances related to toilet training)	*Constipation.*	1. *Diet.* 2. Child withholding due to history of one or two painful, *hard bowel movements.* 3. *Psychological* causation: child withholds from parents to *express anger, opposition,* or passage through a very *independent* developmental stage.	Evaluate *diet* and consistency of stools. Fecal softener may be prescribed if necessary. In all cases, *help parent avoid making* an issue of constipation with the child. Enemas are *contraindicated.* If child is withholding, *work with parents* around not forcing rigid toilet training on child. Most children are more cooperative about *toilet training* at 18–24 mo.
		Encopresis (soiling).	Child's expression of anger or hostility. It is usually directed toward the parent with whom the child is experiencing conflict and is rarely physiological.	Medical evaluation, then assessment and intervention in the child-parent relationship. Therapy for child and parent may be indicated.
		Enuresis Ordinarily refers to wetting while asleep (nocturnal enuresis), though some children who are enuretic wet themselves during the day also. Enuresis is a *symptom,* not a diagnosis or disease entity.	1. *Faulty toilet training* (especially if child wets during the day also) or 2. *Psychological stress.* 3. *Physiological* etiology, such as genitourinary (GU) tract infections or CNS disease, is rare. The child *under 4 yr* old is usually *not* considered enuretic but is included in this section because bladder training is part of toilet training. Etiology is uncertain.	Many approaches have been tried with varying degrees of success. These include *fluid restriction, behavioral intervention* (in which a buzzer wakes the child when the child starts to wet), and psychotherapy. *Educating parents in bladder training* techniques and attitudes can help solve the problem on a *primary* level. It is important when working with children who are enuretic or their parents to *suggest* ways to help the child *overcome feelings of shame and guilt.* These feelings are often exacerbated by parents who are well-meaning but misguided.
	Excessive rebelliousness	Frequent temper tantrums, fighting, destruction of toys and other objects, consistent oppositional behavior.	1. Fear caused by inconsistency in handling the child, the setting of rigid limits, or the parents' refusal or inability to set limits, which can all create insecurity and fear in the child. 2. Excessive rebelliousness, usually indicating a child who is *frightened;* should not be confused with expression of negativism normal at around age 2, which is a necessary (though trying) developmental stage.	The nurse should offer parent counseling if necessary. When working with the child, the nurse needs to be receptive and sympathetic while establishing and maintaining firm limits.

Table 10.10

Emotional Disturbances in Children—cont'd

Stage	Disturbance	Assessment: Symptoms or Characteristics	Analysis: Behavior Related To:	Plan/Implementation
	Excessive conformity	Lack of spontaneity, anxious desire always to please all adult authority figures, timidity, refusal to assert own needs, passivity.	1. Very rigid control established in an attempt to handle fears. 2. Harsh *toilet training,* resulting in a child who is overcompliant. These children need help as much as children who are overrebellious, but they get it less frequently because their behavior is not a "problem"—that is, it is not difficult for parents to tolerate.	Excessive conformity can lead to *compulsive, ritualistic, or obsessive behavior later.* The nurse needs to be able to identify such a child, then work with the child and parents to encourage *self-expression* in the child. Referral for psychotherapy may be necessary to help the child deal with repressed anger.
Oedipal (3–6 yr)	Excessive fears	Child will be frightened even in nonthreatening situations. *Nightmares and other sleep disturbances* occur. Usually, child will be very "clingy" with parents in an attempt to gain reassurance.	*Anxiety* as the causative factor. Anxiety can be induced by many things, such as: 1. Parental *failure to set appropriate limits.* 2. *Physical or psychological abuse.* 3. *Illness.* 4. Fear of *mutilation.* 5. *Imaginary* worries that are common at this age (e.g., a 4-yr-old who is suddenly afraid of the dark, or dogs, or fire engines is not necessarily suffering from excessive fears).	If possible, identify and deal with the factors that are producing the anxiety. Offer child calm reassurance. *Night-light and open doors* can help allay night fears, but *counsel parents* that it is unwise to allow the child to sleep with the parents, because it may make the child feel that the oedipal retaliation has succeeded. With the child who is hospitalized, the nurse needs to be aware of and work with the mutilation fears common at this age. Fears around certain procedures (e.g., injections) can often be resolved by helping the child *play out fears.*
	Excessive masturbation	Touching and fondling of genitals excessively, sometimes in a preoccupied or absent-minded manner.	1. *Insecurity.* 2. Exploration and stimulation of the genital area, which is *normal* and common in this age group. However, if it is compulsive, the behavior is a signal that the child is *insecure.* 3. Occasionally, a *specific fear.* For example, a boy viewing an infant sister's genitals may have castration fears. These can be dealt with directly.	*Assess* the child's masturbating activity. When does it occur and why? Then help the child develop other *strategies* for defense with anxiety. *Answer questions about sexuality* in an open manner. *Counsel parents* that *threats and shaming are contraindicated,* and help parents deal with *their* feelings about masturbation.
	Regression	Resumption of activities (such as *thumb sucking, soiling and wetting, baby talk*) characteristic of earlier developmental levels.	1. Child's attempt to regain a more comfortable, previous level of development in response to a *threatening* situation (such as a new infant), or 2. A response to difficulty resolving oedipal *conflicts.*	*Counsel parents* not to make an issue of behavior. Offer child emotional support and acceptance, though not approval of regressive behavior.

Continued

Table 10.10

Emotional Disturbances in Children—cont'd

Stage	Disturbance	Assessment: Symptoms or Characteristics	Analysis: Behavior Related To:	Plan/Implementation
	Stuttering	Articulation difficulty characterized by many stops and repetitions in speech pattern.	1. Anxiety 2. Frustration. 3. Insecurity. 4. Excitement. Stuttering usually occurs when the affected child feels *anxious, frustrated, insecure,* or *excited.* Parental concerns and attention to stuttering focuses attention on it and increases anxiety. The origins of stuttering are not understood. It is *common around 2–3 yr of age* and is *not* a cause for concern at that time.	Speech therapy is usually indicated. Psychotherapy may also be indicated, if stuttering is an expression of anxiety and conflict, persisting *beyond age 6.*
Latency (6–12 yr)	**Attention deficit-hyperactivity disorder** (age of onset can occur in preschool children)	Both hyperactivity and hyperkinesis are occasionally observed in school-age children; characterized by a *short attention span*, restlessness, distractibility, and *impulsivity.*	1. An *organic disturbance* of the *CNS,* of uncertain origin, as the basis of *hyperkinesis.* Because the primary symptom—difficulty with attention span—is the same as that presented by the child who is hyperactive, the child who is hyperactive is frequently and incorrectly labeled hyperkinetic. 2. Attempts by child who is *hyperactive* to *control* anxiety through *reducement* (and can attend when interested or relaxed). Does not fit smoothly into environment, but problem may be with the environment *rather* than the child. In other words, the school situation requires a high degree of conformity. The child who does not fit the mold is *not* necessarily emotionally disturbed.	For the child who is *hyperkinetic,* psychopharmaceutical intervention—*Ritalin, Concerta* (long-acting), *Dexedrine,* or *Adderall* (long-acting). Psychotherapy and special education classes may also be indicated. *Ritalin* is also frequently prescribed for the child who is *hyperactive*—which raises the issue of whether an individual should be medicated to fit more smoothly into the environment. Drastic improvement in school performance can be seen with behavioral therapy and medication. Therapy can help the child who is hyperactive *decrease anxiety* and *increase self-esteem,* thus reducing the symptoms.
	Attention deficit disorder (age of onset can occur throughout adolescence)	Characterized by: a short attention span, distractibility, and subjective feelings of restlessness without hyperactivity.	*Difficulty* with *schoolwork.* Child frequently considered unmotivated or not intelligent.	Psychopharmaceutical intervention—*Ritalin, Concerta* (long-acting), *Dexedrine,* or *Adderall* (long-acting)—can drastically increase the attention span. Therapy and behavior modification: work on task for short periods; increase physical energy outlets; tutoring; structure; homework; organizational skills.

Table 10.10

Emotional Disturbances in Children—cont'd

Stage	Disturbance	Assessment: Symptoms or Characteristics	Analysis: Behavior Related To:	Plan/Implementation
	Withdrawal	Reduced body movement and verbalization, lack of close relationships, *detachment,* timidity, and seclusiveness.	Need to withdraw as a defensive behavior, through which the child controls anxiety by *reducing contact* with the outer world. Like the child who is overcompliant, the child who is withdrawn frequently is not identified as needing help because this behavior is not a "problem."	Offer *positive reinforcement* when child is more active. Help child *assert* self and *experience success* at certain tasks. The nurse needs to work with parents who are overprotective. Therapy may be useful to work through anxiety and provide child with a chance to form a *trusting* relationship with another.
	Psychophysiological symptoms	The child experiences physical symptoms (such as *vomiting, headaches, eczema, asthma, colitis*) with no apparent physiological cause.	*Conversion* of anxiety into physical symptoms.	After medical evaluation has established lack of physiological etiology, psychotherapy is usually indicated. Family therapy may be treatment of choice because *dysfunctional interpersonal family dynamics* are common in these cases. The nurse can also provide the child with a healthy interpersonal relationship. Nurses are frequently in a position to talk to parents and teachers about the importance of mental health counseling for children with physical symptoms.
	Separation anxiety disorders (school "phobia")	Sudden and seemingly inexplicable fear of going to school. These children often do not know what it is they fear at school. Frequently occurs *after an illness* and absence from school or birth of sibling.	An *acute anxiety reaction related to separation* from home (not actually a phobia).	If the child is allowed to stay home, the dread of returning to school usually increases. The child and parent should have psychiatric intervention quickly (before the problem becomes worse) to help the child separate from the parent.
	Learning disabilities	Failure or difficulty in learning at school	1. Emotional disorders, which cause school failure. 2. Feelings of *inferiority, discouragement,* and loss of confidence from school failure. Learning disabilities may be caused by many factors or combinations of factors, including *anxiety, poor sensory or sensorimotor integration, dyslexia, receptive aphasia.*	A comprehensive evaluation is essential. Ideally, this would include assessments by a pediatric neurologist, a mental health worker such as a psychiatric nurse or psychiatrist, a learning disabilities teacher specialist, and possibly an occupational therapist trained to work with sensory integration. Treatment is then based on the specific problem or problems.

Continued

Table 10.10

Emotional Disturbances in Children—cont'd

Stage	Disturbance	Assessment: Symptoms or Characteristics	Analysis: Behavior Related To:	Plan/Implementation
	Conduct disorders	Behavior that is nonproductive; that is repeated in spite of threats, punishments, or rational argument; and that usually leads to punishment. Persistent *stealing and truancy* are examples.	*Conflicts* that are expressed and communicated through behavior rather than verbally. Child knows what he or she is doing but is unaware of the underlying motivations for the problem behavior.	Counseling or therapy for the child by a child psychiatric nurse or other mental health worker can allow the child to resolve the basic conflict, thus making the problem behavior unnecessary.

Adapted from Wilson, HS, & Kneisl, CR: *Psychiatric Nursing,* ed 3. Addison-Wesley, Redwood City, CA. (out of print)

socially acceptable forms, prepare them for traumatic events, and develop skills.

G. Children who are physically or emotionally ill regress, giving up previously useful habits.

H. Adolescents have special problems relating to need for *control* versus need to *rebel, dependency* versus *interdependency,* and search for *identity* and *self-realization.*

I. Adolescents often *act out* their underlying feelings of insecurity, rejection, deprivation, and low self-esteem.

J. Strong feelings may be evoked in nurses working with children; these feelings should be expressed, and each nurse should be supported by team members.

II. ASSESSMENT *of selected disorders:*

A. *Autistic spectrum disorders* (previously called childhood schizophrenia; most common form of *pervasive developmental disorders* [PDDs])—**assessment** (before age 3):

1. Disturbance in how perceptual information is processed *(sensory integrative dysfunction)*; normal abilities present.
   a. Behave *as though they cannot* hear, see, etc.
   b. Do *not react to external* stimulus.
   c. Sensory defensiveness:
      (1) Might dislike specific food textures or temperatures.
      (2) Covers ears in response to loud noises.
      (3) Can't concentrate if there are competing noises in environment.
      (4) Might dislike riding or climbing on play equipment.
      (5) Doesn't like people standing too close or being touched.
      (6) Stimuli might be interpreted as threatening or anxiety provoking.
      (7) Responds in an exaggerated manner (cries, is negative, resistant, or rigid) when a situation makes it difficult for child to process.
   d. Low muscle tone results in inability to maintain stable positions or postures (e.g., standing on one leg); avoids gross and fine motor movement.
2. Lack of self-awareness as a unified whole—may not relate bodily needs or parts as extension of themselves.
3. Severe difficulty in *social interaction* and *communicating* with others—may be mute or echolalic and isolated.
4. Bizarre *restricted* and *repetitive* postures and gestures (banging head, rocking back and forth), and routines.
5. Disturbances in learning: difficulties in understanding and using language.
6. *Etiology* is unknown; but generally accepted that irregularities in brain structure or function may be congenital or acquired.
7. *Prognosis* depends on severity of symptoms and age of onset (can exhibit any combination of symptoms and behaviors).

B. *Other pervasive developmental disorders* include: *Asperger's disorder* (speak at normal pace and have normal intelligence, but have stunted social skills, limited and obsessive interests), *childhood disintegration disorder (CDD),* and *Rett's disorder.* Characteristics:

1. Hyperactivity.
2. Explosive outbursts.
3. Distractibility.
4. Impulsiveness.
5. Perceptual difficulties (visual distortions, such as figure-ground distortion and mirror reading; body-image problems; difficulty in telling left from right).
6. Receptive or expressive language problems.

C. *Elimination disorders* (functional enuresis)—related to feelings of insecurity due to unmet needs of attention and affection; important to preserve their self-esteem.

D. *Separation anxiety disorders of childhood* (school phobias)—anxiety about school is accompanied by physical distress. Usually observed with fear of leaving home, rejection by mother, fear of loss of mother, or history of separation from mother in early years.

E. *Conduct disorders*—include lying, stealing, running away, truancy, substance abuse, sexual delinquency, vandalism, fire setting, and criminal gang activity; chief motivating force is either overt or covert hostility; history of disturbed parent-child relations.

III. ANALYSIS/NURSING DIAGNOSIS:

A. *Altered feeling states:* anxiety, fear, hostility related to personal vulnerability and poorly developed or inappropriate use of defense mechanisms.

B. *Risk for self-mutilation* related to disturbance in self-concept, abnormal response to sensory input, and history of abuse.

C. *Altered interpersonal processes:*

1. *Impaired verbal communication* related to cerebral deficits, withdrawal into self, inability to trust other.
2. *Altered conduct/impulse processes:* aggressive, violent behaviors toward self, others, environment related to feelings of distrust and altered judgment.
3. *Dysfunctional behaviors:* age-inappropriate behaviors, bizarre behaviors; disorganized and unpredictable behaviors related to inability to discharge emotions verbally.
4. *Impaired social interaction:* social isolation/withdrawal related to feelings of suspicion and mistrust, lack of bonding, inadequate sensory stimulation.

D. *Personal identity disturbance* related to lack of development of trust, organic brain dysfunction, maternal deprivation.

E. *Altered parenting* related to ambivalent or dissonant family relationships and failure of child to meet role expectations.

F. *Sensory/perceptual alterations:* altered attention related to disturbed mental activities.

G. *Altered cognition process:* altered decision making, judgment, knowledge, and learning processes; altered thought content and processes related to perceptual or cognitive impairment and emotional dysfunctioning.

IV. NURSING CARE PLAN/IMPLEMENTATION in mental and emotional disorders in children and adolescents:

A. *General goals:* corrective behavior—*behavior modification.*

B. Help children gain self-awareness.

C. Provide *structured* environment to orient children to reality.

D. Impose *limits* on destructive behavior toward themselves or others without rejecting the children.

1. *Prevent* destructive behavior.
2. *Stop* destructive behavior.
3. *Redirect* nongrowth behavior into constructive channels.

E. Be *consistent.*

F. Meet *developmental and dependency* needs.

G. Recognize and encourage each child's strengths, growth behavior, and reverse regression.

H. Help these children reach the next step in social growth and development scale.

I. Use play and projective media to aid working out feelings and conflicts and in making contact.

J. Offer support to parents and strengthen the parent-child relationship.

K. *Health teaching:* teach parents methods of behavior modification.

V. EVALUATION/OUTCOME CRITERIA:

A. Destructive behavior is inhibited.

B. Demonstrates age-appropriate behavior on developmental scale.

Midlife Crisis: Phase-of-Life Problems

Midlife crisis is a time period that marks the passage between early maturity and middle age.

I. ASSESSMENT:

A. Commonly occurs between ages 35 and 45.

B. Preoccupied with *visible* signs of aging, own mortality.

C. *Feelings: urgency* that time is running out ("last chance") for career achievement and unmet goals; *boredom* with present, *ambivalence, frustration, uncertainty* about the future.

D. Time of *reevaluation:*

1. Reassess: meaning of time and parental role (omnipotence as a parent is challenged).
2. Reexamine and contemplate change in career, marriage, family life.

E. *Personality changes* may occur. *Women:* traditional definitions of femininity may be challenged as become more assertive. *Men:* may be more introspective, sensitive to emotions, make external changes (younger mate, improve looks, new sports activity), mood swings.

F. Presence of *helpful elements* necessary to turn life's obstacles into opportunities.

1. Willingness to take risks.
2. Strong support system.
3. Sense of purpose.
4. Accumulated wisdom.

MENTAL HEALTH

II. ANALYSIS/NURSING DIAGNOSIS:

A. *Self-esteem disturbance (low self-esteem)* related to loss of youth, faltering physical powers, and facing discrepancy between youthful ambitions and actual achievement (no longer a promising person with potential).

B. *Altered role performance (role reversal)* related to parents who previously provided security and comfort but now need care.

C. *Altered feeling processes (depression)* related to disappointments and diminished optimism as life is reconsidered in light of the reality of aging and death.

III. NURSING CARE PLAN/IMPLEMENTATION—*long-term goal:* help individual to rebuild life structure.

A. Help client reappraise meaning of own life in terms of past, present, and future, and integrate aspects of time. Encourage introspection and reflection with questions:

1. What have I done with my life?
2. What do I really get from and give to my spouse, children, friends, work, community, and self?
3. What are my strengths and liabilities?
4. What have I done with my early dream, and do I want it now?

B. Assist client to complete *four major tasks:*

1. Terminate era of early adulthood by *reappraising* life goals identified and achieved during this era.
2. Initiate movement into middle adulthood by beginning to make *necessary changes* in *unsuccessful* aspects of the current life while trying out new choices.
3. Cope with *polarities* that divide life.
4. Directly confront *death of own parents.*

C. *Health teaching:* stress-management techniques; how to do self-assessment of aptitudes, interests; how to plan for retirement, aloneness, and use of increased leisure time; dietary modification and exercise program.

IV. EVALUATION/OUTCOME CRITERIA:

A. Gives up *idealized* self of early 20s for more *realistically* attainable self.

1. Talks *less* of early *hopes of eminence* and *more* on modest goal of *competence.*
2. Shifts values from sexuality to platonic relationships: replaces romantic dreams with *satisfying* friendships and companionships.
3. Modifies early illusions about own capacities.
4. Shifts values away from physical attractiveness and strength to *intellectual* abilities.

B. Comes to accept that life is finite and reconciles what *is* with what *might have been;* appreciates everyday human experience rather than glamour or power.

C. Through self-confrontation, self-discovery, and change, experiences time of restabilization; is reinvigorated, adventuresome.

D. Develops *alternative* abilities that release new energies.

E. Tries *less* to please everyone; others' opinions less important.

F. Makes more efficient and well-seasoned decisions from well-developed sense of judgment.

Mental Health Problems of the Geriatric Client

In general, problems affecting the elderly are *similar* to those affecting persons of *any* age. This section highlights the *differences* from the viewpoint of etiology, frequency, and prognosis.

I. CONCEPTS AND PRINCIPLES RELATED TO MENTAL HEALTH PROBLEMS OF THE GERIATRIC CLIENT:

A. The elderly *do* have capacity for growth and change.

B. Human beings, regardless of age, need sense of future and *hope* for things to come.

C. An inalienable right of all individuals should be to make or participate in all decisions concerning themselves and their possessions as long as they can.

D. Physical disability due to the aging process may enforce dependency, which may be unacceptable to elderly clients and may evoke feelings of anger and ambivalence.

E. In an attempt to *reduce feelings of loss,* elderly clients may *cling to concrete things* that most represent, in a *symbolic* sense, all that has been significant to them.

F. As memory diminishes, *familiar objects* in environment and *familiar routines* are important in helping *to keep clients oriented* and in contact with reality.

G. *Familiarity of environment brings security;* routines bring a sense of security about what is to happen.

H. If individuals feel unwanted, they may tell *stories* about their *earlier* achievements.

I. Many of the traits in the elderly result from *cumulative* effect of *past* experiences of frustrations and *present* awareness of limitations rather than from any primary consequences of physiological deficit.

II. ASSESSMENT:

A. *Psychological characteristics of the geriatric client:*

1. Increasingly *dependent* on others, not only for physical needs but also for emotional security.
2. Concerns focus more and more *inward,* with narrowed outside interests.
   a. Decreased emotional energy for concern with social problems unless these issues affect them.

b. Tendency to *reminisce.*
c. May appear selfish and unsympathetic.
3. Sources of pleasure and gratification are more childlike: *food, warmth, and affection,* for example.
a. Tangible and frequent evidence of affection is important (e.g., letters, cards, and visits).
b. May hoard articles.
4. *Attention span and memory are short;* may be forgetful and *accuse others of stealing.*
5. Deprivation of any kind is *not* tolerated:
a. Easily frustrated.
b. Change is poorly tolerated; need to have favorite chairs and established daily routine, for example.
6. Main *fears* in the aged include fear of *dependency,* chronic *illness, loneliness, boredom,* fear of being unloved, forgotten, *deserted* by those close to them, fear of *death;* fear of *loss of control* of one's own life; a failing *cognition;* loss of *purpose* and productivity.
7. *Nocturnal delirium* may be due to problems with night vision and inability to perceive *spatial* location.

B. *Psychiatric problems in aging:*
1. *Loneliness*—related to *loss* of mate, diminishing circle of friends and family through death and geographic separation, *decline* in physical energy, loss of work (*retirement*), sharp loss of income, and loss of a lifelong lifestyle.
2. *Insomnia*—pattern of sleep changes in significant ways: disappearance of *deep* sleep, frequent *awakening, daytime* sleeping.
3. *Hypochondriasis*—anxiety may shift from concern with finances, job, or social prestige to concern about own bodily function.
4. *Depression*—common problem in the aging, with a *high suicide rate;* partly because of bodily changes that influence the *self-concept,* the older person may direct *hostility toward self* and therefore may be subject to feelings of depression and loneliness.
5. *Senility—four early symptoms:*
a. Change in attention span.
b. Memory loss for *recent* events and *names.*
c. Altered intellectual capacity.
d. Diminished ability to respond to others.

C. *Successful aging:*
1. Being able to *perceive* signs of aging and limitations resulting from the aging process.
2. *Redefining* life in terms of effects on social and physical aspects of living.
3. Seeking *alternatives* for meeting needs and finding sources of pleasure.
4. Adopting a *different outlook* about self-worth.
5. *Reintegrating* values with goals of life.

D. *Causative factors* of mental disorder in the aging client related to:
1. *Nutritional* problems and *physical ill health* related to *acute and chronic illness:*
a. Cardiovascular diseases (heart failure, stroke, hypertension).
b. Respiratory infection.
c. Cancer.
d. Alcohol dependence and abuse.
e. Dentition problems.
2. Faulty adaptation related to *physical* changes of aging (e.g., depression, hypochondriases).
3. Problems related to *loss, grief, and bereavement.*
4. *Retirement* shock related to loss of status and financial security.
5. Social isolation and loneliness related to *inadequate sensory stimulation.*
6. *Environmental change* (relocation within a community or from home to institution): loss of family, privacy.
7. *Hopelessness, helplessness* related to condition and circumstances.
8. *Altered body image* (negative) related to aging process.
9. Depression related to *helplessness, inability to express anger.*

III. ANALYSIS/NURSING DIAGNOSIS:

A. *Self-esteem disturbance* related to body image disturbance and altered family role.
B. *Impaired social interaction* related to social isolation and environmental changes.
C. *Dysfunctional grieving* related to loss and bereavement.
D. *Altered feeling states and spiritual distress* related to hopelessness, anxiety, fear, powerlessness.
E. *Altered physical regulation processes* related to physical ill health.
F. *Sleep pattern disturbance* related to insomnia and altered sleep/arousal patterns.

IV. NURSING CARE PLAN/IMPLEMENTATION:

A. *Long-term goal:* to help reduce hopelessness and helplessness.
B. *Short-term goal:* to focus on ego assets.
C. Help elderly *preserve* what facet of life they can and *regain* that which has already been lost.
1. Help *minimize regression* as much as possible.
2. Help retain their *adult* status.
3. Help preserve their *self-image* as useful individuals.
4. Identify and *preserve their abilities* to perform, emphasizing what they *can* do.

D. Attempt to *prevent* loss of dignity and loss of worth—address them by titles, not "Gramps," "sweetie," or "honey."

MENTAL HEALTH

E. *Reduce* feelings of *alienation* and loneliness. Provide *sensory* experiences for those with visual problems:
   1. Let them *touch* objects of various textures and consistencies.
   2. Encourage heightened *use of remaining senses* to make up for those that are diminished or lost.

F. *Reduce* depression and feelings of isolation.
   1. Allow time to *reminisce.*
   2. *Avoid changes* in surroundings or routine.

G. *Protect* from rush and excitement.
   1. Use simple, unhurried conversation.
   2. Allow *extra* time to organize thoughts.

H. Be sensitive to *concrete* things they may want to *keep.*

I. *Health teaching:*
   1. How to keep track of time (e.g., by marking off days on a calendar), to promote orientation.
   2. How to keep track of medications.
   3. Exercises to promote blood flow.
   4. *Retirement counseling:*
      a. Obtaining satisfaction from leisure time.
      b. Nurturing relationships with younger generations.
      c. Adjusting to changes: physical health, retirement, loss of loved ones.
      d. Developing connections with own age group.
      e. Taking on new social roles.
      f. Maintaining a satisfactory and appropriate living situation.
      g. Coping with dependence on others, especially one's children.

V. EVALUATION/OUTCOME CRITERIA:

A. Less confusion and fewer mood swings.
B. Increased interest in activities of daily living and interaction with others.
C. Lessened preoccupation with death, dying, physical symptoms, feelings of sadness.
D. Reduced insomnia and anorexia.
E. Expresses feelings of belonging and being needed.

Alterations in Self-Concept

I. ASSESSMENT:

A. Self-derisive; self-diminution; and self-critical.
B. Denies own pleasure due to need to punish self; doomed to failure.
C. Disturbed interpersonal relationships (cruel, demeaning, exploitive of others; passive-dependent).
D. Exaggerated self-worth or rejects personal capabilities.
E. Feels guilty, worries (nightmares, *phobias, obsessions*).
F. Sets unrealistic goals.
G. Withdraws from reality with intense self-rejection (*delusional, suspicious,* jealous).
H. Views life as either-or, worst-or-best, wrong-or-right.
I. Postpones decisions due to ambivalence (procrastination).
J. Physical complaints (*psychosomatic*).
K. Self-destructive (*substance abuse* or other destructiveness).

II. ANALYSIS/NURSING DIAGNOSIS: *Altered self-concept may be related to:*

A. *Low self-esteem* that is related to parental rejection, unrealistic parental expectations, repeated failures.
B. *Altered personal identity (negative):* self-rejection and self-hate related to unrealistic self-ideals.
C. *Identity confusion* related to role conflict, role overload, and role ambiguity.
D. *Feelings of helplessness, hopelessness,* worthlessness, fear, vulnerability, inadequacy related to extreme *dependency* on others and *lack of personal responsibility.*
E. *Disturbed body image.*
F. Depersonalization.
G. Physiological factors that produce self-concept distortions (e.g., fatigue, oxygen and sensory deprivation, toxic drugs, isolation, biochemical imbalance).

III. NURSING CARE PLAN/IMPLEMENTATION:

A. *Long-term goal:* facilitate client's self-actualization by helping him or her to grow, develop, and realize potential while compensating for impairments.

B. *Short-term goals:*
   1. Expand client's *self-awareness:*
      a. Establish open, trusting relationship to *reduce fear* of interpersonal relationships.
         (1) Offer unconditional acceptance.
         (2) Nonjudgmental response.
         (3) Listen and encourage discussion of thoughts, feelings.
         (4) Convey that client is valued as a person, is responsible for self *and* able to help self.
      b. Strengthen client's capacity for *reality testing, self-control,* and *ego integration.*
         (1) Identify ego strengths.
         (2) Confirm identity.
         (3) Reduce panic level of anxiety.
         (4) Use undemanding approach.
         (5) Accept and clarify communication.
         (6) Prevent isolation.
         (7) Establish simple routine.
         (8) Set limits on inappropriate behavior.
         (9) Orient to reality.
         (10) Activities: gradual increase; provide positive experiences.
         (11) Encourage self-care; assist in grooming.

c. Maximize *participation in decision making* related to self.
   (1) Gradually increase participation in own care.
   (2) Convey expectation of ultimate self-responsibility.

2. Encourage client's *self-exploration.*
   a. Accept client's feelings and assist *self-acceptance* of emotions, beliefs, behaviors, and thoughts.
   b. Help *clarify* self-concept and relationship to others.
      (1) Elicit client's perception of own strengths and weaknesses.
      (2) Ask client to describe: ideal self, how client believes he or she relates to other people and events.
   c. Nurse needs to be aware of *own* feelings as a model of behavior and to limit countertransference.
      (1) Accept own positive and negative feelings.
      (2) Share own perception of client's feelings.
   d. Respond with *empathy,* not sympathy, with the belief that client is subject to own control.
      (1) Monitor sympathy and self-pity by client.
      (2) Reaffirm that client is *not* helpless or powerless but is responsible for own choice of maladaptive or adaptive coping responses.
      (3) Discuss: alternatives, areas of ego *strength,* available coping resources.
      (4) Use family and group support system for self-exploration of client's conflicts and maladaptive coping responses.
3. Assist client in *self-evaluation.*
   a. Help to clearly *define* problem.
      (1) Identify relevant stressors.
      (2) Mutually identify: faulty beliefs, misperceptions, distortions, unrealistic goals, areas of strength.
   b. Explore use of adaptive *and* maladaptive coping responses and their positive and negative *consequences.*
4. Assist client to formulate a *realistic action plan.*
   a. Identify alternative solutions to client's *inconsistent perceptions* by helping him or her to change:
      (1) Own beliefs, ideals, to bring closer to reality.
      (2) Environment, to make consistent with beliefs.
   b. Identify alternative solutions to client's *self-concept not consistent with his or her behavior* by helping him or her to change:
      (1) Own behavior to conform to self-concept.
      (2) Underlying beliefs.
      (3) Self-ideal.
   c. Help client set and clearly define *goals* with *expected concrete* changes. Use role rehearsal, role modeling, and role playing to see practical, reality-based, emotional consequences of each goal.
5. Assist client to become committed to decision to *take necessary action* to replace maladaptive coping responses and maintain adaptive responses.
   a. Provide opportunity for success and give assistance (vocational, financial, and social support).
   b. Provide positive reinforcement; strengths, skills, healthy aspects of client's personality.
   c. Allow enough time for change.
6. *Health teaching:* how to focus on strengths rather than limitations; how to apply reality-oriented approach.

IV. EVALUATION/OUTCOME CRITERIA:

A. Client able to discuss perception of self and accept aspects of own personality.
B. Client assumes increased responsibility for own behavior.
C. Client able to transfer new perceptions into possible solutions, alternative behavior.

MENTAL HEALTH

Sleep Disturbance

I. TYPES OF SLEEP:

A. *Rapid-eye-movement (REM) sleep:* colorful, dramatic, emotional, implausible dreams.
B. *Non-REM sleep—stages:*
1. Stage 1: lasts 30 seconds to 7 minutes—falls asleep, drowsy; easily awakened; fleeting thoughts.
2. Stage 2: more relaxed; no eye movements, clearly asleep but readily awakens; 45% of total sleep time spent in this stage.
3. Stage 3 (delta sleep): deep muscle relaxation; decreased temperature, pulse, respiration.
4. Stage 4 (delta sleep): very relaxed; rarely moves.

C. *Sleep cycle*—common progression of sleep stages:
1. Stages 1, 2, 3, 4, 3, 2, REM, 2, 3, 4, etc.
2. *Delta* sleep most common during first third of night, with *REM* sleep periods increasing in duration during night from 1 to 2 minutes at start to 20 to 30 minutes by early morning.
3. REM sleep varies.
   a. Adolescents spend 30% of total sleep time in REM sleep.
   b. Adults spend 15% of total sleep time in REM sleep.

II. SLEEP DEPRIVATION (DYSSOMNIAS):

A. Assessment:
1. *Non-REM sleep loss:* physical fatigue due to less time spent in normal deep sleep.

2. *REM sleep loss:* psychological effects—irritability, confusion, anxiety, short-term memory loss, paranoia, hallucinations.
3. *Desynchronized sleep:* occurs when sleep shifts more than 2 hours from normal sleep period. Irritability, anoxia, decreased stress tolerance.

B. Analysis/nursing diagnosis: *sleep pattern disturbance* may be related to:
1. Interrupted sleep cycles before 90-minute sleep cycle is completed.
2. Unfamiliar sleeping environment.
3. Alterations in normal sleep/activity cycles (e.g., jet lag).
4. Preexisting sleep deficits before hospital admission.
5. Medications (e.g., alcohol withdrawal or abruptly discontinuing the use of hypnotic or antidepressant medications).
6. Pain.

C. Nursing care plan/implementation:
1. Obtain sleep history as part of nursing assessment. Determine normal sleep hours, bedtime rituals, factors that promote or interrupt sleep.
2. Duplicate normal bedtime rituals when possible.
3. Make *environment* conducive to sleep: lighting, noise, temperature.
   a. Close door, dim lights, turn off unneeded machinery.
   b. Encourage staff to muffle conversation at night.
4. Encourage *daytime* exercise periods.
5. Allow *uninterrupted periods of 90 minutes of sleep.* Group nighttime treatments and observations that require touching the client.
6. *Minimize* use of hypnotic medications.
   a. Substitute back rubs, warm milk, relaxation exercises.
   b. Encourage physician to consider prescribing hypnotics that minimize sleep disruption (e.g., chloral hydrate and flurazepam HCl [Dalmane]).
   c. *Taper* off hypnotics rather than abruptly discontinuing.
7. Observe client while asleep.
   a. Evaluate quality of sleep.
   b. It may be sleep apnea if client is extremely restless and snoring heavily.
8. *Health teaching: avoid* caffeine and hyperstimulation at bedtime; teach how to promote sleep-inducing environment, relaxation techniques.

D. EVALUATION/OUTCOME CRITERIA: verbalizes satisfaction with amount, quality of sleep.

Eating Disorders

Anorexia Nervosa/Bulimia Nervosa

Anorexia nervosa is an illness of starvation related to a severe disturbance of body image and a morbid fear of obesity; it is an eating disorder, usually seen in adolescence, when a person is underweight and emaciated and refuses to eat. It can result in death due to irreversible metabolic processes.

Bulimia nervosa is another type of eating disorder (binge-purge syndrome) also encountered primarily in late adolescence or early adulthood. It is characterized by at least two binge-eating episodes of large quantities of high-calorie food over a couple of hours followed by disparaging self-criticism and depression. Self-induced vomiting, abuse of laxatives, and abuse of diuretics are commonly associated because they decrease physical pain of abdominal distention, may reduce postbinge anguish, and may provide a method of self-control. Bulimic episodes may occur as part of anorexia nervosa, but these clients rarely become emaciated, and not all have a body image disturbance **(Table 10.11).**

I. CONCEPTS AND PRINCIPLES RELATED TO ANOREXIA NERVOSA:

A. *Not* due to lack of appetite or problem with appetite center in hypothalamus.

B. Normal stomach hunger is *repressed, denied, depersonalized;* no conscious awareness of hunger sensation.

II. ASSESSMENT OF ANOREXIA NERVOSA:

A. *Body image disturbance*—delusional, obsessive (e.g., does not see self as thin and is bewildered by others' concern).

B. Usually *preoccupied* with food, yet dreads gaining too much weight. *Ambivalence:* avoids food, hoards food.

C. Feels ineffectual, with low sex drive. *Repudiation of sexuality.*

D. *Pregnancy* fears, including misconceptions of oral impregnation through food.

E. *Self-punitive* behavior leading to starvation; suppression of anger.

F. *Physical signs and symptoms:*
1. Weight loss (20% of previous "normal" body weight).
2. Amenorrhea and secondary sex organ atrophy.
3. *Hyperactivity;* compulsiveness; excessive gum chewing.
4. Constipation.
5. *Hypotension, bradycardia,* hypothermia.
6. Skin: hyperkeratosis, poor turgor, dry.
7. Blood: leukopenia, anemia, hypoglycemia, hypoproteinemia, hypocholesteremia, hypokalemia, hyponatremia, *decreased* magnesium, *decreased* chloride, *increased* BUN; ECG: T-wave inversion.

Table 10.11

Comparison: Anorexia and Bulimia

Signs and Symptoms	Anorexia	Bulimia
Behavioral	• Self-starvation • Rituals regarding food, eating, and weight loss • Behaviors to ↓ weight: purging, exercise, use of laxatives, enemas, and diuretics	• Repetitive secret bingeing and purging • Behaviors to ↓ weight: purging, exercise, use of laxatives, enemas, and diuretics • Fasts to compensate for bingeing
Physical	• Weight loss 15% below ideal • Cachexia (sunken eyes, protruding bones, dry skin) • Amenorrhea • ↓ Pulse, ↓ body temperature • Lanugo on face • Constipation • Sensitivity to cold	• Weight is usually normal; may be ↑ or ↓ • Fluid/electrolyte imbalances (↓ K, metabolic alkalosis, dehydration) • Menstrual irregularities • Dental caries, loss of dental enamel, • ↓ BP, cardiac dysrhythmias, constipation or diarrhea, GERD, parotid enlargement
Psychological	• Appears fat to self • Intense, irrational fear of being fat • Preoccupation with cooking, food, nutrition • Delayed psychosexual development • Perfectionist, high achiever	• Excessive concern about weight, shape, proportions • Lack of control over eating during bingeing • Depression, shame, self-contempt follow bingeing • Mood swings, irritability • Impulsive, extrovert

BP = blood pressure, GERD = gastroesophageal reflux disease.

III. ANALYSIS/NURSING DIAGNOSIS:

A. *Imbalanced nutrition, less than body requirements,* and *fluid volume deficit* related to attempts to vomit food after eating, overuse of laxatives/diuretics, and refusal to eat, related to need to demonstrate control.

B. *Risk for altered physical regulation processes/risk for or actual fluid volume deficit:* amenorrhea related to starvation; hypotension, bradycardia; metabolic alkalosis.

C. *Risk for self-inflicted injury* related to starvation from refusal to eat or ambivalence about food.

D. *Altered eating* related to altered thought processes: binge-purge syndrome.

E. *Body-image disturbance/chronic low self-esteem* related to anxiety over assuming an adult role and concern with sexual identity; unmet dependency needs, personal vulnerability; perceived loss of control in some aspect of life; dysfunctional family system.

F. *Compulsive behaviors* related to need to maintain control of self, represented by losing weight.

IV. NURSING CARE PLAN/IMPLEMENTATION:

A. Help reestablish connections between body sensations (hunger) and responses (eating). Use *stimulus-response conditioning* methods to set up eating regimen.

1. *Weigh* regularly, at same time and with same amount of clothing, with back to scale.
2. Make sure water drinking is *avoided* before weighing.
3. Give one-to-one supervision during and 30 minutes after mealtimes to *prevent* attempts to vomit food.
4. Monitor exercise program and set limits on physical activity.

B. *Monitor* physiological signs and symptoms (amenorrhea, constipation, hypoproteinemia, hypoglycemia, anemia, eroded tooth enamel, inflamed buccal cavity, brittle nails, dull hair, secondary sexual organ atrophy, hypothermia, hypotension, leg cramps and other signs of hypokalemia).

C. *Health teaching:*

1. Explain normal sexual growth and development to improve knowledge deficit and confront sexual fears.
2. Use behavior modification to reestablish awareness of hunger sensation and to relate it to the clock and regular mealtimes.
3. Teach parents skills in communication related to dependence/independence needs of adolescent; allow client to assume control in areas other than dieting, weight loss (e.g., management of daily activities, work, leisure choices).

V. EVALUATION/OUTCOME CRITERIA:

A. Attains and maintains minimal normal weight for age and height.

B. Eats regular meal (standard nutritional diet).

C. No incidence of self-induced vomiting, bulimia, or compulsive physical activity.

D. Acts on increased internal emotional awareness and recognition of body sensation of hunger (i.e., talks about being hungry and feeling hunger pangs).

E. Relates increased sense of effectiveness with less need to control food intake.

Sensory Disturbance

I. TYPES OF SENSORY DISTURBANCE:

A. *Sensory deprivation*—amount of stimuli *less* than required, such as isolation in bed or room, deafness, victim of stroke (brain attack).

B. *Sensory overload*—receives *more* stimuli than can be tolerated (e.g., bright lights, noise, strange machinery, barrage of visitors).

C. *Sensory deficit*—impairment in functioning of sensory or perceptual processes (e.g., blindness, changes in tactile perceptions).

II. ASSESSMENT—based on awareness of behavioral changes:

A. *Sensory deprivation*—boredom, daydreaming, increasing sleep, thought slowness, inactivity, thought disorganization, hallucinations.

B. *Sensory overload*—same as sensory deprivation, plus restlessness and agitation, confusion.

C. *Sensory deficit*—may not be able to distinguish sounds, odors, and tastes or differentiate tactile sensations.

III. ANALYSIS/NURSING DIAGNOSIS: problems related to sensory disturbance:

A. *Altered thought processes.*

B. *Confusion* (acute vs. chronic).

C. *Anger, aggression.*

D. *Body-image disturbance.*

E. *Sleep pattern disturbance.*

IV. NURSING CARE PLAN/IMPLEMENTATION:

A. *Management of existing* sensory disturbances in:

1. *Acute sensory deprivation:*
   a. Increase interaction with staff.
   b. Use TV.
   c. Provide touch.
   d. Help clients choose menus that have aromas, varied tastes, temperatures, colors, textures.
   e. Use light cologne or aftershave lotion, bath powder.
2. *Sensory overload:*
   a. Restrict number of visitors and length of stay.
   b. Reduce noise and lights.
   c. Reduce newness by establishing and following routine.
   d. Organize care to provide for extended rest periods with minimal input.
3. *Sensory deficits:*
   a. Report observations about hearing, vision.
   b. May imply need for new glasses, medical diagnosis, or therapy.

B. *Health teaching: prevention* of sensory disturbance involves *education* of parents during child's growth and development regarding tactile, auditory, and visual stimulation.

1. Hold, talk, and play with infant when awake.
2. Provide bright toys with different designs for children to hold.
3. Change environment.
4. Provide music and auditory stimuli.
5. Give foods with variety of textures, tastes, colors.

V. EVALUATION/OUTCOME CRITERIA:

A. Client is oriented to time, place, person.

B. Little or no evidence of mood or sleep disturbance.

Delirium, Dementia, and Amnestic and Other Cognitive Disorders

These disorders include etiology associated with (1) the *aging process* (dementias arising in the senium or presenium, including primary degenerative dementia of the Alzheimer type and multi-infarct dementia); (2) *substance-related disorders* (e.g., alcohol, barbiturates, opioids, cocaine, amphetamines, PCP, hallucinogens, *cannabis,* nicotine, and caffeine); and (3) general medical conditions.

I. CONCEPTS, PRINCIPLES, AND SUBTYPES:

A. Course may be progressive, with steady deterioration.

B. Alternative pathways and compensatory mechanisms may develop to show a clinical picture of remissions and exacerbations.

C. *Delirium* is characterized by a *disturbance of consciousness* with reduced ability to focus, sustain, or shift attention; and a *change in cognition* (e.g., memory deficit, disorientation [time and place], language disturbance); or *development of perceptual disturbance* (e.g., illusions, hallucinations) that develops over a *short* time (hours or days) and *fluctuates* during the course of the day. *Etiology:* a direct physiological consequence of a general medical condition, substance intoxication or withdrawal, use of a medication, or toxin exposure. *Diagnostic feature:* cannot repeat sequential string of information (e.g., digit span).

D. *Dementia* is characterized by persistent *multiple cognitive deficits* (e.g., aphasia, apraxia, agnosia, disturbance in executive functioning) accompanied by memory impairment and mood and sleep disturbances. *Possible etiology:* vascular dementia, HIV infection, head trauma, Parkinson's disease, Pick's disease, Alzheimer's disease, Huntington's disease, substance induced, toxin exposure, medication, infections, nutritional deficiencies (hypoglycemia), endocrine conditions (hypothyroidism), brain tumors, seizure disorders, hepatic and renal failure; cardiopulmonary insufficiencies; fluid and electrolyte imbalances. *Diagnostic features:* cannot learn (register) new information (e.g., a list of words), or retain, recall, or recognize information.

1. ***Alzheimer's disease:*** progressive; irreversible loss of cerebral function due to cortical atrophy; exists in 2% to 4% of people over age 65 years; may have a genetic component; may begin at ages 40 to 65; may lead to death within 2 years. Average duration from onset of symptoms to death: 8 to 10 years.
   a. Progressive decline in intellectual capacity (recent and remote memory, judgment), affect, and motor coordination (apraxia); loss of social sense; apathy or restlessness.
   b. *Problems with* speech (aphasia), recognition of familiar objects (agnosia), disorientation to self (even parts of *own* body).
   c. Summaries of stages:

Stage 1: Mild

- Patient recognizes a problem
- ↓ Short-term memory, mild ↓ cognition, confusion, hyperalertness
- Anxiety, depression, invents words that have no common meaning (*neologisms*)
- Fills in memory gaps with fabricated facts (*confabulation*)

Stage 2: Moderate

- Intellectual decline continues; language disturbances (*aphasia*)
- ↓ Motor activity (*apraxia*)
- Repetition of same idea in response to different questions (*perseveration*)
- Failure to recognize words/objects (*agnosia*)
- Confusion/irritation at end of day (*sundowning*); sleep disturbances with wandering
- Acting on thoughts/feelings without social control (*disinhibition*)
- Agitation or aggression, illusion, delusion, and hallucinations

Stage 3: Severe

- Totally dependent
- Complete loss of intellectual functioning
- ↓ Bowel/bladder control
- Difficulty swallowing (dysphagia), emaciation
- Immobility leads to pneumonia, urinary tract infections, and pressure ulcers

2. ***Pick's disease:*** unknown cause; may have genetic component. Onset: middle age; women affected more than men. *Pathology:* atrophy in frontal and temporal lobes of brain. Clinical picture similar to Alzheimer's disease.
3. ***Creutzfeldt-Jakob disease:*** uncommon, extremely rapid neurodegeneration caused by transmissible "slow" virus (prion); genetic component in 5% to 15%. Clinical picture: typical dementia, with muscle rigidity, ataxia, involuntary movements. Occurrence: ages 40 to 60 years. Death within 1 year.

E. *Amnestic disorder* is characterized by *severe* memory impairment *without* other significant impairments of cognitive functioning (i.e., without aphasia, apraxia, or agnosia). *Diagnostic features:* memory impairment is always manifested by impairment in the ability to learn *new* information and sometimes problems remembering previously learned information or past events. May result in *disorientation* to place and time, but *rarely* to self. Appears bewildered or befuddled.

1. *Etiology:* due to direct physiological effects of a general medical condition (e.g., physical trauma or vitamin deficiency) or due to persisting effects of a substance (e.g., drug of abuse, a medication, or toxin exposure).
2. Memory disturbance: sufficiently severe to cause marked impairment in social or occupational functioning and represents a significant decline from a previous level of functioning. May require supervised living situation to ensure appropriate feeding and care.
3. Lacks insight into own memory deficit and may explicitly deny the presence of severe memory impairment despite evidence to the contrary.
4. Altered personality function: apathy, lack of initiative, emotional blandness, shallow range of expression.

II. ASSESSMENT:

A. *Most common areas of difficulty* can be grouped under the mnemonic term *JOCAM: J*—judgment, *O*—orientation, *C*—confabulation, *A*—affect, and *M*—memory.

1. *Judgment:* impaired, resulting in socially inappropriate behavior (such as hypersexuality toward inappropriate objects) and inability to carry out activities of daily living.
2. *Orientation:* confused, disoriented; perceptual disturbances (e.g., illusions, misidentification of other persons and objects; misperception to make unfamiliar more familiar; *visual, tactile, and auditory* hallucinations may appear as images and voices or disorganized light and sound patterns). *Paranoid delusions* of persecution.
3. *Confabulation:* common use of this defense mechanism to fill in memory gaps with invented stories.
4. *Affect:* mood changes and unstable emotions; quarrelsome, with outbursts of morbid anger

MENTAL HEALTH

(as in cerebral arteriosclerosis); tearful; withdrawn from social contact; *depression* is a frequent reaction to loss of physical and social function.

5. *Memory:* impaired, especially for names and *recent* events; may compensate by confabulating and by using *circumstantiality and tangential* speaking patterns.

B. *Other areas of difficulty:*

1. *Seizures* (e.g., in Alzheimer's disease and cerebral arteriosclerosis).
2. *Intellectual capacities diminished.*
    a. Difficulty with *abstract* thought.
    b. Compensatory mechanism is to stay with familiar topics; repetition.
    c. Short concentration periods.
3. *Personality changes.*
    a. Loss of ego flexibility; adoption of more rigid attitudes.
    b. *Ritualism* in daily activities.
    c. Hoarding.
    d. Somatic preoccupations (hypochondriases).
    e. *Restlessness,* wandering away.
    f. Impaired impulse control.
    g. *Aphasia* (in severe dementia).
    h. *Apraxia* (inability to carry out motor activities).

C. *Diagnostic tests:*

1. *Neurological* examination: perform maneuvers or answer questions that are aimed at eliciting information about condition of specific parts of brain or peripheral nerves.
    a. Assessment of mental status and alertness.
    b. Muscle strength and reflexes.
    c. Sensory-perceptual.
    d. Language skills.
    e. Coordination.
2. *Laboratory* tests:
    a. *Blood, urine* to test for: infections, hepatic and renal dysfunction, diabetes, electrolyte imbalances, metabolic/endocrine disorders, nutritional deficiencies, and presence of toxic substances (e.g., drugs).
    b. Electroencephalography (EEG) to check brain's electrical activity.
    c. Computed tomography (CT) scan—image of brain size and shape.
    d. Positron emission tomography (PET)—reveals metabolic activity of brain (important for diagnosis of Alzheimer's disease).
    e. Magnetic resonance imaging (MRI)—computerized image of soft tissue, with sharply detailed picture of brain tissues.

III. ANALYSIS/NURSING DIAGNOSIS:

A. *Risk for trauma* related to cognitive deficits (inability to recognize/identify danger in the environment; confusion; impaired judgment) and altered motor behavior (restlessness, hyperactivity, muscular incoordination).

B. *Disturbed thought processes (altered abstract thinking and altered knowledge processes [agnosia])* related to destruction of cerebral tissue, inability to use information to make judgments and transmit messages, and memory deficits.

C. *Sensory/perceptual alterations:* visual, auditory, kinesthetic, gustatory, tactile, olfactory related to neurological deficit.

D. *Sleep pattern disturbance* resulting in disorientation at night, related to confusion; increased aimless wandering (day/night reversal).

E. *Self-care deficit* (feeding, bathing/hygiene, dressing, toileting) related to physical impairments (poor vision, uncoordination, forgetfulness), disorientation, and confusion.

F. *Imbalanced nutrition, more or less than body requirements,* related to confusion.

G. *Total incontinence* related to sensory/perceptual alterations.

H. *Altered attention and memory* related to progressive neurological losses.

I. *Altered conduct/impulse processes* (irritability and aggressiveness) related to neurological impairment.

J. *Impaired communication* related to poverty of speech and withdrawal behavior, progressive neurological losses, and cerebral impairment.

K. *Caregiver role strain* related to long-term illness and complexity of home care needs.

L. *Relocation stress syndrome* related to separation from support systems, physical deterioration, and changes in daily routine.

IV. NURSING CARE PLAN/IMPLEMENTATION

(see also interventions in **III. Confusion/Disorientation, pp. 741–742**):

A. *Long-term goal:* minimize regression related to memory impairment.

B. *Short-term goal:* provide structure and consistency to increase security.

C. Make *brief, frequent* contacts, because attention span is short.

D. Allow clients *time* to talk and to complete projects.

E. Stimulate *associative* patterns to improve recall (by repeating, summarizing, and focusing).

F. Allow clients to *review* their lives and focus on the past.

G. Use *concrete* questions in interviewing.

H. *Reinforce* reality-oriented comments.

I. Keep environment structured the *same* as much as possible (e.g., same room and placement of furniture); *routine* is important to diminish stress.

J. Recognize the importance of *compensatory* mechanisms (e.g., confabulation) to increase self-esteem; build psychological reserve.

K. Give recognition for each accomplishment.
L. Use *recreational* and physical therapy.
M. *Health teaching:* give *specific* instructions for diet, medication (e.g., tacrine [Cognex], donepezil [Aricept] for improving cognition), and treatment; how to use many sensory approaches to learn new information; how to use existing knowledge, old learning, and habitual approaches to deal with new situations.

V. EVALUATION/OUTCOME CRITERIA:
A. Symptoms occur *less* frequently and are less severe in areas of: emotional lability and appropriateness; false perceptions; self-care ability; disorientation, memory, and judgment; and decision making.
B. Client is able to preserve optimum level of functioning and independence while allowing basic needs to be met.
C. Stays relatively calm and noncombative when upset or fearful.
D. Accepts own irritability and frustrations as part of illness.
E. Asks for assistance with self-care activities.
F. Knows and adheres to daily routine; knows own nurse, location of room, bathroom, clocks, calendars.
G. Uses supportive community services.

Substance-Related Disorders

I. DEFINITION: ingesting in any manner a chemical that has an effect on the body.

II. GENERAL ASSESSMENT:
A. *Behavioral* changes exist while under the influence of substance.
B. Engages in regular *use* of substance.
1. *Substance abuse:*
   a. Pattern of *pathological* use (i.e., day-long intoxication; inability to stop use, even when contraindicated by serious physical disorder; overpowering need or desire to take the drug despite legal, social, or medical problems); daily need of substance for functioning; repeated medical complications from use.
   b. *Interference* with social, occupational functioning.
   c. Willingness to obtain substance by any means, including illegal.
   d. Pathological use for more than 1 month.
2. *Substance dependence:*
   a. More severe than substance abuse; body *requires* substance to continue functioning.
   b. Physiological dependence (i.e., either develops a *tolerance*—must increase dose to obtain desired effect—or has *physical withdrawal symptoms* when substance intake is reduced or stopped).
   c. Person feels it is impossible to get along without drug.

C. Effects of substance on *central nervous system (CNS).*

III. GENERAL ANALYSIS: only in recent years has substance abuse been viewed as an illness rather than moral delinquency or criminal behavior. The disorders are very complex and little understood. There are physiological, psychological, and social aspects to their causality, dynamics, symptoms, and treatment, where personality disorder has a major part.
A. *Physiological aspects*—current unproven theories include "allergic" reaction to alcohol, disturbance in metabolism, genetic susceptibility to dependency, and hypofunction of adrenal cortex. There are *organic effects* of chronic excessive use.
B. *Psychological aspects*—disrupted parent-child relationship and family dynamics; deleterious effect on ego function.
C. *Social and cultural aspects*—local customs and attitudes vary about what is excessive.
D. *Maladaptive behavior related to:*
1. Low self-esteem.
2. Anger.
3. Denial.
4. Rationalization.
5. Social isolation.
6. A rigid pattern of coping.
7. Poorly defined philosophy of life, values, mores.

E. *Nursing diagnosis* in **acute phase of abuse, intoxication:**
1. *Risk for ineffective breathing patterns* related to pneumonia caused by aspiration, malnutrition; depressed immune system; or overdose.
2. *Risk for decreased cardiac output* related to effect of substances on cardiac muscle; electrolyte imbalance.
3. *Risk for injury* related to impaired coordination, disorientation, and altered judgment (worse at night).
4. *Risk for violence:* self-directed or directed at others, related to misinterpretation of stimuli and feelings of suspicion or distrust of others.
5. *Sensory/perceptual alterations:* visual, kinesthetic, tactile, related to intake of mind-altering substances.
6. *Altered nutrition,* less than body requirements.
7. *Altered thought processes* (delusions, incoherence) related to misinterpretation of stimuli due to severe panic and fear.
8. *Sleep pattern disturbance* related to mind-altering substance.
9. *Ineffective individual coping* related to inability to tolerate frustration and to meet basic needs

or role expectations, resulting in unpredictable behaviors.

10. *Noncompliance* with abstinence and supportive therapy, related to inability to stop using substance because of dependence and refusal to alter lifestyle.
11. *Impaired communication* related to mental confusion or CNS depression due to substance use.
12. *Impaired health maintenance management* related to failure to recognize that a problem exists and inability to take responsibility for health needs.

Alcohol Use Disorders: Alcohol Abuse and Dependence

I. DEFINITIONS:

A. *Alcohol dependence* is a primary and chronic disorder that is progressive and often fatal, in which the individual is unable, for physical or psychological reasons or both, to refrain from frequent consumption of alcohol in quantities that produce intoxication and disrupt health and ability to perform daily functions.

B. *Alcohol abuse* is a separate diagnosis, and is defined as a maladaptive pattern of use with one or more of the following over a 1-year period:

1. Repeated alcohol consumption that results in an inability to fulfill obligations at home, school, or work.
2. Repeated alcohol consumption when it could be physically dangerous (e.g., driving a car).
3. Repeated alcohol-related legal problems (e.g., arrests).
4. Continued drinking despite interpersonal or social problems caused or made worse by drinking.

II. CONCEPTS AND PRINCIPLES RELATED TO ALCOHOL ABUSE AND DEPENDENCE:

A. Alcohol affects cerebral cortical functions:

1. Memory.
2. Judgment.
3. Reasoning.

B. Alcohol is a *depressant:*

1. Relaxes the individual.
2. Lessens use of repression of unconscious conflict.
3. Releases inhibitions, hostility, and primitive drives.

C. Drinking represents a tension-reducing device and a relief from feelings of insecurity. Strength of drinking habit equals degree of anxiety and frustration intolerance.

D. Alcohol dependence is not a *symptom* but rather a disease in itself.

E. Underlying fear and anxiety, associated with inner conflict, motivate the person who is alcoholic to drink.

F. People with alcohol use disorder can *never* be cured to drink normally; cure is to be a "sober alcoholic," with total abstinence.

G. The spouse of the person with alcohol use disorder often unconsciously contributes to the drinking behavior because of own emotional needs (*co-alcoholic* or *codependent*).

H. Intoxication occurs with a blood-alcohol level of 0.08% or above. *Signs of intoxication* are:

1. Incoordination.
2. Slurred speech.
3. Dulled perception.

I. Tolerance occurs with alcohol dependence. Increasing amounts of alcohol must be consumed to obtain the desired effect.

III. ASSESSMENT:

A. *Vicious cycle*—(a) low tolerance for coping with frustration; tension, *guilt* and shame, resentment; (b) uses alcohol for relief; (c) new problems created by drinking; (d) new anxieties; and (e) more drinking.

B. Coping mechanisms used: *denial, rationalization, projection.*

C. *Complications of abuse and dependence.*

1. ***Alcohol withdrawal delirium (delirium tremens [DTs])* (Fig. 10.5)**—result of nutritional deficiencies and toxins; requires sedation and constant watchfulness against unintentional suicide and convulsions.
   a. *Impending* signs relate to *CNS*—marked nervousness and restlessness, increased irritability; gross tremors of hands, face, lips; weakness; also *cardiovascular*—increased blood pressure, tachycardia, diaphoresis, dysrhythmias; *depression; gastrointestinal*—nausea, vomiting, anorexia.
   b. *Actual—serious* symptoms of mental confusion, convulsions, hallucinations (visual, olfactory, auditory, tactile). Without treatment, *15% to 25%* may die due to cardiac dysrhythmias, respiratory arrest, severe dehydration, massive infection.
2. ***Wernicke's syndrome***—a neurological disturbance manifested by confusion, ataxia, eye movement abnormalities, and memory impairment. Other problems include:
   a. Disturbed vision (diplopia).
   b. Wandering mind.
   c. Stupor and coma.
3. ***Alcohol amnestic syndrome (Korsakoff's syndrome)***—degenerative neuritis due to *thiamine* deficiency.
   a. Impaired thoughts.
   b. Confusion, loss of sense of time and place.
   c. Use of confabulation to fill in severe recent memory loss.
   d. Follows episode of *Wernicke's encephalopathy.*

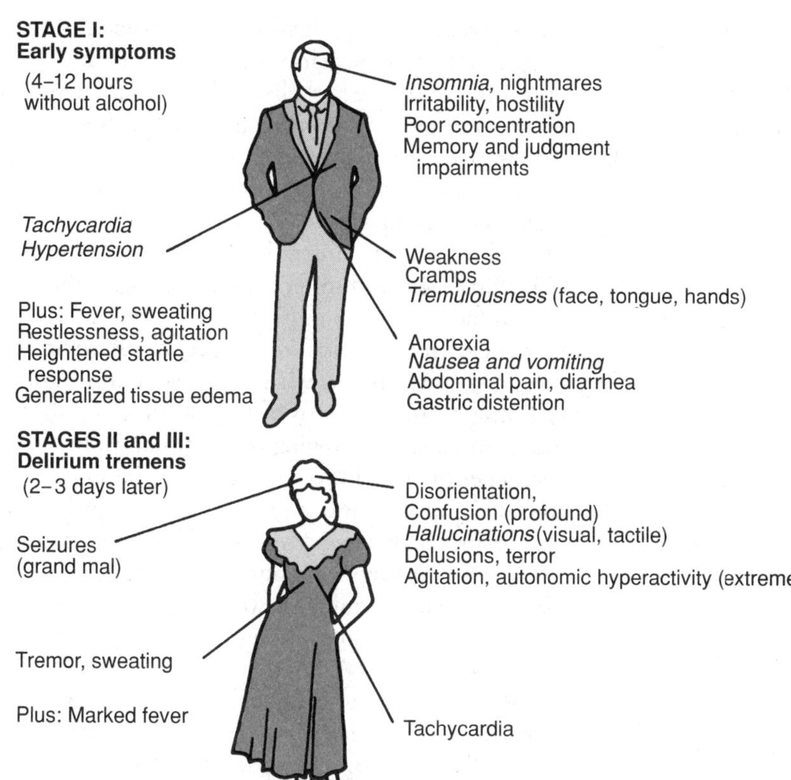

Figure 10.5 Symptoms associated with alcohol withdrawal. (Adapted from Wilson, HS, & Kneisl, CR: *Psychiatric Nursing,* ed 2. Addison-Wesley, Menlo Park, CA. [out of print])

4. *Polyneuropathy*—weak, irregular, rapid peripheral pulses; sensory and motor nerve endings are involved, causing pain, itching, and loss of limb control.
5. Related concerns—chronic heart failure (generalized tissue edema), *gastritis, esophageal varices, cirrhosis, pancreatitis, diabetes,* pneumonia, REM sleep deprivation, *malnutrition,* cancer of mouth, pharynx, and larynx.

D. Diagnostic tests:

1. *Blood tests:*
   a. *Complete blood count (CBC): decreased* hemoglobin/hematocrit (Hgb/Hct) to detect iron-deficiency anemia or acute/chronic GI bleeding; *increased* white blood cell (WBC) count (infection); *decreased* WBC count (if immunosuppressed).
   b. *Glucose:* hyperglycemia/hypoglycemia may be present (pancreatitis, malnutrition, or depletion of liver glycogen stores).
   c. *Electrolytes: decreased* potassium and magnesium.
   d. *Liver function tests* are classic toxic markers that alcohol use leaves on body: *increased* creatine phosphokinase (CPK), lactate dehydrogenase (LDH), aspartate aminotransferase (AST), alanine aminotransferase (ALT), and amylase (liver or pancreatic problem).
   e. *Nutritional tests: decreased* albumin and total protein; *decreased* vitamins A, C, D, E, K, and B (malnutrition/malabsorption).
2. *Urinalysis:* infection; ketones due to breakdown of fatty acids in malnutrition (pseudodiabetic condition).
3. *Chest x-ray:* rule out right lower lobe pneumonia (related to malnutrition, depressed immune system, aspiration).
4. *ECG:* dysrhythmias, cardiomyopathies, or ischemia due to direct effect of alcohol on the cardiac muscle or conduction system, as well as effects of electrolyte imbalance.
5. *Other screening studies* (e.g., hepatitis, HIV, tuberculosis [TB]): dependent on general condition, individual risk factors, and care setting.

IV. ANALYSIS/NURSING DIAGNOSIS:

A. *Risk for injury (self-directed violence):* tendency for *self-destructive* acts related to intake of mind-altering substances and chronic low self-esteem.

B. *Altered nutrition, less than body requirements,* related to a lack of interest in food, interference with absorption/metabolism of nutrients and amino acids.

C. *Ineffective individual coping: denial/defensive coping* related to tendency to be domineering and critical, with difficulties in *interpersonal* relationships.

D. *Conflict with social order* related to extreme dependence coupled with resentment of *authority.*
E. *Spiritual distress* or general dissatisfaction with life related to feelings of powerlessness, *low frustration* tolerance, and demand for immediate need satisfaction.
F. *Dysfunctional behaviors/sexual dysfunction* related to tendency for *excess* in work, sex, recreation, marked *narcissistic* behavior.
G. *Social isolation* related to use of coping mechanisms that are primarily *escapist.*
H. *Knowledge deficit* (learning need) regarding condition, prognosis, treatment, self-care, discharge needs.

V. NURSING CARE PLAN/IMPLEMENTATION:

A. *Detoxification phase*—maintain physiological stability.
1. *Administer adequate sedation* to control anxiety, insomnia, agitation, tremors.
2. *Administer anticonvulsants* to prevent *withdrawal seizures* (diazepam [Valium], chlordiazepoxide [Librium], phenobarbital, magnesium sulfate).
3. *Control nausea and vomiting* to avoid massive GI bleeding or rupture of esophageal varices (antiemetics, antacids).
4. *Assess for* hypertension, tachycardia, increased temperature, Kussmaul's respirations.
5. *Assess fluid and electrolyte balance* for dehydration (may need IV fluids) or overhydration (may need a diuretic).
6. *Reestablish proper nutrition: high protein* (as long as no severe liver damage), carbohydrate, *thiamine, vitamins B complex and C.*
7. *Promote client safety—provide quiet, calm, safe environment:* bedrest *with rails,* and head of bed *elevated;* well-lit room to reduce illusions; constant supervision and reassurance about fears and hallucinations; assess depression for suicide potential.

B. *Recovery-rehabilitation phase:* encourage participation in *group* activities; *avoid sympathy* when client tends to rationalize behavior and seeks special privileges—use acceptance and a *nonjudgmental,* consistent, firm, but kind approach; *avoid:* scorn, contempt, and moralizing or punitive and rejecting behaviors; do *not* reinforce feelings of worthlessness, self-contempt, hopelessness, or low self-esteem.

C. *Problem behaviors:*
1. *Manipulative*—be firm and consistent; *avoid* "bid for sympathy."
2. *Demanding*—set limits.
3. *Acting out*—set limits, enforce rules and regulations, strengthen impulse control and ability to delay gratification.
4. *Dependency*—place responsibility on client; *avoid* giving advice.
5. *Superficiality*—help client make realistic self-appraisals and expectations in lieu of grandiose promises and trite verbalizations; encourage formation of lasting interpersonal relationships.

D. *Common reactions among staff:*
1. Disappointment—instead, set realistic goals, take one step at a time.
2. Moral judgment—instead, support each other.
3. Hostility—instead, offer support to each other when feeling frustrated from lack of results.

E. Refer client from hospital to *community resources* for follow-up treatment with social, economic, and psychological problems, as well as to self-help groups, to reduce "revolving door" situation in which client comes in, is treated, goes out, and comes in again the next night.
1. *Alcoholics Anonymous (AA)*—a self-help group of addicted drinkers who confront, instruct, and support fellow drinkers in their efforts to stay sober 1 day at a time through fellowship and acceptance.
2. *Al-Anon*—support group for *families* of clients with alcohol use disorder. *Alateen*—support group for *teenagers* when parent is alcoholic.
3. *Aversion therapy*—client is subjected to revulsion-producing or pain-inducing stimuli at the same time he or she takes a drink, to establish alcohol rejection behavior. Most common is disulfiram *(Antabuse),* a drug that works by blocking an enzyme that helps metabolize alcohol. It produces intense headache, severe flushing, extreme nausea, vomiting, palpitations, hypotension, dyspnea, and blurred vision when alcohol is consumed while person is taking this drug.
4. *Other drug therapy*—naltrexone (ReVia) is a drug that works by blocking endorphin receptors and interfering in alcohol-induced brain reward circuitry that is involved in good feelings people get from drinking.
   a. *Benefit:* reduces alcohol relapse and decreases total amount of drinking per day.
   b. Dose: 50 mg PO/day.
   c. Common side effects: transitory dizziness, diarrhea, nausea. Does not have extreme side effects of Antabuse.
5. *Group psychotherapy*—the goals of group psychotherapy are for the client to give up alcohol as a tension reliever, identify cause of stress, build different means for coping with stress, and accept drinking as a serious symptom.

F. *Health teaching:* teach improved coping patterns to tolerate increased stress; teach substitute tension-reducing strategies; prepare in advance for difficult, painful events; teach how to reduce irritating or frustrating environmental stress; teach (in simple terms) the physiological effects of alcohol abuse on the body.

VI. EVALUATION/OUTCOME CRITERIA: complications prevented, resolved; everyday living patterns are restructured for a satisfactory life without alcohol; demonstrates feelings of increased self-worth, confidence, and reliance.

Other Substance-Related Disorders

I. CONCEPTS AND PRINCIPLES:

A. *Three* interacting key factors give rise to dependence—*psychopathology* of the individual; frustrating *environment;* and *availability* of powerful, addicting, and temporarily satisfying drug.

B. According to conditioning principles, substance abuse and dependence proceed in *several phases:*

1. *Use* of sedatives-hypnotics, CNS stimulants, hallucinogens, and narcotics for relief from daily tensions and discomforts or anticipated withdrawal symptoms.
2. Habit is *reinforced* with each relief by drug use.
3. Development of *dependency*—drug has less and less efficiency in reducing tensions.
4. Dependency is further reinforced as addict *fails* to maintain adequate drug intake—increase in frequency and duration of periods of tension and discomfort.

II. ASSESSMENT:

A. Abuse:

1. *Hallucinogens* (lysergic acid diethylamide [LSD], marijuana, ecstasy, STP, PCP, peyote): euphoria and rapid mood swings, flight of ideas; perceptual impairment, feelings of omnipotence, "bad trip" (panic, loss of control, paranoia), flashbacks, suicide.
2. *CNS stimulants* (*amphetamines* and *cocaine* abuse): euphoria, hyperactivity, hyperalertness, irritability, persecutory delusions; insomnia, anorexia → weight loss; tachycardia; tremulousness; hypertension; hyperthermia → convulsions.
3. *Narcotics* (*opium* and its derivatives morphine, heroin, codeine, meperidine HCl [Demerol]): used by "snorting," "skin popping," and "mainlining." May lead to abscesses and hepatitis. Decreased pain response, respiratory depression; apathy, detachment from reality; impaired judgment; loss of sexual activity; pinpoint pupils.
4. *Sedatives-hypnotics (barbiturate abuse)*: similar to alcohol-induced behavior (e.g., euphoria) followed by depression, hostility; decreased inhibitions; impaired judgment; staggering gait; slurred speech; drowsiness; poor concentration; progressive respiratory depression.

B. *Withdrawal symptoms:*

1. *Narcotics* (e.g., heroin): begin within 12 hours of last dose, peak in 24 to 36 hours, subside in 72 hours, and disappear in 5 to 6 days.
   a. Pupil *dilation.*
   b. Muscle: twitches, tremors, aches, pains.
   c. Gooseflesh (piloerection).
   d. *Lacrimation, rhinorrhea, sneezing, yawning.*
   e. *Diaphoresis,* chills.
   f. Potential for fever.
   g. *Vomiting,* abdominal distress.
   h. Dehydration.
   i. Rapid weight loss.
   j. Sleep disturbance.
2. *Barbiturates:* may be gradual or abrupt ("cold turkey"); latter is dangerous or *life-threatening;* should be hospitalized.
   a. *Gradual* withdrawal reaction from barbiturates:
      (1) Postural hypotension.
      (2) Tachycardia.
      (3) Elevated temperature.
      (4) Insomnia.
      (5) Tremors.
      (6) Agitation, restlessness.
   b. *Abrupt* withdrawal from barbiturates:
      (1) Apprehension.
      (2) Muscular weakness.
      (3) Tremors.
      (4) Postural hypotension.
      (5) Twitching.
      (6) Anorexia.
      (7) *Grand mal seizures* (a.k.a. generalized seizures).
      (8) *Psychosis-delirium.*
3. *Amphetamines:* depression, lack of energy, somnolence.
4. *Marijuana:* psychological dependency includes craving the "high," and irritability without the drug. Physical withdrawal occurs with heavy daily use; symptoms include: insomnia, anxiety, and loss of appetite.

C. *Difference* between alcohol and other abused substances (e.g., opioid).

1. Other abused substances may need to be obtained by illegal means, making it a legal and criminal problem as well as a medical and social problem; *not* so with alcohol abuse and dependency.
2. Opium and its derivatives *inhibit* aggression; whereas alcohol *releases* aggression.
3. As long as the client is on large enough doses to avoid withdrawal symptoms, abuser of narcotics, sedatives, or hypnotics is comfortable and functions well; whereas chronically intoxicated abuser of alcohol *cannot* function normally.

4. Direct physiological effects of long-term opioid abuse and dependence on other abused substances are much *less critical* than those with chronic alcohol dependence.

III. ANALYSIS/NURSING DIAGNOSIS:

A. *Risk for altered physical regulation processes* (cardiac, circulatory, gastrointestinal, sleep pattern disturbance) related to use of mind-altering drugs.

B. *Risk for injury* due to *altered judgment* related to misinterpretation of sensory stimuli and low frustration tolerance.

C. *Altered conduct/impulse processes* related to rebellious attitudes toward authority.

D. *Altered social interaction* (manipulation, dependency) related to hostility and personal insecurity.

E. *Altered feeling states* (denial) related to underlying self-doubt and personal insecurity.

IV. NURSING CARE PLAN/IMPLEMENTATION: generally the same as in treating antisocial personality and alcohol abuse and dependence.

A. Maintain *safety* and optimum level of *physical* comfort. Supportive physical care: vital signs, nutrition, hydration, seizure precautions.

B. *Assist with medical treatment* and offer support and *reality orientation* to reduce feelings of panic.

1. *Detoxification (or dechemicalization)*—give medications according to detoxification schedule.
2. *Withdrawal*—may be gradual (barbiturates, hypnotics, tranquilizers) or abrupt ("cold turkey" for heroin). Observe for symptoms and report immediately.
3. *Methadone (Dolophine)*—person must have been dependent on narcotics at least 2 years and have failed at other methods of withdrawal before admission to program of readdiction by methadone.
   a. *Characteristics:*
      (1) Synthetic.
      (2) Appeases desire for narcotics without producing euphoria of narcotics.
      (3) Given by mouth.
      (4) Distributed under federal control (**N**arcotic **A**ddict **R**ehabilitation **A**ct).
      (5) Given with urinary surveillance.
   b. *Advantages:*
      (1) Prevents narcotic withdrawal reaction.
      (2) Tolerance not built up.
      (3) Person remains out of prison.
      (4) Lessens perceived need for heroin or morphine.

C. *Participation in group therapy—goals:* peer pressure, support, and identification.

D. *Rehabilitation phase:*

1. Refer to halfway house and group living.
2. Support *employment* as therapy (work training).
3. Expand client's *range of interests* to relieve characteristic boredom and stimulus hunger.
   a. Provide *structured* environment and planned routine.
   b. Provide educational therapy (academic and vocational).
   c. Arrange activities to include current events discussion groups, lectures, drama, music, and art appreciation.

E. Achieve role of *stabilizer and supportive* authoritative figure; this can be achieved through frequent, regular contacts with the same client.

F. *Health teaching:* how to cope with pain, fatigue, and anxiety without drugs.

V. EVALUATION/OUTCOME CRITERIA: replaces addictive lifestyle with self-reliant behavior and a plan formulated to maintain a substance-free life.

Anxiety

Anxiety is a subjective warning of danger in which the specific nature of the danger is usually not known. It occurs when a person faces a new, unknown, or untried situation. Anxiety is also felt when a person perceives threat in terms of past experiences. It is a general concept underlying most disease states. In its milder form, anxiety can contribute to learning and is necessary for problem-solving. In its severe form, anxiety can impede a client's treatment and recovery. The general feelings elicited on all levels of anxiety are nervousness, tension, and apprehension.

It is essential that nurses recognize their own sources of anxiety and behavior in response to anxiety, as well as help clients recognize the manifestations of anxiety in themselves.

I. ASSESSMENT:

A. *Physiological* manifestations:

1. Increased heart rate and palpitations.
2. Increased rate and depth of respiration.
3. Increased urinary frequency and diarrhea.
4. Dry mouth.
5. Decreased appetite.
6. Cold sweat and pale appearance.
7. Increased menstrual flow.
8. Increased or decreased body temperature.
9. Increased or decreased blood pressure.
10. Dilated pupils.

B. *Behavioral* manifestations—stages of anxiety **(Fig. 10.6):**

1. *Mild anxiety:*
   a. Increased perception (visual and auditory).
   b. Increased awareness of meanings and relationships.
   c. Increased alertness (notice more).
   d. Ability to use problem-solving process.

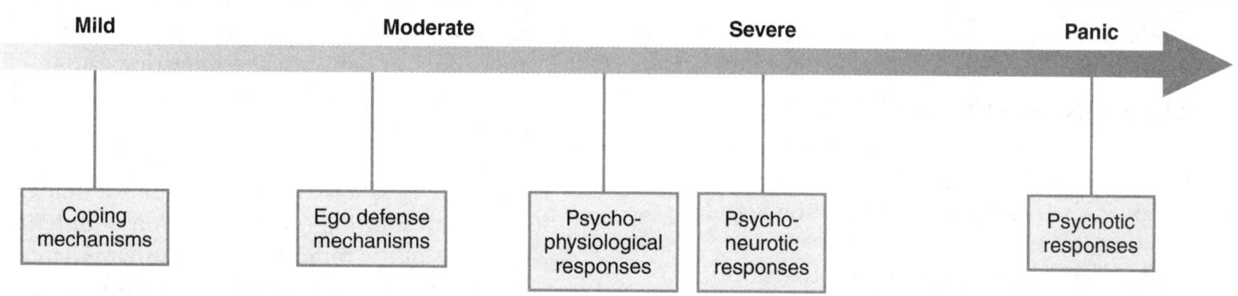

Figure 10.6 Adaptation responses to anxiety on a continuum.

2. *Moderate anxiety:*
   a. Selective inattention (e.g., may not hear someone talking).
   b. Decreased perceptual field.
   c. Concentration on relevant data; "tunnel vision."
   d. Muscular tension, perspiration, GI discomfort.
3. *Severe anxiety:*
   a. Focus on many fragmented details.
   b. Physical and emotional discomfort (headache, nausea, dizziness, dread, horror, trembling).
   c. Not aware of total environment.
   d. Automatic behavior aimed at getting immediate relief instead of problem-solving.
   e. Poor recall.
   f. Inability to see connections between details.
   g. Drastically reduced awareness.
4. *Panic state of anxiety:*
   a. Increased speed of scatter; does not notice what goes on.
   b. Increased distortion and exaggeration of details.
   c. Feeling of terror.
   d. Dissociation (hallucinations, loss of reality, and little memory).
   e. Inability to cope with any problems; no self-control.

C. *Reactions in response to anxiety:*
1. *Fight:*
   a. Aggression.
   b. Hostility, derogation, belittling.
   c. Anger.
2. *Flight:*
   a. Withdrawal.
   b. Depression.
3. *Somatization* (psychosomatic disorder).
4. *Impaired cognition:* blocking, forgetfulness, poor concentration, errors in judgment.
5. *Learning* about or searching for causes of anxiety, and identifying behavior.

II. ANALYSIS/NURSING DIAGNOSIS: *Anxiety related to*:

A. *Physical causes:* threats to biological well-being (e.g., sleep disturbances, interference with sexual functioning, food, drink, pain, fever).

B. *Psychological causes: disturbance in self-esteem* related to:
1. Unmet wishes or expectations.
2. Unmet needs for prestige and status.
3. *Impaired adjustment:* inability to cope with environment.
4. *Altered role performance:* not using own full potential.
5. *Altered meaningfulness:* alienation.
6. *Conflict with social order:* value conflicts.
7. Anticipated disapproval from a significant other.
8. *Altered feeling states: guilt.*

III. NURSING CARE PLAN/IMPLEMENTATION:

A. *Moderate to severe anxiety:*
1. Provide *motor outlet* for tension energy, such as working at a simple, concrete task, walking, crying, or talking.
2. Help clients *recognize* their anxieties by talking about how they are behaving and by exploring their underlying feelings.
3. Help clients *gain insight* into their anxieties by helping them to understand how their behavior has been an expression of anxiety and to recognize the threat that lies behind this anxiety.
4. Help clients *cope* with the threat behind their anxieties by reevaluating the threats and learning new ways to deal with them.
5. *Health teaching:*
   a. Explain and offer hope that emotional pain will decrease with time.
   b. Explain that some tension is normal.
   c. Explain how to channel emotional energy into activity.
   d. Explain need to recognize highly stressful situations and to recognize tension within oneself.

B. *Panic state:*
1. Give simple, clear, *concise* directions.
2. *Avoid* decision making by client. Do *not* try to reason with client, because he or she is irrational and cannot cooperate.
3. *Stay* with client.
   a. Do *not* isolate.
   b. *Avoid* touching.

4. Allow client to seek *motor* outlets (walking, pacing).
5. *Health teaching:* advise activity that requires no thought.

IV. EVALUATION/OUTCOME CRITERIA:

A. Uses more positive thinking and problem-solving activities and is less preoccupied with worrying.
B. Uses values clarification to resolve conflicts and establish realistic goals.
C. Demonstrates regained perspective, self-esteem, and morale; expresses feeling more in control, more hopeful.
D. Fewer or absent physical symptoms of anxiety.

Patterns of Adjustment (Defense Mechanisms)

Defense mechanisms (ego defense mechanisms or mental mechanisms) consist of all the *coping* means used unconsciously by individuals to seek relief from emotional conflict and *to ward off excessive anxiety.*

I. DEFINITIONS

blocking a disturbance in the rate of speech when a person's thoughts and speech are proceeding at an average rate but are suddenly and completely interrupted, perhaps even in the middle of a sentence. The gap may last from several seconds up to a minute. Blocking is often a part of the thought disorder found in *schizophrenic* disorders.

compensation making up for real or imagined handicap, limitation, or lack of gratification in one area of personality by overemphasis in another area to counter the effects of failure, frustration, and limitation (e.g., the person who is blind compensates by increased sensitivity in hearing; the student who is unpopular compensates by becoming an outstanding scholar; men who are small compensate for short stature by demanding a great deal of attention and respect; a nurse who does not have optimal manual dexterity chooses to go into psychiatric nursing).

confabulating filling in gaps of memory by inventing what appear to be suitable memories as replacements. This symptom may occur in various *amnestic disorders* but is most often seen in *Korsakoff's syndrome* (deterioration due to alcohol) and in *dementia.*

conversion psychological difficulties are translated into physical symptoms ***without conscious*** will or knowledge (e.g., pain and immobility on moving your writing arm the day of the examination).

denial an intolerable thought, wish, need, or reality factor is disowned automatically (e.g., a student, when told of a failing grade, acts as if he never heard of such a possibility).

displacement transferring the emotional component from one idea, object, or situation to another, more acceptable one. Displacement occurs because these are painful or dangerous feelings that cannot be expressed toward the original object (e.g., kicking the dog after a bad day at school or work; anger with a clinical instructor gets transferred to a classmate who was late to meet you for lunch).

dissociation splitting off or separation of differing elements of the mind from each other. There can be separation of ideas, concepts, emotions, or experiences from the rest of the mind. Dissociated material is deeply repressed and becomes encapsulated and inaccessible to the rest of the mind. This usually occurs as a result of some very painful experience (e.g., split of affect from idea in *anxiety disorders* and *schizophrenia).*

fixation a state in which personality development is arrested in one or more aspects at a level short of maturity (e.g., "She is anally fixated" [controlling, stingy, holding onto things and memories]).

idealization overestimation of some admired aspect or attribute of another person (e.g., "She was a perfect human being").

ideas of reference fixed, false ideas and interpretations of external events as though they had direct reference to self (e.g., client thinks that TV news announcer is reporting a story about client).

identification the wish to be like another person; situation in which qualities of another are unconsciously transferred to oneself (e.g., boy identifies with his father and learns to become a man; a woman may fear she will die in childbirth because her mother did; a student adopts attitudes and behavior of her favorite teacher).

introjection incorporation into the personality, without assimilation, of emotionally charged impulses or objects; a quality or an attribute of another person is taken into and made part of self (e.g., a girl in love introjects the personality of her lover into herself—his ideas become hers, his tastes and wishes are hers; this is also seen in *severe depression* following death of someone close—client may assume many of deceased's characteristics; similarly, working in a psychiatric unit with a suicidal person brings out depression in the nurse).

isolation temporary or long-term splitting off of certain feelings or ideas from others; separating emotional and intellectual content (e.g., talking emotionlessly about a traumatic accident).

projection attributes and transfers own feelings, attitudes, impulses, wishes, or thoughts to another person or object in the environment, especially when ideas or impulses are too painful to be acknowledged as belonging to oneself (e.g., in *hallucinations* and *delusions* by people who use/abuse alcohol; or,

"I flunked the course because the teacher doesn't know how to teach"; "I hate him" reversed into "He hates me"; or a student impatiently accusing an instructor of being intolerant).

rationalization justification of behavior by formulating a logical, socially approved reason for past, present, or proposed behavior. Commonly used, conscious or unconscious, with false or real reason (e.g., after losing a class election, a student states that she really did not want all the extra work and is glad she lost).

reaction formation going to the opposite extreme from what one wishes to do or is afraid one might do (e.g., being overly concerned with cleanliness when one wishes to be messy; being a mother who is overly protective through fear of own hostility to child; or showing great concern for a person whom you dislike by going out of your way to do special favors).

regression when individuals fail to solve a problem with the usual methods at their command, they may resort to modes of behavior that they have outgrown but that proved successful at an earlier stage of development; retracing developmental steps; going back to earlier interests or modes of gratification (e.g., a senior nursing student about to graduate becomes dependent on a clinical instructor for directions).

repression involuntary exclusion of painful and unacceptable thoughts and impulses from awareness. *Forgetting* these things solves the situation by not solving it (e.g., by not remembering what was on the difficult examination after it was over).

sublimation channeling a destructive or instinctual impulse that cannot be realized into a *socially acceptable,* practical, and less dangerous outlet, with some relation to the original impulse for emotional satisfaction to be obtained (e.g., sublimation of sexual energy into other creative activities [art, music, literature], or hostility and aggression into sports or business competition; or a person who is infertile puts all energies into pediatric nursing).

substitution when individuals cannot have what they wish and accept something else in its place for symbolic satisfaction (e.g., pin-up pictures in absence of sexual object; or a person who failed an RN examination signs up for an LVN/LPN examination).

suppression a deliberate process of blocking from the conscious mind thoughts, feelings, acts, or impulses that are undesirable (e.g., "I don't want to talk about it," "Don't mention his name to me," or "I'll think about it some other time"; or willfully refusing to think about or discuss disappointment with examination results).

symbolism sign language that stands for related ideas and feelings, conscious and unconscious. Used extensively by children, people from primitive cultures, and clients who are psychotic. There is meaning attached to this sign language that makes it very important to the individual (e.g., a student wears dark, somber clothing to the examination site).

undoing a mechanism against anxiety, usually unconscious, designed to negate or neutralize a previous act (e.g., Lady Macbeth's attempt to wash her hands [of guilt] after the murder). A repetitious, symbolic acting out, in reverse of an unacceptable act already completed. Responsible for *compulsions* and magical thinking.

II. CHARACTERISTICS of defense mechanisms:

A. Defense mechanisms are used to some degree by everyone occasionally; they are normal processes by which the ego reestablishes equilibrium—unless they are used to an extreme degree, in which case they interfere with maintenance of self-integrity.

B. Much overlapping:
1. Same behavior can be explained by more than one mechanism.
2. May be used in combination (e.g., isolation and repression, denial and projection).

C. Common defense mechanisms compatible with mental well-being:
1. Compensation.
2. Compromise.
3. Identification.
4. Rationalization.
5. Sublimation.
6. Substitution.

D. Typical defense mechanisms in:
1. *Paranoid disorders*—denial, projection.
2. *Dissociative disorders*—denial, repression, dissociation.
3. *Obsessive-compulsive behaviors*—displacement, reaction formation, isolation, denial, repression, undoing.
4. *Phobic disorders*—displacement, rationalization, repression.
5. *Conversion disorders*—symbolization, dissociation, repression, isolation, denial.
6. *Major depression*—displacement.
7. *Bipolar disorder, manic episode*—reaction formation, denial, projection, introjection.
8. *Schizophrenic disorders*—symbolization, repression, dissociation, denial, fantasy, regression, projection, isolation.
9. *Dementia*—regression.

III. CONCEPTS AND PRINCIPLES RELATED TO DEFENSE MECHANISMS:

A. Unconscious process—defense mechanisms are used as a substitute for more effective problem-solving behavior.

B. *Main functions*—increase *self-esteem; decrease,* inhibit, minimize, alleviate, avoid, or eliminate *anxiety;*

maintain feelings of personal worth and adequacy and soften failures; *protect the ego; increase security.*

C. *Drawbacks*—involve high degree of self-deception and reality distortion; may be maladaptive because they superficially eliminate or disguise conflicts, leaving conflicts unresolved but still influencing behavior.

IV. NURSING CARE PLAN/IMPLEMENTATION with defense mechanisms:

A. Accept defense mechanisms as normal, but not when overused.

B. Look beyond the behavior to the need that is expressed by the use of the defense mechanism.

C. Discuss alternative defense mechanisms that may be more compatible with mental health.

D. Assist the person to translate defensive thinking into nondefensive, direct thinking; a problem-solving approach to conflicts minimizes the need to use defense mechanisms.

Anxiety Disorders (Anxiety and Phobic Neuroses)

I. DEFINITION: emotional illnesses characterized by *fear* and *autonomic nervous system symptoms* (palpitations, tachycardia, dizziness, tremor); related to *intrapsychic conflict* and psychogenic origin where instinctual impulse (related to sexuality, aggression, or dependence) may be in conflict with the ego, superego, or sociocultural environment; related to sudden object loss.

An *anxiety disorder* is a mild to moderately severe functional disorder of personality in which *repressed* inner conflicts between drives and fears are manifested in behavior patterns, including *generalized anxiety* and *phobic, obsessive-compulsive disorders.* (Other related disorders are *dissociative, conversion,* and *hypochondriasis.*)

II. GENERAL CONCEPTS AND PRINCIPLES RELATED TO ANXIETY DISORDERS:

A. Behavior may be an attempt to "bind" anxiety: to *fix* it in some particular area (hypochondriasis) or to *displace* it from the rest of personality (phobic, conversion, and dissociative disorders—amnesia, fugue, obsessive-compulsive disorders).

B. *Purpose of symptoms:*

1. To intensify *repression* as a defense.
2. To exhibit some repressed content in *symbolic* form.

III. GENERAL ASSESSMENT OF ANXIETY DISORDERS:

A. Uses behavior to *avoid* tense situations.

B. Frightened, suggestible.

C. Prone to *minor* physical complaints (e.g., fatigue, headaches, and indigestion) and reluctance to admit recovery from physical illnesses.

D. Attitude of martyrdom.

E. Often feels helpless, insecure, inferior, inadequate.

F. Uses *repression, displacement,* and *symbolism* as key defense mechanisms.

Anxiety Disorders

I. *GENERALIZED ANXIETY DISORDER (GAD):*

A. Assessment:

1. Persistent, diffuse, free-floating, painful anxiety for at least 1 month; not supported by imminent threat or danger. More than everyday worry.
2. Motor tension, autonomic hyperactivity.
3. Hyperattentiveness expressed through vigilance and scanning and avoidance, with minimal risk-taking.

B. Analysis/nursing diagnosis:

1. *Anxiety/powerlessness: excessive worry* related to real or perceived threat to security, unmet needs.
2. *Altered attention* related to overwhelming anxiety out of proportion to actual situation.
3. *Fear* related to sudden object loss.
4. *Guilt* related to inability to meet role expectations.
5. *Risk for alteration in self-concept* related to feelings of inadequacy and worries about own competence.
6. *Altered role performance* related to inadequate support system.
7. *Impaired social interaction* related to use of avoidance in tense situations.
8. *Distractibility* related to pervasive anxiety.
9. *Hopelessness* related to feelings of inadequacy.
10. *Sleep pattern disturbance.*

C. Nursing care plan/implementation:

1. Fulfill needs as promptly as possible.
2. Listen attentively.
3. Stay with client.
4. *Avoid* decision making and competitive situations.
5. Promote rest; decrease environmental stimuli.
6. *Health teaching:* teach steps of anxiety reduction.

D. Evaluation/outcome criteria: symptoms are diminished.

II. *PANIC DISORDER:*

A. Assessment:

1. Three acute, terrifying panic attacks within 3-week period, *unrelated* to marked physical exertion, life-threatening situation, presence of organic illness, or exposure to specific phobic stimulus.
2. Discrete periods of apprehension, fearfulness (lasting from few moments to an hour).
3. *Mimics cardiac* disease: dyspnea, chest pain, smothering or choking sensations, palpitations, tachycardia, dizziness, fainting, sweating.

4. Feelings of unreality, paresthesias.
5. Hot, cold flashes and dilated pupils.
6. Trembling, sense of impending doom and death, fear of becoming insane.

B. Analysis/nursing diagnosis:

1. *Ineffective individual coping* related to undeveloped interpersonal processes.
2. *Altered comfort pattern:* distress, anxiety, fear related to threat to security.
3. *Decisional conflict* related to apprehension.
4. *Altered thought processes* related to impaired concentration.

C. Nursing care plan/implementation:

1. Rule out physiological cuases (e.g., myocardial infarction).
2. *Reduce immediate anxiety* to more moderate and manageable levels.
   a. Stay *physically close* to reduce feelings of alienation and terror.
   b. *Communication approach:* calm, serene manner; short, simple sentences; firm voice to convey that nurse will provide external controls.
   c. *Physical environment:* remove to smaller room to minimize stimuli.
3. Provide *motor outlet* for diffuse energy generated at high anxiety levels (e.g., moving furniture, scrubbing floors).
4. Administer *antianxiety medications* as ordered.
5. *Health teaching:* recommend more effective methods of coping; let client know that panic is time-limited and highly treatable.

D. Evaluation/outcome criteria: can endure anxiety while searching out its causes.

III. OBSESSIVE-COMPULSIVE DISORDER:

A. Assessment—chief characteristic: fear that client can harm someone or something.

1. *Obsessions*—recurrent, persistent, unwanted, involuntary, senseless *thoughts, images, ideas,* or *impulses* that may be trivial or morbid (e.g., fear of germs, doubts as to performance of an act, thoughts of hurting family member, death, suicide; vague fear that "something bad may happen" if routine activities are not done "correctly").
2. *Compulsions*—uncontrollable, persistent urge to perform repetitive, stereotyped *behaviors* that provide relief from unbearable anxiety (e.g., hand washing, counting, touching, checking and rechecking doors to see if locked, elaborate dressing and undressing rituals, excessive collecting, always doing things in "sets," avoiding certain numbers).

B. Analysis/nursing diagnosis:

1. *Ineffective individual coping* related to:
   a. *Intellectualization and avoidance* of awareness of feelings.
   b. Limited ability to express emotions (may be disguised or delayed).
   c. Exaggerated feelings of *dependence and helplessness.*
   d. High need to *control* self, others, and environment.
   e. Rigidity in thinking and behavior.
   f. Poor ability to tolerate anxiety and depression.
2. *Social isolation* related to:
   a. Resentment.
   b. Self-doubt.
   c. Exclusion of pleasure.

C. Nursing care plan/implementation:

1. *Accept* rituals permissively (e.g., excessive hand washing); stopping ritual will increase anxiety.
2. *Avoid* criticism or "punishment," making demands, or showing impatience with client.
3. *Allow* extra time for slowness and client's need for precision.
4. *Protect* from rejection by *others.*
5. *Protect* from *self-inflicted* harmful acts.
6. Engage in nursing therapy *after* the ritual is over, when client is most comfortable.
7. *Limit and redirect* client's actions into substitute outlets.
8. *Health teaching:* teach how to prevent health problems related to rituals (e.g., use rubber gloves, hand lotion).

D. Evaluation/outcome criteria: avoids situations that increase tension and thus reduces need for ritualistic behavior as outlet for tension.

IV. PHOBIC DISORDERS—intense, *irrational, persistent* specific fear in response to *external* object, activity, or situation (e.g., *agoraphobia*—fear of being alone or in public places; *claustrophobia*—fear of closed places; *acrophobia*—fear of heights; *simple phobias* such as *mysophobia*—fear of germs; *social phobias:* fear of situations that may be humiliating or embarrassing). *Dynamics: displacement* of anxiety from original source onto avoidable, *symbolic,* external, and specific object (or activity or situation); that is, phobias help person control intensity of anxiety by providing specific object to attach it to, which he or she can then avoid.

A. Assessment: same as for anxiety symptoms; fear that someone or something will harm them.

B. Analysis/nursing diagnosis: *social isolation;* avoidance; irrational *fear* out of proportion to actual danger; *defensive coping* with high need to control self, others, environment.

C. Nursing care plan/implementation: promote psychological and physical calm.

1. *Use systematic desensitization:* never force contact with feared object or situation.
2. *Health teaching:* progressive relaxation, meditation, biofeedback training, or other behavioral conditioning techniques.

MENTAL HEALTH

D. Evaluation/outcome criteria: phobia is eliminated (i.e., able to come into contact with feared object with lessened degree of anxiety).

V. *ACUTE STRESS DISORDER AND POSTTRAUMATIC STRESS DISORDER:*

A. Assessment:

1. *Acute stress disorder:* symptoms occur *within 1 month* of extreme stressor.
2. *Posttraumatic stress disorder (PTSD):* symptoms occur *after* 1 month.
3. Precipitant: severe, threatening, terrifying traumatic event (natural or man-made disaster) that is not an ordinary occurrence (e.g., rape, fire, flood, earthquake, tornado, bombing, torture, kidnapping).
4. Self-report of reexperiencing incident; intrusive memories (e.g., "flashbacks").
5. Numb, unresponsive, detached, estranged reaction to external world (unable to feel tenderness, intimacy).
6. Change in sleep pattern (insomnia, recurrent dreams, nightmares), memory loss, hyperalertness (startle response).
7. Guilt rumination about survival.
8. Avoids activities reminiscent of trauma; phobic responses.
9. Difficulty with task completion and concentration.
10. Depression.
11. Increased irritability may result in unpredictable, explosive outbursts.
12. Impulsive behavior, sudden lifestyle changes.

B. Analysis/nursing diagnosis:

1. *Posttrauma response* related to overwhelming traumatic event.
2. *Anxiety* (severe to panic)/*fear* related to memory of environmental stressor, threat to self-concept, negative self-talk.
3. *Risk for violence directed at self/others* related to a startle reaction, use of drugs to produce a psychic numbing.
4. *Sleep pattern disturbance* related to fear and rumination.
5. *Decisional conflict (impaired decision making)* related to perceived threat to personal values and beliefs.
6. *Guilt* related to lack of social support system.
7. *Altered feeling states:* emotional lability related to diminished sense of control over self and environment.

C. Nursing care plan/implementation:

1. Crisis counseling (listen with concern and empathy).
   a. Ease way for client to *talk out* the experience and express fear.
   b. Help client to become aware and accepting of what happened.
2. *Health teaching:* suggest how to resume concrete activity and reconstruct life with available social, physical, and emotional resources. Help make contact with friends, relatives, and other resources.

D. Evaluation/outcome criteria: can cry and express anger, loss, frustration, and despair; begins process of social and physical reconstruction.

Dissociative Disorders (Hysterical Neuroses, Dissociative Type)

I. ASSESSMENT:

A. *Dissociative amnesia:* partial or total inability to recall the past; occurs during highly stressful events; client may have conscious desire to escape but be unable to accept escape as a solution; uses *repression.*

B. *Dissociative fugue:* client not only forgets but also *flees* from stress.

C. *Dissociative identity disorder:* client exhibits two or more complete personality systems, each very different from the other; alternates from one personality to the other without awareness of change (*one* personality *may* be aware of others); each personality has well-developed emotions and thought processes that are in conflict; uses *repression.*

D. *Depersonalization disorder:* loss of sense of self; feeling of self-estrangement (as if in a dream); fear of going insane.

II. ANALYSIS/NURSING DIAGNOSIS:

A. Sudden *alteration in:*

1. *Memory (short-* and *long-term memory loss:* cannot recall important personal events) related to repression.
2. *Personal and social identity* (amnesia: forgets own identity; becomes another identity) related to intense anxiety, childhood trauma/abuse, threat to physical integrity, underdeveloped ego.

B. *Sensory/perceptual alteration* of external environment related to repression and escapism.

C. *Confusion* related to use of repression.

D. *Spiritual despair* related to conversion of conflict into physical or mental flights.

E. *Altered meaningfulness* (hopelessness, helplessness, powerlessness) related to lack of control over situation.

III. NURSING CARE PLAN/IMPLEMENTATION:

A. *Remove* client from immediate environment to reduce pressure.

B. *Alleviate* symptoms using behavior modification strategies.

C. *Divert* attention to topics other than symptoms (not remembering names, addresses, and events).
D. Encourage *socialization* rather than isolation.
E. *Avoid* sympathy, pity, and oversolicitous approach.
F. *Health teaching:* teach families to avoid reinforcing dissociative behavior; teach client problem-solving, with goal of minimizing stressful aspects of environment.

IV. EVALUATION/OUTCOME CRITERIA: recall returns to conscious awareness; anxiety kept within manageable limits.

Somatoform Disorders

I. MAIN CHARACTERISTIC: involuntary, physical symptoms *without* demonstrable organic findings or identifiable physiological bases; involve psychological factors or nonspecific conflicts.

II. GENERAL ASSESSMENT:

A. *Precipitant:* major emotional, interpersonal stress.
B. Occurrence of secondary gain from illness.

III. GENERAL ANALYSIS/NURSING DIAGNOSIS:

A. *Fear* related to loss of dependent relationships.
B. *Powerlessness* related to chronic resentment over frustration of dependency needs.
C. *Altered feeling states:* inhibition of anger, which is discharged physiologically and is related to control of anxiety.
D. *Impaired judgment* related to denial of existence of any conflicts or relationship to physical symptoms.
E. *Altered role performance:* regression related to not having dependency needs met.

Somatization Disorder

Repeated, multiple, vague or exaggerated physical complaints of several years' duration *without* identifiable physical cause; clients constantly seek medical attention, undergo numerous tests; at risk for unnecessary surgery or drug abuse.

A. Assessment:

1. Onset and occurrence—teen years, more common in women.
2. Reports illness most of life.
   a. *Neuromuscular* symptoms—fainting, seizures, dysphagia, difficulty walking, back pain, urinary retention.
   b. *Gastrointestinal* symptoms—nausea, vomiting, flatus, food intolerance, constipation or diarrhea.
   c. *Female reproductive* symptoms—dysmenorrhea, hyperemesis gravidarum.
   d. *Psychosexual* symptoms—sexual indifference, dyspareunia.
   e. *Cardiopulmonary* symptoms—palpitations, shortness of breath, chest pain.
   f. *Rule out:* multiple sclerosis, systemic lupus erythematosus (SLE), porphyria, hyperparathyroidism.
3. Appears anxious and depressed.

B. Analysis/nursing diagnosis:

1. *Anxiety* (severe) related to threat to security, unmet dependency needs, and inability to meet role expectations.
2. *Self-care deficit* related to development of physical symptoms to escape stressful situations.
3. *Impaired social interaction* related to inability to accept that physical symptoms lack a physiological basis; preoccupation with self and physical symptoms, chronic pain; rejection by others.
4. *Body-image disturbance and altered role performance* related to passive acceptance of disabling symptoms.

Conversion Disorder (Hysterical Neuroses, Conversion Type)

Sudden symptoms of *symbolic* nature developed under *extreme* psychological stress (e.g., war, loss, natural disaster) that *disappear* through hypnosis.

A. Assessment:

1. *Neurological* symptoms—paralysis, aphonia, tunnel vision, seizures, blindness, paresthesias, anesthesias.
2. *Endocrinological* symptoms—pseudocyesis.
3. Hysterical, dependent *personality profile:* exhibitionistic dress and language; self-indulgent; suggestible; impulsive and global impressions and hunches; little capacity to concentrate, integrate, and organize thoughts or plan action or outcomes; little concern for symptoms, despite severe impairment ("la belle indifference").

B. Analysis/nursing diagnosis:

1. Prolonged *loss or alteration of physiological processes* related to severe psychological stress and conflict that results in disuse, atrophy, contractures. *Primary gain*—internal conflict or need is kept out of awareness; there is a close relationship in time between stressor and occurrence of symbolic symptoms.
2. *Impaired social interaction:* chronic sick role related to attention seeking.
3. *Noncompliance* with expected routines related to *secondary gain*—avoidance of upsetting situation, with support obtained from others.
4. *Impaired adjustment* related to *repression* of feelings through somatic symptoms, *regression, denial* and *isolation,* and *externalization.*
5. *Ineffective individual coping* (e.g., daydreaming, fantasizing, superficial warmth and seductiveness related to inability to control symptoms

voluntarily or to explain them by known physical disorder).

Hypochondriasis (Hypochondriacal Neurosis)

Exaggerated concern for one's physical health; *unrealistic* interpretation of signs or sensations as abnormal; *preoccupation with fear* of having serious disease, *despite* medical reassurance of no diagnosis of physical disorder.

A. Assessment:

1. Preoccupation with symptoms: sweating, peristalsis, heartbeat, coughing, muscular soreness, skin eruptions.
2. Occurs in both men and women in adolescence, 30s or 40s, and elders.
3. History of long, complicated shopping for doctors and refusal of mental health care.
4. *Organ neurosis* may occur (e.g., cardiac neurosis).
5. Personality trait: *compulsive.*
6. Prevalence of anxiety and depression.
7. *Controls* relationships through physical complaints.

B. Analysis/nursing diagnosis:

1. *Personal identity disturbance* related to perception of self as ill in order to meet needs for dependency, attention, affection.
2. Displaced *anxiety* related to inability to verbalize feelings.
3. *Fear* related to not being believed.
4. *Powerlessness* related to feelings of insecurity.
5. *Altered role performance:* disruption in work and interpersonal relations related to regression and need gratification through preoccupation with fantasized illness; and related to control over others through physical complaints.

IV. GENERAL NURSING CARE PLANS/IMPLEMENTATION for somatoform disorders:

A. *Long-term goals:*

1. Develop interests *outside* of self. Introduce to new activities and people.
2. Facilitate experiences of increased feelings of *independence.*
3. Increase *reality perception* and *problem-solving ability.*
4. Emphasize *positive* outlook and promote positive thinking. Reassure that symptoms are anxiety related, not a result of physical disease.
5. Develop mature ways for meeting *affection* needs.

B. *Short-term goals:*

1. *Prevent* anxiety from mounting and becoming uncontrollable by recognizing symptoms, for early intervention.
2. *Environment:* warm, caring, supportive interactions; instill hope that anxiety can be mastered.
3. Encourage client to *express* somatic concerns verbally. Encourage awareness of body processes.
4. Provide *diversional* activities.
5. Develop ability to relax rather than ruminate or worry. Help find palliative relief through anxiety reduction (slower breathing, exercise).

C. *Health teaching:*

1. Relaxation training as self-help measures.
2. Increase knowledge of appropriate and correct information on physiological responses that accompany anxiety.

V. GENERAL EVALUATION/OUTCOME CRITERIA:

A. Does not isolate self.
B. Discusses fears, concerns, conflicts that are self-originated and not likely to be serious.
C. Decides which aspects of situation can be overcome and ways to meet conflicting obligations.
D. Looks for things of importance and value.
E. Deliberately engages in new activities other than ruminating or worrying.
F. Talks self out of fears.
G. Decrease in physical symptoms; is able to sleep, feels less restless.
H. Makes fewer statements of feeling helpless.
I. Can freely express angry feelings in *overt* way and not through symptoms.

Other Conditions in which Psychological Factors Affect Medical Conditions (Psychophysiological Disorders)

This group of disorders occurs in various organs and systems, whereby emotions are expressed by affecting body organs.

I. CONCEPTS AND PRINCIPLES RELATED TO PSYCHOLOGICAL FACTORS AFFECTING PHYSICAL CONDITIONS:

A. Majority of organs involved are usually under control of *autonomic* nervous system.
B. Defense mechanisms

1. *Repression or suppression* of unpleasant emotional experiences.
2. *Introjection*—illness seen as punishment.
3. *Projection*—others blamed for illness.
4. *Conversion*—physical symptoms rather than underlying emotional stresses are emphasized.

C. Clients often exhibit the following underlying *needs in excess:*

1. Dependency.
2. Attention.

3. Love.
4. Success.
5. Recognition.
6. Security.

D. Need to distinguish between:

1. Factitious disorders—deliberate, *conscious* exhibit of physical or psychological illness to avoid an uncomfortable situation.
2. *Conversion disorder*—affecting *sensory* and skeletal-muscular systems that are usually under *voluntary* control; generally *non–life-threatening;* symptoms are symbolic solution to anxiety; *no* demonstrable *organic* pathology.
3. *Psychological factors affecting physical condition* (e.g., psychophysiological disorders); under *autonomic* nervous system control; structural *organic* changes; may be life threatening.

E. A *decrease in emotional security* tends to produce an *increase in symptoms.*

F. When treatment is confined to physical symptoms, emotional problems are *not* usually relieved.

II. ASSESSMENT OF PHYSIOLOGICAL FACTORS:

A. Persistent psychological factors may produce structural *organic* changes resulting in *chronic diseases,* which may be *life-threatening* if untreated.

B. *All* body systems are affected:

1. Skin (e.g., pruritus, acne, dermatitis, herpes, psoriasis).
2. Musculoskeletal (e.g., *backache,* muscle cramps).
3. Respiratory (e.g., *asthma,* hiccups, hay fever).
4. Gastrointestinal (e.g., obesity, *ulcers,* ulcerative colitis, irritable bowel syndrome, gastroesophageal reflux disease, constipation, diarrhea, nausea and vomiting).
5. Cardiovascular (e.g., cardiospasm, angina, paroxysmal tachycardia, *migraines,* palpitations, hypertension, coronary heart disease).
6. Genitourinary (e.g., impotence, enuresis, amenorrhea, dysuria, *dysmenorrhea*).
7. Endocrine (e.g., hypoglycemia, hyperglycemia, hyperthyroidism).
8. Nervous system (e.g., general fatigue, anorexia, exhaustion).
9. Cancer.
10. Autoimmune disease (e.g., multiple sclerosis, systemic lupus erythematosus, rheumatoid arthritis).

III. ANALYSIS/NURSING DIAGNOSIS: *ineffective individual coping* related to inappropriate need-gratification through illness (actual illness used as means of meeting needs for attention and affection). Absence of life experiences that gratify needs for attention and affection.

IV. NURSING CARE PLAN/IMPLEMENTATION in disorders in which psychological factors affect physical conditions:

A. *Long-term goal: release* of feelings through verbalization.

B. *Short-term goals:*

1. Take care of *physical* problems during acute phase.
2. *Remove* client from anxiety-producing stimuli.

C. Prompt attention in meeting clients' *basic needs,* to gratify appropriate needs for dependency, attention, and security.

D. Maintain an attitude of *respect and concern;* clients' pains and worries are very real and upsetting to them; do *not* belittle the symptoms. Do *not* say, "There is nothing wrong with you" because emotions do in fact cause somatic disabilities.

E. *Treat organic* problems as necessary, but without undue emphasis (i.e., do *not* reinforce preoccupation with bodily complaints).

F. Help clients *express their feelings,* especially anger, hostility, guilt, resentment, or humiliation, which may be related to such issues as sexual difficulties, family problems, religious conflicts, and job difficulties. Help clients recognize that, when stress and anxiety are not released through some channel such as verbal expression, the body will release the tension through *"organ language."*

G. Provide *outlets* for release of tensions and diversions from preoccupation with physical complaints.

1. Provide social and recreational activities to decrease time for preoccupation with illness.
2. Encourage clients to use physical and intellectual capabilities in constructive ways.

H. *Protect* clients from any disturbing stimuli; help the healing process in the acute phase of illnesses (e.g., myocardial infarct).

I. Help clients feel *in control* of situations and be as independent as possible.

J. Be *supportive;* assist clients to bear painful feelings through a helping relationship.

K. *Health teaching:*

1. Teach how to express feelings.
2. Teach more effective ways of responding to stressful life situations.
3. Teach the family supportive relationships.

V. EVALUATION/OUTCOME CRITERIA: can verbalize feelings more fully.

Schizophrenia and Other Psychotic Disorders

Schizophrenia is a group of interrelated symptoms with a number of common features involving disorders of *mood, thought content, feelings, perception,* and *behavior.* The term means "splitting of the mind," alluding to the discrepancy between the content of *thought processes* and their emotional expression; this should *not* be confused with "multiple personality" (dissociative reaction).

Half of the clients in mental hospitals are diagnosed as schizophrenic; many more with schizophrenic disorder live in the community. The onset of symptoms for this disorder generally occurs between 15 and 27 years of age.

Genetics and neurochemical imbalances of dopamine and serotonin play a significant role in the etiology of schizophrenia. Clients with schizophrenia have larger brain ventricles, and the prefrontal cortex and limbic cortex are not fully developed. Whether the brain structure changes cause the disorder or are a result of the chemical changes that occur with schizophrenia remains unclear. Other causal theories include prenatal exposure to the influenza virus.

I. COMMON SUBTYPES OF SCHIZOPHRENIA (without clear-cut differentiation):

disorganized type disordered, thinking ("word salad"), *inappropriate affect* (blunted, silly), regressive behavior, incoherent speech, preoccupied and withdrawn.

catatonic type disorder of muscle tension, with rigidity, *waxy flexibility, posturing, mutism, violent rage* outbursts, negativism, and frenzied activity. Marked decrease in involvement with environment and in spontaneous movement.

paranoid type disturbed perceptions leading to disturbance in thought content of *persecutory, grandiose,* or hostile nature; *projection* is key mechanism, with religion a common preoccupation.

residual continued difficulty in thinking, mood, perception, and behavior after schizophrenic episode.

undifferentiated type unclassifiable schizophrenic-like disturbance with mixed symptoms of delusions, hallucinations, incoherence, gross disorganization.

II. CONCEPTS AND PRINCIPLES RELATED TO SCHIZOPHRENIC DISORDERS:

A. *General:*

1. *Symbolic* language used expresses life, pain, and progress toward health; all symbols used have meaning.
2. *Physical care* provides media for relationship; nurturance may be initial focus.
3. *Consistency, reliability,* and *empathic* understanding build trust.
4. *Denial, regression,* and *projection* are key defense mechanisms.
5. Felt anxiety gives rise to distorted thinking.
6. Attempts to engage in verbal communication may result in tension, apprehensiveness, and defensiveness.
7. Person *rejects real world* of painful experiences and *creates fantasy* world through illness.

B. *Withdrawal:*

1. Withdrawal from and resistance to forming relationships are attempts to reduce anxiety related to:
   a. Loss of ability to experience satisfying human relationships.
   b. Fear of rejection.
   c. Lack of self-confidence.
   d. Need for protection and restraint against potential destructiveness of *hostile* impulses (toward self and others).
2. *Ambivalence* results from need to *approach* a relationship and need to *avoid* it.
   a. Cannot tolerate swift emotional or physical closeness.
   b. Needs more time than usual to establish a relationship; time to test sincerity and interest of nurse.
3. Avoidance of client by others, especially staff, will reinforce withdrawal, thereby creating problem of mutual withdrawal and fear.

C. *Hallucinations:*

1. It is possible to replace hallucinations with satisfying interactions.
2. Person can relearn to focus attention on real things and people.
3. Hallucinations originate during *extreme* emotional stress when unable to cope.
4. Hallucinations are very real to client.
5. Client will react as the situation is perceived, *regardless* of reality or consensus.
6. Concrete experiences, *not* argument or confrontation, will correct sensory distortion.
7. Hallucinations are *substitutes* for human relations.
8. Purposes served by or expressed in falsification of reality:
   a. Reflection of problem in inner life.
   b. Statement of criticism, censure, self-punishment.
   c. Promotion of self-esteem.
   d. Satisfaction of instinctual strivings.
   e. Projection of unacceptable unconscious content in disguised form.
9. Perceptions *not* as *totally* disturbed as they seem.
10. Client attempts to restructure reality through hallucinations to *protect remaining ego integrity.*
11. Hallucinations may result from a variety of psychological and biological conditions (e.g., extreme fatigue, drugs, pyrexia, organic brain disease).
12. Person who hallucinates needs to feel free to describe his or her perceptions if he or she is to be understood by the nurse.

III. ASSESSMENT OF SCHIZOPHRENIC DISORDERS:

A. Some clinicians prefer to describe signs and symptoms of schizophrenia as "positive" or "negative."

1. **"Positive" symptoms:** reflect an *excess* or distortion of normal functions; are associated with *normal* brain structures on CT scans, with *relatively good* responses to treatment.
   a. *Delusions* (see definitions in **B.** following)
      (1) Persecution.
      (2) Grandeur.
      (3) Ideas of reference.
      (4) Somatic.
   b. *Hallucinations* (see descriptions in **B.** following)
      (1) Auditory.
      (2) Visual.
      (3) Olfactory.
      (4) Gustatory.
      (5) Tactile.
   c. *Disorganized thinking/speech* (see descriptions in **B.** following; see also **Glossary**)
      (1) Associative looseness.
      (2) Clang associations.
      (3) Word salad.
      (4) Incoherence.
      (5) Neologisms.
      (6) Concrete thinking.
      (7) Echolalia.
      (8) Tangentiality.
      (9) Circumstantiality.
   d. *Disorganized behavior*
      (1) Appearance: disheveled.
      (2) Behavior: restless agitated; inappropriate sexual behavior.
      (3) Waxy flexibility.
2. **"Negative" symptoms: four A's** reflect a loss or diminution of normal functions; CT scans often show structural brain abnormalities, with poor response to treatment.
   a. **A***ffective flattening*
      (1) Facial expression: unchanged.
      (2) Eye contact: poor.
      (3) Body language: reduced.
      (4) Emotional expression: diminished.
      (5) Affect: inappropriate.
   b. **A***logia* (poverty of speech)
      (1) Responses: brief, empty.
      (2) Speech: decreased content and fluency.
   c. **A***volition/***A***pathy*
      (1) Grooming/hygiene: impaired.
      (2) Activities: little or no interest (in work or other activities).
      (3) Inability to initiate goal-oriented actions.
   d. **A***nhedonia*
      (1) Absence of pleasure in social activities.
      (2) Diminished interest in intimacy/sexual activities.
   e. *Social withdrawal* (see **C.** following)

B. Eugene Bleuler described four classic and primary symptoms as the **"four A's"**:

1. *Associative looseness*—impairment of logical thought progression, resulting in confused, bizarre, and abrupt thinking. *Neologisms*—making up new words or condensing words into one.
2. *Affect*—exaggerated, apathetic, blunt, flat, inappropriate, inconsistent feeling tone that is communicated through face and body posture.
3. *Ambivalence*—simultaneous, conflicting feelings or attitudes toward person, object, or situation; *need-fear* dilemma.
   a. Stormy outbursts.
   b. Poor, weak interpersonal relations.
   c. Difficulty even with simple decisions.
4. *Autism—withdrawal* from external world; preoccupation with fantasies and idiosyncratic thoughts.
   a. *Delusions*—false, fixed beliefs, not corrected by logic; a defense against intolerable feeling. The two most common delusions are:
      (1) *Delusions of grandeur*—conviction in a belief related to being famous, important, or wealthy.
      (2) *Delusions of persecution*—belief that one's thoughts, moods, or actions are controlled or influenced by strange forces or by others.
   b. *Hallucinations*—false sensory impressions without observable external stimuli.
      (1) *Auditory*—affecting hearing (e.g., hears voices).
      (2) *Visual*—affecting vision (e.g., sees snakes).
      (3) *Tactile*—affecting touch (e.g., feels electric charges in body).
      (4) *Olfactory*—affecting smell (e.g., smells rotting flesh).
      (5) *Gustatory*—affecting taste (e.g., food tastes like poison).
   c. *Ideas of reference*—clients interpret cues in the environment as having reference to them. Ideas *symbolize guilt, insecurity,* and *alienation;* may become delusions, if severe.
   d. *Depersonalization*—feelings of strangeness and unreality about self or environment or both; difficulty in differentiating boundaries between self and environment.

C. *Prodromal or residual symptoms:*
   1. Social isolation, *withdrawal; regression:* **extreme** *withdrawal* and social isolation.
   2. Marked impairment in *role* functioning (e.g., as student, employee).
   3. Markedly *peculiar* behavior (e.g., collecting garbage).
   4. Marked impairment in personal *hygiene.*
   5. *Affect:* blunt, inappropriate.
   6. *Speech:* vague, overelaborate, circumstantial, metaphorical.
   7. *Thinking:* bizarre ideation or magical thinking (e.g., ideas of reference, "others can feel my feelings").
   8. Unusual *perceptual* experiences (e.g., sensing the presence of a force or person not physically there).

D. Rule out general medical conditions/substances that may cause psychotic symptoms.
   1. *Neurological* conditions: neoplasms, cardiovascular disease, epilepsy, Huntington's disease, deafness, migraine headaches, CNS infections.
   2. *Endocrine* conditions: hypothyroidism or hyperthyroidism, hypoparathyroidism or hyperparathyroidism, hypoadrenocorticism.
   3. *Metabolic* conditions: hypoxia, hypoglycemia, hypercarbia.
   4. *Autoimmune* disorders: SLE.
   5. *Other conditions:* hepatic or renal disease.
   6. *Substances: drugs of abuse* (alcohol, amphetamines, cannabis, cocaine, hallucinogens, inhalants); anesthetics; chemotherapeutic agents; corticosteroids; *toxins* (nerve gases, carbon monoxide, carbon dioxide, fuel or paint, insecticides).

IV. ANALYSIS/NURSING DIAGNOSIS:

A. *Sensory/perceptual alterations* related to inability to define reality and distinguish the real from the unreal (hallucinations, illusions) and misinterpretation of stimuli, disintegration of ego boundaries.

B. *Altered thought processes* related to intense anxiety and blocking (delusions), ambivalence or conflict.

C. *Risk for violence to self or others* related to fear and distortion of reality.

D. *Altered communication process* with inability to *verbally* express needs and wishes related to difficulty with processing information and unique patterns of speech.

E. *Self-care deficit* with *inappropriate* dress and poor physical hygiene related to perceptual or cognitive impairment or immobility.

F. *Altered feeling states* related to anxiety about others (*inappropriate emotions*).

G. *Altered judgment* related to lack of trust, fear of rejection, and doubts regarding competence of others.

H. *Altered self-concept* related to *feelings of inadequacy* in coping with the real world.

I. *Body-image disturbance* related to inappropriate use of defense mechanisms.

J. *Disorganized behaviors:* impaired relatedness to others, related to withdrawal, distortions of reality, and lack of trust.

K. *Diversional activity deficit* related to personal ambivalence.

V. NURSING CARE PLAN/IMPLEMENTATION IN SCHIZOPHRENIC DISORDERS:

A. *General:*
   1. Set *short-term* goals, realistic to client's levels of functioning.
   2. Use *nonverbal* level of communication to demonstrate concern, caring, and warmth, because client often distrusts words.
   3. Set climate for free expression of *feelings* in whatever mode, without fear of retaliation, ridicule, or rejection.
   4. Seek client out in his or her own fantasy world.
   5. Try to understand meaning of symbolic language; help client to communicate less symbolically.
   6. Provide *distance,* because client needs to feel safe and to observe nurses for sources of threat or promises of security.
   7. Help client tolerate nurses' presence and learn to *trust* nurses enough to move out of isolation and share painful and often unacceptable (to client) feelings and thoughts.
   8. Anticipate and accept negativism; do *not* personalize.
   9. *Avoid* joking, abstract terms, and figures of speech when client's thinking is literal.
   10. Give antipsychotic medications.

B. *Withdrawn behavior:*
   1. *Long-term goal:* develop satisfying interpersonal relationships.
   2. *Short-term goal:* help client feel safe in *one-to-one* relationship.
   3. Seek client out at every chance, and establish some bond.
      a. Stay with client, in silence.
      b. Initiate talk when he or she is ready.
      c. Draw out, but do *not* demand, response.
      d. Do *not* avoid the client.
   4. Use *simple language, specific words.*
   5. Use an *object or activity* as medium for relationship; initiate activity.
   6. Focus on *everyday* experiences.
   7. *Delay* decision making.
   8. *Accept one-sided* conversation, with silence from the client; *avoid* pressuring to respond.

9. Accept the client's outward attempts to respond and inappropriate social behavior, without remarks or disdain; teach social skills.
10. *Avoid* making demands on client or exposing client to failure.
11. *Protect* from persons who are aggressive and from impulsive attacks on self and others.
12. Attend to *nutrition, elimination, exercise,* hygiene, and signs of physical illness.
13. Add structure to the day; tell him or her, "This is your 9 a.m. medication."
14. *Health teaching:* assist family to understand client's needs, to see small sign of progress; teach client to perform simple tasks of self-care to meet own biological needs.

C. *Hallucinatory behavior:*

1. *Long-term goal:* establish satisfying relationships with *real* persons.
2. *Short-term goal:* interrupt *pattern* of hallucinations.
3. Provide a *structured* environment with routine activities. Use *real* objects to keep client's interest or to stimulate new interest (e.g., in painting or crafts).
4. *Protect* against injury to self and others resulting from "voices" client thinks he or she hears.
5. *Short, frequent* contacts initially, increasing social interaction gradually (one person → small groups).
6. Ask person to describe experiences as hallucinations occur.
7. *Respond to anything real* the client says (e.g., with acknowledgment or reflection). Focus more on *feelings,* not on delusional, hallucinatory content.
8. *Distract* client's attention to something real when he or she hallucinates.
9. *Avoid* direct confrontation that voices are coming from client himself or herself; do *not* argue, but listen.
10. *Clarify* who "they" are:
    a. Use personal pronouns, *avoid* universal and global pronouns.
    b. Nurse's own language must be clear and unambiguous.
11. Use one sentence, ask only one question, at a time.
12. Encourage *consensual validation.* Point out that experience is not shared by you; voice doubt.
13. *Health teaching:*
    a. Recommend more effective ways of coping (e.g., consensual validation).
    b. Advise that highly emotional situations be avoided.
    c. Explain the causes of misperceptions.
    d. Recommend methods for reducing sensory stimulation.

VI. EVALUATION/OUTCOME CRITERIA:

A. Small behavioral changes occur (e.g., eye contact, better grooming).
B. Evidence of beginning trust in nurse (keeping appointments).
C. Initiates conversation with others; participates in activities.
D. Decreases amount of time spent alone.
E. Demonstrates appropriate behavior in public places.
F. Articulates relationship between feelings of discomfort and autistic behavior.
G. Makes positive statements.

Delusional (Paranoid) Disorders

Paranoid disorders have a concrete and pervasive delusional system, usually *persecutory. Projection* is a chief defense mechanism of this disorder.

I. CONCEPTS AND PRINCIPLES RELATED TO PARANOID DISORDERS:

A. Delusions are attempts to cope with stresses and problems.
B. May be a means of allegorical or symbolic communication and of testing others for their trustworthiness.
C. Interactions with others and activities interrupt delusional thinking.
D. To establish a rational therapeutic relationship, gross distortions, misorientation, misinterpretation, and misidentification need to be overcome.
E. People with delusions have extreme need to maintain self-esteem.
F. False beliefs cannot be changed without first changing experiences.
G. A delusion is held because it *performs a function.*
H. When people who are experiencing delusions become at ease and comfortable with people, delusions will not be needed.
I. Delusions are misjudgments of reality based on a series of mental mechanisms: (a) *denial,* followed by (b) *projection* and (c) *rationalization.*
J. There is a *kernel of truth* in delusions.
K. Behind the anger and suspicion in a person who is paranoid, there is a person who is *lonely* and *terrified* and who *feels vulnerable* and *inadequate.*

II. ASSESSMENT of paranoid disorders:

A. Chronically *suspicious,* distrustful (thinks "people are out to get me").
B. Distant, but *not* withdrawn.
C. Poor insight; blames others (*projects*).
D. Misinterprets and *distorts reality.*
E. Difficulty in admitting own errors; takes pride in intelligence and in being correct (superiority).

F. Maintains false persecutory belief despite evidence or proof (may refuse food and medicine, insisting he or she is poisoned).
G. Literal thinking (*rigid*).
H. Dominating and provocative.
I. Hypercritical and intolerant of others; *hostile,* quarrelsome, and aggressive.
J. *Very sensitive* in perceiving minor injustices, errors, and contradictions.
K. Evasive.

III. ANALYSIS/NURSING DIAGNOSIS:

A. *Altered thought processes* related to lack of insight, conflict, increased fear and anxiety.
B. *Severe anxiety* related to projection of threatening, aggressive impulses and misinterpretation of stimuli.
C. *Ineffective individual coping* (misuse of power and force) related to lack of trust, fear of close human contact.
D. *Impaired cognitive functioning* related to rigidity of thought.
E. *Chronic low self-esteem* related to feelings of inadequacy, powerlessness.
F. *Impaired social interaction* related to lack of tender, kind feelings, feelings of grandiosity or persecution.

IV. NURSING CARE PLAN/IMPLEMENTATION in paranoid disorders:

A. *Long-term goals:* gain clear, correct perceptions and interpretations through corrective experiences.
B. *Short-term goals:*
   1. Help client recognize distortions, misinterpretations.
   2. Help client feel safe in exploring reality.
C. Help client learn to *trust self;* help to develop self-confidence and ego assets through positive reinforcement.
D. Help to *trust others.*
   1. Be consistent and honest at all times.
   2. *Do not whisper, act secretive, or laugh with others* in client's presence when he or she cannot hear what is said.
   3. Do *not* mix medicines with food.
   4. Keep promises.
   5. Let client know ahead of time what he or she can expect from others.
   6. Give *reasons* and careful, complete, and *repetitive* explanations.
   7. Ask permission to contact others.
   8. Consult client first about all decisions concerning him or her.
E. Help to *test reality.*
   1. Present and repeat reality of the situation.
   2. Do *not* confirm or approve distortions.
   3. Help client accept responsibility for own behavior rather than project.
   4. *Divert* from delusions to reality-centered focus.
   5. Let client know when behavior does not seem appropriate.
   6. Assume nothing and leave no room for assumptions.
   7. *Structure* time and activities to limit delusional thought, behavior.
   8. Set limit for *not* discussing delusional content.
   9. Look for underlying needs expressed in delusional content.
F. Provide *outlets* for anger and aggressive drives.
   1. Listen matter-of-factly to angry outbursts.
   2. *Accept* rebuffs and abusive talk as symptoms.
   3. *Do not* argue, disagree, or debate.
   4. *Allow* expression of negative feelings without fear of punishment.
G. Provide *successful group experience.*
   1. *Avoid competitive* sports involving *close physical* contact.
   2. Give recognition to skills and work well done.
   3. Use *managerial* talents.
   4. Respect client's intellect and engage him or her in activities with others requiring *intellect* (e.g., chess, puzzles, Scrabble).
H. *Limit* physical contact.
I. *Health teaching:* teach a more rational basis for deciding whom to trust by identifying behaviors characteristic of trusting and people who are trustworthy.

V. EVALUATION/OUTCOME CRITERIA: able to differentiate people who are trustworthy from untrustworthy; growing self-awareness, and able to share this awareness with others; accepting of others without need to criticize or change them; is open to new experiences; able to delay gratification.

Personality Disorders

Subtypes of personality disorders include *borderline, paranoid, schizoid, schizotypal, obsessive-compulsive, antisocial, histrionic, narcissistic, avoidant,* and *dependent personalities.* A *personality disorder* is a syndrome in which the person's inner difficulties are revealed through general behaviors and by a pattern of living that seeks *immediate gratification of impulses* and instinctual needs without regard to society's laws, mores, and customs and *without censorship* of personal conscience. *Borderline* and *antisocial personality* disorders are the most significant in interactions with the nurse.

Borderline personality disorder is a subtype in which the client is unstable in many areas: she or he has unstable but intense interpersonal relationships, *impulsive* and unpredictable behavior, wide *mood swings,* chronic feelings of boredom or emptiness, intolerance of being alone, and uncertainty about identity, and is physically *self-damaging.*

I. CONCEPTS AND PRINCIPLES RELATED TO ANTISOCIAL PERSONALITY DISORDERS:

A. One defense against severe anxiety is "acting out," or dealing with distressful feelings or issues through action.

B. Faulty or arrested emotional development in preoedipal period has interfered with development of adequate social control or superego.

C. Because there is a malfunctioning or *weakened superego,* there is little internal demand and therefore no tension between ego and superego to evoke guilt feelings.

D. The defect is *not* intellectual; person shows *lack of moral responsibility, inability to control emotions* and impulses, and *deficiency in normal feeling* responses.

E. "Pleasure principle" is dominant.

F. Initial stage of treatment is most crucial; treatment situation is very threatening because it mobilizes client's anxiety, and client ends treatment abruptly. Key underlying emotion: *fear of closeness,* with threat of *exploitation, control,* and *abandonment.*

II. ASSESSMENT of antisocial personality disorders:

A. Onset *before* age 15.

B. History of behavior that *conflicts with society:* truancy, expulsion, or suspension from school for misconduct; delinquency, thefts, vandalism, running away from home; persistent lying; repeated substance abuse; initiating fights; fire starting and cruelty to animals; chronic violation of rules at home or school; school grades below IQ level.

C. Inability to sustain consistent *work* behavior (e.g., frequent job changes or absenteeism).

D. Lack of ability to function as parent who is *responsible* (evidence of child's malnutrition or illness due to lack of minimal hygiene standards; failure to obtain medical care for child who is seriously ill; failure to arrange for caregiver when parent is away from home).

E. Failure to accept *social norms* with respect to *lawful* behavior (e.g., thefts, multiple arrests).

F. Inability to maintain enduring *intimate* relationship (e.g., multiple relations, desertion, multiple divorces); lack of respect or loyalty.

G. *Irritability* and *aggressiveness* (spouse, child abuse; repeated physical fights).

H. Failure to honor *financial* obligations.

I. Failure to *plan ahead.*

J. *Disregard for truth* (lying, "conning" others for personal gain).

K. *Recklessness* (driving while intoxicated, recurrent speeding).

L. *Violating* rights of others.

M. Does not appear to profit from experience; *repeats* same punishable or antisocial behavior; usually does not feel guilt or depression.

N. Exhibits *poor judgment;* may have intellectual, but not emotional, insight to guide judgments. Inadequate problem-solving and reality testing.

O. Uses *manipulative* behavior patterns in treatment setting (see **VIII. Manipulation, pp. 745–747**).

1. Demands and controls.
2. Pressures and coerces, threatens.
3. Violates rules, routines, procedures.
4. Requests special privileges.
5. Betrays confidences and lies.
6. Ingratiates.
7. Monopolizes conversation.

III. ANALYSIS/NURSING DIAGNOSIS in personality disorders:

A. *Ineffective individual coping* related to:

1. Inability to tolerate frustration (altered conduct/impulse processes).
2. Verbal, nonverbal manipulation (*lying*).
3. Destructive behavior toward self (e.g., in borderline personality disorder) or others.
4. Cognitive distortions (e.g., overuse of denial, projection, rationalization, intellectualization, persecutory thoughts).
5. Inability to learn from experience.

B. *Personal identity disturbance* related to:

1. *Self-esteem disturbance* as evidenced by grandiosity, depression, extreme mood changes.
2. Lack of: responsibility, accountability, commitment, tolerance of rejection.
3. Distancing relationships.

C. *Social intrusiveness* related to fear of real or potential loss.

D. *Noncompliance* related to excess need for independence.

IV. NURSING CARE PLAN/IMPLEMENTATION in personality disorders:

A. *Long-term goal:* help person accept responsibility and consequences of own actions.

B. *Short-term goal: minimize manipulation* and acting out.

C. Set *fair, firm, consistent limits and follow through on consequences* of behavior; let client know what she or he can expect from staff and what the unit's regulations are, as well as the consequences of violations. Be explicit.

D. *Avoid* letting staff be played against one another by a particular client; staff should present a unified approach.

E. Nurses should *control* their *own* feelings of anger and defensiveness aroused by any person's manipulative behavior.

F. Change focus when client persists in raising inappropriate subjects (such as personal life of a nurse).

G. Encourage expression of *feelings* as an alternative to acting out.

H. Aid client in realizing and accepting responsibility for own actions and *social responsibility* to others.

I. Use group therapy as a means of *peer control* and multiple feedback about behavior.

J. *Health teaching:* teach family how to use behavior modification techniques to reward client's acceptable behavior (i.e., when he or she accepts responsibility for own behavior, is responsive to rights of others, adheres to social and legal norms).

V. EVALUATION/OUTCOME CRITERIA: less use of lying, blaming others for own behavior; more evidence of following rules; less impulsive, explosive behavior.

Mood Disorders

Mood disorders include (1) *depressive disorders* and (2) *bipolar disorders.* Bipolar disorders are further divided into (a) *manic,* (b) *depressed,* (c) *mixed,* or (d) *cyclothymia.* The mood disturbance may occur in a number of patterns of severity and duration, alone or in combination, where client feels extreme sadness and guilt, withdraws socially, expresses self-deprecatory thoughts (*major depression*), or experiences an elevated, expansive mood with hyperactivity, pressured speech, inflated self-esteem, and decreased need for sleep (*manic episode or disorder*).

Another specific mood disorder is *dysthymic* disorder (depressive neuroses), in which there is a chronic mood disturbance involving a depressed mood or loss of interest and pleasure in all usual activities, but not of sufficient severity or duration to be classified as a *major depressive episode.* **Table 10.12** *summarizes* the main points of *difference between the two types of depression.*

These affective disorders should be *distinguished from grief.* Grief is *realistic* and proportionate to what has been *specifically* lost and involves *no loss of self-esteem.* There is a *constant* feeling of sadness over a period of 3 to 12 months or longer, with good reality contact (no delusions) (see **Fig. 10.3** comparing normal grief reaction and symptoms of clinical depression).

Major Depressive Disorder

I. CONCEPTS AND PRINCIPLES:

A. Self-limiting factors—most depressions are self-limiting disturbances, making it important to look for a change in functioning and behavior.

B. *Theories of cause of depression:*

1. Aggression turned inward—*self-anger.*
2. Response to separation or object *loss.*
3. *Genetic* or *neurochemical* basis—impaired neurotransmission system, especially serotonin regulation.
4. *Cognitive*—negative mindset of hopelessness toward self, world, future; overgeneralizes; focuses on single detail rather than whole picture; draws conclusions on inadequate evidence.
5. *Personality*—negative self-concept, low self-esteem affects belief system and appraisal of stressors; ambivalence, guilt, feeling of failure.

Table 10.12

Comparison of the Two Different Types of Depressive Disorders

Dimension	Major Depressive Disorder—Melancholic Type	Dysthymic Disorder
Cause	Primary disturbance in structure and function of brain and nervous system	Severe, prolonged stress, unresolved conflicts; chronic anxiety, fears, anger
Onset	Rapid and *without* apparent cause	Gradual
Form of depression	Restlessness and agitation, *or* psychomotor retardation; severe; tends to be *worse in morning* and better in evening	Mixed; mild to severe; unpredictable mood; usually optimistic in morning and *depressed in evening*
Sleep	Insomnia after being awakened; early-morning awakening	Easily awakened, but goes back to deep sleep in morning
Appetite	Anorexia leading to weight *loss*	Varied (anorexia leading to compulsive eating)
Activity	Chronically tired; needs structure at all times	Occasional energy bursts (feels embarrassed at lack of energy)
Self-esteem	Very low	Fluctuates from high to low
Fears	Intense fear of being alone	Multiple fears about present and future
Decision making	Totally indecisive	OK on minor decisions; indecisive on important decisions
Memory	Poor	Unreliable
Contact with reality	Poor; paranoid, self-deprecatory delusions, distorted judgment	Varies

6. *Learned helplessness*—dependency; environment cannot be controlled; powerlessness.
7. *Behavioral*—loss of positive reinforcement; lack of support system.
8. *Integrated*—interaction of chemical, experiential, and behavioral variables acting on diencephalon.

C. Levels of depression **(Fig. 10.7).**

II. GENERAL ASSESSMENT:

A. *Physical:* early-morning awakening, *insomnia* at night, increased need for sleep during the day, fatigue, constipation, *anorexia* with weight loss, loss of sexual interest, *psychomotor retardation,* physical complaints, amenorrhea.

B. *Psychological:* inability to remember, decreased *concentration,* slowing or blocking of thought, all-or-nothing thinking, *less interest in* and involvement with external world and own appearance, feeling worse at certain times of day or after any sleep, difficulty in enjoying activities, monotonous voice, *repetitive* discussions, *inability to make decisions* due to ambivalence, impaired coping with practical problems.

C. *Emotional:* loss of self-esteem, feelings of *hopelessness* and *worthlessness,* shame and self-derogation due to *guilt, irritability,* despair and *futility* (leading to *suicidal* thoughts), alienation, *helplessness,* passivity, avoidance, *inertia,* powerlessness, denied anger; uncooperative, tense, crying, demanding, *dependent* behavior, and negativistic.

III. ANALYSIS/NURSING DIAGNOSIS:

A. *Risk for violence* toward self (suicide) related to inability to verbalize emotions.

B. *Sleep pattern disturbance* (insomnia or excessive sleep) related to unresolved fears and anxieties, biochemical alterations (decreased serotonin).

C. *Impaired social interaction/social isolation/withdrawal* related to decreased energy/inertia, inadequate personal resources, absence of significant purpose in life.

D. *Altered nutrition* (anorexia) related to lack of interest in food.

E. *Self-care deficit* related to disinterest in activities of daily living.

F. *Chronic low self-esteem* with self-reproaches and blame related to feelings of inadequacy.

G. *Altered feeling states and meaning patterns* (sadness, loneliness, apathy) related to overwhelming feeling of unworthiness, hopelessness, and *dysfunctional grieving.*

IV. NURSING CARE PLAN/IMPLEMENTATION:

A. Promote sleep and food intake: take nursing measures to ensure the *physical* well-being of the client.

B. Provide steady company to assess *suicidal* tendencies and to diminish feelings of loneliness and alienation.

1. Build trust in a one-to-one relationship.
2. Interact with client on a nonverbal level if that is his or her immediate mode of communication; this will promote feelings of being recognized, accepted, and understood.
3. Focus on *today,* not the past or far into the future.
4. Reassure that present state is temporary and that he or she will be protected and helped.

C. Make the *environment* nonchallenging and nonthreatening.

1. Use a kind, firm attitude, with warmth.
2. See that client has favorite foods; respond to other wishes and likes.
3. Protect from overstimulation and coercion.

D. Postpone client's *decision making* and resumption of duties.

1. Allow *more time* than usual to complete activity (dressing, eating) or thought process and speech.
2. Structure the environment for client to help reestablish a set schedule and predictable *routine* during ambivalence and problems with decisions.

E. *Provide nonintellectual activities* (e.g., sanding wood); *avoid* activities such as chess and crossword puzzles, because thinking capacity at this time tends to be circular.

MENTAL HEALTH

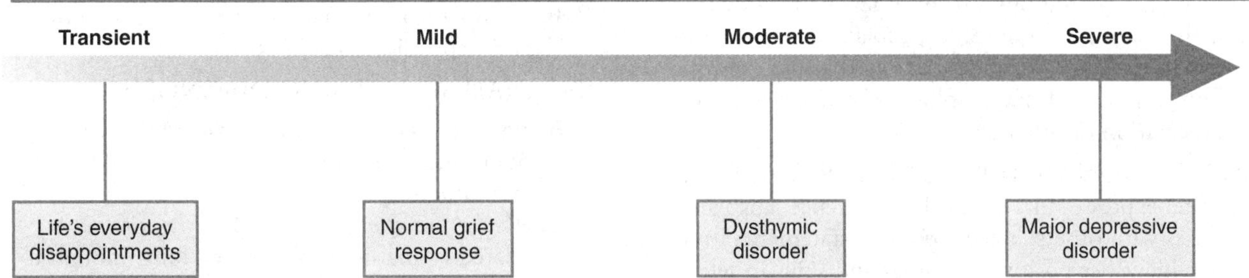

Figure 10.7 Levels of depression.

F. Encourage expression of emotions: denial, hopelessness, helplessness, guilt, regret; provide *outlets for anger* that may be underlying the depression; as client becomes more verbal with anger and recognizes the origin and results of anger, help client resolve feelings—allow client to complain and be *demanding* in initial phases of depression.
G. Discourage *redundancy in speech and thought:* redirect focus from a monologue of painful recounts to an appraisal of more neutral or positive attributes and aspects of situations.
H. Encourage client to *assess own* goals, unrealistic expectations, and perfectionist tendencies.
   1. May need to change goals or give up some goals that are incompatible with abilities and external situations.
   2. Assist client to recapture what was lost through substitution of goals, sublimation, or relinquishment of unrealistic goals—reanchor client's self-respect to other aspects of his or her existence; help him or her free self from *dependency* on one person or single event or idea.
I. Indicate that success is possible and not hopeless.
   1. Explore what steps client has taken to achieve goals and suggest new or alternative ones.
   2. Set *small, immediate goals* to help attain mastery.
   3. Recognize client's efforts to mobilize self.
   4. Provide positive reinforcement for client through exposure to activities in which client can experience a sense of *success, achievement, and completion* to build *self-esteem* and self-confidence.
   5. Help client experience *pleasure;* help client start good relationships in social setting.
J. *Long-term goal:* to encourage interest in external surroundings, outside of self, to increase and strengthen social relationships.
   1. Encourage purposeful activities.
   2. Let client advance to activities at own pace (graded task assignments).
   3. Gradually encourage activities with others.
   4. Cognitive restructuring: changing negative thoughts to positive ones.
K. *Health teaching:* explain need to recognize highly stressful situation and fatigue as stress factor; advise that negative responses from others be regarded with minimum significance; explain need to maintain positive self-attitude; advise occasional respite from responsibilities; emphasize need for realistic expectation of others.

V. EVALUATION/OUTCOME CRITERIA: performs self-care; expresses increased self-confidence; engages in activities with others; accepts positive statements from others; identifies positive attributes and skills in self.

Bipolar Disorders

Bipolar disorders are major emotional illnesses characterized by mood swings, alternating from depression to elation, with periods of relative normality between episodes. Most persons experience a *single* episode of manic or depressed type; some have *recurrent* depression or recurrent mania or *mixed.* There is increasing evidence that a biochemical disturbance may exist and that most individuals with manic episodes eventually develop depressive episodes.

I. CONCEPTS AND PRINCIPLES RELATED TO BIPOLAR DISORDERS:
A. The psychodynamics of manic and depressive episodes are related to hostility and guilt.
B. The struggle between unconscious impulses and moral conscience produces feelings of *hostility, guilt,* and *anxiety.*
C. To relieve the internal discomfort of these reactions, the person *projects* long-retained hostile feelings onto others or onto objects in the environment during *manic* phase; during *depressive* phase, hostility and guilt are *introjected* toward self.
D. Demands, irritability, sarcasm, profanity, destructiveness, and threats are signs of the *projection of hostility;* guilt is handled through *persecutory delusions and accusations.*
E. Feelings of inferiority and fear of rejection are handled by being light and amusing.
F. Both phases, though appearing distinctly different, have the *same objective: to gain attention, approval, and emotional support.* These objectives and behaviors are unconsciously determined by the client; this behavior may be either biochemically determined or *both biochemically* and *unconsciously* determined.

II. ASSESSMENT of bipolar disorders:
A. Manic and depressed types are *opposite* sides of the *same* disorder.
   1. Both are disturbances of mood and self-esteem.
   2. Both have underlying aggression and hostility.
   3. Both are intense.
   4. Both are self-limited in duration.
B. Comparison of behaviors associated with mania and depression (**Table 10.13**).

III. ANALYSIS/NURSING DIAGNOSIS:
A. *Risk for violence directed at others/self* related to poor judgment, impulsiveness, irritability, manic excitement.
B. *Altered nutrition, less than body requirements,* related to inability to sit down long enough to eat, metabolic expenditures.

Table 10.13

Behaviors Associated with Mania and Depression

Mania (Periods of Predominantly and Persistently Elevated, Expansive, or Irritable Mood)	Depression (Loss of Interest or Pleasure in Usual Activities)
Affect	
Lack of shame or guilt; inflated self-esteem; euphoria; intolerance of criticism	Anger, anxiety, apathy, denial, delusions of guilt, helplessness, feelings of doom, hopelessness, loneliness, low self-esteem (self-degradation)
Physiology	
Insomnia; inadequate nutrition, weight loss	Insomnia; anorexia, constipation, indigestion, nausea, vomiting → weight loss
Cognition	
Denial of realistic danger *Thoughts:* flight of ideas, loose associations; illusions, delusions of grandeur; lack of judgment; distractibility	Ambivalence, confusion, inability to concentrate, self-blame; loss of interest and motivation; self-destructive (preoccupied with suicide)
Behavior	
Hyperactivity (social, sexual, work) → irrationality, aggressiveness, sarcasm, exhibitionism, and acting out in behavior and dress Hostile, arrogant, argumentative, demanding, and controlling *Speech:* rapid, rhyming, punning, witty, pressured	Altered activity level, social isolation, substance abuse, overdependency, underachievement, inability to care for self, *psychomotor retardation*

C. *Sleep pattern disturbance:* lack of sleep and rest related to restlessness, hyperactivity, emotional dysfunctioning, lack of recognition of fatigue.
D. *Self-care deficits* related to altered motor behavior due to anxiety.
E. *Sensory/perceptual alterations (overload)* related to endogenous chemical alteration, sleep deprivation.
F. *Altered feeling state* (anger), *judgment, thought content* (magical thinking), *thought processes* (altered concentration and problem-solving) related to disturbance in self-concept.
G. *Altered feeling processes* (mood swings).
H. *Altered attention:* hyperalertness.
I. *Impaired social interaction* related to internal and external stimuli (overload, underload).
J. *Impaired verbal communication:* flight of ideas and racing thoughts.

IV. NURSING CARE PLAN/IMPLEMENTATION:

A. *Manic:*

1. Prevent *physical* dangers stemming from suicide and exhaustion—promote rest, sleep, and intake of nourishment.
   a. Use *suicide* precautions.
   b. Reduce outside stimuli or remove to quieter area.
   c. *Diet:* provide *high-calorie beverages, finger foods* within sight and reach.
2. Attend to client's personal care.
3. Absorb with understanding and without reproach behaviors such as talkativeness, provocativeness, criticism, sarcasm, dominance, profanity, and dramatic actions.
   a. Allow, postpone, or partially fulfill demands and freedom of expression *within limits* of ordinary social rules, comfort, and safety of client and others.
   b. Do *not* cut off manic stream of talk, because this increases anxiety and need for release of hostility.
4. Constructively utilize excessive energies with *activities* that do *not* call for concentration or follow-through.
   a. Outdoor walks, gardening, putting, and ball tossing are therapeutic.
   b. Exciting, disturbing, and highly *competitive* activities should be *avoided.*
   c. Creative occupational therapy activities promote release of hostile impulses, as does creative writing.
5. Give benzodiazepines and/or atypical antipsychotics (e.g., aripiprazole [Abilify]) for rapid stabilization of acute mania, as ordered until lithium affects symptoms *(3 weeks);* then give lithium carbonate as ordered. An anticonvulsant (e.g., valproic acid [Depakote]) may be used as an alternative treatment for mood stabilization.
6. Help client to recognize and express *feelings* (denial, hopelessness, anger, guilt, blame, helplessness).
7. Encourage realistic self-concept.
8. *Health teaching:* how to monitor effects of lithium; instructions regarding salt intake.

B. *Depressed:*

1. Take routine *suicide* precautions.
2. Give attention to *physical* needs for food and sleep and to hygiene needs. Prepare warm baths and hot beverages to aid sleep.
3. Initiate *frequent* contacts:
   a. *Do not allow long periods of silence* to develop or client to remain withdrawn.
   b. Use a kind, understanding, but emotionally neutral approach.

MENTAL HEALTH

4. *Allow dependency* in severe depressive phase. Because dependency is one of the underlying concerns with persons who are depressed, if nurse allows dependency to occur as an initial response, he or she must plan for resolution of the dependency toward himself or herself as an example for the client's other dependent relationships.
5. Slowly repeat simple, direct information.
6. *Assist in daily decision making* until client regains self-confidence.
7. Select *mild* exercise and diversionary *activities* instead of stimulating exercise and competitive games, because they may overtax physical and emotional endurance and lead to feelings of inadequacy and frustration.
8. Give antidepressive drugs.
9. *Health teaching:* how to make simple decisions related to health care.

V. EVALUATION/OUTCOME CRITERIA:

A. *Manic:* speech and activity are slowed down; affect is less hostile; able to sleep; able to eat with others at the table.

B. *Depressed:* takes prescribed medications regularly. Does not engage in self-destructive activities. Able to express feelings of anger, helplessness, hopelessness.

Psychiatric Emergencies*

I. DEFINITION: sudden onset (days or weeks, not years) of unusual (for that individual), disordered (without pattern or purpose), or socially inappropriate behavior caused by emotional or physiological situation. Examples include: suicidal feelings or attempts, overdose, acute psychotic reaction, acute alcohol withdrawal, acute anxiety.

II. GENERAL CHARACTERISTICS:

A. Assessment: the presence of great distress without reasonable explanation; *extreme* behavior in comparison with antecedent event.

1. *Fear*—related to a *particular* person, activity, or place.
2. *Anxiety*—fearful feeling without any obvious reason, *not* specifically related to a particular person, activity, or place (e.g., adolescent turmoil).
3. *Depression*—continual pessimism, easily moved to tears, hopelessness, and isolation (e.g., student despondency around examination time, middle-age crisis, elderly who feel hopelessness).
4. *Mania*—unrealistic optimism.
5. *Anger*—many events seen as deliberate insults.
6. *Confusion*—diminished awareness of who and where one is; memory loss.
7. *Loss of reality contact*—hallucinations or delusion (as in acute psychosis).
8. *Withdrawal*—neglect or giving away of belongings and neglect of appearance; loss of interest in activities; apathy.

B. Analysis/nursing diagnosis: *ineffective individual coping* related to degree of seriousness:

1. *Life-threatening emergencies*—violence toward self or others (e.g., suicide, homicide).
2. *Serious emergencies*—confused and unable to care for or protect self from dangerous situations (as in substance abuse).
3. *Potentially serious emergencies*—anxious and in pain; disorganized behavior; can become worse or better (as in grief reaction).

C. General nursing care plan/implementation:

1. *Remove* from stressful situation and persons.
2. Engage in *dialogue* at a nonthreatening distance, to offer help.
3. Use *calm, slow, deliberate* approach to relieve stress and disorganization.
4. *Explain* what will be done about the problem and the likely outcome.
5. *Avoid* using force, threat, or counterthreat.
6. Use *confident, firm, reasonable* approach.
7. Encourage client to relate.
8. Elicit *details.*
9. Encourage *ventilation* of feelings without interruption.
10. Accept distortions of reality *without arguing.*
11. Give form and *structure* to the conversation.
12. Contact significant others to gain information and to be with client, including previous therapist.
13. Treat emergency as *temporary* and *readily resolved.*
14. Check every half hour if cannot remain with client.

III. CATEGORIES OF PSYCHIATRIC EMERGENCIES:

A. *Acute nonpsychotic reactions,* such as acute anxiety attack or panic reaction (for symptoms, see **Anxiety, p. 770,** and **Anxiety Disorders [Anxiety and Phobic Neuroses], pp. 774–776**).

1. **Assessment** includes differentiating hyperventilation that is anxiety-connected from asthma, angina, and heart disease.
2. **Nursing care plan/implementation** in hyperventilation syndrome—*goal:* prevent paresthesia, tetanic contractions, disturbance in awareness; reassure client that vital organs are not impaired.
   a. Increase CO_2 in lungs by rebreathing from paper bag.
   b. Minimize secondary gains; *avoid* reinforcing behavior.
   c. *Health teaching:* demonstrate how to slow down breathing rate.

*Adapted from Aguilera, D, & Messick, J: *Crisis Intervention,* ed 5. Mosby, St. Louis. (out of print)

3. **Evaluation/outcome criteria:** respirations slowed down; no evidence of effect of hyperventilation.

B. *Delirium*—conditions produced by changes in the cerebral chemistry or tissue by metabolic toxins, direct trauma to the brain, drug effects, or withdrawal.

1. *Acute alcohol intoxication* (see also **Alcohol Use Disorders: Alcohol Abuse and Dependence, pp. 766–769**).
   a. **Assessment:** signs of head or other injury (past and recent), emotional lability, memory defects, loss of judgment, disorientation.
   b. **Nursing care plan/implementation:**
      (1) Observe, monitor *vital signs.*
      (2) *Prevent aspiration* of vomitus by positioning.
      (3) *Decrease* environmental stimuli:
         (a) Place in quiet area of emergency department.
         (b) Speak and handle calmly.
      (4) Give medication (benzodiazepines) to control agitation.
   c. **Evaluation/outcome criteria:** oriented to time, place, person; appears calmer.
2. *Hallucinogenic drug intoxication*—LSD, mescaline, amphetamines (e.g. speed), cocaine, scopolamine, and belladonna.
   a. **Assessment:**
      (1) Perceptual and cognitive distortions (e.g., feels heart stopped beating).
      (2) Anxiety (apprehension → panic).
      (3) Subjective feelings (omnipotence → worthlessness).
      (4) Interrelationship of dose, potency, setting, expectations and experiences of user.
      (5) Eyes: *red*—marijuana; *dilated*—LSD, mescaline, belladonna; *constricted*—heroin and derivatives.
   b. **Nursing care plan/implementation:**
      (1) "Talk down."
         (a) Establish *verbal* contact, attempt to have client verbally express what is being experienced.
         (b) *Environment*—few people, normal lights, calm, supportive.
         (c) Allay fears.
         (d) Encourage to keep eyes *open.*
         (e) Have client focus on *inanimate* objects in room as a bridge to reality contact.
         (f) Use simple, *concrete, repetitive* statements.
         (g) *Repetitively* orient to time, place, and temporary nature.
         (h) Do *not* moralize, challenge beliefs, or probe into lifestyle.
         (i) Emphasize confidentiality.
      (2) *Medication (minor tranquilizer or benzodiazepines):*
         (a) Allay anxiety.
         (b) Reduce aggressive behavior.
         (c) Reduce suicidal potential; check client every 5 to 15 minutes.
         (d) *Avoid* anticholinergic crisis (precipitated by use of phenothiazines, belladonna, and scopolamine ingestion) with 2 to 4 mg IM or PO of physostigmine salicylate.
      (3) *Hospitalization:* if hallucinations, delusions last more than 12 to 18 hours; if client has been injecting amphetamines for extended time; if client is paranoid and depressed.
   c. **Evaluation/outcome criteria:** less frightened; oriented to time, place, person.
3. *Acute delirium*—seen in postoperative electrolyte imbalance, systemic infections, renal and hepatic failure, oversedation, metastatic cancer.
   a. **Assessment:**
      (1) Disorientation regarding time, at night.
      (2) Hallucinations, delusions, illusions.
      (3) Alterations in mood.
      (4) Increased emotional lability.
      (5) Agitation.
      (6) Lack of cooperation.
      (7) Withdrawal.
      (8) Sleep pattern reversal.
      (9) Alterations in food intake.
   b. **Nursing care plan/implementation:**
      (1) Identify and remove *toxic* substance.
      (2) Reality orientation—well-lit room; constant attendance to *repetitively* inform of place and time and to *protect* from injury to self and others.
      (3) Simplify environment.
      (4) *Avoid* excessive medication and restraints; use low-dose phenothiazines; do *not* give barbiturates or sedatives (these increase agitation, confusion, disorientation).
   c. **Evaluation/outcome criteria:** oriented to time, place, person; cooperative; less agitated.

C. *Acute psychotic reactions*—disorders of mood or thinking characterized by hallucinations, delusions, excessive euphoria (mania), or depression.

1. *Acute schizophrenic reaction* (see also **Schizophrenia and Other Psychotic Disorders, pp. 779–783**).
   a. **Assessment:**
      (1) History of previous hospitalization, illicit drug ingestion; use of major tranquilizers and recent withdrawal from them or alcohol.
      (2) Auditory hallucinations and delusions.
      (3) Violent, assaultive, suicidal behavior directed by auditory hallucinations.

MENTAL HEALTH

(4) Assault, withdrawal, and panic related to paranoid delusions of persecution; fear of harm.
(5) Disturbance in mental status (associative thought disorder).

b. **Nursing care plan/implementation** (see also **II. C. Hallucinations, p. 780):**
(1) Hospitalization.
(2) Medication: phenothiazines or atypical antipsychotics.
(3) *Avoid* physical restraints or touch when fears and delusions of sexual attack exist.
(4) Allow client to *diffuse* anger and intensity of panic through talk.
(5) Use simple, *concrete* terms, *avoid* figures of speech or content subject to multiple interpretations.
(6) Do *not* agree with reality distortions; point out that client's thoughts are difficult to understand but you are willing to listen.

c. **Evaluation/outcome criteria:** does not hear frightening voices; less fearful and combative behavior.

2. *Manic reaction* (see also **Bipolar Disorders, pp. 788–790**).

a. **Assessment:**
(1) History of depression requiring antidepressants.
(2) *Thought disorder* (flight of ideas, delusions of grandeur).
(3) *Affect* (elated, irritable, irrational anger).
(4) *Speech* (loud, pressured).
(5) *Behavior* (rapid, erratic, chaotic).

b. **Nursing care plan/implementation:**
(1) Hospitalization to protect from injury to self and others.
(2) Medication: *lithium carbonate.* An atypical antipsychotic may be used as an adjunct medication for acute mania.
(3) Same as for acute schizophrenic reaction, *except do not encourage talk,* because of need to decrease stimulation.
(4) Provide food and fluids that can be consumed while "on the go."

c. **Evaluation/outcome criteria:** speech and activity slowed down; thoughts less disordered.

D. *Homicidal or assaultive reaction*—seen in acutely drug-intoxicated, delirious, paranoid, acutely excited manic, or acute anxiety-panic conditions.

1. **Assessment:** history of obvious antisocial behavior, paranoid psychosis, previous violence, sexual conflict, rivalry, substance abuse, recent moodiness, and withdrawal.

2. **Nursing care plan/implementation:**
a. Physically restrain if client has a weapon; use group of trained people to help.
b. Allow person to "save face" in giving up weapon.
c. *Separate* from intended victims.
d. Approach: calm, unhurried; *one person* to offer support and reassurance; use clear, unambiguous statements.
e. Immediate and rapid admission procedures.
f. Observe for *suicidal* behavior that may follow homicidal attempt.

3. **Evaluation/outcome criteria:** client regains impulse control.

E. *Suicidal ideation*—seen in anxiety attacks, substance intoxication, toxic delirium, schizophrenic auditory hallucinations, and depressive reactions.

1. **Concepts and principles related to suicide:**

a. *Based on social theory:* suicidal tendency is a result of collective social forces rather than isolated individual motives (Durkheim's *Le Suicide*).
(1) Common factor: increased *alienation* between person and social group; psychological isolation, called "anomie," when links between groups are weakened.
(2) "Egoistic" suicide: results from lack of integration of individual with others.
(3) "Altruistic" suicide: results from insufficient individualization.
(4) *Implication:* increase group cohesiveness and mutual interdependence, making group more coherent and consistent in fulfilling needs of each member.

b. *Based on symbolic interaction theory:*
(1) Person evaluates self according to *others' assessment.*
(2) Thus, suicide stems from *social rejection* and disrupted social relations.
(3) Perceived failure in relationships with others may be inaccurate but seen as real by the individual.
(4) *Implication:* need to recognize difference in perception of alienation between own viewpoint and those of others.

c. *Based on psychoanalytic theory:*
(1) Suicide stems mainly from the individual, with external events only as precipitants.
(2) There is a strong life urge in people.
(3) *Universal death instinct* is always present (Freud).
(4) Person may be balancing life wishes and death wishes. When self-preservation instincts are diminished, death instincts may find direct outlet via suicide.
(5) When *love instinct* is frustrated, *hate* impulse takes over (Menninger).
(a) Desire to kill → desire to be killed → desire to kill oneself.

(b) Suicide may be an act of extreme hostility, manipulation, and revenge to elicit guilt and remorse in significant others.
(c) Suicide may also be act of self-punishment to handle own guilt or to control fate.

d. *Based on synthesis of social and psychoanalytic theories:*
(1) Suicide is seen as *running away* from an intolerable situation to interrupt it, rather than *running to* something more desirable.
(2) Process *defined in operational terms* involves:
(a) Despair over inability to cope.
(b) Inability to feel hope or adequacy.
(c) Frustration with others when others cannot fill needs.
(d) Rage and aggression experienced toward significant other is turned inward.
(e) Psychic blow acts as precipitant.
(f) Life seen as harder to cope with, with no chance of improvement in life situation.
(g) *Implication:* persons who experience suicidal impulses can gain a certain amount of control over these impulses through the support they gain from meaningful relationships with others.

e. *Based on crisis theory (Dublin):* concept of emotional disequilibrium:
(1) Everyone at some point in life is in a crisis, with temporary inability to solve problems or to master the crisis.
(2) Usual coping mechanisms do not function.
(3) Person unable to relate to others.
(4) Person searches consciously and unconsciously for useful coping techniques, with suicide as one of various solutions.
(5) With inadequate communication of needs and isolation, suicide is possible.

f. *Based on the view that suicide is an individual's personal reaction and decision, a final response to own situation:*
(1) *Process* of anger turned inward → self-inflicted, destructive action.
(2) *Definition* of concept in operational steps:
(a) Frustration of individual needs → anger.
(b) Anger turned inward → feelings of guilt, despair, depression, incompetence, hopelessness, and exhaustion.
(c) Stress felt and perceived as unbearable and overwhelming.
(d) Attempt to communicate hopelessness and defeat to others.
(e) Others do not provide hope.
(f) Sudden change in behavior, as noted when depression appears to lift, may indicate *danger,* as person has more energy to act on suicidal thoughts and feelings.
(g) Decision to end life → plan of action → self-induced, self-destructive behavior.
(3) May be *pseudosuicide* attempts, where there is no actual or realistic desire to achieve finality of death. Intentions or causes may be:
(a) "Cry for help," where nonlethal attempt notifies others of deeper intentions.
(b) Desire to *manipulate* others.
(c) Need for *attention and pity.*
(d) Self-punishment.
(e) Symbol of *utter frustration.*
(f) Wish to *punish* others.
(g) *Misuse* of alcohol and other drugs.
(4) Other reasons for self-destruction, where the individual *gives his or her life* rather than takes it, include:
(a) Strong parental love that can overcome fear and instinct of self-preservation to save child's life.
(b) "Sacrificial death" during war, such as kamikaze pilots in World War II.
(c) Submission to death for religious beliefs (martyrdom).

2. **Assessment of suicide:**
a. *Assessment of risk regarding statistical probability of suicide—composite picture:* male, older than 45 years, unemployed, divorced, living alone, depressed (weight loss, somatic delusions, sleep disturbance, preoccupied with suicide), history of substance abuse and suicide within family.
b. Eleven *factors* to predict potential suicide and assess risk:
(1) *Age, sex, and race*—teenage and young adult (ages 15 to 24), older age; more women make attempts; more men complete suicide act. *Highest risk:* older women rather than young boys; older men rather than young girls. Suicide occurs in all races and socioeconomic groups.
(2) *Recent stress* related to *loss*—family problems: death, divorce, separation, alienation; financial pressures; loss of job; loss of status; failing grades.
(3) *Clues to suicide:* suicidal thoughts are usually time limited and do not last forever. Early assessment of behavioral and verbal clues is important.*
(a) *Verbal clues—direct:* "I am going to shoot myself." *Indirect:* "It's more

*Adapted from the *classic* article in *Am J Nurs* 65(5).

MENTAL HEALTH

than I can bear." *Coded:* "This is the last time you'll ever see me." "I want you to have my coin collection."

(b) *Behavioral clues—direct:* trial run with pills or razor, for example. *Indirect:* sudden lifting of depression, buying a casket, giving away cherished belongings, putting affairs in order, writing a will.

(c) *Syndromes—dependent-dissatisfied:* emotionally dependent but dislikes dependent state, irritable, helpless. *Depressed:* detachment from life; feels life is a burden; hopelessness, futility. *Disoriented:* delusions or hallucinations, confusion, delirium tremens, organic brain syndromes. *Willful-defiant:* active need to direct and control environment and life situation, with low frustration tolerance and rigid mind-set, rage, shame.

(4) *Suicide plan*—the *more details* about method, timing, and place, and preoccupation with thoughts of suicide plan, the *higher* the risk.

(5) *Previous suicidal behavior*—history of prior attempt increases risk. Eight out of 10 suicide attempts give verbal and behavioral warnings as listed previously.

(6) *Medical and psychiatric status*—chronic ailments, terminal illness, and pain increase suicidal risk; people with bipolar disorder, and when emerging from depression.

(7) *Communication*—the more disorganized thinking, anxious, hostile, and withdrawn and apathetic, the greater the potential for suicide, unless extreme psychomotor retardation is present.

(8) *Style of life*—high risks include *substance abusers*, those with sexual identity conflicts, unstable relationships (personal and job related). Suicidal tendencies are not inherited but learned from family and other interpersonal relationships.

(9) *Alcohol*—can reinforce helpless and hopeless feelings; may be *lethal* if *used with barbiturates;* can decrease inhibitions, result in impulsive behavior.

(10) *Resources*—the *fewer* the resources, the *higher* the suicide potential. Examples of resources: family, friends, colleagues, religion, pets, meaningful recreational outlets, satisfying employment.

(11) *Stigma*—unwilling to seek help because of stigma attached to mental illness, substance abuse, and/or suicidal thoughts.

c. Assess *needs* commonly communicated by individuals who are suicidal:
   (1) To trust.
   (2) To be accepted.
   (3) To bolster self-esteem.
   (4) To "fit in" with groups.
   (5) To experience success and interrupt the failure syndrome.
   (6) To expand capacity for pleasure.
   (7) To increase autonomy and sense of self-mastery.
   (8) To work out an acceptable sexual identity.

3. **Analysis/nursing diagnosis:** *risk for suicide* related to:
   a. Feelings of *alienation.*
   b. Feelings of *rejection.*
   c. Feelings of *hopelessness, despair.*
   d. Feelings of *frustration and rage.*

4. **Nursing care plan/implementation:**
   a. *Long-term goals:*
      (1) Increase client's self-reliance.
      (2) Help client achieve more realistic and positive feelings of self-esteem, self-respect, acceptance by others, and sense of belonging.
      (3) Help client experience success, interrupt failure pattern, and expand views about pleasure.
   b. *Short-term goals:*
      (1) Medical: assist as necessary with gastric lavage; provide respiratory and vascular support; assist in repair of inflicted wounds.
      (2) Provide a safe environment for protection from self-destruction until client is able to assume this responsibility.
      (3) *Allow outward* and *constructive* expression of hostile and aggressive feelings.
      (4) Provide for physical needs.
   c. *Suicide precautions* to institute under emergency conditions:
      (1) One-to-one supervision at *all* times for maximum precautions; check whereabouts every 15 minutes, if on basic suicide precautions.
      (2) Before instituting these measures, explain to client what you will be doing and why; physician must also explain; document this explanation.
      (3) Do *not* allow client to leave the unit for tests, procedures.
      (4) Look through client's *belongings with* the client and remove any potentially harmful objects (e.g., pills, knife, gun, matches, belts, razors, glass, tweezers).
      (5) Allow visitors and phone calls, but maintain one-to-one supervision during visits.

(6) Check that visitors do not leave potentially harmful objects in the client's room.
(7) Serve meals in an isolation meal tray that contains no glass or metal silverware.
(8) Do *not* discontinue these measures without an order.

d. *General approaches:*
(1) *Observe* closely at all times to assess suicide potential.
(2) *Be available.*
(a) Demonstrate concern, acceptance, and respect for client as a person.
(b) Be sensitive, warm, and consistent.
(c) Listen with empathy.
(d) *Avoid* imposing your own feelings of reality on client.
(e) *Avoid* extremes in your own mood when with client (especially exaggerated cheerfulness).
(3) *Focus directly* on client's self-destructive ideas.
(a) Reduce alienation and immobilization by discussing this "taboo" topic.
(b) Acknowledge suicidal threats with calmness and without reproach—do *not* ignore or minimize threat.
(c) *Find out details* about suicide plan and reduce environmental hazards.
(d) Help client verbalize aggressive, hostile, and hopeless *feelings.*
(e) *Explore death fantasies*—try to take "romance" out of death.
(4) Acknowledge that suicide is one of several options and that there are alternatives.
(5) *Make a contract* with the client, and structure a plan of alternatives for coping when next confronted with the need to commit suicide (e.g., the client could call someone, express feeling of anger outwardly, or ask for help).
(6) Point out client's *self-responsibility* for suicidal act.
(a) *Avoid* manipulation by client who says, "You are responsible for stopping me from killing myself."
(b) Emphasize protection against self-destruction *rather than* punishment.
(7) *Support* the part of the client that wants to live.
(a) Focus on *ambivalence.*
(b) Emphasize meaningful past relationships and events.
(c) Look for reasons left for wanting to live. Elicit what is meaningful to the client at the moment.
(d) Point out effect of client's death on others.
(8) *Remove sources of stress.*
(a) Decrease uncomfortable feelings of *alienation* by initiating one-to-one interactions.
(b) Make all *decisions* when client is in severe depression.
(c) Progressively let client make simple decisions: what to eat, what to watch on TV, etc.
(9) *Provide hope.*
(a) Let client know that problems can be solved with help.
(b) Bring in new resources for help.
(c) Talk about likely changes in client's life.
(d) Review past effective coping behaviors.
(10) *Provide with opportunity to be useful.* Reduce self-centeredness and brooding by planning diversional activities within the client's capabilities.
(11) *Involve as many people as possible.*
(a) Gradually bring in others (e.g., other therapists, friends, staff, clergy, family, coworkers).
(b) Prevent staff "burnout," found when only one nurse is working with client who is suicidal.
(12) *Health teaching:* teach client and staff principles of crisis intervention and resolution. Teach new coping skills.

5. **Evaluation/outcome criteria:** physical condition is stabilized; client able to verbalize feelings rather than acting them out.

Crisis Intervention

Crisis intervention is a type of brief psychiatric treatment in which individuals or their families are helped in their efforts to forestall the process of mental decompensation in reaction to severe emotional stress by direct and immediate supportive approaches.

I. DEFINITION OF CRISIS: sudden event in one's life that disturbs homeostasis, during which usual coping mechanisms cannot resolve the problem. Types of crisis:

A. *Maturational* (internal): see Erik Erikson's eight stages of developmental crises anticipated in the development of the infant, child, adolescent, and adult (see **Chapter 5**).

MENTAL HEALTH

B. *Situational* (external): occurs at any time (e.g., loss of job, loss of income, death of significant person, illness, hospitalization).

C. *Catastrophic* (external): can occur at anytime (e.g., natural disasters and terrorist attacks).

II. CONCEPTS AND PRINCIPLES RELATED TO CRISIS INTERVENTION:

A. Crises are turning points where changes in behavior patterns and lifestyles can occur; individuals in crisis are most amenable to altering old and unsuccessful coping mechanisms and are most likely to learn new and more functional behaviors.

B. Social milieu and its structure are contributing factors in both the development of psychiatric symptoms and eventual recovery from them.

C. If crisis is handled effectively, the person's mental stability will be maintained; individual may return to a precrisis state or better.

D. If crisis is not handled effectively, individual may progress to a worse state with exacerbations of earlier conflicts; future crises may not be handled well.

E. There are a number of universal developmental crisis periods (maturational crises) in every individual's life.

F. Each person tries to maintain equilibrium through use of adaptive behaviors.

G. When individuals face a problem they cannot solve, tension, anxiety, narrowed perception, and disorganized functioning occur.

H. *Immediate relief* of symptoms produced by crisis is more urgent than *exploring* their cause.

III. CHARACTERISTICS OF CRISIS INTERVENTION:

A. Acute, sudden onset related to a stressful precipitating event of which individual is aware but which immobilizes previous coping abilities.

B. Responsive to brief therapy with focus on immediate problem.

C. Focus shifted from the psyche in the individual to the *individual in the environment;* deemphasis on intrapsychic aspects.

D. Crisis period is *time limited* (usually up to 6 weeks).

IV. NURSING CARE PLAN/IMPLEMENTATION IN CRISES:

A. General goals:

1. *Avoid* hospitalization if possible.
2. Return to precrisis level and preserve ability to function.
3. Assist in problem-solving, with *here-and-now* focus.

B. *Assess* the crisis:

1. Identify stressful *precipitating* events: duration, problems created, and degree of significance.
2. Assess *suicidal and homicidal risk.*
3. Assess amount of *disruption* in individual's life and effect on significant others.
4. Assess *current coping skills,* strengths, and general level of functioning.

C. *Plan* the intervention:

1. Consider *past coping* mechanisms.
2. Propose *alternatives* and untried coping methods.

D. *Implementation:*

1. Help client relate the crisis event to current feelings.
2. Encourage expression of all feelings related to disruption.
3. Explore past coping skills and *reinforce adaptive* ones.
4. Use all means available in *social network* to take care of client's *immediate needs* (e.g., significant others, law enforcement agencies, housing, welfare, employment, medical, and school).
5. Set limits.
6. *Health teaching:* teach additional problem-solving approaches.

V. EVALUATION/OUTCOME CRITERIA:

A. Client returns to precrisis level of functioning.

B. Client learns new, more effective coping skills.

C. Client can describe realistic plans for future in terms of own perception of progress, support system, and coping mechanisms.

Selected Specific Crisis Situations: Problems Related to Abuse/Violence

I. DOMESTIC VIOLENCE*:

A. Characteristics:

1. *Victims:* feel helpless, powerless to prevent assault; blame themselves; ambivalent about leaving the relationship.
2. *Abusers:* often blame the victims; have poor impulse control; use power (physical strength or weapon) to threaten and subject victims to their assault.
3. *Cycle* of stages, with increase in severity of the battering:
   a. *Buildup of tension* (through verbal abuse): abuser is often drinking or taking other drugs; victim blames self.
   b. *Physical abuse:* abuser does not remember brutal beating; victim is in shock and detached ("honeymoon" phase).
   c. *Calm:* abuser "makes up," apologizes, and promises "never again"; victim believes and forgives the abuser, and feels loved.

*Source: © Lagerquist, S: In *NurseNotes Psychiatric-Mental Health.* A.T.I.

B. Risk factors:

1. *Learned responses:* abuser and victim have had past experience with violence in family; victim has "learned helplessness."
2. Women who are *pregnant* and those with one or more *preschool children,* who see no alternative to staying in the battering relationship.
3. Women who *fear* punishment from the abuser.

C. Assessment:

1. Injury to parts of body, especially face, head, genitals (e.g., welts, bruises, fracture of nose).
2. Presents in the emergency department with report of "accidental injury."
3. Severe anxiety.
4. Depression.

D. Analysis/nursing diagnosis:

1. *Risk for injury* related to physical harm.
2. *Posttraumatic response* related to assault.
3. *Fear* related to threat of death or change in health status.
4. *Pain* related to physical and psychological harm.
5. *Powerlessness* related to interpersonal interaction.
6. *Ineffective individual coping* related to situational crisis.
7. *Spiritual distress* related to intense suffering and challenged value system.

E. Nursing care plan/implementation:

1. Provide safe environment; refer to community resources for shelter.
2. Treat physical injuries.
3. Document injuries.
4. Supportive, nonjudgmental approach: identify woman's strengths; help her to accept that she cannot control the abuser; encourage description of home situation; help her to see choices.
5. Encourage individual and family therapy for victim and abuser.

F. Evaluation/outcome criteria:

1. Physical symptoms have been treated.
2. Discusses plans for safety (for self and any children) to protect against further injury.

II. RAPE-TRAUMA SYNDROME:

A. Definition: forcible perpetration of an act of sexual intercourse on the body of an unwilling person.

B. Assessment:

1. *Signs of physical trauma*—physical findings of entry.
2. *Symptoms of physical trauma*—verbatim statements regarding type of sexual attack.
3. *Signs of emotional trauma*—tears, hyperventilation, extreme anxiety, withdrawal, self-blame, anger, embarrassment, fears, sleeping and eating disturbances, desire for revenge.
4. *Symptoms of emotional trauma*—statements regarding method of force used and threats made.

C. Analysis/nursing diagnosis: *rape-trauma syndrome* related to phases of response to rape:

1. *Acute response:* volatility, disorganization, disbelief, shock, incoherence, agitated motor activity, nightmares, guilt (feels that should have been able to protect self), phobias (crowds, being alone, sex).
2. *Outward coping:* denial and suppression of anxiety and fear (silent rape syndrome), feelings appear controlled.
3. *Integration and resolution:* confronts anger with attacker; realistic perspective.

D. Nursing care plan/implementation in counseling victims of rape. **Figure 10.8** is a summary of self-care decisions a victim faces the first night following a sexual assault.

1. Overall goals:
   a. Protect legal (forensic) evidence.
   b. Acknowledge feelings.
   c. Face feelings.
   d. Resolve feelings.
   e. Maintain and restore *self-respect, dignity, integrity,* and *self-determination.*
2. Work through issues:
   a. Handle *legal* matters and police contacts.
   b. Clarify facts.
   c. Assist medical examiner in collecting DNA evidence.
   d. Get *medical* attention if needed.
   e. Notify *family and friends.*
   f. Understand emotional reaction.
   g. Attend to *practical* concerns.
   h. Evaluate need for psychiatric consultations.
3. *Acute phase:*
   a. Decrease victim's stress, anxiety, fear.
   b. Seek medical care.
   c. Increase self-confidence and self-esteem.
   d. Identify and accept feelings and needs (to be in control, cared about, to achieve).
   e. Reorient perceptions, feelings, and statements about self.
   f. Help resume normal lifestyle.
4. *Outward coping phase:*
   a. Remain available and supportive.
   b. Reflect words, feelings, and thoughts.
   c. Explore real problems.
   d. Explore alternatives regarding contraception, legal issues.
   e. Evaluate response of family and friends to victim and rape.
5. *Integration and resolution phase:*
   a. Assist exploration of feelings (anger) regarding attacker.
   b. Explore feelings (guilt and shame) regarding self.
   c. Assist in making own decisions regarding health care.

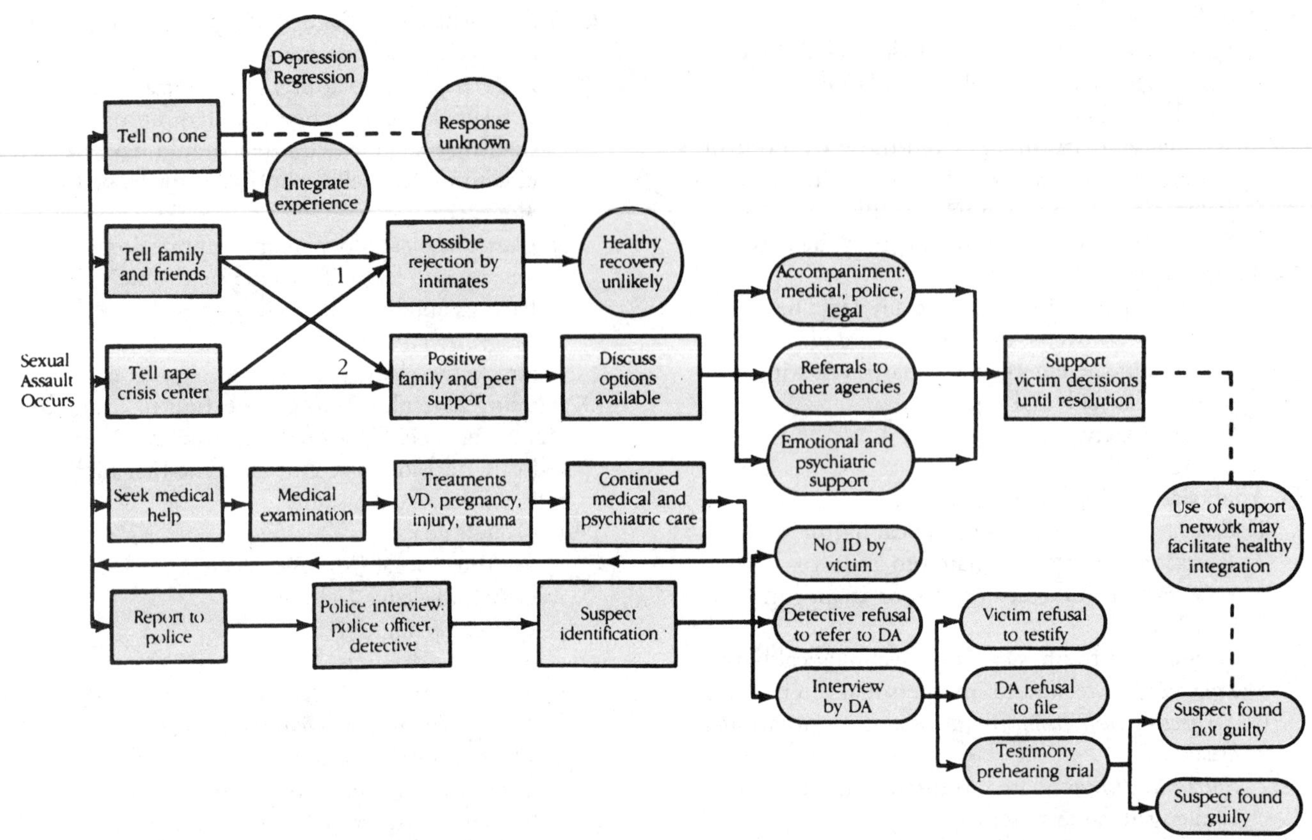

Figure 10.8 Victim decisions following a sexual assault. (From Violence Intervention and Prevention Services at the YWCA of Greater Harrisburg, PA.)

6. Maintain confidentiality and neutrality—facilitate person's own decision.
7. Search for alternatives to giving advice.
8. *Health teaching:*
   a. Explain procedures and services to victim.
   b. Counsel to avoid isolated areas and being helpful to strangers.
   c. Counsel where and how to resist attack (scream, run unless assailant has weapon).
   d. Teach what to do if pregnancy or STI is outcome.

E. Evaluation/outcome criteria: little or no evidence of possible long-term effects of rape (guilt, shame, phobias, denial).

III. CHILD WHO IS VICTIM OF VIOLENCE:

A. Assessment—clues to the identification of a child who is a victim of violence.*

1. Clues in the *history:*
   a. Significant *delay* in seeking medical care.
   b. Major *discrepancies* in the history:
      (1) Discrepancy between different people's versions of the story.
      (2) Discrepancy between the history and the observed injuries.
      (3) Discrepancy between the history and the child's developmental capabilities.
   c. History of multiple emergency department visits for various injuries.
   d. A story that is *vague* and *contradictory.*
2. Clues in the *physical examination:*
   a. Child who seems withdrawn, apathetic, and *does not cry* despite the injuries.
   b. Child who *does not turn to parents for comfort;* or unusual desire to please parent; unusual fear of parent(s).
   c. *Child who is poorly nourished* and *poorly cared for.*
   d. The presence of *bruises: multiple bruises,* welts, and abrasions, especially around the trunk and buttocks; lesions resembling bites or fingernail marks; *old bruises in addition to fresh ones* **(Table 10.14).**
   e. The presence of *suspicious burns:*
      (1) Cigarette burns.
      (2) Scalds without splash marks or involving the buttocks, hands, or feet but sparing skinfolds.
      (3) Rope marks.

*Adapted from Caroline, N: *Emergency Care in the Streets,* ed 5. Little, Brown, Boston (out of print)

Table 10.14

Estimation of Time at Which Soft Tissue Injury Occurred

Injury Occurred	Color
0–2 hr	No discoloration (may have edema and pain)
1–5 days	Red/blue
5–7 days	Green
7–10 days	Yellow
10–14 days	Brown

f. Clues in parent behavior—exaggerate care and concern.
g. X-rays: old fractures or dislocation, especially in child under 3 years.

B. Analysis/nursing diagnosis:
1. Same as for *domestic violence* (see **pp. 796–797**).
2. *Altered parenting* related to poor role model/identity, unrealistic expectations, presence of stressors and lack of support.
3. *Low self-esteem* related to deprivation and negative feedback.

C. Nursing care plan/implementation:
1. Same as for *domestic violence.*
2. Report suspected child abuse to appropriate source.
3. Conduct assessment interview in private, with child and parent separated.
4. Be supportive and nonjudgmental.

D. Evaluation/outcome criteria:
1. Same as *domestic violence.*
2. Child safety has been ensured.
3. Parent(s) or caregivers have agreed to seek help.

IV. SEXUAL ABUSE OF CHILDREN:

A. Assessment—characteristic behaviors:
1. *Relationship* of offender to victim: many filling paternal role (uncle, grandfather, cousin) with repeated, unquestioned access to the child.
2. Methods of *pressuring* victim into sexual activity: offering material goods, misrepresenting moral standards ("it's OK"), exploiting need for human contact and warmth.
3. Method of pressuring victim to *secrecy* (to conceal the act) is inducing fear of punishment, not being believed, rejection, being blamed for the activity, abandonment.
4. Disclosure of sexual activity via:
   a. Direct visual or verbal confrontation and *observation* by others.
   b. *Verbalization* of act by victim.
   c. *Visible clues:* excess money and candy, new clothes, pictures, notes; enlarged vaginal or rectal orifice; stains and/or blood on underwear.
   d. *Signs and symptoms:* bedwetting, excessive bathing, tears, avoiding school, somatic distress (*GI and urinary* tract pains). Genital irritation (itching, bruised, bleeding, pain); unusual sexual behavior.
   e. Overly solicitous parental attitude toward child.

B. Analysis/nursing diagnosis:
1. *Altered protection* related to inflicted pain.
2. *Risk for injury* related to neglect, abuse.
3. *Personal identity disturbance* related to abuse as child and feeling guilty and responsible for being a victim.
4. *Ineffective individual coping* related to high stress level.
5. *Sleep pattern disturbance* related to traumatic sexual experiences.
6. *Ineffective family coping.*
7. *Altered family processes* related to use of violence.
8. *Altered parenting* related to violence.
9. *Powerlessness* related to feelings of being dependent on abuser.
10. *Social isolation/withdrawal* related to shame about family violence.
11. *Risk for altered abuse response patterns.*

C. Nursing care plan/implementation:
1. Establish safe environment and the termination of trauma.
2. Encourage child to verbalize feelings about incident to dispel tension built up by secrecy.
3. Ask child to draw a picture or use dolls and toys to show what happened.
4. Observe for symptoms over a period of time.
   a. *Phobic* reactions when seeing or hearing offender's name.
   b. *Sleep pattern* changes, recurrent dreams, nightmares.
5. Look for *silent reaction* to being an accessory to sex (i.e., child keeping burden of the secret activity within self); help deal with unresolved issues.
6. Establish therapeutic alliance with parent who is abusive.
7. *Health teaching:*
   a. Teach child that his or her body is private and to inform a responsible adult when someone violates privacy without consent.
   b. Teach adults in family to respond to victim with sensitivity, support, and concern.

D. Evaluation/outcome criteria:
1. Child's needs for affection, attention, personal recognition, or love met without sexual exploitation.

2. Perpetrator accepts therapy.
3. Conspiracy of silence is broken.

E. Summary: signs that are common to both *physical* and *sexual abuse:*
1. Parental behaviors:
   a. Blaming child or sibling for injury.
   b. Anger (rather than providing comfort) toward child for injury.
   c. Hostility toward health-care providers.
   d. Exaggeration or absence of response from parent regarding child's injury.
2. Child (toddler or preschooler):
   a. No protest when parent leaves.
   b. Shows preference for health-care provider over parent.
   c. Signs of "failure to thrive" syndrome.
3. Other signs:
   a. History: inconsistent with stages of growth and development.
   b. Inconsistent details of injury between one person and another.

V. ELDER ABUSE/NEGLECT:

A. Definition: battering, psychological abuse, sexual assault, or any act or omission by personal caregiver, family, or legal guardian that results in harm or threatened harm.

B. Concepts, principles, and characteristics:
1. Elders who are currently being abused often abused their abusers—their offspring. Violence is a learned behavior.
2. *Victim characteristics:* diminished self-esteem, feeling responsibility for the abuse, isolated.
3. *Abuser characteristics:* usually has physical or psychosocial stressors related to marital or fiscal difficulties; substance abuse.
4. *Legal:* most states have mandatory laws to report elder abuse, although many cases are not reported because of shame, fear of more abuse, cultural/religious beliefs, optimism, loyalty, financial dependency.
5. Types of abuse:
   a. *Financial* abuse (e.g., fraudulent monetary schemes, theft [money, property, or both]).
   b. *Neglect* (e.g., withholding food, water, medications; no provision for assistive devices [dentures, hearing aids, glasses, canes], adequate heating).
   c. *Psychological* abuse (e.g., verbal abuse, yelling, harsh commands, insults, threats, ignoring, social isolation, and withholding affection).
   d. *Physical* abuse (e.g., beating, shoving, bruising, subconjunctival hemorrhage; physical restraints, rape).

C. Assessment:
1. *Risk factors:*

Victim:	*Abuser:*
• Poor health	• Substance abuse
• Isolated	• Stressful life events
• Impaired memory, thinking	• Interpersonal problems
← Hx: Mental illness →	
← Hx: Family violence →	
← Financial difficulties →	
← Dependency →	
← Share living space →	

2. *Behavioral clues:* agitation, anger, denial, fear, poor eye contact; confusion, depression, withdrawal, unbelievable stories about causes of injuries.
3. *Physical indicators:* weight loss; dehydration; unexplained cuts, welts, burns, bruises, puncture wounds; untreated injuries, fractures, contractures; unkempt; noncompliance with medical plan of care; severe skin breakdown.
4. *Financial matters* (e.g., recent changes in will; unusual banking activity; missing checks, personal belongings; forged signatures; unwillingness to spend money on the elder).

D. Analysis/nursing diagnosis:
1. *Risk for injury* related to neglect, abuse.
2. *Fear.*
3. *Powerlessness* related to dependency on abuser.
4. *Unilateral neglect.*
5. *Spiritual distress.*
6. *Altered family processes* related to use of violence.
7. *Caregiver role strain.*

E. Nursing care plan/implementation:
1. *Primary prevention:*
   a. Early case-finding; early treatment.
   b. Referral to community services for caregiver (e.g., respite care) before serious abuse occurs.
2. *Secondary prevention:*
   a. Report case to law enforcement agencies.
   b. Provide elder with phone number for confidential hotline.
   c. Plan for safety of elder (e.g., shelter).
3. *Tertiary prevention:*
   a. Counseling, support, and self-help groups for victim.
   b. Legal action against abuser.

F. Evaluation/outcome criteria:
1. Elder develops trust in caregivers, without fear of further abuse.
2. Spiritual well-being is enhanced, with diminished feelings of guilt, hopelessness, and powerlessness.

TREATMENT MODES

Milieu Therapy

Milieu therapy consists of treatment by means of controlled modification of the client's environment to promote positive living experiences.

I. CONCEPTS AND PRINCIPLES RELATED TO MILIEU THERAPY:

A. Everything that happens to clients from the time they are admitted to the hospital or treatment setting has a potential that is either therapeutic or antitherapeutic.

1. Not only the therapists but all who come in contact with the clients in the treatment setting are important to the clients' recovery.
2. Emphasis is on the social, economic, and cultural dimension, the interpersonal climate, and the physical environment.

B. Clients have the right, privilege, and responsibility to make decisions about daily living activities in the treatment setting.

II. CHARACTERISTICS of milieu therapy:

A. Friendly, warm, trusting, secure, supportive, comforting atmosphere throughout the unit.

B. An optimistic attitude about prognosis of illness.

C. Attention to comfort, food, and daily living needs; help with resolving difficulties related to tasks of daily living.

D. Opportunity for clients to take responsibility for themselves and for the welfare of the unit in gradual steps.

1. Client government.
2. Client-planned and client-directed social activities.

E. Maximum individualization in dealing with clients, especially regarding treatment and privileges in accordance with clients' needs.

F. Opportunity to live through and test out situations in a realistic way by providing a setting that is a microcosm of the larger world outside.

G. Opportunity to discuss interpersonal relationships in the unit among clients and between clients and staff (decreased social distance between staff and clients).

H. Program of carefully selected resocialization activities to prevent regression.

III. NURSING CARE PLAN/IMPLEMENTATION in milieu therapy:

A. *New structured relationships*—allow clients to develop new abilities and use past skills; support them through new experiences as needed; help build liaisons with others; set limits; help clients modify destructive behavior; encourage group solutions to daily living problems.

B. *Managerial*—inform clients about expectations; preserve orderliness of events.

C. *Environmental manipulation*—regulate the outside environment to alter daily surroundings.

1. Geographically move clients to units more conducive to their needs.
2. Work with families, clergy, employers, etc.
3. Control visitors for the benefit of the client.

D. *Team approach* uses the milieu to meet each client's needs.

IV. EVALUATION/OUTCOMES CRITERIA:

A. *Physical dimension:* order, organization.

B. *Social dimension:* clarity of expectations, practical orientation.

C. *Emotional dimension:* involvement, support, responsibility, openness, valuing, accepting.

MENTAL HEALTH

Behavior Modification

Behavior modification is a therapeutic approach involving the application of learning principles so as to change maladaptive behavior.

I. DEFINITIONS:

conditioned avoidance (also ***aversion therapy***) a technique whereby there is a purposeful and systematic production of strongly unpleasant responses in situations to which the client has been previously attracted but now wishes to avoid.

desensitization frequent exposure in small but gradually increasing doses of anxiety-evoking stimuli until undesirable behavior disappears or is lessened (as in phobias).

token economy desired behavior is reinforced by rewards, such as candy, money, and verbal approval, used as tokens.

operant conditioning a method designed to elicit and reinforce desirable behavior (especially useful in mental retardation).

positive reinforcement giving rewards to elicit or strengthen selected behavior or behaviors.

II. OBJECTIVES AND PROCESS OF TREATMENT in behavior modification:

A. Emphasis is on changing unacceptable, overt, and observable behavior to that which is acceptable; emphasis is on changed way of *acting* first, not of thinking.

B. Mental health team determines behavior to change and treatment plan to use.

C. Therapy is based on the knowledge and application of *learning* principles, that is, *stimulus-response;* the unlearning, or *extinction,* of undesirable behavior; and the *reinforcement* of desirable behavior.

D. Therapist identifies what events are important in the life history of the client and arranges situations in which the client is therapeutically confronted with them.

E. Two primary aspects of behavior modification:

1. *Eliminate* unwanted behavior by *negative reinforcement* (removal of an aversive stimulus, which acts to reinforce the behavior) and *ignoring* (withholding positive reinforcement).
2. *Create* acceptable new responses to an environmental stimulus by *positive* reinforcement.

F. Useful with: children who are disturbed, victims of rape, dependent and manipulative behaviors, eating disorders, obsessive-compulsive disorders, sexual dysfunction.

III. ASSUMPTIONS OF BEHAVIORAL THERAPY:

A. Behavior is what an organism does.

B. Behavior can be observed, described, and recorded.

C. It is possible to predict the conditions under which the same behavior may recur.

D. Undesirable social behavior is not a symptom of mental illness but is behavior that can be modified.

E. Undesirable behaviors are learned disorders that relate to acute anxiety in a given situation.

F. Maladaptive behavior is learned in the same way as adaptive behavior.

G. People tend to behave in ways that "pay off."

H. *Three ways* in which behavior can be reinforced:

1. *Positive* reinforcer (adding something pleasurable).
2. *Negative* reinforcer (removing something unpleasant).
3. *Adverse* stimuli (punishing).

I. If an undesired behavior is ignored, it will be extinguished.

J. Learning process is the same for all; therefore, all conditions (except organic) are accepted for treatment.

IV. NURSING CARE PLAN/IMPLEMENTATION in behavior modification:

A. Find out what is a "reward" for the person.

B. Break the goal down into small, successive *steps.*

C. Maintain *close* and continual observation of the selected behavior or behaviors.

D. Be *consistent* with on-the-spot, immediate intervention and correction of undesirable behavior.

E. Record focused observations of behavior frequently.

F. Participate in close teamwork with the *entire* staff.

G. Evaluate procedures and results continually.

H. *Health teaching:* teach preceding steps to colleagues and family.

V. EVALUATION/OUTCOME CRITERIA: acceptable behavior is increased and maintained; undesirable behavior is decreased or eliminated.

Activity Therapy

Activity therapy consists of a variety of recreational and vocational activities (recreational therapy [RT]; occupational therapy [OT]; and music, art, and dance therapy) designed to test and examine social skills and serve as adjunctive therapies.

I. CONCEPTS AND PRINCIPLES RELATED TO ACTIVITY THERAPY:

A. Socialization counters the regressive aspects of illness.

B. Activities must be selected for specific psychosocial reasons to achieve specific effects.

C. Nonverbal means of expression as an additional behavioral outlet add a new dimension to treatment.

D. Sublimation of sexual drives is possible through activities.

E. Indications for activity therapy: clients with *low self-esteem* who are socially *unresponsive.*

II. CHARACTERISTICS OF ACTIVITY THERAPY:

A. Usually planned and coordinated by other team members, such as the recreational therapists or music therapists.

B. Goals:

1. Encourage socialization in community and social activities.
2. Provide pleasurable activities.
3. Help client release tensions and express feelings.
4. Teach new skills; help client find new hobbies.
5. Offer graded series of experiences, from passive spectator role and vicarious experiences to more direct and active experiences.
6. Free or strengthen physical and creative abilities.
7. Increase self-esteem.

III. NURSING CARE PLAN/IMPLEMENTATION in activity therapy:

A. Encourage, support, and cooperate in client's participation in activities planned by the adjunct therapists.

B. Share knowledge of client's illness, talents, interests, and abilities with others on the team.

C. *Health teaching:* teach client necessary skills for each activity (e.g., sports, games, crafts).

IV. EVALUATION/OUTCOME CRITERIA: client develops occupational and leisure-time skills that will help provide a smoother transition back to the community.

Group Therapy

Group therapy is a treatment modality in which two or more clients and one or more therapists interact in a helping process to relieve emotional difficulties, increase self-esteem and insight, and improve behavior in relations with others.

I. CONCEPTS AND PRINCIPLES RELATED TO GROUP THERAPY:

A. People's problems usually occur in a social setting; thus they can best be evaluated and corrected in a social setting. **Table 10.15** is a summary of curative factors.

B. *Not* all are amenable to group therapies. For example:
1. Brain damaged.
2. Acutely suicidal.
3. Acutely psychotic.
4. Persons with very passive-dependent behavior patterns.
5. Acutely manic.

C. It is best to match group members for *complementarity in behaviors* (verbal with nonverbal, withdrawn with outgoing) but for *similarity in problems* (obesity, predischarge group, clients with cancer, prenatal group) to facilitate empathy in the sharing of experiences and to heighten group identification and cohesiveness.

D. Feelings of *acceptance,* belonging, respect, and comfort develop in the group and facilitate change and health.

E. In a group, members can *test reality* by giving and receiving *feedback.*

F. Clients have a chance to experience in the group that they are not alone (concept of *universality*).

G. Expression and *ventilation* of strong emotional feelings (anger, anxiety, fear, and guilt) in the safe setting of a group is an important aspect of the group process aimed at health and change.

H. The group setting and the *interactions* of its members may provide *corrective emotional experiences* for its members. A key mechanism operating in groups is *transference* (strong emotional attachment of one member to another member, to the therapist, or to the entire group).

I. To the degree that people modify their behavior through corrective experiences and identification with others rather than through personal-insight analysis, group therapy may be of special advantage over individual therapy, in that the possible number of interactions is greater in the group and the patterns of behavior are more readily observable.

J. There is a higher client-to-staff ratio, and it is thus less expensive.

II. GENERAL GROUP GOALS:

A. Provide opportunity for self-expression of ideas and feelings.

B. Provide a setting for a variety of relationships through group interaction.

C. Explore current behavioral patterns with others and observe dynamics.

D. Provide peer and therapist support and source of strength for the individuals to modify present behavior and try out new behaviors; made possible through development of identity and group identification.

E. Provide on-the-spot, multiple feedback (i.e., incorporate others' reactions to behavior), as well as give feedback to others.

F. Resolve dynamics and provide insight.

III. NURSING CARE PLAN/IMPLEMENTATION in group setting:

A. Nurses need to fill different roles and functions in the group, depending on the type of group, its size, its aims, and the stage in the group's life cycle. The multifaceted roles may include:
1. Catalyst.
2. Transference object (of client's positive or negative feelings).

Table 10.15

Curative Factors of Group Therapy

Factor	Definition
Instilling of hope	Imbuing the client with optimism for the success of the group therapy experience.
Universality	Disconfirming the client's sense of aloneness or uniqueness in misery or hurt
Imparting of information	Giving didactic instruction, advice, or suggestions
Altruism	Finding that the client can be of importance to others; having something of value to give
Corrective recapitulation of the primary family group	Reviewing and correctively reliving early familial conflicts and growth-inhibiting relationships
Development of socializing techniques	Acquiring sophisticated social skills, such as being attuned to process, resolving conflicts, and being facilitative toward others
Imitative behavior	Trying out bits and pieces of the behavior of others and experimenting with those that fit well
Interpersonal learning	Learning that the client is the author of his or her interpersonal world and moving to alter it
Group cohesiveness	Being attracted to the group and the other members with a sense of "we"-ness rather than "I"-ness
Catharsis	Being able to express feelings
Existential factors	Being able to "be" with others; to be a part of a group

Adapted from Wilson, HS, & Kneisl, CR: *Psychiatric Nursing,* ed 3. Addison-Wesley, Redwood City, CA. (out of print)

3. Clarifier.
4. Interpreter of "here and now."
5. Role model and resource person.
6. Supporter.

B. During the *first sessions*, explain the purpose of the group, go over the "contract" (structure, format, and goals of sessions), and facilitate introductions of group members.

C. In *subsequent sessions*, promote greater group cohesiveness.

1. Focus on *group concerns* and group process rather than on intrapsychic dynamics of individuals.
2. Demonstrate nonjudgmental acceptance of behaviors within the limits of the group contract.
3. Help group members handle their anxiety, especially during the initial phase.
4. Encourage members who are silent to interact at their level of comfort.
5. Encourage members to interact verbally without dominating the group discussion.
6. Keep the focus of discussion on related themes; *set limits and interpret group rules.*
7. Facilitate sharing and *communication* among members.
8. Provide *support* to members as they attempt to work through anxiety-provoking ideas and feelings.
9. Set the expectation that the members are to take responsibility for carrying the group discussion and exploring issues on their own.

D. *Termination phase:*

1. Make early preparation for group termination (endpoint should be announced at the first meeting).
2. Anticipate common reactions from group members to separation anxiety and help each member to work through these reactions:
   a. Anger.
   b. Acting out.
   c. Regressive behavior.
   d. Repression.
   e. Feelings of abandonment.
   f. Sadness.

IV. EVALUATION/OUTCOME CRITERIA:

A. *Physical:* shows improvement in daily life activities (eating, rest, work, exercise, recreation).

B. *Emotional:* asks for and accepts feedback; states feels good about self and others.

C. *Intellectual:* is reality oriented; greater awareness of self, others, environment.

D. *Social:* willing to take a risk in trusting others; sharing self; reaching out to others.

Reality Orientation and Resocialization

Table 10.16 lists the differences between these two modes of therapy.

Table 10.16

Differences Between Reality Orientation and Resocialization

Reality Orientation	Resocialization
1. Maximum use of assets.	1. Reality living situation in a community.
2. Structured.	2. Unstructured.
3. Refreshments *may* be served.	3. Refreshments served.
4. Constant reminders of who the clients are, where they are, and why and what is expected of them.	4. Reliving happy experiences; encouragement to participate in home activities.
5. *Group size:* 3–5, depending on degree and level of confusion or disorientation.	5. *Group size:* 5–17, depending on mental and physical capabilities.
6. *Meetings:* 30 minutes daily, same time and place.	6. *Meetings:* 3 times per week for 30 minutes to 1 hour.
7. Planned topics: reality-centered objects.	7. *No* planned topic; group-centered feelings.
8. *Role of leader:* eliciting response of participants.	8. *Role of leader:* clarification and interpretation.
9. Periodic reality-orientation test of participants' level of confusion.	9. Periodic progress note of participants' enjoyment and improvements.
10. *Emphasis:* time, place, person orientation.	10. Any topic freely discussed.
11. Use of mind function still intact.	11. Rely on memories and experiences.
12. Participant is greeted *by name,* thanked for coming, extended a handshake or other physical contact.	12. Participant greeted on arrival, thanked, extended a handshake on leaving.
13. Conducted by trained aides and activity assistants.	13. Conducted by RN, LPN/LVN, aides, program assistants.

Adapted from *the classic article* by Barns, E, Sack, A, & Shore, H: *Gerontologist* 13:513, 1973.

Family Therapy

Family therapy is a process, method, and technique of psychotherapy in which the focus is not on an individual but on the total family as an interactional system (see also **Major Theoretical Models, pp. 713–714**).

I. DEVELOPMENTAL TASKS OF NORTH AMERICAN FAMILY (Duvall, 1971):

A. *Physical maintenance*—provide food, shelter, clothing, health care.
B. *Resource allocation* (physical and emotional)—allocate material goods, space, and facilities; give affection, respect, and authority.
C. *Division of labor*—decide who earns money, manages household, cares for family.
D. *Socialization*—guidelines to control food intake, elimination, sleep, sexual drives, and aggression.
E. *Reproduction, recruitment, release of family member*—give birth to, or adopt, children; rear children; incorporate in-laws, friends, etc.
F. *Maintenance of order*—ensure conformity to norms.
G. *Placement of members in larger society*—interaction in school, community, etc.
H. *Maintenance of motivation and morale*—reward achievements, develop philosophy for living; create rituals and celebrations to develop family loyalty. Show acceptance, encouragement, affection; meet crises of individuals and family.

II. BASIC THEORETICAL CONCEPTS RELATED TO FAMILY THERAPY:

A. The ill family member (called the *identified client*), by symptoms, sends a message about the "illness" of the family as a *unit.*
B. *Family homeostasis* is the means by which families attempt to maintain the status quo.
C. *Scapegoating* is found in families who are disturbed and is usually focused on one family member at a time, with the intent to keep the family in line.
D. Communication and behavior by some family members bring out communication and behavior in other family members.
1. Mental illness in the identified client is almost always accompanied by emotional illness and disturbance in other family members.
2. Changes occurring in one member will produce changes in another; that is, if the identified client improves, another identified client may emerge, or family may try to place original person back into the role of the identified client.

E. Human communication is a key to emotional stability and instability—to normal and abnormal health. *Conjoint* family therapy is a communication-centered approach that looks at interactions between family members.
F. *Double bind* is a "damned if you do, damned if you don't" situation; it results in helplessness, insecurity; anxiety; fear, frustration, and rage.
G. *Symbiotic tie* usually occurs between one parent and a child, hampering individual ego development and fostering strong dependence and identification with the parent (usually the mother).
H. *Three basic premises* of communication*:
1. One cannot *not* communicate; that is, silence is a form of communication.
2. Communication is a *multilevel* phenomenon.
3. The message sent is *not* necessarily the *same* message that is received.

I. Indications for family therapy:
1. Marital conflicts.
2. Severe sibling conflicts.
3. Cross-generational conflicts.
4. Difficulties related to a transitional stage of family life cycle (e.g., retirement, new infant, death).
5. *Dysfunctional family patterns:* mother who is overprotective and father who is distant, with child who is timid or destructive, teenager who is acting out; overfunctioning "superwife" or "superhusband" and the spouse who is underfunctioning, passive, dependent, and compliant; child with poor peer relationships or academic difficulties.

III. FAMILY ASSESSMENT should consider the following factors:

A. *Family assessment: cultural profile* (see also **Chapter 3**)†:
1. *Communication style:*
   a. Language and dialect preference (understand concept, meaning of pain, fever, nausea).
   b. Nonverbal behaviors (meaning of bowing, touching, speaking softly, smiling).
   c. Social customs (acting agreeable or pleasant to avoid the unpleasant, embarrassing).
2. *Orientation:*
   a. Ethnic identity and adherence to traditional habits and values.
   b. Acculturation: extent.
   c. Value orientations:
      (1) *Human nature:* evil, good, both.
      (2) *Relationship between humans and nature:* subjugated, harmony, mastery.
      (3) *Time:* past, present, future.
      (4) *Purpose of life:* being, becoming, doing.
      (5) *Relationship to one another:* lineal, collateral, individualistic.

---

*Adapted from Watzlawick, P: *An Anthology of Human Communication.* Science and Behavior Books, Palo Alto, CA. (out of print)

†Adapted from the *classic* work by Fong, C: Ethnicity and nursing practice. *Topics Clin Nurs* 7(3):4, with permission of Aspen Publishers, Inc. © 1985.

3. *Nutrition:*
   a. Symbolism of food.
   b. Preferences, taboos.
4. *Family relationships:*
   a. Role and position of women, men, aged, boys, girls.
   b. Decision-making styles/areas: finances, child rearing, health care.
   c. Family: nuclear, extended, or tribal.
   d. Matriarchal or patriarchal.
   e. Lifestyle, living arrangements (crowded; urban/rural; ethnic neighborhood or mixed).
5. *Health beliefs:*
   a. Alternative health care: self-care, folk medicine; cultural healer: herbalist, medicine man, curandero.
   b. Health crisis and illness beliefs concerning causation: germ theory, maladaptation, stress, evil spirits, yin/yang imbalance, envy and hate.
   c. Response to pain, hospitalization: stoic endurance, loud cries, quiet withdrawal.
   d. Disease predisposition:
      (1) *African Americans:* sickle cell anemia; cardiovascular disease, brain attack (stroke), hypertension; high infant mortality rate; diabetes.
      (2) *Asians:* lactose intolerance, myopia.
      (3) *Latinos:* cardiovascular, diabetes, cancer, obesity, substance abuse, TB, AIDS, suicide, homicide.
      (4) *Native Americans:* high infant and maternal mortality rates, cirrhosis, fetal alcohol abnormalities, pancreatitis, malnutrition, TB, alcoholism.
      (5) *Jews:* Tay-Sachs disease.

B. *Family as a social system:*
1. Family as responsive and contributing unit within network of other social units.
   a. Family boundaries—permeability or rigidity.
   b. Nature of input from other social units.
   c. Extent to which family fits into cultural mold and expectations of larger system.
   d. Degree to which family is considered deviant.
2. Roles of family members:
   a. Formal roles and role performance (father, child, etc.).
   b. Informal roles and role performance (scapegoat, controller, follower, decision maker).
   c. Degree of family agreement on assignment of roles and their performance.
   d. Interrelationship of various roles—degree of "fit" within total family.
3. Family rules:
   a. Family rules that foster stability and maintenance.
   b. Family rules that foster maladaptation.
   c. Conformity of rules to family's lifestyle.
   d. How rules are modified; respect for difference.
4. Communication network:
   a. How family communicates and provides information to members.
   b. Channels of communication—who speaks to whom.
   c. Quality of messages—clarity or ambiguity.

C. *Developmental stage of family:*
1. Chronological stage of family.
2. Problems and adaptations of transition.
3. Shifts in role responsibility over time.
4. Ways and means of solving problems at earlier stages.

D. *Subsystems operating within family:*
1. Function of family alliances in family stability.
2. Conflict or support of other family subsystems and family as a whole.

E. *Physical and emotional needs:*
1. Level at which family meets essential physical needs.
2. Level at which family meets social and emotional needs.
3. Resources within family to meet physical and emotional needs.
4. Disparities between individual needs and family's willingness or ability to meet them.

F. *Goals, values, and aspirations:*
1. Extent to which family members' goals and values are articulated and understood by all members.
2. Extent to which family values reflect resignation or compromise.
3. Extent to which family will permit pursuit of individual goals and values.

G. *Socioeconomic factors* (see list in **Table 10.9, p. 733**).

IV. NURSING CARE PLAN/IMPLEMENTATION in family therapy:

A. Establish a family *contract* (who attends, when, duration of sessions, length of therapy, fee, and other expectations).

B. Encourage family members to identify and clarify own *goals.*

C. *Set ground rules:*
1. Focus is on the family as a whole unit, *not* on the identified client.
2. *No* scapegoating or punishment of members who "reveal all" should be allowed.
3. Therapists should *not* align themselves with issues or individual family members.

D. *Use self* to empathetically respond to family's problems; share own emotions openly and directly; function as a role model of interaction.

E. Point out and encourage the family to *clarify* unclear, inefficient, and ambiguous family communication patterns.

F. Identify family *strengths.*

G. Listen for repetitive interpersonal *themes, patterns,* and *attitudes.*

H. *Attempt to reduce guilt and blame* (important to neutralize the scapegoat phenomenon).

I. Present possibility of *alternative* roles and rules in family interaction styles.

J. *Health teaching:* teach clear communication to all family members.

V. EVALUATION/OUTCOME CRITERIA: each person clearly speaks for self; asks for and receives feedback; communication patterns are clarified; family problems are delineated; members more aware of each other's needs.

Electroconvulsive Therapy

Electroconvulsive therapy (ECT) is a physical treatment that induces grand mal (generalized) convulsions by applying electric current to the head. It is also called electric shock therapy (EST).

I. CHARACTERISTICS of electroconvulsive therapy:

A. Usually used in treating: major depression with severe suicide risk, extreme hyperactivity, severe catatonic stupor, or those with bipolar affective disorders not responsive to psychotropic medication.

B. Consists of a series of treatments (6 to 25) over a period of time (e.g., 3 times per week).

C. Person is asleep through the procedure and for 20 to 30 minutes afterward.

D. Convulsion may be seen as a series of minor, jerking motions in extremities (e.g., toes). Spasms are reduced by use of muscle-paralyzing drugs.

E. Confusion is present for 30 minutes after treatment.

F. Induces loss of memory for *recent* events.

II. VIEWS CONCERNING SUCCESS of electroconvulsive therapy:

A. Posttreatment sleep is the "curative" factor.

B. Shock treatment is seen as punishment, with an accompanying feeling of absolution from guilt.

C. Chemical alteration of thought patterns results in memory loss, with decrease in redundancy and awareness of painful memories.

III. NURSING CARE PLAN/IMPLEMENTATION in electroconvulsive therapy:

A. *Always* tell the client of the treatment.

B. Inform client about temporary memory loss for recent events after the treatment.

C. *Pretreatment care:*

1. Take vital signs.
2. See to client's toileting.
3. Remove: client's dentures, eyeglasses or contact lenses, and jewelry.
4. NPO for 8 hours beforehand.
5. *Atropine sulfate* subcutaneously 30 minutes before treatment to decrease bronchial and tracheal secretions.
6. Anesthetist gives anesthetic and muscle relaxant IV (succinylcholine chloride [*Anectine*]) and oxygen for 2 to 3 minutes and inserts airway. Often all three are given close together—anesthetic first, followed by another syringe with *Anectine* and atropine sulfate. Electrodes and treatment must be given within 2 minutes of injections, because *Anectine* is very short acting (2 minutes).

D. *During the convulsion,* the nurse must make sure the person is in a safe position to avoid dislocation and compression fractures (although *Anectine* is given to prevent this).

E. *Care during recovery stage:*

1. Put up side rails while client is confused; *side* position.
2. Take blood pressure, pulse (check for bradycardia), and respirations.
3. Stay until person awakens, responds to questions, and can care for self.
4. Orient client to time and place and inform that treatment is over when awakens.
5. Offer support to help client feel more secure and relaxed as the confusion and anxiety decrease.
6. Medication for nausea and headache, prn.

F. *Health teaching:* teach family members what to expect of client after ECT (confusion, headache, nausea); how to reorient the client.

IV. EVALUATION/OUTCOME CRITERIA: feelings of worthlessness, helplessness, and hopelessness seem diminished.

Complementary and Alternative Medicine (CAM)

(Also see **Appendix E** for specific conditions in which CAM can be integrated into the treatment plan.)

I. DEFINITIONS:

A. *Complementary therapy*—used to *supplement or augment* conventional therapy (e.g., use of guided imagery, music and relaxation techniques for pain control in combination with drug therapy).

B. *Alternative therapy*—generally used *instead* of conventional treatment (e.g., use of acupuncture instead of analgesic).

II. BASIC BELIEFS AND ASSUMPTIONS about health, health care:

A. Diseases are *complex, multifaceted* states of imbalance and require an approach that uses *several* strategies for facilitating healing.

B. Individuals can facilitate their own healing process by engaging their *inner resources* and becoming active participants in promoting their health.

C. Holistic nursing can be a major provider of CAM, with an underlying philosophy of *caring* and *healing.*

1. Use of an approach to the care of others that facilitates the integration, harmony, and balance of body, mind, and spirit.
2. Focus is on the *whole* person in the process of healing.
3. Experience of illness is an opportunity for growth that invites reflection on important dimensions of their lives and to make changes that encourage a more balanced and integrated state of being. *Emphasis* on: self-responsibility and self-care.
4. Client-nurse relationship is *reciprocal* where each benefits from the interaction and grows in self-awareness.

III. AREAS OF PRACTICE WITHIN CAM:

A. Mind-body interventions.

B. Bioelectromagnetic applications in medicine.

C. Manual healing methods.

D. Pharmacological and biological treatments.

E. Herbal medicine (see **Chapters 8** and **9** and **Appendix E**).

F. Diet and nutrition in the prevention and treatment of chronic disease.

IV. EXAMPLES OF WELL-KNOWN ALTERNATIVE AND COMPLEMENTARY THERAPIES:

A. *Natural healing:*

1. Aquatherapy.
2. Aromatherapy.
3. Color therapy.
4. Homeopathy.

B. *Plant therapy:*

1. Flower essence therapy.
2. Herbal medicine.

C. *Nutrition and diet:*

1. Diet therapies (see **Chapter 9**).
2. Naturopathic medicine.

D. *Mobility and posture:*

1. Dance therapy.
2. Rolfing.
3. Yoga.

E. *The mind:*

1. Meditation.
2. Music therapy.
3. Visualization, guided imagery.
4. Humor therapy.
5. Pet therapy.

F. *Massage and touch:*

1. Massage therapy.
2. Reflexology.
3. Energy field therapies, including therapeutic touch.

G. *Eastern therapies:*

1. Acupuncture.
2. Acupressure.
3. Shiatsu.
4. Chinese herbal medicine.

V. IMPLICATIONS FOR NURSING:

A. Familiarize yourself with one or two basic therapies (e.g., massage, music, or guided imagery).

B. Try to eliminate own preconceived ideas.

C. Get adequate instruction before using any CAM with clients.

D. Ask clients if they use any CAM and their response to them.

E. *Health teaching:* Nurses can discuss and do teaching based on scientific research about effectiveness of each therapy when clients seek information about alternative and complementary therapies (because they are *noninvasive*, *holistic* [encompass mind and spirit], and *less* expensive) (see **Appendix E**). For example:

1. *Physical tension and anxiety*—can be decreased with meditation combined with guided imagery.
2. Effect of coronary heart disease—can be reversed with carefully planned nutrition, exercise, and meditation (Dr. Dean Ornish's plan).
3. Coordination—can be improved with yoga.
4. Blood pressure and stress—can be lowered and reduced with massage.
5. Apical heart rate—can be reduced; peripheral blood flow—can be increased with music.
6. Pain in arthritic joints and back—can be relieved by localized healing touch techniques.
7. Headache pain and breaking up congestion—can be aided by healing touch.
8. Prepare client for pre- and postoperative energy and recovery—can be aided by relaxation and energy-balancing methods.

GLOSSARY

affect *feeling* or *mood* communicated through the face and body posture. Can be blunted, blocked, flat, inappropriate, or displaced.

ambivalence coexisting *contradictory* (positive and negative) emotions, desires, or attitudes toward an object or person (e.g., love-hate relationship).

anhedonia inability to experience any pleasure.

amnesia loss of memory due to physical or emotion trauma.

anxiety state of uneasiness or response to a *vague,* unspecific danger cued by a threat to some value that the individual holds essential to existence (or by a threat of loss of control); the danger may be *real or imagined. Physiological* manifestations are increased pulse, respiration, and perspiration, with feeling of "butterflies."

associative looseness speaks with unconnected topics (e.g., "no one needs a bus; we all have heaven here"); disorganized thoughts and verbalizations.

autism self-preoccupation and absorption in fantasy, as found with schizophrenia, with a complete *exclusion of reality* and loss of interest in and appreciation of others.

catatonia type of schizophrenia characterized by muscular rigidity; alternates with periods of excitability.

circumstantiality doesn't reach a main point because speaks with too many unnecessary details.

clang association speaks in rhymes in nonsensical pattern.

compulsion an insistent, repetitive, intrusive, and unwanted urge to perform an *act* that is contrary to ordinary conscious wishes or standards.

concrete thinking difficulty with abstract concepts (e.g., "It's raining cats and dogs").

conflict emotional struggle resulting from *opposing* demands and drives of the id, ego, and superego.

coping mechanism a conscious action mobilized by a person to deal with stressful events. Coping mechanisms can be effective or ineffective.

cyclothymia alterations in moods of elation and sadness, with mood swings out of proportion to apparent stimuli.

defense mechanism device used to ward off anxiety or uncomfortable thoughts and feelings; an activity of the ego that operates outside of awareness to hold impulses in check that might cause conflict (e.g., repression, regression).

delusion a false fixed *belief,* idea, or group of ideas that are contrary to what is thought of as real and that cannot be changed by logic; arise out of the individual's needs and are maintained in spite of evidence or facts (e.g., grandeur and persecution).

depression morbid sadness or dejection accompanied by feelings of hopelessness, inadequacy, and unworthiness. *Distinguished from grief,* which is realistic and in proportion to loss.

disorientation loss of awareness of the position of self in relation to time, place, or person.

echolalia automatic repetition of heard *phrases or words.*

echopraxia automatic repetition of observed *movements.*

ego the "I," "self," and "person" as distinguished from "others"; that part of the personality, according to Freudian theory, that *mediates* between the primitive, pleasure-seeking, instinctual drives of the id and the self-critical, prohibitive, restraining forces of the superego; that aspect of the psyche that is *conscious* and most in touch with external reality and is directed by the *reality principle;* the part of the personality that has to make the *decision.* Most of the ego is conscious and represents the *thinking-feeling* part of a person. The *compromises* worked out on an unconscious level help to resolve intrapsychic conflict by keeping thoughts, interpretations, judgments, and behavior practical and efficient.

electroshock electroshock treatment (EST) or electroconvulsive treatment (ECT) is the treatment of certain psychiatric disorders (best suited for *depression*) by therapeutic administration of regulated electrical impulses to the brain to produce convulsions.

empathy an objective awareness of another's thoughts, feelings, or behaviors and their meaning and significance; intellectual identification versus emotional identification (sympathy).

euphoria exaggerated feeling of physical and emotional well-being *not* related to external events or stimuli.

flight of ideas a *thought disorder* in which one thought moves rapidly to another without reaching a main idea or point, as in manic behavior. The next sentence may be triggered by a word in the previous sentence or by something in the environment.

fugue dissociative state involving amnesia and actual *physical flight.*

hallucination *false sensory* perception in the absence of an actual external stimulus. May be due to chemicals or inner needs and may occur in any of the five senses (auditory and visual are most common). Seen in *psychosis* and *acute* and *chronic* brain disorder.

hypochondriasis state of morbid preoccupation about one's health (somatic concerns).

id psychoanalytic term for that division of the psyche that is unconscious, contains instinctual primitive drives that lead to immediate gratification, and is dominated by the *pleasure principle.* The id wants what it wants when it wants it.

illusion misinterpretation of a real, external sensory stimulus (e.g., a person may see a shadow on the floor and think it is a hole).

insanity *legal* term for mental defect or disease that is of sufficient gravity to bring person under special legal restrictions and immunities.

labile unstable and rapidly shifting (referring to emotions).

manipulation process of influencing another to meet one's own needs, *regardless* of the other's needs.

mental retardation term for mental deficiency or deficit in normal development of intelligence that makes intellectual abilities lower than normal for chronological age. May result from a condition present at birth, from injury during or after birth, or from disease after birth.

mutism inability or refusal to speak.

narcissism *exaggerated self-love* with all attention focused on own comfort, pleasure, abilities, appearance, etc.

neologism a newly coined word or condensed combination of several words not readily understood by others but with symbolic meaning for the person with *schizophrenia.*

neurosis *an older* term for mild to moderately severe illness in which there is a disorder of feeling or behavior but no gross mental disorganization, delusions, or hallucinations, as in serious psychoses. Typical reactions include disproportionate *anxiety, phobias,* and *obsessive-compulsive behavior.*

obsession persistent, unwanted, and uncontrollable *urge* or *idea* that *cannot* be banished by logic or will.

organic psychosis mental disease resulting from defect, damage, infection, tumor, or other *physical cause* that can be *observed* in the body tissues.

paranoid adjective indicating feelings of suspicion and persecution; one type of schizophrenia.

perseveration repeats same word or idea in response to different questions.

personality disorder broad category of illnesses in which inner difficulties are revealed not by specific symptoms but by *antisocial* behavior.

phobia *irrational, persistent,* abnormal, *morbid,* and unrealistic dread of external object or situation displaced from unconscious conflict.

premorbid personality state of an individual's personality *before* the onset of an illness.

psyche synonymous with mind or the *mental and emotional* "self."

psychoanalysis theory of human development and behavior, method of research, and form of treatment described by Freud that attributes abnormal behavior to repressions in the unconscious mind. Treatment involves dream interpretation and free association to bring into awareness the origin and effects of unconscious conflicts in order to eliminate or diminish them.

psychodrama a therapeutic approach that involves a structured, dramatized, and directed *acting out* of emotional problems and troubled interactions by the client in order to gain insight into individual's own difficulties.

psychogenic symptoms or physical disorders caused by emotional or mental factors, as opposed to organic.

psychopath *older,* inexact term for one of a variety of *personality disorders* in which person has poor impulse control, releasing tension through immediate action, without social or moral conscience.

psychosis severe emotional illness characterized by a disorder of *thinking, feeling, and action* with the following symptoms: loss of contact, denial of reality, bizarre thinking and behavior, perceptual distortion, delusions, hallucinations, and regression.

regression primary ego defense mechanism of retreat to earlier level of development, with childlike mannerisms and comfort techniques.

schizoid form of personality disorder characterized by shyness, introspection, introversion, withdrawal, and aloofness.

schizophrenia severe functional mental illness characterized in general by a disorder in perception, thinking, feeling, behavior, and interpersonal relationships.

sociopathic pertaining to a disorder of behavior in which a person's feelings and behavior are asocial, with impaired judgment and inability to profit from experience; the intellect remains intact. This term is often used interchangeably with "antisocial personality."

soma term meaning the body or *physical* aspects.

superego in psychoanalysis, that part of the mind that incorporates the parental or societal values, ethics, and standards. It guides, restrains, criticizes, and punishes. It is unconscious and learned and is sometimes equated with the term *conscience.*

tangentiality speaks on unrelated topics without getting to the point.

transference unconscious projections of feelings, attitudes, and wishes that were originally associated with early significant others onto persons or events in the present; may be positive or negative transference.

waxy flexibility psychomotor underactivity in which the individual maintains the posture in which he or she is placed.

word salad meaningless and random mixture of phrases and words without any logical connection often seen in *schizophrenic* behavior (e.g., "the rid jams frost wool mix").

Questions

Select the one answer that is best for each question, unless otherwise directed.

1. A nurse assesses a school-age child who asks questions and can associate subjects with concepts. In which stage of development is this child?
   1. Industry.
   2. Intuitive.
   3. Sensorimotor.
   4. Concrete.

2. A nurse observes a client on a locked mental health unit who is manifesting behaviors consistent with the mastery of Maslow's level of safety and security. Which behavior is this client most likely exhibiting?
   1. Attending medication information sessions and maintaining the unit garden.
   2. Joining group therapy sessions and agreeing to seek aftercare.
   3. Responding to limit setting and requesting anxiolytics.
   4. Eating meals with other clients in the quiet room.

3. An adult client, who is petitioning for release from a legal hold on a mental health unit, demonstrates care and consideration for other clients, complies with unit rules, and attends regular group meetings. According to Maslow, what level(s) has the client mastered? *Select all that apply.*
   1. Safety and security.
   2. Self-esteem.
   3. Self-actualization.
   4. Self-preservation.
   5. Love and belonging.

4. An adolescent client, admitted for depression due to peer pressures and substance use, is unable to contract for safety. A nurse should recognize that this client is in Erikson's developmental stage of:
   1. *Identity vs. role diffusion.*
   2. *Industry vs. inferiority.*
   3. *Intimacy vs. isolation.*
   4. *Ideality vs. reality.*

5. A client is on lithium for management of bipolar disorder. Which signs and symptoms should indicate to a nurse that the client is at risk for severe toxicity?
   1. Lethargy and motor weakness.
   2. Hand tremors.
   3. Tardive dyskinesia.
   4. Pruritus.

6. A client's spouse reveals ongoing infidelity in their relationship. A nurse identifies that this client is at increased risk for:
   1. Ineffective protection.
   2. Pain.
   3. Injury.
   4. Knowledge deficit.

7. A nurse assesses an adolescent client in a psychiatric emergency department for suicidal ideation. The client's parents are preoccupied with divorce proceedings. Which problem should the nurse suspect that this client is experiencing?
   1. Oppositional defiant disorder related to parental separation.
   2. Acute traumatic stress disorder related to family stress.
   3. Mood disorder related to role reversal.
   4. Adjustment disorder related to parental separation.

8. Clients who are dependent on alcohol and experience withdrawal are at risk for physical problems. Which independent nursing actions should be conducted during the detoxification phase when caring for this client? *Select all that apply.*
   1. Assess vital signs every 4 hours and as needed.
   2. Place the client on seizure and fall precautions.
   3. Administer benzodiazepines and anticonvulsants.
   4. Increase the intravenous rate to match serum sodium levels.
   5. Restrain the client if hallucinations are present.

9. A physician orders trihexyphenidyl (Artane) 4 mg at bedtime to relax a client's rigid muscles. The elixir is dispensed as 2 mg/5 mL. A nurse should correctly instruct the client to take _______ teaspoons of this medication. *Fill in the blank.*

10. The client is prescribed risperidone (Risperdal) at discharge for treatment of bipolar disorder. A nurse should recognize that more teaching is needed when the client states:
    1. "I will call the physician if I have unusual movements."
    2. "I will not stop the medication when my voices have gone away."
    3. "I will pay close attention to my weight increases."
    4. "I will have my liver panel drawn every month."

11. A client, who has had several verbal outbursts and is pacing around a psychiatric unit, is at risk for assaultive behavior. Which verbal response by a nurse is most appropriate?
    1. "Do not get agitated; everything is safe here."
    2. "Please take a time-out in your room."
    3. "If you don't follow the rules, you will be put in seclusion."
    4. "Let me take your blood pressure. I think you are having a lot of anxiety."

12. A client, who is severely depressed, is unable to contract for safety. Which nurse would be most appropriate to care for this client?
    1. A charge RN with 17 years' experience in a psychiatric/mental health unit who routinely takes a one- or two-client assignment.
    2. An experienced medical-surgical float nurse who assists in break relief.
    3. A new graduate RN who has not cared for a client experiencing severe depression.
    4. An RN with 3 years' experience in a psychiatric/mental health unit who has been on leave for 2 months.

13. A client on a medical-surgical unit is recovering from a suicide attempt and is now stable and anticipating discharge to an outpatient program. Which staff nurse is most appropriate to assign to this client?
    1. The LPN/LVN with 5 years' experience, supervised by an experienced nurse.
    2. The nurse who is assigned to a client who is high acuity.
    3. The RN with 3 years' experience who is assigned to admit and discharge clients.
    4. The RN who is a preceptor to the new graduate nurse who has 3 weeks of experience.

14. A nurse is conducting a health program regarding grief at a local community center. Considering the concepts related to loss, which client is most likely to experience an unsuccessful grief response?
    1. The adolescent who is irritable and testing limits with authority.
    2. The spouse who returns to work, but sobs daily during breaks.
    3. The young child experiencing the sudden death of a parent.
    4. The middle-aged adult who develops a gastric ulcer.

15. A nurse is caring for a client who is diagnosed with psychogenic diabetes insipidus. Which laboratory value is most indicative of this condition?
   1. Serum glucose of 65 mg/dL.
   2. Serum Na of 130 mEq/L.
   3. Serum Na of 300 mEq/L.
   4. Serum glucose of 129 mg/dL.

16. A client's family reports clinical manifestations of hyperactivity, delusions of grandeur, impaired judgment, and inability to sit still during a meal. Which diagnosis should a nurse suspect?
   1. Attention deficit-hyperactivity disorder (ADHD).
   2. Attention deficit disorder (ADD).
   3. Psychosis.
   4. Mania.

17. A nurse assess a client suspected of taking opiates. Which pupil size/shape represents opiate intoxication?
   1.

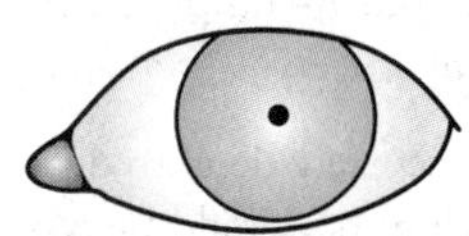

   2.

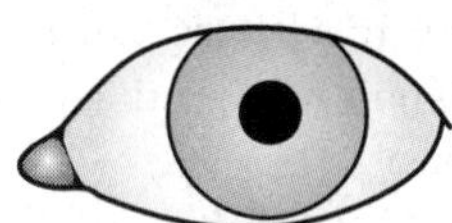

   3.

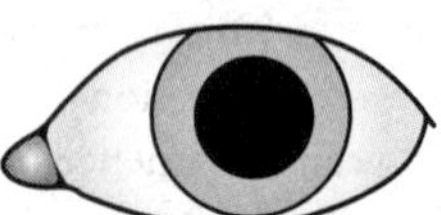

   4.

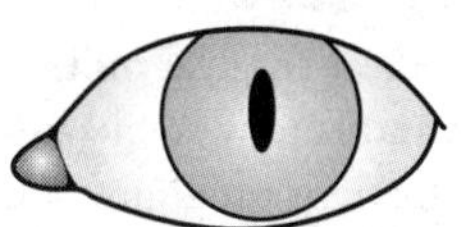

18. A physician orders a maintenance IV of 5% dextrose in normal saline (D_5NS) at 125 mL/hr for a client who is in alcohol withdrawal. In addition to the maintenance IV, the client is also receiving thiamine 30 mg IV, three times a day in 50-mL bags. A nurse calculates that this client's total parenteral intake is ________ mL/24 hr. *Fill in the blank.*

19. A nurse's *priority* related to clients who are experiencing clinical manifestations of borderline personality disorder should be to:
   1. Increase therapeutic communication when the client exhibits intrusiveness.
   2. Set limits when the client exhibits threats of self-damaging behaviors.
   3. Engage in one-to-one discussions about childhood experiences.
   4. Employ behavior modification using covert techniques.

20. A client was recently diagnosed with depression related to loss of a spouse. The client describes thinking constantly about the relationship and dreams of reconciliation even though the spouse is deceased. A nurse should document this as:
   1. Omnipotence.
   2. Isolation of affect.
   3. Fantasy.
   4. Regression.

21. A client is 1 day postoperative for a stereotactic brain procedure for relief of compulsive behavior. For which complication should a nurse observe this client?
   1. Altered level of consciousness.
   2. Immobility.
   3. Electrolyte imbalance.
   4. Infection.

22. An adolescent client is diagnosed with anorexia nervosa and discloses an incestuous relationship. Which is a nurse's most therapeutic response?
   1. "Tell me more about what happened when you were younger."
   2. "You will be okay, just keep on talking."
   3. "What kind of comfort food do you want tonight?"
   4. "Can you tell me how you feel about what happened?"

23. A registered nurse (RN) can best demonstrate empathy by:
   1. Revealing personal experiences with similar issues.
   2. Conveying genuine understanding of the client's problems.
   3. Identifying behavioral problems.
   4. Advising the client about better communication techniques.

24. In attempting to reduce acting-out behaviors by a child in a pediatric psychiatric unit, a brief therapeutic hold is implemented. An RN knows that a therapeutic hold means:
   1. Involuntary confinement of a child in a locked room for no more than 30 minutes.
   2. Physically holding a child, up to 30 minutes, to assist the child to calm down.
   3. Placement of a papoose-like device on a child who is out of control and acting out.
   4. Use of a padded room to confine a child who cannot behave in the therapeutic milieu.

25. A psychiatric nurse is assigned to care for multiple clients. Which client should the nurse assess *first?*
   1. The client with auditory hallucinations, who is responding to the voices with laughter.
   2. The client with hallucinations, who has increased blood pressure and heart rate.
   3. The client with suicidal ideations, who has a nonlethal plan.
   4. The client with superficial self-inflicted wounds to the wrists and arms.

26. In evaluating a client's understanding of divalproex sodium (Depakote) during discharge teaching, a nurse should identify that the client requires additional teaching if the client states:
   1. "I will need to get my complete blood count tested frequently."
   2. "I will take this medication the same time each day."
   3. "I will report any unusual bleeding to my doctor."
   4. "It is important to use sunscreen when taking this medication."

27. Which actions should a nurse include when developing a care plan for a client with problems associated with body image disturbance? *Select all that apply.*
   1. Provide the client with detailed plans for the future.
   2. Support the client with a realistic appraisal of the situation.
   3. Explore the client's strengths and available resources.
   4. Encourage the client to focus on the specific limitations.
   5. Teach the client about expected changes in functioning.

28. Considering the development of egocentrism, which clients are most likely to experience egocentrism? *Select all that apply.*
   1. The adolescent with addiction to weight loss products.
   2. The infant fixated on the black-and-white figures.
   3. The elderly client with a history of substance abuse.
   4. The hospitalized toddler having a tantrum.
   5. The adult client with depression who is finding support from others.

29. A nurse is required to provide limit setting on a pediatric mental health unit. What are the most important concepts related to limit setting? *Select all that apply.*
   1. Provide unit information to clients upon admission.
   2. Remove all contraband and employ frequent inspections.
   3. Stop destructive behavior immediately.
   4. Reinforce dependent behaviors with earned privileges.
   5. Engage in playful experiences to foster social growth.

30. A nurse is caring for a client who is experiencing serotonin syndrome. Which serotonergic drugs should a nurse recognize as possibly contributing to this problem? *Select all that apply.*
   1. Duloxetine (Cymbalta).
   2. Fluoxetine (Prozac).
   3. Aripiprazole (Abilify).
   4. Haloperidol (Haldol).
   5. Paroxetine (Paxil).

31. A client with antisocial personality disorder has been acting very manipulative. Which actions by a nurse will help to reduce the manipulative behaviors? *Select all that apply.*
   1. Develop a list of realistic goals with the client.
   2. Accept small tokens of appreciation as collaboration.
   3. Maintain consistent limit setting.
   4. Place the client on the "problem" board to modify behaviors.
   5. Evaluate actions, the consequences, and successes.

32. A nurse has just received morning report and is organizing and prioritizing the client assignment. *Prioritize* the nurse's actions by placing each client in the correct order.
   ________ 1. The client with depression scheduled for discharge to the partial care program in 3 hours.
   ________ 2. The client who is in alcohol withdrawal with a serum sodium of 150 mEq/L.
   ________ 3. The client with an anxiety disorder complaining of chest discomfort.
   ________ 4. The client with aphasia requesting a piece of writing paper.

33. A nurse is reviewing the laboratory values for a group of clients in a psychiatric emergency department. *Prioritize* each laboratory result from most to least important to report to a physician.
   ________ 1. The client taking clozapine (Clozaril) with a WBC count of <3000/mm^3.
   ________ 2. The client with bipolar disorder and a lithium level of 1.6 mEq/L.
   ________ 3. The client with a blood alcohol level of 0.08%.
   ________ 4. The client with schizoaffective disorder and a potassium level of 6.0 mEq/L.

34. A client was admitted yesterday with a diagnosis of acute traumatic stress disorder. What should a nurse expect this client's assessment to reveal? *Select all that apply.*
   1. Increased intimacy.
   2. Amnesia.
   3. Flashbacks.
   4. Expressions of guilt.
   5. Sleep disturbances.

35. Which clinical manifestations should a nurse recognize as being related to the "negative" symptoms associated with a schizophrenic client? *Select all that apply.*
   1. Brief, empty responses.
   2. Clang associations.
   3. Inappropriate sexual behaviors.
   4. Poor eye contact.
   5. Somatic delusions.

36. A client, who is manic, is at risk for nutritional deficits. Which nutritional products should the nurse encourage this client to select? *Select all that apply.*
   1. Fresh fruits and vegetables.
   2. Protein booster shake.
   3. Bean and cheese mini-tacos.
   4. Chocolate ice cream sundae.
   5. Sweetened iced coffee drink.

QUESTIONS

37. A manic client's temperature readings were 37.0°C, 38.2°C, 38.1°C, and 37.5°C. A nurse calculates that the client's mean temperature over the past 24 hours was _______ °C. *Fill in the blank* using one decimal place.

38. A physician prescribes haloperidol decanoate (Haldol Decanoate) 0.5 mg IM to a client diagnosed with schizophrenia. Haldol Decanoate is available as a 2-mg/mL solution for IM injection. In order to administer the correct dosage, a nurse should inject _______ mL intramuscularly. *Fill in the blank.*

39. The parent of the client with attention deficit-hyperactivity disorder (ADHD) is receiving discharge teaching for methylphenidate (Ritalin). A nurse evaluates that the parent is in need of additional teaching when the parent states: *Select all that apply.*
1. "I must give my child the medication 30 minutes before meals."
2. "My child will need to take this medication in the morning."
3. "I would know that it indicates tolerance if my child gains weight."
4. "It is best for my child to avoid caffeine with this medication."
5. "This CNS depressant should not be combined with other CNS depressants."

40. A client diagnosed with manic-depressive disorder is prescribed lithium PO 1,200 mg to be given in divided doses twice daily. The dosage on hand is 300 mg per tablet. In order to administer the correct dose, a nurse should give the client _______ tablets every 12 hours. *Fill in the blank.*

41. A clinical nurse specialist describes behavior modification techniques to a group of new graduates. Which therapies should the clinical nurse specialist include in this description? *Select all that apply.*
1. Free association.
2. Cognitive-based therapy.
3. Desensitization.
4. Token economy.
5. Occupational therapy.

42. A client, who abuses alcohol, is at risk for injury during the detoxification phase of alcohol withdrawal. Which physician order for this client should the nurse question?
1. Apply soft wrist restraints as needed.
2. Bedrest with side rails up.
3. Maintain IV D_5 0.45% NS at 100 mL/hr.
4. Baseline ECG.

43. A client is responding with hostility to staff and other clients. A nurse's *priority* diagnosis for this client should be:
1. Distorted sensory perception.
2. Impaired social interaction.
3. Risk for violence.
4. Impaired thought processes.

44. When caring for a client who has been raped, which action should a nurse take *first?*
1. Explore legal issues and prosecution.
2. Acknowledge client's anxiety and fear.
3. Explore client's feelings about recovery.
4. Introduce defensive tactics.

45. A primary prevention measure that should be implemented by a nurse when working with clients who are at risk for elder abuse is:
1. Reporting a case to law enforcement officials.
2. Referring caregivers to community resources.
3. Offering counseling to the victim.
4. Providing the elder with hotline numbers.

46. A nurse suspects that a client may be experiencing anorexia nervosa. Which statement by the client's family supports the nurse's suspicion?
1. "She spends so much time in the bathroom."
2. "She plans the meals and counts calories."
3. "She has stopped menstruating."
4. "She is always oversalting her foods."

47. A long-term care client, diagnosed with Alzheimer's disease, is having difficulties with changes in daily routine and attempts to call family members at all hours and is no longer able to walk unassisted. Which problem should a nurse document as *priority?*
1. Relocation stress syndrome.
2. Altered attention and memory.
3. Sensory/perceptual alterations.
4. Risk for trauma.

48. A client, who has abused alcohol for 20 years, is admitted to a rehabilitation unit. Which laboratory values should a nurse expect to find?
1. Decreased total protein and increased albumin.
2. Increased blood alcohol levels and impaired reflexes.
3. Increased LDH and amylase and decreased albumin.
4. Decreased potassium and increased magnesium.

49. Which nursing assessments should indicate to a nurse that a newly admitted client is in amphetamine withdrawal?
1. Apprehension, tremors, and psychosis-delirium.
2. Insomnia, anxiety, and loss of appetite.
3. Vomiting, tremors, and diaphoresis.
4. Depression, lack of energy, and somnolence.

50. A client whispers, "The spiders are coming out of the vents; we need to move." Which response by a nurse demonstrates the therapeutic technique of focusing on reality?
1. "I didn't understand you. Can you repeat that?"
2. "That's strange. I don't see any spiders."
3. "What did you see?"
4. "That must be frightening to think that."

Answers/Rationales/Tips

1. CORRECT ANSWER: 2. Answer 1 is incorrect because this concept relates to Erikson's theory. **Answer 2 is correct because the school-age child in the intuitive stage asks questions, uses symbols, and can associate subjects with concepts. Answer 3** is incorrect because this is the stage that Piaget relates to infants and toddlers. **Answer 4** is incorrect because this is the stage Piaget relates to the older child who has more advanced cognitive processes.

■ **TEST-TAKING TIP:** ***Eliminate Answer 1 because it is the wrong theorist. Eliminate Answers 3 and 4 because these relate to preschool-age children.***

Content Area: Mental Health, Child Health; ***Integrated Process:*** Nursing Process, Assessment; ***Cognitive Level:*** Application; ***Client Need/Subneed:*** Health Promotion and Maintenance/Developmental Stages and Transitions

2. CORRECT ANSWER: 3. Answer 1 is incorrect because these behaviors are consistent with working toward self-esteem. **Answer 2** is incorrect because this reflects the client who is mastering love and belonging. **Answer 3 is correct because safety and security are evident when the client feels safe with structure and avoids harm. Answer 4** is incorrect because the client has just achieved meeting physiological needs.

■ **TEST-TAKING TIP:** ***Eliminate Answers 1 and 2 because these are at a higher level of Maslow's hierarchy. Eliminate Answer 4 because this is at the lowest level of Maslow's hierarchy. Remember the pyramid and each level.***

Content Area: Mental Health, Growth and Development; ***Integrated Process:*** Nursing Process, Assessment; ***Cognitive Level:*** Application; ***Client Need/Subneed:*** Psychosocial Integrity/Mental Health Concepts

3. CORRECT ANSWERS: 1, 5. Answer 1 is correct because the client is meeting basic physiological needs. Answer 2 is incorrect because the client has not mastered this level. **Answer 3** is incorrect because the client has not mastered the previous level and therefore cannot reach Maslow's next level. **Answer 4** is incorrect because this is not a concept associated with Maslow's hierarchy of needs. **Answer 5 is correct because the client is achieving love and belonging. The client has developed a positive sense of self, but has not mastered the level of self-esteem.**

■ **TEST-TAKING TIP:** ***Eliminate Answers 2 and 3 because the client has not mastered these higher levels. Eliminate Answer 4 because this isn't a concept related to Maslow' theory at all. Remember the pyramid and each level.***

Content Area: Mental Health, Growth and Development; ***Integrated Process:*** Nursing Process, Assessment; ***Cognitive Level:*** Application; ***Client Need/Subneed:*** Psychosocial Integrity/Mental Health Concepts

4. CORRECT ANSWER: 1. Answer 1 is correct because the adolescent develops intense concern over peer influences and is at risk for developing role diffusion (e.g., acting out with substance abuse). Answer 2 is incorrect because this is a developmental level reflecting *later* childhood. **Answer 3** is incorrect because this is a developmental level experienced by the *young adult.* **Answer 4** is incorrect as this is *not* a level described by Erikson.

■ **TEST-TAKING TIP:** ***Eliminate Answers 2 and 3 because, according to Erikson, these are not the developmental levels of an adolescent. Eliminate Answer 4 because this is not a developmental level related to Erikson or any other theorist.***

Content Area: Mental Health, Child Health, Growth and Development; ***Integrated Process:*** Nursing Process, Assessment; ***Cognitive Level:*** Application; ***Client Need/Subneed:*** Psychosocial Integrity/Mental Health Concepts

5. CORRECT ANSWER: 1. Answer 1 is correct because motor weakness and lethargy are early signs of toxicity. Answer 2 is incorrect because this is an initial side effect and should diminish with time. **Answer 3** is incorrect because tardive dyskinesia is a result related to prolonged use of neuroleptics, not lithium. **Answer 4** is incorrect because this is an expected mild side effect or an allergic reaction.

■ **TEST-TAKING TIP:** ***Eliminate Answers 2 and 4 because these are more mild side effects of lithium. Eliminate Answer 3 because this is an adverse effect of neuroleptics.***

Content Area: Mental Health, Pharmacology; ***Integrated Process:*** Nursing Process, Assessment; ***Cognitive Level:*** Application; ***Client Need/Subneed:*** Physiological Integrity/Pharmacological and Parenteral Therapies/Adverse Effects/Contraindications/Interactions

6. CORRECT ANSWER: 3. Answer 1 is incorrect as this nursing diagnosis is not necessarily risk related. Ineffective protection would be a problem if the client were immunocompromised, which is not known at this time. **Answer 2** is incorrect because, although the client may experience pain, it is not a common problem with sexually transmitted infections. **Answer 3 is correct because, if sexual encounters were unprotected, this may place the client at risk for sexually transmitted infections, which could lead to injury, permanent dysfunction, and possible infection-related problems. Answer 4** is incorrect because, even though knowledge deficit about sexually transmitted infections is likely, it is not a priority.

■ **TEST-TAKING TIP:** ***Eliminate Answers 1, 2, and 4 because these are*** not risk-related ***nursing diagnoses. Remember: priority problems are those that pose a threat to the client's homeostasis.***

Content Area: Mental Health, Adult Health, Sexually Transmitted Infections; ***Integrated Process:*** Nursing Process, Analysis; ***Cognitive Level:*** Application; ***Client Need/Subneed:*** Safe and Effective Care Environment/Safety and Infection Control/Standard/Transmission-based/Other Precautions

ANSWERS

7. CORRECT ANSWER: 4. Answer 1 is incorrect because oppositional defiant disorder is characterized by defiant behaviors (e.g., truancy and lying) and opposition to authority. **Answer 2** is incorrect because this disorder is characterized by intrusive thoughts, memories that are emotionally painful, and increased anxiety. **Answer 3** is incorrect because the client is not having role reversal issues (e.g., taking on the role of one or both parents). **Answer 4 is correct because this is a typical disorder experienced by adolescents whose parents are experiencing marital problems; suicidal ideation is short-lived and usually related to separation or divorce.**

■ **TEST-TAKING TIP:** *Answers 1 and 2 are incorrect because the situation does not suggest these issues at all. Answer 3 is close, but still incorrect because the adolescent is not switching roles with either parent.*

Content Area: Mental Health, Anxiety; ***Integrated Process:*** Nursing Process, Analysis; ***Cognitive Level:*** Application; ***Client Need/Subneed:*** Psychosocial Integrity/Stress Management

8. CORRECT ANSWERS: 1, 2. Answer 1 is correct because the client may experience increases in vital signs (e.g., pulse and blood pressure). Answer 2 is correct because it is important to place the client on seizure precautions as these occur during withdrawal. The nurse must place the client on fall precautions to prevent injury if the client becomes confused. Answer 3 is incorrect because this action requires a physician's order. **Answer 4** is incorrect because this action requires a physician's order. **Answer 5** is incorrect because this action requires a physician's order.

■ **TEST-TAKING TIP:** *Remember independent nursing actions (e.g., vital signs and all precautions) do not require a physician's order.*

Content Area: Mental Health, Substance Abuse; ***Integrated Process:*** Nursing Process, Implementation; ***Cognitive Level:*** Application; ***Client Need/Subneed:*** Psychosocial Integrity/ Chemical and Other Dependencies

9. CORRECT ANSWER: 2 tsp. Use this calculation:

$$\frac{4\text{ mg}}{2\text{ mg}} \times 5\text{ mL} = 10\text{ mg} \rightarrow \text{convert to teaspoons}$$
$$(5\text{ mg} = 1\text{ tsp}) \rightarrow 10\text{ mg} = 2\text{ tsp}$$

■ **TEST-TAKING TIP:** *Always check medication calculations twice before administering a medication.*

Content Area: Mental Health, Pharmacology; ***Integrated Process:*** Nursing Process, Implementation; ***Cognitive Level:*** Analysis; ***Client Need/Subneed:*** Physiological Integrity/ Pharmacological and Parenteral Therapies/Dosage Calculation

10. CORRECT ANSWER: 4. Answer 1 is incorrect because it *is* important that the client report this problem to the physician. **Answer 2** is incorrect because the client *does* need to take the medication even if target symptoms are relieved. **Answer 3** is incorrect because weight increase *can* occur with this medication. **Answer 4 is correct because it is not routine for the client using risperidone (Risperdal) to have liver function tests performed.**

■ **TEST-TAKING TIP:** *The best answer is the one that is* not *correct.*

Content Area: Mental Health, Pharmacology; ***Integrated Process:*** Nursing Process, Evaluation; ***Cognitive Level:*** Analysis; ***Client Need/Subneed:*** Physiological Integrity/Pharmacological and Parenteral Therapies/Medication Administration

11. CORRECT ANSWER: 2. Answer 1 is incorrect because the nurse is offering false reassurance. **Answer 2 is correct because, at the client's increasing level of anxiety, the client can only understand simple, short phrases. Answer 3** is incorrect because the nurse's response is inappropriate because it challenges the client and is threatening. **Answer 4** is incorrect because the nurse's response is inappropriate because it doesn't address the verbal outburst, and the action of taking the client's blood pressure places the nurse's safety at risk.

■ **TEST-TAKING TIP:** *As anxiety levels increase, the client's ability to process information decreases. Choose the most specific intervention. Eliminate the two "negative" options (Answer 1 "not", Answer 3 "don't").*

Content Area: Mental Health, Anxiety; ***Integrated Process:*** Communication and Documentation; ***Cognitive Level:*** Application; ***Client Need/Subneed:*** Psychosocial Integrity/ Mental Health Concepts

12. CORRECT ANSWER: 4. Answer 1 is incorrect because the nurse who has charge nurse responsibilities may not be able to keep a client in constant view. **Answer 2** is incorrect because the nurse has experience as a medical-surgical float nurse but may not have been consistently assigned to the mental health unit. **Answer 3** is incorrect because the new graduate may not be qualified to care for a client at risk for self-harm, due to lack of experience. **Answer 4 is correct because the nurse is experienced in working with clients who are at risk for self-harm.**

■ **TEST-TAKING TIP:** *Eliminate Answers 1, 2, and 3 because these place the client's safety at risk. Always think safety first.*

Content Area: Mental Health, Management of Care; ***Integrated Process:*** Nursing Process, Analysis; ***Cognitive Level:*** Analysis; ***Client Need/Subneed:*** Safe and Effective Care Environment/ Management of Care/Delegation

13. CORRECT ANSWER: 1. Answer 1 is correct because this client is stable. Answer 2 is incorrect because this nurse will need to care for a client who requires the nurse's time and attention. **Answer 3** is incorrect because the nurse will be focused on specific tasks related to admissions and discharges. **Answer 4** is incorrect because the new graduate nurse is inexperienced (e.g., new to the medical-surgical unit) with medical-surgical clients who have complex diagnoses (e.g., the client recovering from a suicide is in need of psychosocial interventions with which the nurse may not be familiar).

■ **TEST-TAKING TIP:** *Remember that the LPN/LVN can care for a client who is stable with predictable outcomes.*

Content Area: Mental Health, Management of Care; ***Integrated Process:*** Nursing Process, Analysis; ***Cognitive Level:*** Analysis;

Client Need/Subneed: Safe and Effective Care Environment/ Management of Care/Delegation

14. CORRECT ANSWER: 3. Answer 1 is incorrect because the adolescent is displaying normal and expected behaviors consistent with loss. **Answer 2** is incorrect because the adult is resuming work, and sobbing is an expected grief response if it does not interrupt daily function. **Answer 3 is correct because a young child who has experienced a sudden loss has more risk factors than other age groups. Answer 4** is incorrect because development of physiological problems is consistent with loss and does not necessarily result in an unresolved grief response.
■ **TEST-TAKING TIP:** *Adolescents and adults are more capable of resolving issues and problems than children.*
Content Area: Mental Health, Grief; *Integrated Process:* Nursing Process, Analysis; *Cognitive Level:* Analysis; *Client Need/Subneed:* Psychosocial Integrity/Grief and Loss

15. CORRECT ANSWER: 3. Answer 1 is incorrect because serum glucose levels are not indicative laboratory values for diabetes insipidus. **Answer 2** is incorrect because serum sodium is not decreased with diabetes insipidus. **Answer 3 is correct because serum sodium is elevated with diabetes insipidus. Answer 4** is incorrect because serum glucose levels are not laboratory values for diabetes insipidus.
■ **TEST-TAKING TIP:** *Think: sodium makes the client insipidus. Look for the highest sodium level.*
Content Area: Adult Health, Endocrine; *Integrated Process:* Nursing Process, Analysis; *Cognitive Level:* Application; *Client Need/Subneed:* Physiological Integrity/Reduction of Risk Potential/Laboratory Values

16. CORRECT ANSWER: 4. Answer 1 is incorrect because clinical manifestations for ADHD do not include delusions of grandeur. **Answer 2** is incorrect because clinical manifestations of ADD do not include delusions of grandeur. **Answer 3** is incorrect because psychosis involves hallucinations. **Answer 4 is correct because these are typical signs of mania distinguished by the delusions of grandeur.**
■ **TEST-TAKING TIP:** *Although hyperactivity may be a key symptom in all four options, delusions of grandeur are specific for manic behavior.*
Content Area: Mental Health, Mood Disorders; *Integrated Process:* Nursing Process, Analysis; *Cognitive Level:* Application; *Client Need/Subneed:* Psychosocial Integrity/Mental Health Concepts

17. CORRECT ANSWER: 1. Answer 1 is correct because pinpoint pupils are indicative of opiate use. Answer 2 is incorrect because the pupil size is within *normal* range. **Answer 3** is incorrect because this pupil is *dilated,* which is consistent with *amphetamine* abuse. **Answer 4** is incorrect because the abnormal shape of the pupil may indicate *optic surgery,* not opiate abuse.
■ **TEST-TAKING TIP:** *Opiates cause pupil constriction compared to amphetamines, which cause dilation.*
Content Area: Mental Health, Substance Abuse; *Integrated Process:* Nursing Process, Assessment; *Cognitive Level:* Application; *Client Need/Subneed:* Physiological Integrity/Reduction of Risk Potential/System Specific Assessments

18. CORRECT ANSWER: 3,150 mL. Use this calculation:
125 mL × 24 = 3,000 mL
50 mL × 3 = 150 mL
3,000 mL + 150 mL = 3,150 mL
■ **TEST-TAKING TIP:** *Multiply volume and time for each solution and then add the products together.*
Content Area: Mental Health, Pharmacology; *Integrated Process:* Nursing Process, Implementation; *Cognitive Level:* Analysis; *Client Need/Subneed:* Physiological Integrity/Pharmacological and Parenteral Therapies/Parenteral/Intravenous Therapies

ANSWERS

19. CORRECT ANSWER: 2. Answer 1 is incorrect because it is important to set limits with negative behaviors rather than having therapeutic communication sessions. **Answer 2 is correct because the client who is borderline *may* demonstrate a need for attention and break unit-based rules (e.g., hiding contraband), which could lead to behaviors that are dangerous (e.g., self-mutilation). The nurse reinforces expected behaviors through setting limits. Answer 3** is incorrect because it is not therapeutic to probe into the client's childhood experiences at this time, as it will not help to correct destructive or self-damaging behavior. **Answer 4** is incorrect because it creates a lack of trust and is not therapeutic to use any covert (i.e., hidden) tactics to change the client's behavior.
■ **TEST-TAKING TIP:** *Remember the clinical manifestations of the borderline client. These clients are very manipulative and require firm limits.*
Content Area: Mental Health, Borderline Disorder; *Integrated Process:* Nursing Process, Planning; *Cognitive Level:* Application; *Client Need/Subneed:* Psychosocial Integrity/Mental Health Concepts

20. CORRECT ANSWER: 3. Answer 1 is incorrect because omnipotence is when a person acts as if more important than others with power over others (e.g., the spouse feels the ability to control the situation through power and persuasion of others). **Answer 2** is incorrect because isolation of affect is experienced when the client separates feelings from thoughts or ideas (e.g., feels no emotion when thinking of a sad loss). **Answer 3 is correct because the client is "dreaming" and experiencing the ego defense mechanism of fantasy to cope with the anxiety associated with the loss of a spouse. Fantasy is a break from reality. Answer 4** is incorrect because regression occurs when the client exhibits behaviors from an earlier stage of development (e.g., an adult who behaves in an immature manner, such as clutching a stuffed animal, when dealing with stressful situations such as loss).
■ **TEST-TAKING TIP:** *Note the key word "dreams," which is related to fantasy.*
Content Area: Mental Health, Anxiety—Coping Mechanisms; *Integrated Process:* Communication and Documentation; *Cognitive Level:* Application; *Client Need/Subneed:* Psychosocial Integrity/Grief and Loss

21. CORRECT ANSWER: 1. Answer 1 is correct because a client who has stereotactic brain surgery has had an invasive neurosurgical procedure that places the client at risk for increased intracranial pressure, exhibited by a decreasing level of consciousness. **Answer 2** is incorrect because immobility is not a common problem associated with this procedure. Clients are usually up and out of bed within hours of the procedure. **Answer 3** is incorrect because it is unlikely that the client will experience problems with electrolyte imbalances in 1 day. **Answer 4** is incorrect because signs and symptoms of infection will not likely manifest by the first postoperative day.

■ **TEST-TAKING TIP:** *Think "priority" and think what problem is likely to occur within 24 hours after this neurosurgical procedure. Also think: brain = level of consciousness.*

Content Area: Mental Health—Neurological; ***Integrated Process:*** Nursing Process, Assessment; ***Cognitive Level:*** Application; ***Client Need/Subneed:*** Physiological Integrity/Reduction of Risk Potential/Potential for Complications of Diagnostic Tests/Treatments/Procedures

22. CORRECT ANSWER: 4. **Answer 1** is incorrect because it is a nontherapeutic approach and the nurse is probing for a factual account about a past event. **Answer 2** is incorrect because it is a nontherapeutic approach and the nurse is using false reassurance. **Answer 3** is incorrect because it is a nontherapeutic approach and the nurse switches focus to food, away from feelings. Answer 4 is correct because the nurse is using a therapeutic approach by encouraging expression of feelings.

■ **TEST-TAKING TIP:** *Focus on feelings (Answer 4) rather than facts (Answer 1).*

Content Area: Mental Health, Therapeutic Communication; ***Integrated Process:*** Communication and Documentation; ***Cognitive Level:*** Analysis; ***Client Need/Subneed:*** Psychosocial Integrity/Therapeutic Communications

23. CORRECT ANSWER: 2. **Answer 1** is incorrect because the statement is a sympathetic, not empathetic, response. Answer 2 is correct because the intent is for the client to feel that the nurse understands the client's experiences and conveys this back to the client. **Answer 3** is incorrect because empathy does not include problem identification. **Answer 4** is incorrect because giving advice is not a therapeutic approach.

■ **TEST-TAKING TIP:** *Empathy = "understanding."*

Content Area: Mental Health, Therapeutic Communication; ***Integrated Process:*** Caring; ***Cognitive Level:*** Application; ***Client Need/Subneed:*** Psychosocial Integrity/Therapeutic Communications

24. CORRECT ANSWER: 2. **Answer 1** is incorrect because this is not therapeutic and can place the client at a risk for injury if left unattended in a room by self. Answer 2 is correct as this is a desired and recognized therapeutic pediatric hold. The nurse implements this type of hold when a client is acting out and in danger of hurting self or others. The therapeutic hold is brief—no longer than 30 minutes—and is used specifically to calm down a child who is out of control. **Answer 3** is incorrect because this type of hold is dangerous and has been found to lead to asphyxiation (e.g., restricting respirations). **Answer 4** is incorrect because it is not considered a therapeutic hold; rather it is confinement to a designated area and not effective to help calm a client.

■ **TEST-TAKING TIP:** *Note the key word "hold"; all other responses relate to confinement.*

Content Area: Mental Health, Child Health—Restraint, Acting Out; ***Integrated Process:*** Nursing Process, Implementation; ***Cognitive Level:*** Comprehension; ***Client Need/Subneed:*** Safe and Effective Care Environment/Safety and Infection Control/Use of Restraints/Safety Devices

25. CORRECT ANSWER: 2. **Answer 1** is incorrect because the client is not in immediate danger of self-inflicted harm. Answer 2 is correct because this client has a risk of cardiovascular problems and may need medical attention. **Answer 3** is incorrect because the client does not have a *lethal* plan. **Answer 4** is incorrect because these superficial wounds are not immediately life-threatening.

■ **TEST-TAKING TIP:** *Note the key word "first." Think ABCs (circulation); the nurse's priority is based on an immediate threat to the client's safety and physiological integrity.*

Content Area: Mental Health, Management of Care; ***Integrated Process:*** Nursing Process, Analysis; ***Cognitive Level:*** Analysis; ***Client Need/Subneed:*** Safe and Effective Care Environment/Management of Care/Establishing Priorities

26. CORRECT ANSWER: 1. Answer 1 is correct because the client will need liver function tests, *not* a complete blood count, due to Depakote use and the potential to cause liver damage. **Answer 2** is incorrect because the client *will* need to take the medication the same time each day to maintain therapeutic levels. **Answer 3** is incorrect because this medication *can* alter liver function and clotting factors. **Answer 4** is incorrect because the client *does* understand that Depakote increases sun sensitivity.

■ **TEST-TAKING TIP:** *The best answer is the wrong statement.*

Content Area: Mental Health, Pharmacology; ***Integrated Process:*** Nursing Process, Evaluation; ***Cognitive Level:*** Analysis; ***Client Need/Subneed:*** Physiological Integrity/Pharmacological and Parenteral Therapies/Expected Effects/Outcomes

27. CORRECT ANSWERS: 2, 3, 5. **Answer 1** is incorrect because it is inappropriate for the nurse to predict what the future will hold for the client. The client needs to problem-solve, with the encouragement of the nurse, to gain self-sufficiency and empowerment over the situation. Answer 2 is correct because the nurse should plan to support the client by encouraging the client to apply a practical problem-solving approach. Answer 3 is correct because the nurse should explore the client's strengths and resources to assist the client to explore his or her own positive assets and seek help from others to focus on positive coping strategies. **Answer 4** is incorrect because the nurse needs to help the client view self as a total person, not focus on *only* the limitations. **Answer 5 is correct because the nurse should teach the client about expected changes in functioning. It is the nurse's role to teach the client about limitations and abilities (e.g., how to be mobile when a limb has been amputated) within the context of changes in the body.**

■ **TEST-TAKING TIP:** *Eliminate the options that are unrealistic for the client with body image disturbances (e.g., the nurse should not overload with detailed plans for the future; and it is a negative focus to talk about limitations).*

Content Area: Mental Health, Body Image; *Integrated Process:* Nursing Process, Planning; *Cognitive Level:* Application; *Client Need/Subneed:* Physiological Integrity/Physiological Adaptation/Alterations in Body Systems

28. CORRECT ANSWERS: 1, 3, 4. Answer 1 is correct because the adolescent experiences a surge in egocentrism (e.g., self-focus on meeting own needs). The adolescent is overly concerned with the self-image and the presentation of self to others. **Answer 2** is incorrect because the infant has not developed a fully formed ego (e.g., does not recognize a separation from self and the environment). **Answer 3 is correct because the client who is advancing in age experiences another resurgence of egocentrism related to deficits in bodily function and performance (e.g., is slower, decreased in stamina). The elder becomes aware of declining physical and mental functioning, which can result in use/abuse of substances to cope. Answer 4 is correct because toddlerhood is when the ego is developed and focus on self and meeting own needs is first experienced. The toddler begins to interact with others and the environment and reacts in defending the ego through acting-out behaviors.** **Answer 5** is incorrect because the adult is coping through reaching out to others, meeting needs through the assistance and feedback from a group.

■ **TEST-TAKING TIP:** *Consider the age and eliminate any answer that does not typically relate to self-focus.*

Content Area: Mental Health, Growth and Development; *Integrated Process:* Nursing Process, Analysis; *Cognitive Level:* Application; *Client Need/Subneed:* Health Promotion and Maintenance/Developmental Stages and Transitions

29. CORRECT ANSWERS: 1, 3, 5. Answer 1 is correct because giving information regarding unit rules and expected behavior informs the client that structure and adherence to standards is enforced and defiance will result in consequences (e.g., withholding a privilege). **Answer 2** is incorrect because, although it is important to remove all contraband (e.g., sharp objects) and maintain safety, frequent random inspections of clients' personal space *may* lead to mistrust of staff and more limit testing (e.g., breaking rules). **Answer 3 is correct because stopping destructive behavior immediately is important in maintaining the limits and reinforces the rule that the behavior is not tolerated.** **Answer 4** is incorrect because it is important to foster *independence* with rewards (e.g., privileges), especially when associated with the client taking responsibility for actions, leading to increased self-control. **Answer 5 is correct because, when the nurse engages in play therapy with the young client, this therapy is *often* very effective in reducing stress and gives the nurse the opportunity to role model appropriate behaviors that are expected.**

■ **TEST-TAKING TIP:** *Note the key words "limit setting" and select responses that are related.*

Content Area: Mental Health, Child Health, Play Therapy; *Integrated Process:* Nursing Process, Planning; *Cognitive Level:* Analysis; *Client Need/Subneed:* Psychosocial Integrity/Mental Health Concepts

30. CORRECT ANSWERS: 1, 2, 5. Answer 1 is correct because duloxetine (Cymbalta) is a serotonin-norepinephrine reuptake inhibitor that can lead to serotonin syndrome (e.g., uncoordinated movements, diarrhea, or tremors). Answer 2 is correct because fluoxetine (Prozac) is a selective serotonin reuptake inhibitor that can lead to serotonin syndrome. **Answer 3** is incorrect because aripiprazole (Abilify) is an antipsychotic and does not inhibit the reuptake of serotonin. **Answer 4** is incorrect because haloperidol (Haldol) is an antipsychotic and does not inhibit the reuptake of serotonin. **Answer 5 is correct because paroxetine (Paxil) is a selective serotonin reuptake inhibitor that can lead to serotonin syndrome.**

■ **TEST-TAKING TIP:** *Remember the medications that affect serotonin end in "ine."*

Content Area: Mental Health, Pharmacology; *Integrated Process:* Nursing Process, Implementation; *Cognitive Level:* Application; *Client Need/Subneed:* Physiological Integrity/Pharmacological and Parenteral Therapies/Adverse Effects/Contraindications/Interactions

31. CORRECT ANSWERS: 1, 3, 5. Answer 1 is correct because the client works with the nurse to develop goals that are realistic and attainable, aimed at improving self-esteem and redirecting the use of manipulation. **Answer 2** is incorrect because this will encourage even more manipulative behaviors. **Answer 3 is correct because it is important to be firm and consistent in reinforcing unit rules. When undesirable behavior occurs and there are reliable and repeated negative consequences, manipulative behaviors are *likely* to decrease. This builds trust in the client that the staff will be consistent in providing support.** **Answer 4** is incorrect because pointing out a client as a problem is a negative technique and a breach of confidentiality. **Answer 5 is correct because the client needs feedback regarding behavior that is positive and negative. This gives the nurse the opportunity to reinforce positive actions.**

■ **TEST-TAKING TIP:** *Eliminate all answers that are negative approaches to correcting behavior.*

Content Area: Mental Health, Common Behavioral Problems; *Integrated Process:* Nursing Process, Planning; *Cognitive Level:* Application; *Client Need/Subneed:* Psychosocial Integrity/Behavioral Interventions

32. CORRECT ANSWERS: 3, 4, 2, 1. Answer 3 is correct because the nurse should assess the third client with the chest discomfort *first* as this client is at greatest risk for a potentially life-threatening condition. Answer 4 is correct because the nurse will be able to assess the fourth client *second*, quickly checking in with the client and providing the requested item if the care plan allows. Answer 2 is correct because the nurse will assess the second client experiencing a problem with homeostasis *third*, and will need to assess for signs and symptoms associated with hypernatremia. Answer 1 is correct because the nurse will assess the first client, who is being discharged, *last*. More tasks and teaching are required with the process, and the nurse will be able complete these actions as a last priority.

■ TEST-TAKING TIP: *In ranking which client to assess from first to fourth priority, the nurse always considers physiological safety first, customer service second, non–life-threatening concerns third and the client who has needs that can be met later (e.g., discharge or teaching) last.*

Content Area: Mental Health, Management of Care; *Integrated Process:* Nursing Process, Planning; *Cognitive Level:* Analysis; *Client Need/Subneed:* Safe and Effective Care Environment/ Management of Care/Establishing Priorities

33. CORRECT ANSWERS: 4, 1, 2, 3. Answer 4 is correct because the nurse would report the laboratory value of the fourth client with a potassium level of 6.0 mEq/L *first* because this is a critical value (e.g., dysrhythmias) and needs to be reported immediately to the physician. Answer 1 is correct because the nurse would report the first client with the WBC count at <3,000/mm^3 *second* because the client who is taking clozapine (Clozaril) is at risk for agranulocytosis (e.g., neutropenia). Answer 2 is correct because the nurse would attend to the second client with the lithium level of 1.6 mEq/L *third* because this is just over the therapeutic level (1.5 mEq/L) and the client could experience more severe side effects (e.g., marked tremor). Answer 3 is correct because the nurse would prioritize the third client with the blood alcohol level of 0.08% *last* because the level does show intoxication, but it is not at a dangerous level (e.g., 0.30%).

■ TEST-TAKING TIP: *Remember priorities and to rank according to a threat to the client's physiological integrity.*

Content Area: Mental Health, Management of Care; *Integrated Process:* Nursing Process, Planning; *Cognitive Level:* Analysis; *Client Need/Subneed:* Safe and Effective Care Environment/ Management of Care/Establishing Priorities

34. CORRECT ANSWERS: 3, 4, 5. **Answer 1** is incorrect because the client is likely to experience a *decrease* in feelings of intimacy. **Answer 2** is incorrect because the client usually does *not* have amnesia, but rather experiences intrusive thoughts of the events in the form of flashbacks. Answer 3 is correct because the client experiencing acute traumatic stress disorder will have flashbacks (e.g., repetitive intrusive images) of the traumatic event. Answer 4 is correct because the client often expresses guilt and shame over the event. Answer 5 is correct because the client has disturbed sleep patterns during this phase.

■ TEST-TAKING TIP: *Think of acute anxiety and eliminate signs and symptoms that are not related to increases in anxiety.*

Content Area: Mental Health, Anxiety; *Integrated Process:* Nursing Process, Assessment; *Cognitive Level:* Application; *Client Need/Subneed:* Psychosocial Integrity/Mental Health Concepts

35. CORRECT ANSWERS: 1, 4. Answer 1 is correct because the client with negative symptoms has diminished functions systematically (e.g., withdrawn, mute, and psychomotor retardation) and a flattened or inappropriate affect. **Answer 2** is incorrect because this is a clinical manifestation of positive symptoms (e.g., inappropriate and bizarre verbal communication). **Answer 3** is incorrect because inappropriate behaviors (e.g., an excess of normal behaviors) are clinical manifestations of positive symptoms. Answer 4 is correct because the client is exhibiting negative symptoms, which include poor eye contact. **Answer 5** is incorrect because excessive delusional thoughts (e.g., the client may believe himself or herself to be afflicted with a terminal illness when there is no medical evidence) are clinical manifestations of positive symptoms related to schizophrenia.

■ TEST-TAKING TIP: *Remember: positive symptoms are behaviors that are added on to the client and negative symptoms are those that taken away.*

Content Area: Mental Health, Schizophrenia; *Integrated Process:* Nursing Process, Assessment; *Cognitive Level:* Comprehension; *Client Need/Subneed:* Physiological Integrity/Physiological Adaptation/Pathophysiology

36. CORRECT ANSWERS: 2, 3. **Answer 1** is incorrect because, while nutritious, fresh fruit and vegetables may *not* be taken in *sufficient* quantities to attain a minimum caloric intake (e.g., 2,200 to 2,900 kcal/day) while the client is *on-the-run*. Answer 2 is correct because this is a high-calorie supplement that is easy for the client who is manic to consume in a short period of time. Answer 3 is correct because this type of food can be consumed quickly and is high in calories and nutrients (e.g., protein and carbohydrates). **Answer 4** is incorrect because the client who is manic usually doesn't sit down to eat, which is needed when eating a sundae. **Answer 5** is incorrect because the client should avoid products that contain caffeine (caffeine products are stimulants, which can increase activity and cause appetite suppression).

■ TEST-TAKING TIP: *Best food items: high carbohydrate, high calorie, high protein.*

Content Area: Mental Health, Manic Disorder; *Integrated Process:* Nursing Process, Implementation; *Cognitive Level:* Application; *Client Need/Subneed:* Physiological Integrity/Basic Care and Comfort/Nutrition and Oral Hydration

37. CORRECT ANSWER: 37.7°C. Use this calculation:
37.0°C + 38.2°C + 38.1°C + 37.5°C = 150.8°C ÷ 4 = 37.7°C

■ TEST-TAKING TIP: *To find the mean, add all values and then divide by the number of values listed.*

Content Area: Adult Health, Vital Signs; *Integrated Process:* Nursing Process, Analysis; *Cognitive Level:* Analysis; *Client Need/Subneed:* Physiological Integrity/Reduction of Risk Potential/Vital Signs Changes/Abnormalities

38. CORRECT ANSWER: 0.25 mL. Use this calculation:
0.5 mg/2 mg × 1 mL = 0.25 mL

■ TEST-TAKING TIP: *Remember "desired over have."*

Content Area: Mental Health, Pharmacology; *Integrated Process:* Nursing Process, Analysis; *Cognitive Level:* Analysis; *Client Need/Subneed:* Physiological Integrity/Pharmacological and Parenteral Therapies/Dosage Calculation

39. CORRECT ANSWERS: 1, 5. **Answer 1 is correct because methylphenidate (Ritalin) is a stimulant and has an appetite suppression effect. It is best to administer the medication after meals to avoid problems with decreased appetite.** Answer 2 is incorrect because methylphenidate (Ritalin) is a CNS stimulant and should be taken at least 6 hours before bedtime to prevent insomnia. Answer 3 is incorrect because a sign of tolerance with this medication *is* weight gain. Answer 4 is incorrect because caffeine would create a synergistic effect (e.g., increased activity and diminished attention span) when used with this medication and should be avoided. **Answer 5 is correct because methylphenidate (Ritalin) is *not* a CNS depressant (it is classified as a stimulant).**

■ TEST-TAKING TIP: *Eliminate those responses that are not related to stimulants. The best answers are the wrong options (e.g., where more teaching is needed).*

Content Area: Mental Health, Pharmacology; *Integrated Process:* Nursing Process, Evaluation; *Cognitive Level:* Analysis; *Client Need/Subneed:* Physiological Integrity/Pharmacological and Parenteral Therapies/Medication Administration

40. CORRECT ANSWER: 2 tablets. Use this calculation:
1,200 mg/300 mg × 1 tablet = 4 tablets total ÷ 2 = 2 tablets twice daily or every 12 hours.

■ TEST-TAKING TIP: *Read the question carefully. Remember, the request is for* **divided doses.**

Content Area: Mental Health, Pharmacology; *Integrated Process:* Nursing Process, Analysis; *Cognitive Level:* Analysis; *Client Need/Subneed:* Physiological Integrity/Pharmacological and Parenteral Therapies/Dosage Calculation

41. CORRECT ANSWERS: 3, 4. Answer 1 is incorrect because it is related to psychoanalytic therapy. Answer 2 is incorrect because it is used to change negative thought patterns to positive ones. **Answer 3 is correct because desensitization involves a behavior change. Desensitization, with repeated exposure to provoking stimuli, reduces the client's anxiety and undesirable behaviors (e.g., severe or panic level anxiety). Answer 4 is correct because a token economy approach uses rewards for desired behavior.** Answer 5 is incorrect because it is related to activity-based therapies that improve daily functioning.

■ TEST-TAKING TIP: *Note the key word "behavior." Select those options that involve behavior changes.*

Content Area: Mental Health, Treatment Modes; *Integrated Process:* Teaching and Learning; *Cognitive Level:* Application; *Client Need/Subneed:* Psychosocial Integrity/Behavioral Interventions

42. CORRECT ANSWER: 1. **Answer 1 is correct because it is inappropriate for the physician to order restraints *as needed* for any client.** Answer 2 is incorrect because this *is* an appropriate order for a client detoxifying from alcohol due to the client's potential for confusion and a fall risk. Answer 3 is incorrect because this *is* an appropriate order for a client detoxifying from alcohol due to dehydration related to alcohol intake. Answer 4 is incorrect because this *is* an appropriate order for a client detoxifying from alcohol due to withdrawal complications related to increases in heart rate and risk for dysrhythmias.

■ TEST-TAKING TIP: *Restraints are never ordered on a prn basis; least restrictive approaches need to be tried first.*

Content Area: Mental Health, Substance Abuse; *Integrated Process:* Nursing Process, Analysis; *Cognitive Level:* Application; *Client Need/Subneed:* Safe and Effective Care Environment/Management of Care/Advocacy

43. CORRECT ANSWER: 3. Answer 1 is incorrect because the client may have distorted perceptions or thoughts (e.g., thinking others are out to harm the client), but these may not necessarily lead to a safety issue to self or others. Answer 2 is incorrect because the client's problems with social interaction are not a priority because safety is more important to establish at this time. **Answer 3 is most correct because a client who is full of intense anger and rage may pose a safety issue for others.** Answer 4 is incorrect because the client may have altered thoughts (e.g., believing one is related to royalty). Hostility and threat to others is a priority.

■ TEST-TAKING TIP: *Priority is the key, and safety is a priority.*

Content Area: Mental Health, Common Behavioral Problems; *Integrated Process:* Nursing Process, Analysis; *Cognitive Level:* Analysis; *Client Need/Subneed:* Psychosocial Integrity/Sensory/Perceptual Alterations

44. CORRECT ANSWER: 2. **Answer 1** is incorrect because the nurse would assist the client to explore legal issues (e.g., prosecution) *after* the medical evidence is collected and initial trauma has passed. **Answer 2 is correct because it may be difficult for the client to process any information the nurse will be giving until anxiety is reduced and the client's feelings are acknowledged.** **Answer 3** is incorrect because the nurse would explore feelings (e.g., plans for the future) with the client *after* anxiety is lessened and coping behaviors are improved (e.g., increased control over fear and acceptance of what happened). **Answer 4** is incorrect because this is an issue that can be addressed much later in the rape-trauma syndrome.

■ **TEST-TAKING TIP:** *Note the clue regarding which nursing action to take "first."*

Content Area: Mental Health, Rape, Sexual Abuse; *Integrated Process:* Nursing Process, Implementation; *Cognitive Level:* Analysis; *Client Need/Subneed:* Psychosocial Integrity/Stress Management

45. CORRECT ANSWER: 2. **Answer 1** is incorrect because this is a *secondary* prevention measure. **Answer 2 is correct because of the problems associated with role strain, stress, and taxed coping behaviors; the caregiver needs support (e.g., through individual or group therapy, education, and respite) to prevent elder abuse.** **Answer 3** is incorrect because this is a *tertiary* measure. **Answer 4** is incorrect because this is a *secondary* prevention measure.

■ **TEST-TAKING TIP:** *Primary prevention occurs before there is a problem.*

Content Area: Mental Health, Prevention—Caregiver Strain; *Integrated Process:* Nursing Process, Implementation; *Cognitive Level:* Application; *Client Need/Subneed:* Safe and Effective Care Environment/Management of Care/Referrals

46. CORRECT ANSWER: 2. **Answer 1** is incorrect because this is more typical of the client with bulimia. **Answer 2 is the most correct answer because clients with anorexia nervosa tend to obsess about food, meals, and calories.** **Answer 3** is incorrect because menstruation is not a behavior but a sign of an endocrine effect. **Answer 4** is incorrect because this is not a common behavior for a client with anorexia nervosa.

■ **TEST-TAKING TIP:** *Eliminate Answers 1 and 4 because these relate to bulimia. Eliminate Answer 3 because the stem asks for a* behavior *related to anorexia nervosa.*

Content Area: Mental Health, Eating Disorder; *Integrated Process:* Nursing Process, Assessment; *Cognitive Level:* Application; *Client Need/Subneed:* Psychosocial Integrity/ Sensory/Perceptual Alterations

47. CORRECT ANSWER: 1. **Answer 1 is correct because the client is having difficulties with separation from the usual support system, is experiencing physical problems, and cannot cope with changes in routine.** **Answer 2** is incorrect because the client is experiencing more than just memory or attention problems. **Answer 3** is incorrect because the client is not experiencing *sensory/perceptual* alterations (e.g., hearing or visual changes) at this time. **Answer 4** is incorrect because the client is having *mobility* problems (e.g., weakness) but is not a risk for trauma at this time.

■ **TEST-TAKING TIP:** *When all are correct, choose the answer that includes the other options too, although at a later time.*

Content Area: Mental Health, Older Adult; *Integrated Process:* Communication and Documentation; *Cognitive Level:* Analysis; *Client Need/Subneed:* Psychosocial Integrity/Sensory/Perceptual Alterations

48. CORRECT ANSWER: 3. **Answer 1** is incorrect because the laboratory values would reflect a *decrease* in albumin, not an increase, because impaired liver function decreases albumin synthesis. **Answer 2** is incorrect because, by the time the client arrives at rehab, the blood alcohol level would be low to zero. **Answer 3 is correct because these are common laboratory values for liver impairment when someone is a long-term abuser of alcohol.** **Answer 4** is incorrect because the magnesium would be *decreased,* not increased, because of inadequate intake of nutrients during alcohol consumption and impaired transport of nutrients related to a lack of the liver enzymes.

■ **TEST-TAKING TIP:** *Think impaired liver function as a long-term effect of alcohol abuse.*

Content Area: Mental Health, Substance Abuse; *Integrated Process:* Nursing Process, Assessment; *Cognitive Level:* Application; *Client Need/Subneed:* Physiological Integrity/ Reduction of Risk Potential/Laboratory Values

49. CORRECT ANSWER: 4. **Answer 1** is incorrect because these symptoms are related to barbiturate withdrawal. **Answer 2** is incorrect because these are signs of amphetamine abuse but could also be signs of marijuana withdrawal. **Answer 3** is incorrect because these are withdrawal symptoms associated with opiates. **Answer 4 is correct because depression, lack of energy, and somnolence are signs of withdrawal from amphetamines. The body responds to the sudden lack of amphetamine with symptoms similar to depression.**

■ **TEST-TAKING TIP:** *Think about the opposite of being "up" (amphetamines are "uppers").*

Content Area: Mental Health, Substance Abuse; *Integrated Process:* Nursing Process, Assessment; *Cognitive Level:* Application; *Client Need/Subneed:* Psychosocial Integrity/ Chemical and Other Dependencies

50. CORRECT ANSWER: 2. **Answer 1** is incorrect because the nurse is using the technique of giving feedback and asking for restatement, which is not therapeutic at this time because the client needs reality orientation first. **Answer 2 is correct because the nurse is expressing doubt about an unreal perception.** **Answer 3** is incorrect because the nurse is encouraging clarification of an experience before providing reality orientation, which then needs to be followed by acknowledgement of the client's feelings. **Answer 4** is incorrect because the nurse needs to first provide reality orientation, not focus on feelings.

■ **TEST-TAKING TIP:** *Choose feedback (Answer 2) before* feelings *(Answer 4) or before facts (Answer 3) or feedback by nurse and request for repetition by client (Answer 1). Think of the three "Fs": feedback, then feelings, then fact.*

Content Area: Mental Health, Therapeutic Communication; ***Integrated Process:*** Nursing Process, Implementation; ***Cognitive Level:*** Application; ***Client Need/Subneed:*** Psychosocial Integrity/Sensory/Perceptual Alterations

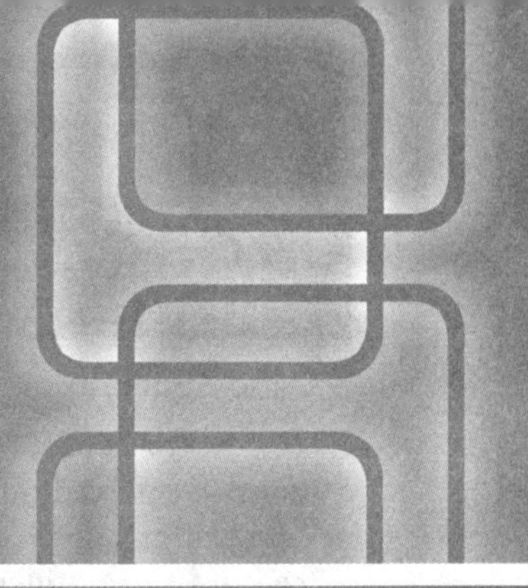

CHAPTER 11

Reduction of Risk Potential

Common Procedures: Diagnostic Tests, Oxygen Therapy, and Hands-on Nursing Care

Janice Lloyd McMillin • Robyn Marchal Nelson

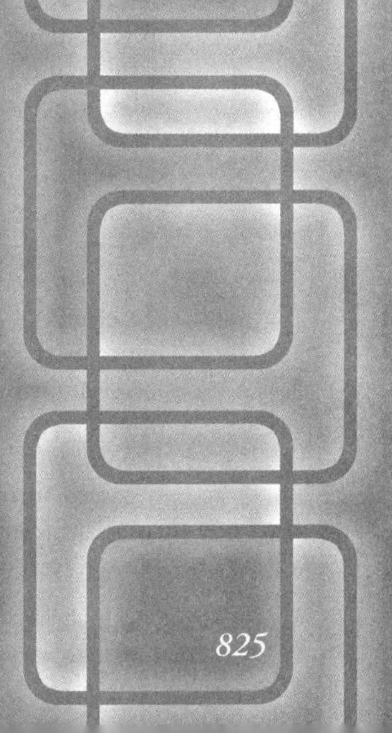

COMMON DIAGNOSTIC PROCEDURES

See also **Appendix A** for blood and urine laboratory tests.

I. NONINVASIVE DIAGNOSTIC PROCEDURES are those procedures that provide an indirect assessment of organ size, shape, and/or function; these procedures are considered safe, are easily reproducible, require less complex equipment for recording, and generally do not require the written consent of the client or guardian.

A. General nursing responsibilities:

1. Reduce client's anxieties and provide emotional support by:
   a. Explaining purpose and procedure of test.
   b. Answering questions regarding safety of the procedure, as indicated.
   c. Remaining with client during procedure when possible.
2. Use procedures in the collection of specimens that avoid contamination and facilitate diagnosis—clean-catch urine and sputum specimens after deep breathing and coughing, for example.

B. Graphic studies of heart and brain:

1. *Electrocardiogram (ECG, also known as EKG)*—graphic record of electrical activity generated by the heart during depolarization and repolarization; *used to:* diagnose abnormal cardiac rhythms and coronary heart disease.
2. *Echocardiography* (ultrasound cardiography)—graphic record of motions produced by cardiac structures as high-frequency sound vibrations are echoed through chest wall into the heart; transesophageal echocardiography produces a clearer image, particularly in clients who are obese, barrel-chested, or with chronic obstructive pulmonary disease (COPD); *used to:* demonstrate valvular or other structural deformities, detect pericardial effusion, diagnose tumors and cardiomegaly, or evaluate prosthetic valve function.
3. *Phonocardiogram*—graphic record of heart sounds; *used to:* keep a permanent record of client's heart sounds before and after cardiac surgery.
4. *Electroencephalogram (EEG)*—graphic record of the electrical potentials generated by the physiological activity of the brain; *used to:* detect surface lesions or tumors of the brain and presence of epilepsy.
5. *Echoencephalogram*—beam of pulsed ultrasound is passed through the head, and returning echoes are graphically recorded; *used to:* detect shifts in cerebral midline structures caused by subdural hematomas, intracerebral hemorrhage, or tumors.

C. Roentgenological studies (x-ray)

1. *Chest—used to:* determine size, contour, and position of the heart; size, location, and nature of pulmonary lesions; disorders of thoracic bones or soft tissue; diaphragmatic contour and excursion; pleural thickening or effusions; and gross changes in the caliber or distribution of pulmonary vasculature.
2. *Kidney, ureter, and bladder (KUB)—used to:* determine size, shape, and position of kidneys, ureters, and bladder.
3. *Mammography*—examination of the breast with or without the injection of radiopaque substance into the ducts of the mammary gland; *used to:* determine the presence of tumors or cysts. *Client preparation: no* deodorant, perfume, powders, or ointment in underarm area on day of x-ray. May be uncomfortable due to pressure on the breast.
4. *Skull*—outline configuration and density of brain tissues and vascular markings; *used to:* determine the size and location of intracranial calcifications, tumors, abscesses, or vascular lesions.

D. Roentgenological studies (fluoroscopy)—require the ingestion or injection of a radiopaque substance to visualize the target organ.

1. *Additional nursing responsibilities* may include:
   a. Administration of *enemas or cathartics* before the procedure and a laxative after.
   b. Keeping the client *NPO* 6 to 12 hours before examination; check with physician regarding oral medications.
   c. Ascertaining client's *history of allergies* or allergic reactions (e.g., iodine, seafood).
   d. Observing for *allergic* reactions to contrast medium following procedure.
   e. Providing *fluid* and *food* following procedure, to counteract dehydration.
   f. Observing *stool* for color and consistency until barium passes.
2. Common fluoroscopic examinations:
   a. ***Upper GI***—ingestion of barium sulfate or meglumine diatrizoate (Gastrografin, a white, chalky, radiopaque substance), followed by fluoroscopic and x-ray examination; *used to* determine:
      (1) Patency and caliber of *esophagus;* may also detect esophageal varices.
      (2) Mobility and thickness of *gastric* walls, presence of ulcer craters, filling defects due to tumors, pressures from outside the stomach, and patency of pyloric valve.
      (3) Rate of passage in small bowel and presence of structural abnormalities.

b. ***Lower GI***—rectal instillation of barium sulfate followed by fluoroscopic and x-ray examination; *used to:* determine contour and mobility of colon and presence of any space-occupying tumors; perform before upper GI.

Client preparation: explain purpose; *no food after evening meal* the evening before test; *stool softeners, laxatives, enemas, and suppositories* to cleanse the bowel before the test; *NPO after midnight* before test; oral medications *not* permitted day of test. *After completion of examination:* food, *increased liquid* intake, and rest; *laxatives for at least 2 days* or until stools are normal in color and consistency.

c. *Cholecystogram* (done if gallbladder not seen with ultrasound)—ingestion of organic iodine contrast medium Telepaque (iopanoic acid), or Oragrafin (preparation of calcium or sodium salt of ipodate), followed in 12 hours by x-ray visualization; gallbladder disease is indicated with *poor* or no visualization of the bladder; accurate only if GI and liver function is intact; perform before barium enema or upper GI.

Client preparation: explain purpose; administer large amount of *water* with contrast capsules; *low-fat meal* evening *before* x-ray; *oral laxative or stool softener after meal; no food* allowed after contrast capsules; water, tea, or coffee, with *no* cream or sugar usually allowed. *After completion of examination:* fluids, food, and rest; observe for any signs of allergy to contrast medium.

d. *Cholangiogram*—intravenous injection of a radiopaque contrast substance, followed by fluoroscopic and x-ray examination of the bile ducts; failure of the contrast medium to pass certain points in the bile duct pinpoints *obstruction.*

e. *Intravenous urography (IVU) or pyelography (IVP)*—injection of a radiopaque contrast medium, followed by fluoroscopic and x-ray films of kidneys and urinary tract; *used to:* identify lesions in kidneys and ureters and provide a rough estimate of kidney function.

f. *Cystogram*—instillation of radiopaque medium through a catheter into the bladder; *used to:* visualize bladder wall and evaluate ureterovesical valves for reflux.

g. *Phlebography* (lower limb venography)—determines patency of the tibial-popliteal, superficial femoral, common femoral, and saphenous veins. A contrast medium is injected into the superficial and/or deep veins of the involved extremity, followed by x-rays, while the leg is placed in a variety of positions; *used to:* detect deep vein thrombosis (DVT) and to select a vein for use in arterial bypass grafting; localized clotting may result.

E. **Computed tomography (CT)**—an x-ray beam sweeps around the body, allowing measurement of various tissue densities; provides clear radiographic definition of structures that are not visible by other techniques, permitting earlier diagnosis and treatment and more effective and efficient follow-up. Initial scan may be followed by "contrast enhancement" using an injection of an intravenous contrast agent (iodine), followed by a repeat scan.

Client preparation: instructions for eating before test vary. Clear liquids up to 2 hours before are usually permitted.

F. **Positron emission tomography (PET)**—A radionuclide-based imaging technique. Tracers given IV or by inhalation; rarely intra-arterial. Metabolic and physiological changes are produced by strokes, brain tumors, epilepsy, mental illnesses such as schizophrenia and bipolar disorder, and Parkinson's disease. PET measures blood flow, glucose metabolism, and oxygen extraction. *Useful in:* diagnosing myocardial flow deficits and evaluating successful thrombolysis, outcomes of bypass surgery, and percutaneous transluminal coronary angioplasty (PTCA).

Client preparation: fast for 4 hours. Injection of radioactive tracers that emit signals. Must remain motionless for 45 minutes. Scanner is quiet.

G. **Magnetic resonance imaging (MRI)**—noninvasive, non-ionic technique produces cross-sectional images by exposure to magnetic energy sources. Provides superior contrast of soft tissue, including healthy, benign, and malignant tissue, along with veins and arteries; uses no contrast medium. Takes 30 to 90 minutes to complete; client must *remain still* for periods of 5 to 20 minutes at a time—equipment often very noisy.

Client preparation: client can take food and medications except for low abdominal and pelvic studies (food/fluids withheld 4 to 6 hours to decrease peristalsis). *Restrictions:* clients who have metal implants, permanent pacemakers, or implanted medication pumps such as insulin, or who are pregnant or on life support systems. Clients who are obese may not be able to have full-body MRI because they may not fit in the scanner tunnel. Clients who are claustrophobic may need distraction (e.g., music) or may be referred to a facility that has an MRI chamber that is more open.

H. **Multiple gated acquisition (MUGA) scan**—also known as blood pool imaging. Red blood cells

(RBCs) are tagged with a radioactive isotope. A computer-operated camera takes sequential pictures of actual heart wall motion; *complement* to cardiac catheterization; *used to:* determine valvular effectiveness, follow progress of heart disease, diagnose cardiac aneurysms, detect coronary artery disease, determine effects of cardiovascular drug therapy. No special preparation. Painless, except for injections. Wear *gloves* if contact with client urine occurs within 24 hours after scan.

I. Ultrasound (sonogram)—scanning by ultrasound is used to diagnose disorders of the thyroid, kidney, liver, uterus, gallbladder, and fetus and the intracranial structures in the neonate. It is *not* useful when visualization through air or bone is required (lung studies). In some agencies, the sonogram has taken the place of the oral cholecystogram in diagnosing gallbladder disease, bile duct distention, and calculi.

Client preparation is minimal—for example, NPO for at least 8 hours for gallbladder studies. No x-rays. Thirty-two ounces of water PO 30 minutes *before* studies of lower abdomen or uterus.

J. Pulmonary function studies:

1. *Ventilatory studies*—utilization of a spirometer to determine how well the lung is ventilating.
   a. *Vital capacity (VC)*—largest amount of air that can be expelled after maximal inspiration.
      (1) *Normally* 4,000 to 5,000 mL.
      (2) *Decreased* in restrictive lung disease.
      (3) May be normal, slightly increased, or decreased in chronic obstructive lung disease.
   b. *Forced expiratory volume (FEV)*—percentage of vital capacity that can be forcibly expired in 1, 2, or 3 seconds.
      (1) *Normally* 81% to 83% in 1 second, 90% to 94% in 2 seconds, and 95% to 97% in 3 seconds.
      (2) *Decreased* values indicate expiratory airway obstruction.
   c. *Maximum breathing capacity (MBC)*—maximum amount of air that can be breathed in and out in 1 minute with maximal rate and depth of respiration.
      (1) Best overall measurement of ventilatory ability.
      (2) *Reduced* in restrictive and chronic obstructive lung disease.
2. *Diffusion studies*—measure the rate of exchange of gases across alveolar membrane. Carbon monoxide single-breath, rebreathing, and steady-state techniques—used because of special affinity of hemoglobin for carbon monoxide; *decreased* when fluid is present in alveoli or when alveolar membranes are thick or fibrosed.

K. Sputum studies:

1. Gross sputum evaluations—collection of sputum samples to ascertain quantity, consistency, color, and odor.
2. *Sputum smear*—sputum is smeared thinly on a slide so that it can be studied microscopically; *used to:* determine cytological changes (malignant cells) or presence of pathogenic bacteria (e.g., tubercle bacilli).
3. *Sputum culture*—sputum samples are implanted or inoculated into special media; *used to:* diagnose pulmonary infections.
4. *Gastric lavage or analysis*—insertion of a nasogastric tube into the stomach to siphon out swallowed pulmonary secretions; *used to:* detect organisms causing pulmonary infections; especially useful for detecting tubercle bacilli in children.

L. Examination of gastric contents:

1. *Gastric analysis*—aspiration of the contents of the fasting stomach for analysis of free and total acid.
   a. Gastric acidity is generally *increased* in presence of duodenal ulcer.
   b. Gastric acidity is usually *decreased* in pernicious anemia, cancer of the stomach.
2. Stool specimens—*examined for:* amount, consistency, color, character, and melena; *used to:* determine presence of urobilinogen, fat, nitrogen, parasites, and other substances.

M. Thermography—a picture of the surface temperature of the skin using infrared photography (nonionizing radiation) detects the circulation pattern of areas in the breasts. Tumors produce more heat than normal breast tissue. Useful with *large* tumors, but may not detect small or deep lesions. Requires expensive equipment and is difficult to interpret accurately.

N. Doppler ultrasonography—*used to:* measure blood flow in the major veins and arteries. The transducer of the test instrument is placed on the skin, sending out bursts of ultra-high-frequency sound. The ratio of ankle to brachial systolic pressure (API $\geq$ 1) provides information about vascular insufficiency. Sound varies with respiration and the Valsalva maneuver. No discomfort to the client.

O. Caloric stimulation test—*used to:* evaluate the vestibular portion of the eighth cranial nerve, identify the impairment or loss of thermally induced nystagmus. Reflex eye movements (nystagmus) result in response to cold or warm irrigations of the external auditory canal if the nerve is intact. A *diminished or absent* response occurs with Ménière's disease or acoustic neuroma. Nausea, vomiting, or dizziness can be precipitated by the test.

P. 24-hour urine collection—a true and accurate evaluation of kidney function, primarily glomerular filtration. Substances excreted by the kidney are excreted at different rates, amounts, and times of day or night. Timed urine collection is done for *protein, creatinine, electrolytes, urinary steroids,* etc. A large container is used with or without preservative. Label with client name, type of test, and exact time test starts and ends. Not usually necessary to measure urine. Have client void, discard urine; test starts at this time. Have client void as close to the end of the 24-hour period as possible. If refrigeration is required, urine may be stored in iced container.

Q. Glucose testing—to detect disorder of glucose metabolism, such as diabetes.

1. *Fasting blood sugar (FBS):* blood sample is drawn after a 12-hour fast (usually overnight). Water is allowed. If diabetes is present, value will be 126 mg/dL or greater.
2. *2-hour postprandial blood sugar (PPBS):* blood is taken after a meal. For best results, client should be on a high-carbohydrate diet for 2 to 4 days before testing. Client fasts overnight, eats a high-carbohydrate breakfast; blood sample is drawn 2 hours after eating. Client should rest during 2-hour interval. Smoking and coffee may increase glucose level.
3. *Glucose tolerance test (GTT):* done when sugar in urine, or FBS or 2-hour PPBS, is not conclusive. A timed test, usually 2 hours. A high-carbohydrate diet is eaten 3 days before test. Blood is drawn after overnight fast. Client drinks a very sweet glucose liquid. All of the solution must be taken. Blood and urine samples usually taken at 30 minutes, 1 hour, 2 hours, and sometimes 3 hours after drinking solution. Blood glucose peaks in 30 to 60 minutes, and returns to normal, usually within 3 hours.

II. INVASIVE DIAGNOSTIC PROCEDURES—

procedures that directly record the size, shape, or function of an organ and that are often complex or expensive or require utilization of highly trained personnel; these procedures may result in morbidity and occasionally death of the client and therefore require the written consent of the client or guardian.

A. General nursing responsibilities:

1. *Before procedure:* institute measures to provide for client's safety and emotional comfort.
   a. Have client sign permit for procedure.
   b. Ascertain and report any client history of allergy or allergic reactions.
   c. Explain procedure briefly, and accurately advise client of any possible sensations, such as flushing or a warm feeling, as when a contrast medium is injected.
   d. Keep client NPO 6 to 12 hours before procedure if anesthesia is to be used.
   e. Allow client to verbalize concerns, and note attitude toward procedure.
   f. Administer preprocedure sedative, as ordered.
   g. If procedure done at bedside:
      (1) Remain with client, offering frequent reassurance.
      (2) Assist with optional positioning of client.
      (3) Observe for indications of complications—shock, pain, or dyspnea.
2. *After procedure:* institute measures to avoid complications and promote physical and emotional comfort.
   a. Observe and record vital signs.
   b. Check injection, cutdown, or biopsy sites for bleeding, infection, tenderness, or thrombosis.
      (1) Report untoward reactions to physician.
      (2) Apply warm compresses to ease discomfort, as ordered.
   c. If topical anesthetic is used during procedure (e.g., gastroscopy, bronchoscopy), do *not* give food or fluid until gag reflex returns.
   d. Encourage relaxation by allowing client to discuss experience and verbalize feelings.

B. Procedures to evaluate the cardiovascular system:

1. *Angiocardiography*—intravenous injection of a radiopaque solution or contrast medium for the purpose of studying its circulation through the client's heart, lungs, and great vessels; *used to:* check the competency of heart valves, diagnose congenital septal defects, detect occlusions of coronary arteries, confirm suspected diagnoses, and study heart function and structure before cardiac surgery.
2. *Cardiac catheterization*—insertion of a radiopaque catheter into a vein to study the heart and great vessels.
   a. *Right-heart catheterization*—catheter is inserted through a cutdown in the antecubital vein into the superior vena cava, through the right atrium and ventricle, and into the pulmonary artery.
   b. *Left-heart catheterization*—catheter may be passed retrograde to the left ventricle through the brachial or femoral artery; it can be passed into the left atrium after right-heart catheterization by means of a special needle that punctures the septa; or it may be passed directly into the left ventricle by means of a posterior or anterior chest puncture.
   c. Cardiac catheterizations are *used to:*
      (1) Confirm diagnosis of heart disease and determine the extent of disease.
      (2) Determine existence and extent of congenital abnormalities.

(3) Measure pressures in the heart chambers and great vessels.
(4) Obtain estimate of cardiac output.
(5) Obtain blood samples to measure oxygen content and determine presence of cardiac shunts.

d. *Specific nursing interventions:*
(1) *Preprocedure client teaching:*
(a) Fatigue due to lying still for 3 hours or more is a common complaint.
(b) Some fluttery sensations may be felt—occur as catheter is passed backward into the left ventricle.
(c) Flushed, warm feeling may occur when contrast medium is injected.
(2) *Postprocedure observations:*
(a) Monitor ECG pattern for arrhythmias.
(b) Check extremities for color and temperature, peripheral pulses (femoral and dorsalis pedis) for quality.

3. *Angiography (arteriography)*—injection of a contrast medium into the arteries to study the vascular tree; *used to:* determine obstructions or narrowing of peripheral arteries.
4. *Pericardiocentesis (pericardial aspiration)*—puncture of the pericardial sac is performed to remove fluid accumulating with pericardial effusion. The goal is to *prevent* cardiac tamponade (compression of the heart).

Nursing interventions: monitor ECG and central venous pressure (CVP) during the procedure, have resuscitative equipment ready. Head of bed elevated to *45 to 60 degrees.* Maintain peripheral IV with saline or glucose. *Following the procedure:* monitor BP, CVP, and heart sounds for recurrence of tamponade (pulsus paradoxus).

C. Procedures to evaluate the respiratory system:

1. *Pulmonary circulation studies—used to:* determine regional distribution of pulmonary blood flow.
a. *Lung scan*—injection of radioactive isotope into the body, followed by lung scintiscan, which produces a graphic record of gamma rays emitted by the isotope in lung tissues; *used to:* determine lung perfusion when space-occupying lesions or pulmonary emboli and infarction are suspected.
b. *Pulmonary angiography*—x-ray visualization of the pulmonary vasculature after the injection of a radiopaque contrast medium; *used to:* evaluate pulmonary disorders (e.g., pulmonary embolism, lung tumors, aneurysms, and changes in the pulmonary vasculature due to such conditions as emphysema or congenital defects).
2. *Bronchoscopy*—introduction of a special lighted instrument (bronchoscope) into the trachea and bronchi; *used to:* inspect tracheobronchial tree for pathological changes, remove tissue for cytological and bacteriological studies, remove foreign bodies or mucous plugs causing airway obstruction, assess functional residual capacity of diseased lung, and apply chemotherapeutic agents.
a. *Prebronchoscopy nursing interventions:*
(1) Oral hygiene.
(2) Postural drainage is indicated.
b. *Postbronchoscopy nursing interventions:*
(1) Instruct client *not* to swallow oral secretions but to let saliva run from side of mouth.
(2) Save expectorated sputum for laboratory analysis, and observe for frank bleeding.
(3) NPO until gag reflex returns.
(4) Observe for subcutaneous emphysema and dyspnea.
(5) Apply ice collar to reduce throat discomfort.
3. *Thoracentesis*—needle puncture through the chest wall and into the pleura; *used to:* remove fluid and occasionally air from the pleural space.
a. *Nursing interventions before* thoracentesis:
(1) *Position:* high-Fowler's position or sitting up on edge of bed, with feet supported on chair to facilitate accumulation of fluid in the base of the chest.
(2) If client is unable to sit up—turn onto *unaffected* side.
(3) Evaluate continually for signs of shock, pain, cyanosis, increased respiratory rate, and pallor.

D. Procedures to evaluate the renal system:

1. *Renal angiogram*—small catheter is inserted into the femoral artery and passed into the aorta or renal artery, radiopaque fluid is instilled, and serial films are taken.
a. *Used to:* diagnose renal hypertension and pheochromocytoma and differentiate renal cysts from renal tumors.
b. *Postangiogram nursing actions:* check pedal pulse for signs of decreased circulation.
2. *Cystoscopy*—visualization of bladder, urethra, and prostatic urethra by insertion of a tubular, lighted, telescopic lens (cystoscope) through the urinary meatus.
a. *Used to:* directly inspect the bladder; collect urine from the renal pelvis; obtain biopsy specimens from bladder and urethra; remove calculi; and treat lesions in the bladder, urethra, and prostate.
b. *Nursing interventions following* procedure:
(1) Observe for urinary retention.
(2) Warm sitz baths to relieve discomfort.

3. *Renal biopsy*—needle aspiration of tissue from the kidney for the purpose of microscopic examination.

E. Procedures to evaluate the digestive system:

1. *Celiac angiography, hepatoportography, and umbilical venography*—injection of a contrast medium into the portal vein or related vessel; *used to:* determine patency of vessels supplying target organ or detect lesions in the organs that distort the vasculature.
2. *Esophagoscopy and gastroscopy*—visualization of the esophagus, the stomach, and sometimes the duodenum by means of a lighted tube inserted through the mouth.
3. *Proctoscopy*—visualization of rectum and colon by means of a lighted tube inserted through the anus.
4. *Peritoneoscopy*—direct visualization of the liver and peritoneum by means of a peritoneoscope inserted through an abdominal stab wound.
5. *Liver biopsy*—needle aspiration of tissue for the purpose of microscopic examination; *used to:* determine tissue changes, facilitate diagnosis, and provide information regarding a disease course.

   Nursing interventions: place client on *right side* and position pillow for pressure, to prevent bleeding.
6. *Paracentesis*—needle aspiration of fluid from the peritoneal cavity; *used to:* relieve excess fluid accumulation or for diagnostic studies.
   a. *Specific nursing interventions before paracentesis:*
      (1) Have client void—to prevent possible injury to bladder during procedure.
      (2) *Position*—sitting up on side of bed, with feet supported by chair.
      (3) Check vital signs and peripheral circulation frequently throughout procedure.
      (4) Observe for signs of hypovolemic shock—may occur due to fluid shift from vascular compartment following removal of protein-rich ascitic fluid.
   b. *Specific nursing interventions following paracentesis:*
      (1) Apply pressure to injection site and cover with sterile dressing.
      (2) Measure and record amount and color of ascitic fluid; send specimens to laboratory for diagnostic studies.
7. *Small-bowel biopsy*—a specimen is obtained by passing a tube through the oral cavity and is microscopically examined for changes in cellular morphology.

   Nursing interventions: no food or fluids 8 hours before procedure. Obtain written consent. Remove dentures if present. Monitor vital signs before, during, and after procedure for indications of hemorrhage. Procedure takes approximately 1 hour.

F. Procedures to evaluate the reproductive system in women:

1. *Culdoscopy*—surgical procedure in which a culdoscope is inserted into the posterior vaginal cul-de-sac; *used to:* visualize uterus, fallopian tubes, broad ligaments, and peritoneal contents.
2. *Hysterosalpingography*—x-ray examination of uterus and fallopian tubes following insertion of a radiopaque substance into the uterine cavity; *used to:* determine patency of fallopian tubes and detect pathology in uterine cavity.
3. *Breast biopsy*—needle aspiration or incisional removal of breast tissue for microscopic examination; *used to:* differentiate among benign tumors, cysts, and malignant tumors in the breast.
4. *Cervical biopsy and cauterization*—removal of cervical tissue for microscopic examination and cautery; *used to:* control bleeding or obtain additional tissue samples.
5. *Uterotubal insufflation (Rubin's test)*—injection of carbon dioxide into the cervical canal; *used to:* determine fallopian tube patency.

G. Procedures to evaluate the neuroendocrine system:

1. *Radioactive iodine uptake test (iodine-131 [^{131}I] uptake)*—ingestion of a tracer dose of ^{131}I, followed in 24 hours by a scan of the thyroid for amount of radioactivity emitted.
   a. *High* uptake indicates hyperthyroidism.
   b. *Low* uptake indicates hypothyroidism.
2. *Eight-hour intravenous ACTH test*—administration of 25 units of adrenocorticotropic hormone (ACTH) in 500 mL of saline over an 8-hour period.
   a. *Used to:* determine function of adrenal cortex.
   b. 24-hour urine specimens are collected, before and after administration, for measurement of 17-ketosteroids and 17-hydroxycorticosteroids.
   c. In *Addison's* disease, urinary output of steroids does *not increase* following administration of ACTH; *normally* steroid excretion *increases threefold to fivefold* following ACTH stimulation.
   d. In *Cushing's* syndrome, hyperactivity of the adrenal cortex *increases* the urine output of steroids in the second urine specimen *10-fold.*
3. *Cerebral angiography*—fluoroscopic visualization of the brain vasculature after injection of a contrast medium into the carotid or vertebral arteries; *used to:* localize lesions (tumors, abscesses, intracranial hemorrhages, and occlusions) that are large enough to distort cerebrovascular blood flow.

4. *Myelogram*—through a lumbar puncture needle, a contrast medium is injected into the subarachnoid space of the spinal column to visualize the spinal cord; *used to:* detect herniated or ruptured intervertebral disks, tumors, or cysts that compress or distort spinal cord.

   Nursing interventions: elevate head of bed with water-soluble contrast; *flat* with oil contrast; check for bladder distention with metrizamide (water soluble); vital signs every 4 hours for 24 hours.
5. *Brain scan*—intravenous injection of a radioactive substance, followed by a scan for emission of radioactivity.
   a. *Increased* radioactivity at site of abnormality.
   b. *Used to:* detect brain tumors, abscesses, hematomas, and arteriovenous malformations.
6. *Lumbar puncture*—puncture of the lumbar subarachnoid space of the spinal cord with a needle to withdraw samples of cerebrospinal fluid (CSF); *used to:* evaluate CSF for infections and determine presence of hemorrhage. *Not* done if increased intracranial pressure (ICP) suspected.

H. Procedures to evaluate the skeletal system. *Arthroscopy*—examination of a joint through a fiberoptic endoscope called an arthroscope. Usually done in the operating room (same-day surgery) under aseptic conditions using a local anesthetic, although a general anesthetic may be used. A tourniquet is used to reduce blood flow to the area while the scope is introduced through a cannula. Saline is used as the viewing medium. Biopsy or removal of loose bodies from the joint may be done. A compression dressing (e.g., Ace bandage) is applied. Restrictions vary according to surgeon preference and nature of procedure. Weight-bearing may be immediate or restricted for 24 hours. Teach client to observe for signs of infection.

DIAGNOSTIC TESTS TO EVALUATE FETAL WELL-BEING

Table 11.1

Diagnostic Tests to Evaluate Fetal Well-Being

Test	Implications of Results	Risks
Nonstress Test (NST)		
Requires electronic fetal monitoring	*Reactive test*—indicate intact central nervous system (CNS).	Noninvasive procedures
Correlates fetal movements with fetal heart rate (FHR) and intact fetal CNS; 90% of gross fetal movements associated with accelerations of the FHR	*Nonreactive test*—does not meet criteria for reactivity. May indicate fetal jeopardy.	No known contraindications
Breast Stimulation Stress Test (BSST)		
Can be performed by stimulation of nipples until contraction occurs	Contractions can be stimulated	May be contraindicated in preterm gestation
Contraction Stress Test (CST)		
Correlates fetal heart rate response to induced uterine contractions; indicator of *uteroplacental insufficiency*	Increased doses of oxytocin are administered to stimulate uterine contractions. Interpretation: • *Negative results* indicates absence of abnormal deceleration with all contractions. Reassurance that the fetus is likely to survive if labor occurs in 1 week. • *Positive results* indicate abnormal FHR decelerations with contractions. May indicate *uteroplacental insufficiency* and that the fetus is at increased risk for perinatal morbidity and death.	Invasive procedure Risk for uterine hyperstimulation and jeopardy to the fetus

Table 11.1

Diagnostic Tests to Evaluate Fetal Well-Being—cont'd

Test	Implications of Results	Risks
Ultrasound		
Passage of high-frequency sound waves through uterus to obtain data regarding fetal growth, placental position, placental detachment, and uterine cavity; can be done abdominally or vaginally	May be *used for:* pregnancy confirmation, fetal viability, estimation of fetal age, placental location, placental abruption, detection of fetal abnormalities, identification of multiple gestation, and confirmation of fetal death.	Noninvasive procedure Inconclusive evidence of harmful effects on humans
Biophysical Profile (BPP)		
Assessment of five fetal biophysical variables: *tone, breathing movements, gross body movement, amniotic fluid volume (AFV),* and *FHR reactivity* (monitored by nonstress test [NST]); first four variables assessed by *ultrasound;* score of 2 assigned to each normal finding, and 0 to each abnormal; maximum score: 10	*Used to*: assess the fetus at risk for intrauterine compromise. • *Normal* fetal biophysical activities indicate that the CNS is functional and the fetus is not hypoxemic. • *Abnormal* findings with oligohydramnios indicate fetal jeopardy (acidosis and impending death) and necessity for **immediate** delivery. • Normal: 8–10 (if AFV adequate). • Equivocal: 6. • Abnormal: <4.	Noninvasive procedure No known contraindications
Amniocentesis		
Invasive procedure for amniotic fluid analysis; needle placed through abdominal wall to obtain designated amount of fluid for examination; ultrasound *always precedes* this procedure; possible after 14 weeks of gestation	Amniotic fluid (fetal cells) might be analyzed for chromosomal studies to detect: aberrations, inborn errors of metabolism; determine fetal lung maturity, presence of isoimmune disease, α-fetoprotein (AFP) levels for determination of neural tube defects, and presence of meconium.	Complications: <1%, but risks might include: onset of contractions; infections; placental, cord, fetal, or bladder puncture • Fetomaternal hemorrhage with possible Rh isoimmunization • Mothers who are Rh-negative should receive RhoGAM following the procedure
Percutaneous Umbilical Blood Sampling (PUBS; also called cordocentesis)		
Technique used to obtain pure fetal blood from the umbilical cord while the fetus is in utero; *ultrasound* done first to locate umbilical cord, then a needle is inserted through the maternal abdomen and into the fetal umbilical vein; done in *second and third trimesters;* a paralytic agent, such as Pavulon, may be given to prevent fetal movement during the procedure	*Indications* for fetal blood sampling: • Rapid fetal karyotyping. • Diagnosis of fetal infection. • Platelet disorders. • Fetal blood grouping. • Diagnosis and treatment of isoimmunization. • Fetal metabolic disorders. • Fetal blood transfusion. • Administration of fetal medications.	Overall fetal loss risk <2%; complication rate after PUBS: <0.5% *Complications* include: failure to obtain sample, bleeding, premature rupture of membranes, chorioamnionitis, fetal bradycardia, Rh isoimmunization (women who are Rh-negative are given RhoGAM).
Chorionic Villus Sampling (CVS)		
Involves obtaining a small sample of chorionic villi from edge of developing placenta between 10 and 12 weeks of gestation; can be accomplished either transcervically or transabdominally; use sterile procedure; chorionic tissue aspirated into a syringe	Because chorionic villi originate in zygote, they reflect the genetic makeup of the fetus. *Indications for CVS:* • Advanced maternal age (>35 years). • Biochemical and molecular assays for infections. • Assays for metabolic disorders.	Vaginal bleeding, spontaneous abortion (SAB), rupture of membranes, limb anomalies (increased risk if done <10 weeks of gestation); intrauterine infection, Rh isoimmunization (women who are Rh-negative are given RhoGAM)

DIAGNOSTIC TESTS

NEWBORN SCREENING PROCEDURES

Table 11.2

Newborn Screening Procedures

Test	Implications of Results	Nursing Priorities
Cord blood type, group, and Coombs' test	Sample of cord blood is collected at delivery to determine newborn's *blood type* and *group* (Rh positive or negative). Coombs' test is done, especially for those whose mothers have type O or Rh-negative blood, or for neonates who are considerably jaundiced. Direct Coombs' test will determine *if antibodies* are present in the neonate's blood.	1. Review prenatal record to determine risk for ABO and Rh incompatibility. 2. Assess for jaundice. Age of the neonate in hours or days at the onset of jaundice is essential to diagnose underlying clinical causes. 3. Provide support and information to the family regarding screening procedures.
Phenylketonuria (PKU)	PKU is an autosomal recessive disease of protein synthesis in which the blood level of the amino acid phenylalanine becomes very high; the disorder results in *mental retardation*. If test is positive, retardation can be prevented through dietary control. Test is done with blood sample from neonate's heel 24–36 hours after having milk. Usually repeat screening recommended, especially if discharged early.	1. Review family history for incidence of inborn errors of metabolism. 2. Observe neonate for: lethargy, apnea, poor feeding, poor muscle tone, jaundice, enlarged tongue, diarrhea, and unusual (musty) body odor. 3. Provide support and information regarding screening procedures. Stress importance of follow-up testing.
Hypothyroidism	Mass neonatal screening for hypothyroidism is a cost-effective measure for preventing mental retardation caused by thyroid dysfunction. Sample of neonate's blood is taken for analysis (may be done with PKU analysis).	1. Review family history for thyroid dysfunction. 2. Provide support and information regarding screening procedures.
Galactosemia	Galactosemia is an autosomal recessive disease in which the inborn error of metabolism involves the body's inability to convert galactose to glucose. Surplus of galactose causes *liver* and *brain damage*. May be done with blood sample for PKU.	1. Review family history for incidence of inborn errors of metabolism. 2. Provide support and information to the family regarding screening procedures.
Sickle cell disease	Sickle cell is an autosomal recessive disorder occurring in certain ethnic groups, most commonly African American. Other ethnic origins may include: Mediterranean, Caribbean, Arabian, East Indian, and South and Central American. Disease is marked by crescent-shaped RBCs caused by defective hemoglobin. Severe, life-threatening attacks (crises) begin in childhood (fever and abdominal pain). Blood sample is taken after birth.	1. Review family history for autosomal blood disorders, especially if member of high-risk ethnic group. 2. Provide support and information to parents regarding genetic screening. 3. Provide support and information to the family.
Tay-Sachs disease	Tay-Sachs disease (TSD) is an autosomal recessive disease characterized by the *absence* of the enzyme hexosaminidase A (Hex-A). Especially common in people with eastern European (Ashkenazi) Jewish descent. Without Hex-A, a lipid GM_2 ganglioside accumulates abnormally in cells, especially in the nerve cells of the brain. The destructive process begins in the fetus early in pregnancy, although the disease is not clinically apparent until the child is several months old. By the time a child with TSD is 3 or 4 years old, the nervous system is badly affected. Even with the best of care, all children with classical TSD die early in childhood, usually by age 5.	1. Review family history for autosomal disorders, especially if member of high-risk ethnic group. 2. Provide information about carrier screening. 3. Provide support and information for the family.

OXYGEN THERAPY

I. PURPOSE—to relieve hypoxia and provide adequate tissue oxygenation.

II. CLINICAL INDICATIONS:

A. Any client who is likely to have significant *shunt* from:
1. Fluid in the alveoli.
   a. Pulmonary edema.
   b. Pneumonia.
   c. Near-drowning.
   d. Chest trauma.
2. Collapsed alveoli (atelectasis).
   a. Airway obstruction.
      (1) Any client who is unconscious.
      (2) Choking.
   b. Failure to take deep breaths.
      (1) Pain (rib fracture).
      (2) Paralysis of the respiratory muscles (spine injury).
      (3) Depression of the respiratory center (head injury, drug overdose).
   c. Collapse of an entire lung (pneumothorax).
3. Other gases in the alveoli.
   a. Smoke inhalation.
   b. Toxic inhalations.
   c. Carbon monoxide poisoning.
4. Respiratory arrest.

B. Cardiac arrest.
C. Shock.
D. Shortness of breath.
E. Signs of respiratory insufficiency.
F. Breathing fewer than 10 times per minute.
G. Chest pain.
H. Stroke.
I. Anemia.
J. Fetal decelerations during labor.

III. PRECAUTIONS:

A. Clients with COPD should receive oxygen at *low* flow rates (usually 1 to 3 L/min), to prevent inhibition of hypoxic respiratory drive.

B. *Excessive* amounts of oxygen for prolonged periods of time will cause *retrolental fibroplasia* and blindness in infants who are premature.

C. Oxygen delivered *without* humidification will result in drying and irritation of respiratory mucosa, decreased ciliary action, and thickening of respiratory secretions.

D. Oxygen supports combustion, and *fire* is a potential hazard during its administration.
1. Ground electrical equipment.
2. Prohibit smoking.
3. Institute measures to decrease static electricity.

E. *High* flow rates of oxygen delivered by ventilator or cuffed tracheostomy and endotracheal tubes can produce signs of *oxygen toxicity* in 24 to 48 hours:
1. Cough, sore throat, decreased vital capacity, and substernal discomfort.
2. Pulmonary manifestations due to:
   a. Atelectasis.
   b. Exudation of protein fluids into alveoli.
   c. Damage to pulmonary capillaries.
   d. Interstitial hemorrhage.

IV. OXYGEN ADMINISTRATION:

A. Oxygen is dispensed from cylinder or piped-in system.

B. Methods of delivering oxygen:
1. **Nasal prongs/cannula.**
   a. Comfortable and simple, and allows client to move about in bed.
   b. Delivers 25% to 40% oxygen at flow rates of 4 to 6 L/min.
   c. Difficult to keep in position unless client is alert and cooperative.
2. Jet mixing **Venturi mask.**
   a. Allows for accurate delivery of prescribed concentration of oxygen.
   b. Delivers 24% to 50% oxygen at flow rates of 4 to 8 L/min.
   c. Useful in long-term treatment of *COPD.*
3. **Simple O_2 face mask.**
   a. Poorly tolerated—used for short periods of time; feeling of "suffocation."
   b. Delivers 50% to 60% oxygen at flow rates of 8 to 12 L/min.
   c. Significant rebreathing of carbon dioxide at low oxygen flow rates.
   d. Hot—may produce *pressure sores* around nose and mouth.
4. **Continuous positive airway pressure (CPAP) mask.**
   a. Increases pulmonary volume; opens alveoli; may improve ventilation-perfusion (V/Q) mismatch.
   b. Used with *sleep apnea* with or without O_2 source.
5. **Non-rebreather reservoir mask.**
   a. Reservoir bag has one-way valve preventing the client from exhaling back into the bag.
   b. Oxygen flow rate prevents collapse of bag during inhalation.
   c. Delivers 90% to 95% oxygen at flow rates of 10 to 12 L/min.
   d. Ideal for *severe hypoxia,* but client may complain of feelings of suffocation.

6. **T-tube.**
   a. Provides humidification and enriched oxygen mixtures to *tracheostomy* or *endotracheal tube.*
   b. Delivers up to 100% oxygen at flow rates at least twice the minute ventilation.
   c. Refer to **Table 11.3** for summary of oxygen delivery equipment.

V. INTUBATION AND MECHANICAL VENTILATION:

A. *Indications:*
1. Apnea.
2. Inadequate upper airway or inability to clear secretions.
3. Worsening respiratory acidosis ($Paco_2$ greater than 50 mm Hg) and hypoventilation.
4. Pao_2 less than 55 mm Hg.
5. Absent gag reflex.
6. Heavy sedation or paralysis.
7. Imminent respiratory failure (respiratory rate less than 8 to 10 breaths/min or greater than 30 to 40 breaths/min).
8. Chest wall trauma.
9. Profound shock.
10. Controlled hyperventilation (e.g., increased ICP).

B. *Types of positive-pressure ventilators:*
1. *Pressure cycled*—gas flows into the client until a predetermined airway pressure is reached. Tidal volume is not constant.
2. *Time cycled*—gas flows for a certain percentage of time during ventilatory cycle.
3. *Volume cycled*—most common ventilators used; tidal volume is determined, and a fixed volume is delivered with each breath.

C. *Ventilator modes:*
1. *Controlled*—machine delivers a breath at a fixed rate regardless of client's effort or demands.
2. *Assist-controlled*—machine senses a client's efforts to breathe and delivers a fixed tidal volume with each effort.
3. *Intermittent mandatory ventilation (IMV)*—breaths are delivered by the machine, but the client may also breathe spontaneously without machine assistance.
4. *Pressure support*—client breathes spontaneously and determines ventilator rate. Tidal volume determined by inflation pressure and client's lung-thorax compliance.

D. *Minute ventilation*—determined by the respiratory rate and the tidal volume. A respiratory rate of 10 to 15 breaths/min is considered appropriate. Close monitoring is required to achieve desired (not necessarily normal) $Paco_2$.

E. *Positive end-expiratory pressure* (PEEP)—maintenance of positive airway pressure at the end of expiration. Applied in the form of continuous positive airway pressure (CPAP) for the client breathing spontaneously or continuous positive-pressure ventilation (CPPV) for the client receiving mechanical breaths. Applied in 3- to 5-cm H_2O increments. Levels greater than 10 to 15 cm H_2O are associated with *cardiovascular dysfunction* and *hemodynamic* compromise.

Table 11.3

Summary: Oxygen Delivery Equipment

O_2	Flow Rate Delivered	Percent O_2
Nasal cannula*	1–6 L/min	24%–44%
Simple mask	6–10 L/min	35%–55%
Non-rebreather mask	6–15 L/min	50%–90%
Venti mask (Venturi)	3–15 L/min	24%–50%
Bag-valve mask (ambu bag)	15 L/min	100% with reservoir

*Nasal cannulas should be humidified when they are used for an extended time.
From Myers, E: *RNotes.* FA Davis, Philadelphia, 2010.

HANDS-ON NURSING CARE

Positioning the Client

Positioning of the client for specific surgical conditions is detailed in **Table 11.4.** Various common client positions are illustrated in **Figure 11.1.**

Commonly Used Tubes

Table 11.5 provides a review of the use of common tubes. A chest drainage system is illustrated in **Figure 11.2.**

Colostomy Care

Tables 11.6 and **11.7** provide information on emptying and changing a colostomy appliance.

Basic Prosthetic Care

Information on the care of dentures is provided in **Table 11.8. Table 11.9** lists steps in caring for an artificial eye, and information on caring for a hearing aid is provided in **Table 11.10.**

Bladder Training

Table 11.11 provides information on bladder training.

Table 11.4

Positioning the Client for Specific Surgical Conditions

Surgical Condition	Key Points	Rationale
Amputation: lower extremity	*No* pillows under stump after first 24 hr; turn client *prone* several times a day	Prevents flexion deformity of the limb
Appendicitis: ruptured	Keep in *Fowler's* position—*not* flat in bed	Keeps infection from spreading upward in the peritoneal cavity
Burns (extensive)	Usually *flat* for first 24 hr	Potential problem is hypovolemia, which will be more symptomatic in a sitting position
Cast, extremity	Keep extremity *elevated*	Prevents edema
Craniotomy	Head *elevated* with supratentorial incision; *flat* with cerebellar or brainstem incision	Reduces cerebral edema, which contributes to increased intracranial pressure
Flail chest	Position on *affected* side	Reduces the instability of the chest wall that is causing the paradoxical respiratory movements
Gastric resection	Lie down *after* meals	May be useful in preventing dumping syndrome
Hiatal hernia (*before* repair)	Head of bed *elevated* on shock blocks	Prevents esophageal irritation from gastric regurgitation
Hip prosthesis	1. Keep affected leg in *abduction* (splint or pillow between legs) 2. *Avoid* adduction and flexion of the hip 3. Use trochanter roll along outside of femur anterior joint capsule incision to keep affected leg turned slightly *inward;* no trochanter roll with posterior joint capsule incision as leg is turned slightly *outward*	If affected hip is flexed and allowed to adduct and internally rotate, the head of the femur may be displaced from the socket
Laminectomy; fusion	*Avoid* twisting motion when getting out of bed, ambulating	Prevents any shearing force on the spine
Liver biopsy	Place on *right* side, and position pillow for pressure	Prevents bleeding
Lobectomy	Do *not* put in Trendelenburg position. Position of comfort—sides, back	Pushes abdominal contents against diaphragm; may cause respiratory embarrassment
Mastectomy	1. Do *not* abduct arm first few days 2. Elevate hand and arm *higher* than shoulder if lymph glands removed	Puts tension on suture line Prevents lymphedema
Pneumonectomy	Turn *only* toward operative side for short periods; *no* extreme lateral positioning	1. Gives unaffected lung room for full expansion 2. Prevents mediastinal shift 3. In case of bleeding, there will be no drainage into the unaffected bronchi
Pneumothorax	Semi-Fowler's	Gives optimal chest expansion
Radium implantation in cervix	Bedrest—usually may *elevate* head to 30 degrees	*Must* keep radium insert positioned correctly
Respiratory distress	*Orthopnea* position usually desirable	Allows for maximum expansion of lungs
Retinal detachment	1. Affected area toward bed—*complete bedrest* 2. No *sudden* movements of head 3. *Face down* if gas bubble in place	1. Gravity may help retina fall in place; prevents further tearing 2. Any sudden increase in intraocular pressure may further dislodge retina
Traction		
Straight traction	Check specific orders about how much head may be elevated	Body is used as the countertraction—this must not be less than the pull of the traction
Balanced suspension	May give client more freedom to move about than in straight traction	In balanced suspension, additional weights supply countertraction
Client who is unconscious	Turn on side with head slightly *lowered*—"coma" position	1. Important to let secretions drain out by gravity 2. *Must* prevent aspiration

Continued

POSITIONING

Table 11.4

Positioning the Client for Specific Surgical Conditions—cont'd

Surgical Condition	Key Points	Rationale
Vascular		
Iliofemoral bypass; arterial insufficiency	1. Do *not* elevate legs 2. *Avoid* hip flexion—walk or stand, but do *not* sit	1. Arterial flow is helped by gravity 2. Flexion of the hip compresses the vessels of the extremity
Vein strippings; vein ligations	1. Keep legs *elevated* 2. Do *not* stand or sit for long periods	1. Prevents venous stasis 2. Prevents venous pooling

Source: Jane Vincent Corbett, RN, MS, EdD, Professor Emerita, School of Nursing, University of San Francisco. Used with permission.

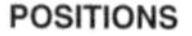

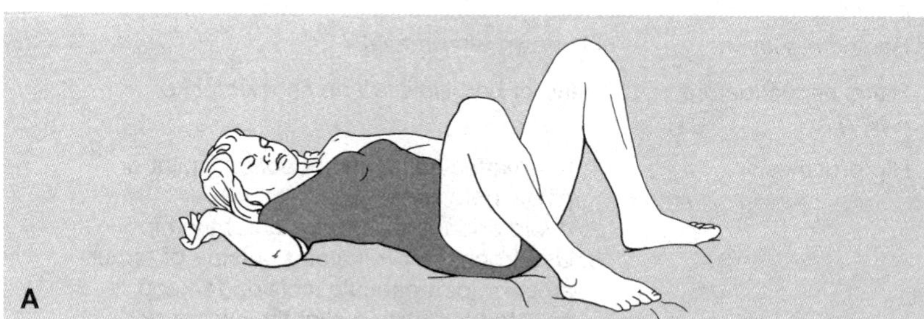

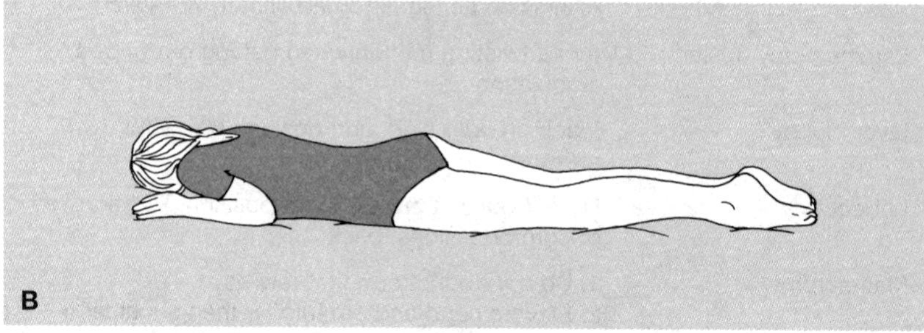

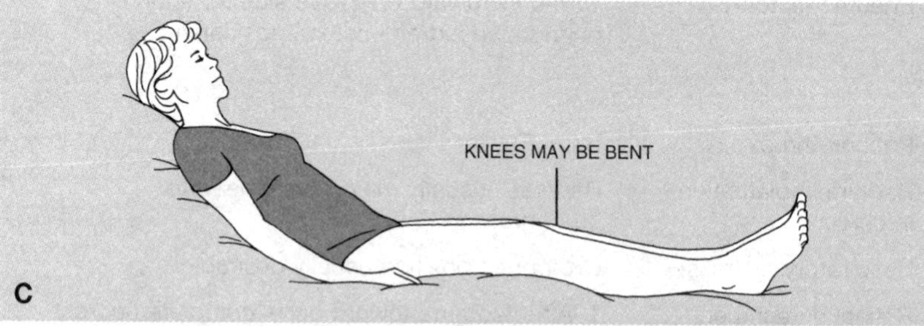

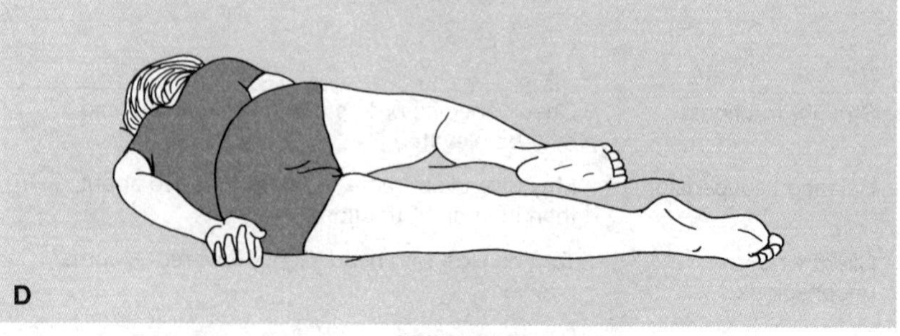

Figure 11.1 Common client positions. ***(A)* Dorsal recumbent (back-lying), legs up**—used in gynecological and obstetrical procedures such as forceps delivery or vaginal examination; **legs down**—for comfort and following spinal anesthesia. ***(B)* Prone**—may be used in clients who are unconscious to promote drainage from mouth and prevent flexion contractures. ***(C)* Fowler's—semi-sitting; 45 to 60 degrees; knees may or may not be bent.** Facilitates breathing and drainage. ***(D)* Sims'**—position of choice for enemas and rectal examination, prevents aspiration in clients who are unconscious, comfortable sleeping position for women who are pregnant.

POSITIONS

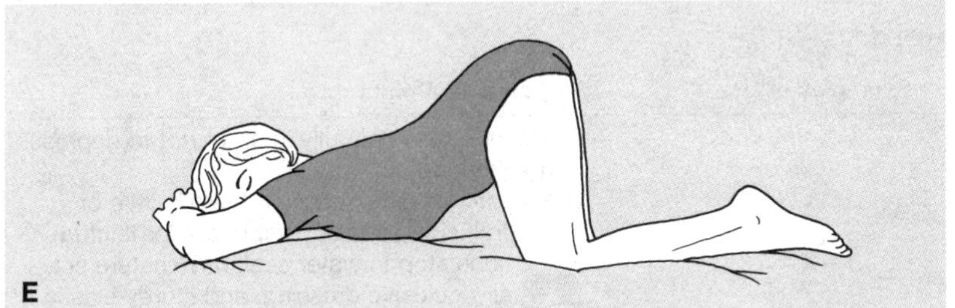

KNEE-CHEST OR GENUPECTORAL POSITION

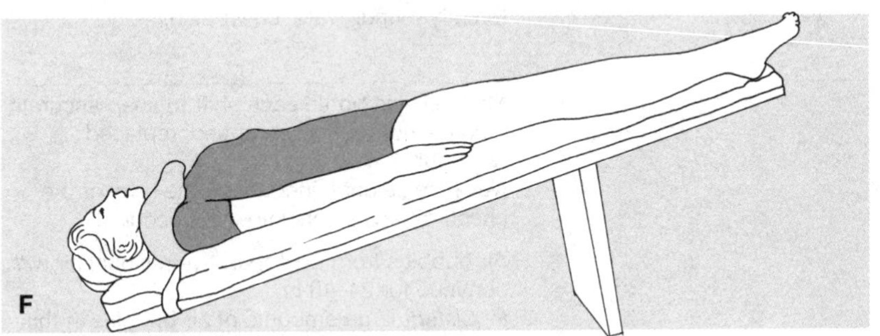

TRENDELENBURG POSITION

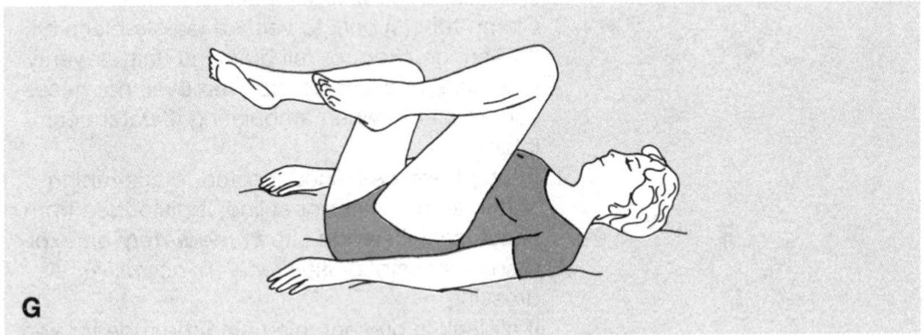

LITHOTOMY OR DORSOSACRAL POSITION

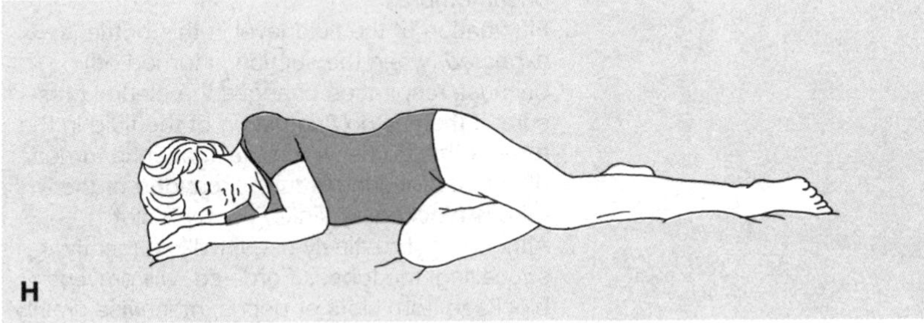

RIGHT LATERAL RECUMBENT POSITION

Figure 11.1—cont'd ***(E)* Knee-chest or genupectoral**—used for gynecological and obstetrical conditions such as impacted fetal head or transverse presentation. ***(F)*** **Trendelenburg**—used in abdominal surgery. **Modified Trendelenburg (torso flat and feet elevated)** preferred in shock. ***(G)*** **Lithotomy or dorsosacral**—used in genital tract operations and vaginal hysterectomy. ***(H)*** **Right lateral recumbent**—side-lying, relieves pressure on sacrum and heels.

Table 11.5

Review of the Use of Common Tubes

Tube or Apparatus	Purpose	Examples of Use	Key Nursing Points
Chest tubes	1. *Anterior tube* drains mostly air from pleural space 2. *Posterior tube* drains mostly fluid from pleural space	1. *Thoracotomy* 2. *Open heart surgery* 3. *Spontaneous pneumothorax* 4. *Traumatic pneumothorax*	1. *See* Key Points for each of the three entries under Drainage system, **p. 840** 2. *Sterile* technique is used when changing dressings around the tube insertions 3. Fowler's *position* to facilitate air and fluid removal 4. Cough, deep breathe q1h; splint chest; medicate for pain

Continued

Table 11.5

Review of the Use of Common Tubes—cont'd

Tube or Apparatus	Purpose	Examples of Use	Key Nursing Points
	3. Removal of fluid and air from pleural space is necessary to reestablish negative intrapleural pressure		5. Manage pain carefully in order *not* to depress respirations 6. Prepare for removal when there is little or no drainage, air leak disappears, or fluctuations stop in water seal; have suture set, air-occlusive dressing, and sturdy elastic tape ready; medicate for pain before removal; monitor breathing after removal (breath sounds, rate, chest pain)
Drainage system (see Fig. 11.2, p. 843)			
#1: drainage compartment	Collect drainage		1. Mark level in bottle each shift to keep accurate record—*not* routinely emptied; replaced when full 2. ***Never*** raise container above the level of the chest; otherwise backflow will occur
#2: water-seal chamber	Water seal prevents flow of atmospheric air into pleural space; essential to prevent recollapse of the lung		1. Air bubbles from postoperative residual air *will* continue for 24–48 hr 2. *Persistent* large amounts of air bubbles in this compartment indicate an *air leak* between the alveoli and the pleural space 3. Clamp tube(s) *only* to verify a leak; replace a broken, cracked, or full drainage unit; or verify readiness of client for tube removal; not necessary to clamp when ambulating if water seal intact 4. If tube becomes disconnected, place tubing end in sterile water or saline; if dislodged from chest, seal insertion site ***immediately*** on expiration if possible; use *sterile air-occlusive* dressing 5. If air leak is present, clamping the tube for very long (more than 10 sec) may cause a tension pneumothorax 6. Fluctuation of the fluid level in this bottle is *expected* (when the suction is turned off) because respiration changes the pleural pressure: if there is *no fluctuation* of the fluid in the tube of this bottle (when the suction is turned off), either the lung is fully expanded or the tube is blocked by kinking or by a clot 7. Although not routinely used, milking (gently squeezing) the tubes, if ordered, will prevent blockage from clots or debris; otherwise gravity drainage is sufficient to maintain patency 8. Drainage of more than 100 mL in 1 hr should be ***reported*** to physician
#3: suction control—connected to wall suction	Level of the column of water (i.e., 15–20 cm) is used to control the amount of suction applied to the chest tube—if the water evaporates to only *10 cm* depth, this will be the *maximum* suction generated by the wall suction		1. Air *should continuously bubble* through this compartment when the suction is on; the bubbles are from the atmosphere—not the client; when the wall suction is turned higher, the bubbling will increase, but the increased pulling of air is from the atmosphere and *not* from the pleural space 2. Because the level of H_2O determines the maximum negative pressure that can be obtained, make sure the water does *not* evaporate—keep filling the bottle to keep the ordered level; if there is *no* bubbling of air through this container, the wall suction is *too low*

TUBES

Table 11.5

Review of the Use of Common Tubes—cont'd

Tube or Apparatus	Purpose	Examples of Use	Key Nursing Points
Heimlich flutter valve	1. Has a one-way valve so fluids and air can drain out of the pleural space but cannot flow back 2. Eliminates the need for water seal—no danger when tube is unclamped below the valve	Same as for other chest tubes	1. Can be connected to suction if ordered 2. Sometimes can just drain into portable bag so client is more mobile
Tracheostomy tube	1. Maintains patent airway and promotes better O_2-CO_2 exchange 2. Makes removal of secretions by suctioning easier 3. Cuff on trach is necessary if need air-tight fit for assisted ventilation	1. *Acute respiratory distress* due to poor ventilation 2. *Severe burns of head and neck* 3. *Laryngectomy* (trach is permanent)	1. Use oxygen *before* and *after* each suctioning 2. Humidify oxygen 3. *Sterile* technique in suctioning; clean technique at home 4. Cleanse inner cannula as needed–only leave out 5–10 min 5. Hemostat handy if outer cannula is expelled—have obturator taped to bed and another trach set handy 6. Cuff **must** be deflated periodically to prevent necrosis of mucosa, unless low-pressure cuff used
Penrose drain	Soft collapsible latex rubber drain inserted to drain serosanguineous fluid from a surgical site; usually brought out to the skin via a stab wound	*Bowel resection*	1. Expect drainage to progress from serosanguineous to more serous 2. *Sterile* technique when changing dressing—do often 3. Physician will advance tube a little each day
Nasogastric (NG) tubes			
Levin tube and small-bore feeding tubes	1. Inserted into stomach to decompress by removing gastric contents and air—prevents any buildup of gastric secretions, which are continuous 2. Used when stomach must be washed out *(lavage)* 3. Used for feedings when client is unable to swallow *(gavage)*	1. Any abdominal or other *surgery after which peristalsis is absent* for a few days 2. *Overdoses* 3. *Gastrointestinal hemorrhage* 4. *Cancer of the esophagus* 5. *Early postoperative care for client who had a laryngectomy or radical neck dissection*	1. Connect to *low* intermittent suction 2. Irrigate prn with normal saline or puffs of air 3. Clean, but *not* sterile, procedure 4. Mouth care needed 5. Report "***coffee ground***" material (digested blood) 6. For overdose, stomach is pumped out as ***rapidly*** as possible 7. For hemorrhage, tepid normal saline may be used to lavage 8. Critical to make sure tube still in stomach *before* beginning feeding; listen for air passing into stomach, and if possible aspirate gastric contents; small-bore tubes require placement check by x-ray 9. Follow feeding with some water to rinse out the tube 10. Clamp tube when ambulating 11. With larger-bore tubes, determine residuals and withhold feeding if large residuals obtained
Salem sump	Double-lumen tube with vent to *protect gastric mucosa* from trauma of suctioning	Same as Levin tube	1. Irrigate vent (blue tubing) with air only 2. *See* Levin tube

Continued

Table 11.5

Review of the Use of Common Tubes—cont'd

Tube or Apparatus	Purpose	Examples of Use	Key Nursing Points
Gastrostomy tube	1. Inserted into stomach via abdominal wall 2. May be used for decompression 3. Used *long term for feedings*	Conditions affecting *esophagus* in which it is impossible to insert a nasogastric tube	1. Principles of tube feedings same as with Levin nasogastric tube, *except* no danger that tube is in trachea 2. If permanent, tube may be replaceable
Miller-Abbott tube Cantor tube	Longer than Levin tube—has mercury or air in bags so tube can be used to *decompress the lower intestinal tract*	1. *Small-bowel obstructions* 2. *Intussusception* 3. *Volvulus*	1. Care similar to that for Levin NG tube—irrigated 2. Connected to suction, *not* sterile technique 3. Orders will be written on how to advance the tube, gently pushing tube a few inches each hour; client position may affect advancement of tube 4. X-rays determine the desired location of tube
T-tube	To *drain bile* from the common bile duct *until* edema has subsided	*Cholecystectomy* when a common duct exploration (CDE) or choledochostomy was also done	1. Bile drainage is influenced by *position* of the drainage bag 2. Clamp tube as ordered to see if bile will flow into duodenum normally
Hemovac	A type of closed-wound drainage connected to suction—used to *drain a large amount of* serosanguineous drainage from under an incision	1. *Mastectomy* 2. *Total hip procedures* 3. *Total knee procedures*	1. May compress unit, and have portable vacuum or connect to wall suction 2. Small drainage tubes may get clogged—physician may irrigate these at times
Jackson Pratt	1. A method of *closed-wound suction* drainage—indicated when tissue displacement and tissue trauma may occur with rigid drain tubes (e.g., Hemovac) 2. *See* Hemovac	1. *Neurosurgery* 2. *Neck surgery* 3. *Mastectomy* 4. *Total knee and hip replacement* 5. *Abdominal surgery* 6. *Urological procedures*	1. Empty reservoir when full, to prevent loss of wound drainage and back-contamination 2. *See* Hemovac.
Three-way Foley	To provide avenues for *constant irrigation and constant drainage* of the urinary bladder	1. Transurethral resection (TUR) 2. *Bladder* infections	1. Watch for blocking by clots—causes bladder spasms 2. Irrigant solution often has *antibiotic* added to normal saline or sterile water 3. *Sterile* water rather than normal saline may be used for lysis of clots
Suprapubic catheter	To *drain bladder* via an opening through the abdominal wall above the pubic bone	*Suprapubic* prostatectomy	May have orders to irrigate prn or continuously
Ureteral catheter	To *drain urine* from the pelvis of one kidney, or for *splinting* ureter	1. Cystoscopy for diagnostic workups 2. *Ureteral surgery* 3. *Pyelotomy*	1. ***Never*** clamp the tube—pelvis of kidney only holds 4–8 mL 2. Use ***only*** 5 mL sterile normal saline if ordered to irrigate

Note: This review focuses on care of tubes, not on total client care.
Source: Jane Vincent Corbett, RN, MS, EdD, Professor Emerita, School of Nursing, University of San Francisco. Used with permission.

TUBES

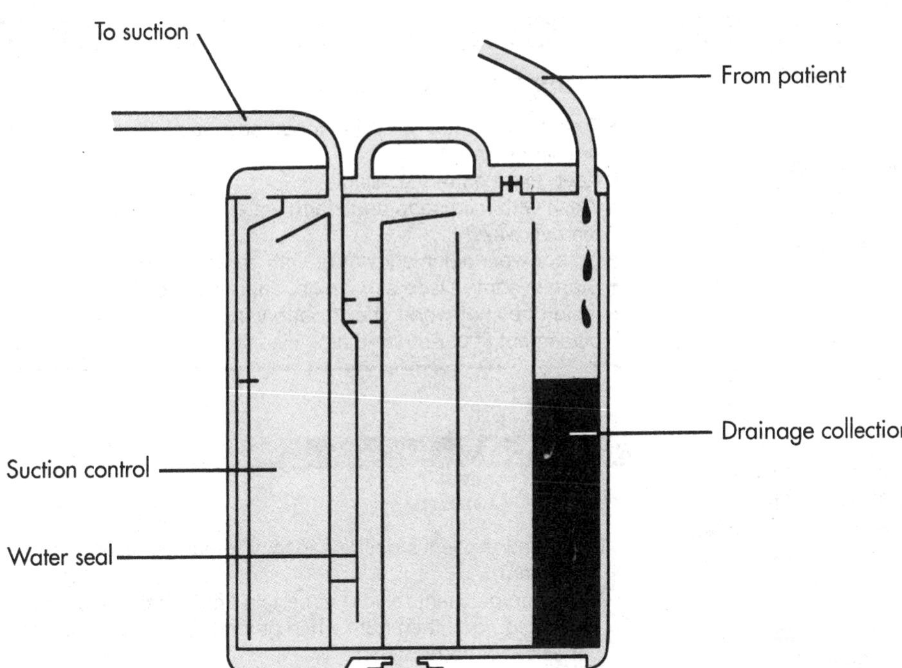

Figure 11.2 **Chest drainage system.**

Table 11.6

Emptying Colostomy Appliance

Check for drainage in appliance at least twice during each shift. If drainage present (diarrhea-type stool):

Do	Do Not
1. Unclamp the bottom of bag.	Remove appliance each time it needs emptying.
2. Drain into bedpan.	
3. Use a squeeze-type bottle filled with warm water to rinse inside of appliance.	
4. Clean off clamp if soiled.	
5. Put a few drops of deodorant in appliance if not odor-proof.	Use any materials that could irritate bowel.
6. Fasten bottom of appliance securely (fold bag over clamp 2–3 times before closing).	
7. Check for leakage under appliance every 2–4 hours.	
8. Communicate with client while attending to appliance.	Ignore client's needs.

Table 11.7

Changing Colostomy Appliance

Gather equipment: gloves, skin prep packet, colostomy appliance measured to fit stoma properly (if new surgical stoma, it will continue to shrink with the healing process; use stoma measuring guide), skin barrier, warm water and soap, face cloth/towel, plastic bag for disposal of old equipment. Remember that bowel is very fragile; also, working near bowel increases peristalsis, and feces and flatulence may be expelled.

Do	Do Not
1. Remove old appliance carefully, pulling from area with least drainage to area with most drainage.	1. Tear appliance quickly from skin.
2. Wash skin area with soap and water.	2. Wash stoma with soap; put anything dry onto stoma.
3. Observe skin area for potential breakdown.	3. Irritate skin or stoma.
4. Use packet of skin prep on the skin around the stoma; allow skin prep solution to dry on skin before applying colostomy appliance.	4. Put skin prep solution onto stoma; it will cause irritation.
5. Apply skin barrier you have measured and cut to size.	5. Make opening too large (increases risk of leakage).

Continued

Table 11.7

Changing Colostomy Appliance—cont'd

Do	Do Not
6. Put appliance on so that the bottom of the appliance is easily accessible for emptying (e.g., if client is out of bed most of the time, put the bottom facing the feet; if client is in bed most of the time, have bottom face the side); picture-frame the adhesive portion of the appliance with 1-inch tape.	6. Have appliance attached so client cannot be involved in own care.
7. Put a few drops of deodorant in appliance if not odor-proof.	7. Use any materials that would irritate bowel.
8. Use clamp to fasten bottom of appliance.	
9. Talk to client (or communicate in best way possible for client) during and after procedure.	9. *Avoid* conversation/ eye contact.
10. Use good hand-washing technique.	10. Contaminate other incisions.

Table 11.8

Care of Dentures

- Wear gloves.
- If client cannot remove own dentures, grasp upper plate at the front teeth and move up and down gently to release suction.
- Lift the lower plate up one side at a time.
- Use extreme care not to damage dentures while cleaning.
- Use tepid, *not* hot, water to clean.
- *Avoid* soaking for long periods of time.
- Inspect for sharp edges.
- Do oral cavity assessment.
- Replace moistened dentures in client's mouth.
- Use appropriately labeled container for storage when dentures are to remain out of client's mouth.

Table 11.9

Caring for an Artificial Eye

- With gloved hand, pull lower eyelid down over the infraorbital bone and exert pressure below the eyelid.
- Pressure will make the eye prosthesis pop out.
- Handle eye prosthesis carefully.
- Using *aseptic* technique, cleanse socket with saline-moistened gauze, stroking from inner to outer canthus.
- Wash the prosthesis in warm normal saline.
- To reinsert, gently pull the client's lower lid down, raise the upper lid if necessary, slip the saline-moistened eye prosthesis gently into the socket, and release the lids.

Table 11.10

Caring for a Hearing Aid

- Turn off aid when not using (open case at night to prevent draining battery).
- Keep extra battery available.
- Wash with mild soap and warm water; use pipe cleaner to remove wax.
- Do *not* wear aid in shower or with ear infection.
- Store in same place every night and away from pets.
- If aid does not work: check battery insertion, on-off switch, placement (if ear-molded aid), cleanliness.

Table 11.11

Bladder Training

1. Determine client's desire/capacity to participate in such a program.
2. Encourage client to void at certain times throughout the day (e.g., q2h then q3h, when getting up in morning, after meals, before bedtime).
3. Do *not* decrease fluid intake (would put client at risk for infection).
4. Encourage client to resist voiding when bladder is not full (use a technique such as counting while voiding and trying to increase that number to a desired level).
5. Encourage client to ask for assistance when needed, to avoid falls when attempting to get to toilet alone while unsteady on feet.
6. Respond to requests for assistance.
7. *Decrease caffeine* and *alcohol* in diet.
8. Monitor for skin breakdown in clients who are incontinent.
9. Have client practice Kegel exercises to improve tone and function of pelvic floor.
10. Refer to physical therapist who specializes in this area, if necessary.

Bowel Training

Table 11.12 provides information on bowel training.

Table 11.12

Bowel Training

1. Verify that the client is not impacted.
2. Determine client's desire/capacity to participate in the program.
3. Determine normal bowel habits.
4. Increase fiber and fluids in the diet.
5. Establish a routine: same time each day.
6. Give stool softener; cathartic, or suppository as ordered.
7. Offer client a hot drink before set time for defecation.
8. Provide time and privacy.

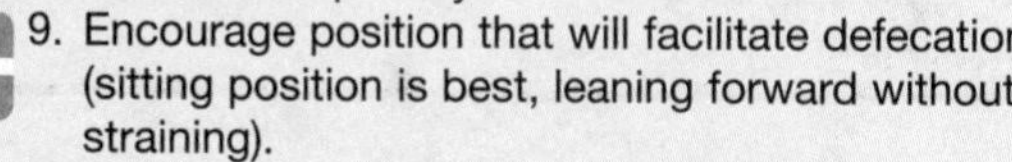

9. Encourage position that will facilitate defecation (sitting position is best, leaning forward without straining).
10. Document interventions that are successful.

Questions

Select the one answer that is best for each question, unless otherwise directed.

1. Oxygen therapy is ordered to assist the client with breathing. Which principle should guide a nurse in managing the delivery of oxygen to an elderly client with emphysema?
   1. O_2 should be high (6–8 L) since hypoxemia is the stimulus to breathe.
   2. O_2 should be high since the stimulus to breathe is the high PCO_2.
   3. O_2 should be low (2–3 L) since the stimulus to breathe is the low PO_2.
   4. O_2 should be low since the stimulus to breathe is the high PCO_2

2. If fluctuation (tidaling) in the water-seal compartment of a closed chest drainage system has stopped, a nurse should:
   1. Increase wall suction above 20 cm H_2O pressure.
   2. Raise the apparatus above the chest to move the fluid.
   3. Ask the client to cough and deep breathe.
   4. Vigorously strip the tube to dislodge the clot.

3. Which nursing measures are aspects of proper tracheostomy care? *Select all that apply.*
   1. Securing the twill tape ties on the side of the neck.
   2. Cleaning or changing the inner cannula at least once a day.
   3. Inflating the tracheostomy cuff before tracheostomy care.
   4. Using peroxide and sterile saline to clean around the stoma.
   5. Suctioning when secretions or adventitious breath sounds are present.
   6. Ensuring a means of communication with the client.

4. Which nursing actions are appropriate following a liver biopsy? *Select all that apply.*
   1. Place client in supine, semi-Fowler's position.
   2. Immediately assist client to turn on right side.
   3. Check ammonia level every hour for 4 hours.
   4. Check vital signs every 10–15 minutes for 1–2 hours.
   5. Place a pillow under the right costal margin.
   6. Instruct the client to avoid heavy lifting for 1 week after biopsy.

5. Which nursing actions should be completed before a physician performs a thoracentesis? *Select all that apply.*
   1. Assessing the client for any allergy to local anesthetics.
   2. Teaching the client to do pursed-lip breathing during the procedure.
   3. Placing the client in an upright sitting position leaning forward, if able.
   4. Placing the client in a prone position with the side with the affected lung on a pillow.
   5. Making sure that the consent form is signed and in the chart.
   6. Telling the client not to expect discomfort.

6. What should *alert* a nurse to a possible problem with a client who is on a mechanical ventilator?
   1. Loud beeping when the respiratory therapist is suctioning the client.
   2. A client is using accessory muscles while on the ventilator.
   3. Bronchovesicular breath sounds are heard on auscultation.
   4. Water is collecting in the ventilator tubing.

7. A client is scheduled for an ultrasound to rule out bile duct obstruction. What preparation is required for an ultrasound test?
   1. NPO for 48 hours.
   2. Explanation about the procedure.
   3. Enemas until clear.
   4. Pain meds and sedation.

8. A nurse is assessing a client who had an esophagogastroduodenoscopy. The *first* priority for the nurse should be:
   1. Checking for bowel sounds.
   2. Giving warm gargles for a sore throat.
   3. Administering pain medication.
   4. Monitoring for return of the gag reflex.

9. Gallstones can be diagnosed and sometimes removed by endoscopic retrograde cholangiopancreatography (ERCP). Preparation of a client scheduled for this procedure should include:
   1. Planning for a 2- to 3-day hospitalization.
   2. Drinking 500 mL of dye-containing juice 30 minutes beforehand.
   3. Receiving sedative but not general anesthesia.
   4. Planning on a 5- to 10-minute procedure.

10. A client will return to the floor from the postanesthesia care unit (PACU) following a laparoscopic cholecystectomy when:
    1. The oral airway is removed.
    2. Pain is controlled.
    3. The client can move both legs.
    4. The client is awake with stable vital signs.

11. Discharge teaching for the client following a laparoscopic cholecystectomy includes:
    1. Take a shower but do not soak in the bathtub.
    2. Change wet-to-dry dressings 2 times a day.
    3. Milk any clots from the bile drainage tube every 2 hours.
    4. Remain on bedrest for 3 days.

12. A client with cystic fibrosis is to receive chest physiotherapy. When should a nurse plan to give this treatment?
    1. One hour before lunch.
    2. One half-hour after breakfast.
    3. Every 4 hours.
    4. After receiving pain medication.

QUESTIONS

13. A nurse is preparing a client for an elective electrical cardioversion. What should be included in this client's teaching?
   1. General anesthesia will be used during the procedure.
   2. Digoxin is given 48 hours before cardioversion.
   3. Analgesia and sedation are given before the procedure.
   4. Following the procedure, the client will remain hospitalized for 24 hours.

14. A client is scheduled for a cholecystogram. In preparation for the test, a nurse should ask the client about allergies to:
   Select all that apply.
   1. Eggs.
   2. Organ meats.
   3. Clams.
   4. Shrimp.
   5. Crab.
   6. Latex.

15. A client has a T-tube inserted in the surgical wound following a cholecystectomy. The *most important* nursing function in managing this tube is:
   1. Recording the quantity and color of drainage.
   2. Changing the dressing every shift.
   3. Preventing the tube from kinking.
   4. Teaching the client about the reason for the tube.

16. A client reports pain in the right shoulder following a laparoscopic cholecystectomy. A nurse explains that the pain is related to:
   1. Migration of the gas used to insufflate the abdomen during the procedure.
   2. Nerve irritation from the leakage of bile.
   3. Strain on the shoulder due to a right side-lying position during the procedure.
   4. Referred pain from an obstructed common bile duct.

17. Which assessment would be most appropriate for a nurse to make during peritoneal dialysis while the solution is dwelling within the abdomen?
   1. Assessing for urticaria.
   2. Observing respiratory status.
   3. Checking capillary refill.
   4. Monitoring electrolyte status.

18. Radioactive iodine (^{131}I) is administered to a client with hyperthyroidism to:
   1. Limit thyroid hormone absorption by the sympathetic nervous system.
   2. Limit secretion of thyroid hormone by destroying thyroid tissue.
   3. Stimulate circulating thyroid hormone for use by the body.
   4. Reduce the symptoms of CHF caused by excess thyroid hormone.

19. A radioactive iodine (^{131}I) treatment has just been completed. Knowing the excretion and effect of ^{131}I, a nurse should:
   1. Inform the client that there is little danger of exposing others to radiation.
   2. See that the urine is collected in a leakproof container.
   3. Always wear a radiation detection badge when near the client.
   4. Avoid prolonged contact with the client for 6 days after the treatment.

20. A client with intractable ascites from liver failure has a transjugular intrahepatic portosystemic shunt (TIPS). For which common complication should a nurse assess the client?
   1. Ankle edema.
   2. Angina.
   3. Increased blood pressure.
   4. Change in mental status.

21. The best nursing action to reduce an allergic response in a client who is latex-sensitive is to:
   1. Use contact isolation.
   2. Do frequent hand washing.
   3. Use cloth, plastic, or vinyl products.
   4. Expose client to repeated low-dose latex.

22. A nurse should anticipate that the chest tube for a client recovering from a pneumothorax will be removed when:
   1. Chest drainage decreases to 50 mL in 24 hours.
   2. Chest x-ray shows atelectasis has resolved.
   3. Water-seal chamber no longer fluctuates with breathing.
   4. Breath sounds are present bilaterally in apical lobes.

23. An RN observes a nursing student collecting a wound culture specimen from a client's surgical site. The RN determines that the nursing student is using the correct technique when:
   1. The wound is irrigated before collecting the specimen.
   2. The wound is swabbed from the center outward.
   3. The dry, crusty area around the wound is swabbed.
   4. Drainage from the dressing is swabbed.

24. A nurse observes a medical student preparing to insert a central venous catheter. The nurse would know that the insertion technique was correct if, after cleansing the site:
   1. The catheter was immediately inserted.
   2. Sterile gauze was used to dry the site.
   3. Insertion occurred after the site dried thoroughly.
   4. The catheter was inserted 2 minutes later.

25. Maximal barrier precautions prior to insertion of a central venous catheter should include:
   Select all that apply.
   1. Hand hygiene.
   2. Sterile gown.
   3. Surgical cap and mask.

4. Sterile gloves.
5. Draping of patient's entire body.
6. Prophylactic antibiotics.

26. The staff nurse is observing the student teaching the client about collecting a 24-hour urine test after discharge. The student understands the collection process if the student's teaching includes:
1. Urine collection container must be kept on ice the whole 24-hour period.
2. Need to void, discard the urine, and then start the 24-hour time period.
3. The importance of recording the urine volume each time client voids.
4. The need to increase oral fluid intake during the 24-hour collection period.

27. A client's wife tells a nurse that her husband snores loudly when sleeping, then he actually stops breathing. The nurse informs the client's wife that a physician can order a sleep study and he may need to use:
1. A negative pressure ventilation device such as a pneumo-wrap.
2. A time-cycled ventilator that will deliver a set volume of air.
3. A continuous positive airway pressure (CPAP) device.
4. A preset intermittent mandatory ventilation mask.

28. A nurse tells a client that, after total knee replacement surgery, a continuous passive motion (CPM) device will be used. Which statement by the nurse should be included in the client education?
1. The device will generally be applied immediately after surgery and used continuously when in bed.
2. The device will be applied every 2 hours while the client is awake.
3. The device will be used until the limb can extend 10 degrees and flex 50 degrees.
4. There is no weight-bearing until the desired degree of extension or flexion is achieved.

29. The spouse of a client who had a transurethral resection of the prostate (TURP) 24 hours ago is upset because the irrigation seems to be increasing the client's pain. Which is the best response by a nurse?
1. "I will stop the bladder irrigation and the pain should subside."
2. "I will add a local anesthetic to the irrigant to treat the pain."
3. "Perhaps you should go home and get some rest."
4. "The rate of the irrigant can be slowed when the drainage is pale pink."

30. A nurse is concerned that the results of a client's recent arterial blood gas (ABG) analysis may be inaccurate. Which factors may affect the accuracy of ABG results? *Select all that apply.*
1. Creatinine level of client that continues to rise.
2. Client has been increasingly more confused.
3. Sample was drawn 15 minutes after suctioning.
4. Absence of an air bubble in the ABG.
5. Sample returned to the lab an hour after it was drawn.
6. Sample drawn from peripherally inserted central catheter (PICC).

31. A client presents to an emergency department complaining of pain on the left side and shortness of breath. Vital signs are: BP 140/80 mm Hg; P 110, and R 44. The client's ABG results are: pH 7.5, $Paco_2$ 30 mm Hg; and Hco_3 22 mEq/L, Sao_2 86%, Pao_2 64 mm Hg. A nurse should recognize that these symptoms are consistent with:
1. Possible trauma to the chest wall.
2. Possible pneumonia.
3. Possible pulmonary embolism.
4. Possible acute pulmonary edema.

32. A client with ascites as a result of hepatitis C is in the emergency department complaining of abdominal discomfort. A paracentesis has been ordered. Nursing actions would include:
Select all that apply.
1. Having the client void before the procedure.
2. Observing for possible increase in blood pressure during the procedure.
3. Positioning the client in semi-Fowler's, head of bed elevated 30 degrees.
4. Applying pressure to the injection site following the procedure.
5. Allowing fluid to drain from catheter for 24 hours.
6. Measuring and recording amount of fluid removed.

33. Which nursing actions would most likely help prevent the development of ventilator-associated pneumonia (VAP) in a client who is mechanically ventilated? *Select all that apply.*
1. Oral hygiene every 2 hours.
2. Elevation of the head of bed at least 20 degrees.
3. Proper hand hygiene between clients.
4. Routinely remove condensation from ventilator tubing.
5. Change ventilator tubing every 12 hours.

34. Following a cardiac catheterization for recurrent angina, a 76-year-old client with a history of hypertension and type 2 diabetes, has had no urine output since the catheterization 16 hours before. Laboratory results revealed: Na^+ 134 mEq/L, Cl^- 96 mEq/L, K^+ 6.4 mEq/L, BUN 71 mg/dL, and creatinine 4.0 mg/dL. Which factors are most likely contributing to this client's condition? *Select all that apply.*
1. IV 0.45% NS at 125 mL/hr
2. Prophylactic tobramycin (Nebcin) given during the procedure.
3. Client age.
4. Possible history of renal insufficiency.
5. Recurrent angina.
6. Risk of cardiac catheterization.

35. In which situations would it be appropriate for a critical care nurse to use intra-arterial monitoring access to meet the client's needs? *Select all that apply.*
1. To do daily blood draws for studies in a client with pancreatitis in acute pain.
2. To do frequent arterial blood gases for a client in acute respiratory failure.
3. When additional access is needed to administer blood products for hypovolemia.
4. To administer vasoactive medication to treat cardiogenic shock.
5. To do continuous monitoring of blood pressure in a client with malignant hypertension.

36. The neurological assessment of a client diagnosed with a ruptured cerebral aneurysm reveals the client is unresponsive to verbal stimuli, occasionally moans and, when painful stimuli are applied, decerebrate posturing and partial eye openings are noted. A nurse assesses that this client should receive of score of ________ on the Glasgow Coma Scale (GCS). *Fill in the blank.*

37. Which statements by a client prior to a cardiac catheterization would require a nurse to take further action? *Select all that apply.*
1. "My kidney doctor has been suggesting I have this done for a year."
2. "I haven't had anything to eat since dinner last night."
3. "The last time I had a catheterization I had respiratory problems."
4. "I am glad I can go home right after the procedure."
5. "During the procedure I will feel warm all over."

38. Following a left pneumonectomy, the optimal position for a client would be:
1. In a high Fowler's position.
2. Supine with a pillow under the right shoulder.
3. Supine with a pillow under the left shoulder.
4. Left side-lying to promote expansion of right lung.

39. An RN draws an arterial blood gas sample from a client. The correct action to prevent bleeding at the site is to:
1. Apply direct pressure for 2 minutes.
2. Leave the tourniquet in place for 3 minutes.
3. Secure an ice pack over the site to cause arterial constriction.
4. Apply a vascular closure device to the site.

40. A client has just returned from having a femoral arteriogram. The *first* assessment by a nurse should be:
1. Vital signs.
2. Bowel sounds.
3. Groin area.
4. Respiratory status.

41. A client has just returned from the operating room following a hip replacement. The *most important* nursing assessment over the next 8 hours is:
1. Bleeding from the surgical site.
2. Respiratory status.
3. Urinary output.
4. Circulation and sensation on the operative side.

42. A client, who is 23 years old, gravida 2, para 0, had a miscarriage at 6 weeks' gestation last year. She presents for her first prenatal appointment at 12 weeks' gestation. She is having blood drawn for routine prenatal screening. Which laboratory result would indicate a risk to the fetus for erythroblastosis fetalis?
1. Low α-fetoprotein.
2. Blood type B–, antibody +.
3. Lecithin/sphingomyelin ratio of 2:1.
4. Blood type O+, antibody –.

43. A client, who is 15 years old, gravida 1, para 0 at 26 weeks of gestation, is admitted to an obstetrics unit with a diagnosis of mild preeclampsia. She has a blood pressure of 138/88 mm Hg and 1+ protein on urine dipstick. Which assessment finding should indicate to a nurse that the client's condition is getting severe?
1. 2+ deep tendon reflexes.
2. BP of 140/90 mm Hg.
3. 3+ urine protein on dipstick.
4. 2+ dependent edema.

44. A nurse is performing a postpartum assessment on a client who is gravida 2, para 1 and delivered 6 hours ago by vacuum extraction with a fourth-degree laceration. The nurse notes that the fundus is firm, 2 fingerbreadths above the level of the umbilicus, and displaced to the right. Which action should the nurse take next?
1. Assess the blood pressure for hypotension.
2. Check the client for bladder distention.
3. Determine whether an oxytocic drug was given.
4. Massage the fundus to expel small clots.

45. A client, who is 27 years old, gravida 1, para 0, presents to a labor and delivery unit in active labor at 38 weeks' gestation. During the initial vaginal examination, a nurse notes a papular lesion on her left labia minora. Which action should the nurse take *first?*
1. Document the finding.
2. Continue routine labor care as ordered by the physician.
3. Prepare the client for a cesarean section.
4. Report the finding to the physician.

46. A client, who is 27 years old, presents to the gynecology clinic for her yearly screening examination. She is diagnosed with human papillomavirus (HPV). A nurse should recognize that this client is at increased risk for developing which illness?
1. Hodgkin's lymphoma.
2. Cervical cancer.

3. Multiple myeloma.
4. Ovarian cancer.

47. During an initial interview, a client reports that she has a lesion on the perineum. Further investigation reveals a small blister on the vulva that is painful to touch. A nurse understands that the most likely source of the lesion is:
1. Syphilis.
2. Condylomata.
3. Gonorrhea.
4. Herpes.

48. A client, who is gravida 3, para 2, has elected to have epidural anesthesia to relieve labor pain. About 5 minutes after the epidural is placed, a nurse notes the following vital signs: blood pressure is 80/30 mm Hg, pulse is 80, respiration 18, and temperature 99.0°F. Which nursing intervention is most appropriate?
1. Place the client in Trendelenburg position.
2. Decrease the rate of IV infusion.
3. Administer oxygen per nasal cannula.
4. Increase the rate of the IV infusion.

49. A client, who is gravida 3, para 1 at 37 weeks' gestation, is dilated to 5 cm, 100% effaced, and at a –2 station. A physician performs an amniotomy to augment the progress of labor. After an amniotomy, which should a nurse assess *first?*
1. Degree of cervical dilation.
2. Fetal heart tones.
3. Client's vital signs.
4. Client's level of discomfort.

50. A 34-year-old client, who is gravida 1, para 0, comes in for a routine prenatal visit. A physician orders a routine prenatal blood panel. The client asks a nurse why her physician has recommended a multiple marker screen. The nurse should explain that the physician has recommended the test:
1. To screen for spinal cord defects.
2. To screen for cardiovascular defects.
3. To comply with state law.
4. To screen for age-related conditions.

51. An 18-year-old client, who is gravida 4, para 0, has been treated for sickle cell anemia since age 5. She is admitted to labor and delivery at 37 weeks' gestation in the latent phase of labor with spontaneous rupture of membranes. Which client need should a nurse anticipate?
1. Fluid restriction.
2. Supplemental oxygen.
3. Blood transfusion.
4. Delivery by cesarean section.

52. A 34-year-old client, who is gravida 4, para 2, has gestational diabetes that is controlled by diet. At 38 weeks' gestation, a physician orders an ultrasound for estimated fetal weight and amniotic fluid index. To prepare for the ultrasound, a nurse instructs the client to:
1. Increase fluid intake.
2. Withhold food for 8 hours.
3. Administer an enema.
4. Limit ambulation.

53. A 22-year-old client with a history of perinatal substance abuse is scheduled for biweekly nonstress tests. The client asks why she has to come twice a week for nonstress tests. A nurse knows that teaching has been successful when the client states:
1. "The test is to tell if my baby's lungs are mature."
2. "The test is to measure the well-being of the baby."
3. "The test measures the number of baby's kicks."
4. "The test shows the effect of contractions on the baby's heart rate."

54. During surgery, a client received spinal anesthesia 4 hours ago. The client reports severe incisional pain. BP is 90/70 mm Hg, P is 108, T is 99°F (37.2°C), and R is 30. The skin is pale. The dressing is dry and intact. The most appropriate nursing intervention is to:
1. Call the physician and report the findings.
2. Medicate the client for pain, as ordered.
3. Reposition the client.
4. Open the IV to run at a rapid rate.

55. Following insertion of a pacemaker, a nurse should instruct a client to avoid:
1. Cellular phones.
2. Contact sports.
3. Cordless phones.
4. Microwave ovens.

56. The most common cause of an increase in a hemoglobin (Hgb) value is:
1. Dehydration.
2. Infection.
3. Malnutrition.
4. Antibiotic use.

57. Which client should the nurse assess *first* following report?
1. A client with a BUN of 28 mg/dL, creatinine of 1.1 mg/dL.
2. A client with a total calcium level of 9.2 mg/dL.
3. A client with a prothrombin time of 36 seconds.
4. A client with a Hgb of 15 gm/dL.

58. Following colostomy-reversal surgery, a client refuses to wear the prescribed antiembolic stockings. A prophylactic heparin dose was not given because the order was unclear. Admission BP was 130/80 mm Hg; pulse 106. Morphine was given for pain. The next morning the BP is 88/60 mm Hg and the pulse is 140. Pain level is 5/10. The correct action by a nurse would be:
1. Check pulse oximetry and breath sounds.
2. Give morphine as prescribed for pain.
3. Check for a positive Homans' sign.
4. Notify the physician of the BP changes.

59. Client assessment for pain should include a general history, clinical examination, and a pain history. A nurse knows that the most reliable indication of pain severity is:
1. Responsiveness to ordered drugs.
2. Client's self-report.
3. Duration of the pain.
4. Presence of facial grimaces.

60. Which change in a vital sign should a nurse note that is specific to neurogenic shock in a client who has a spinal cord injury?
1. Bradycardia.
2. Hypotension.
3. Tachycardia
4. Hyperthermia.

61. A nurse should instruct a client with edema from venous stasis to avoid:
Select all that apply.
1. Crossing the legs while sitting.
2. Keeping the legs in a dependent position.
3. Elevating the legs whenever possible.
4. Taking frequent hot baths.
5. Wearing support hose when sleeping.
6. Walking every day.

62. A client's laboratory results reveal: Hct 52, K^+ 5.0, BUN 35, creatinine 1.1. Vital signs are: BP 102/60 mm Hg, P 124, R 20, T 38.7°C, and O_2 Sat 96%. A possible explanation of these findings would be:
1. Volume overload following rehydration.
2. Dehydration from an elevated temperature.
3. Development of renal failure.
4. Worsening hypoxemia.

63. A client who has had a stroke begins to exhibit symptoms of syndrome of inappropriate antidiuretic hormone (SIADH). Which laboratory findings should be expected with SIADH? *Select all that apply.*
1. Increased urine sodium.
2. Increased urine concentration.
3. Decreased serum sodium.
4. Decreased serum osmolarity.
5. Decreased urine sodium.

64. A nursing student asks an RN for an example of an arterial blood gas result that demonstrates compensation for acidosis has occurred. The correct pH example would be:
1. pH = 7.36; $Paco_2$ = 33; HCO_3 = 20.
2. pH = 7.30; $Paco_2$ = 60; HCO_3 = 28.
3. pH = 7.46; $Paco_2$ = 34; HCO_3 = 22.
4. pH = 7.44; $Paco_2$ = 48; HCO_3 = 30.

65. A nurse is caring for a client who had a recent myocardial infarction (MI). During the cardiac assessment, a new murmur is noted. What question should the nurse ask the client *first?*
1. "Are you currently having chest pain?"
2. "Did you recently walk to the bathroom?"
3. "Have you ever been told you had a murmur?"
4. "Do you feel short of breath?"

66. A client who has diabetes is admitted to a hospital with a blood glucose of over 500, and states that the diabetic diet and exercise plan has been followed faithfully. The result of the $HgbA_{1c}$ is 10. The best interpretation by a nurse would be:
1. This is normal, nothing to worry about.
2. This is just slightly above normal for a person who is nondiabetic.
3. This is below normal.
4. This is very high and the client needs to be honest with the medical team.

67. When evaluating the laboratory results of a client who is diabetic, which test should a nurse review for the best indication of compliance with the diabetic regimen?
1. Urine dipstick for sugar and acetone.
2. Finger stick blood glucose.
3. Random blood glucose.
4. Hemoglobin A_{1c}.

68. A large, red area is noted over a client's right greater trochanter. To differentiate between simple redness and a Stage I decubitus ulcer, a nurse should:
1. Note if the redness lasts longer than 30 minutes.
2. Press on the intact skin to see if it blanches.
3. Look for areas of blistering.
4. Check for subcutaneous tissue breakdown.

69. A nurse prepares to suction the tracheostomy tube of a 15-month-old child. What steps should the nurse take in completing this procedure? *Select all that apply.*
1. Select vacuum pressure between 60 and 100 mm Hg.
2. Suction for 10 seconds.
3. Insert suction catheter so that the tip passes beyond the carina.
4. Wash hands.
5. Hyperventilate the child with 100% oxygen via resuscitation bag.
6. Remove sterile 8- or 10-French suction catheter from package.

70. A nurse prepares to obtain a blood sample from a preschooler who is hospitalized. Which steps should the nurse take to complete this procedure? *Select all that apply.*
1. Tell the child what will happen in simple terms.
2. Use a 25- or 27-gauge needle.
3. Have parents gently restrain child if necessary.
4. Keep venipuncture equipment hidden from view prior to the procedure.
5. Obtain the specimen from the child's dominant side, if possible.
6. Allow the child to be distracted in the playroom during the procedure.

71. A camp nurse is reviewing the intake forms of the school-age children in attendance. Which children should the nurse recognize as having an increased risk for infection? *Select all that apply.*

1. Child with a seizure disorder.
2. Child with sickle cell anemia.
3. Child with type 1 diabetes.
4. Child with juvenile idiopathic arthritis.
5. Child with food allergies.
6. Child with a history of cleft lip and palate.

72. A nurse is performing discharge teaching with the parents of a newborn diagnosed with Down syndrome. Which statements by the parents should indicate to the nurse that teaching has been effective? *Select all that apply.*

1. "We are having a big welcome home party for the baby tomorrow."
2. "We should pay close attention to any cold-like symptoms."
3. "Our child will reach developmental milestones about 2 years after peers."
4. "An appointment with an audiologist is important."
5. "We will keep the baby's head elevated after feedings."

73. A child is seen in an emergency department for possible leukemia. Which laboratory values should a nurse expect to be abnormal? *Select all that apply.*

1. WBC.
2. BUN.
3. RBC.
4. PLT.
5. Na.
6. Hgb.

Answers/Rationales/Tips

1. CORRECT ANSWER: 3. Answer 1 is incorrect because setting the O_2 level above 2 to 3 L will *diminish* the stimulus to breathe. **Answer 2** is incorrect because the stimulus to breathe in a client with COPD is the *low* Po_2. **Answer 3 is correct because the client with emphysema (COPD) will stop breathing if O_2 is set too high. Answer 4** is incorrect because the stimulus to breathe in the client with COPD is *not* CO_2 but a *low* Po_2.

■ **TEST-TAKING TIP:** *The stimulus to breathe in the client with emphysema is a* low O_2; *raising the* Po_2 *will* depress *the respiratory drive.*

Content Area: Geriatrics, Respiratory; ***Integrated Process:*** Nursing Process, Analysis; ***Cognitive Level:*** Application; ***Client Need/Subneed:*** Safe and Effective Care Environment/ Safety and Infection Control/Safe Use of Equipment

2. CORRECT ANSWER: 3. Answer 1 is incorrect because the *level* of wall suction *does not* affect the water seal. This pressure enhances drainage. **Answer 2** is incorrect because closed chest drainage should *always remain below* the level of the heart. **Answer 3 is correct because this will change the intrapleural pressure and reestablish suctioning. Answer 4** is incorrect because stripping a chest tube may *cause trauma* to the lung.

■ **TEST-TAKING TIP:** *Remember that the water seal fluctuates with changes in the intrathoracic pressure from breathing.*

Content Area: Adult Health, Respiratory; ***Integrated Process:*** Nursing Process, Implementation; ***Cognitive Level:*** Application; ***Client Need/Subneed:*** Physiological Integrity/Reduction of Risk Potential/Potential for Complications of Diagnostic Tests/Treatments/Procedures

3. CORRECT ANSWERS: 1, 2, 4, 5, 6. Answer 1 is correct because positioning the ties on the side of the neck makes it easier and safer to change. Answer 2 is correct because secretions will accumulate on the cannula and need daily cleaning. Answer 3 is incorrect because the cuff should have already been inflated to stabilize the tracheostomy tube. **Answer 4 is correct because these solutions are effective in removing the remaining secretions, and reduce the risk of infection. Answer 5 is correct because accumulated secretions interfere with gas exchange. Answer 6 is correct because the inability to make credible speech sounds may be frustrating to the client and increase anxiety. If possible, it is best to establish an alternate means (flash cards, dry erase board) before the tracheostomy.**

■ **TEST-TAKING TIP:** *Use a true-or-false approach to each option. Consider options that are safe and effective care.*

Content Area: Adult Health, Respiratory; ***Integrated Process:*** Nursing Process, Implementation; ***Cognitive Level:*** Analysis; ***Client Need/Subneed:*** Physiological Integrity/Reduction of Risk Potential/Therapeutic Procedures

4. CORRECT ANSWERS: 2, 4, 5, 6. Answer 1 is incorrect because this position will not put pressure on the biopsy site, which is needed to prevent bleeding. **Answer 2 is correct because right-side positioning exerts pressure on the liver and reduces the chance for bleeding. Answer 3** is incorrect because the risk following a biopsy is bleeding. **Answer 4 is correct because there is a risk of bleeding and a change in vital signs would alert the nurse to bleeding. Answer 5 is correct because the pillow adds direct pressure to the biopsy side and increases comfort. Answer 6 is correct because lifting or straining may lead to bleeding.**

■ **TEST-TAKING TIP:** *With any biopsy, think about preventing bleeding and observing for signs of bleeding.*

Content Area: Adult Health, Gastrointestinal; ***Integrated Process:*** Nursing Process, Implementation; ***Cognitive Level:*** Application; ***Client Need/Subneed:*** Physiological Integrity/ Reduction of Risk Potential/Potential for Complications of Diagnostic Tests/Treatments/Procedures

5. CORRECT ANSWERS: 1, 3, 5. Answer 1 is correct because a local anesthetic will be used to minimize pain to the puncture site. **Answer 2** is incorrect because the reason for the thoracentesis is fluid in the pleural space, *not* in the *lung*. Answer 3 is correct because this position drops the diaphragm and allows for easier access to the pleural space. **Answer 4** is incorrect because upright and leaning forward is the optimal position. Answer 5 is correct because the client needs to have been informed of the risks before the procedure is started. **Answer 6** is incorrect because there is some discomfort, although use of the local anesthetic reduces the pain.

■ TEST-TAKING TIP: *Think client safety before, during, and after the procedure.*

Content Area: Adult Health, Respiratory; ***Integrated Process:*** Nursing Process, Implementation; ***Cognitive Level:*** Application; ***Client Need/Subneed:*** Physiological Integrity/Reduction of Risk Potential/Therapeutic Procedures

ANSWERS

6. CORRECT ANSWER: 2. **Answer 1** is incorrect because an alarm sounds whenever the client is disconnected or the pressure drops (as with suctioning). This alarm can be silenced. Answer 2 is correct because use of accessory muscles indicates the client has to work to breathe. **Answer 3** is incorrect because bronchovesicular breath sounds are *normal*. **Answer 4** is incorrect because water collects in the ventilator tube and requires periodic draining. Unless excessive in volume, or unless it pours into the client's endotracheal tube, it does *not* represent a client problem.

■ TEST-TAKING TIP: *Look for the option that describes a client in distress.*

Content Area: Adult Health, Respiratory; ***Integrated Process:*** Nursing Process, Analysis; ***Cognitive Level:*** Application; ***Client Need/Subneed:*** Physiological Integrity/Reduction of Risk Potential/Therapeutic Procedures

7. CORRECT ANSWER: 2. **Answer 1** is incorrect because NPO for 6 hours is sufficient to promote good visualization for the study. Answer 2 is correct because all procedures should be explained prior to being done on a client. **Answer 3** is incorrect because it is *not* necessary to clear out the lower gut in order to evaluate the gallbladder. **Answer 4** is incorrect because an ultrasound is *noninvasive,* and does *not* necessitate pain medications and sedation.

■ TEST-TAKING TIP: *Eliminate the three options that are* not necessary. *The best answer is appropriate for all diagnostic tests.*

Content Area: Adult Health, Gastrointestinal; ***Integrated Process:*** Nursing Process, Implementation; ***Cognitive Level:*** Comprehension; ***Client Need/Subneed:*** Physiological Integrity/Reduction of Risk Potential/Therapeutic Procedures

8. CORRECT ANSWER: 4. **Answer 1** is incorrect because the scope passes through the lumen of the upper GI tract. *Alteration* in bowel sounds would *not* be expected. **Answer 2** is incorrect because the throat may be sore from the tube as the anesthetic wears off. *Avoid* putting anything in the mouth *until* the gag reflex returns. **Answer 3** is incorrect because pain medications would have been given *during* the procedure, but *after* the procedure is completed, continued pain would *not* be *expected.* Answer 4 is correct because, to pass the scope down through the esophagus, the gag reflex is suppressed by spraying an anesthetic on the back of the throat. After the procedure, nothing should be taken orally until the gag reflex has returned.

■ TEST-TAKING TIP: *What is safest for the client?*

Content Area: Adult Health, Gastrointestinal; ***Integrated Process:*** Nursing Process, Implementation; ***Cognitive Level:*** Application; ***Client Need/Subneed:*** Physiological Integrity/Reduction of Risk Potential/Diagnostic Tests

9. CORRECT ANSWER: 3. **Answer 1** is incorrect because generally no more than *one* overnight stay is required. **Answer 2** is incorrect because dye will be *injected during* the procedure, but is *not* taken *orally beforehand.* A client will be NPO. Answer 3 is correct because a sedative is given for this procedure, which does not require general anesthesia. ERCP permits direct visualization of structures and requires multiple position changes. **Answer 4** is incorrect because this procedure generally takes about *1 hour.*

■ TEST-TAKING TIP: *Eliminate the three options that involve specific* time *frames (i.e., 2 to 3 days, 30 minutes, 5 to 10 minutes). Select the one option that is different.*

Content Area: Adult Health, Gastrointestinal; ***Integrated Process:*** Nursing Process, Planning; ***Cognitive Level:*** Application; ***Client Need/Subneed:*** Physiological Integrity/Reduction of Risk Potential/Diagnostic Tests

10. CORRECT ANSWER: 4. **Answer 1** is incorrect because an oral airway can be removed when the client is awake enough to prevent tongue obstruction of the airway. A client should *remain* in PACU until it is determined that the client is stable and not at risk of having to return to the operating room. **Answer 2** is incorrect because pain control is *not* a criterion for discharge from the PACU to the floor. Medical-surgical nurses can manage pain on the floor. **Answer 3** is incorrect because moving both legs is a sign that spinal anesthesia has worn off. This client will have had *general* anesthesia for a laparoscopic cholecystectomy. Answer 4 is correct because, in the PACU, the client recovers from anesthesia. This surgery will have been done using general anesthesia, so the client should be awake. Vital signs are typically measured every 15 minutes, so after about an hour, stability can be determined and the client discharged to an area with less frequent monitoring.

■ TEST-TAKING TIP: *Safety of the client is most important. A client should not be returned to the floor until stable.*

Content Area: Adult Health, Gastrointestinal; ***Integrated Process:*** Nursing Process, Analysis; ***Cognitive Level:*** Application;

Client Need/Subneed: Physiological Integrity/Reduction of Risk Potential/Diagnostic Tests

11. CORRECT ANSWER: 1. Answer 1 is correct because, while it is important to keep the skin clean, soaking in a tub can soften the skin closure and allow microbes to enter the wound. It is better to suggest that the client take a *shower* rather than a bath. **Answer 2** is incorrect because, unless there have been complications, the client will have four small closed wounds, and will *not* need wet-to-dry dressing changes. **Answer 3** is incorrect because, unless there were complications, the client will have four small closed wounds and will *not* have a *drainage tube.* **Answer 4** is incorrect because *mobility* is very important for the client in the postoperative period to prevent risks such as blood clots and infections.

■ TEST-TAKING TIP: *Look for the option that is different than the other choices. Only one is consistent with the advantages of the laparoscopic approach—four less than 1/2-inch incisions that didn't need wet-to-dry dressings or a drainage tube or 3 days of bedrest.*

Content Area: Adult Health, Gastrointestinal; *Integrated Process:* Teaching and Learning; *Cognitive Level:* Application; *Client Need/Subneed:* Health Promotion and Maintenance/ Self-care

12. CORRECT ANSWER: 1. Answer 1 is correct because chest physiotherapy includes postural drainage and chest percussion and vibration. A full stomach would interfere with the effectiveness of the treatment, and vomiting and aspiration could occur. **Answer 2** is incorrect because a full stomach would *interfere* with the effectiveness of the treatment, and vomiting and aspiration could occur. **Answer 3** is incorrect because chest physiotherapy would normally be a *daily* (once a day) treatment. **Answer 4** is incorrect because there is *no* expectation of pain with cystic fibrosis.

■ TEST-TAKING TIP: *Eliminate the two answers with "after" and "every 4 hours." Select the answer with the word "before," for a time that would be most effective and not contribute to vomiting.*

Content Area: Adult Health, Respiratory; *Integrated Process:* Nursing Process, Planning; *Cognitive Level:* Application; *Client Need/Subneed:* Physiological Integrity/Reduction of Risk Potential/Therapeutic Procedures

13. CORRECT ANSWER: 3. **Answer 1** is incorrect because the client receives moderate IV sedation (e.g., conscious sedation), *not* general anesthesia. **Answer 2** is incorrect because digoxin is usually *held* for 48 hours before cardioversion to ensure resumption of a normal sinus rhythm. Answer 3 is correct because the client will receive moderate IV sedation as well as an analgesic medication before the procedure. **Answer 4** is incorrect because the length of time after the procedure will *depend* on how rapidly the client recovers from the sedation and analgesia used, as well as the success of the cardioversion.

■ TEST-TAKING TIP: *Eliminate the option that would vary with the client's preprocedure drug therapy (Answer 2) and postprocedure hospitalization (Answer 4). Eliminate the inappropriate anesthesia for this procedure (Answer 1).*

Content Area: Adult Health, Cardiology; *Integrated Process:* Teaching and Learning; *Cognitive Level:* Application; *Client Need/Subneed:* Physiological Integrity/Reduction of Risk Potential/Therapeutic Procedures

14. CORRECT ANSWERS: 3, 4, 5. **Answer 1** is incorrect because an allergy to eggs will *not* increase the risk to the client from the dye used in the test. **Answer 2** is incorrect because organ meats do *not* contain iodine, which is the allergic concern for the client receiving the dye during the test. Answer 3 is correct because clams are a shellfish and an allergy to shellfish would increase the risk that the client would have an allergic reaction to the dye used during the test. Answer 4 is correct because shrimp are a shellfish and an allergy to shrimp would increase the likelihood that the client would have an allergic reaction to the dye used during the test. Answer 5 is correct because crab is a shellfish and an allergy to shellfish would increase the risk that the client would have an allergic reaction to the dye used during the test. **Answer 6** is incorrect because the risk to the client is the iodine that is found in the dye used in the test. A latex allergy would be important to know; however, the question relates to a risk associated with the *test.*

■ TEST-TAKING TIP: *Think "shellfish" as the possible sources of iodine, which is the* allergic *concern.*

Content Area: Adult Health, Gastrointestinal; *Integrated Process:* Nursing Process, Assessment; *Cognitive Level:* Analysis; *Client Need/Subneed:* Physiological Integrity/Reduction of Risk Potential/Therapeutic Procedures

15. CORRECT ANSWER: 3. **Answer 1** is incorrect because there would be *no drainage* if the tube were kinked. **Answer 2** is incorrect because the dressing should be *left in place,* unless advised by the surgeon to change the dressing. Answer 3 is correct because a T-tube is used when there has been exploration of the common bile duct, which results in swelling. The tube prevents blockage to the flow of bile, and patency of the tube is important to the client's recovery. **Answer 4** is incorrect because the priority and most important nursing action is to ensure that the tube is draining properly.

■ TEST-TAKING TIP: *This question has more than one correct answer. Look for an option that may impact others. A tube that isn't draining (Answer 3) will affect the quantity of drainage (Answer 1), the dryness of the dressing (Answer 2), and the purpose of the tube (Answer 4).*

Content Area: Adult Health, Gastrointestinal; *Integrated Process:* Nursing Process, Implementation; *Cognitive Level:* Analysis; *Client Need/Subneed:* Physiological Integrity/ Reduction of Risk Potential/Therapeutic Procedures

16. CORRECT ANSWER: 1. **Answer 1 is correct because right shoulder pain is normal following the laparoscopy. The client should know this before the procedure is done. A heating pad applied for 15 to 20 minutes every hour helps.** Answer 2 is incorrect because the pain is due to migration of *carbon dioxide,* not bile. Answer 3 is incorrect because the client is *supine* during the procedure, not right side-lying. Answer 4 is incorrect because a laparoscopic cholecystectomy would *not* have been done if exploration of the common bile duct were necessary or a stone were present.

■ TEST-TAKING TIP: *Focus on the two answers (Answers 1 and 3) that state "during the procedure," then eliminate Answer 3 because the position is incorrect.*

Content Area: Adult Health, Gastrointestinal; *Integrated Process:* Teaching and Learning; *Cognitive Level:* Application; *Client Need/Subneed:* Physiological Integrity/Reduction of Risk Potential/Therapeutic Procedures

17. CORRECT ANSWER: 2. Answer 1 is incorrect because the hypertonic solution is *not* associated with allergic reactions. **Answer 2 is correct because 2 to 3 L of fluid is infused into the peritoneum and the fluid may be pressing on the diaphragm.** Answer 3 is incorrect because capillary refill would indicate oxygenation and hypovolemia. Peritoneal dialysis removes fluid more slowly, and sudden volume changes are *unlikely.* Answer 4 is incorrect because peritoneal dialysis takes 36 to 48 hours to correct an electrolyte imbalance.

■ TEST-TAKING TIP: *Think: breathing. Visualize where the fluid is located and potential complications from the pressure of the fluid.*

Content Area: Adult Health, Renal; *Integrated Process:* Nursing Process, Assessment; *Cognitive Level:* Application; *Client Need/Subneed:* Physiological Integrity/Reduction of Risk Potential/Therapeutic Procedures

18. CORRECT ANSWER: 2. Answer 1 is incorrect because the goal of therapy with radioactive iodine is to *destroy* thyroid tissue, not limit absorption. **Answer 2 is correct because the radioactive iodine destroys the overactive thyroid tissue that is causing hyperthyroidism and produces a hypothyroid state.** Answer 3 is incorrect because radioactive iodine *destroys* the thyroid tissue, reducing the amount of circulating thyroid hormone. Answer 4 is incorrect because the action of radioactive iodine is to *destroy* the thyroid tissue. Correcting hyperthyroidism will minimize the cardiac effects that may lead to CHF if there has been no permanent myocardial damage.

■ TEST-TAKING TIP: *Consider which option would stop the problem—destroy the cause.*

Content Area: Adult Health, Endocrine; *Integrated Process:* Nursing Process, Planning; *Cognitive Level:* Comprehension; *Client Need/Subneed:* Physiological Integrity/Reduction of Risk Potential/Therapeutic Procedures

19. CORRECT ANSWER: 1. **Answer 1 is correct because the dose is so low that there is little chance of exposure to others. Avoiding contact with pregnant women and young children, or close contact, such as kissing or dancing cheek to cheek, is often advised for 2 to 3 days after treatment.** Answer 2 is incorrect because there are *no special disposal precautions* needed. Flushing the toilet two to three times after each use for 2 to 3 days is sufficient. Answer 3 is incorrect because the dose is so low that there is *little chance* of exposure to others. A client can return to work the next day after treatment. Answer 4 is incorrect because exposure to others is *not a risk.* However, physicians may recommend avoiding close contact for *2 to 3 days* after treatment.

■ TEST-TAKING TIP: *Choose the option that is different from the others. Only one says there is really nothing to worry about.*

Content Area: Adult Health, Endocrine; *Integrated Process:* Nursing Process, Implementation; *Cognitive Level:* Application; *Client Need/Subneed:* Physiological Integrity/Reduction of Risk Potential/Potential for Complications of Diagnostic Tests/Treatments/Procedures

20. CORRECT ANSWER: 4. Answer 1 is incorrect because the ascites would pull protein from the vascular system, and fluid will move from the vascular system into the peritoneal space. Answer 2 is incorrect because there is a decrease in circulating volume, and the work of the heart will *decrease.* Answer 3 is incorrect because with liver failure there is portal hypertension, but *not* systemic hypertension. **Answer 4 is correct because the purpose of the shunt is to reduce portal hypertension. TIPS is a procedure in which a stent carries blood from the portal vein to the hepatic vein. Consequently, toxic substances reach the brain without being detoxified by the liver.**

■ TEST-TAKING TIP: *Choose the option that is* different *from the others. Three of the choices would be complications of* cardiac *dysfunction.*

Content Area: Adult Health, Gastrointestinal; *Integrated Process:* Nursing Process, Analysis; *Cognitive Level:* Analysis; *Client Need/Subneed:* Physiological Integrity/Reduction of Risk Potential/Potential for Complications of Diagnostic Tests/Treatments/Procedures

21. CORRECT ANSWER: 3. Answer 1 is incorrect because contact isolation is used to prevent transmission of infections, not reduce an allergic response. Answer 2 is incorrect because, unless there is latex on the hands, washing them will *not* reduce the client's allergic response. **Answer 3 is correct because these products avoid exposing a client to something to which he or she is allergic.** Answer 4 is incorrect because sensitization helps with *some* allergies, but repeated exposure to latex has made the allergic response *worse.*

■ TEST-TAKING TIP: *Look for an option that* replaces *a latex product. Latex is found in many products. The best action in the case of allergies is to minimize contact or exposure.*

Content Area: Adult Health, Integumentary; *Integrated Process:* Nursing Process, Implementation; *Cognitive Level:* Application; *Client Need/Subneed:* Physiological Integrity/Reduction of Risk Potential/Potential for Alterations in Body Systems

22. CORRECT ANSWER: 3. **Answer 1** is incorrect because there may have been little drainage if the chest drainage system was removing *air, not blood.* There should be minimal drainage before removal also. **Answer 2** is incorrect because a pneumothorax is a collapse of the *lung,* partial or complete, not a collapse of alveoli. **Answer 3 is correct because the cessation of fluctuation in the water-seal chamber when the chest drainage system is no longer attached to suction is an indication of re-expansion. A chest x-ray would also be indicated. Answer 4** is incorrect because presence of breath sounds would need to be in *all* lobes, and particularly in the area of lung collapse.
■ TEST-TAKING TIP: *Remember the water seal allows air and fluid to escape from the lung. As the client breathes in, the fluid level rises. If that action has stopped, the system may no longer be needed.*
Content Area: Adult Health, Respiratory; ***Integrated Process:*** Nursing Process, Analysis; ***Cognitive Level:*** Analysis; ***Client Need/Subneed:*** Physiological Integrity/Reduction of Risk Potential/Therapeutic Procedures

23. CORRECT ANSWER: 2. **Answer 1** is incorrect because irrigation will *wash away* any organisms that might be present. **Answer 2 is correct because rolling the swab from the center of the wound to the outside of the wound is the correct technique. Organisms that have colonized the wound directly will be collected by this technique. Answer 3** is incorrect because there may be organisms on the outside of the wound that have *not affected* the wound. **Answer 4** is incorrect because a swab from the dressing does *not* reflect what is *actually* present in the wound.
■ TEST-TAKING TIP: *Visualize each option and select the one that will collect only organisms in the wound for the culture specimen.*
Content Area: Adult Health, Integumentary; ***Integrated Process:*** Nursing Process, Evaluation; ***Cognitive Level:*** Analysis; ***Client Need/Subneed:*** Physiological Integrity/Reduction of Risk Potential/Diagnostic Tests

24. CORRECT ANSWER: 3. **Answer 1** is incorrect because the antiseptic that will be used needs to air-dry *before* insertion. **Answer 2** is incorrect because the antiseptic used to clean the site should *air-dry.* **Answer 3 is correct because the site needs to air-dry totally before catheter insertion. Answer 4** is incorrect because the catheter should not be inserted *until* the antiseptic has air-dried totally, not within a specific time frame.
■ TEST-TAKING TIP: *Focus on the three options with time frames: "immediately" (Answer 1), "after" (Answer 3), and "later" (Answer 4). Review aseptic techniques and select "after."*
Content Area: Adult Health, Cardiovascular; ***Integrated Process:*** Nursing Process, Evaluation; ***Cognitive Level:*** Application; ***Client Need/Subneed:*** Physiological Integrity/Reduction of Risk Potential/Therapeutic Procedures

25. CORRECT ANSWERS: 1, 2, 3, 4, 5. **Answer 1 is correct because hand hygiene (hand washing) is a very important barrier to transmission of microorganism. Answer 2 is correct because clothes could be a source of transmission from nurse to client. Answer 3 is correct because hair and nose/mouth could be a source of transmission. Answer 4 is correct because gloves protect both the nurse and client from microorganisms. Answer 5 is correct because draping protects the insertion site. Answer 6** is incorrect because prophylactic drug therapy is *not* a "barrier" precaution.
■ TEST-TAKING TIP: *Choose precautions that prevent transmission of a microorganism.*
Content Area: Adult Health, Cardiovascular; ***Integrated Process:*** Nursing Process, Planning; ***Cognitive Level:*** Application; ***Client Need/Subneed:*** Safe and Effective Care Environment/ Safety and Infection Control/Standard/Transmission-based/ Other Precautions

26. CORRECT ANSWERS: 2. **Answer 1** is incorrect because the collection container *may or may not* need to be kept cold, so saying it *must* is not accurate. **Answer 2 is correct because the 24-hour collection period begins after the client voids and discards the urine. The test measures glomerular filtration of substances such as protein, creatinine, electrolytes, and urinary steroids, which are excreted at different rates, anounts, and times of day. Starting the time after the client voids and discards the urine gives a true picture of filtration during the 24 hours. Answer 3** is incorrect because measuring the urine each time the client voids is usually *not* required. The test measures results for 24 hours, not more frequently. **Answer 4** is incorrect because the test measures *filtration* of substances. There is no need to increase oral intake but rather maintain a healthy intake of fluids (e.g., 8 glasses daily).
■ TEST-TAKING TIP: *Choose the option that perpares the client to* start *the test.*
Content Area: Adult Health, Renal; ***Integrated Process:*** Nursing Process, Evaluation; ***Cognitive Level:*** Application; ***Client Need/Subneed:*** Physiological Integrity/Reduction of Risk Potential/Diagnostic Tests

27. CORRECT ANSWER: 3. **Answer 1** is incorrect because negative pressure on the external chest does not require intubation and will *not keep* the airway open during sleep, which is needed. **Answer 2** is incorrect because this type of ventilator controls inspiration, *not expiration,* which is the problem. **Answer 3 is correct because CPAP is used to prevent airway collapse associated with obstruction during sleep. Answer 4** is incorrect because this is a *ventilator* mode that provides a *combination* of mechanical and spontaneous breaths.
■ TEST-TAKING TIP: *Three of the options are artificial ventilation systems. The problem is with the airway.*
Content Area: Adult Health, Respiratory; ***Integrated Process:*** Teaching and Learning; ***Cognitive Level:*** Application; ***Client Need/Subneed:*** Physiological Integrity/Reduction of Risk Potential/Therapeutic Procedures

28. CORRECT ANSWER: 1. Answer 1 is correct because the device is best applied after surgery and may be used for up to 6 weeks as prescribed. **Answer 2** is incorrect because the device is used *most* of the time when in bed. **Answer 3** is incorrect because this amount of flexion and extension are prescribed initially, progressing to *90* degrees of flexion with full extension, which is 0 degrees. **Answer 4** is incorrect because the client *will* be assisted out of bed the evening of or day after surgery with a knee immobilizer, and *prescribed* weight-bearing.

■ **TEST-TAKING TIP:** *Note the same word "continuously" in the* correct *answer and the name of the device, "continuous passive motion."*

Content Area: Adult Health, Musculoskeletal; ***Integrated Process:*** Teaching and Learning; ***Cognitive Level:*** Application; ***Client Need/Subneed:*** Physiological Integrity/Reduction of Risk Potential/Therapeutic Procedures

29. CORRECT ANSWER: 4. **Answer 1** is incorrect because the nurse *cannot* stop the irrigation without an order. **Answer 2** is incorrect because the nurse does *not* have the authority to add an anesthetic. The pain is likely from spasms, which are treated with belladonna or opiate suppositories. **Answer 3** is incorrect because the response does *not* address the spouse's concern. Answer 4 is correct because the purpose of the irrigant is to prevent clots. A pale pink would indicate that bleeding is diminishing.

■ **TEST-TAKING TIP:** *Choose the answer that gives information to reduce anxiety.*

Content Area: Adult Health, Genitourinary; ***Integrated Process:*** Communication and Documentation; ***Cognitive Level:*** Application; ***Client Need/Subneed:*** Physiological Integrity/ Reduction of Risk Potential/Potential for Complications of Diagnostic Tests/Treatments/Procedures

30. CORRECT ANSWERS: 3, 5, 6. **Answer 1** is incorrect because kidney function would affect acid-base balance, but the technique for drawing the sample affects the accuracy of the results or values. **Answer 2** is incorrect because confusion does *not affect* the accuracy of the sample. Answer 3 is correct because blood gases should be drawn at *least 20* minutes after suctioning because suctioning removes oxygen. **Answer 4** is incorrect because there *should not* be an air bubble in the sample. A bubble would affect the accuracy. Answer 5 is correct because the blood gas sample should be placed on *ice* and returned to the laboratory as *quickly* as possible. Answer 6 is correct because blood from a PICC line is *venous* blood, not arterial.

■ **TEST-TAKING TIP:** *Look for the options that describe possible errors in collection or handling of the* sample. *Note the word "sample" in the three correct answers.*

Content Area: Adult Health, Hematological; ***Integrated Process:*** Nursing Process, Analysis; ***Cognitive Level:*** Application; ***Client Need/Subneed:*** Physiological Integrity/Reduction of Risk Potential/Laboratory Values

31. CORRECT ANSWER: 3. **Answer 1** is incorrect because chest trauma would likely result in respiratory *acidosis* (pH below 7.35 and CO_2 above 45), *not* alkalosis. **Answer 2** is incorrect because pneumonia would likely result in respiratory acidosis (pH below 7.35 and CO_2 above 45), *not* alkalosis. Answer 3 is correct because the *ABGs show respiratory alkalosis* (pH above 7. 45 and CO_2 below 35) and a problem with hypoxemia (O_2 Sat below 96%) from rapid respirations. The vital signs and symptoms are consistent with a pulmonary embolism, which interferes with exchange of O_2. Client hyperventilates, blowing off CO_2. **Answer 4** is incorrect because pulmonary edema would likely result in respiratory acidosis (pH below 7.35 and CO_2 above 45), *not* alkalosis.

■ **TEST-TAKING TIP:** *Eliminate those conditions that produce respiratory acidosis.*

Content Area: Adult Health, Respiratory; ***Integrated Process:*** Nursing Process, Analysis; ***Cognitive Level:*** Analysis; ***Client Need/Subneed:*** Physiological Integrity/Reduction of Risk Potential/Laboratory Values

32. CORRECT ANSWERS: 1, 4, 6. Answer 1 is correct because emptying the bladder before the procedure will reduce the risk of damage to the bladder when the needle is inserted into the peritoneal cavity to drain the fluid. **Answer 2** is incorrect because the client may experience *low* blood pressure and should be monitored for signs of hypovolemic shock during the procedure. This is due to the shift of fluid from the vascular space as the protein-rich ascitic fluid is removed. **Answer 3** is incorrect because the desired position is *sitting* on the *side* of the bed with *feet supported by a chair.* If large amounts of fluid are to be removed, the client might be flat. Answer 4 is correct because applying pressure to stop any bleeding following removal of the needle is important. The insertion site should be covered with a sterile dressing. **Answer 5** is incorrect because a paracentesis usually takes *20 to 30 minutes* and the physician is present during the procedure. The needle is *not* left in place for 24 hours. Answer 6 is correct because the amount and color of the ascitic fluid is documented and a specimen is sent to the laboratory for analysis before discarding the rest of the fluid.

■ **TEST-TAKING TIP:** *Use a true-and-false approach to choosing the correct answers. Visualize a needle in the abdomen and fluid draining out.*

Content Area: Adult Health, Gastrointestinal; ***Integrated Process:*** Nursing Process, Implementation; ***Cognitive Level:*** Application; ***Client Need/Subneed:*** Physiological Integrity/ Reduction of Risk Potential/Potential for Complications of Diagnostic Tests

33. CORRECT ANSWERS: 1, 3, 4. Answer 1 is correct because frequent oral hygiene prevents the pooling of oral secretions, which may lead to aspiration. **Answer 2** is incorrect because the head of the bed should be elevated to at least *30 to 45* degrees, unless contraindicated, to prevent gastric reflux, which can cause

VAP. Answer 3 is correct because washing hands before and after every contact with clients prevents cross-contamination of microorganisms. Answer 4 is correct because draining the condensation prevents the potential for aspiration of the collected fluid. **Answer 5** is incorrect because changing the ventilator tubing has *not* been shown to prevent VAP.

■ TEST-TAKING TIP: ***Think about basic care and the prevention of aspiration and infection.***

Content Area: Adult Health, Respiratory; ***Integrated Process:*** Nursing Process, Implementation; ***Cognitive Level:*** Analysis; ***Client Need/Subneed:*** Physiological Integrity/Reduction of Risk Potential/Potential for Complications of Diagnostic Tests/Treatments/Procedures

34. CORRECT ANSWERS: 2, 3, 4, 6. **Answer 1** is incorrect because IV hydration is known to *prevent* renal damage from the contrast medium that was used during the catheterization. Answer 2 is correct because the client is likely to have decreased renal function because of hypertension and diabetes. Aminoglycoside antibiotics are known to be nephrotoxic. Answer 3 is correct because the glomerular filtration rate decreases with advancing age and may be a contributing factor to the elevated creatinine level. Answer 4 is correct because the client has hypertension and diabetes, which increase the risk of impaired renal function as indicated by the elevated creatinine and blood urea nitrogen (BUN) levels. **Answer 5** is incorrect because angina is *not* contributing to the renal *dysfunction.* Answer 6 is correct because the contrast medium used during cardiac catheterization is nephrotoxic.

■ TEST-TAKING TIP: ***Select options that are*** contraindicated—***what would make the client worse?***

Content Area: Geriatric, Renal; ***Integrated Process:*** Nursing Process, Analysis; ***Cognitive Level:*** Analysis; ***Client Need/Subneed:*** Physiological Integrity/Reduction of Risk Potential/Laboratory Values

35. CORRECT ANSWERS: 2, 4, 5. **Answer 1** is incorrect because the drawing of venous blood samples (daily) would *not* be an appropriate use of an arterial line. A venous access should be established for the client. Answer 2 is correct because arterial blood gas sticks are *painful.* Using the arterial port would be appropriate for clients requiring frequent collection of samples. **Answer 3** is incorrect because arterial lines are not routinely used as an infusion port. A venous access should be established, and only if a venous port cannot be established would the arterial port be used. Arterial ports may be used in neonates/pediatrics or for the delivery of chemotherapy with specific tumors. Answer 4 is correct because a client who is receiving a vasoactive drug would need *continuous* monitoring of blood pressure, which is an appropriate use of an intra-arterial line. Answer 5 is correct because *continuous* monitoring of blood pressure is an appropriate use of an intra-arterial line.

■ TEST-TAKING TIP: ***Think of cardiovascular and respiratory conditions.***

Content Area: Adult Health, Cardiovascular; ***Integrated Process:*** Nursing Process, Analysis; ***Cognitive Level:*** Analysis; ***Client Need/Subneed:*** Physiological Integrity/Reduction of Risk Potential/Therapeutic Procedures

36. CORRECT ANSWER: 6. Using the GCS, this client receives 2 points for opening eyes to painful stimuli, 2 points for extensor posturing, and 2 points for incomprehensible sounds. Total score is 6 out of 15.

■ TEST-TAKING TIP: ***Normal response is 15 and no response is 3. The GCS is used to evaluate ability to open eyes, respond verbally, and move normally, primarily in clients with trauma or stroke.***

Content Area: Adult Health, Neurological; ***Integrated Process:*** Nursing Process, Assessment; ***Cognitive Level:*** Analysis; ***Client Need/Subneed:*** Physiological Integrity/Reduction of Risk Potential/Diagnostic Tests

37. CORRECT ANSWERS: 1, 3, 4. Answer 1 is correct because the presence of renal dysfunction should be known before a cardiac catheterization, which increases the risk of renal failure from the dye. The nurse needs to be sure whether the history includes possible renal dysfunction. **Answer 2** is incorrect because the client *would* be NPO prior to the procedure to prevent vomiting and possible aspiration. Answer 3 is correct because the history of a possible adverse response should be reviewed further. Answer 4 is correct because discharge will be determined by the client's status after the procedure and no bleeding at the catheter insertion site. **Answer 5** is incorrect because feeling warm *is* an expected response to the contrast media.

■ TEST-TAKING TIP: ***Select responses that indicate an ongoing or past problem.***

Content Area: Adult Health, Cardiovascular; ***Integrated Process:*** Nursing Process, Evaluation; ***Cognitive Level:*** Analysis; ***Client Need/Subneed:*** Physiological Integrity/Reduction of Risk Potential/Diagnostic Tests

38. CORRECT ANSWER: 1. Answer 1 is correct because high Fowler's and turned slightly on the operative side promotes ventilation in the remaining lung. **Answer 2** is incorrect because the supine positioning is incorrect, although the pillow under the right shoulder is appropriate. **Answer 3** is incorrect because supine does *not* facilitate ventilation of the remaining lung. The client can be positioned on the operative side with a pillow under the right shoulder. **Answer 4** is incorrect because this positioning will contribute to *mediastinal* shift to the operative side.

■ TEST-TAKING TIP: ***Visualize the surgery. The left lung is removed and the chest cavity on the left is empty. Only one lung remains. Next, eliminate the two options with "supine."***

Content Area: Adult Health, Respiratory; ***Integrated Process:*** Nursing Process, Implementation; ***Cognitive Level:*** Application; ***Client Need/Subneed:*** Physiological Integrity/Reduction of Risk Potential/Potential for Complications of Diagnostic Tests/Treatments/Procedures

39. CORRECT ANSWER: 1. **Answer 1 is correct because 2 minutes is usually long enough to stop the bleeding.** **Answer 2** is incorrect because a tourniquet is *not needed* when drawing blood from an artery. **Answer 3** is incorrect because *direct pressure* is needed with an artery. **Answer 4** is incorrect because a vascular closure device is used following cardiac catheterization, *not* blood gases.

■ **TEST-TAKING TIP:** ***Pressure is the usual way to stop bleeding. Eliminate the three options with measures that are not needed (tourniquet, ice, vascular closure).***

Content Area: Adult Health, Vascular; ***Integrated Process:*** Nursing Process, Implementation; ***Cognitive Level:*** Application; ***Client Need/Subneed:*** Physiological Integrity/Reduction of Risk Potential/Potential for Complications of Diagnostic Tests/Treatments/Procedures

40. CORRECT ANSWER: 3. **Answer 1** is incorrect because vital signs are important, but they are *not* the *first* assessment. **Answer 2** is incorrect because the procedure should *not interfere* with the normal bowel sounds. **Answer 3 is correct because there is a higher incidence of bleeding and hematoma formation in the groin, where the procedure was performed, due to high pressure in the femoral artery.** **Answer 4** is incorrect because respiratory status is important, but *not* the *first* assessment.

■ **TEST-TAKING TIP:** ***Think: ABCs as priority. There is no reason to suspect Airway or Breathing problems; therefore, the priority is Circulation (bleeding).***

Content Area: Adult Health, Vascular; ***Integrated Process:*** Nursing Process, Assessment; ***Cognitive Level:*** Application; ***Client Need/Subneed:*** Physiological Integrity/Reduction of Risk Potential/Potential for Complications of Diagnostic Tests/Treatments/Procedures

41. CORRECT ANSWER: 2. **Answer 1** is incorrect because, while it is important to observe for bleeding, the first concern in the immediate postoperative period is the development of respiratory problems. **Answer 2 is correct because the client's respiratory status needs to be monitored closely for the prolonged effects of general anesthesia used during major surgery.** **Answer 3** is incorrect because, while urinary output also needs to be monitored, the lingering effects of general anesthesia on the respiratory system are minimized with coughing and deep breathing in the early postoperative period. **Answer 4** is incorrect because, while this also needs to be monitored, respiratory status is *more imminently life-threatening.*

■ **TEST-TAKING TIP:** ***Use the "B" in the ABCs (airway, breathing, circulation) here when setting priorities for this client. The question asks for the*** **most important** ***assessment,*** **not the only** ***assessment . . . most life-threatening.***

Content Area: Adult Health, Musculoskeletal; ***Integrated Process:*** Nursing Process, Assessment; ***Cognitive Level:*** Analysis; ***Client Need/Subneed:*** Physiological Integrity/Reduction of Risk Potential/Potential for Complications from Surgical Procedures and Health Alterations

42. CORRECT ANSWER: 2. **Answer 1** is incorrect because α-fetoprotein (AFP) is drawn in the *second* trimester around *18 weeks'* gestation. Low AFP may indicate *Down* syndrome. **Answer 2 is correct because this client has a positive (+) antibody screen indicating antibodies are present. The antibodies formed by a mother can cause erythroblastosis fetalis. Blood and Rh typing and antibody screening can alert the physician to the possible development of this condition.** **Answer 3** is incorrect because the lecithin/sphingomyelin ratio is obtained from *amniotic fluid analysis* and indicates *fetal lung maturity.* This test is not performed in the first trimester of pregnancy. **Answer 4** is incorrect because the antibody screen is negative, indicating that the client has *not* developed antibodies that can cause erythroblastosis fetalis.

■ **TEST-TAKING TIP:** ***Remember: if a woman is Rh negative and antibody +, the fetus is at risk for developing Rh incompatibility and possibly erythroblastosis fetalis. Eliminate Answers 1 and 3 because they do not test for erythroblastosis fetalis.***

Content Area: Maternity, Antepartum; ***Integrated Process:*** Nursing Process, Analysis; ***Cognitive Level:*** Application; ***Client Need/Subneed:*** Physiological Integrity/Reduction of Risk Potential/Laboratory Values

43. CORRECT ANSWER: 3. **Answer 1** is incorrect because *normal* deep tendon reflexes *are* 2+. **Answer 2** is incorrect because a blood pressure reading of 140/90 mm Hg indicates *mild* preeclampsia. Severe preeclampsia is when *diastolic* blood pressures consistently *exceed* 110 mm Hg. **Answer 3 is correct because 3+ urine protein on dipstick is a symptom of severe preeclampsia and would indicate that the client's condition is worsening.** **Answer 4** is incorrect because *dependent* edema is a *normal* finding of pregnancy. Edema of the hands or face or pitting edema indicates a worsening of the disease.

■ **TEST-TAKING TIP:** ***The key to this question is remembering that the most important difference between mild and severe preeclampsia is the amount of*** **proteinuria.**

Content Area: Maternity, Antepartum; ***Integrated Process:*** Nursing Process, Assessment; ***Cognitive Level:*** Analysis; ***Client Need/Subneed:*** Physiological Integrity/Reduction of Risk Potential/System Specific Assessments

44. CORRECT ANSWER: 2. **Answer 1** is incorrect because hypotension is a *late* sign of postpartum hemorrhage. **Answer 2 is correct because the likely reason for the fundus to be higher than expected and deviated to the right is bladder distention. If the bladder is not emptied, a postpartum hemorrhage can occur.** **Answer 3** is incorrect because the likely reason for the fundus to be higher than expected and deviated to the right is *bladder distention.* Administration of oxytocic agents will *not* resolve her bladder distention. **Answer 4** is incorrect because massaging the fundus to expel small clots will *not resolve* her bladder distention.

■ **TEST-TAKING TIP:** ***The key to this question is that the fundus is deviated to the right. This finding is very common in bladder distention.***

Content Area: Maternity, Postpartum; *Integrated Process:* Nursing Process, Implementation; *Cognitive Level:* Analysis; *Client Need/Subneed:* Physiological Integrity/Reduction of Risk Potential/Potential for Complications from Surgical Procedures and Health Alterations

45. CORRECT ANSWER: 4. **Answer 1** is incorrect because documenting the finding is *not the first* action to take when a client with active herpes is in active labor and needs a cesarean section. **Answer 2** is incorrect because a papular lesion is consistent with genital herpes, and needs to be reported to the physician. **Answer 3** is incorrect because the physician needs to be informed and the lesion should be evaluated to determine if it is herpes before proceeding with any other procedure. Active genital herpes requires a cesarean delivery, but the physician needs to make a final decision. Preparing her for a cesarean before the physician evaluates the client is not appropriate. **Answer 4 is correct because a papular lesion is consistent with genital herpes and needs to be reported to the physician first before proceeding with any other assessment or treatment.**

■ TEST-TAKING TIP: *An unidentified lesion in the vaginal area should be reported to the physician as soon as possible to avoid possible transmission of herpes. Note that only one option has "report to the physician."*

Content Area: Maternity, Intrapartum; *Integrated Process:* Nursing Process, Implementation; *Cognitive Level:* Analysis; *Client Need/Subneed:* Safe and Effective Care Environment/Safety and Infection Control/Standard/Transmission-based/Other Precautions

46. CORRECT ANSWER: 2. **Answer 1** is incorrect because an increased risk of Hodgkin's lymphoma is associated with *Epstein-Barr virus* (EBV), *not* HPV. **Answer 2 is correct because HPV has been associated with an increased risk of developing cervical cancer.** **Answer 3** is incorrect because there are *no infections* that are associated with an increased risk of multiple myeloma. **Answer 4** is incorrect because HPV is *not associated* with an increased risk of ovarian cancer.

■ TEST-TAKING TIP: *Two of the options (Answers 1 and 3) are cancers having to do with the blood system. Since this question is talking about a gynecological condition (HPV), eliminate those two answers.*

Content Area: Adult Health, Genitourinary; *Integrated Process:* Nursing Process, Analysis; *Cognitive Level:* Application; *Client Need/Subneed:* Physiological Integrity/Reduction of Risk Potential/Potential for Complications from Surgical Procedures and Health Alterations

47. CORRECT ANSWER: 4. **Answer 1** is incorrect because syphilis infections have a chancre, a *painless* ulceration formed during the primary stage of syphilis. **Answer 2** is incorrect because condylomata are genital warts, *not* lesions. **Answer 3** is incorrect because, with gonorrhea infections, the initial symptoms in women include a *painful* or burning sensation when urinating or a yellowish vaginal discharge, *not* a lesion. **Answer 4 is correct because a small blister on the vulva that is painful to touch is consistent with herpes.**

■ TEST-TAKING TIP: *The only sexually transmitted infection that has a painful lesion is herpes.*

Content Area: Adult Health, Genitourinary; *Integrated Process:* Nursing Process, Analysis; *Cognitive Level:* Comprehension; *Client Need/Subneed:* Safe and Effective Care Environment/Safety and Infection Control/Standard/Transmission-based/Other Precautions

48. CORRECT ANSWER: 4. **Answer 1** is incorrect because placing the client in the Trendelenburg position will *not resolve* her hypotension. The Trendelenburg position provides *no benefit* for the client to reverse her low blood pressure, and should *not be used* during pregnancy as a treatment for low blood pressure. **Answer 2** is incorrect because decreasing the rate of IV infusion will make the hypotension *worse.* Decreased intravascular volume may *add to the client's hypotension.* **Answer 3** is incorrect because administering oxygen per nasal cannula will *not resolve* her hypotension. Hyperoxygenation of the client can increase oxygen perfusion to the fetus, but will *do nothing* to reverse the woman's low blood pressure. **Answer 4 is correct because the appropriate intervention for the client's hypotension is a fluid bolus.**

■ TEST-TAKING TIP: *This question is asking for the intervention to resolve the hypotension caused by the epidural. Eliminate the interventions that would not resolve the hypotension. Focus on two options that are opposites of each other (Answer 2, "decrease the rate" and Answer 4, "increase the rate").*

Content Area: Maternity, Intrapartum; *Integrated Process:* Nursing Process, Implementation; *Cognitive Level:* Analysis; *Client Need/Subneed:* Physiological Integrity/Reduction of Risk Potential/Vital Signs Changes/Abnormalities

49. CORRECT ANSWER: 2. **Answer 1** is incorrect because the physician usually examines the cervix directly before the amniotomy. The nurse does not need to reevaluate the cervix. **Answer 2 is correct because, with amniotomy, there is a chance of prolapsed umbilical cord, and that results in fetal bradycardia. Assessing the fetal heart tones is the nurse's most important action.** **Answer 3** is incorrect because the maternal vital signs are *not affected* by the amniotomy, and do not need to be evaluated directly after amniotomy. **Answer 4** is incorrect because the client's level of discomfort may increase after amniotomy, but pain is *not the most important* evaluation.

■ TEST-TAKING TIP: *When prioritizing nursing actions, the first priority should be to assess the fetal heart rate because it is directly affected by rupturing the amniotic sac. Note that three options relate to the woman, and one to the fetus. Select the option that is different.*

Content Area: Maternity, Intrapartum; *Integrated Process:* Nursing Process, Assessment; *Cognitive Level:* Analysis; *Client Need/Subneed:* Physiological Integrity/Reduction of Risk Potential/Diagnostic Tests

50. CORRECT ANSWER: 1. **Answer 1 is correct because the multiple marker screen can screen for certain spinal column defects.** **Answer 2** is incorrect because the multiple marker screen is *not primarily* a screen for cardiovascular defects; it can screen for *Down* syndrome, which can have associated cardiac defects. **Answer 3** is incorrect because it is a state law to *offer* the screening, *not* a state law to *mandate* that the test be performed. **Answer 4** is incorrect because the screen is offered *to all* women who are pregnant regardless of age.

■ **TEST-TAKING TIP:** *It's important to understand the difference between a screening test and a diagnostic test.* Screening *tests are offered to* all *pregnant women to help evaluate their risk for certain birth defects, but they* cannot diagnose *a birth defect. The multiple marker screen is a screening test, not a diagnostic test.*

Content Area: Maternity, Antepartum; *Integrated Process:* Teaching and Learning; *Cognitive Level:* Application; *Client Need/Subneed:* Physiological Integrity/Reduction of Risk Potential/Diagnostic Tests

51. CORRECT ANSWER: 2. **Answer 1** is incorrect because proper *hydration* is important during labor. There is no reason for fluid restriction. **Answer 2 is correct because supplemental oxygen is needed to compensate for the decreased oxygen-carrying capacity of sickling cells.** **Answer 3** is incorrect because a blood transfusion is usually *not* required *unless* there is a significant blood loss during delivery. *Prophylactic* blood transfusions are *not* recommended. **Answer 4** is incorrect because there is a *higher risk in operative* deliveries, especially of blood loss. Unless an operative delivery is obstetrically indicated, a *vaginal* delivery is the *preferred* method of delivery.

■ **TEST-TAKING TIP:** *The question states the client has been treated for sickle cell anemia, but does* not *state she has a current sickle cell* crisis. *Management of a sickle cell* crisis *may include blood transfusion (Answer 3).*

Content Area: Maternity, Intrapartum; *Integrated Process:* Nursing Process, Planning; *Cognitive Level:* Application; *Client Need/Subneed:* Physiological Integrity/Reduction of Risk Potential/Potential for Alterations in Body Systems

52. CORRECT ANSWER: 1. **Answer 1 is correct because the bladder should be full to lift the uterus and fetus out of the pelvis in order to obtain good measurements.** **Answer 2** is incorrect because a pelvic ultrasound does *not* require the client to be without food for the examination. **Answer 3** is incorrect because a pelvic ultrasound does *not* require the client to have an enema for the examination. **Answer 4** is incorrect because limiting ambulation has *nothing* to do with preparing for a pelvic ultrasound.

■ **TEST-TAKING TIP:** *When considering radiological examinations and the proper preparation, think about the purpose of the examination and what structures are being examined. For a fetal ultrasound, good visualization is important; therefore, the bladder must be full.*

Content Area: Maternity, Intrapartum; *Integrated Process:* Nursing Process, Implementation; *Cognitive Level:* Application; *Client Need/Subneed:* Physiological Integrity/Reduction of Risk Potential/Diagnostic Tests

53. CORRECT ANSWER: 2. **Answer 1** is incorrect because a nonstress test does *not* measure *lung* maturity; a nonstress test (NST) measures the *fetal heart rate* in response to the fetus' movements. **Answer 2 is correct because the purpose of a nonstress test is to measure the well-being of the fetus.** **Answer 3** is incorrect because a nonstress test (NST) measures the fetal heart rate *in response to the fetus' movements.* It is *not* a measure of the *number* of fetal kicks. **Answer 4** is incorrect because a nonstress test *does not* show the effect of contractions or stress on the fetus.

■ **TEST-TAKING TIP:** *Eliminate Answer 4 because it does* not *meet the definition of nonstress; contractions are* not *a part of an NST. Select the option that is a* general *measure ("well-being"), not lungs or number of kicks.*

Content Area: Maternity, Intrapartum; *Integrated Process:* Nursing Process, Evaluation; *Cognitive Level:* Analysis; *Client Need/Subneed:* Physiological Integrity/Reduction of Risk Potential/Diagnostic Tests

54. CORRECT ANSWER: 2. **Answer 1** is incorrect because the client should be medicated *first,* and then if BP and pulse do not change, the physician should be contacted. **Answer 2 is correct because the postoperative pain is most likely causing the vital sign changes.** **Answer 3** is incorrect because the only position that would improve the BP would be to elevate the legs, which would be *contraindicated* following spinal anesthesia. **Answer 4** is incorrect because the problem is *not hypovolemia.*

■ **TEST-TAKING TIP:** *Keep It Simple (K.I.S.)—This client is in pain → give medication for pain. Recognize the effects of pain on vital signs.*

Content Area: Adult Health, Pain Control; *Integrated Process:* Nursing Process, Implementation; *Cognitive Level:* Application; *Client Need/Subneed:* Physiological Integrity/Reduction of Risk Potential/Vital Signs Changes/Abnormalities

55. CORRECT ANSWER: 2. **Answer 1** is incorrect because cellular phones should be *held 6 to 12* inches away from the pacemaker. **Answer 2 is correct because contact sports could dislodge the pacing electrodes.** **Answer 3** is incorrect because pacemaker technology allows the client to *safely* use household electronics. **Answer 4** is incorrect because pacemaker technology allows the client to *safely use* household electronics previously not allowed.

■ **TEST-TAKING TIP:** *Look for the option that is different from the others . . . . sports versus electronics (phones and ovens).*

Content Area: Adult Health, Cardiovascular; *Integrated Process:* Teaching and Learning; *Cognitive Level:* Comprehension; *Client Need/Subneed:* Physiological Integrity/Reduction of Risk Potential/Potential for Alterations in Body Systems

56. CORRECT ANSWER: 1. **Answer 1 is correct because hemoglobin responds to changes in hydration. Dehydration would result in hemoconcentration and elevated hemoglobin.** **Answer 2** is incorrect because infection does *not* influence the hemoglobin level. **Answer 3** is incorrect because malnutrition would most likely cause a *decrease,* not an increase, in hemoglobin from inadequate iron intake. **Answer 4** is incorrect because antibiotic therapy effectiveness would affect the white blood cell count, *not* Hgb.

■ TEST-TAKING TIP: ***Remember that hemoglobin, hematocrit, and blood urea nitrogen will reflect the hydration status.***

Content Area: Adult Health, Hematological; ***Integrated Process:*** Nursing Process, Implementation; ***Cognitive Level:*** Comprehension; ***Client Need/Subneed:*** Physiological Integrity/Reduction of Risk Potential/Laboratory Values

57. CORRECT ANSWER: 3. **Answer 1** is incorrect because the creatinine level, which indicates renal function, is within *normal* limits (0.7 to 1.4 mg/dL). The BUN is elevated, which could indicate possible fluid volume deficit, and *further assessment* will be needed. **Answer 2** is incorrect because the calcium level is within *normal* limits (8.6 to 10.2 mg/dL). **Answer 3 is correct because the normal prothrombin time is 9.5 to 12 seconds. If anticoagulation is desired, the level is usually 1½ to 2 times the normal. This value puts the client at serious risk for bleeding.** **Answer 4** is incorrect because the Hgb is within *normal* limits for both men and women.

■ TEST-TAKING TIP: ***Know the normal values for common laboratory tests.***

Content Area: Adult Health, Hematological; ***Integrated Process:*** Nursing Process, Analysis; ***Cognitive Level:*** Analysis; ***Client Need/Subneed:*** Physiological Integrity/Reduction of Risk Potential/Laboratory Values

58. CORRECT ANSWER: 1. **Answer 1 is correct because this client is at high risk for pulmonary emboli. Assess for additional signs before calling the physician.** **Answer 2** is incorrect because the pain is *not severe* enough to cause the vital sign changes. Note that morphine *was* given; additional morphine is not indicated. **Answer 3** is incorrect because the risk is pulmonary emboli, *not* thrombophlebitis. **Answer 4** is incorrect because the physician will *need additional* data that the nurse needs to provide first.

■ TEST-TAKING TIP: ***In 24 hours ("the next morning") the risk is pulmonary emboli, not thrombophlebitis. Therefore, do additional* respiratory *assessments, not assessments for inflammation ("-itis").***

Content Area: Adult Health, Respiratory; ***Integrated Process:*** Nursing Process, Implementation; ***Cognitive Level:*** Application; ***Client Need/Subneed:*** Physiological Integrity/Reduction of Risk Potential/Vital Signs Changes/Abnormalities

59. CORRECT ANSWER: 2. **Answer 1** is incorrect because the effectiveness of drugs *varies* from client to client. **Answer 2 is correct because pain is what the client reports it to be: severe, unrelenting, or relieved. Pain is now considered as the fifth vital sign.** **Answer 3** is incorrect because duration (how long the pain has persisted) is *not* an indication of severity, which can be mild, moderate, severe, or excruciating. **Answer 4** is incorrect because *cultural* norms may *alter* expressions of pain. The stereotypical "stoic Asian" may not show an expression recognized by others as pain.

■ TEST-TAKING TIP: ***The question asks for the most reliable indication—what the client says!***

Content Area: Adult Health, Pain Control; ***Integrated Process:*** Nursing Process, Analysis; ***Cognitive Level:*** Application; ***Client Need/Subneed:*** Physiological Integrity/Reduction of Risk Potential/Vital Signs Changes/Abnormalities

60. CORRECT ANSWER: 1. **Answer 1 is correct because there is a loss of autonomic nervous system function below the level of injury—pulse decreases, which is unique to spinal cord injury.** **Answer 2** is incorrect because hypotension is *not specific* to spinal cord injury. **Answer 3** is incorrect because the loss of autonomic nervous system function causes bradycardia. **Answer 4** is incorrect because an abrupt onset of fever may occur, but hyperthermia is *not specific* to neurogenic shock. Fever is present in *septic* shock.

■ TEST-TAKING TIP: ***Look for opposites: tachycardia (Answer 3) versus bradycardia (Answer 1). Typical vital sign changes with shock include tachycardia, so that it* isn't specific *to one type of shock as this question asks.***

Content Area: Adult Health, Neurological; ***Integrated Process:*** Nursing Process, Assessment; ***Cognitive Level:*** Application; ***Client Need/Subneed:*** Physiological Integrity/Reduction of Risk Potential/Vital Signs Changes/Abnormalities

61. CORRECT ANSWERS: 1, 2, 4. **Answer 1 is correct because crossing the legs impedes circulation. Answer 2 is correct because maintaining a dependent position increases edema.** **Answer 3** is incorrect because elevating the legs above the heart *will* decrease edema. **Answer 4 is correct because hot or warm water causes vasodilation, decreases venous return, and increases edema.** **Answer 5** is incorrect because wearing support hose *increases* venous return and *decreases* edema. **Answer 6** is incorrect because walking increases muscle tone and *increases* venous return.

■ TEST-TAKING TIP: ***The key word in the stem is "avoid." Consider how each option would affect venous return.***

Content Area: Adult Health, Vascular; ***Integrated Process:*** Teaching and Learning; ***Cognitive Level:*** Analysis; ***Client Need/Subneed:*** Physiological Integrity/Reduction of Risk Potential/Potential for Alterations in Body Systems

62. CORRECT ANSWER: 2. **Answer 1** is incorrect because the laboratory findings and vital signs are *not* consistent with volume overload. **Answer 2 is correct because the findings indicate hemoconcentration from dehydration.** **Answer 3** is incorrect because the creatinine value is within *normal* limits, and is the more specific indicator of renal function. **Answer 4** is incorrect because the O_2 saturation is within *normal* limits.

■ TEST-TAKING TIP: ***Only one vital sign is of concern: T 38.7°C = fever → dehydration.***

Content Area: Adult Health, Hematological; ***Integrated Process:*** Nursing Process, Analysis; ***Cognitive Level:*** Analysis; ***Client Need/Subneed:*** Physiological Integrity/Reduction of Risk Potential/Laboratory Values

63. CORRECT ANSWERS: 1, 2, 3, 4. Answer 1 is correct because in SIADH urine output is decreased, the urine becomes more concentrated and the urine Na^+ increases. Answer 2 is correct because in SIADH urine output is decreased and the osmolarity of the urine increases (i.e., the urine becomes more concentrated). Answer 3 is correct because fluid is retained, causing hemodilution and a low serum sodium. Answer 4 is correct because in SIADH the fluid retention causes hemodilution and a decrease in the serum osmolarity. **Answer 5** is incorrect because in SIADH the urine becomes more concentrated and the urine sodium concentration increases.

■ **TEST-TAKING TIP:** *Look at the relationship between the serum (i.e., blood) level and* urine *level—if one goes up, the other goes down.*

Content Area: Adult Health, Renal; ***Integrated Process:*** Nursing Process, Analysis; ***Cognitive Level:*** Analysis; ***Client Need/Subneed:*** Physiological Integrity/Reduction of Risk Potential/Laboratory Values

64. CORRECT ANSWER: 1. Answer 1 is correct because compensation is evident when the pH is within the normal range (7.35 to 7.45) and one of the other components is outside of normal. Both the bicarbonate (normal is 22 to 26) and CO_2 (normal: 35 to 45) are below the normal range. **Answer 2** is incorrect because this sample is *outside* the normal range, so that compensation has not occurred. **Answer 3** is incorrect because the pH is *outside* the normal range of 7.35 to 7.45. **Answer 4** is incorrect because the pH in this sample is within the normal range, but on the *alkaline* side, not the acidotic side.

■ **TEST-TAKING TIP:** *Look for the pH to be within normal limits (7.35 to 7.45).*

Content Area: Adult Health, Acid-Base; ***Integrated Process:*** Teaching and Learning; ***Cognitive Level:*** Analysis; ***Client Need/Subneed:*** Physiological Integrity/Reduction of Risk Potential/Laboratory Values

65. CORRECT ANSWER: 2. **Answer 1** is incorrect because murmurs are created by turbulent flow of blood. They do *not* cause chest pain. **Answer 2 is correct because murmurs occur when blood flow through a normal cardiac structure is increased with activity.** **Answer 3** is incorrect because the answer to the question would *not explain* the development of the murmur. **Answer 4** is incorrect because murmurs are *not* associated with shortness of breath.

■ **TEST-TAKING TIP:** *Focus on activity as a cause for a murmur that was not previously present.*

Content Area: Adult Health, Cardiovascular; ***Integrated Process:*** Nursing Process, Assessment; ***Cognitive Level:*** Analysis; ***Client Need/Subneed:*** Physiological Integrity/Reduction of Risk Potential/System Specific Assessments

66. CORRECT ANSWER: 4. **Answer 1** is incorrect because the desired level for the $HgbA_{1c}$ is below 7. **Answer 2** is incorrect because a $HgbA_{1c}$ of 6 would be consistent with a blood sugar of 138, and that would be normal for a person who has diabetes. **Answer 3** is incorrect because a $HgbA_{1c}$ of 5 or less would be below normal. **Answer 4 is correct because a $HgbA_{1c}$ of 5 is a blood sugar of approximately 100. A $HgbA_{1c}$ below 7 is desired. A $HgbA_{1c}$ of 10 reflects lack of glycemic control.**

■ **TEST-TAKING TIP:** *Three of the options focus on "normal," "slightly above normal," and "below normal." Choose the option that is different from the others ("very high"). $HgbA_{1c}$ is the best indication of glycemic control (below 7 is desired).*

Content Area: Adult Health, Endocrine; ***Integrated Process:*** Nursing Process, Analysis; ***Cognitive Level:*** Analysis; ***Client Need/Subneed:*** Physiological Integrity/Reduction of Risk Potential/Laboratory Values

67. CORRECT ANSWER: 4. **Answer 1** is incorrect because sugar and acetone are indicators of what the blood glucose is at *one* point in time only. **Answer 2** is incorrect because blood glucose from a finger stick is only an indicator of what the blood glucose is at *one* point in time. **Answer 3** is incorrect because random blood glucose is only an indicator of what the blood glucose is at *one* point in time. **Answer 4 is correct because this test gives an average of the client's blood glucose for the past 90 days rather than just 1 day or one point in time.**

■ **TEST-TAKING TIP:** *Eliminate the options that can be used at the bedside and are random measures of blood sugar. Hemoglobin A_{1c} is done in a laboratory.*

Content Area: Adult Health, Endocrine; ***Integrated Process:*** Nursing Process, Analysis; ***Cognitive Level:*** Application; ***Client Need/Subneed:*** Physiological Integrity/Reduction of Risk Potential/Laboratory Values

68. CORRECT ANSWER: 2. **Answer 1** is incorrect because the redness of a stage I ulcer does not last, but *progresses* to a *dusky blue-gray* color. If it is simple redness, it will *resolve* in less than 30 minutes. **Answer 2 is correct because the redness of a stage I ulcer does not blanch with pressure, whereas simple redness will blanch.** **Answer 3** is incorrect because blisters are a sign of a *stage II* pressure ulcer. **Answer 4** is incorrect because subcutaneous tissue breakdown occurs with a *stage II* pressure ulcer.

■ **TEST-TAKING TIP:** *The question asks for the sign that may be indicative of stage I ulcer.*

Content Area: Adult Health, Integumentary; ***Integrated Process:*** Nursing Process, Assessment; ***Cognitive Level:*** Application; ***Client Need/Subneed:*** Physiological Integrity/Reduction of Risk Potential/System Specific Assessments

69. CORRECT ANSWERS: 1, 4, 5, 6. Answer 1 is correct because the nurse should select the appropriate amount of suction, which is between 60 and 100 mm Hg. Selecting less suction would not remove secretions and applying greater than 100 mm Hg of suction may cause trauma to the tissues. **Answer 2** is incorrect because the child should be suctioned for *no longer* than 5 seconds. **Answer 3** is incorrect because the tip of the suction catheter should be inserted no further than the end of the tracheostomy tube, or to a maximum of 0.5 cm past the end of the tube. Inserting the catheter past the carina could damage the tracheobronchial wall, sending the catheter down one side of the bronchial tree. **Answer 4 is correct because the nurse should first wash hands to prevent infection. Answer 5 is correct because the nurse should oxygenate the child prior to suctioning and immediately after suctioning. Answer 6 is correct because the nurse should remove the catheter from the package and have it ready for suctioning. Additionally, the nurse should select a small catheter for suctioning, such as an 8 or 10 French.**

■ **TEST-TAKING TIP:** *Pay close attention to the age of the client in the question stem. A 15-month-old child requires* less *vacuum pressure and a* smaller *catheter than an older child or adult.*

Content Area: Child Health, Respiratory; *Integrated Process:* Nursing Process, Implementation; *Cognitive Level:* Application; *Client Need/Subneed:* Physiological Integrity/Reduction of Risk Potential/Therapeutic Procedures

70. CORRECT ANSWERS: 1, 2, 3, 4. Answer 1 is correct because the child should be informed about the procedure in a way that the child can understand. Answer 2 is correct because a 25- or 27-gauge needle is small, making it best suited for obtaining a blood sample from a preschooler who has small veins. Answer 3 is correct because the parents should be encouraged to participate in the procedure by helping the child to hold still, using gentle restraint such as hugging. Answer 4 is correct because the child will become less anxious if the nurse does not show the needle and other equipment during the preparatory period. **Answer 5** is incorrect because the sample should be obtained from the child's *nondominant* side. **Answer 6** is incorrect because painful procedures should not be performed in the playroom.

■ **TEST-TAKING TIP:** *Do not assume that the correct responses are not already in the proper order (1, 2, 3, 4).*

Content Area: Child Health, Hematological; *Integrated Process:* Nursing Process, Implementation; *Cognitive Level:* Application; *Client Need/Subneed:* Physiological Integrity/Reduction of Risk Potential/Therapeutic Procedures

71. CORRECT ANSWERS: 2, 3, 4. **Answer 1** is incorrect because a seizure disorder does *not* increase the risk for infection. **Answer 2 is correct because a child with sickle cell anemia has decreased oxygen-carrying capacity of the blood, increasing the risk for infection. Answer 3 is correct because a child with diabetes has increased circulating blood glucose levels, which can lead to the growth and proliferation of bacteria. Answer 4 is correct because a child with juvenile idiopathic arthritis is likely to take corticosteroid medication, which may mask infection.** **Answer 5** is incorrect because food allergies do *not* increase the risk for infection. **Answer 6** is incorrect because having a history of cleft lip and palate does *not* increase the risk for infection.

■ **TEST-TAKING TIP:** *Recall that disorders of the blood, as well as diseases that require medications affecting the immune system, may increase the risk for infection.*

Content Area: Child Health, Infectious Disease; *Integrated Process:* Nursing Process, Analysis; *Cognitive Level:* Analysis; *Client Need/Subneed:* Physiological Integrity/Reduction of Risk Potential/Potential for Alterations in Body Systems

72. CORRECT ANSWERS: 2, 4, 5. **Answer 1** is incorrect because this statement indicates teaching has *not* been effective, since the parents have failed to understand that the infant is at high risk for infection. **Answer 2 is correct because the child with Down syndrome is at increased risk for respiratory infection.** **Answer 3** is incorrect because this statement indicates teaching has *not* been effective, since children with Down syndrome may never reach some developmental milestones as a result of mental retardation. **Answer 4 is correct because hearing deficits are common in children with Down syndrome. Answer 5 is correct because these children are at increased risk for aspiration and should be positioned to prevent this complication related to oral feedings.**

■ **TEST-TAKING TIP:** *Select the answers that* are *correct; eliminate the answers that are* not *correct.*

Content Area: Child Health, Neurological; *Integrated Process:* Nursing Process, Evaluation; *Cognitive Level:* Analysis; *Client Need/Subneed:* Physiological Integrity/Reduction of Risk Potential/Potential for Complications from Surgical Procedures and Health Alterations

73. CORRECT ANSWERS: 1, 3, 4, 6. Answer 1 is correct because leukemia causes a decrease in white blood cells (WBCs). **Answer 2** is incorrect because the nurse should not expect abnormal BUN in a child with a new diagnosis of leukemia since the disease affects bone marrow function, not kidney function. **Answer 3 is correct because leukemia causes a decrease in red blood cells (RBCs). Answer 4 is correct because leukemia causes a decrease in platelets (PLTs).** **Answer 5** is incorrect because the nurse should not expect abnormal sodium in a child with a new diagnosis of leukemia. Sodium is a good indicator of fluid status and not indicative of bone marrow functioning. **Answer 6 is correct because leukemia causes a decrease in hemoglobin.**

■ **TEST-TAKING TIP:** *Leukemia affects bone marrow function. The bone marrow is responsible for hematopoiesis; therefore, select laboratory values that measure the primary blood components of red cells, white cells, and platelets.*

Content Area: Child Health, Hematological; *Integrated Process:* Nursing Process, Evaluation; *Cognitive Level:* Application; *Client Need/Subneed:* Physiological Integrity/Reduction of Risk Potential/Laboratory Values

CHAPTER 12

Final Tests 1 and 2

Sally Lambert Lagerquist • Janice Lloyd McMillin • Robyn Marchal Nelson • Denise Wall Parilo • Kathleen E. Snider • Janis Ryan Wisherop

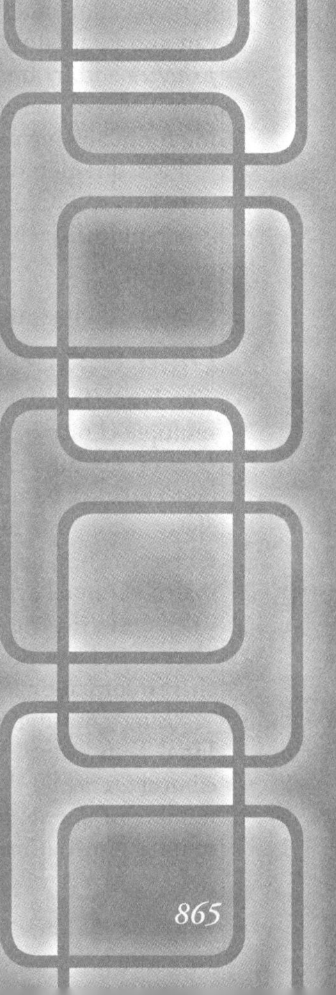

Introduction

What is Final Test 1?

Final Test 1 is a *follow-up assessment* tool designed to assess areas of improvement from your initial self-assessment using the **Pre-tests.** Take **Final Test 1** immediately after reading the specific *content* areas related to your individual problem areas as identified by the **Pre-tests.** Determine that you are now able to meet the goal of 80% correct answers in this integrated examination, which also includes 15% in alternate item format.

After taking **Final Test 1,** use the units in this book again to fill in any "gaps" this test reveals in your preparation. Then take **Final Test 2** to assess your readiness for the NCLEX-RN®.

What is Final Test 2?

Final Test 2 is a multiple-choice examination with 4, 5, or 6 options, which also includes 26% in alternate item format, designed to assess your baseline nursing knowledge and evaluate your ability to apply that knowledge to various clinical situations and to items presented in a simulated NCLEX-RN® examination. Self-analysis of your scores will help you prioritize what to study by identifying your individual problem areas.

Written to reflect the content framework and the purpose of the NCLEX-RN® Text Plan (to measure a candidate's ability to practice safely and effectively as a Registered Nurse in an entry-level position), **Final Test 2** can be used as preparation and review for the licensure examination. It can also be used for review by ***nurses returning to active practice*** and by **international nurses** who are *graduates of nursing schools* outside of the United States and are preparing for qualifying examinations.

Each question on **Final Test 2** was field tested in a pilot test given to NCLEX-RN® candidates representing a wide geographic distribution, as well as various types of nursing programs.

Selection of Content and Distribution of the Questions

The **Final Tests** are composed of 150 content-integrated, multiple-choice questions, most with four answer options. *One* of the answers is most complete and therefore the best choice. The other three answers (distractors) are not always wrong but are usually not as complete or as important as the best answer. In addition, 31 alternate item format questions have been added to these tests, where you will be asked to *select all that apply* from 5 to 6 options, place in order of priority/sequence, fill in the blank, use the chart information, and locate the area/spot on the diagram.

Using a nursing process framework, the questions on the **Final Tests** reflect nursing situations that involve different clinical areas and diagnoses. As on the NCLEX-RN®, the number of questions for each content area varies. The percentage distribution of items in these tests related to client needs follows the NCLEX-RN® blueprint (see **Table 1.1** in **Chapter 1,** Orientation and Pre-Test, for percentages).

Based on the blueprint for the *Test Plan for the National Council Licensure Examination* (NCLEX-RN®) published by the National Council of State Boards of Nursing, Inc., the **Final Tests** assess your knowledge, skills, and abilities in the **four** broad areas of *client needs:* Safe, Effective Care Environment (SECE), Physiological Integrity (PhI), Psychosocial Integrity (PsI), and Health Promotion and Maintenance (HPM); and **six** *client subneeds* (Management of Care, Safety and Infection Control, Basic Care and Comfort, Physiological Adaptation, Reduction of Risk Potential, and Pharmacological and Parenteral Therapies). Each question in the **Final Tests** has been classified according to the above categories and according to clinical area, as well as cognitive level and integrated process.

Timing

Allow about 1 minute per question. Time yourself and plan to complete each of the 75-question tests in no more than 1 hour and 15 to 30 minutes. Simulate test-taking conditions by having uninterrupted time of 1 hour and 30 minutes.

Test Results

When you check your answers, keep track not only of how many are incorrect, but also how many are incorrect in *each category* of client needs/subneeds and content area.

Suggestions for Further Study

You can use your test results, in combination with the following Appendices following Chapter 12, to assess your NCLEX-RN® strengths and weaknesses.

When you have problems with NCLEX®-relevant content/subject areas:	Refer to Appendix:
A. Client needs (4 broad categories and 6 client subneeds)	
1. Use the index to *content* to locate pages in this book where the specific subjects/topics will be found	F, H
2. Use the index to *practice questions that cover these content areas*	G

You now have an individualized evaluation with which to develop your plan for what you need to study and where to find the material for further study. Our good wishes for your success!

Final Test 1

Questions

Select the one answer that is best for each question, unless otherwise directed.

1. A Hispanic client, who is gravida 5, para 4, notices small bluish marks with indistinct edges on her newborn's

buttocks and lower back. The most appropriate response by the nurse would be to:
1. Call child protective services to remove the baby from an abusive environment.
2. Reassure her that it is a normal finding in darker skinned infants.
3. Measure the size of the mark and document it.
4. Call the physician to report the finding.

2. During the physical assessment of a client diagnosed with a right tension pneumothorax, a nurse would expect to find:
Select all that apply.
1. Tracheal shift to the left.
2. Tracheal shift to the right.
3. Decreased breath sounds on the right side.
4. Subcutaneous emphysema on the left chest.
5. Increased breath sounds on the left side.
6. Point of Maximum Impulse (PMI) shifted further to the left of midline.

3. A 24-year-old client, who is gravida 3, para 2 at 28 weeks' gestation with hypothyroidism, asks a nurse if she will still need to take thyroid medication during the pregnancy. The nurse' best response should be based on the knowledge that:
1. During pregnancy, a woman's metabolism slows down, and it is more difficult to maintain thyroid regulation.
2. The thyroid medication will be stopped during pregnancy because the fetus' thyroid produces a thyroid-stimulating hormone.
3. The dosage may have to be increased as much as 50% during pregnancy.
4. Fetal brain development will be affected if thyroid medication is continued during pregnancy.

4. Following application of a cast to immobilize a closed fracture of the humerus, a client returns to an emergency department. A nurse suspects compartment syndrome when the client reports:
Select all that apply.
1. Urine has become dark reddish-brown.
2. Radial pulse in the arm is diminished.
3. Swelling has decreased in the arm.
4. Pain distal to the fracture site has increased.
5. Oxycodone prescribed for pain is not working.
6. Fingers distal to the fracture are warm.

5. A toddler with leukemia is hospitalized for fever and neutropenia. Which physician order should a nurse question?
1. Tylenol PR q4h prn fever.
2. Limit visitors.
3. NS bolus × 1.
4. Daily G-CSF SQ.

6. A neonatal nurse is performing the initial assessment on a neonate. The neonate was delivered by vacuum extraction at 39 weeks' gestation. Which finding would be considered "normal" for this infant at 1 minute of age?
1. Acrocyanosis.
2. Absence of tone.
3. Icteric skin.
4. An apical pulse of 100.

7. Surgery has been delayed for a client with Graves' disease. The correct nursing actions while waiting for the operating room to call should be:
Select all that apply.
1. Pad the side rails of the bed as the risk of seizures may increase.
2. Offer the client a high-protein meal supplement to prevent hypoglycemia.
3. Offer mouth care as NPO status may cause oral dryness.
4. Anticipate the cleansing enema order will need to be repeated.
5. Monitor the client closely for a positive Chvostek's sign.
6. Apply artificial tears to prevent eye irritation.

8. A male neonate is delivered by cesarean section at 36 weeks' gestation. A neonatal nurse is performing a newborn assessment and notes the presence of hypospadias. Which statement to the mother best describes hypospadias?
1. The penis is smaller and shorter.
2. The urethral opening is absent.
3. The urethra opens on the dorsal side of the penis.
4. The urethra opens on the ventral side of the penis.

9. A client with benign prostatic hypertrophy (BPH) asks a nurse what can be done to manage the symptoms. The correct response by the nurse would be:
1. "There is really nothing that can be done except surgical removal of the prostate."
2. "Increase the amount of zinc in your diet."
3. "Herbal therapy such as saw palmetto may improve urinary flow."
4. "Vitamin E will reduce the size of the prostate."

10. A client, who is gravida 3, para 2, is admitted to labor and delivery. A sterile vaginal examination reveals that the client's cervix is 9 to 10 cm dilated, 100% effaced, and a +2 station. Which action should the nurse take *first?*
1. Administer IV pain relief.
2. Prepare the client for delivery.
3. Administer fluid bolus.
4. Place client in knee-chest position.

11. An 18-year-old client is having her first gynecological examination. She asks a nurse about a pill for birth control. Which nursing statement about oral contraceptive agents is correct?
1. Oral contraceptives are the best choice with just a few minor side effects.
2. Most women stop taking oral contraceptives because they cause severe nausea.
3. Oral contraceptives inhibit ovulation and change the consistency of cervical mucus.
4. These drugs can be made more effective by monitoring basal body temperature.

12. During the assessment of a client who is in labor, a nurse notes that the fetal heart tones are loudest in the upper right quadrant. The infant is most likely in which position?
   1. Right sacrum anterior presentation.
   2. Right occipital anterior presentation.
   3. Left sacrum anterior presentation.
   4. Left occipital transverse presentation.

13. During a physical assessment of a client with cardiac tamponade, a nurse should expect to find:
   Select all that apply.
   1. A widened pulse pressure.
   2. Jugular venous distention (JVD).
   3. Loud heart sounds.
   4. Bounding pulses.
   5. Muffled heart sounds.

14. A client, who is gravida 1, para 0, is attending a prenatal breastfeeding class. Which statement by the client should indicate to a nurse that additional teaching is needed?
   1. "If I get sore nipples, I can use expressed breast milk to relieve the pain."
   2. "I will follow a strict schedule for breastfeeding, every 3 hours."
   3. "I will avoid giving my baby a pacifier for the first 4 to 6 weeks after birth."
   4. "I will wear a supportive nursing bra."

15. Which situation could lead to metabolic acidosis in a client?
   1. Frequent vomiting.
   2. Nasogastric suctioning.
   3. Hyperventilation.
   4. ASA overdose.

16. A nurse is working with the parents of an infant who has just died of sudden infant death syndrome (SIDS). What interventions by the nurse would be most appropriate?
   Select all that apply.
   1. Ask the hospital chaplain to bring the family a bible.
   2. Advise the family to not bring siblings to see the child who has died.
   3. Explain that autopsies must be performed on all suspicious deaths.
   4. Place a sign on the child's room door requesting visitors to first check in at the nurse's station.
   5. Give parents written information regarding SIDS.
   6. Ask parents to wait before touching the infant.

17. A client, who is a gravida 1, para 0, delivers a 9-pound, 8-ounce baby using vacuum extraction after a 2-hour second stage of labor. The client has a fourth-degree laceration. Which medication should the nurse anticipate administering to this client?
   1. Dulcolax suppository.
   2. Docusate sodium.
   3. Methylergonovine maleate.
   4. Carboprost tromethamine.

18. The client's arterial blood gases (ABGs) are: pH 7.32; $Paco_2$ 48 mm Hg, and HCO_3 25 mEq/L. A nurse should anticipate that an appropriate order for this client will be:
   1. Incentive spirometer to be used hourly.
   2. O_2 via mask with a rebreather mask.
   3. Antianxiety medication to slow respiratory rate.
   4. Sodium bicarbonate IV to raise the pH.

19. A 14-year-old client, who is gravida 1, para 0 at 11 weeks' gestation, is at her first prenatal visit. To provide anticipatory guidance for this client, the nurse should assess:
   1. The client's attitude about the pregnancy.
   2. Whether the client used birth control methods.
   3. The client's feelings about future children.
   4. The client's knowledge of the symptoms of preterm labor.

20. A nursing student asks an RN to explain the results of a client's arterial blood gases. The results are: pH 7.43; $Paco_2$ 30 mm Hg; and HCO_3 18 mEq/L. The nurse knows the client's acid-base status is:
   1. Uncompensated respiratory acidosis.
   2. Compensated respiratory alkalosis.
   3. Uncompensated metabolic alkalosis.
   4. Compensated metabolic acidosis.

21. A client, who is gravida 4, para 3 at 38 weeks' gestation, is entering the second stage of labor. Which *essential* action should a nurse perform at this time?
   1. Prepare the client for an emergency cesarean section.
   2. Administer 10 units oxytocin IM.
   3. Administer 800 mcg misoprostol rectally.
   4. Notify the physician of the client's vaginal exam.

22. The night before surgery, a client is given pentobarbital sodium (Nembutal) for sleep, with an order to repeat. One hour later the client is still unable to sleep. What should the nurse do *next?*
   1. Give the second dose of pentobarbital sodium.
   2. Prepare a glass of warm milk.
   3. Rub the client's back until relaxed.
   4. Explore the client's feelings about surgery.

23. A client, who is gravida 2, para 1, delivered an 8-pound baby 24 hours ago. The client's blood type is B negative and the fetus is B positive. A physician orders an injection of Rho(D) immune globulin. A nurse understands that the Rho(D) immune globulin should be administered to this client to:
   1. Inactivate the fetal Rh antigens.
   2. Prevent the formation of Rh antigens.
   3. Provide immunity against Rh isoenzymes.
   4. Convert the Rh factor from negative to positive.

24. A client with a history of type 1 diabetes has not been eating or taking insulin for 3 days because of "feeling poorly." The client is confused, respirations are 32, and breath odor is fruity. The serum glucose is 620 mg/dL.

A nurse should know that the correct action for this client is:
1. Rapid rehydration with NS at 1 L/hr per order.
2. Regular insulin IV 5 units/hr in D_5NS per order.
3. Begin 40% O2 per order.
4. Begin infusion of sodium bicarbonate per order.

25. A Caucasian, male neonate is delivered at 33 weeks' gestation due to premature, preterm rupture of membranes and a maternal fever. A nurse is performing an initial assessment of the neonate. The nurse should expect to find the presence of:
1. Scrotal rugae.
2. Mongolian spots.
3. Desquamation.
4. Vernix caseosa.

26. A client has a pressure ulcer that extends into the dermis and subcutaneous tissue. Which stage of pressure ulcer formation should a nurse document?
1. I.
2. II.
3. III.
4. IV.

27. A school nurse is creating a plan to educate teenagers against the use of smokeless tobacco. What informational strategy would be best suited for the target population?
1. Invite adults who were former users of smokeless tobacco to give presentations regarding how to quit.
2. Create brochures that report the latest statistics regarding the link with cancer and dental complications.
3. Run a series of anti-smokeless tobacco advertisements in the school newspaper.
4. Display informational posters that carry images of former users' faces disfigured by oral cancer.

28. A neonate is delivered by cesarean section at 39 weeks' gestation. The neonate has an Apgar score of 9 at 5 minutes. A nurse should be aware that the most likely cause for subtraction of one point is:
1. The neonate has low blood glucose.
2. The neonate has bradycardia.
3. The neonate has acrocyanosis.
4. The neonate has decreased tone.

29. A client, who is admitted in hypertensive crisis, has a blood pressure of 246/128 mm Hg. Which findings in the client's history should a nurse identify as being related to complications of hypertension?
Select all that apply.
1. History of brain attack (stroke).
2. Elevated blood urea nitrogen.
3. Bilateral glaucoma.
4. Left ventricular hypertrophy.
5. Intermittent claudication.

30. A client, who is gravida 4, para 3, delivered a "fetal demise" last year. A physician orders a contraction stress test (CST) for this client at 38 weeks' gestation. A nurse is aware that a contraction stress test is ordered for this client to:
1. Determine lung maturity.
2. Measure the fetal activity.
3. Check the fetal oxygen reserve.
4. Measure the amniotic fluid.

31. A nurse should determine a client with type 2 diabetes needs additional teaching if which statement is made?
1. "When I am sick, my blood sugar needs to be checked more often."
2. "As a diabetic, going barefoot is unwise."
3. "The goal for my HgbA1c is less than 8."
4. "Losing weight will likely affect my insulin needs."

32. A 43-year-old client delivers a neonate with Down syndrome at 37 weeks' gestation. A nurse performs a routine assessment on the neonate. Which finding should the nurse report immediately to a physician?
1. Simian crease.
2. Brachycephaly.
3. Cyanosis after feeding.
4. Hypotonicity.

33. A 30-year-old client has been trying to conceive for about a year. A physician prescribes clomiphene citrate. A nurse is teaching the client about the drug's potential side effects. Which statement, if made by the client, would indicate that the teaching was effective?
1. "I have a possibility of having more than one fetus."
2. "I have an increased chance of spontaneous abortion."
3. "I have an increased risk of Down syndrome."
4. "I should take this medication throughout my pregnancy."

34. A client, who is gravida 5, para 4, delivers an 11-pound, 4-ounce neonate at 38 weeks' gestation. The client has been noncompliant with her insulin administration for gestational diabetes and her blood sugar has been poorly controlled throughout this pregnancy. Which nursing intervention is the most important for the neonate?
1. Administer a bolus of 50 grams of glucose IV.
2. Begin formula feedings immediately after birth.
3. Check heel stick blood sugar.
4. Administer 10 units of insulin subcutaneously.

35. Over the past 36 hours following open heart surgery, a client has become increasingly restless and agitated, and demands that "the bird" be removed from the room. Which factors are most likely contributing to this client's mental status?
Select all that apply.
1. Administration of norepinephrine (Levophed) IV for low blood pressure.
2. Visitors have been limited in the ICU.
3. Visual hallucinations.
4. Status post open heart surgery.
5. Frequent interruptions for lab tests and procedures.

36. A neonate is born at 39 weeks' gestation and is exclusively breastfed. Which finding by a nurse is considered "normal" in a neonate of this gestation during the first few days after birth?
1. Birth weight of 4,000 to 4,500 grams.
2. Weight gain of 5% to 10% from birth weight.
3. Weight loss of 5% to 10% from birth weight.
4. Birth weight of 2,000 to 2,500 grams.

37. Which side effect(s) from the combination therapy of isoniazid and rifampin should a client report *immediately?*
1. Paleness of conjunctiva and oral mucosa.
2. Dark urine and pale-colored stool.
3. Blood in the urine.
4. Decrease in hearing ability.

38. A child is admitted for suspicion of Reye syndrome. A nurse understands that symptoms of Reye syndrome follow a timeline. Which manifestations support the nurse's suspicion? *Select all that apply.*
1. Behavioral changes and agitation.
2. Administration of acetaminophen.
3. Coma.
4. Decreased PTT.
5. Decreased intracranial pressure.
6. Viral illness.

39. An emergency department nurse assess a client, who is gravida 2, para 0 at 8 weeks' gestation, with a history of pelvic inflammatory disease. The nurse suspects a diagnosis of ectopic pregnancy. Which signs or symptoms would be consistent with this diagnosis?
1. Positive pregnancy test, shoulder pain, and copious vaginal bleeding.
2. Hyperemesis, hypertension, and moderate vaginal bleeding.
3. Amenorrhea, abdominal pain, and hypotension.
4. Copious vaginal discharge, weight loss, and positive pregnancy test.

40. Which signs and symptoms are often seen in a person with active tuberculosis?
1. Fatigue, night sweats, low-grade fever.
2. Weight gain, cough, purulent sputum.
3. High fever; dry, hacking cough.
4. Malaise, epistaxis, headache.

41. A home health nurse visits a client 10 days after delivery. The client is breastfeeding her infant. The nurse's assessment includes pain, redness, and swelling of the client's left breast. The nurse suspects that the client has developed mastitis. The nurse's teaching plan for the client with mastitis should include:
1. Wearing a tight-fitting bra for good support.
2. Stopping breastfeeding permanently.
3. Avoiding breastfeeding on the affected side.
4. Taking analgesics for pain relief.

42. A nurse should know that the oxygen flow rate set for clients with emphysema is usually low because:
1. Low flow rates enhance ventilation-perfusion (V/Q) ratios.
2. Higher flow rates can depress the hypoxic drive.
3. Low flow rates are palliative and relieve anxiety.
4. O2 prevents compensatory respiratory alkalosis.

43. A 23-year-old client has missed two menstrual periods and decides to visit a prenatal clinic to see if she is pregnant. Besides amenorrhea, the client tells a nurse that she has experienced breast tenderness, nausea and vomiting, urinary frequency, and fatigue. The nurse determines that the client has been experiencing symptoms of pregnancy that are classified as:
1. Predictive.
2. Presumptive.
3. Probable.
4. Positive.

44. The best indication of dehydration in a client who is 85 years old would be changes in:
1. Urine output.
2. Skin turgor.
3. Hemoglobin (Hgb) levels.
4. BP.

45. A client, who is gravida 4, para 3, delivered a 7-pound, 3-ounce neonate at 38 weeks' gestation about 24 hours ago. Upon assessment, where should a nurse expect to palpate the client's fundus?
1. At the level of the symphysis pubis.
2. Midway between the umbilicus and the symphysis.
3. At the level of the xyphoid process.
4. At the level of the umbilicus.

46. What should a nurse watch for in a client with autonomic dysreflexia following a cervical spinal cord injury?
1. Severe hypertension.
2. Sudden hypotension.
3. Tachycardia.
4. Cheyne-Stokes breathing.

47. A client, who is gravida 1, para 0, asks a nurse about how to get back into shape after the birth of her child. The nurse instructs the client about a variety of exercises including Kegel exercises. The client asks about the purpose for the Kegel exercises. Which explanation should the nurse give?
1. To relieve lower back pain.
2. To strengthen the perineal muscles.
3. To tone the abdominal muscles.
4. To prevent urinary retention.

48. A possible complication from a carotid endarterectomy performed for transient ischemic attacks is:
1. Hypoglossal nerve damage.
2. Trouble speaking.
3. Lymph tissue compression.
4. Visual impairment.

49. Which action by a nurse would be most helpful in preparing a 2-year-old child for immunization?
   1. Show a video of a child receiving an immunization.
   2. Offer to provide a toy afterward if the child does not cry.
   3. Give the child a choice of two injection sites.
   4. Have the parents discuss the procedure the night before.

50. A client who is pregnant asks a nurse about when she should be able to hear her baby's heart sounds at her physician's appointment. The nurse tells her that fetal heart tones can *first* be heard using a Doppler at approximately:
   1. 6 weeks' gestation.
   2. 12 weeks' gestation.
   3. 18 weeks' gestation.
   4. 22 weeks' gestation.

51. The correct technique for administration of phenytoin (Dilantin), 300 mg IV, would be:
   1. Diluted in 300 mL of 5% dextrose in water (D_5W).
   2. Rapid IV push over 1 minute.
   3. Slowly over 5 to 6 hours.
   4. Direct IV over 6 to 8 minutes.

52. A client, who is gravida 1, para 0, is attending her initial prenatal visit. The client asks a nurse if it is safe to have sexual intercourse during pregnancy. Which is the best response by the nurse?
   1. "During pregnancy, it is best to engage in oral sex only."
   2. "Although interest in sex may change during pregnancy, intercourse is safe during an uncomplicated pregnancy."
   3. "Sexual intercourse is only safe after the first trimester of pregnancy."
   4. "Sexual intercourse should be avoided during the last trimester of pregnancy."

53. During cardiac resuscitation for ventricular fibrillation, which drug would a nurse most likely prepare *first?*
   1. Atropine.
   2. Epinephrine.
   3. Amiodarone.
   4. Lidocaine.

54. A nurse assesses a client who is 13 years old and 28 weeks pregnant. For which complication is this adolescent client at an increased risk?
   1. Gestational diabetes.
   2. Vulvar varicosities.
   3. Placenta previa.
   4. Iron-deficiency anemia.

55. A client, who is gravida 6, para 5, presents to an obstetric clinic 6 weeks after giving birth. She has decided to use the rhythm method as her choice for natural family planning. Which client statement should indicate to a nurse that the teaching about the rhythm method has been successful?
   1. "It is important to take my temperature at about the same time every morning before getting out of bed."
   2. "When my temperature remains elevated for 5 days, ovulation has occurred."
   3. "I can take my temperature when I wake up in the morning after I get out of bed."
   4. "I will take my temperature every evening before I go to bed."

56. A primiparous client at 20 weeks' gestation reports symptoms of thick white vaginal discharge and intense itching. A wet mount specimen reveals a diagnosis of *Candida albicans.* The client asks a nurse what she can do to prevent future infections. Which response by the nurse is most accurate?
   1. "Eat a serving of live-culture yogurt daily."
   2. "Douche with vinegar and water after intercourse."
   3. "Douche with live-culture yogurt daily."
   4. "Take antibiotics as ordered until all are gone."

57. The desired outcome following hydrocortisone injection for rheumatoid arthritis is to:
   1. Reduce synovial fluid.
   2. Reduce joint pain.
   3. Correct joint deformity.
   4. Reverse cartilage erosion.

58. A primiparous client at 26 weeks' gestation presents to a prenatal clinic with concerns about her symptoms of nosebleeds, nasal stuffiness, and slight bilateral hearing loss. She asks a nurse about the cause of her symptoms. Which explanation by the nurse is most accurate?
   1. "This sounds like you have a bad cold. You need to take a decongestant."
   2. "These symptoms are common in pregnancy because pregnancy hormones cause increased blood flow, which causes head congestion."
   3. "These are symptoms of a major problem. You need to be referred to a specialist."
   4. "This sounds like the symptoms of a sinus infection. You need to take antibiotics and decongestants."

59. The desired clinical outcome of pseudoephedrine (Sudafed) is:
   1. Termination of paroxysmal atrial tachycardia (PAT).
   2. Reduction of intraocular pressure.
   3. Relief of upper airway congestion.
   4. Prolongation of local anesthesia.

60. A nurse observes a group of preschool children playing at a day-care facility. What play practices should the nurse recognize as characteristic of children in this stage of development? *Select all that apply.*
   1. Boys and girls like to play dress-up.
   2. Games are highly competitive.
   3. Pairs of children play next to but not with one another.
   4. Small groups of children are seen playing "house."
   5. Children prefer to play with members of the same gender.
   6. Some children have an imaginary playmate.

61. A client, who is 18 years old and primigravida, is attending a prenatal class on pregnancy discomforts and breastfeeding. Which statement, if given by the client, should indicate to a nurse that further teaching is needed?
1. "My areolas will get smaller and lighter in color."
2. "My breasts may feel lumpy and get larger."
3. "My breasts may be tender and swollen."
4. "The nipples will get darker and more erect."

62. How many drops per minute should an IV run to deliver 75 mL/hr (drop factor = 15 gtt/mL)?
1. 15 gtt/min.
2. 19 gtt/min.
3. 17 gtt/min.
4. 22 gtt/min.

63. A 39-year-old career woman is pregnant for the first time. She is attending her first prenatal visit at 10 weeks' gestation and tells a nurse that her pregnancy was planned, but that she is feeling like maybe this was not such a good idea at this stage in her life. Which response by the nurse would be most appropriate?
1. "These are unnatural feelings. You should be happy to be pregnant."
2. "Maybe you should consider abortion since you feel this way."
3. "Many women have mixed emotions when they are first pregnant."
4. "Don't worry, you'll feel differently once the baby is born."

QUESTIONS

64. Which change in fluid or electrolyte status would a nurse identify as being consistent with syndrome of inappropriate antidiuretic hormone (SIADH)?
1. Serum sodium of 150 mEq.
2. Urine output of 2,500 mL/24 hr.
3. Urine specific gravity of 1.036.
4. Presence of edema.

65. A client, who is gravida 5, para 2 at 41 weeks' gestation, is in active labor. She is having contractions every 2 to 3 minutes and they are moderate in intensity. Her cervix is 6 cm dilated, 90% effaced, and a -1 station. The fetal heart rate (FHR) baseline is 120 with moderate long-term variability, no accelerations in the past 30 minutes, and three late decelerations noted within the last 15 minutes. Which nursing action is most appropriate?
1. Encourage the client to ambulate.
2. Position the client on her back so the monitor strip is more accurate.
3. Turn the client to her left side.
4. Prepare for an emergency cesarean section.

66. A client with a history of a myocardial infarction (MI) reports calf pain. What should a nurse assess *first?*
1. Ability to complete a stress test.
2. Effects of climbing a flight of stairs.
3. Information related to the precipitating event.
4. Response to dorsiflexion of the foot.

67. A client, who is 41 years old, gravida 3, para 2, is 8 weeks pregnant. She presents to an emergency department for right-sided, severe abdominal pain. Upon assessment, her temperature is 98.9°F, blood pressure is 60/40 mm Hg, pulse is 126, and respirations 22. Based on these assessment findings, a nurse should suspect that this client probably has:
1. Ruptured appendix.
2. Threatened spontaneous abortion.
3. Ruptured ectopic pregnancy.
4. Missed abortion.

68. A client is to receive 40 units of insulin per hour IV using a microdrip. Insulin in a concentration of 2 U/mL is available. A nurse correctly calculates that _______ gtt/min should be infused. *Fill in the blank.*

69. A client is attending a childbirth preparation class. The topic of the class is the process of labor and pain relief. Which statement by the client should indicate to a nurse that more teaching is needed?
1. "The first stage of labor is the onset of labor through complete dilation of the cervix."
2. "The first phase of labor is cervical dilation through the delivery of the placenta."
3. "The fourth stage of labor is the delivery of the placenta through complete stabilization of the mother."
4. "The third stage of labor is birth through the delivery of the placenta."

70. What time of day would a nurse expect to see signs of hypoglycemia in a client following NPH insulin given at 7:30 a.m.?
1. 8:00 a.m. to 11:00 a.m.
2. 2:00 p.m. to 5:00 p.m.
3. 8:00 p.m. to 11:00 p.m.
4. 2:00 a.m. to 5:00 a.m.

71. Which documentation would be appropriate by a nurse who suspects child abuse or neglect? *Select all that apply.*
1. Child states, "My little brother hit me."
2. Mother appears stressed by hospital environment.
3. Parents do not take interest in caring for child.
4. Child's height-weight ratio is below 5th percentile.
5. Parent reports that the child has not seen a physician for 1 year.
6. When asked by physician about bruising, child refused to answer.

72. A nurse is teaching basic infant care to a group of first-time parents before their discharge from a hospital. A client asks about the proper method of bathing her infant. The nurse should explain that a sponge bath is recommended during the first 2 weeks of life because:
1. New parents need time to learn how to hold the baby.
2. The umbilical cord needs time to separate.

3. Newborn skin is easily traumatized by washing.
4. The chance of chilling the baby outweighs the benefits of bathing.

73. A client, who is 15 years old, gravida 1, para 0, is admitted to a labor and delivery unit with a diagnosis of HELLP syndrome. Which laboratory finding, associated with HELLP syndrome should be of greatest concern to a nurse?
 1. Elevated blood glucose.
 2. Elevated platelet count.
 3. Elevated creatinine clearance.
 4. Elevated liver enzymes.

74. Which imbalance is a client recovering from hyperglycemia at greatest risk of developing?
 1. Hypoglycemia.
 2. Hypokalemia.
 3. Hyponatremia.
 4. Hypocalcemia.

75. A client, who is gravida 2, para 1, is admitted at 34 weeks' gestation with severe preeclampsia. A nurse is assessing the client's deep tendon reflexes. Which method should the nurse use to elicit the biceps reflex?
 1. Placing the thumb on the tendon in the antecubital space and tapping the thumb briskly with the reflex hammer.
 2. Suspending the client's arm at the elbow, using an open hand, while tapping the back of the client's elbow.
 3. Instructing the client to dangle her legs as the nurse strikes the tendon below the patella with the blunt side of the reflex hammer.
 4. Instructing the client to place her arms loosely at her side as the nurse strikes the tendon just above the wrist.

Answers/Rationales/Tips

1. CORRECT ANSWER: 2. **Answer 1** is incorrect because the mark is not a bruise or a sign of abuse, and does not need to be reported to child protective services. **Answer 2 is correct because the mark is a mongolian spot, a normal variant in darker-skinned infants.** **Answer 3** is incorrect because the size of the mongolian spot(s) is not usually documented since they are *normal,* and do *not change* in size during hospitalization. **Answer 4** is incorrect because mongolian spots are *normal.* There is no need to call and report to the physician.

■ TEST-TAKING TIP: *Mongolian spots are sometimes* **mistaken** *for bruises, but are normal findings. Eliminate the alternatives that suggest it is abnormal.*

Content Area: Child Health, Newborn; ***Integrated Process:*** Nursing Process Implementation; ***Cognitive Level:*** Application; ***Client Need/Subneed:*** Health Promotion and Maintenance/ Ante/Intra/Postpartum and Newborn Care

2. CORRECT ANSWERS: 1, 3, 6. **Answer 1 is correct because, during a tension pneumothorax, thoracic structures are pushed toward the opposite side.** **Answer 2** is incorrect because thoracic structures are pushed toward the opposite side of the problem. Since **Answer 1** is correct, this answer is wrong. **Answer 3 is correct because pneumothorax causes partial or total collapse of the lung; therefore, breath sounds would be diminished or absent.** **Answer 4** is incorrect because, if present, the subcutaneous emphysema would be in the *affected* side (i.e., right side). **Answer 5** is incorrect because the pressure on the nonaffected side might result in a *decrease,* or *no* change, in breath sounds. **Answer 6 is correct because thoracic structures, including the heart, would shift to the left.**

■ TEST-TAKING TIP: *Look for key words in the options and ask if those findings would occur if the pressure were on the right side.*

Content Area: Adult Health, Respiratory; ***Integrated Process:*** Nursing Process, Analysis; ***Cognitive Level:*** Analysis; ***Client Need/Subneed:*** Physiological Integrity/Physiological Adaptation/Pathophysiology

3. CORRECT ANSWER: 3. **Answer 1** is incorrect because a woman's metabolism *speeds* up, not slows down during pregnancy. **Answer 2** is incorrect because a fetus is *entirely dependent* on the mother for thyroid hormone until the fetus' own thyroid gland can start to function. This usually does not occur until about 12 weeks. The client still needs to take thyroid medication during the remainder of the pregnancy, even though the fetus is producing some thyroid hormone on its own. The fetus needs the thyroid hormone, and fetal production of thyroid hormone is not a reason to stop the client from taking her replacement. **Answer 3 is correct because women who are on thyroid hormone replacement *before* pregnancy should also be tested to make certain that their levels are appropriate. During pregnancy, the medication dose required may increase by up to 50%. Increases may be required as early as in the first trimester.** **Answer 4** is incorrect because fetal brain development will be affected *if* thyroid medication is *not continued* during pregnancy. The babies of mothers who were hypothyroid in the first part of pregnancy, but adequately treated, exhibited slower motor development than the babies of mothers who had normal thyroid function. However, during the later part of pregnancy, hypothyroidism in the mother can lead to intellectual impairment in the baby.

■ TEST-TAKING TIP: *When the answers have multiple parts, all the parts must be true for the answer to be true. Be careful when reading these types of questions; read all the way through the option.*

Content Area: Maternity, Intrapartum; ***Integrated Process:*** Nursing Process, Analysis; ***Cognitive Level:*** Application; ***Client Need/Subneed:*** Health Promotion and Maintenance/ Ante/Intra/Postpartum and Newborn Care

4. CORRECT ANSWERS: 1, 2, 4, 5. Answer 1 is correct because myoglobin is released from the damaged muscle and excreted in the urine, which makes it dark reddish-brown. Answer 2 is correct because circulation is decreased and radial pulse diminishes as intracompartmental pressure increases. **Answer 3** is incorrect because a decrease in swelling would *decrease* intracompartmental pressure and symptoms. **Answer 4 is correct because this is a characteristic symptom. A hallmark sign is when pain intensifies with passive range of motion. Answer 5 is correct because *despite* opioids the pain increases.** **Answer 6** is incorrect because increased intracompartmental pressure decreases circulation, so that fingers distal to the fracture would be cool, not warm.

■ **TEST-TAKING TIP:** *Look for symptoms of* ineffective *circulation.*

Content Area: Adult Health, Musculoskeletal; ***Integrated Process:*** Nursing Process, Analysis; ***Cognitive Level:*** Analysis; ***Client Need/Subneed:*** Physiological Integrity/Physiological Adaptation/Alterations in Body Systems

5. CORRECT ANSWER: 1. Answer 1 is correct because *rectal* medications should be avoided since they pose the risk of trauma to the rectum, which could lead to further infection. A toddler should be able to take Tylenol (acetaminophen) *elixir* for fever. **Answer 2** is incorrect because a child who is neutropenic *should* have limited visitation due to the high risk for infection. **Answer 3** is incorrect because the child is at risk for dehydration and *should* be well hydrated, which may necessitate a fluid bolus. **Answer 4** is incorrect because, although needle punctures of the skin should be avoided in the neutropenic child, granulocyte colony-stimulating factor (G-CSF) is not contraindicated and *is* given to increase the child's white blood cell count.

■ **TEST-TAKING TIP:** *The stem asks for "what order should be questioned." The child with neutropenia who has a fever is at greatest risk for infection. Question any order where the risk for infection outweighs a possible benefit.*

Content Area: Child Health, Hematological; ***Integrated Process:*** Nursing Process, Analysis; ***Cognitive Level:*** Analysis; ***Client Need/Subneed:*** Physiological Integrity/Reduction of Risk Potential/Potential for Alterations in Body Systems

6. CORRECT ANSWER: 1. Answer 1 is correct because acrocyanosis is cyanosis of the fingers and toes, and is a normal finding for the first few hours after delivery. **Answer 2** is incorrect because absence of tone is *not a normal* finding. A floppy baby at 1 minute of age may be indicative of depression after delivery. **Answer 3** is incorrect because icteric skin, also referred to as jaundice, is *not a normal* finding *immediately* after delivery. **Answer 4** is incorrect because an apical pulse of 100 is *bradycardia* and *not* a *normal* finding at 1 minute of age.

■ **TEST-TAKING TIP:** *Eliminate the obvious* abnormal *findings in a 1-minute-old infant: absence of tone, icteric skin, and bradycardia.*

Content Area: Child Health, Newborn; ***Integrated Process:*** Nursing Process, Assessment; ***Cognitive Level:*** Application; ***Client Need/Subneed:*** Health Promotion and Maintenance/Ante/Intra/Postpartum and Newborn Care

7. CORRECT ANSWERS: 3, 6. **Answer 1** is incorrect because there is *no* risk of seizures with hyperthyroidism. **Answer 2** is incorrect because the client is *NPO* to prevent potential vomiting and aspiration during surgery. **Answer 3 is correct because prolonged NPO status will increase dryness of the mouth. Oral care increases client comfort.** **Answer 4** is incorrect because a cleansing enema is required *only* for *GI* surgery. **Answer 5** is incorrect because Chvostek's sign occurs with *hypocalcemia, not* hyperthyroidism. Postoperatively this would be part of the assessment. **Answer 6 is correct because hyperthyroidism may cause exophthalmos and drops would be soothing.**

■ **TEST-TAKING TIP:** *Think about client comfort measures during the wait.*

Content Area: Adult Health, Endocrine; ***Integrated Process:*** Nursing Process, Implementation; ***Cognitive Level:*** Analysis; ***Client Need/Subneed:*** Physiological Integrity/Basic Care and Comfort/Personal Hygiene

8. CORRECT ANSWER: 4. **Answer 1** is incorrect because a smaller and shorter penis is called a *micropenis.* **Answer 2** is incorrect because absence of a urethral opening is *not* a hypospadias. **Answer 3** is incorrect because, when the urethra is open on the dorsal side of the penis, it is called an *epispadias.* **Answer 4 is correct because a hypospadias is when the urethra opens on the ventral side of the penis.**

■ **TEST-TAKING TIP:** *Focus on the two options that are similar and remember the difference between the dorsal and ventral; picture the hypospadias and choose that location (ventral).*

Content Area: Child Health, Newborn; ***Integrated Process:*** Nursing Process, Implementation; ***Cognitive Level:*** Comprehension; ***Client Need/Subneed:*** Physiological Integrity/Physiological Adaptation/Pathophysiology

9. CORRECT ANSWER: 3. **Answer 1** is incorrect because dietary changes such as decreasing fats and increasing fruits *may* reduce symptoms. Reducing meat and dairy intake decreases hormone stimulation. **Answer 2** is incorrect because zinc has been shown to delay the development of BPH, but not reverse or manage the symptoms. **Answer 3 is correct because saw palmetto has been shown to improve urine flow by blocking the ability of dihydrotestosterone (DHT) to stimulate prostate cell growth.** **Answer 4** is incorrect because vitamin E has *not* been shown to reduce the size.

■ **TEST-TAKING TIP:** *Review the nutritional therapies for BPH.*

Content Area: Adult Health, Genitourinary; ***Integrated Process:*** Communication and Documentation; ***Cognitive Level:*** Application; ***Client Need/Subneed:*** Health Promotion and Maintenance/Health and Wellness

10. CORRECT ANSWER: 2. **Answer 1** is incorrect because this client is a multipara and is very close to delivery. Administration of IV pain relief is not a priority, and is *not* appropriate *immediately before* delivery. **Answer 2 is correct because this client is a multipara and is very close to delivery. Preparing the client for delivery is the most important nursing action at this time.** **Answer 3** is incorrect because there are no risk factors or problems that indicate that this client needs a fluid bolus. **Answer 4** is incorrect because there is *no* indication for placing this client in knee-chest position. This position is used for *cord prolapse, not* for delivery.

■ TEST-TAKING TIP: *The most important factor to consider is the* **number of previous** *deliveries. If the client is having her first baby, the priorities may be different than with the third baby. Clients who are multiparous usually deliver more quickly than the clients who are primigravida.*

Content Area: Maternity, Intrapartum; ***Integrated Process:*** Nursing Process, Implementation; ***Cognitive Level:*** Application; ***Client Need/Subneed:*** Health Promotion and Maintenance/ Ante/Intra/Postpartum and Newborn Care

11. CORRECT ANSWER: 3. **Answer 1** is incorrect because oral contraceptives may not be the best choice for this client. This response has nothing to do with indicating that teaching has been correct. Teaching should include information that taking oral contraceptives increases the chance of blood clots, which can be life-threatening. **Answer 2** is incorrect because most women do *not* stop taking oral contraceptives due to nausea. The nausea is usually not severe enough to cause women to stop taking the contraceptive. **Answer 3 is correct because oral contraceptives do inhibit ovulation and change the consistency of cervical mucus. The hormones prevent ovulation and affect the color and consistency of cervical mucus.** **Answer 4** is incorrect because oral contraceptives *suppress* ovulation. The basal body temperature is *not* an indicator of ovulation when a woman is taking *oral* contraceptives, and cannot be used to increase the effectiveness of oral contraceptives.

■ TEST-TAKING TIP: *Teaching a client that a particular contraceptive is the best choice is* **not therapeutic or appropriate.** *Look for the option that gives the current information about the effects of the drug, not incorrect information (Answers 2 and 4).*

Content Area: Women's Health, Family Planning; ***Integrated Process:*** Teaching and Learning; ***Cognitive Level:*** Application; ***Client Need/Subneed:*** Health Promotion and Maintenance/ Lifestyle Choices

12. CORRECT ANSWER: 1. **Answer 1 is correct because right sacrum anterior (RSA) means that the fetal sacrum is closest to the mother's symphysis and rotated slightly to the mother's right; therefore, the heart tones would be loudest in the upper right quadrant.** **Answer 2** is incorrect because a right occipital anterior presentation would have loudest fetal heart tones in the *lower right* quadrant. **Answer 3** is incorrect because in a left sacrum anterior presentation the fetal sacrum is closest to the mother's symphysis and rotated slightly to the *mother's left;* therefore, the heart tones would be loudest in the *upper left* quadrant. **Answer 4** is incorrect because a left occipital transverse presentation would have loudest fetal heart tones in the *lower left* quadrant.

■ TEST-TAKING TIP: *Divide the maternal abdomen into four quadrants. Hearing the heart tones loudest in the upper quadrant is usually associated with breech presentation; note the word "sacrum."*

Content Area: Maternity, Intrapartum; ***Integrated Process:*** Nursing Process, Assessment; ***Cognitive Level:*** Application; ***Client Need/Subneed:*** Health Promotion and Maintenance/ Ante/Intra/Postpartum and Newborn Care

13. CORRECT ANSWERS: 2, 5. **Answer 1** is incorrect because the failing heart cannot maintain a normal cardiac output and the pulse pressure narrows, not widens. Hypotension is one of the three classic indications of cardiac tamponade called *Beck's triad.* **Answer 2 is correct because increased intracardiac pressure causes impaired filling of the right atrium, resulting in JVD. JVD is one of the three indicators of cardiac tamponade known as Beck's triad.** **Answer 3** is incorrect because contractility is hindered, and heart sounds are *muffled* from the fluid in the pericardium, not loud. **Answer 4** is incorrect because the impaired cardiac contractility diminishes cardiac output. **Answer 5 is correct because muffled heart sounds occur due to fluid inside the pericardium. Muffled heart sounds are one of the three indicators of cardiac tamponade known as Beck's triad.**

■ TEST-TAKING TIP: *Correct options describe cardiac compromise and* Beck's triad*—JVD, muffled heart sounds, and hypotension.*

Content Area: Adult Health, Cardiovascular; ***Integrated Process:*** Nursing Process, Assessment; ***Cognitive Level:*** Application; ***Client Need/Subneed:*** Physiological Integrity/Physiological Adaptation/Pathophysiology

14. CORRECT ANSWER: 2. **Answer 1** is incorrect because expressed breast milk or lanolin *can* be used to relieve pain of sore nipples. **Answer 2 is correct because babies who are breastfed should be on a *demand* schedule, feeding an average of 8 to 12 times in a 24-hour period.** **Answer 3** is incorrect because avoiding a pacifier during the first 4 to 6 weeks while breastfeeding is being established *helps* to avoid nipple confusion and prevent reinforcing non-nutritive sucking. **Answer 4** is incorrect because wearing a supportive bra *helps* reduce pain associated with engorgement.

■ TEST-TAKING TIP: *This question is asking which of the options is* **not a correct statement.** *Restate the question to answer the question correctly.*

Content Area: Maternity, Antepartum; ***Integrated Process:*** Nursing Process, Evaluation; ***Cognitive Level:*** Analysis; ***Client Need/Subneed:*** Health Promotion and Maintenance/ Ante/Intra/Postpartum and Newborn Care

15. CORRECT ANSWER: 4. **Answer 1** is incorrect because gastric acid *lost* from vomiting will cause metabolic *alkalosis.* **Answer 2** is incorrect because gastric acid is lost with nasogastric suctioning and metabolic alkalosis will result. **Answer 3** is incorrect because hyperventilation either would cause respiratory alkalosis (CO_2 below 35), or would be the compensatory response to a metabolic acidosis—not the cause. **Answer 4 is correct because acetylsalicylic acid (ASA) is an acid compound.**

■ TEST-TAKING TIP: *Look for an option that adds acid to the body.*

Content Area: Adult Health, Fluid and Electrolyte Imbalances; *Integrated Process:* Nursing Process, Analysis; *Cognitive Level:* Application; *Client Need/Subneed:* Physiological Integrity/ Physiological Adaptation/Fluid and Electrolyte Imbalances

16. CORRECT ANSWERS: 4, 5. **Answer 1** is incorrect because the parents should be made aware of the religious resources available, allowing them to choose when and if they would like this kind of assistance. **Answer 2** is incorrect because siblings should be permitted to see the child who has died if they want to. A nurse should refer the parents to the Child Life Specialist, who is an excellent resource for understanding child bereavement. **Answer 3** is incorrect because, although an autopsy will be conducted, describing the child's death as suspicious at this time may be hurtful to parents. **Answer 4 is correct because parents should be allowed to grieve in privacy, allowing visitors at their own discretion. Answer 5 is correct because parents may have additional needs once they return home. They may not be able to process or remember verbal information given in the hospital.** **Answer 6** is incorrect because parents may want to and should be encouraged to talk to and touch the child who has died.

■ TEST-TAKING TIP: *Note the time frame in the stem of the question: "just died."*

Content Area: Child Health, End-of-life; *Integrated Process:* Nursing Process, Implementation; *Cognitive Level:* Application; *Client Need/Subneed:* Psychosocial Integrity/End-of-Life Care

17. CORRECT ANSWER: 2. **Answer 1** is incorrect because *rectal* medications should be *avoided* when the client has a fourth-degree laceration. **Answer 2 is correct because having a bowel movement can be painful after a fourth-degree laceration. Docusate sodium is a stool softener that can make the bowel movements less painful.** **Answer 3** is incorrect because methylergonovine maleate is a drug used for controlling *postpartum hemorrhage,* and has *nothing* to do with fourth-degree lacerations. **Answer 4** is incorrect because carboprost tromethamine is a drug used for controlling postpartum hemorrhage, and has *nothing* to do with fourth-degree lacerations.

■ TEST-TAKING TIP: *Two of the medications are used for postpartum hemorrhage, not for treating fourth-degree lacerations. Eliminate those options because both drugs have similar uses, and therefore cannot be the correct answer.*

Content Area: Maternity, Postpartum; *Integrated Process:* Nursing Process, Implementation; *Cognitive Level:* Application; *Client Need/Subneed:* Physiological Integrity/Basic Care and Comfort/Elimination

18. CORRECT ANSWER: 1. **Answer 1 is correct because the ABGs show respiratory acidosis (pH below 7.35 and CO_2 above 45), which would be decreased with effective deep breathing.** **Answer 2** is incorrect because, with a rebreather mask, the client rebreathes CO_2, increasing the CO_2 level even more. **Answer 3** is incorrect because the respiratory acidosis may be due to hypoventilation and a decreased respiratory rate. Slowing the respiratory rate would not be desirable. **Answer 4** is incorrect because IV sodium bicarbonate is *not indicated* for respiratory acidosis. Increasing the pH does not correct the respiratory problem. Drugs that improve breathing would be indicated.

■ TEST-TAKING TIP: *Choose an option that will "blow off" CO_2.*

Content Area: Adult Health, Acid-Base Balance; *Integrated Process:* Nursing Process, Analysis; *Cognitive Level:* Analysis; *Client Need/Subneed:* Physiological Integrity/Physiological Adaptation/Fluid and Electrolyte Imbalances

19. CORRECT ANSWER: 1. **Answer 1 is correct because the client's attitude about the pregnancy is the primary concern during the first trimester. Plans for termination or continuation of the pregnancy should be discussed to provide anticipatory guidance for this client.** **Answer 2** is incorrect because birth control methods are *not* the *primary* concern for this client during the first trimester of pregnancy. **Answer 3** is incorrect because the client's feeling about future pregnancies is *not the primary* concern for this *adolescent* client during the first trimester of pregnancy. **Answer 4** is incorrect because the client's knowledge of the symptoms of preterm labor is important during the *second* and *third* trimester, *not* during the first trimester.

■ TEST-TAKING TIP: *The key concept in this question is the* first trimester. *The first trimester consideration is mainly how the client is feeling about the* pregnancy. *Because she can choose to terminate the pregnancy, her feelings about the pregnancy and plans for the pregnancy are the primary concerns.*

Content Area: Maternity, Antepartum; *Integrated Process:* Nursing Process, Assessment; *Cognitive Level:* Application; *Client Need/Subneed:* Health Promotion and Maintenance/ Ante/Intra/Postpartum and Newborn Care

20. CORRECT ANSWER: 2. **Answer 1** is incorrect because the pH is within normal limits, which indicates compensation. **Answer 2 is correct because the pH is within normal limits, which reflects compensation. The body never overcompensates; therefore, the problem is an alkalosis because the pH is on the alkaline side of 7.4 and the CO_2 is low.** **Answer 3** is incorrect because the pH is within normal limits, which indicates compensation. **Answer 4** is incorrect because the pH shows compensation for an alkalosis problem, *not* acidosis. ABG values in the stem of the question show a respiratory problem because the CO_2 is low. If it were a metabolic problem, the HCO_3 would be above 26.

■ TEST-TAKING TIP: *Remember that the body never overcorrects when the pH returns from an acidosis or alkalosis. Interpret pH first.*

Content Area: Adult Health, Acid-Base; *Integrated Process:* Nursing Process, Analysis; *Cognitive Level:* Application; *Client Need/Subneed:* Physiological Integrity/Physiological Adaptation/Fluid and Electrolyte Imbalances

21. CORRECT ANSWER: 4. **Answer 1** is incorrect because there is *nothing* in the question that indicates a need for an emergency cesarean section. The second stage of labor is from complete dilation to delivery of the neonate. **Answer 2** is incorrect because administering oxytocin IM is appropriate *after delivery of the placenta* to contract the uterus and decrease bleeding. **Answer 3** is incorrect because administering a large dose of misoprostol rectally is appropriate *after delivery of the placenta to control postpartum hemorrhage.* **Answer 4 is correct because the second stage of labor is the pushing stage, and a client who is a multipara usually delivers without a long second stage. The nurse should notify the physician of the results of the cervical examination and the need for the physician to come for delivery.**

■ TEST-TAKING TIP: *Remember the four stages of labor and the three phases of the first stage of labor. The important consideration is that the client is a multipara, and the second stage is usually shortened.*

Content Area: Maternity, Intrapartum; *Integrated Process:* Nursing Process, Implementation; *Cognitive Level:* Application; *Client Need/Subneed:* Health Promotion and Maintenance/ Ante/Intra/Postpartum and Newborn Care

22. CORRECT ANSWER: 4. **Answer 1** is incorrect because the second dose, although ordered, does not treat the presurgical anxiety. **Answer 2** is incorrect because the client may be NPO. **Answer 3** is incorrect because the question asks for a priority. Although not incorrect, this option does not address the suspected anxiety. **Answer 4 is correct because, given the data, presurgical anxiety is suspected. The client needs an opportunity to talk about concerns related to surgery before further actions (which may mask the anxiety) are taken.**

■ TEST-TAKING TIP: *Look for patterns—only one answer explores feelings about surgery.*

Content Area: Mental Health, Anxiety; *Integrated Process:* Nursing Process, Analysis; *Cognitive Level:* Application; *Client Need/Subneed:* Psychosocial Integrity/Stress Management

23. CORRECT ANSWER: 1. **Answer 1 is correct because Rh_0(D) immune globulin contains anti-Rh antibodies that work by destroying the fetal blood cells in the mother's blood before her body can react to them, inactivating the fetal antigens.** **Answer 2** is incorrect because Rh_0(D) immune globulin prevents formation of Rh *antibodies, not* the antigens. The fetal red blood cells contain the antigens; the mother's body develops antibodies to those antigens if Rh_0(D) immune globulin is not given. **Answer 3** is incorrect because Rh_0(D) immune globulin does *not* provide immunity. There is no immunity that develops to the fetal antigens. **Answer 4** is incorrect because Rh_0(D) immune globulin does not convert the client's blood from negative to positive. It is not possible to change the Rh factor from negative to positive.

■ TEST-TAKING TIP: *Remember the difference between an antigen and an antibody. The fetal red blood cells contain antigens; the mother's body will develop antibodies against the exposure to the antigen.*

Content Area: Maternity, Postpartum; *Integrated Process:* Nursing Process, Analysis; *Cognitive Level:* Application; *Client Need/Subneed:* Physiological Integrity/Pharmacological and Parenteral Therapies/Expected Effects/Outcomes

24. CORRECT ANSWER: 2. **Answer 1** is incorrect because hydration *alone* is not the correct action. An insulin drip is needed. **Answer 2 is correct because the client needs insulin and fluids to correct the hyperglycemia (serum glucose of 620 mg/dL) and dehydration that occurs with diabetic ketoacidosis (DKA).** **Answer 3** is incorrect because the rapid respirations are compensation for the metabolic acidosis (Kussmaul's breathing). The respirations will slow as the diabetic ketoacidosis is corrected. **Answer 4** is incorrect because the *first* action is an *insulin* drip and *hydration.* IV bicarbonate may be given for severe acidosis, but the pH is not known here.

■ TEST-TAKING TIP: *Recognize the characteristic signs and symptoms of diabetic ketoacidosis.*

Content Area: Adult Health, Endocrine; *Integrated Process:* Nursing Process, Analysis; *Cognitive Level:* Analysis; *Client Need/Subneed:* Physiological Integrity/Physiological Adaptation/Medical Emergencies

25. CORRECT ANSWER: 4. **Answer 1** is incorrect because scrotal rugae do not develop until after about *37 weeks* of gestation. They would not be present at 33 weeks' gestation. **Answer 2** is incorrect because mongolian spots are not commonly found in neonates who are Caucasian; however, they are frequently found in neonates who are darker skinned. **Answer 3** is incorrect because desquamation is found when the vernix has absorbed and the skin begins to peel, usually indicative of a *postmature* neonate. **Answer 4 is correct because vernix caseosa is very apparent in a preterm fetus at 33 weeks' gestation.**

■ TEST-TAKING TIP: *There are two key points: a neonate who is male and 33 weeks' gestation. Eliminate the options that are not found in an infant who is preterm or an infant who is Caucasian. The preterm rupture and fever have nothing to do with the options and are, therefore, distracters.*

Content Area: Maternity, Postpartum; *Integrated Process:* Nursing Process, Assessment; *Cognitive Level:* Application; *Client Need/Subneed:* Health Promotion and Maintenance/ Ante/Intra/Postpartum and Newborn Care

26. CORRECT ANSWER: 3. **Answer 1** is incorrect because with stage I there are only *superficial* changes in the skin. **Answer 2** is incorrect because a stage II pressure ulcer is *confined* to the *top* layer of the skin. **Answer 3 is correct because a stage III pressure ulcer extends past the top layer of the skin.** **Answer 4** is incorrect because a stage IV pressure ulcer extends into the *muscle* and bone.

■ **TEST-TAKING TIP:** *Eliminate the two extremes: I and IV—from the superficial layer to the deepest layer affected. Decide whether it affects the top layer or past the top layer.*

Content Area: Adult Health, Integumentary; *Integrated Process:* Nursing Process. Analysis; *Cognitive Level:* Application; *Client Need/Subneed:* Physiological Integrity/Physiological Adaptation/Alterations in Body Systems

27. CORRECT ANSWER: 4. **Answer 1** is incorrect because teenagers respond better to peers than adults. **Answer 2** is incorrect because creating the brochures does not ensure their distribution to the target audience. Teenagers are also not likely to believe that they are at risk despite the statistical evidence. **Answer 3** is incorrect because simply telling teenagers not to use smokeless tobacco is not likely to be effective. Adolescents have a strong need to be independent with little desire to follow health-care directives given by adults. **Answer 4 is correct because the posters would demonstrate how smokeless tobacco use can affect an individual's appearance as well as cause serious health complications. Additionally, the posters would be visible for a sustained period of time.**

■ **TEST-TAKING TIP:** *Recall that teenagers are most concerned with how they* appear *to others, especially their peer group. Prevention efforts that emphasize the effects on* physical appearance *are likely to be more effective than those that discuss potential long-term health consequences. Reading (Answers 2 and 3) and hearing (Answer 1) are not as effective as seeing an image (Answer 4).*

Content Area: Child Health, Respiratory; *Integrated Process:* Nursing Process, Planning; *Cognitive Level:* Analysis; *Client Need/Subneed:* Health Promotion and Maintenance/ Principles of Teaching and Learning

28. CORRECT ANSWER: 3. **Answer 1** is incorrect because low blood glucose is *not* one of the parameters for Apgar scoring. **Answer 2** is incorrect because bradycardia would be a *one-* or *two-point* deduction in the Apgar scoring, *in addition* to the subtraction of a point for the acrocyanosis, leaving a *7* or *8 Apgar* score. **Answer 3 is correct because acrocyanosis (blue color of hands and feet in most infants usually for the first few hours after birth) is a normal finding for a neonate at 5 minutes of age. The acrocyanosis would lead to subtracting a point from the Apgar score. An Apgar score of 9 at 5 minutes is normal in a healthy neonate.** **Answer 4** is incorrect because decreased tone would *subtract a point in addition* to the presence of acrocyanosis, giving an *8 Apgar* score at 5 minutes.

■ **TEST-TAKING TIP:** *Even though 10 is the highest Apgar score, the acrocyanosis effectively makes 9 the best score for a neonate. Note that three of the options are ↓: blood glucose (low), heart rate (*brady*), tone (decreased). Choose the option that is different, that is, not "low."*

Content Area: Child Health, Newborn; *Integrated Process:* Nursing Process, Assessment; *Cognitive Level:* Application; *Client Need/Subneed:* Health Promotion and Maintenance/ Ante/Intra/Postpartum and Newborn Care

29. CORRECT ANSWERS: 1, 4, 5. Answer 1 is correct because untreated hypertension increases the risk of stroke. **Answer 2** is incorrect because elevated *creatinine* levels indicate renal dysfunction, *not* blood urea nitrogen (BUN). **Answer 3** is incorrect because an increase in systemic blood pressure does *not* cause glaucoma, which is related to increased intraocular pressure, *not* blood pressure. **Answer 4 is correct because left ventricular hypertrophy indicates prolonged or untreated hypertension. Answer 5 is correct because hypertension increases the risk of peripheral arterial disease.**

■ **TEST-TAKING TIP:** *Look for* cardiovascular *complications.*

Content Area: Adult Health, Cardiovascular; *Integrated Process:* Nursing Process, Analysis; *Cognitive Level:* Analysis; *Client Need/Subneed:* Physiological Integrity/Physiological Adaptation/Pathophysiology

30. CORRECT ANSWER: 3. **Answer 1** is incorrect because an *amniocentesis* is required to check fetal lung maturity, using analysis of amniotic fluid. Fetal monitoring *cannot* determine lung maturity. **Answer 2** is incorrect because the purpose of a CST is to check the fetal oxygen reserve. A *daily fetal kick count* is used to measure the fetal activity. **Answer 3 is correct because the test uses a fetal monitor to watch the baby's response to contractions. A healthy fetus in good condition will tolerate the mild stress caused by contractions without difficulty. However, a fetus who is getting barely enough oxygen may have late decelerations, where the baby's heart slows down from the stress of the contraction, then recovers back to baseline after a few moments. In this way, a CST is able to check fetal oxygen reserve.** **Answer 4** is incorrect because an *ultrasound* is required to measure the amniotic fluid; fetal monitoring *cannot* determine amniotic fluid volume.

■ **TEST-TAKING TIP:** *Electronic fetal monitoring can only determine fetal well-being; it cannot evaluate amniotic fluid or lung development. Eliminate those options that cannot evaluate fetal monitoring.*

Content Area: Maternity, Antepartum; *Integrated Process:* Nursing Process, Analysis; *Cognitive Level:* Application; *Client Need/Subneed:* Physiological Integrity/Reduction of Risk Potential/Diagnostic Tests

31. CORRECT ANSWER: 3. **Answer 1** is incorrect because clients with diabetes *do* need to test their glucose more often when ill. **Answer 2** is incorrect because diabetes leads to peripheral neuropathies and diminished sensation in the feet. People with diabetes may not be aware of injury to the feet. **Answer 3 is correct because the goal for the $HgbA_{1c}$ is less than 7.0.** **Answer 4** is incorrect because weight loss *has* been shown to *decrease* the need for insulin.

■ **TEST-TAKING TIP:** *Look for an incorrect statement by the client.*

Content Area: Adult Health, Endocrine; *Integrated Process:* Nursing Process, Evaluation; *Cognitive Level:* Analysis; *Client Need/Subneed:* Health Promotion and Maintenance/Self-care

32. CORRECT ANSWER: 3. **Answer 1** is incorrect because a simian crease is a *normal* finding in a neonate with Down syndrome, and does *not* need to be reported to the physician. **Answer 2** is incorrect because brachycephaly is a *normal* finding in a neonate with Down syndrome, and does *not* need to be reported to the physician. **Answer 3 is correct because cyanosis after feeding may be indicative of a heart defect. Since heart defects are common in neonates with Down syndrome, it needs to be reported immediately to the physician.** **Answer 4** is incorrect because hypotonicity is a *normal* finding in a neonate with Down syndrome, and does *not* need to be reported to the physician.

■ **TEST-TAKING TIP:** *Restate the question: Which option is not a normal finding in Down syndrome? Any cyanosis, other than acrocyanosis, should be reported immediately to the physician.*

Content Area: Child Health, Newborn; *Integrated Process:* Nursing Process, Assessment; *Cognitive Level:* Application; *Client Need/Subneed:* Physiological Integrity/Physiological Adaptation/Alterations in Body Systems

33. CORRECT ANSWER: 1. **Answer 1 is correct because clomiphene citrate may result in multiple births (e.g., twins, triplets) due to the stimulation of ovulation, when more than one egg may be released and fertilized.** **Answer 2** is incorrect because clomiphene citrate stimulates *ovulation;* it does *not* result in an *increased risk of miscarriage.* **Answer 3** is incorrect because clomiphene citrate stimulates ovulation; it does *not* have an effect on the incidence of *spontaneous trisomy* 21. **Answer 4** is incorrect because clomiphene citrate *must not* be used during pregnancy.

■ **TEST-TAKING TIP:** *Drugs used for fertility treatments have an increased risk of multiple gestation. Eliminate the options that suggest the drugs increase the chance of teratogenic effects (e.g., miscarriage, trisomy 21).*

Content Area: Women's Health, Family Planning; *Integrated Process:* Nursing Process, Evaluation; *Cognitive Level:* Analysis; *Client Need/Subneed:* Physiological Integrity/Pharmacological and Parenteral Therapies/Expected Effects/Outcomes

34. CORRECT ANSWER: 3. **Answer 1** is incorrect because checking heel stick blood sugar is the first intervention. Further interventions may be necessary, but administering a bolus of 50 grams of glucose would *not* be the *proper* dosage. The correct dose is 0.20 grams of glucose/kg (i.e., 2 mL/kg) of IV 10% glucose, given over 1 to 2 minutes. **Answer 2** is incorrect because checking heel stick blood sugar is the first intervention. Based on the results, formula feeding may be necessary, but not necessarily started immediately after birth. The neonate may be able to breastfeed first, depending on the blood sugar. **Answer 3 is correct because checking heel stick blood sugar is the first intervention. Based on the results, further interventions may be necessary. Specific intervention will depend on the blood sugar value.** **Answer 4** is incorrect because neonates of clients with diabetes experience hypoglycemia, and administering insulin would make hypoglycemia worse.

■ **TEST-TAKING TIP:** *Remember: if a client has diabetes, the increased blood sugar in the mother triggers increased insulin production in the fetus, and the neonate will be hypoglycemic after birth. Select a* data-gathering *type of intervention (Answer 3) before an* implementation *option, even if the dosage in Answer 1 were correctly stated (which it wasn't).*

Content Area: Child Health, Newborn; *Integrated Process:* Nursing Process, Implementation; *Cognitive Level:* Application; *Client Need/Subneed:* Physiological Integrity/Reduction of Risk Potential/Diagnostic Tests

35. CORRECT ANSWERS: 1, 2, 4, 5. **Answer 1 is correct because delirium may be related to the use of vasoactive drugs.** **Answer 2 is correct because delirium may be caused by a combination of factors, including sensory deprivation from the restriction of familiar visitors.** **Answer 3** is incorrect because the hallucinations are a *symptom, not* the cause. **Answer 4 is correct because delirium can be related to major surgery.** **Answer 5 is correct because delirium may occur from sleep deprivation and sensory overload.**

■ **TEST-TAKING TIP:** *Choose causes, not symptoms.*

Content Area: Adult Health, Neurological; *Integrated Process:* Nursing Process, Analysis; *Cognitive Level:* Application; *Client Need/Subneed:* Physiological Integrity/Physiological Adaptation/Alterations in Body Systems

36. CORRECT ANSWER: 3. **Answer 1** is incorrect because birth weight of 4,000 to 4,500 grams is considered *macrosomia* and *large* for gestational age, *not* a *normal* finding in a 39-week-gestation neonate. **Answer 2** is incorrect because weight gain of 5% to 10% in an infant who is exclusively breastfed is *not* a normal finding. Neonates usually lose 5% to 10% of their birth weight and regain it by 2 weeks after birth. **Answer 3 is correct because weight loss of 5% to 10% from birth weight is normal for neonates the first few days after birth, *not* weight gain.** **Answer 4** is incorrect because birth weight of 2,000 to 2,500 grams is considered *small* for gestational age, *not* a normal finding in a 39-week-gestation neonate.

■ **TEST-TAKING TIP:** *Know the normal range of weight at birth for a full-term infant as well as the parameters for small and large for gestational age. Is it weight gain or weight loss? Breastfed neonates* lose *about 5% to 10% of their birth weight.*

Content Area: Child Health, Newborn; *Integrated Process:* Nursing Process, Assessment; *Cognitive Level:* Application; *Client Need/Subneed:* Health Promotion and Maintenance/Ante/Intra/Postpartum and Newborn Care

37. CORRECT ANSWER: 2. Answer 1 is incorrect because these symptoms would be indicative of *anemia.* **Answer 2 is correct because antifungal agents can cause liver damage, which results in obvious jaundice and the disruption of normal bile flow. Answer 3** is incorrect because blood in the urine would indicate a *bladder* or *kidney* problem, which is *not* a side effect of these drugs. **Answer 4** is incorrect because ototoxicity more often occurs from *other* antituberculosis drugs in the aminoglycoside classification (e.g., streptomycin), although ototoxicity can occur from isoniazid or rifampin.

■ **TEST-TAKING TIP:** ***Recognize expected outcomes of therapy, including serious side effects.***

Content Area: Adult Health, Infectious Disease; ***Integrated Process:*** Nursing Process, Assessment; ***Cognitive Level:*** Application; ***Client Need/Subneed:*** Physiological Integrity/Pharmacological and Parenteral Therapies/Adverse Effects/Contraindications/Interactions

38. CORRECT ANSWERS: 1, 3, 6. Answer 1 is correct because often the first symptoms are behavioral changes such as lethargy, confusion, and combativeness. Answer 2 is incorrect because the administration of acetylsalicylic acid (aspirin) during viral illness, *not* acetaminophen (Tylenol), is associated with Reye syndrome. **Answer 3 is correct because coma is a late symptom of Reye syndrome. Answer 4** is incorrect because the child with Reye syndrome is likely to experience *elevated* partial thromboplastin time (PTT) as a result of liver damage. **Answer 5** is incorrect because intracranial pressure *increases* during Reye syndrome. **Answer 6 is correct because the syndrome does not occur unless the child first has a viral illness.**

■ **TEST-TAKING TIP:** ***When answering this question, categorize symptoms as early or late, and then break it down further by looking at which symptom precedes another.***

Content Area: Child Health, Neurological; ***Integrated Process:*** Nursing Process, Analysis; ***Cognitive Level:*** Analysis; ***Client Need/Subneed:*** Physiological Integrity/Physiological Adaptation/Pathophysiology

39. CORRECT ANSWER: 3. Answer 1 is incorrect because, although a positive pregnancy test and shoulder pain would be consistent with ectopic pregnancy, *copious vaginal bleeding* would *not* be a sign of ectopic pregnancy; it would be a sign of *spontaneous abortion.* **Answer 2** is incorrect because hyperemesis, hypertension, and moderate vaginal bleeding would be signs of a *hydatidiform mole, not* ectopic pregnancy. **Answer 3 is correct because amenorrhea is a possible sign of pregnancy, abdominal pain can be a sign of tubal pregnancy, and hypotension can be a sign of internal bleeding as a result of a ruptured ectopic pregnancy. Answer 4** is incorrect because copious vaginal discharge, weight loss, and positive pregnancy test would be consistent with *first-trimester* pregnancy, *not* ectopic pregnancy.

■ **TEST-TAKING TIP:** ***Ectopic pregnancy symptoms also include signs of shock due to internal bleeding with decreased blood pressure and increased heart rate.***

Content Area: Maternity, Antepartum; ***Integrated Process:*** Nursing Process, Assessment; ***Cognitive Level:*** Application; ***Client Need/Subneed:*** Physiological Integrity/Physiological Adaptation/Alterations in Body Systems

40. CORRECT ANSWER: 1. Answer 1 is correct because the presenting symptoms are vague and "flu-like." Initially, they are nagging and less acute. Answer 2 is incorrect because weight gain and purulent sputum are *not* characteristic of active tuberculosis (although cough would be a presenting symptom). **Answer 3** is incorrect because the high fever would likely be associated with a more acute condition (although cough would be a tempting choice). **Answer 4** is incorrect because the headache and nosebleed cannot be linked to the disease pathology.

■ **TEST-TAKING TIP:** ***The key word is*** **often**—***three of the choices have incorrect signs and symptoms (purulent sputum, high fever, nosebleed).***

Content Area: Adult Health, Infectious Disease; ***Integrated Process:*** Nursing Process, Assessment; ***Cognitive Level:*** Application; ***Client Need/Subneed:*** Physiological Integrity/Physiological Adaptation/Pathophysiology

41. CORRECT ANSWER: 4. Answer 1 is incorrect because a tight-fitting bra can increase pain and blockage of milk ducts. A *loose-fitting* bra or no bra would relieve the pressure on the affected area. **Answer 2** is incorrect because there is *no reason to stop* breastfeeding and it can actually makes the mastitis worse, leading to an abscess that may need to be surgically drained. **Answer 3** is incorrect because not feeding on the affected side would actually make the mastitis *worse,* leading to an abscess that may need to be surgically drained. **Answer 4 is correct because acetaminophen and/or ibuprofen are safe to take while breastfeeding. *Unrelieved* pain not only decreases the ability to produce milk, but suppresses the body's ability to fight infection.**

■ **TEST-TAKING TIP:** ***Mastitis treatment is the same as that for engorgement, only more urgent. Consider the same interventions as for engorgement. Eliminate two of the options (Answers 2 and 3) that "stop" or "avoid" breastfeeding.***

Content Area: Maternity, Postpartum; ***Integrated Process:*** Teaching and Learning; ***Cognitive Level:*** Application; ***Client Need/Subneed:*** Physiological Integrity/Physiological Adaptation/Alterations in Body Systems

42. CORRECT ANSWER: 2. Answer 1 is incorrect because the V/Q abnormality is related to the disease process and *cannot be corrected with* O_2. **Answer 2 is correct because clients with emphysema suffer from chronically high** CO_2 **levels, so the normal** CO_2 **stimulus is ineffective.**

ANSWERS

The stimulus is the low O_2—a hypoxic drive. **Answer 3** is incorrect because it does not answer the question. Supplemental O_2 is not curative; it does make the client feel better, which may be palliative, but the choice of a flow rate is purposeful. **Answer 4** is incorrect because the compensation that occurs in response to respiratory acidosis is a *metabolic* alkalosis.

■ TEST-TAKING TIP: *Selecting the correct answer requires knowing the stimulus to breathe in emphysema. Focus on the one option that states an undesirable effect ("depress the hypoxic drive").*

Content Area: Adult Health, Respiratory; ***Integrated Process:*** Nursing Process, Planning; ***Cognitive Level:*** Application; ***Client Need/Subneed:*** Physiological Integrity/Reduction of Risk Potential/Therapeutic Procedures

43. CORRECT ANSWER: 2. **Answer 1** is incorrect because there are *no* "predictive" signs of pregnancy; it is a made-up term. Answer 2 is correct because presumptive signs/symptoms of pregnancy include: absent menstrual periods (amenorrhea), nausea and/or vomiting ("morning sickness"), unexplained fatigue, the frequent need to urinate, breast tenderness and changes, excessive salivation (ptyalism), skin changes, and a sensation of movement in the abdomen (quickening). **Answer 3** is incorrect because probable signs of pregnancy include: positive pregnancy test (presence of human chorionic gonadotropin detected by blood or urine test); softening of cervix at 6 to 8 weeks (Goodell's sign); bluish coloration of cervix, vagina, and vulva at 6 to 8 weeks (Chadwick's sign); enlarged abdomen; Braxton Hicks contractions; and passive movement of the fetus during an examination (ballottement). **Answer 4** is incorrect because positive signs of pregnancy include: fetal heart sounds heard by Doptone or Doppler, fetus visible on ultrasound, fetal movements felt by caregiver, and fetus visible on x-ray, magnetic resonance imaging (MRI) or other diagnostic imaging device. (Note: X-ray, MRI and other imaging devices are *not* recommended during pregnancy.)

■ TEST-TAKING TIP: *Presumptive signs are the* earliest *signs and symptoms of pregnancy, but some symptoms can be explained by other conditions. Probable signs are usually signs of pregnancy, but may be false or explained by other conditions. Positive signs are those that cannot be explained by any other condition than pregnancy.*

Content Area: Maternity, Antepartum; ***Integrated Process:*** Nursing Process, Analysis; ***Cognitive Level:*** Application; ***Client Need/Subneed:*** Health Promotion and Maintenance/Ante/Intra/Postpartum and Newborn Care

44. CORRECT ANSWER: 1. Answer 1 is correct because the normal frequency, quantity, and characteristics of urine (specific gravity) would be the best choice. (Daily weight would be a better choice, if included.) **Answer 2** is incorrect because the *normal* aging process decreases the amount of water in the skin. **Answer 3** is incorrect because hematocrit (Hct), *not* Hgb, responds to changes in hydration. **Answer 4** is incorrect because elderly clients are likely to have some degree of hypertension, which would make a change in BP *less reliable.*

■ TEST-TAKING TIP: *Select the one* **least** *effected by changes of* **aging.**

Content Area: Geriatrics, Fluid and Electrolyte Imbalances; ***Integrated Process:*** Nursing Process, Assessment; ***Cognitive Level:*** Application; ***Client Need/Subneed:*** Physiological Integrity/Reduction of Risk Potential/System Specific Assessments

45. CORRECT ANSWER: 4. **Answer 1** is incorrect because the fundus does not descend to the level of the symphysis pubis until about *the 10th postpartum day.* **Answer 2** is incorrect because the fundus *immediately after* delivery is contracted to the level halfway between the umbilicus and the symphysis. But by *24 hours* after delivery, the fundus rises to the *level of the umbilicus,* and then decreases about a fingerbreadth per day after delivery. **Answer 3** is incorrect because the xyphoid process is approximately where the fundus is found *before* delivery. Answer 4 is correct because the fundus would be about the level of the umbilicus 24 hours after delivery. It rises up about 1 cm above the umbilicus about 12 hours after delivery. Then at 24 hours after delivery it is back to the level of the umbilicus, and then decreases about a fingerbreadth per day after delivery.

■ TEST-TAKING TIP: *Focus on the anatomical landmarks of the symphysis and the xyphoid process. Eliminate the option that is not consistent with a 24-hours-postdelivery fundus.*

Content Area: Maternity, Postpartum; ***Integrated Process:*** Nursing Process, Assessment; ***Cognitive Level:*** Application; ***Client Need/Subneed:*** Health Promotion and Maintenance/Ante/Intra/Postpartum and Newborn Care

46. CORRECT ANSWER: 1. Answer 1 is correct because there is a sudden onset of severe hypertension (300 mm Hg systolic), headache, and diaphoresis from some stimulus such as a distended bladder or fecal impaction. **Answer 2** is incorrect because the client experiences severe *hypertension.* **Answer 3** is incorrect because the pulse is usually *bradycardic.* **Answer 4** is incorrect because the Cheyne-Stokes pattern is associated with abnormal CO_2-O_2 tensions in the blood or certain neurological conditions.

■ TEST-TAKING TIP: *Look for contradictory options—* **hypo-** *or* **hyper-**. *Know the effect of the autonomic system on vital signs.*

Content Area: Adult Health, Neurological; ***Integrated Process:*** Nursing Process, Assessment; ***Cognitive Level:*** Application; ***Client Need/Subneed:*** Physiological Integrity/Physiological Adaptation/Pathophysiology

47. CORRECT ANSWER: 2. Answer 1 is incorrect because Kegel exercises *do not target* the muscles of the lower *back.* Doing this exercise would *not* help lower back pain. **Answer 2 is correct because the goal of Kegel exercises is to improve muscle tone by strengthening the pubococcygeus muscles of the pelvic floor. This helps the muscles to regain the strength they had before childbirth. Answer 3** is incorrect because Kegel exercises *do not target* the muscles of the *abdomen.* Doing this exercise would *not* help strengthen those muscles. **Answer 4** is incorrect because Kegel exercises *can help* with urinary incontinence, but performing these exercises does *not prevent* urinary retention.

■ **TEST-TAKING TIP:** ***Know which muscles Kegel exercises are designed to strengthen. Exercises are designed to tone and strengthen muscles; therefore, eliminate options that do not address muscle toning or strengthening (Answers 1 and 4). Eliminate Answer 3 because it focuses on abdominal, rather than pubococcygeus, muscles.***

Content Area: Maternity, Postpartum; ***Integrated Process:*** Teaching and Learning; ***Cognitive Level:*** Application; ***Client Need/Subneed:*** Health Promotion and Maintenance/ Health and Wellness

48. CORRECT ANSWER: 2. Answer 1 is incorrect because cranial nerve XII is not in close proximity to the carotid artery. **Answer 2 is correct because the vagus nerve (cranial nerve X) can be damaged during surgical retraction. Other complications include hemorrhage and neurological impairment. Answer 3** is incorrect because any compression or swelling that may occur would most likely be due to interstitial edema from trauma, not lymph node enlargement. **Answer 4** is incorrect because visual damage would be associated with damage to cranial nerve II, III, IV, or VI; none of these cranial nerves is affected by the procedure.

■ **TEST-TAKING TIP:** ***Use the process of elimination and consider how close the surgical site is to the area damaged.***

Content Area: Adult Health, Vascular; ***Integrated Process:*** Nursing Process, Analysis; ***Cognitive Level:*** Application; ***Client Need/Subneed:*** Physiological Integrity/Reduction of Risk Potential/Potential for Complications from Surgical Procedures and Health Alterations

49. CORRECT ANSWER: 3. Answer 1 is incorrect because having a toddler watch a video of what is about to happen may increase the child's anxiety, especially when the video shows the needle. **Answer 2** is incorrect because children should be given permission to cry if they want to. It is more helpful to tell children that they should hold still but can cry if desired. **Answer 3 is correct because a toddler would best respond to the nurse who allows a choice of injection sites. Giving the child a choice provides a sense of control during this stressful situation. Answer 4** is incorrect because discussing the procedure the night before may increase the child's anxiety and cause the child to resist going to the immunization clinic the day of the procedure.

■ **TEST-TAKING TIP:** ***The growth and development stage of a toddler calls for the development of autonomy. By allowing options when they are available, the toddler is better able to express autonomous choice.***

Content Area: Child Health, Growth and Development; ***Integrated Process:*** Nursing Process, Implementation; ***Cognitive Level:*** Application; ***Client Need/Subneed:*** Health Promotion and Maintenance/Developmental Stages and Transitions

50. CORRECT ANSWER: 2. Answer 1 is incorrect because, at 6 weeks' gestation, the fetal heart is beating, but the Doppler is *unable* to detect the fetal heart tones. **Answer 2 is correct because fetal heart tones can first be heard using a Doppler at about 11 to 12 weeks' gestation. Answer 3** is incorrect because the Doppler is able to *first* detect fetal heart tones at 11 to 12 weeks; by 18 weeks, they are *easily* heard. **Answer 4** is incorrect because the Doppler is able to first detect fetal heart tones at 11 to 12 weeks; by 22 weeks, they are *easily* heard and the *client can also* usually feel fetal movement by this time point in gestation.

■ **TEST-TAKING TIP:** ***The question asks when the heart tones can first be heard. The question requires careful reading to choose the correct response. Generally, it is best to avoid options with extreme numbers (i.e., 6 weeks and 22 weeks).***

Content Area: Maternity, Antepartum; ***Integrated Process:*** Teaching and Learning; ***Cognitive Level:*** Application; ***Client Need/Subneed:*** Health Promotion and Maintenance/ Ante/Intra/Postpartum and Newborn Care

51. CORRECT ANSWER: 4. Answer 1 is incorrect because the drug is *incompatible* in D_5W. NaCl 0.9% should be used for dilution. **Answer 2** is incorrect because the rate is *too rapid.* It should be given no faster than over 6 minutes. **Answer 3** is incorrect because the infusion should be completed within *4 hours.* **Answer 4 is correct because phenytoin (Dilantin) may be given via direct IV no faster than 50 mg/min. If diluted, use saline.**

■ **TEST-TAKING TIP:** ***Eliminate: large volume (Answer 1), too fast (Answer 2), and too slow (Answer 3). Think safety.***

Content Area: Adult Health, Neurological; ***Integrated Process:*** Nursing Process, Implementation; ***Cognitive Level:*** Application; ***Client Need/Subneed:*** Physiological Integrity/Pharmacological and Parenteral Therapies/Medication Administration

52. CORRECT ANSWER: 2. Answer 1 is incorrect because this response is giving an *opinion* not based on correct information about sexual intercourse during pregnancy. **Answer 2 is correct because sexual intercourse is safe for an uncomplicated pregnancy. This answer gives the best information about sexual relations during pregnancy. Answer 3** is incorrect because this is inaccurate information about sex being only safe after the first trimester; this response implies that sexual intercourse can lead to a problem such as miscarriage. **Answer 4** is incorrect because there is *no reason* to avoid sexual relations during the last trimester in a low-risk pregnancy.

■ **TEST-TAKING TIP:** *One of the responses includes the word "only," which usually can be eliminated as an incorrect answer.*

Content Area: Maternity, Antepartum; ***Integrated Process:*** Nursing Process, Implementation; ***Cognitive Level:*** Application; ***Client Need/Subneed:*** Health Promotion and Maintenance/Ante/Intra/Postpartum and Newborn Care

53. CORRECT ANSWER: 2. **Answer 1** is incorrect because atropine is used to treat *bradycardia.* **Answer 2 is correct because the first-line drug for ventricular fibrillation according to advanced cardiac life support protocol is epinephrine, a sympathomimetic.** **Answer 3** is incorrect because antidysrhythmics such as amiodarone are given *after* vasopressors (epinephrine) have been given and may have not worked. **Answer 4** is incorrect because lidocaine is *not* the first-line drug; it is used *if* ventricular fibrillation is still present after defibrillation.

■ **TEST-TAKING TIP:** *Know expected outcomes of drug classifications.*

Content Area: Adult Health, Cardiac; ***Integrated Process:*** Nursing Process, Implementation; ***Cognitive Level:*** Analysis; ***Client Need/Subneed:*** Physiological Integrity/Pharmacological and Parenteral Therapies/Expected Effects/Outcomes

54. CORRECT ANSWER: 4. **Answer 1** is incorrect because, although *adolescent pregnancy* has been linked to poor maternal weight gain, premature birth, preeclampsia, and sexually transmitted infections (STIs), it is not linked to a higher incidence of gestational diabetes. Gestational diabetes is usually higher in particular ethnic groups, such as Asian American, Native American, African American, and Hispanic. **Answer 2** is incorrect because adolescent pregnancy is not a risk factor for the development of vulvar varicosities. Having varicose veins *prior* to pregnancy may increase the chance of developing vulvar varicosities in pregnancy. **Answer 3** is incorrect because placenta previa is associated with *over* 30 years of age, previous cesarean delivery, previous placenta previa, and a high number of closely spaced pregnancies. **Answer 4 is correct because iron-deficiency anemia is defined as hemoglobin below 11 grams. Anemia is more likely to occur in adolescent pregnancy. Adolescent pregnancy has also been linked to poor maternal weight gain, premature birth, preeclampsia, and STIs.**

■ **TEST-TAKING TIP:** *Think about the fact that anemia is a common adolescent problem due to increased need of iron for growth and the sometimes poor eating habits of adolescents. Pregnancy would increase the chance for anemia.*

Content Area: Maternity, Antepartum; ***Integrated Process:*** Nursing Process, Assessment; ***Cognitive Level:*** Application; ***Client Need/Subneed:*** Physiological Integrity/Reduction of Risk Potential/Potential for Complications from Surgical Procedures and Health Alterations

55. CORRECT ANSWER: 1. **Answer 1 is correct because taking the temperature at the same time every day before getting out of bed is essential for determining the true basal body temperature. Successful natural family planning is dependent on accurate basal body temperature.** **Answer 2** is incorrect because it is too late for natural family planning to be effective, as ovulation has already occurred. For most women, 96° to 98° is considered normal prior to ovulation, and 97° to 99° after ovulation. By charting the differences, in 0.1° increments, ovulation can be determined to have taken place. Typically, a rise of at least 0.4° to 0.6° will take place at ovulation, though for *different women* the temperature increases may be *sudden or gradual.* Ovulation has already occurred when the temperature is elevated for 5 days. **Answer 3** is incorrect because basal body temperature needs to be taken at the same time every day *before* any activity, even getting out of bed. **Answer 4** is incorrect because basal body temperature needs to be taken in the *morning,* at same time every day and before activity. In the evening, the results will *not* be predictive of ovulation.

■ **TEST-TAKING TIP:** *Three of the options deal with temperature* taking. *Eliminate the option that does not address the method and timing of temperature taking. Of the options remaining, accurate temperature monitoring at the same time, in the* morning before *getting out of bed, is crucial to successful natural family planning.*

Content Area: Women's Health, Family Planning; ***Integrated Process:*** Nursing Process, Evaluation; ***Cognitive Level:*** Analysis; ***Client Need/Subneed:*** Health Promotion and Maintenance/Lifestyle Choices

56. CORRECT ANSWER: 1. **Answer 1 is correct because evidence suggests that ingestion of live-culture yogurt may decrease the incidence of vaginal yeast infections.** **Answer 2** is incorrect because, although douching with vinegar and water decreases the vaginal pH and inhibits the growth of yeast cells, douching is *not* recommended *in pregnancy.* **Answer 3** is incorrect because, even though douching with live-culture yogurt decreases vaginal pH and inhibits the growth of yeast, douching is *not* recommended *in pregnancy.* **Answer 4** is incorrect because a ntibiotic therapy is *not effective in preventing* yeast infections, and can actually *increase* the incidence of vaginal yeast infections.

■ **TEST-TAKING TIP:** *Two of the options are similar ("douche" in Answers 2 and 3) and involve a practice that is not recommended in pregnancy; therefore, eliminate these options.*

Content Area: Maternity, Intrapartum Infection; ***Integrated Process:*** Nursing Process, Implementation; ***Cognitive Level:*** Application; ***Client Need/Subneed:*** Health Promotion and Maintenance/Self-Care

ANSWERS

57. CORRECT ANSWER: 2. **Answer 1** is incorrect because the fluid is *not* removed. **Answer 2 is correct because clients with rheumatoid arthritis have joint swelling, thickening of the synovial membrane, and pain. The anti-inflammatory action of the steroid will hopefully reduce swelling and decrease pain.** **Answer 3** is incorrect because joint deformity, if present, will *not* be reversed. **Answer 4** is incorrect because any erosion, if present, will *not* be reversed.

■ **TEST-TAKING TIP:** *Look for the most comprehensive answer—the other three choices cause pain.*

Content Area: Adult Health, Musculoskeletal; *Integrated Process:* Nursing Process, Evaluation; *Cognitive Level:* Comprehension; *Client Need/Subneed:* Physiological Integrity/Pharmacological and Parenteral Therapies/Expected Effects/Outcomes

58. CORRECT ANSWER: 2. **Answer 1** is incorrect because these symptoms are a result of increased estrogen levels that cause the congestion, and will *not* be relieved by a decongestant. **Answer 2 is correct because the elevated levels of estrogen during pregnancy cause an increased blood flow in the upper respiratory tract. Nasal stuffiness, some hearing loss, and nosebleeds are common during pregnancy.** **Answer 3** is incorrect because these are *normal* pregnancy symptoms; a referral to a specialist is *not* necessary. **Answer 4** is incorrect because these symptoms are a *normal* part of pregnancy. Decongestants and antibiotics are *not* needed.

■ **TEST-TAKING TIP:** *Three options state that there is a problem. One option states that it is "normal"; select the option that is different. Remember that the normal symptoms of pregnancy do not require any medical interventions. Education and reassurance are the appropriate interventions.*

Content Area: Maternity, Intrapartum; *Integrated Process:* Teaching and Learning; *Cognitive Level:* Application; *Client Need/Subneed:* Health Promotion and Maintenance/Ante/Intra/Postpartum and Newborn Care

59. CORRECT ANSWER: 3. **Answer 1** is incorrect because the drug increases heart rate, which would not help PAT. Phenylephrine (Sinex) is used for PAT. **Answer 2** is incorrect because phenylephrine, *not* pseudoephedrine, reduces intraocular pressure. **Answer 3 is correct because pseudoephedrine (Sudafed) is a familiar over-the-counter (OTC) allergy or cold preparation used for upper respiratory congestion. The drug has both alpha and beta effects, which also can cause hypertension, increased cardiac stimulation, increased respirations, erratic behavior, and delirium.** **Answer 4** is incorrect because phenylephrine, *not* pseudoephedrine, prolongs anesthetic effects.

■ **TEST-TAKING TIP:** *Know expected outcomes of common OTC preparations.*

Content Area: Adult Health, Respiratory; *Integrated Process:* Nursing Process, Evaluation; *Cognitive Level:* Comprehension; *Client Need/Subneed:* Physiological Integrity/Pharmacological and Parenteral Therapies/Expected Effects/Outcomes

60. CORRECT ANSWERS: 1, 4, 6. **Answer 1 is correct because this is characteristic of preschool children's play.** **Answer 2** is incorrect because this is characteristic of *school-age* children. **Answer 3** is incorrect because this is characteristic of *toddlers.* **Answer 4 is correct because this is characteristic of preschool children's play.** **Answer 5** is incorrect because this is characteristic of *school-age* children. **Answer 6 is correct because this is characteristic of preschool children's play.**

■ **TEST-TAKING TIP:** *Preschool children like to imitate their parents. Look for activities that accomplish this task, such as playing dress-up and playing house.*

Content Area: Child Health, Growth and Development; *Integrated Process:* Nursing Process. Assessment; *Cognitive Level:* Comprehension; *Client Need/Subneed:* Health Promotion and Maintenance/Developmental Stages and Transitions

61. CORRECT ANSWER: 1. **Answer 1 is correct because pregnancy causes the areolas to darken and enlarge.** **Answer 2** is incorrect because breast enlargement *is* caused by the influence of progesterone and estrogen. Nodularity is caused by an increase in the size of the mammary glands during the second trimester. **Answer 3** is incorrect because breast tenderness and swelling *are* very common findings in pregnancy. **Answer 4** is incorrect because pregnancy *does* cause darkening of the pigment in the nipples, and causes them to become more erectile.

■ **TEST-TAKING TIP:** *The key to this type of question is focusing on the answer that is incorrect, requiring the nurse to do additional teaching.*

Content Area: Maternity, Intrapartum; *Integrated Process:* Nursing Process, Evaluation; *Cognitive Level:* Application; *Client Need/Subneed:* Health Promotion and Maintenance/Health Promotion Programs

62. CORRECT ANSWER: 2. **Answer 1** is incorrect because, using the formula, the hourly rate times the drop factor divided by 60 should equal 19. **Answer 2 is correct because the formula to determine the correct rate is $(75 \times 15)/60 = 19$ gtt/min.** **Answer 3** is incorrect because the solution, using the formula of hourly rate times the drop factor divided by 60, is 19. **Answer 4** is incorrect because the calculation is 19, based on the formula of hourly rate times the drop factor divided by 60.

■ **TEST-TAKING TIP:** *Memorize the formula for IV rate calculation.*

Content Area: Adult Health, Pharmacology; *Integrated Process:* Nursing Process, Implementation; *Cognitive Level:* Analysis; *Client Need/Subneed:* Physiological Integrity/Pharmacological and Parenteral Therapies/Dosage Calculation

63. CORRECT ANSWER: 3. **Answer 1** is incorrect because ambivalent feelings about pregnancy are common in all women. In addition, this response is a *block to therapeutic communication.* The nurse is telling the client how she "should" feel, rather than validating her feelings. **Answer 2** is incorrect because even women with a desired pregnancy have ambivalent feelings. Such feelings do not necessarily mean the woman desires an abortion. In addition, this response is a *block to therapeutic communication.* The nurse is suggesting a treatment rather than validating the client's feelings. **Answer 3 is correct because ambivalence is a normal response experienced by any individual preparing for a new role, especially an older primigravida.** **Answer 4** is incorrect because love does not necessarily instantly happen right after birth, especially in a first pregnancy. It may take time for such feelings to grow. The nurse is using a trite cliché.

■ **TEST-TAKING TIP:** *Eliminate the options that are not examples of therapeutic communication, or suggest treatment to a client who has feelings that are a normal part of the first pregnancy in the first trimester.*

Content Area: Maternity, Antepartum; ***Integrated Process:*** Communication and Documentation; ***Cognitive Level:*** Application; ***Client Need/Subneed:*** Psychosocial Integrity/ Therapeutic Communications

64. CORRECT ANSWER: 3. **Answer 1** is incorrect because the increase in intravascular volume causes a *hemodilution* of the serum sodium. **Answer 2** is incorrect because output is *decreased,* not increased. **Answer 3 is correct because, in SIADH, there is an increase in the antidiuretic hormone, which results in increased total body water and hyponatremia. Urine is *concentrated* and volume is decreased.** **Answer 4** is incorrect because intravascular volume and weight increase, but there is *no* interstitial edema.

■ **TEST-TAKING TIP:** *Look for key words in the stem—* **inappropriate** *ADH means too much ADH.*

Content Area: Adult Health, Fluid and Electrolyte Imbalances; ***Integrated Process:*** Nursing Process, Analysis; ***Cognitive Level:*** Application; ***Client Need/Subneed:*** Physiological Integrity/ Physiological Adaptation/Fluid and Electrolyte Imbalances

65. CORRECT ANSWER: 3. **Answer 1** is incorrect because ambulation is encouraged in the presence of a *reassuring* fetal monitor tracing. Late decelerations are caused by decreased uteroplacental perfusion and are a *non-reassuring pattern.* **Answer 2** is incorrect because positioning the client in a supine position causes compression of the major vessels of the pelvis. This position will *compromise* placental perfusion and contribute to fetal distress. **Answer 3 is correct because late decelerations are caused by decreased uteroplacental perfusion. Turning a woman on her side increases placental perfusion and subsequent fetal oxygenation. This position change may end the late decelerations.** **Answer 4** is incorrect because the fetus still has oxygen reserve as evidenced by moderate baseline variability. An emergency operative delivery is *not yet required.*

■ **TEST-TAKING TIP:** *Remember the physiology of different types of decelerations and the interventions that are needed to relieve them. Late decelerations require immediate intervention to prevent compromise of fetal oxygen perfusion.*

Content Area: Maternity, Intrapartum; ***Integrated Process:*** Nursing Process, Implementation; ***Cognitive Level:*** Analysis; ***Client Need/Subneed:*** Health Promotion and Maintenance/ Ante/Intra/Postpartum and Newborn Care

66. CORRECT ANSWER: 4. **Answer 1** is incorrect because a stress test would *not* be indicated if a *thrombosis* is suspected. **Answer 2** is incorrect because assessing whether or not stair climbing elicits pain would *not* help the nurse determine the possible presence of a venous thrombosis. **Answer 3** is incorrect because *verbal* information would *not* help the nurse to determine the possible presence of a venous thrombosis. **Answer 4 is correct because, in a client with a history of MI, there is always a risk of thrombophlebitis from immobility or arrhythmias. If Homans' sign (dorsiflexion of the foot) is negative, the nurse can proceed with other assessments.**

■ **TEST-TAKING TIP:** *Thrombophlebitis is the concern. Look for a* **nursing action** *(e.g., testing for Homans' sign) that is the* **first step** *in the nursing process and assess for a thrombosis.*

Content Area: Adult Health, Cardiovascular; ***Integrated Process:*** Nursing Process, Assessment; ***Cognitive Level:*** Analysis; ***Client Need/Subneed:*** Physiological Integrity/Reduction of Risk Potential/System Specific Assessments

67. CORRECT ANSWER: 3. **Answer 1** is incorrect because the client has a *normal* temperature; a fever would be present with a ruptured appendix. **Answer 2** is incorrect because the client would have *vaginal bleeding* if she had a threatened spontaneous abortion. **Answer 3 is correct because ruptured ectopic pregnancy is consistent with the assessment findings. The client has blood loss internally and her vital signs reflect shock due to hypovolemia. Advanced maternal age is a risk factor for ectopic pregnancy.** **Answer 4** is incorrect because a missed abortion is a fetus that has died and is retained. This client has *none* of the symptoms of a missed abortion.

■ **TEST-TAKING TIP:** *Look at the client's vital signs; they indicate changes associated with acute blood loss. Look for the condition that involves significant blood loss.*

Content Area: Maternity, Antepartum; ***Integrated Process:*** Nursing Process, Analysis; ***Cognitive Level:*** Analysis; ***Client Need/Subneed:*** Physiological Integrity/Physiological Adaptation/Medical Emergencies

68. CORRECT ANSWER: 1. 20 mL/hr times 60 divided by 60 = 20 gtt/min.

■ **TEST-TAKING TIP:** *Memorize the IV calculation formula.* ***Hint:*** *When using 60-gtt/mL tubing, the mL/hr is the same as the drops/min (20 mL/hr = 20 gtt/min).*

Content Area: Adult Health, Endocrine; ***Integrated Process:*** Nursing Process, Analysis; ***Cognitive Level:*** Analysis; ***Client Need/Subneed:*** Physiological Integrity/Pharmacological and Parenteral Therapies/Dosage Calculation

69. CORRECT ANSWER: 2. Answer 1 is incorrect because the first stage of labor *is* the onset of labor through complete dilation of the cervix. **Answer 2 is correct because the first stage of labor is the onset of labor through complete cervical dilation. The first phase of the first stage of labor is the latent phase of labor, characterized by 0 to 3 cm of cervical dilation. Answer 3** is incorrect because the fourth stage of labor *is* the delivery of the placenta through complete stabilization of the mother. **Answer 4** is incorrect because the third stage of labor *is* birth through the delivery of the placenta.

■ **TEST-TAKING TIP:** *Note that the stem asks for the* **incorrect** *statement. Remember that there are four stages of labor, but only the first stage has phases: latent, active, and transition.*

Content Area: Maternity, Antepartum; *Integrated Process:* Nursing Process, Evaluation; *Cognitive Level:* Application; *Client Need/Subneed:* Health Promotion and Maintenance/ Ante/Intra/Postpartum and Newborn Care

70. CORRECT ANSWER: 2. Answer 1 is incorrect because this time period would be more likely with regular or *fast-acting* insulin. **Answer 2 is correct because NPH is an *intermediate*-acting insulin with peak effects between 6 and 12 hours after administration. Answer 3** is incorrect because this time period would be more likely with *long-acting* insulin. **Answer 4** is incorrect because this time period would be more likely with *long-acting* insulin.

■ **TEST-TAKING TIP:** *Recognize expected effects—look for an* **intermediate** *time period.*

Content Area: Adult Health, Endocrine; *Integrated Process:* Nursing Process, Analysis; *Cognitive Level:* Analysis; *Client Need/Subneed:* Physiological Integrity/Pharmacological and Parenteral Therapies/Medication Administration

71. CORRECT ANSWERS: 1, 4, 5, 6. Answer 1 is correct because the nurse charts the child's words exactly as they were spoken, using quotes. Answer 2 is incorrect because the nurse is charting a personal interpretation of the mother's reaction to the environment. Additionally, many parents are stressed in the hospital environment, making this charting entry of questionable value. **Answer 3** is incorrect because this is a vague description and is a subjective interpretation. A better entry would be to describe a specific event such as the parent failing to visit during the child's hospitalization. **Answer 4 is correct because this is an objective piece of data that is easily measured. Answer 5 is correct because the nurse reports a period of time as stated by the parents. Answer 6 is correct because this succinctly describes the interaction between physician and child.**

■ **TEST-TAKING TIP:** *When charting, the nurse should always strive for objective language by stating facts in measurable and precise phrases. Subjective language introduces the nurse's bias and must be avoided.*

Content Area: Child Health, Abuse; *Integrated Process:* Communication and Documentation; *Cognitive Level:* Application; *Client Need/Subneed:* Psychosocial Integrity/ Abuse/Neglect

72. CORRECT ANSWER: 2. Answer 1 is incorrect because, although new parents do need time to learn how to hold the baby, this is not a reason for delaying the tub bath. **Answer 2 is correct because the cord needs to dry and fall off before immersing a newborn in a tub bath. There is a higher risk of infection and delayed cord separation if the newborn is given a tub bath while the cord is still attached. Answer 3** is incorrect because newborn skin in a full-term infant is *very resistant* to trauma caused by proper washing technique. **Answer 4** is incorrect because, once the neonate's temperature has stabilized, giving a sponge bath will *not* cause unnecessary chilling.

■ **TEST-TAKING TIP:** *The question is asking about what significant event that happens during the first 2 weeks of life would be affected by exposure to water . . . . cord separating!*

Content Area: Child Health, Newborn; *Integrated Process:* Teaching and Learning; *Cognitive Level:* Comprehension; *Client Need/Subneed:* Health Promotion and Maintenance/ Ante/Intra/Postpartum and Newborn Care

73. CORRECT ANSWER: 4. Answer 1 is incorrect because elevated blood glucose is associated with *gestational diabetes.* **Answer 2** is incorrect because decreased platelet count, *not elevated* platelet count, is found in HELLP syndrome. **Answer 3** is incorrect because the creatinine clearance is *decreased* in HELLP syndrome. **Answer 4 is correct because HELLP syndrome stands for hemolysis, elevated liver enzymes, and low platelet count. Elevated hepatic enzymes are associated with HELLP syndrome.**

■ **TEST-TAKING TIP:** *Remembering what the acronym HELLP means will give information about the changes that occur with this variant of preeclampsia.*

Content Area: Maternity, Intrapartum; *Integrated Process:* Nursing Process, Analysis; *Cognitive Level:* Application; *Client Need/Subneed:* Physiological Integrity/Reduction of Risk Potential/Potential for Complications from Surgical Procedures and Health Alterations

74. CORRECT ANSWER: 2. Answer 1 is incorrect because, before the client experiences hypoglycemia, the potassium level drops below normal. **Answer 2 is correct because, as glucose moves back into the cell with insulin treatment, potassium moves back into the cell, causing a low serum level and a risk of hypokalemia. Answer 3** is incorrect because a client who is hyperglycemic and in ketoacidosis is usually dehydrated, so serum sodium is *elevated,* and then returns to normal. **Answer 4** is incorrect because low calcium is *not* associated with hyperglycemia.

ANSWERS

Low calcium occurs from accidental removal of the parathyroid glands or with renal dysfunction.

■ TEST-TAKING TIP: ***Hypoglycemia is too obvious. Remember that*** K^+ ***moves with glucose into the cell.***

Content Area: Adult Health, Fluid and Electrolyte Imbalances; ***Integrated Process:*** Nursing Process, Analysis; ***Cognitive Level:*** Comprehension; ***Client Need/Subneed:*** Physiological Integrity/Physiological Adaptation/Fluid and Electrolyte Imbalances

75. CORRECT ANSWER: 1. Answer 1 is correct because this is the correct method to elicit the biceps reflex. **Answer 2** is incorrect because this describes eliciting the *triceps* reflex. **Answer 3** is incorrect because this describes eliciting the *knee* reflex. **Answer 4** is incorrect because this describes eliciting the *wrist* reflex.

■ TEST-TAKING TIP: ***Picturing the method and what part of the body is being described will help eliminate the wrong answers.***

Content Area: Maternity, Antepartum; ***Integrated Process:*** Nursing Process, Implementation; ***Cognitive Level:*** Application; ***Client Need/Subneed:*** Health Promotion and Maintenance/Techniques of Physical Assessment

Final Test 2

Questions

Select the one answer that is best for each question, unless otherwise directed.

1. A 25-year-old client is being seen in a clinic for the first time for possible osteoarthritis. Which statement by the client would be consistent with an *early* symptom of arthritis?

1. "When I get up in the morning, I feel stiff."
2. "I am concerned that my fingers are looking deformed."
3. "Look how blue the skin is over my knuckles."
4. "My lower back is constantly in pain."

2. A child is admitted to the hospital for suspicion of leukemia. Which test is needed to confirm the suspected diagnosis?

1. White blood cell count.
2. Bone marrow biopsy.
3. Spinal tap.
4. Platelet count.

3. A client, who is a 16-year-old primigravida and 34 weeks pregnant, is complaining of constantly feeling tired. Which assessment should lead a nurse to suspect that the client's blood volume has increased?

1. Increased hemoglobin.
2. Hypercalcemia.
3. Decreased hematocrit.
4. Hyperkalemia.

4. In a closed chest drainage system, which area regulates the amount of suction?

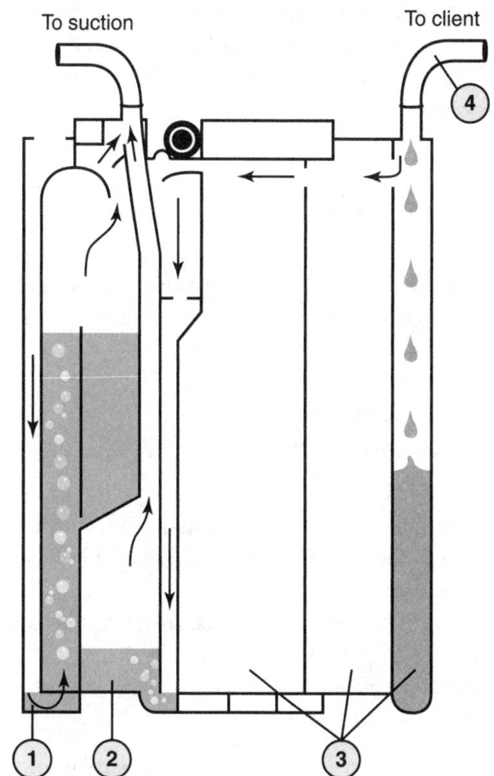

1. Chamber 1.
2. Chamber 2.
3. Chamber 3.
4. Tube to the client.

5. A newborn suspected of having Down syndrome is held in the nursery for observation. For what acute health problems should a nurse observe? *Select all that apply.*

1. Congenital heart disease.
2. Mental retardation.
3. Cleft palate.
4. Infertility.
5. Tracheoesophageal fistula.
6. Respiratory distress.

6. A 28-year-old client is admitted to an intensive care unit (ICU) following a construction accident. Which assessment finding requires an *immediate* response by a nurse?

1. Extremities warm and dry.
2. Temperature 100°F (37.8°C).
3. Urinary output 100 mL/hr.
4. Extremity capillary refill 5 seconds.

7. Following the diagnosis of hemophilia after the birth of their first baby boy, a nurse should immediately counsel the parents regarding the need for:

1. Genetic counseling.
2. Involvement in a support group.
3. Involvement with a comprehensive health-care team.
4. Couples' counseling.

8. A 37-year-old client, who is a multipara, delivered an 8-pound, 9-ounce infant about 24 hours ago. A nurse is performing a routine assessment of the client's lower extremities for the possible development of thrombophlebitis. For which sign should the nurse assess?
   1. Chadwick's sign.
   2. Homans' sign.
   3. Hegar's sign.
   4. Goodell's sign.

9. A client with acute viral hepatitis has a serum bilirubin of 3.6 mg/dL on admission. A nurse should expect the client to report:
   1. Dark orange urine.
   2. Tar-colored bowel movements.
   3. A high fever for several days.
   4. Red, irritated eyes.

10. A child has ingested a toxic amount of aspirin. Which order written by a pediatrician should a nurse question?
   1. Administer activated charcoal following the lavage.
   2. Prepare for possible hemodialysis.
   3. Warming blanket as needed.
   4. Have vitamin K on hand.

11. A client has just been weaned from ventilation therapy. While working closely with a respiratory therapist, what other member of the health team should be consulted *first?*
   1. Dietitian, because high carbohydrate intake increases carbon dioxide production.
   2. Social worker, to initiate appropriate case management.
   3. Speech therapist, to help in resuming oral communication.
   4. Physical therapist, to improve strength in leg muscles for ambulation.

12. A toddler with hemophilia strikes the right knee against a coffee table. A nurse could best evaluate the effectiveness of the teaching the mother received regarding the early signs of hemarthrosis when the mother reports:
   1. Epistaxis.
   2. Spontaneous hematuria.
   3. Stiffness, tingling, and aching in the involved joint, followed by a decrease in ability to move the joint.
   4. Warmth, redness, and swelling in the involved joint with a considerable loss of movement.

13. A client, who is gravida 6, para 2, is attending her regular prenatal appointment. She complains to a nurse about pain from her hemorrhoids. The nurse knows additional teaching would be required if the client states:
   1. "I should avoid getting constipated."
   2. "I can use hemorrhoid cream and witch hazel pads for relief."
   3. "I can take warm sitz baths frequently."
   4. "I should stop taking my iron supplements."

14. Which nursing diagnosis reflects the basic rationale for symptoms in a client with acute respiratory distress syndrome (ARDS)?
   1. Ineffective breathing pattern.
   2. High risk for infection.
   3. Impaired gas exchange.
   4. Activity intolerance.

15. A parent of a child who ingested a toxic dose of acetaminophen (Tylenol) refuses to allow a nurse to administer *N*-acetylcysteine (Mucomyst) because "it smells spoiled." A nurse should correctly:
   1. Withhold the dose.
   2. Request that another dose be sent to the pediatric unit by the pharmacy.
   3. Discard the dose and prepare another dose.
   4. Discuss the medication with the parents.

16. Following external radiation, a client reports dry, irritated skin in the treatment area. Additional teaching by a nurse would be needed if the client says:
   Select all that apply.
   1. "Ice relieves the itching and redness."
   2. "I found a nonmedicated, fragrance-free lotion."
   3. "The sunlamp feels good and seems to help."
   4. "I have been washing the site with tap water."
   5. "My mother always said warm water and alcohol would toughen the skin."
   6. "I would like to scratch the site but I don't."

17. The parents of a child newly diagnosed with hemophilia ask, "Why do we have to learn how to give the medicine?" A nurse's best response would be:
   1. "It will promote immediacy of treatment."
   2. "It will provide for less disruption of family life."
   3. "It will result in fewer missed school days."
   4. "It will enhance your child's sense of self-esteem and independence."

18. A client, who is gravida 4, para 1, is admitted for preterm labor at 32 weeks' gestation. She is 1 cm dilated, 90% effaced, and a +1 station. A nurse is monitoring her preterm labor using an external fetal monitor. Which statement, if made by the client, should indicate to the nurse that further teaching is needed?
   1. "I'll need to lie flat on my back to monitor the contractions."
   2. "I can expect to be checked frequently while I am wearing the monitor."
   3. "I can lie in a comfortable position, but I should avoid lying on my back."
   4. "I know that the external monitor will show how my baby is responding to the contractions."

19. A nurse is assessing a client for bowel sounds following abdominal surgery. In which quadrant is the nurse most likely to hear bowel sounds, if they are present?

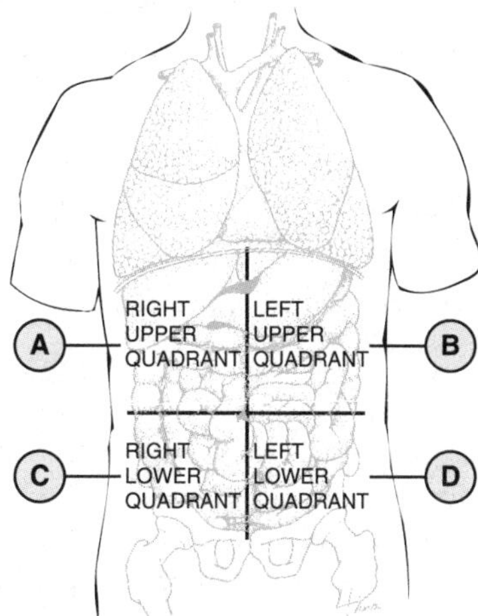

1. A.
2. B.
3. C.
4. D.

20. A nurse is counseling a group of parents of young children regarding the prevention of iron poisoning. The nurse should correctly inform the parents to:
1. Not purchase multivitamins that contain iron.
2. Not purchase iron tablets that look like candy.
3. Keep the tablets in a high place.
4. Keep syrup of ipecac in a locket medicine cabinet.

21. A nurse is to give meperidine (Demerol) 75 mg IV and scopolamine 0.3 mg IV preoperatively to a client with a history of glaucoma. Which action should be taken by the nurse?
1. Give the drugs as ordered.
2. Teach the client the side effects.
3. Dim the lights and raise side rails after injection.
4. Do not give the drugs and call the physician.

22. Prior to administering a dose of theophylline, a nurse checks a child's serum theophylline level and notes that it is 14.2 mcg/mL. What should the nurse do? *Select all that apply.*
1. Withhold the medication and notify the pediatrician.
2. Administer the medication as ordered.
3. Note the serum theophylline level on the Medication Administration Record (MAR).
4. Circle the theophylline dose on the Medication Administration Record (MAR) as being "withheld."

23. A client, who is gravida 3, para 1, is at 29 weeks' gestation. Upon examination, her cervix is 2 cm dilated, 40% effaced, and a –2 station. A physician admits the client for preterm labor. What is an appropriate nursing intervention for this client?
1. Perform a nipple stimulation stress test to evaluate fetal well-being.
2. Encourage adequate hydration.
3. Administer misoprostol to decrease contractions.
4. Encourage ambulation to prevent thrombophlebitis.

24. A client has just been extubated. Which assessment by a nurse should indicate signs of laryngeal edema?
1. Diffuse, wheezing breath sounds.
2. Arterial blood gases show a P_{CO_2} of 52 mm Hg and P_{O_2} of 90%.
3. Pulse oximeter of 91% with cool extremities.
4. High-pitched crowing sounds on inspiration.

25. A nurse is teaching a parent about childhood poisonings. The nurse should instruct the parent that the *first* action to take is to:
1. Call the Poison Control Center for instructions.
2. Attempt to reach the child's pediatrician.
3. Follow the instructions on the label of the substance that the child has ingested.
4. Treat the child's obvious signs and symptoms.

26. A client is diagnosed with heart failure and has an ejection fraction of 30% and is receiving an angiotensin-converting enzyme (ACE) inhibitor. Which finding would be an expected drug effect?
1. Increases cardiac preload.
2. Decreases cardiac afterload.
3. Discontinues the need for diuretics.
4. Promotes diuresis.

27. A nurse instructs the parents of an infant with developmental dysplasia of the hip in the care for a Pavlik harness. Instructions to prevent skin breakdown from the harness should include:
Select all that apply.
1. Put an undershirt under the chest straps of the harness.
2. Put kneesocks under the foot and leg pieces of the harness.
3. Apply lotion and powder under the straps of the harness.
4. Massage skin under the straps of the harness.

28. A 41-year-old client, who is gravida 4, para 2, is 37 weeks pregnant. She states to a nurse that her varicose veins are intolerable and she would like the physician to induce her labor. The best suggestion for the nurse to give the client would be:
1. "You should wear knee-high support hose daily."
2. "Increasing your dairy intake can provide some relief."
3. "You should try nipple stimulation to try and start your labor."
4. "You can try lying down with your feet elevated."

29. A nurse should know that an important aspect of the care following surgery for glaucoma includes:
1. Coughing and deep breathing to prevent atelectasis.
2. Rest for 24 hours, then a return to normal activities.
3. No food for 24 hours, or until bowel sounds return.
4. Increased fluids to promote filtration of aqueous humor.

30. Which orders, regarding a 2-month-old infant born to a mother who is HBsAg– (hepatitis B surface antigen negative), should a nurse question during the infant's well-baby checkup?
1. "Administer HepB immunization #2 today."
2. "Administer DTaP immunization #1 today."
3. "Administer Hib immunization #1 today."
4. "Withhold HepB immunization #2 today."

31. A client is started on a regular diet following gastric surgery. According to the chart, the client receives the following for lunch. How many milliliters of fluid should a nurse record on the client's intake record?

8 oz of apple juice
1 cup of herb tea
½ turkey sandwich on white bread
½ cup of orange gelatin with mandarin oranges
2 cookies
½ cup of cottage cheese

1. 100 mL.
2. 300 mL.
3. 450 mL.
4. 600 mL.

32. A child with osteomyelitis of the tibia is hospitalized. The nurse's *priority* instruction to the parents would be to:
1. Let the parents know that the child's appetite will return as the acute symptoms recede.
2. Maintain adequate nutrition for the child to aid healing.
3. Keep the child from weight-bearing on the affected limb until healing is well underway.
4. Allow the child to move about on a gurney or in a wheelchair when bedrest is no longer necessary.

33. A client, who is a primigravida about 8 weeks pregnant, has been experiencing abdominal cramping, bright red vaginal spotting, and passing some small clots. A sterile speculum examination in a physician's office reveals cervical dilation. A nurse determines that this client is most likely experiencing:
1. Inevitable abortion.
2. Complete abortion.
3. Missed abortion.
4. Threatened abortion.

34. A client is scheduled for a bilateral herniorrhaphy. Teaching about preparation of the skin before surgery should include:
1. The need to shave the skin from nipple level to groin.
2. Shaving or clipping depends on the amount of body hair.
3. Just the area around the umbilicus will be shaved.
4. Shaving will be done by the client at home.

35. The parents of a child recently diagnosed with Legg-Calvé-Perthes disease ask a nurse, "Why does our child have to be in bed for so long?" The nurse's most factual response is because bedrest:
1. Reduces the inflammation and restores motion.
2. Prevents weight-bearing in the affected limb.
3. Prevents onset of degenerative arthritis.
4. Allows for recovery from the trauma that caused the disease.

36. An older client in a long-term care facility reports severe pain in the groin while walking to the activities center. The *first* action by a nurse should be to:
1. Give Tylenol as ordered.
2. Suspect a fracture and eliminate weight-bearing.
3. Question the client further about the pain.
4. Offer the client a walker to provide support.

37. While a school-age child is on bedrest for Legg-Calvé-Perthes disease, a nurse's *priority* intervention would be to encourage the school-age child to:
1. Keep in contact with classmates.
2. Learn to tolerate immobility.
3. Learn to correctly apply the prescribed braces.
4. Begin a hobby.

38. A client, who is gravida 3, para 1, is at 41 weeks' gestation. The client is 6 cm dilated, 80% effaced, and a –1 station. A nurse is assessing the client's fetal monitor tracing. Which assessment should indicate to the nurse that the fetus is in distress?
1. Decelerations in the fetal heart rate during contractions that end when the contraction is over.
2. An increase in the fetal heart rate during a vaginal examination.
3. A uniform decrease in the heart rate that begins after each contraction for the past four contractions.
4. Lack of meconium staining after the amniotic membranes have ruptured.

39. A physician orders heparin 900 units/hr IV for a client. The pharmacy sends a solution that has 25,000 units of heparin in 500 mL D_5W. A nurse calculates that the client should receive the IV heparin at a rate of _______ mL/hr. *Fill in the blank.*

40. An adolescent with juvenile idiopathic arthritis states to a nurse, "I don't feel any better since I started the NSAIDs a week ago." The nurse's most accurate response would be:
1. "You need to advance to the slower-acting antirheumatic drugs."
2. "You need to give aspirin another try."
3. "You need a course of corticosteroids."
4. "You need another 2 weeks of NSAIDs."

QUESTIONS

41. A week after chemotherapy, a client's absolute neutrophil count (ANC) is $300/mm^3$.
Which nursing interventions are appropriate? *Select all that apply.*
1. Apply gloves while hands are still damp from washing.
2. Use an alcohol-based hand wash.
3. Remove fresh flowers from the room.
4. Triple-wash all fresh vegetables.
5. Avoid fresh unpeeled fruits.
6. Place in same room with another client who is free of airborne infections.

42. An adolescent with juvenile idiopathic arthritis has daytime sleepiness. The nurse would encourage: *Select all that apply.*
1. Scheduling 8 to 10 hours of nighttime sleep.
2. Use of a firm mattress.
3. Daytime naps.
4. Implementing relaxation techniques prior to bedtime.

43. On her first postpartum day, a woman who is diabetic has been eating a full diet, and her insulin was reduced to one third of the dosage received during pregnancy. Which sign(s) and/or symptom(s) would indicate that the client is experiencing hyperglycemia? *Select all that apply.*
1. Profuse perspiration.
2. Irritability.
3. Flushed face.
4. Headache.
5. Rapid pulse.
6. Deep, rapid respirations.

44. A client with acute pancreatitis and fluid volume deficit is in an ICU. Which assessment finding should a nurse report to a physician?
1. Urine output of 35 mL/hr.
2. CVP of 12 mm Hg.
3. Cardiac output of 5 L/min.
4. Decreased pain in the fetal position.

45. The parents of an infant in a hip spica cast who is being treated for developmental dysplasia of the hip inform the nurse that they are having difficulty with positioning the infant. A nurse should suggest that they try: *Select all that apply.*
1. Supine position with the head elevated.
2. "Football" hold, with the infant facing the parent, with the legs behind the parent.
3. Upright position on the parent's lap, with the infant's legs on either side of the parent's legs.
4. Prone position on the floor.

46. A client with acute pancreatitis reports numbness with circumoral tingling and muscle cramps. Which nursing intervention is most appropriate?
1. Assess for hypocalcemia.
2. Request an order for a serum sodium test.
3. Assess for hypoglycemia.
4. Check the chart for a current dose of furosemide (Lasix).

47. A nurse notes that a 2-week-old infant with a cyanotic heart defect and mild congestive heart failure has an apical pulse rate of 100 beats/min. Which action should the nurse take?
1. Withhold the digoxin because the heart rate is too low.
2. Notify the pediatrician immediately.
3. Administer the medication as scheduled.
4. Retake the apical pulse in 1 hour.

48. A nurse performs an assessment on a newborn, 39 weeks' gestation, with Apgar scores of 8 and 9. Which findings are not "normal" in a newborn of this gestational age? *Select all that apply.*
1. A slight heart murmur heard at 6 hours of age.
2. Overlapping skull bones.
3. Bluish hue of fingers and toes.
4. Slightly incurving pinnae.
5. Expiratory grunting with respirations.

49. A client is admitted with acute pancreatitis after a holiday celebration including excessive food and alcohol. Which assessment finding reflects this diagnosis?
1. Hyperactive bowel sounds.
2. Sudden onset of continuous epigastric and back pain.
3. Moist crackles in both lung fields.
4. Elevated temperature and BP.

50. A nurse prepares to teach the parents of a newborn infant with an unrepaired cardiac defect about the side effects of digoxin. Which side effects of digoxin should the nurse include in the teaching plan? *Select all that apply.*
1. Dysrhythmias.
2. Yellow-green visual halos.
3. Bradycardia.
4. Vomiting.

51. A client is admitted for a cholecystectomy because of cholelithiasis. A nurse notes that the serum amylase report shows a level of 900 units/L. Which action should the RN take?
1. Prepare the client for surgery.
2. Assess the client for jaundice.
3. Check the RBC, Hgb, and Hct reports.
4. Call and report the findings to the physician.

52. The pediatrician assesses a child with an acute episode of hemophilia that involves the lower extremities Which pediatrician's order should a nurse question?
1. Active range-of-motion exercises twice daily.
2. Passive range-of-motion exercises twice daily.
3. May use wrist splints at night.
4. May use ankle splints at night.

53. A physician orders 6 mg of betamethasone IM for a client in preterm labor. The vial contains 2 mg/2 mL. The nurse should administer _______ mL of betamethasone. *Fill in the blank.*

54. A client with chronic pancreatitis is placed on pancrelipase (Pancrease) three times daily. What information is essential to teach with this medication?
1. Observe for diarrhea.
2. Take the medication with meals.
3. Chew tablets, or allow enteric-coated tablets to dissolve in the mouth.
4. Take the medication every 8 hours.

55. An adolescent with acne is placed on a course of tetracycline. What important environmental controls should a nurse emphasize to the adolescent when teaching the adolescent about the medication? *Select all that apply.*
1. Wearing a hat.
2. Wearing long-sleeved shirts.
3. Wearing sunglasses.
4. Applying sunscreen.
5. Wearing heavy socks.

56. When explaining the purpose of radiation to a client with multiple myeloma, which treatment goal should be described?
1. Enhancing the effects of chemotherapy.
2. Killing metastatic cells.
3. Shrinking invasive tumor masses.
4. Preventing invasion of bone by cells.

57. An infant receives an engraved pewter rattle as a gift. A nurse correctly teaches the parents that this gift should be:
1. Returned to the sender.
2. Displayed in a locked cabinet.
3. Utilized by the infant.
4. Utilized by the infant when the parents are present.

58. A woman, who is 36 weeks pregnant, is admitted directly from clinic with a blood pressure of 146/98 mm Hg, puffy face and hands, and "awful headaches and problems seeing." The admission note states: "Admit for preeclampsia." Which nursing orders should not be implemented? *Select all that apply.*
1. Up as desired, activities as desired.
2. Assess deep tendon reflexes, and amount and distribution of edema on every shift.
3. Admission and daily weight.
4. Test urine for protein every 4 hours.
5. Intake and output on every shift.

59. Upon a client's admission for extracapsular fracture of the left femur, how should a nurse expect the extremity to appear?
1. Shorter than the other leg.
2. Internally rotated.
3. Blanched over the fracture site.
4. To have footdrop.

60. Which activity should a nurse counsel an adolescent with severe hemophilia to not participate in?
1. Walking.
2. Jogging.
3. Bowling.
4. Soccer.

61. Which statement correctly describes the four-point gait that should be used when partial weight-bearing is permitted?
1. Move both crutches and the weaker leg forward at the same time.
2. Move the left crutch and the right foot forward together.
3. Move the right crutch ahead, then follow with the left foot.
4. Move both crutches forward together, then swing legs through.

62. A child receives a dose of atropine. A nurse should anticipate that the expected effect of the medication would require that the nurse monitor the child's:
Select all that apply.
1. Heart rate.
2. Behavior.
3. Blood pressure.
4. Temperature.
5. Respirations.

63. A nurse is observing a primigravida client admitted in active labor. Which observation would be the most reliable guide to assess the progression of the client's labor?
1. Vaginal discharge that is increasing.
2. Breathing that is becoming more rapid.
3. Contractions that are getting more intense.
4. Cervix that is progressively dilating.

64. To prevent contractures, in which position should a nurse place a client 72 hours after an above-the-knee amputation?
1. Sitting in a reclining chair twice a day.
2. Supine with the stump elevated at least 30 degrees.
3. Side-lying, alternating left and right sides.
4. Lying on the abdomen several times daily.

65. A nurse prepares to administer 0.3 mL of a medication intramuscularly to a 4-month-old infant. Which equipment should the nurse collect? *Select all that apply and place in sequential order.*
1. 3-mL syringe with a 23-gauge needle.
2. 1-mL syringe with a 25-gauge needle.
3. Alcohol pad.
4. Cotton ball and bandage.

66. Which choice best describes the pain associated with a duodenal ulcer?
    1. Dull, epigastric pain that occurs one-half hour after eating.
    2. Sharp, intermittent pain in the left upper quadrant.
    3. Gnawing, epigastric pain 1 to 3 hours after eating.
    4. Continuous, dull pain in the right lower quadrant.

67. Before administering gentamicin to a child, a nurse should check the results of the child's:
    Select all that apply.
    1. Abdominal and chest x-rays.
    2. Renal function tests.
    3. Auditory tests.
    4. Complete blood count and platelet count.

68. A client, 28 weeks' gestation, is having uterine contractions every 3 minutes lasting 60 seconds. Her physician orders a tocolytic and a steroid. The order reads: "Give 0.25 mg of terbutaline SQ now and 6 mg of Celestone IM now." The vial of terbutaline is labeled 5 mg per 5 mL, and the vial of Celestone is labeled 2 mg per mL. The nurse should administer _______ mL of terbutaline and _______ mL of Celestone to the client. *Fill in the blanks.*

69. What physical assessment data should a nurse consider typical for a client during an acute attack of Ménière's disease?
    1. Jerking eye movements, high BP, tachycardia.
    2. Difficulty ambulating, normal BP, tachycardia.
    3. Jerking eye movements, normal vital signs.
    4. Difficulty ambulating, high BP, tachycardia.

70. Following a mastoidectomy, which changes should a nurse anticipate if cranial nerve VII was damaged? *Select all that apply.*
    1. Drooling and drooping of the mouth.
    2. Sagging of the face on the operative side.
    3. Inability to close eyelid on operative side.
    4. Inability to open eyelid on operative side.

71. In assisting a physician to perform a thoracentesis, how should the nurse position a client with pleural effusion of the left lung?
    1. Supine with the left arm extended over the head.
    2. Sitting at the side of the bed with both arms resting on a locked over-the-bed table.
    3. High Fowler's position with both arms resting on pillows.
    4. Semi-Fowler's position tilted on the right side.

72. A client, who is gravida 6, para 5, has a sudden urge to push. A nurse performs a sterile vaginal examination and finds that the cervix is completely dilated and the fetus is at a +2 station. Which nursing intervention is *most important* at this time?
    1. Call the physician to come for delivery and place the client in high Fowler's position.
    2. Call the physician for delivery, and then put pressure against the fetus' head until the physician arrives for delivery.
    3. Call the physician for delivery, and then gently pull on the fetus' head until it is delivered.
    4. Call the physician for delivery, apply gentle pressure to the perineum and guide the fetus' head as it is delivered.

73. A client needs prophylaxis for group B β-hemolytic streptococcus. A physician orders 2.5 million units of penicillin G to be administered IV every 4 hours. A nurse has a 5-million-unit vial of penicillin powder that needs to be reconstituted with diluent. The directions state 10 mL of sterile saline should be used to reconstitute the antibiotic. The nurse should draw up _______ mL of diluent and administer _______ mL of reconstituted solution. *Fill in the blanks.*

74. Which over-the-counter (OTC) medications should a nurse instruct a client with glaucoma to avoid?
    1. NSAIDs.
    2. Salicylates.
    3. Antacids.
    4. Antihistamines.

75. A client, who is a 38-year-old gravida 4, para 2, has an ultrasound at 34 weeks' gestation, which reveals a marginal placenta previa. The client has some bright red spotting, but no contractions or abdominal pain. A nurse should anticipate that the expected management for a client with marginal placenta previa will be:
    1. Limiting activity to bedrest, with bathroom privileges.
    2. Preparing for an immediate cesarean delivery.
    3. Doing a contraction stress test for fetal well-being.
    4. Inducing labor with misoprostol.

Answers/Rationales/Tips

1. CORRECT ANSWER: 1. Answer 1 is correct because morning stiffness usually lasts less than 30 minutes and decreases with movement. Pain and functional impairment are also manifestations of osteoarthritis. **Answer 2** is incorrect because deformities of hands and feet are common in *rheumatoid* arthritis. **Answer 3** is incorrect because, if swelling is present, the joints may be *reddened* and warm, *not* blue. **Answer 4** is incorrect because this may be due to *muscle* strain rather than arthritis, as arthritis in the lumbar region develops more slowly.

■ **TEST-TAKING TIP:** *Look for an* **early** *indication.*

Content Area: Adult Health, Musculoskeletal; *Integrated Process:* Nursing Process, Evaluation; *Cognitive Level:* Application; *Client Need/Subneed:* Physiological Integrity/Physiological Adaptation/Alterations in Body Systems

2. CORRECT ANSWER: 2. **Answer 1** is incorrect because, although the white blood cell count is low in a child with leukemia, this alone is *insufficient* to diagnose leukemia. **Answer 2 is correct because the diagnosis of leukemia is confirmed by assessing the bone marrow through a needle biopsy.** **Answer 3** is incorrect because a spinal tap is *part of* the diagnostic assessment but this laboratory test alone is *insufficient* to diagnose leukemia. **Answer 4** is incorrect because, although the platelet count is low in a child with leukemia, this laboratory test alone is *insufficient* to diagnose leukemia.

■ **TEST-TAKING TIP:** *The question asks for the test that will* **confirm** *a* **diagnosis** *of leukemia, not symptoms. Since leukemia is a disease of the bone marrow, a biopsy is the best answer.*

Content Area: Child Health, Hematological; *Integrated Process:* Nursing Process, Analysis; *Cognitive Level:* Comprehension; *Client Need/Subneed:* Physiological Integrity/Reduction of Risk Potential/Diagnostic Tests

3. CORRECT ANSWER: 3. **Answer 1** is incorrect because increased hemoglobin is indicative of dehydration or third spacing of fluid that is common in *preeclampsia. Decreased* hemoglobin is associated with increased blood volume. **Answer 2** is incorrect because hypercalcemia is associated with *dehydration, not* increased blood volume. **Answer 3 is correct because decreased hematocrit is an indicator of increased blood volume, which is normal in pregnancy and peaks between 32 and 34 weeks' gestation.** **Answer 4** is incorrect because hyperkalemia is associated with *dehydration, not* increased blood volume.

■ **TEST-TAKING TIP:** *Remember the association of increase/decrease: ↑ blood volume resulting in ↓ hemoglobin and ↓ hematocrit. Blood volume increase in pregnancy does not increase all the components equally; for example, hemoglobin and hematocrit decrease with increased blood volume.*

Content Area: Maternity, Antepartum; *Integrated Process:* Nursing Process, Assessment; *Cognitive Level:* Analysis; *Client Need/Subneed:* Physiological Integrity/Reduction of Risk Potential/System Specific Assessments

4. CORRECT ANSWER: 1. Chamber 1 is the suction control chamber (or in a three-bottle system, the third bottle in the sequence from the client). The amount of water in this chamber controls the amount of pressure being exerted.

■ **TEST-TAKING TIP:** *Picture the device. Client drainage is* **closest** *to the client; suction is* **farthest** *from the client.*

Content Area: Adult Health, Respiratory; *Integrated Process:* Nursing Process, Analysis; *Cognitive Level:* Comprehension; *Client Need/Subneed:* Physiological Integrity/Reduction of Risk Potential/Therapeutic Procedures

5. CORRECT ANSWERS: 1, 3, 5, 6. Answer 1 is correct because children with Down syndrome have a greater incidence of congenital heart disease. A nurse should observe for symptoms of a cardiac defect (e.g., murmur, pallor, and hypoxemia). **Answer 2** is incorrect because, although children with Down syndrome have varying degrees of retardation, this is *not* a problem in the newborn period. **Answer 3 is correct because children with Down syndrome have a greater incidence of cleft palate. A nurse should assess the oral cavity for structural abnormality.** **Answer 4** is incorrect because, although children with Down syndrome are likely to be infertile, this is *not* a problem in the newborn period. **Answer 5 is correct because children with Down syndrome have a greater incidence of tracheoesophageal fistula. A nurse should observe if the child chokes or becomes hypoxic during feedings. Answer 6 is correct because children with Down syndrome have floppy airways and are prone to aspiration and respiratory infection.**

■ **TEST-TAKING TIP:** *The key words in the stem of the question are "newborn" and "acute."*

Content Area: Child Health, Neurological; *Integrated Process:* Nursing Process, Analysis; *Cognitive Level:* Application; *Client Need/Subneed:* Physiological Integrity/Physiological Adaptation/Pathophysiology

6. CORRECT ANSWER: 4. **Answer 1** is incorrect because warm and dry indicates *perfusion.* **Answer 2** is incorrect because this is *not* a *significant* elevation. **Answer 3** is incorrect because this is within the *normal* range. **Answer 4 is correct because this is too slow and peripheral blood flow is sluggish, indicating impaired circulation. Normal reperfusion occurs in 3 seconds.**

■ **TEST-TAKING TIP:** *Three options are "OK" findings; one option is not an "OK" sign. Use a process of elimination to narrow down the options to the one that is a problem finding.*

Content Area: Adult Health, Cardiovascular; *Integrated Process:* Nursing Process, Analysis; *Cognitive Level:* Application; *Client Need/Subneed:* Physiological Integrity/Reduction of Risk Potential/Potential for Alterations in Body Systems

7. CORRECT ANSWER: 1. Answer 1 is correct because genetic counseling is essential as soon as possible after the diagnosis. This will determine if the hemophilia is an X-linked recessive disorder or a gene mutation and assist the parents to determine the desirability of future pregnancies. **Answer 2** is incorrect because this is *not* an *immediate* concern. Involvement in a support group is an excellent nursing intervention, but can safely be delayed for a period of time. **Answer 3** is incorrect because this is *not* an *immediate* concern. Involvement with a comprehensive health-care team (e.g., pediatricians, hematologists, orthopedists, nurses, social workers, and physical therapists) will happen as the infant's needs for such referrals occur. **Answer 4** is incorrect because this is *not* an *immediate* concern. Unlike many other disorders in which both parents carry the trait, the feeling of responsibility usually rests with the mother, and this can affect the couple's relationship. Couples' counseling should take place *after* the determination of the cause of the hemophilia is made.

■ **TEST-TAKING TIP:** *Determining the cause of the hemophilia is the* **first** *action needed; it will guide the timing of all other interventions. When all four answers are correct, select the most* **immediate** *need; see the word "immediately" in the stem.*

Content Area: Child Health, Hematological; ***Integrated Process:*** Nursing Process, Implementation; ***Cognitive Level:*** Application; ***Client Need/Subneed:*** Safe and Effective Care Environment/ Management of Care/Establishing Priorities

8. CORRECT ANSWER: 2. **Answer 1** is incorrect because Chadwick's sign is a bluish discoloration of the *cervix and vagina,* classically associated with *pregnancy.* **Answer 2 is correct because Homans' sign is pain in the back of the calf or knee when the foot is dorsiflexed, and is typically associated with thrombosis in veins of the calf.** **Answer 3** is incorrect because Hegar's sign is a softening of the lower uterine segment just above the cervix, seen as a *probable sign of pregnancy.* **Answer 4** is incorrect because Goodell's sign is the softening of the cervix seen as early as *6 weeks' gestation* and is a *probable* sign of pregnancy.

■ **TEST-TAKING TIP:** *Three of the options (Answers 1, 3, and 4) are pregnancy-related conditions. Eliminate those options since the focus is on* **postpartum.**

Content Area: Maternity, Postpartum; ***Integrated Process:*** Nursing Process, Assessment; ***Cognitive Level:*** Application; ***Client Need/Subneed:*** Physiological Integrity/Reduction of Risk Potential/System Specific Assessments

9. CORRECT ANSWER: 1. Answer 1 is correct because, when total bilirubin is elevated (normal 0 to 0.9 mg/dL), bilirubin is excreted in the urine, which becomes deep orange and foamy. **Answer 2** is incorrect because the bowel movements are clay-colored with liver disease. Tar-colored stools would be seen with *GI* bleeding or *iron* supplements. **Answer 3** is incorrect because, if there are symptoms *other* than jaundice, they would be flu-like with maybe a fever. **Answer 4** is incorrect because, if the eyes were involved, the *sclera* would be *yellow* (jaundiced), not red.

■ **TEST-TAKING TIP:** *Look for an option that could be due to excessive bilirubin: ↑ serum bilirubin resulting in ↑ urine color.*

Content Area: Adult Health, Gastrointestinal; ***Integrated Process:*** Nursing Process, Analysis; ***Cognitive Level:*** Application; ***Client Need/Subneed:*** Physiological Integrity/ Physiological Adaptation/Pathophysiology

10. CORRECT ANSWER: 3. **Answer 1** is incorrect because administering activated charcoal following the lavage *is* correct protocol when dealing with aspirin overdosages. There is no need for the nurse to question this order. **Answer 2** is incorrect because hemodialysis *may be used* in severe cases of aspirin overdosages. There is no need for the nurse to question this order. **Answer 3 is correct because hyperthermia is associated with toxic ingestions of aspirin. Therefore, external cooling (such as a cooling blanket) rather than warming is indicated.** **Answer 4** is incorrect because vitamin K *may be needed* to control the bleeding associated with aspirin overdosages. There is no need for the nurse to question this order.

■ **TEST-TAKING TIP:** *The stem asks for an order that is "not OK." Think of all of the possible side effects of aspirin overdosage and note what three options* **are** *correct protocol.*

Content Area: Child Health, Poisoning; ***Integrated Process:*** Nursing Process, Evaluation; ***Cognitive Level:*** Application; ***Client Need/Subneed:*** Safe and Effective Care Environment/ Safety and Infection Control/Error Prevention

11. CORRECT ANSWER: 1. Answer 1 is correct because nutrition plays an essential role in respiratory care. The increased carbon dioxide production from a high carbohydrate intake would promote hypercapnea and respiratory acidosis, adding to the pulmonary workload. **Answer 2** is incorrect because, although essential to the management of care, it is *not a priority* at this stage of respiratory transition. **Answer 3** is incorrect because the neural and muscle control of speech has *not been affected;* therefore, retraining is not necessary. **Answer 4** is incorrect at this point because, although ambulation improves circulation, the respiratory adaptation and workload of breathing are the *priority* for this client.

■ **TEST-TAKING TIP:** *Think* **priority** *and the nursing concept of* **adaptation** *during the weaning process.* **Short-term** *interventions (Answer 1) have the priority over long-term management (Answers 2 and 4); Answer 3 is inappropriate. Because the focus of the question is the respiratory system, choose the option that relates to respiration (i.e., carbon dioxide).*

Content Area: Adult Health, Respiratory; ***Integrated Process:*** Nursing Process, Planning; ***Cognitive Level:*** Application; ***Client Need/Subneed:*** Safe and Effective Care Environment/ Management of Care/Collaboration with Interdisciplinary Team

12. CORRECT ANSWER: 3. Answer 1 is incorrect because, while epistaxis may occur following an injury, it is *not as frequent* as other kinds of hemorrhage. **Answer 2** is incorrect because, while spontaneous hematuria is not uncommon and may occur following an injury, it is *not as frequent* as other kinds of hemorrhage. **Answer 3 is correct because early signs of hemarthrosis include a feeling of stiffness, tingling, and aching in the involved joint, followed by a decrease in ability to move the joint. Answer 4** is incorrect because, while warmth, redness, and swelling in the involved joint are common signs and symptoms of a hemarthrosis, considerable loss of movement would be a *later* clinical manifestation.

■ **TEST-TAKING TIP:** *Key focus is in the word "early" in the stem; also think of frequency; therefore, you can eliminate Answers 1 and 2.*

Content Area: Child Health, Hematological; ***Integrated Process:*** Nursing Process, Evaluation; ***Cognitive Level:*** Analysis; ***Client Need/Subneed:*** Physiological Integrity/Physiological Adaptation/Pathophysiology

13. CORRECT ANSWER: 4. Answer 1 is incorrect because the client *should* avoid getting constipated to reduce straining during a bowel movement. **Answer 2** is incorrect because the client *can* use hemorrhoid cream and witch hazel pads for relief. **Answer 3** is incorrect because the client *can* take warm sitz baths frequently to relieve the pain. **Answer 4 is correct because the client *should not* stop taking iron supplements to relieve pain from hemorrhoids. Since iron can be constipating, the client should be given instructions to increase fiber and fluid intake to avoid constipation.**

■ **TEST-TAKING TIP:** *This question asks for the* incorrect *response.*

Content Area: Maternity, Antepartum; ***Integrated Process:*** Nursing Process, Evaluation; ***Cognitive Level:*** Analysis; ***Client Need/Subneed:*** Physiological Integrity/Basic Care and Comfort/Elimination

14. CORRECT ANSWER: 3. Answer 1 is incorrect because, although there are symptoms of ineffective breathing pattern, it is the *sequela* from the impaired gas exchange. **Answer 2** is incorrect because an infection is a *risk or precipitating factor* for ARDS. The question asks for the *rationale* for the impaired gas exchange. **Answer 3 is correct because ARDS affects the arterial-alveolar capillary membrane gas exchange. The basic pathophysiology in ARDS is alveolar capillary damage, decreased surfactant, and the resultant noncardiogenic pulmonary edema. As a result, carbon dioxide cannot be eliminated, oxygen cannot be absorbed, and severe hypoxemia and acidosis result. Answer 4** is incorrect because, although activity intolerance is present, it is due to the hypoxia from protein accumulation in the alveoli. The RN must monitor the arterial blood gases to assess levels of hypercapnea and hypoxemia.

■ **TEST-TAKING TIP:** *When all options appear relevant, choose the one that addresses the key term (i.e., "basic rationale"). Answers 1, 2, and 4 are more the* result *rather than the* cause *of the symptoms. Choose the broader answer (Answer 3) that encompasses another* related *answer (Answer 1).*

Content Area: Adult Health, Respiratory; ***Integrated Process:*** Nursing Process, Analysis; ***Cognitive Level:*** Analysis; ***Client Need/Subneed:*** Physiological Integrity/Physiological Adaptation/ Pathophysiology

15. CORRECT ANSWER: 4. Answer 1 is incorrect because a total of 1 loading dose followed by 17 maintenance doses of *N*-acetylcysteine (Mucomyst) *must* be given in order for the medication to be effective. Withholding the medication will not accomplish this goal. **Answer 2** is incorrect because another dose of *N*-acetylcysteine (Mucomyst) will have the *same* odor. **Answer 3** is incorrect because discarding the dose and preparing another dose will *not change* the odor of *N*-acetylcysteine (Mucomyst). **Answer 4 is correct because *N*-acetylcysteine (Mucomyst) has an offensive odor (e.g., "rotten eggs"), but this is a normal side effect of the medication and does not interfere with the medication's efficacy. The parents should be informed of these characteristics and encouraged to allow the nurse to administer the medication to the child.**

■ **TEST-TAKING TIP:** *Since there are a limited number of antidotes for poisons/overdosages, the parents' involvement is important to ensure that this antidote will be given.*

Content Area: Child Health, Poisoning; ***Integrated Process:*** Nursing Process, Implementation; ***Cognitive Level:*** Application; ***Client Need/Subneed:*** Psychosocial Integrity/Behavioral Interventions

16. CORRECT ANSWERS: 1, 3, 5. Answer 1 is correct because ice should *not* be used. It limits circulation and can cause *thermal damage*. Answer 2 is incorrect because this type of lotion *is* appropriate and will provide relief. **Answer 3 is correct because a sunlamp may cause *thermal burn* to the area. Answer 4** is incorrect because gentle washing and drying will *not cause* further damage. **Answer 5 is correct because alcohol would *sting* and *further* irritate the skin. Answer 6** is incorrect because scratching would cause further damage and lead to infection.

■ **TEST-TAKING TIP:** *Note that the question asks for what is* not *OK; therefore, choose actions that would cause further skin irritation or damage such as options that imply cold (Answer 1), heat (Answer 3), and irritation (Answer 5).*

Content Area: Adult Health, Integumentary; ***Integrated Process:*** Nursing Process, Evaluation; ***Cognitive Level:*** Application; ***Client Need/Subneed:*** Physiological Integrity/Physiological Adaptation/Alterations in Body Systems

17. CORRECT ANSWER: 1. Answer 1 is correct because immediate treatment of bleeding may help to promote a more rapid recovery with a decreased likelihood of complications. Answer 2 is incorrect because, while it is appropriate, it is *not* the *priority* rationale for teaching parents home care for hemophilia. **Answer 3** is incorrect because, while it is appropriate, it is *not* the *priority* rationale for teaching parents home care for hemophilia.

Answer 4 is incorrect because, while it is appropriate, it is *not* the *priority* rationale for teaching parents home care for hemophilia.

■ **TEST-TAKING TIP:** *The key word in the best answer is "immediacy."*

Content Area: Child Health, Hematological; ***Integrated Process:*** Teaching and Learning; ***Cognitive Level:*** Application; ***Client Need/Subneed:*** Physiological Integrity/Reduction of Risk Potential/Potential for Complications from Surgical Procedures and Health Alterations

18. CORRECT ANSWER: 1. Answer 1 is correct because women who are pregnant should avoid lying directly on their backs. A right or left tilt is the correct position during pregnancy, to avoid vena cava compression. **Answer 2** is incorrect because the nurse *will* check on the client frequently while she is wearing the monitor to ensure fetal well-being, as well as to determine the frequency and duration of any contractions. **Answer 3** is incorrect because women who are pregnant *should* avoid lying directly on the back. A right or left tilt is the correct position during pregnancy, to avoid vena cava compression. The client should lie in whatever position is comfortable, except on the back. **Answer 4** is incorrect because the monitor *is* used to ensure the fetal well-being, as well as to determine the frequency and duration of any contractions.

■ **TEST-TAKING TIP:** *Read the question carefully; it is asking which statement is incorrect, meaning that the nurse would need to do further teaching.*

Content Area: Maternity, Intrapartum; ***Integrated Process:*** Nursing Process, Evaluation; ***Cognitive Level:*** Analysis; ***Client Need/Subneed:*** Physiological Integrity/Reduction of Risk Potential/Potential for Complications from Surgical Procedures and Health Alterations

19. CORRECT ANSWER: 3. Following abdominal surgery and general anesthesia, bowel sounds may not return for 48 hours. If they are present, they will be heard in the lower right quadrant over the area of the ileocecal valve, where the small and large intestines join.

■ **TEST-TAKING TIP:** *General anesthesia paralyzes gastric motility. Think proximal to distal for the return of function.*

Content Area: Adult Health, Gastrointestinal; ***Integrated Process:*** Nursing Process, Assessment; ***Cognitive Level:*** Application; ***Client Need/Subneed:*** Physiological Integrity/Reduction of Risk Potential/System Specific Assessments

20. CORRECT ANSWER: 2. Answer 1 is incorrect because it is not reasonable or realistic. Many young children *will require* multivitamins that contain iron. The key is to prevent the young child from gaining access to the iron tablets, rather than to not purchase the required medication. **Answer 2 is correct because iron tablets resemble candy (e.g., M&Ms) and present a special temptation to a young child who cannot differentiate between medication and candy.** **Answer 3** is incorrect because the parents *should* be informed of the need to keep the tablets in a high place that is also *locked.* A curious young child can access even high places if given enough time to do so. **Answer 4** is incorrect because syrup of ipecac (a powerful emetic) is *no* longer recommended as a poison intervention in the home (American Academy of Child Health, 2003). One reason for this is the increased number of medications for which inducing emesis is contraindicated; another is the possibility of abuse by individuals with eating disorders.

■ **TEST-TAKING TIP:** *Focus on the "don't buy" options here and select the simple obvious (candy) answer. Children cannot correctly differentiate between substances. Therefore, remove any substance that the child might identify as "OK" but would present a danger.*

Content Area: Child Health, Poisoning; ***Integrated Process:*** Teaching and Learning; ***Cognitive Level:*** Application; ***Client Need/Subneed:*** Safe and Effective Care Environment/ Safety and Infection Control/Error Prevention

21. CORRECT ANSWER: 4. Answer 1 is incorrect because scopolamine should *not* be given. **Answer 2** is incorrect because it indicates that the drugs were given, whereas scopolamine is *contraindicated.* **Answer 3** is incorrect because the drugs should *not* be given. (These actions would be appropriate if the drugs *were* given.) **Answer 4 is correct because clients with glaucoma should not receive anticholinergic drugs (e.g., scopolamine), which dilate the pupils and increase intraocular pressure.**

■ **TEST-TAKING TIP:** *Look for a pattern—three choices relate to giving the drug and one raises concern.*

Content Area: Adult Health, Sensory; ***Integrated Process:*** Nursing Process, Analysis; ***Cognitive Level:*** Analysis; ***Client Need/Subneed:*** Physiological Integrity/Pharmacological and Parenteral Therapies/Contraindications

22. CORRECT ANSWERS: 2, 3. Answer 1 is incorrect because the serum theophylline level should range from 10 to 20 mcg/mL. There is *no need to withhold* the medication because the medication level is safe. **Answer 2 is correct because the serum theophylline level should range from 10 to 20 mcg/mL. It is safe to administer the medication to the child. Answer 3 is correct because the nurse should note the child's serum theophylline level on the Medication Administration Record (MAR) next to the dose and time to validate that it is safe to administer the medication to the child. It is the *first* action that the nurse should take. *Documentation* of a safe medication level always takes place prior to administration of the medication.** **Answer 4** is incorrect because the medication level is safe and there is *no need to withhold* the medication.

■ **TEST-TAKING TIP:** *Two options say "don't give" (i.e., withhold) while two options say "give" (administer). Select the two options that say "give" because the blood level is within normal range. The priority is to* note *the blood level, then* give *the medication.*

Content Area: Child Health, Respiratory; ***Integrated Process:*** Nursing Process, Evaluation; ***Cognitive Level:*** Analysis; ***Client Need/Subneed:*** Physiological Integrity/Reduction of Risk Potential/Laboratory Value

23. CORRECT ANSWER: 2. **Answer 1** is incorrect because a nipple stimulation test will result in contractions, the *opposite* of expected management. A nonstress test and amniotic fluid index are appropriate for fetal surveillance. **Answer 2 is correct because dehydration can lead to preterm labor contractions. Encouraging adequate hydration can decrease mild uterine irritability.** **Answer 3** is incorrect because misoprostol *stimulates* contractions; it is not a tocolytic. **Answer 4** is incorrect because, although ambulation can prevent thrombophlebitis, *sequential compression* devices are more appropriate for this client.

■ TEST-TAKING TIP: *Since this client would most likely be on bedrest, with treatment aimed to decrease contractions, eliminate Answer 4 because ambulation may increase contractions and is not an appropriate intervention for preterm labor. Eliminate Answers 1 and 3 also because the actions are likely to stimulate contractions.*

Content Area: Maternity, Intrapartum; *Integrated Process:* Nursing Process, Implementation; *Cognitive Level:* Application; *Client Need/Subneed:* Physiological Integrity/Reduction of Risk Potential/Potential for Alterations in Body Systems

24. CORRECT ANSWER: 4. **Answer 1** is incorrect because diffuse, wheezing breath sounds reflect bronchoconstriction, *not* laryngeal edema. **Answer 2** is incorrect because arterial blood gases are *not* used to diagnose laryngeal edema. The alteration in vocal cord sounds is the *first* indication. The normal P_{CO_2} is 35 to 45 mm Hg. A P_{CO_2} of 52 mm Hg reflects *respiratory acidosis.* A P_{O_2} of 90% at normal altitude is considered low-normal. **Answer 3** is incorrect because a pulse oximetry reading reflects oxygen perfusion of the red blood cells. It may be decreased by severe vasoconstriction from decreased temperature, shock, or bleeding. It will *not* reflect the status of the larynx *unless* there is airway obstruction. **Answer 4 is correct because the high-pitched crowing sounds, or stridor, are indications of edema of the larynx. Clients with this sign must be watched for obstruction and the need for possible re-intubation. Recognition of early signs of edema of the larynx prevents respiratory complications from occurring.**

■ TEST-TAKING TIP: *Focus on* early signs. *Vocal (laryngeal) sounds (Answer 4) would be the first, specific, and early sign of obstruction; all others are respiratory signs that would* follow. *Focus on the two answers that relate to nursing assessment of breath sounds. Select the answer that is a* specific *sign of obstruction.*

Content Area: Adult Health, Respiratory; *Integrated Process:* Nursing Process, Assessment; *Cognitive Level:* Analysis; *Client Need/Subneed:* Physiological Integrity/Physiological Adaptation/Medical Emergencies

25. CORRECT ANSWER: 4. **Answer 1** is incorrect because *immediate* first aid and life support measures should be the parent's first action. Once the child's status is determined, the Poison Control Center should be contacted. **Answer 2** is incorrect because *immediate* first aid and life support measures should be the parent's first action. Once the child's status is determined, the parent can begin trying to reach the child's pediatrician. **Answer 3** is incorrect because immediate first aid and life support measures should be the parent's first action. Following the instructions on the label of the substance that the child has ingested is not recommended. The instructions are usually for an *adult* rather than for a child; following these adult instructions could lead to additional harm to the child. **Answer 4 is correct because the first and most important principle in dealing with a poisoning is to treat the child's signs and symptoms (e.g., assess for shock or absence of respiratory function). The nurse should teach the parent basic first aid and life support measures to begin immediately upon discovering that the child has ingested a poison.**

■ TEST-TAKING TIP: *Treat the child first and the poison second. Select a here-and-now direct action for the child, not "call" or read the label.*

Content Area: Child Health, Poisoning; *Integrated Process:* Teaching and Learning; *Cognitive Level:* Comprehension; *Client Need/Subneed:* Physiological Integrity/Physiological Adaptation/Medical Emergencies

26. CORRECT ANSWER: 2. **Answer 1** is incorrect because the action of ACE inhibitors is to decrease venous return (decrease preload) as a result of vasodilation. **Answer 2 is correct because ACE inhibitors (potent vasodilators) are used to lower the BP by decreasing both cardiac afterload and workload, actions that are essential for a client with a low ejection fraction. A systolic BP of 90 mm Hg would be acceptable in these clients as long as they remain asymptomatic.** **Answer 3** is incorrect because the use of an ACE inhibitor decreases aldosterone formation and sodium is excreted by the kidney along with water, and potassium increases, which may be a serious side effect. **Answer 4** is incorrect because ACE inhibitors actually have a diuretic action. In heart failure, they improve the ejection fraction by reducing venous volume and arterial pressure.

■ TEST-TAKING TIP: *Because ACE inhibitors are not diuretics, first eliminate the two options pertaining to diuretic/diuresis. Know the action of ACE inhibitors. When unsure, eliminate Answers 1 and 3 as undesirable actions for a client with congestive heart failure; Answer 4 is not the action of an antihypertensive. Note two contradictory options: "increase" (Answer 1) versus "decrease" (Answer 2). Select the logical choice of "decreases cardiac afterload."*

Content Area: Adult Health, Cardiovascular; *Integrated Process:* Nursing Process, Analysis; *Cognitive Level:* Comprehension; *Client Need/Subneed:* Physiological Integrity/Pharmacological and Parenteral Therapies/Expected Effects/Outcomes

27. CORRECT ANSWERS: 1, 2, 4. **Answer 1 is correct because putting an undershirt under the chest straps of the harness prevents the straps from rubbing the skin and causing skin breakdown. Answer 2 is correct because putting socks under the foot and leg pieces of the harness prevents the straps from rubbing the skin and causing skin breakdown.** **Answer 3** is incorrect because lotion and powder applied under the straps of the harness can "cake" and irritate the skin and cause skin breakdown. **Answer 4 is correct because massaging healthy skin under the straps of the harness once a day stimulates circulation and prevents skin breakdown.**

■ TEST-TAKING TIP: ***Remember that, when caring for infants/children, powder is rarely used because of its tendency to accumulate and "cake" and lead to skin irritation and breakdown.***

Content Area: Child Health, Musculoskeletal; ***Integrated Process:*** Teaching and Learning; ***Cognitive Level:*** Application; ***Client Need/Subneed:*** Physiological Integrity/Basic Care and Comfort/Assistive Devices

28. CORRECT ANSWER: 4. **Answer 1** is incorrect because knee-high support hose can *worsen* the varicose veins. *Full-length* support hose can *decrease* the pain associated with varicose veins. **Answer 2** is incorrect because increasing dairy intake will *not* decrease the pain associated with varicose veins. Increasing calcium intake can provide some relief from leg cramps, but the question is about varicose veins, and calcium (e.g., dairy) does not help varicose vein pain. **Answer 3** is incorrect because the nurse should *not* give advice regarding labor stimulation. Nipple stimulation causes uncontrolled release of oxytocin, which can lead to hyperstimulation of the uterus and fetal distress. **Answer 4 is correct because lying down with the feet elevated can provide some relief *for* pain caused by varicose veins. Having varicose veins is usually not an indication for induction of labor.**

■ TEST-TAKING TIP: ***The word "should" indicates advice or opinion and should be eliminated. The question did not ask what the nurse should advise the client to do. The word "try" indicates a suggestion by the nurse.***

Content Area: Maternity, Antepartum; ***Integrated Process:*** Nursing Process, Implementation; ***Cognitive Level:*** Application; ***Client Need/Subneed:*** Physiological Integrity/Reduction of Risk Potential/Potential for Complications of Diagnostic Tests/Treatments/Procedures

29. CORRECT ANSWER: 2. **Answer 1** is incorrect because *no general anesthesia* was used. The procedure is done under *local* anesthetic. **Answer 2 is correct because activity following the filtering procedure is liberal. Unless contraindicated, the client may resume normal activities. The client should avoid any activity that increases pressure in the eye.** **Answer 3** is incorrect because *no general anesthesia,* which affects bowel sounds, was used. **Answer 4** is incorrect because the movement of aqueous humor is influenced by *drugs* that cause dilation and constriction, *not* increasing fluids.

■ TEST-TAKING TIP: ***When selecting the best action for this client, you need to know the type of anesthesia used. Answers 1 and 3 are not relevant to local anesthesia.***

Content Area: Adult Health, Sensory; ***Integrated Process:*** Nursing Process, Planning; ***Cognitive Level:*** Application; ***Client Need/Subneed:*** Physiological Integrity/Reduction of Risk Potential/Potential for Complications from Surgical Procedures

30. CORRECT ANSWER: 4. **Answer 1** is incorrect because an infant born to a mother who has HBsAg– should have received the first HepB (hepatitis B) immunization *soon (if not immediately) after birth and before hospital discharge.* The HepB immunization series would thus be on schedule; the second immunization should be given between 1 and 4 months of age, and the third immunization should be given between 6 and 18 months of age. There is *no* need for the nurse to question this order. **Answer 2** is incorrect because the first DTaP (diphtheria and tetanus toxoids and acellular pertussis) immunization *should* be given at 2 months of age. There is *no* need for the nurse to question this order. **Answer 3** is incorrect because the first Hib (*Haemophilus influenzae* type b) immunization *should* be given at 2 months of age. There is in *no* need for the nurse to question this order. **Answer 4 is correct because an infant born to a HBsAg– mother would not have any active immunity to the disease and *should* receive the immunization on schedule. The nurse *should* question this order.**

■ TEST-TAKING TIP: ***Three of the responses require that the nurse* give *an immunization; one response does* not. *Select the response that is* different. *Know the immunization schedule and what effect, if any, the mother's immune status has on the infant's immunization schedule.***

Content Area: Child Health, Immunizations; ***Integrated Process:*** Nursing Process, Analysis; ***Cognitive Level:*** Analysis; ***Client Need/Subneed:*** Health Promotion and Maintenance/Immunizations

31. CORRECT ANSWER: 4. There are 30 mL in 1 ounce; 8 ounces in a cup; 4 ounces in ½ cup. Thus, 8 ounces of apple juice is 240 mL, 1 cup of tea is 240 mL, and ½ cup of gelatin is 120 mL, totaling 600 mL.

■ TEST-TAKING TIP: ***Know the basic conversions for liquid measures.***

Content Area: Adult Health, Diet; ***Integrated Process:*** Nursing Process, Implementation; ***Cognitive Level:*** Analysis; ***Client Need/Subneed:*** Physiological Integrity/Basic Care and Comfort/Nutrition and Oral Hydration

32. CORRECT ANSWER: 3. **Answer 1** is incorrect because, while it is valid that the child's appetite will return as the acute symptoms recede, it is *not* the nurse's priority instruction. Prevention of a pathologic fracture from weight-bearing on the affected limb is the nurse's priority instruction to the parent. **Answer 2** is incorrect because, while it is valid that adequate nutrition must be maintained to aid healing, it is *not* the nurse's priority instruction. Prevention of a pathological fracture from weight-bearing on the affected limb is the nurse's priority instruction to the parent. **Answer 3 is correct because weight-bearing on the affected limb is not permitted until healing is well underway. This is done to prevent a pathological fracture.** **Answer 4** is incorrect because, while it is valid that moving about on a gurney or in a wheelchair will be permitted when bedrest is no longer necessary, it is *not* the nurse's priority instruction. Prevention of a pathological fracture from weight-bearing on the affected limb is the nurse's priority instruction to the parent.

■ **TEST-TAKING TIP:** *When caring for a child with osteomyelitis, prevention of complications is always the nurse's priority teaching intervention. A pathological fracture could be a serious complication from inappropriate/early weight-bearing on the affected limb.*

Content Area: Child Health, Musculoskeletal; ***Integrated Process:*** Teaching and Learning; ***Cognitive Level:*** Analysis; ***Client Need/Subneed:*** Physiological Integrity/Basic Care and Comfort/Mobility/Immobility

33. CORRECT ANSWER: 1. **Answer 1 is correct because the symptoms of an inevitable abortion are abdominal cramping, bright red vaginal spotting, passing clots, and cervical dilation.** **Answer 2** is incorrect because the symptoms of a complete abortion are cramping, bleeding and the passage of the *products* of conception. **Answer 3** is incorrect because a missed abortion happens when the fetus has died and is not passed. There is *no* cramping, bleeding, or passage of clots. **Answer 4** is incorrect because the symptoms of a threatened abortion are cramping and bleeding, but *not cervical dilation.*

■ **TEST-TAKING TIP:** *Types of abortions sound like the symptoms. Inevitable abortion cannot be stopped; threatened abortion has* some *signs, and complete abortion is when all the products of conception are passed.*

Content Area: Maternity, Antepartum; ***Integrated Process:*** Nursing Process, Analysis; ***Cognitive Level:*** Application; ***Client Need/Subneed:*** Physiological Integrity/Physiological Adaptation/Alterations in Body Systems

34. CORRECT ANSWER: 2. **Answer 1** is incorrect because the torso is no longer shaved. Only the areas where incisions will be made may be shaved to avoid potential skin cuts or abrasions. **Answer 2 is correct because skin preparation for a hernia repair may include the client scrubbing with an antispetic sponge (Hibiclens) for several days before surgery. Hair removal is usually done in the operating room (OR), and whether clipped or shaved depends on the amount of hair.** **Answer 3** is incorrect because the area shaved will depend on the surgical approach. The umbilicus may be shaved by the client at home plus shaving or clipping in the OR. **Answer 4** is incorrect because shaving or clipping in the groin will be done in the OR. The client may be asked to remove excess hair from the umbilicus.

■ **TEST-TAKING TIP:** *Choose an option that minimizes the potential for skin cuts or abrasions that could lead to infection.*

Content Area: Adult Health, Integumentary; ***Integrated Process:*** Nursing Process, Planning; ***Cognitive Level:*** Application; ***Client Need/Subneed:*** Physiological Integrity/Reduction of Risk Potential/Therapeutic Procedures

35. CORRECT ANSWER: 1. **Answer 1 is correct because initial therapy is rest and non–weight-bearing in order to reduce the inflammation and restore motion. There will be other treatment modalities used in arresting this disease, but the first action is aimed at reducing the inflammation and restoring motion through rest and non–weight-bearing.** **Answer 2** is incorrect because, while preventing weight-bearing in the affected limb is desirable, it is *not* the *initial* therapy. This treatment modality includes braces or casts and is initiated *later* in the plan of care. **Answer 3** is incorrect because, while preventing the onset of degenerative arthritis is desirable, it is *not* the *initial* therapy. This complication of the disease is usually a *later finding* in children over 10 years of age who also had a delayed diagnosis of the disease. **Answer 4** is incorrect because, while trauma can be the cause of some cases of the disease, the actual cause of the disease is *unknown.*

■ **TEST-TAKING TIP:** *In the initial stage, priority is to ↓ inflammation. Know the four stages of Legg-Calvé-Perthes disease in order to answer this question correctly.*

Content Area: Child Health, Musculoskeletal; ***Integrated Process:*** Teaching and Learning; ***Cognitive Level:*** Application; ***Client Need/Subneed:*** Physiological Integrity/Basic Care and Comfort/Mobility/Immobility

36. CORRECT ANSWER: 2. **Answer 1** is incorrect because the *cause* of pain needs to be first *assessed* before medicating. **Answer 2 is correct because severe groin or hip pain is a common complaint of a possible hip fracture when the client is able to bear weight.** **Answer 3** is incorrect because eliminating weight-bearing would be the first priority to prevent further trauma to the joint, then this would be the *next* action. **Answer 4** is incorrect because a walker still requires the client to use *both* legs.

■ **TEST-TAKING TIP:** *If the symptom is groin pain while walking—think hip and eliminate weight-bearing.*

Content Area: Geriatrics, Musculoskeletal; ***Integrated Process:*** Nursing Process, Implementation; ***Cognitive Level:*** Application; ***Client Need/Subneed:*** Physiological Integrity/Basic Care and Comfort/Mobility/Immobility

37. CORRECT ANSWER: 4. **Answer 1** is incorrect because, while keeping in contact with classmates is desirable, it will not assist the school-age child to achieve the developmental milestone of industry like beginning a hobby will. **Answer 2** is incorrect because, while learning to tolerate immobility is desirable, it is an *unrealistic* expectation of a child in this age group. This is essentially a well child who must remain inactive for a prolonged period of time. Beginning a hobby will help the time pass more quickly. **Answer 3** is incorrect because, while learning to correctly apply the prescribed braces is desirable, it will be *accomplished after* the period of bedrest. This is essentially a well child who must remain inactive for a prolonged period of time. Beginning a hobby will help the time pass more quickly. **Answer 4 is correct because the school-age child is in the developmental stage of industry, and enforced long-term bedrest interferes with the achievement of this milestone. Assembling collections, building models, engaging in crafts, and the like will fulfill the child's need for a creative outlet and assist in achieving the desired milestone.**

■ **TEST-TAKING TIP:** *Relate achievement of the child's developmental task (industry) to the consequences of the disease process (bedrest). Choose an option that is something pleasurable and can be done at will.*

Content Area: Child Health, Musculoskeletal; ***Integrated Process:*** Nursing Process, Implementation; ***Cognitive Level:*** Application; ***Client Need/Subneed:*** Health Promotion and Maintenance/Developmental Stages and Transitions

38. CORRECT ANSWER: 3. Answer 1 is incorrect because decelerations in the fetal heart rate during contractions that end when the contraction is over are either early decelerations or variable decelerations; *neither pattern is indicative of fetal distress.* **Answer 2** is incorrect because an increase in the fetal heart rate during a vaginal examination indicates *fetal well-being* and is a reassuring sign. **Answer 3 is correct because a uniform decrease in the heart rate that begins after each contraction for the past four contractions describes late decelerations, which is an indication of fetal distress. Answer 4** is incorrect because lack of meconium staining is *normal, not* an indication of fetal distress.

■ **TEST-TAKING TIP:** *When the question describes a fetal monitor pattern, try drawing out the described pattern.*

Content Area: Maternity, Intrapartum; ***Integrated Process:*** Nursing Process, Analysis; ***Cognitive Level:*** Application; ***Client Need/Subneed:*** Physiological Integrity/Reduction of Risk Potential/Vital Signs Changes/Abnormalities

39. CORRECT ANSWER: 18. The solution contains 50 units/mL. It is a simple matter to divide 900 units/hr of heparin by 50 units/mL to obtain the hourly flow rate:

$$\frac{\textbf{900 units/hr}}{\textbf{50 units/mL}} = \textbf{18 mL/hr}$$

■ **TEST-TAKING TIP:** *The first step in completing this calculation is to determine how many units of heparin are in each mL of IV fluid.*

Content Area: Adult Health, Hematological; ***Integrated Process:*** Nursing Process, Analysis; ***Cognitive Level:*** Analysis; ***Client Need/Subneed:*** Physiological Integrity/Pharmacological and Parenteral Therapies/Dosage Calculation

40. CORRECT ANSWER: 4. Answer 1 is incorrect because, while 65% of all children with juvenile idiopathic arthritis will require a slower-acting antirheumatic drug (SAARD), it is usually begun *after* a trial on the nonsteroidal anti-inflammatory drugs (NSAIDs). It may then be used in *conjunction* with the NSAIDs. Additional time is required to evaluate the effectiveness of the NSAID. **Answer 2** is incorrect because, while aspirin (acetylsalicylic acid [ASA]) was once the initial drug of choice in the treatment of juvenile idiopathic arthritis, it is now *seldom* used in children. It has been replaced with other more effective, less toxic medications. **Answer 3** is incorrect because, while corticosteroids are the most potent anti-inflammatory agents, they will not cure arthritis, and the significant *adverse* effects of long-term steroid use are undesirable. **Answer 4 is correct because the child must take a nonsteroidal anti-inflammatory drug (NSAID) for at least 3 weeks before the effectiveness of the medication can be evaluated.**

■ **TEST-TAKING TIP:** *Three options suggest something different to consider; the best option implies "wait." Know the medications and their order of usage associated with juvenile idiopathic arthritis.*

Content Area: Child Health, Musculoskeletal; ***Integrated Process:*** Communication and Documentation; ***Cognitive Level:*** Application; ***Client Need/Subneed:*** Physiological Integrity/Pharmacological and Parenteral Therapies/Expected Effects/Outcomes

41. CORRECT ANSWERS: 2, 3, 5. Answer 1 is incorrect because hands should be *dry* before applying gloves, which are difficult to put on with wet hands. Microorganisms survive better in moist environments. **Answer 2 is correct because this client has few white blood cells (WBCs), and must be protected from infection. Neutrophils make up 55% to 70% of WBCs. An ANC below 1,000/mm^3 places the client at significant risk for infection. Alcohol-based hand cleaners that are at least 60% alcohol eliminate microbes as well as soap and water. Answer 3 is correct because this client has few white blood cells, and must be protected from infection. An ANC below 1,000/mm^3 places the client at high risk for infection. Fresh flowers contain many microbes. Answer 4** is incorrect because this client has few white blood cells, and must be protected from infection. The risk for infection increases as the ANC decreases. Vegetables should be washed and cooked. Triple-washing is *not* necessary. **Answer 5 is correct because this client has few white blood cells, and must be protected from infection. A normal ANC would be 2,000/mm^3 or higher. Most microbes are on the outer surface of the fruit. Fruit must be peeled or cooked. Answer 6** is incorrect because this client has few white cells and must be protected from all sources of infections.

■ **TEST-TAKING TIP:** *Think of actions that reduce the risk of infection. Choose the four options that are precautionary (e.g., wash hands and fresh vegetables; remove flowers; avoid unpeeled fruit).*

Content Area: Adult Health, Hematological; ***Integrated Process:*** Nursing Process, Implementation; ***Cognitive Level:*** Application; ***Client Need/Subneed:*** Safe and Effective Care Environment/Safety and Infection Control/Standard/Transmission-based/Other Precautions

42. CORRECT ANSWERS: 1, 2, 4. Answer 1 is correct because 8 to 10 hours of nighttime sleep is required by all adolescents, especially an adolescent with a chronic disease process. Getting the correct number of nighttime hours of sleep may prevent daytime sleepiness. Answer 2 is correct because a firm mattress will maintain skeletal alignment, which will reduce stiffness and pain and promote nighttime sleep, which may prevent daytime sleepiness. **Answer 3** is incorrect because daytime naps are *discouraged.* The inactivity promotes stiffness, and prolonged naps can interfere with sleepiness at bedtime. Fatigue should be handled with rest rather than sleep. **Answer 4 is correct because implementing relaxation techniques prior to bedtime (listening to music, meditation, etc.) may promote nighttime sleep, which may prevent daytime sleepiness.**

■ **TEST-TAKING TIP:** *Eliminate one obviously incorrect option: sleep in the daytime, which would not help to sleep at night.*

Content Area: Child Health, Musculoskeletal; ***Integrated Process:*** Nursing Process, Implementation; ***Cognitive Level:*** Application; ***Client Need/Subneed:*** Physiological Integrity/Basic Care and Comfort/Rest and Sleep

43. CORRECT ANSWERS: 2, 3, 4, 5, 6. **Answer 1** is incorrect because profuse perspiration or diaphoresis is associated with an insulin reaction or a *low* blood sugar. **Answer 2 is correct because irritability, confusion, and lethargy are associated with high blood sugar levels. Answer 3 is correct because flushing is associated with dehydration, which results from a high blood sugar level. Answer 4 is correct because headache can result from high or low blood sugar levels. Answer 5 is correct because hyperglycemia can lead to hypovolemic shock, with a rapid, thready pulse from severe dehydration. Answer 6 is correct because deep, rapid breathing (Kussmaul's breathing) is an attempt to compensate for the increased carbon dioxide level resulting from ketoacidosis.**

■ **TEST-TAKING TIP:** *Think about the expected changes with sufficient or insufficient glucose levels. Review signs and symptoms of hypoglycemia and hyperglycemia.*

Content Area: Maternity, Postpartum; ***Integrated Process:*** Nursing Process, Assessment; ***Cognitive Level:*** Application; ***Client Need/Subneed:*** Physiological Integrity/Physiological Adaptation/Pathophysiology

44. CORRECT ANSWER: 2. **Answer 1** is incorrect because the urine output is within the *normal* range. **Answer 2 is correct because the normal central venous pressure (CVP) is 0 to 8 mm Hg. A value of 12 mm Hg reflects hypervolemia. The right ventricular function of this client reflects fluid volume overload, and the physician should be alerted.** **Answer 3** is incorrect because the cardiac output is within the *normal* range of 4 to 6 L/min. **Answer 4** is incorrect because this position, as well as leaning forward or sitting, *helps decrease* the pain from acute pancreatitis. The RN should foster a comfortable yet safe position.

■ **TEST-TAKING TIP:** *"Report to a physician" means something is wrong. The question addresses* both *the disease* and *fluid volume. Know normal values (Answers 1 and 3); Answer 2 is the* only abnormal *value. Answer 4 addresses* only *the disease and* not *the fluid volume.*

Content Area: Adult Health, Fluid and Electrolyte Imbalances; ***Integrated Process:*** Nursing Process, Evaluation; ***Cognitive Level:*** Analysis; ***Client Need/Subneed:*** Physiological Integrity/Reduction of Risk Potential/Laboratory Values

45. CORRECT ANSWERS: 1, 2, 3, 4. Answer 1 is correct because this is an appropriate position for an infant in a hip spica cast. It is especially effective when feeding a young infant. Answer 2 is correct because this is an appropriate position for an infant in a hip spica cast. It is especially effective when breastfeeding a young infant. Answer 3 is correct because this is an appropriate position for an infant in a hip spica cast. It is especially effective when feeding a young infant. Answer 4 is correct because this is an appropriate position for an infant in a hip spica cast. It is especially effective when encouraging the infant to play with toys.

■ **TEST-TAKING TIP:** *Visualize each position and then determine that all positions here* are *appropriate for the infant in a hip spica cast and the desired activity (outcome).*

Content Area: Child Health, Musculoskeletal; ***Integrated Process:*** Teaching and Learning; ***Cognitive Level:*** Analysis; ***Client Need/Subneed:*** Physiological Integrity/Basic Care and Comfort/Assistive Devices

46. CORRECT ANSWER: 1. Answer 1 is correct because calcium is lost in the fat necrosis, and saponification (formation of calcium soap) may occur. Circumoral tingling and muscle cramps are early signs of hypocalcemia. Assess for signs of tetany by checking Chvostek's and Trousseau's signs. **Answer 2** is incorrect because these are *not* signs of alteration in the sodium level. **Answer 3** is incorrect because clients would demonstrate hyperglycemia, *not* hypoglycemia. Numbness and circumoral tingling are *not* signs/symptoms relating to serum glucose. **Answer 4** is incorrect because circumoral tingling is *not* a sign of hypokalemia or hyperkalemia, which are related to furosemide (Lasix).

■ **TEST-TAKING TIP:** *Narrow the choice to the two* assessment *options, and select the one that relates to the symptoms in the stem. Choose the answer that addresses* both *complaints. If unsure, use the process of elimination. Muscle cramps do* not *occur with hypoglycemia; Answers 2 and 4 are vague and do* not *relate to circumoral tingling.*

Content Area: Adult Health, Gastrointestinal; ***Integrated Process:*** Nursing Process, Assessment; ***Cognitive Level:*** Application; ***Client Need/Subneed:*** Physiological Integrity/Physiological Adaptation/Fluid and Electrolyte Imbalances

47. CORRECT ANSWER: 1. Answer 1 is correct because a normal heart rate for a 2-week-old infant is 120 to 160 beats per minute. A heart rate of 100 beats per

minute is too low in a 2-week-old infant, and the digoxin should be withheld pending further assessment of the infant. **Answer 2** is incorrect because it is *too soon* to notify the pediatrician. The nurse needs to *further assess* the infant and then notify the pediatrician if it is appropriate. **Answer 3** is incorrect because a heart rate of 100 beats per minute is too low in a 2-week-old infant, and the digoxin should be *withheld* pending further assessment of the infant. **Answer 4** is incorrect because the nurse should revalidate the initial assessment findings in *15 minutes,* prior to proceeding with any additional interventions. *If* the infant's heart rate remains 100 beats per minute, the nurse should continue to withhold the medication and then notify the pediatrician.

■ TEST-TAKING TIP: ***The nurse should withhold the digoxin in an infant in this age group with this diagnosis when the heart rate is 100 beats per minute. Ask yourself: Is there a problem or not? And, if there is a problem, what steps and in what order should the nurse proceed?***

Content Area: Child Health, Cardiovascular; ***Integrated Process:*** Nursing Process, Implementation; ***Cognitive Level:*** Application; ***Client Need/Subneed:*** Physiological Integrity/Pharmacological and Parenteral Therapies/Adverse Effects/Contraindications/Interactions

48. CORRECT ANSWERS: 1, 5. **Answer 1 is correct because a murmur heard after 4 hours can be indicative of a cardiac condition and needs further investigation. Answer 2** is incorrect because overlapping skull bones, called molding, are a *normal* finding in the term infant. **Answer 3** is incorrect because the bluish hue of fingers and toes, called acrocyanosis, is a *normal* part of the infant's transition from intrauterine to extrauterine life. **Answer 4** is incorrect because the pinnae of the ears are *normally* incurving at term. **Answer 5 is correct because grunting with respirations is not a normal finding at 39 weeks' gestation and can be indicative of respiratory distress.**

■ TEST-TAKING TIP: ***Each of the alternatives should be viewed separately, as normal or not normal. Eliminate the normal findings (Answers 2, 3, and 4).***

Content Area: Child Health, Newborn; ***Integrated Process:*** Nursing Process, Assessment; ***Cognitive Level:*** Analysis; ***Client Need/Subneed:*** Health Promotion and Maintenance/Health Screening

49. CORRECT ANSWER: 2. **Answer 1** is incorrect because bowel sounds in acute pancreatitis are usually *diminished or absent.* **Answer 2 is correct because the autodigestion of tissue by the pancreatic enzymes results in pain from inflammation, edema, and possible hemorrhage. Continuous, unrelieved epigastric and/or back pain reflect the inflammatory process in the pancreas. Answer 3** is incorrect because breath sounds may be *decreased or absent* from atelectasis or pleural effusion. **Answer 4** is incorrect because the client becomes hypotensive, *not* hypertensive, due to shock. The temperature becomes elevated because of the acute inflammatory reaction.

■ TEST-TAKING TIP: ***Pancreatitis = Pain (e.g., Answer 2 is an acute inflammatory reaction); therefore Answers 1, 3, and 4 would not apply. Although there may be an elevated temperature (Answer 4), elevated BP would* not *occur.***

Content Area: Adult Health, Gastrointestinal; ***Integrated Process:*** Nursing Process, Assessment; ***Cognitive Level:*** Application; ***Client Need/Subneed:*** Physiological Integrity/Physiological Adaptation/Pathophysiology

50. CORRECT ANSWERS: 1, 3, 4. **Answer 1 is correct because dysrhythmia *is* a side effect that can be assessed in this age group. Answer 2** is incorrect because, while yellow-green visual halos *are* a side effect of digoxin, they *cannot* be assessed in this age group. This would be a side effect of the medication that the nurse would want to teach the parents about when the child is older and can communicate sensations that are being experienced. **Answer 3 is correct because bradycardia *is* a side effect that can be assessed in this age group. Answer 4 is correct because vomiting *is* a side effect that can be assessed in this age group.**

■ TEST-TAKING TIP: ***When all of the responses to a question seem correct, reread the question and note if any of the responses would be impossible due to the child's* age *or* developmental *status. Note a pattern of three objective signs and one subjective sign. Eliminate the one that is* different.**

Content Area: Child Health, Cardiovascular; ***Integrated Process:*** Teaching and Learning; ***Cognitive Level:*** Analysis; ***Client Need/Subneed:*** Physiological Integrity/Pharmacological and Parenteral Therapies/Adverse Effects/Contraindications/Interactions

51. CORRECT ANSWER: 4. **Answer 1** is incorrect because this client has a possible inflammatory process due to obstruction of the pancreatic duct by a gallstone. Surgery should be *postponed* until further evaluation by the physician. **Answer 2** is incorrect because an elevated serum amylase does *not* reflect obstructive jaundice. **Answer 3** is incorrect because the white blood cell (WBC) count, *not* the red blood cell (RBC) count, would be elevated in acute pancreatitis. The hemoglobin and hematocrit will be altered *later* from decreased transferrin and changes in iron absorption. **Answer 4 is correct because cholelithiasis may block the pancreatic duct and initiate pancreatitis. The elevated serum amylase report indicates that the client has pancreatitis and the operation should be canceled because of the *acute inflammatory process.***

■ TEST-TAKING TIP: ***By knowing the normal laboratory values, you can see that there is a problem that must be reported. Know the significance of an elevated serum amylase: Answers 1, 2, and 3 have no relevance to this abnormal laboratory result. If unsure, remember that the* serum bilirubin *reflects jaundice (Answer 2), and the RBC count would reflect* anemia *(Answer 3), leaving the decision to postpone surgery as the only option.***

Content Area: Adult Health, Gastrointestinal; ***Integrated Process:*** Nursing Process, Analysis; ***Cognitive Level:*** Analysis; ***Client Need/Subneed:*** Physiological Integrity/Reduction of Risk Potential/Laboratory Values

52. CORRECT ANSWER: 2. Answer 1 is incorrect because active range-of-motion exercises *are* best so that the child can gauge his or her own pain tolerance. **Answer 2 is correct because passive range-of-motion exercises should never be part of an exercise regimen after an acute episode of hemophilia because the joint capsule could easily be stretched and bleeding could recur. Answer 3** is incorrect because there is *no contraindication* to using wrist splints at night since the child may have sustained previous injuries to, or previous bleeds in, this area of the body. The splints assist in maintaining mobility and provide comfort when the wrists are not in use while asleep at night. **Answer 4** is incorrect because there is *no contraindication* to using ankle splints at night since the child may have sustained previous injuries to, or previous bleeds in, this area of the body. The splints assist in maintaining mobility and provide comfort when the ankles are not in use while asleep at night.

■ **TEST-TAKING TIP:** *Look for what should* not *be ordered. Think active (i.e., the child does it) rather than passive (i.e., done by physical therapist) and what the consequences of each activity could be.*

Content Area: Child Health, Hematological; ***Integrated Process:*** Nursing Process, Evaluation; ***Cognitive Level:*** Application; ***Client Need/Subneed:*** Safe and Effective Care Environment/ Safety and Infection Control/Error Prevention

53. CORRECT ANSWER: 6. Calculate 2 mg/2 mL, reduce to 1 mg/1 mL, and then calculate 6 mg = 6 mL.

■ **TEST-TAKING TIP:** *Be careful when calculating medication dosages. Reduce the fraction, if possible, and make the calculation as easy as possible.*

Content Area: Maternity, Intrapartum; ***Integrated Process:*** Nursing Process, Implementation; ***Cognitive Level:*** Analysis; ***Client Need/Subneed:*** Physiological Integrity/Pharmacological and Parenteral Therapies/Dosage Calculation

54. CORRECT ANSWER: 2. Answer 1 is incorrect because the medication should *decrease* the number and type of bowel movements from malabsorption and steatorrhea. **Answer 2 is correct because pancreatic enzymes must be taken with meals to assist in digestion. Food will protect the enzymes in the medication from destruction by the hydrochloric acid in the stomach, making them available for digestion. Answer 3** is incorrect because enteric-coated tablets should *not* be chewed or dissolved in the mouth. The coating is to protect the medication from gastric enzymes. **Answer 4** is incorrect because the medication should be taken *with meals* to promote the digestion of carbohydrates, fats, and protein.

■ **TEST-TAKING TIP:** *Three of the four options relate to medication administration. In this case, do* not *assume that the odd option is correct.* Time *element is the key here—with meals versus every 8 hours. Note that "three times daily" in the stem refers to three times* with meals *per day, not every 8 hours (Answer 4). Answer 1 is inappropriate because the client has steatorrhea,* not *diarrhea. Answer 3 is contraindicated with any enteric-coated tablet. Answer 4 is inappropriate because pancrelipase (Pancrease) is an enzyme to be taken* with *meals.*

Content Area: Adult Health, Gastrointestinal; ***Integrated Process:*** Teaching and Learning; ***Cognitive Level:*** Application; ***Client Need/Subneed:*** Physiological Integrity/Pharmacological and Parenteral Therapies/Medication Administration

55. CORRECT ANSWERS: 1, 2, 3, 4. Answer 1 is correct because a side effect of tetracycline is photosensitivity/ phototoxicity. The nurse's teaching should include instructing the adolescent to avoid exposure to the sun or to minimize exposure to the sun with the use of a hat. Answer 2 is correct because photosensitivity is a side effect of tetracycline. Wearing long-sleeved shirts will minimize the exposure to the sun. Answer 3 is correct because photosensitivity is a side effect of tetracycline. Wearing sunglasses reduces exposure to the sun. Answer 4 is correct because photosensitivity is a side effect of tetracycline. Applying sunscreen minimizes exposure to the sun. Answer 5 is incorrect because it is not necessary to wear *heavy* socks; just covering exposed parts of skin to protect from sun exposure is important.

■ **TEST-TAKING TIP:** *Note the word "environmental" in the stem of the question; think "outdoors" and then think "sun."*

Content Area: Child Health, Integumentary; ***Integrated Process:*** Nursing Process, Implementation; ***Cognitive Level:*** Application; ***Client Need/Subneed:*** Physiological Integrity/ Pharmacological and Parenteral Therapies/Adverse Effects/ Contraindications/Interactions

56. CORRECT ANSWER: 3. Answer 1 is incorrect because the effects of radiation are distinct from those of chemotherapy. **Answer 2** is incorrect because the *primary* purpose is shrinkage. **Answer 3 is correct because multiple myeloma is a malignancy of the bone and bone marrow; radiation may be used to shrink the size of a tumor that interferes with movement and causes pain. Answer 4** is incorrect because the disease has *already* caused widespread bone destruction before radiation is used.

■ **TEST-TAKING TIP:** *If two choices seem correct (Answers 2 and 3), choose the broadest—shrinkage* will kill *cells (Answer 3).*

Content Area: Adult Health, Oncological; ***Integrated Process:*** Nursing Process, Implementation; ***Cognitive Level:*** Application; ***Client Need/Subneed:*** Physiological Integrity/Physiological Adaptation/Alterations in Body Systems

57. CORRECT ANSWER: 2. Answer 1 is incorrect because, while pewter contains lead and could be a potential exposure to the substance, there is *no need* to return the rattle to the sender. It can safely be displayed in a locked cabinet. **Answer 2 is correct because pewter contains lead. Infants are known to suck on rattles and could be exposed to the lead on a continuous basis. The item should be displayed in a locked cabinet. Answer 3** is incorrect because pewter contains lead and could be a potential exposure to the substance. It *cannot be safely used* by the infant and should instead be displayed in a locked cabinet. **Answer 4** is incorrect because pewter contains lead and could be a potential exposure to the substance. It cannot be safely used by the infant *even* in the presence of the parents, and should instead be displayed in a locked cabinet.

■ TEST-TAKING TIP: *Decide if it is "OK" for the child to use or not use the item. Eliminate Answers 3 and 4 as they mean "use." Remember that lead can be found in multiple "innocent-appearing" sources. Know all of the possible sources of lead, even in gifts.*

Content Area: Child Health, Poisoning; *Integrated Process:* Teaching and Learning; *Cognitive Level:* Application; *Client Need/Subneed:* Safe and Effective Care Environment/ Safety and Infection Control/Handling Hazardous and Infectious Materials

58. CORRECT ANSWER: 1. **Answer 1 is correct because, if possible, women hospitalized for treatment of preeclampsia should be on bedrest in a quiet environment to minimize stimuli.** **Answer 2** is incorrect because the nurse *should* assess the amount and distribution of edema. **Answer 3** is incorrect because weight *is* an indicator of edema and diuresis and *should* be assessed in the woman with preeclampsia. **Answer 4** is incorrect because the presence and amount of protein in the urine *are* important indicators of her status. **Answer 5** is incorrect because I&O relationships *are* important indicators of her status.

■ TEST-TAKING TIP: *This question asks for the* wrong *action. Four of the options* are *appropriate orders; select the one that is not.*

Content Area: Maternity, Intrapartum; *Integrated Process:* Nursing Process, Implementation; *Cognitive Level:* Application; *Client Need/Subneed:* Physiological Integrity/Physiological Adaptation/Illness Management

59. CORRECT ANSWER: 1. **Answer 1 is correct because the affected leg will be shorter and externally rotated. "Extracapsular" means "outside the capsule."** **Answer 2** is incorrect because the leg will be *externally* rotated. **Answer 3** is incorrect because blanching would most likely be seen with *dislocation.* **Answer 4** is incorrect because footdrop would be likely with *muscular* weakness or *neurological* impairment.

■ TEST-TAKING TIP: *Visualize the options to help decide between two choices.*

Content Area: Adult Health, Musculoskeletal; *Integrated Process:* Nursing Process, Assessment; *Cognitive Level:* Application; *Client Need/Subneed:* Physiological Integrity/ Physiological Adaptation/Alterations in Body Systems

60. CORRECT ANSWER: 4. **Answer 1** is incorrect because it is a *noncontact* sport and presents no danger of injury. **Answer 2** is incorrect because it is a *noncontact* sport and presents no danger of injury. **Answer 3** is incorrect because it is a *noncontact* sport and presents no danger of injury. **Answer 4 is correct because it is a contact sport and should be discouraged, as the risk of injury outweighs the physical and psychosocial benefits of participating in this sport. This is especially important in adolescents with severe hemophilia.**

■ TEST-TAKING TIP: *Three answers do not involve contact with others; one does. Select that option. Think "prevent injury and possible bleeding" when answering this question.*

Content Area: Child Health, Hematological; *Integrated Process:* Teaching and Learning; *Cognitive Level:* Analysis; *Client Need/Subneed:* Safe and Effective Care Environment/ Safety and Infection Control/Accident Prevention and Injury Prevention

61. CORRECT ANSWER: 3. **Answer 1** is incorrect because it describes the *three-point* gait. **Answer 2** is incorrect because it describes the *two-point* gait. **Answer 3 is correct because the idea of four points means a crutch, the opposite foot, the other crutch, then the opposite foot. Each moves separately.** **Answer 4** is incorrect because it describes the *swing-through* gait.

■ TEST-TAKING TIP: *Visualize how many "points" (touches) are in each option.*

Content Area: Adult Health, Musculoskeletal; *Integrated Process:* Nursing Process, Analysis; *Cognitive Level:* Comprehension; *Client Need/Subneed:* Physiological Integrity/Basic Care and Comfort/Assistive Devices

62. CORRECT ANSWERS: 1, 2, 3, 4. **Answer 1 is correct because atropine is an anticholinergic medication. It blocks vagal impulses to the myocardium and stimulates the cardioinhibitory center in the medulla, thereby increasing heart rate and cardiac output while decreasing blood pressure as small blood vessels are dilated. Therefore, the nurse should monitor the child's heart rate and blood pressure. Answer 2 is correct because atropine can induce mental confusion/ excitement, especially in children, so the nurse should also monitor the child's behavior. Answer 3 is correct because atropine is an anticholinergic medication that blocks vagal impulses to the myocardium and stimulates the cardioinhibitory center in the medulla, thereby increasing heart rate and cardiac output while decreasing blood pressure as small blood vessels are dilated. Therefore, the nurse should monitor the child's heart rate and blood pressure. Answer 4 is correct because atropine can cause hyperpyrexia (elevated temperature), so the nurse should also monitor the child's temperature.** **Answer 5** is incorrect because cardiac effects are primarily associated with administration of atropine.

■ TEST-TAKING TIP: *Note the use of the words "expected effect" in the question, and answer accordingly.*

Content Area: Child Health, Cardiovascular; *Integrated Process:* Nursing Process, Evaluation; *Cognitive Level:* Application; *Client Need/Subneed:* Physiological Integrity/Pharmacological and Parenteral Therapies/ Expected Effects/Outcomes

63. CORRECT ANSWER: 4. Answer 1 is incorrect because vaginal discharge that is increasing is not a reliable method of assessing progress of labor. The only method for reliably evaluating the progress of labor is a cervical examination. Labor is defined as a change in the cervix. **Answer 2** is incorrect because breathing that is becoming more rapid is not a reliable method of assessing progress of labor. Clients have different pain tolerance, and breathing may change in response to pain; only checking the cervix for a change in dilation is a reliable method to assess the progress of labor. **Answer 3** is incorrect because contractions that are getting more intense is not a reliable method of assessing progress of labor. The definition of labor is a change in the cervix; stronger contractions may lead to a change in the cervix. The intensity of the contractions alone is not indicative of progress in labor. **Answer 4 is correct because a cervix that is progressively dilating is the definition of labor progress.**

■ **TEST-TAKING TIP:** *This question is asking for the definition of progress of labor. Eliminate the answers that do not define labor progress.*

Content Area: Maternity, Intrapartum; ***Integrated Process:*** Nursing Process, Assessment; ***Cognitive Level:*** Application; ***Client Need/Subneed:*** Health Promotion and Maintenance/ Ante/Intra/Postpartum and Newborn Care

64. CORRECT ANSWER: 4. Answer 1 is incorrect because sitting will only increase the likelihood of flexion contractures. **Answer 2** is incorrect because *after 48 hours* the client must *change* from this position (which was indicated initially to reduce edema). **Answer 3** is incorrect because it would not fully extend the leg and hip. **Answer 4 is correct because, at approximately 48 to 72 hours following the procedure, the client must be turned onto the abdomen to prevent flexion contractures.**

■ **TEST-TAKING TIP:** *The priority changes with time:* early *postoperative period—edema;* late *postoperative period—contractures.*

Content Area: Adult Health, Neuromuscular; ***Integrated Process:*** Nursing Process, Implementation; ***Cognitive Level:*** Application; ***Client Need/Subneed:*** Physiological Integrity/ Reduction of Risk Potential/Potential for Alterations in Body Systems

65. CORRECT ANSWERS: 2, 3, 4. Answer 1 is incorrect because a 3-mL syringe does not allow for precise measurement of the small amount of medication that the infant is to receive. In addition, a 23-gauge needle could cause injury as well as unnecessary discomfort to the infant. **Answer 2 is correct because a 1-mL syringe does allow for precise measurement of the small amount of medication that the infant is to receive. In addition, a 25-gauge needle will provide a degree of safety as well as comfort for the infant. Selection of the most appropriate syringe and needle is the *first* action that the nurse should take. Answer 3 is correct because the nurse must cleanse the infant's skin prior to the injection. Working in an organized fashion and visualizing what steps must be performed and in what order to administer the injection makes this the nurse's *second* action. Answer 4 is correct because the nurse must *apply* pressure and then *cover* the injection site after administration of the injection. Working in an organized fashion and visualizing what steps must be performed and in what order to complete the injection makes this the nurse's *third* action.**

■ **TEST-TAKING TIP:** *The nurse should always select the smallest gauge of syringe and needle possible for use in infants; the* larger *the number, the* smaller *the gauge. Think "organization" (i.e., sequence of steps) to give the medication, to* cleanse *the skin, and to* apply pressure *and to* cover.

Content Area: Child Health, Medication Administration; ***Integrated Process:*** Nursing Process, Implementation; ***Cognitive Level:*** Application; ***Client Need/Subneed:*** Safe, Effective Care Environment/Safety and Infection Control/ Safe Use of Equipment

66. CORRECT ANSWER: 3. Answer 1 is incorrect because the timing is *too soon,* although the symptom is appropriate. **Answer 2** is incorrect because the characteristics of the pain are not consistent with an ulcer, but more like those associated with *pancreatitis.* **Answer 3 is correct because the pain is described as aching, burning, cramp-like, and gnawing, occurring at some time after eating, depending on where the ulcer is located. Answer 4** is incorrect because the characteristics and the location are *not* consistent with ulcer pain.

■ **TEST-TAKING TIP:** *Time and location are important.*

Content Area: Adult Health, Gastrointestinal; ***Integrated Process:*** Nursing Process, Assessment; ***Cognitive Level:*** Comprehension; ***Client Need/Subneed:*** Physiological Integrity/Physiological Adaptation/Pathophysiology

67. CORRECT ANSWERS: 2, 3. Answer 1 is incorrect because x-rays would *not* yield *specific* information regarding the appropriateness and safety of administering *any* drug. **Answer 2 is correct because gentamicin can cause renal impairment and acute renal failure; thus baseline renal functions (I&O, daily weights, urine specific gravity, urinalysis, creatinine levels, and blood urea nitrogen) *must* be evaluated prior to administering the medication. Answer 3 is correct because gentamicin can cause hearing loss. Baseline hearing tests should be conducted prior to and at the conclusion of gentamicin therapy. Answer 4** is incorrect because gentamicin usually does *not* cause bone marrow suppression.

■ **TEST-TAKING TIP:** *Know all of the systems that a medication can potentially affect.*

Content Area: Child Health, Renal; ***Integrated Process:*** Nursing Process, Assessment; ***Cognitive Level:*** Analysis; ***Client Need/Subneed:*** Physiological Integrity/Pharmacological and Parenteral Therapies/Adverse Effects/Contraindications/ Interactions

68. **CORRECT ANSWERS: 0.25 and 3.** Concentration of terbutaline 5 mg per 5 mL, reduced down to 1 mg per 1 mL; 0.25 mg of terbutaline is equal to 0.25 mL. Concentration of Celestone is 2 mg per mL; a dose of 6 mg divided by 2 mg/mL is equal to 3 mL.

■ **TEST-TAKING TIP:** *Read the question carefully and calculate the dosages of both medications.*

Content Area: Maternity, Intrapartum; *Integrated Process:* Nursing Process, Analysis; *Cognitive Level:* Analysis; *Client Need/Subneed:* Physiological Integrity/Pharmacological and Parenteral Therapies/Dosage Calculation

69. **CORRECT ANSWER: 3.** **Answer 1** is incorrect because *vital signs* are *normal* in Ménière's disease. **Answer 2** is incorrect because, although ambulating would be difficult with nystagmus, the *pulse* would be *normal.* **Answer 3 is correct because the most objective sign of Ménière's disease is nystagmus, or jerking eye movements. The vital signs are normal in clients with this disease. Ménière's disease affects the inner ear, which would cause the eye movements.** **Answer 4** is incorrect because the *vital signs* are *normal* in Ménière's disease.

■ **TEST-TAKING TIP:** *Know the expected effect of an inner ear problem. Choose the option that is different from the others. Only one option has normal vital signs; the other options have either pulse or BP that is not normal.*

Content Area: Adult Health, Sensory; *Integrated Process:* Nursing Process, Assessment; *Cognitive Level:* Application; *Client Need/Subneed:* Physiological Integrity/Physiological Adaptation/Pathophysiology

70. **CORRECT ANSWERS: 1, 2, 3.** **Answer 1 is correct because these changes *are* associated with cranial nerve VII damage. Answer 2 is correct because these changes *are* associated with cranial nerve VII damage. Answer 3 is correct because these changes *are* associated with cranial nerve VII damage.** **Answer 4** is incorrect because inability to open the eyelid is associated with *cranial nerve III* damage.

■ **TEST-TAKING TIP:** *Narrow the choices to contradictory options—close versus open eyelid. Visualize facial paralysis. You can eliminate the option that is* not *associated with cranial nerve VII by reviewing cranial nerves VII and III.*

Content Area: Adult Health, Neurological; *Integrated Process:* Nursing Process, Evaluation; *Cognitive Level:* Application; *Client Need/Subneed:* Physiological Integrity/Physiological Adaptation/Pathophysiology

71. **CORRECT ANSWER: 2.** **Answer 1** is incorrect because, although this position will promote separation of the ribs, it will *not* promote maximal access to the fluid. **Answer 2 is correct because having the client's pleural cavity in a good vertical, yet safe, comfortable position will achieve maximum access to the pleural fluid. The fluid will gravitate to the lowest point for maximal aspiration.** **Answer 3** is incorrect because there is inadequate exposure for a midaxillary or posterior aspiration of the pleural fluid. It would be the proper position for the insertion of a chest tube for the aspiration of air, as in a pneumothorax. **Answer 4** is incorrect because this position will *not* facilitate maximal drainage.

■ **TEST-TAKING TIP:** *First visualize the positions. Recall that gravity promotes maximal drainage of pleural fluid. Choose the position that will promote the best access and aspiration of pleural fluid (Answer 2); Answer 3 impedes accessibility, and Answers 1 and 4 impede maximal drainage.*

Content Area: Adult Health, Respiratory; *Integrated Process:* Nursing Process, Implementation; *Cognitive Level:* Application; *Client Need/Subneed:* Physiological Integrity /Reduction of Risk Potential/Therapeutic Procedures

72. **CORRECT ANSWER: 4.** **Answer 1** is incorrect because placing the client in high Fowler's position will facilitate the delivery and does *not prevent* perineal tearing during a precipitous delivery. **Answer 2** is incorrect because putting pressure against the fetus' head until the physician arrives for delivery is an *inappropriate* method to manage a precipitous delivery. **Answer 3** is incorrect because gently pulling on the fetus' head until it is delivered is *not* an *appropriate* method for managing a precipitous delivery, and can *cause fetal damage* during delivery. Nurses are expected to prevent damage from a precipitous delivery, but not to facilitate the delivery by pulling on the fetal head. **Answer 4 is correct because calling the physician for delivery, applying gentle pressure to the perineum, and guiding the fetus' head as it is delivered is the proper method for managing a precipitous delivery. By using gentle pressure on the perineum, the head is controlled during delivery, and the chance of perineal tearing is reduced.**

■ **TEST-TAKING TIP:** *Calling the physician is the first thing the nurse should do and is a part of all the answers, but management of a precipitous delivery is the key concept in this question. Controlling the* fetal head, *but not placing pressure against (Answer 2) and not pulling (Answer 3) on the head, during delivery is the* nurse's *responsibility.*

Content Area: Maternity, Intrapartum; *Integrated Process:* Nursing Process, Implementation; *Cognitive Level:* Analysis; *Client Need/Subneed:* Health Promotion and Maintenance/Ante/Intra/Postpartum and Newborn Care

73. **CORRECT ANSWERS: 10 and 5.** The 10-mL total reconstituted solution contains 5 million units; 2.5 million units is half the total amount, or 5 mL of reconstituted solution.

■ **TEST-TAKING TIP:** *Be careful when calculating medication dosages. Reduce the fraction, if possible, and make the calculation as easy as possible.*

Content Area: Adult Health, Infectious Disease, Pharmacology; *Integrated Process:* Nursing Process, Implementation; *Cognitive Level:* Analysis; *Client Need/Subneed:* Physiological Integrity/Pharmacological and Parenteral Therapies/Dosage Calculation

74. CORRECT ANSWER: 4. Answer 1 is incorrect because clients with glaucoma *may* take NSAIDs. **Answer 2** is incorrect because clients with glaucoma *may* take salicylates. **Answer 3** is incorrect because clients with glaucoma *may* take antacids. **Answer 4 is correct because antihistamines cause pupil dilation and should be avoided with glaucoma.**
■ **TEST-TAKING TIP:** ***Use the process of elimination to choose the medication with the potential for risk, which therefore needs to be avoided.***
Content Area: Adult Health, Sensory; ***Integrated Process:*** Nursing Process, Implementation; ***Cognitive Level:*** Application; ***Client Need/Subneed:*** Physiological Integrity/Pharmacological and Parenteral Therapies/Adverse Effects/Contraindications/Interactions

75. CORRECT ANSWER: 1. Answer 1 is correct because, since the client is not having significant active bleeding, the pregnancy can safely be extended by limiting activity to bedrest with bathroom privileges. Answer 2 is incorrect because there is *no immediate need* to perform a cesarean section delivery. The client is hemodynamically stable and can be managed by bedrest. **Answer 3** is incorrect because a contraction stress test for fetal well-being would be *contraindicated* in a client with marginal placenta previa. Contractions can lead to *increased* vaginal bleeding. A *non-stress test is the appropriate* test for fetal well-being in a client with marginal placenta previa. **Answer 4** is incorrect because induction of labor with misoprostol would be *contraindicated* in a client with a marginal placenta previa. Contractions can lead to *increased* vaginal bleeding and *fetal distress.*
■ **TEST-TAKING TIP:** ***Visualize a placenta previa, marginal placenta previa, and partial placenta previa. The varying extent of the placenta covering over the cervix will determine the management.***
Content Area: Maternity, Antepartum; ***Integrated Process:*** Nursing Process, Planning; ***Cognitive Level:*** Application; ***Client Need/Subneed:*** Physiological Integrity/Reduction of Risk Potential/Potential for Alterations in Body Systems

APPENDIX A

Laboratory Values

This chart gives a quick overview of what is normal and the conditions that result in high or low values.

Test	Normal Values	Possible Causes of High or Low Values *May Increase with:*	*May Decrease with:*
Hematology			
Aspartate aminotransferase (AST)—formerly called serum glutamic-oxaloacetic transaminase (SGOT)	*Men:* 10–40 units/L *Women:* 9–25 units/L	Myocardial infarction, cardiac surgery, hepatitis, cirrhosis, trauma, severe burns, progressive muscular dystrophy, infectious mononucleosis, acute renal failure, Reye syndrome, HELLP syndrome	Uremia, chronic dialysis, ketoacidosis
Bleeding time—indication of hemostatic efficiency	1–9 min	Hemorrhagic purpura, acute leukemia, aplastic anemia, DIC, oral anticoagulant therapy, Reye syndrome	
Hematocrit—volume of packed red blood cells/100 mL of blood	*Men:* 45% (40%–50%) *Women:* 40% (38%–47%)	Dehydration, polycythemia, congenital heart disease	Anemia, hemorrhage, leukemia, dietary deficiencies
Hemoglobin—oxygen-combining protein	*Men:* 13.5–18 gm/dL *Women:* 12–16 gm/dL	Same as for Hematocrit	Same as for Hematocrit
Activated partial thromboplastin time (aPTT)—tests coagulation mechanism; stage I deficiencies	*aPTT:* 25–41	Deficiency of factors VIII, IX, X, XI, XII; anticoagulant therapy	Extensive cancer, DIC
Platelets—thrombocytes	150,000–400,000/mm^3	Polycythemia vera, post-splenectomy, anemia, Kawasaki disease	Leukemia, aplastic anemia, cirrhosis, multiple myeloma, chemotherapy, HELLP syndrome
Prothrombin time—tests extrinsic clotting; stages II and III	10–13 sec INR: 2.0–3.0	Anticoagulant therapy, DIC, hepatic disease, malabsorption, Reye syndrome	Digitalis therapy, diuretic reaction, vitamin K therapy
Red blood cell count—number of circulating erythrocytes in 1 microL of whole blood	*Men:* 4.5–6.2 million/microL *Women:* 4.2–5.4 million/microL	Polycythemia vera, anoxia, dehydration	Leukemia, hemorrhage, anemias, Hodgkin's
Sedimentation rate—speed at which red blood cells settle in uncoagulated blood	*Men:* 0–15 mm/hr *Women:* 0–20 mm/hr	Acute bacterial infection, cancer, infectious disease, numerous inflammatory states, rheumatic fever, Kawasaki disease	Polycythemia vera, sickle cell anemia

Continued

Test	Normal Values	Possible Causes of High or Low Values *May Increase with:*	*May Decrease with:*
White blood cell count—number of leukocytes in 1 microL	4.5–11 × 10^3/microL	Leukemia, bacterial infection, severe sepsis, Kawasaki disease	Viral infection, overwhelming bacterial infection, lupus erythematosus, antineoplastic chemotherapy, bone marrow depression
White blood cell differential—enumeration of individual leukocyte distribution			
Neutrophils	56% mean cell count 1800–7800/microL	Bacterial infection, tumor, inflammation, stress, drug reaction, trauma, metabolic disorders	Acute viral infection, anorexia nervosa, radiation therapy, drug induced, alcoholic ingestion
Eosinophils	2.7% cell count 0–450/microL	Allergic disorder, parasitic infestation, eosinophilic leukemia	Acute or chronic stress; excess ACTH, cortisone, or epinephrine; endocrine disorder
Basophils	25–100/microL, or 0–1% cell count 0–200/microL	Myeloproliferative disease, leukemia	Anaphylactic reaction, hyperthyroidism, radiation therapy, infections, ovulation, pregnancy, aging
Lymphocytes	20%–40% cell count 1000–4800/microL	Chronic lymphocytic leukemia, infectious mononucleosis, chronic bacterial infection, viral infection	Leukemia, systemic lupus erythematosus, immune deficiency disorders
Blood Chemistry			
Alkaline phosphatase (ALP)	32–92 units/L	Hyperparathyroidism, Paget's disease, cancer with bone metastasis, obstructive jaundice, cirrhosis, hepatitis A, rickets	Malnutrition, scurvy, celiac disease, chronic nephritis, hypothyroidism, cystic fibrosis
Amylase	80–180 IU/L	Acute pancreatitis, mumps, duodenal ulcer, pancreatic cancer, perforated bowel, renal failure	Advanced chronic pancreatitis, chronic alcoholism
Bilirubin, serum	*Direct:* 0.0–0.4 mg/dL *Indirect:* 0.2–0.8 mg/dL *Total:* 0.3–1.0 mg/dL	Massive hemolysis, low-grade hemolytic disease, cirrhosis, obstructive liver disease, hepatitis, biliary obstruction, neonatal (physiological) jaundice	
B-type natriuretic peptide	Non-CHF *Men:* 10 pg/mL (pg, picogram) *Women:* 17 pg/mL CHF *Men:* 146–928 pg/mL *Women:* 149–858 pg/mL	Heart failure	
Calcium, serum	8.2–10.2 mg/dL	Hyperparathyroidism, multiple myeloma, bone metastasis, bone fracture, thiazide diuretic reaction, milk-alkali syndrome	Hypoparathyroidism, renal failure, pregnancy, massive transfusion
Carbon dioxide	22–30 mEq/L	Emphysema, salicylate toxicity, vomiting	Starvation, diarrhea
Chloride, serum	98–107 mEq/L	Hyperventilation, diabetes insipidus, uremia, cystic fibrosis	Heart failure, pyloric obstruction, hypoventilation, vomiting, chronic respiratory acidosis
Creatine, serum	*Men:* 0.7–1.3 mg/dL *Women:* 0.5–1.0 mg/dL	Chronic glomerulonephritis, nephritis, heart failure, muscle disease	Debilitation, long-term corticosteroid therapy

Test	Normal Values	Possible Causes of High or Low Values *May Increase with:*	*May Decrease with:*
Creatine kinase (CK) (creatine phosphokinase [CPK])	*Men:* 17–148 IU/L *Women:* 10–79 IU/L	Acute myocardial infarction, acute stroke, convulsions, surgery, muscular dystrophy, hypokalemia	Addison's disease
CPK/CK Isoenzymes			
CPK-MM/CK-MM	100%	Muscular dystrophy, delirium tremens, surgery, hypokalemia, crush injuries, hypothyroidism	
CPK-MB/CK-MB	0.6% of total CPK	Acute myocardial infarction, cardiac defibrillation, myocarditis, cardiac ischemia	
CPK-BB/CK-BB	0%	Pulmonary infarction, brain surgery, stroke, pulmonary embolism, seizures, intestinal ischemia	
Fibrinogen, serum	0.2–0.4 gm/100 dL or 200–400 mg/dL	Pneumonia, acute infection, nephrosis, rheumatoid arthritis	Cirrhosis, toxic liver necrosis, anemia, obstetric complications, DIC, advanced carcinoma
Glucose (fasting)	60–110 mg/100 mL (serum)	Acute stress, Cushing's syndrome, hyperthyroidism, acute or chronic pancreatitis, diabetes mellitus, hyperglycemia	Addison's disease, liver disease, reactive hypoglycemia, pituitary hypofunction
Glycosylated hemoglobin ($HgbA_{1c}$)	4.0%–7.0%	Newly diagnosed or poorly controlled diabetes mellitus	Iron-deficiency anemia, chronic blood loss
Iron-binding capacity (total)	218–385 gm/dL	Lead poisoning, hepatic necrosis	
Lactate dehydrogenase (LDH)	60–120 units/mL (Wacker Scale) 150–450 units/mL (Wroblewski)	Myocardial infarction, pernicious anemia, chronic viral hepatitis, pneumonia, pulmonary emboli, stroke, renal tissue destruction, leukemia, non-Hodgkin's lymphoma, shock, trauma, Reye syndrome	
LDH-1	17%–27%		
LDH-2	27%–37%		
LDH-3	18%–25%		
LDH-4	3%–8%		
LDH-5	6%–16%		
Lipids:			
Cholesterol (total serum) Low-density lipoprotein (LDL) High-density lipoprotein (HDL) Triglycerides	<200 mg/dL <130 mg/dL 35–75 mg/dL 40–150 mg/100 mL	Hypercholesterolemia, hyperlipidemia, myocardial infarction, uncontrolled diabetes mellitus, high-cholesterol diet, hypothyroidism, atherosclerosis, stress, familial biliary obstruction, nephrotic syndrome	Malnutrition, cholesterol-lowering medication, anemia, liver disease, hyperthyroidism
Phosphorus, inorganic serum	3.0–4.5 mg/dL	Chronic glomerular disease, hypoparathyroidism, milk-alkali syndrome, sarcoidosis	Hyperparathyroidism, rickets, osteomalacia, renal tubular necrosis, malabsorption syndrome, vitamin D deficiency

Continued

Test	Normal Values	Possible Causes of High or Low Values *May Increase with:*	*May Decrease with:*
Potassium, serum	3.5–5.0 mEq/L	Diabetic ketosis, renal failure, Addison's disease, excessive intake, APSGN	Thiazide diuretics, Cushing's syndrome, cirrhosis with ascites, hyperaldosteronism, steroid therapy, malignant hypertension, poor dietary habits, chronic diarrhea, diaphoresis, renal tubular necrosis, malabsorption syndrome, vomiting
Protein, serum (albumin/globulin)	*Total:* 6.4–8.3 gm/dL *Albumin:* 3.5–5.0 gm/dL *Globulin:* 2.8–4.4 gm/dL	Dehydration, multiple myeloma, APSGN	Chronic liver disease, myeloproliferative disease, burns, nephrotic syndrome, Hirschsprung's disease
Serum glutamic-oxaloacetic transaminase (SGOT)—see AST			
Sodium, serum	136–145 mEq/L	Increased intake, either orally or IV; Cushing's syndrome, excessive sweating, diabetes insipidus, cystic fibrosis	Addison's disease, sodium-losing nephropathy, vomiting, diarrhea, fistulas, tube drainage, burns, renal insufficiency with acidosis, starvation with acidosis, paracentesis, thoracentesis, ascites, heart failure, SIADH
T_3 uptake	24%–34%	Hyperthyroidism, thyroxine-binding globulin (TBG) deficiency	Hypothyroidism, pregnancy, TBG excess
Thyroxine	5–12 mcg/dL	Hyperthyroidism, pregnancy	Hypothyroidism, renal failure
Troponin 1	0–0.5 ng/ml	Acute myocardial infarction	
Urea nitrogen, serum (BUN)	5–20 mg/dL	Acute or chronic renal failure, heart failure, obstructive uropathy, dehydration, HELLP syndrome	Cirrhosis, malnutrition
Uric acid, serum	*Men:* 4.5–8 mg/dL *Women:* 2.5–6.2 mg/dL	Gout, chronic renal failure, starvation, diuretic therapy	
Blood Gases			
Bicarbonate (HCO_3)	21–28 mEq/L	Metabolic alkalosis	Metabolic acidosis
Carbon dioxide pressure (PCO_2), whole blood, arterial	35–45 mm Hg	Primary respiratory acidosis, loss of H^+ through nasogastric suctioning or vomiting	Primary respiratory alkalosis
Oxygen pressure (PO_2), whole blood, arterial	80–100 mm Hg	Oxygen administration in the absence of severe lung disease	Chronic obstructive lung disease, severe pneumonia, pulmonary embolism, pulmonary edema, respiratory muscle disease
pH, serum	7.35–7.45	Metabolic alkalosis–alkali ingestion, respiratory alkalosis–hyperventilation	Metabolic acidosis–ketoacidosis, shock, respiratory acidosis–alveolar hypoventilation

APPENDIX A

Test	Normal Values	Possible Causes of High or Low Values *May Increase with:*	*May Decrease with:*
Immunodiagnostic Studies			
Carcinoembryonic antigen	<2.5 ng/mL	*Cancer* of: colon, lung, metastatic breast, pancreas, stomach, prostate, ovary, bladder, limbs; also neuroblastoma, leukemias, osteogenic carcinoma; *noncancer* conditions such as: hepatic cirrhosis, uremia, pancreatitis, colorectal polyposis, peptic ulcer disease, ulcerative colitis, regional enteritis	
Urinalysis			
pH	4.5–7.8	Metabolic alkalosis	Metabolic acidosis
Specific gravity	1.003–1.029	Dehydration, pituitary tumor, hypotension, APSGN	Distal renal tubular disease, polycystic kidney disease, diabetes insipidus, overhydration
Glucose	Negative	Diabetes mellitus	
Protein	Negative	Nephrosis, glomerulonephritis, lupus erythematosus, preeclampsia	
Casts	0–0.4 hyaline casts per LPF	Nephrosis, glomerulonephritis, lupus erythematosus, infection	
Red blood cells	Negative	Renal calculi, hemorrhagic cystitis, tumors of the kidney, APSGN	
White blood cells	Negative	Inflammation of the kidneys, ureters, or bladder	
Color	Normal yellow, clear	*Abnormal: red to reddish brown*—hematuria; *brown to brownish gray*—bilirubinuria or urobilinuria; *tea colored*—possible obstructive jaundice	*Almost colorless:* chronic kidney disease, diabetes insipidus, diabetes mellitus
Sodium	40–220 mEq/L/24 hr	Salt-wasting renal disease, SIADH, dehydration	Heart failure, primary aldosteronism
Chloride	110–250 mEq/24 hr	Chronic obstructive lung disease, dehydration, salicylate toxicity	Gastric suction, heart failure, emphysema
Potassium	25–125 mEq/L/24 hr	Diuretic therapy	Renal failure
Creatinine clearance	90–139 mL/min		Renal disease
Hydroxycorticosteroids	2–10 mg/24 hr	Cushing's disease	Addison's disease
17-Ketosteroids	*Men:* 4.5–12 mg/24 hr *Women:* 2.5–10 mg/24 hr	Hirsutism, adrenal hyperplasia	Thyrotoxicosis, Addison's disease
Catecholamines (VMA)	*Epinephrine:* <20 mcg/24 hr *Norepinephrine:* <100 mcg/24 hr	Pheochromocytoma, severe anxiety, numerous medications	
Urine Test			
Schilling test	Excretion of 8%–40% or more of test dose should appear in urine		Gastrointestinal malabsorption, pernicious anemia

APPENDIX A

APPENDIX B

Memory Aids

Acid-base—*"RAMS" (Respiratory Alternate, Metabolic Same)*

	Respiratory (Alternate)		Metabolic (Same)	
Acidosis	↓ pH	↑ PCO_2	↓ pH	↓ HCO_3
Alkalosis	↑ pH	↓ PCO_2	↑ pH	↑ HCO_3

Alcohol withdrawal: clinical features—*"HITS"*[a]
- **H**allucinations (visual, tactile)
- **I**ncreased vital signs and insomnia
- **T**remens → delirium tremens (potentially lethal)
- **S**hakes/Sweats/Seizures/Stomach pains (nausea, vomiting)

Angina: precipitating factors—*"three Es"*
- **E**ating
- **E**motion
- **E**xertion (Exercise)

Anorexia nervosa: clinical features—*"$A^2NOREXI^2C$"*[a]
- **A**dolescent women/**A**menorrhea
- **N**GT alimentation (most severe cases)
- **O**bsession with losing weight/becoming fat though underweight
- **R**efusal to eat (≥5% die)
- **E**lectrolyte abnormalities (e.g., ↓ K^+, cardiac arrhythmia)
- ↑ e**X**ercise
- **I**ntelligence often above average/**I**nduced vomiting
- **C**athartic use (and diuretic abuse)

Appendicitis: assessment—*"PAINS"*
- **P**ain (RLQ)
- **A**norexia
- **I**ncreased temperature, WBC (15,000–20,000)
- **N**ausea
- **S**igns (McBurney's, psoas)

[a]Modified from Rogers, PT: *The Medical Student's Guide to Top Board Scores.* Little, Brown, Boston (out of print).

Arterial occlusion: symptoms—*"six Ps"*
- **P**ain
- **P**ale
- **P**ulseless
- **P**aresthesia
- **P**oikilothermic
- **P**aralysis

Blood glucose (rhyme)

Symptom	*Implication*
Cold and **clammy** . . .	give hard **candy**
Hot and **dry** . . .	glucose is **high**

Blood vessels in umbilical cord—*"AVA"*
- **A**rtery
- **V**ein
- **A**rtery

Cancer: early signs—*"CAUTION"*
- **C**hange in bowel or bladder habits
- **A** persistant sore throat
- **U**nusual bleeding or discharge
- **T**hickening or lump
- **I**ndigestion: dysphagia
- **O**bvious change in a wart/mole
- **N**agging cough or hoarseness

Cancer: focus of patient care—*"CANCER"*
- **C**hemotherapy
- **A**ssess body image disturbance (related to alopecia)
- **N**utritional needs when N/V present
- **C**omfort from pain
- **E**ffective response to Tx? (Evaluate)
- **R**est (for patient and family)

Cholecystitis: risk factors—"*five Fs*"
- **F**emale
- **F**at
- **F**orty
- **F**ertile
- **F**air

Cleft lip: nursing care plan (postoperative)—"*CLEFT 2 LIP*"
- **C**rying, minimize
- **L**ogan bow
- **E**lbow restraints
- **F**eed with Breck feeder
- **T**each feeding techniques/**T**wo months of age (average age at repair)
- **L**iquid (sterile water), rinse after feeding
- **I**mpaired feeding (no sucking)
- **P**osition—*never* on abdomen

Cognitive disorders: assessment of difficulties—"*JOCAM*"
- **J**udgment
- **O**rientation
- **C**onfabulation
- **A**ffect
- **M**emory

Coma: causes—"*A²-E³-I-O-U T²IPS²*"[b]
- **A**lcohol, **A**cidosis (hyperglycemic coma)
- **E**pilepsy (also **E**lectrolyte abnormality, **E**ndocrine problem)
- **I**nsulin (hypoglycemic shock)
- **O**verdose (or poisoning)
- **U**remia and other renal problems
- **T**rauma; **T**emperature abnormalities (hypothermia, heat stroke)
- **I**nfection (e.g., meningitis)
- **P**sychogenic ("hysterical coma")
- **S**troke or **s**pace-occupying lesions in the cranium

Complication of severe preeclampsia—"*HELLP*" *syndrome*
- **H**emolysis
- **E**levated **L**iver enzymes
- **L**ow **P**latelet count

Cushing's syndrome: symptoms—"*three Ss*"
- **S**ugar (hyperglycemia)
- **S**alt (hypernatremia)
- **S**ex (excess androgens)

Diabetes: signs and symptoms—"*three Ps*," "*three 'poly's*"
- **P**olydipsia (very thirsty)
- **P**olyphagia (very hungry)
- **P**olyuria (urinary frequency)

[b]Adapted from Caroline, NL: *Emergency Care in the Streets,* ed 5. Little, Brown, Boston (out of print)

Diet: low cholesterol—*avoid the three Cs:*
- **C**ake
- **C**ookies
- **C**ream (dairy, e.g., milk, ice cream)

Dystocia: etiology—"*three Ps*"
- **P**ower
- **P**assageway
- **P**assenger

Dystocia: general aspects (maternal)—"*three Ps*"
- **P**sych
- **P**lacenta
- **P**osition

Episiotomy assessment—"*REEDA*"
- **R**edness
- **E**dema
- **E**cchymosis
- **D**ischarge
- **A**pproximation of skin

Eye medications
- My**d**riatic = **d**ilated pupils
- Mio**t**ic = **t**iny (constricted) pupils

Hypertension: complications—"*four Cs*"
- **CAD** (coronary artery disease)
- **CHF** (congestive heart failure)
- **CRF** (chronic renal failure)
- **CVA** (cardiovascular accident; now called brain attack or stroke)

Hypertension: nursing care plan—"*I TIRED*"
- **I**ntake and output (urine)
- **T**ake blood pressure
- **I**schemia attack, transient (watch for TIAs)
- **R**espiration, pulse
- **E**lectrolytes
- **D**aily weight

Hypoglycemia: signs and symptoms—"*DIRE*"
- **D**iaphoresis
- **I**ncreased pulse
- **R**estless
- **E**xtra hungry

Infections during pregnancy—"*TORCH*"
- **T**oxoplasmosis
- **O**ther (hepatitis B, syphilis, group B beta strep)
- **R**ubella
- **C**ytomegalovirus
- **H**erpes simplex virus

Infections: signs—"*INFE³CT*"
- **I**ncreased—pulse, respiration, WBC
- **N**odes—enlarged
- **F**unction—impaired
- **E³: E**rythema, **E**dema, **E**xudate
- **C**omplaints—discomfort, pain
- **T**emperature—local or systemic

IUD: potential problems with use—*"PAINS"*[c]
Period (menstrual: late, spotting, bleeding)
Abdominal pain, dyspareunia
Infection (abnormal vaginal discharge)
Not feeling well, fever or chills
String missing

Manipulation: nursing plan—promote the "*three Cs*"
Cooperation
Compromise
Collaboration

Medication administration—*"six rights"*
RIGHT medication
RIGHT dosage
RIGHT route
RIGHT time
RIGHT client
RIGHT technique

Melanoma characteristics—*"ABCD"*
Asymmetry
Border
Color
Diameter

Mental retardation: nursing care plan—*"three Rs"*
Regularity (provide routine and structure)
Reward (positive reinforcement)
Redundancy (repeat)

Myocardial infarction: treatment—*"M²ONA"*
MONA greets every M.I.:
Monitor/Morphine
Oxygen
Nitroglycerin
Aspirin

Newborn assessment components—*"APGAR"*
Appearance
Pulse
Grimace
Activity
Respiratory effort

Obstetric (maternity) history—"*GTPAL*"
Gravida
Term
Preterm
Abortions (SAB, TAB)
Living children

Oral contraceptives: signs of potential problems—"*ACHES*"[c]
Abdominal pain (possible liver or gallbladder problem)
Chest pain or shortness of breath (possible pulmonary embolus)
Headache (possible hypertension, brain attack)
Eye problems (possible hypertension or vascular accident)
Severe leg pain (possible thromboembolic process)

Pain: assessment—*"PQRST"*

What	Provokes the pain?
What is the	Quality of the pain?
Does the pain	Radiate?
What is the	Severity of the pain?
What is the	Timing of the pain?

Pain: management—*"ABCDE"*
Ask about the pain
Believe when clients say they have pain
Choices—let clients know their choices
Deliver what you can, when you said you would
Empower/Enable clients' control over pain

Postoperative complications: order—*"four Ws"*
Wind (pulmonary)
Wound
Water (urinary tract infection)
Walk (thrombophlebitis)

Preterm infant: anticipated problems—"*TRIES*"
Temperature regulation (poor)
Resistance to infections (poor)
Immature liver
Elimination problems (necrotizing enterocolitis [NEC])
Sensory-perceptual functions (retinopathy of prematurity [ROP])

Psychotropic medications: common antidepressives (tricyclics)—"*VENT*"
Vivactil
Elavil
Norpramin
Tofranil

Schizophrenia: primary symptoms—*"four As"*
Affect
Ambivalence
Associative looseness
Autism

Sprain: nursing care plan—"*RICE*"
Rest
Ice
Compression
Elevation

Stool assessment—*"ACCT"*
Amount
Color
Consistency
Timing

[c]From Hatcher, RA, et al: *Contraceptive Technology,* ed 16. Irving, New York.

Tracheoesophageal fistula: assessment—*"three Cs"*
Coughing
Choking
Cyanosis

Traction: nursing care plan—*"TRACTION"*
Trapeze bar overhead to raise and lower upper body
Requires free-hanging weights; body alignment
Analgesia for pain, prn
Circulation (check color and pulse)
Temperature (check extremity)
Infection prevention
Output (monitor)
Nutrition (alteration related to immobility)

Transient ischemic attacks: assessment—*"three Ts"*
Temporary unilateral visual impairment
Transient paralysis (one-sided)
Tinnitus = vertigo

Trauma care: complications—*"T²RAUMA"*
Thromboembolism; Tissue perfusion, altered
Respiration, altered
Anxiety related to pain and prognosis
Urinary elimination, altered
Mobility impaired
Alterations in sensory-perceptual functions and skin integrity (infections)

Wernicke-Korsakoff syndrome (alcohol-associated neurological disorder)—*"COAT RACK"*[d]
Wernicke's encephalopathy (acute phase): clinical features:
Confusion
Ophthalmoplegia
Ataxia
Thiamine is an important aspect of Tx
Korsakoff's psychosis (chronic phase): characteristic findings:
Retrograde amnesia (↓ recall of some old memories)
Anterograde amnesia (↓ ability to form new memories)
Confabulation
Korsakoff's psychosis

---

[d]Adapted from Rogers, PT: *The Medical Student's Guide to Top Board Scores.* Little, Brown, Boston (out of print).

APPENDIX C

Common Acronyms and Abbreviations

This list provides a review of what you need to know about acronyms and abbreviations used in charting, verbal directives, and study guides.

a	Before (*ante*)
AAA	Abdominal aortic aneurysm
Ab	Antibody; Abortion
Abd	Abdomen; Abdominal
ABG	Arterial blood gas
ac	Before meals (*ante cibum*)
ACE	Angiotensin-converting enzyme
ACTH	Adrenocorticotropic hormone
ADH	Antidiuretic hormone
ADHD	Attention deficit-hyperactivity disorder
ad lib	As much as desired (*ad libitum*)
ADLs	Activities of daily living
AED	Automatic external defibrillator
AFB	Acid-fast bacillus
Afib	Atrial fibrillation
Aflutter	Atrial flutter
AFP	Alpha-fetoprotein
AG	Antigen
AGA	Average for gestational age
AGE	Acute gastroenteritis
AHF	Antihemophilic factor
AIDS	Acquired immunodeficiency syndrome
AK (or AKA)	Above-the-knee (amputation)
ALL	Acute lymphocytic (lymphoblastic) leukemia
ALS	Amyotrophic lateral sclerosis
AMA	Against medical advice
AML	Acute myelogenous leukemia
Amp	Ampule
ANP	Adult nurse practitioner
ANS	Autonomic nervous system
A&O ×3	Alert, oriented to person, place, time
AP	Anteroposterior; Alkaline phosphatase
aPPT	Activated partial thromboplastin time
APSGN	Acute poststreptococcal glomerulonephritis
ARC	AIDS-related complex
ARDS	Adult respiratory distress syndrome
ARF	Acute renal failure
ARMD	Age-related macular degeneration
AROM	Artificial rupture of membranes
ASA	Acetylsalicylic acid (aspirin)
ASAP	As soon as possible
ASD	Atrial septal defect
AST	Aspartate aminotransferase
AV	Atrioventricular; Arteriovenous; Aortic valve
AVB	Atrioventricular block
AVM	Arteriovenous malformation
AVR	Aortic valve repair
BAC	Blood alcohol concentration
BBT	Basal body temperature
BCLS	Basic cardiac life support
BK (or BKA)	Below-the-knee (amputation)
BM	Bowel movement; Bone marrow
BMA	Bone marrow aspiration
BMI	Body mass index
BMR	Basal metabolic rate
BMT	Bone marrow transplant
BOM	Bilateral otitis media
BP	Blood pressure
BPD	Bronchopulmonary dysplasia

BPH	Benign prostatic hyperplasia
bpm	Beats per minute
BPP	Biophysical profile
BRP	Bathroom privileges
BSE	Breast self-examination
BUN	Blood urea nitrogen
c̄	With (*cum*)
CA	Carcinoma; Cancer
CABG	Coronary artery bypass graft operation (×1, 2, 3, 4: number of grafts)
CAD	Coronary artery disease
CBC	Complete blood count
CCU	Cardiac (intensive) care unit
CD	Communicable disease
CDC	Centers for Disease Control and Prevention
CF	Cystic fibrosis
CHD	Congenital heart disease; Coronary heart disease
CHF	Congestive heart failure
CICU	Cardiac intensive care unit
CMV	Cytomegalovirus
CNS	Central nervous system; Coagulase-negative *Staphylococcus;* Clinical nurse specialist
C/O	Complains of
COA (CoA)	Coarctation of the aorta
COPD	Chronic obstructive pulmonary disease
CP	Cerebral palsy
CPD	Cephalopelvic disproportion
CPK	Creatine phosphokinase (now creatine kinase [CK])
CPR	Cardiopulmonary resuscitation
CRF	Chronic renal failure; Cardiac risk factors
CRP	C-reactive protein
C&S	Culture and sensitivity
CSF	Cerebrospinal fluid
CSM	Circulation, sensory, and motor
CST	Contraction stress test
CT	Computed tomography
CV	Cardiovascular
CVA	Cerebrovascular accident (now called brain attack); Costovertebral angle
CVP	Central venous pressure
Δ	Change (Greek letter delta)
D&C	Dilation and curettage
D&D	Dehydration and diarrhea
DDH	Developmental dysplasia of the hip
D&E	Dilation and evacuation
DI	Diabetes insipidus
DIC	Disseminated intravascular coagulation
Dig	Digitalis
DJD	Degenerative joint disease
DKA	Diabetic ketoacidosis
DM	Diabetes mellitus
DMD	Duchenne's muscular dystrophy
DNR	Do not resuscitate
DOA	Dead on arrival
DOB	Date of birth
DOE	Dyspnea on exertion
DPT	Diphtheria, pertussis, and tetanus
DRG	Diagnosis-related group
DRI	Dietary reference intakes
DTR	Deep tendon reflex
DTs	Delirium tremens
DVT	Deep vein thrombosis
D_5W/D5W	5% dextrose in water
Dx	Diagnosis
ECF	Extended care facility; Extracellular fluid
ECG	Electrocardiogram (purist's version)
Echo	Echocardiogram
ECMO	Extracorporeal membrane oxygenation
ECT	Electroconvulsive therapy (see EST)
ED	Emergency department (commonly called *emergency room*); Erectile dysfunction
EDD	Estimated date of delivery
EEG	Electroencephalogram
EENT	Eye, ear, nose, and throat
EFM	Electronic fetal monitoring
EKG	Electrocardiogram (common version)
EMG	Electromyogram
EMS	Emergency medical service
EMT	Emergency medical technician
ENT	Ear, nose, and throat
EPS	Extrapyramidal symptoms
ER	Emergency room
ESR	Erythrocyte sedimentation rate
EST	Electroshock therapy
ETOH	Alcohol (ethanol)
FAS	Fetal alcohol syndrome
FBS	Fasting blood sugar
FEV_1	Forced expiratory volume in 1 second
FHR	Fetal heart rate
FHT	Fetal heart tones
FNP	Family nurse practitioner
FRC	Functional residual capacity
FSH	Follicle-stimulating hormone
FTT	Failure to thrive
FUO	Fever of unknown origin

FVC	Forced vital capacity
Fx	Fracture
g	Gram
G	Gravida
GABS	Group A beta-hemolytic streptococcus
GB	Gallbladder
GBS	Group B streptococcus; Guillain-Barré syndrome
GC	Gonococcus; Gonorrhea
GCS	Glasgow Coma Scale
G&D	Growth and development
GDM	Gestational diabetes mellitus
GER	Gastroesophageal reflux
GI	Gastrointestinal
gm	Gram
gr	Grain
GTT	Glucose tolerance test
gtt(s)	Drop(s) (*guttae*)
GU	Genitourinary
GYN	Gynecological
HAV	Hepatitis A virus
HBGM	Home blood glucose monitoring
HBV	Hepatitis B virus
HCG	Human chorionic gonadotropin
Hct	Hematocrit
HCV	Hepatitis C virus
HDL	High-density lipoprotein
HEENT	Head, eyes, ears, nose, throat
Hgb	Hemoglobin
$HgbA_{1c}$	Glycosylated hemoglobin
HIB	*Haemophilus influenzae* type B
HIV	Human immunodeficiency virus
HMO	Health maintenance organization
HOB	Head of bed
HPL	Human placental lactogen
HPS	Hypertrophic pyloric stenosis
HPV	Human papillomavirus
HR	Heart rate
HRT	Hormone replacement therapy
HSP	Henoch-Schönlein purpura
HSV	Herpes simplex virus
HTN	Hypertension
Hx	History
ICP	Intracranial pressure
ICU	Intensive care unit
I&D	Incision and drainage
IDDM	Insulin-dependent diabetes mellitus
Ig	Immunoglobulin
IM	Intramuscular
INH	Isoniazid
I/O, I&O	Intake and output
IPPB	Intermittent positive-pressure breathing
IQ	Intelligence quotient
IUD	Intrauterine device
IUFD	Intrauterine fetal death
IV	Intravenous
IVC	Inferior vena cava
IVH	Intraventricular hemorrhage
IVP	Intravenous pyelogram; Intravenous push
JCAHO	Joint Commission on Accreditation of Healthcare Organizations
JIA	Juvenile ideopathic arthritis
JRA	Juvenile rheumatoid arthritis (old term for juvenile ideopathic arthritis)
KD	Kawasaki disease
KUB	Kidneys, ureters, bladder (flat/upright abdominal x-ray)
L&B	Laryngoscopy and bronchoscopy
L-C-P, LCPD	Legg-Calvé-Perthes disease
LDL	Low-density lipoprotein
LFTs	Liver function tests
LGA	Large for gestational age
LGI	Lower gastrointestinal
LLL	Left lower (lung) lobe
LLQ	Left lower quadrant
LMP	Last menstrual period
LOC	Loss of consciousness; Level of consciousness
LPN	Licensed practical nurse
LTB	Laryngotracheobronchitis
LTE	Life-threatening event
LUL	Left upper (lung) lobe
LUQ	Left upper quadrant
LVN	Licensed vocational nurse
MAOI	Monoamine oxidase inhibitor
MAP	Mean arterial pressure
MCL	Midclavicular line
MD	Muscular dystrophy
MDI	Metered-dose inhaler
Med	Medication
mEq	Milliequivalent
MI	Myocardial infarction
mL	Milliliter
MMR	Measles, mumps, rubella
MOM	Milk of magnesia
Mono	Mononucleosis
MR	Mitral regurgitation; Mental retardation

MRI	Magnetic resonance imaging
MRSA	Methicillin-resistant *Staphylococcus aureus*
MVR	Mitral valve repair/replacement
NA	Not applicable
NEC	Necrotizing enterocolitis
NG	Nasogastric
NICU	Neonatal intensive care unit
NIDDM	Non–insulin-dependent diabetes mellitus
NL	Normal
NM	Neuromuscular
NOC	Night (nocturnal)
NPH	Neutral protamine Hagedorn (intermediate-acting insulin)
NPO	Nothing by mouth (*nil per os*)
NS	Normal saline
NSAID	Nonsteroidal anti-inflammatory drug
NSR	Normal sinus rhythm
NST	Nonstress test
NTG	Nitroglycerin
N/V	Nausea, vomiting
NVD	Nausea, vomiting, diarrhea
O_2	Oxygen
OB	Obstetrics
OFTT	Organic failure to thrive
OM	Otitis media
OOB	Out of bed; out of breath
O&P	Ova and parasites
OR	Operating room
OT	Occupational therapy
OTC	Over-the-counter
p	Post (after)
P	Para; Pulse
PA	Posteroanterior; Physician's assistant; Pulmonary artery
PAC	Premature atrial contraction
PACU	Postanesthesia care unit
PAF	Paroxysmal atrial fibrillation
Pao_2	Arterial partial pressure of oxygen
PAO_2	Alveolar oxygen pressure
PAS	Para-aminosalicylic acid
PAT	Paroxysmal atrial tachycardia
pc	After meals (*post cibum*)
PCA	Patient-controlled analgesia (pump); Patient care assistant
PCP	*Pneumocystis* pneumonia; Phencyclidine
PDA	Patent ductus arteriosus
PE	Pulmonary embolus; Pulmonary edema
PEEP	Positive end-expiratory pressure
PERRL(A)	Pupils equally round and reactive to light (and accommodation)
PFTs	Pulmonary function tests
PICU	Pediatric intensive care unit
PID	Pelvic inflammatory disease
PIH	Pregnancy-induced hypertension
PKU	Phenylketonuria
PMI	Point of maximum impulse
PMS	Premenstrual syndrome
PND	Paroxysmal nocturnal dyspnea
PNP	Pediatric nurse practitioner
PO	By mouth (*per os*)
PPD	Purified protein derivative (TB skin test); Percussion and postural drainage
PPHN	Persistent pulmonary hypertension of the newborn
PPO	Preferred provider organization
PQRST	Provoke-quality-radiation-severity-time
prn	When necessary (*pro re nata*)
PSA	Prostate-specific antigen
Pt	Patient
PT	Prothrombin time; Physical therapy
PTA	Prior to admission
PTCA	Percutaneous transluminal coronary angioplasty
PTL	Preterm labor
PTSD	Post-traumatic stress disorder
PTT	Partial thromboplastin time
PUD	Peptic ulcer disease
PVC	Premature ventricular contraction
q	Each, every (*quaque*)
qh	Every hour
R	Respirations
RA	Rheumatoid arthritis; Right atrium
RAD	Reactive airway disease
RBC	Red blood cell
RDA	Recommended daily/dietary allowance
RDS	Respiratory distress syndrome
RHD	Rheumatic heart disease
RLL	Right lower (lung) lobe
RLQ	Right lower quadrant
RML	Right middle (lung) lobe
R/O	Rule out
ROM	Range of motion; Rupture of membranes
ROP	Retinopathy of prematurity
ROS	Review of systems
RR	Respiratory rate
RSV	Respiratory syncytial virus
RT	Respiratory therapy
R/T	Related to
RUL	Right upper (lung) lobe

RUQ Right upper quadrant
Rx Prescription/Therapy/Treatment

s Without (*sine*)
S_1 First heart sound
S_2 Second heart sound
S_3 Third heart sound
S_4 Fourth heart sound
SAB Spontaneous abortion
Sao_2 Arterial blood-oxygen saturation
SBE Subacute bacterial endocarditis
SCA Sickle cell anemia
SGA Small for gestational age
SIADH Syndrome of inappropriate antidiuretic hormone
SICU Surgical intensive care unit
SIDS Sudden infant death syndrome
SL Sublingually
SLE Systemic lupus erythematosus
SNF Skilled nursing facility
SOB Short(ness) of breath
SR Sinus rhythm
SROM Spontaneous rupture of membranes
S/Sx Signs/symptoms
Stat Immediately (*statim*)
STI Sexually transmitted infection
SVD Spontaneous vaginal delivery
Sx Symptoms

T Temperature
T&A Tonsillectomy and adenoidectomy
TAB Therapeutic abortion
TAR Total all routes (intake)
TB Tuberculosis
TCA Tricyclic antidepressant
TEF Tracheoesophageal fistula
TENS Transcutaneous electrical nerve stimulation
TGV Transposition of great vessels
TIA Transient ischemic attack
TKO To keep open
TLC Total lung capacity; Tender loving care; Therapeutic lifestyle change
TOF Tetralogy of Fallot
TOLAC Trial of labor after cesarean section
TORCH Toxoplasmosis, other (hepatitis B, syphilis), rubella, cytomegalovirus, herpes simplex 2
TPA Tissue plasminogen activator
TPN Total parenteral nutrition
TPR Temperature, pulse, respirations
TSE Testicular self-examination
TSH Thyroid-stimulating hormone
TSS Toxic shock syndrome
TURP Transurethral resection of prostate
TV Total volume; Tidal volume
TVH Total vaginal hysterectomy
Tx Treatment

UA Urinalysis
UAP Unlicensed assistive personnel
UDAB Urine drugs of abuse
UGI Upper gastrointestinal
UQ Upper quadrant
URI Upper respiratory infection
UTI Urinary tract infection
UV Ultraviolet

VBAC Vaginal birth after cesarean
VC Vital capacity
VCUG Voiding cystourethrography
VD Venereal disease
VF, Vfib Ventricular fibrillation
VS Vital signs
VSD Ventricular septal defect
VZV Varicella-zoster virus

w/ With
WBC White blood cell; White blood (cell) count
WHO World Health Organization
WIC Women, infants, and children
WNL Within normal limits
w/o Without

APPENDIX D

Quick Guide to Common Clinical Signs

Many clinical signs have been named for the physicians who first described them, or the phenomena they resemble. Following is a list of 34 *of the most common clinical signs* for use as a quick reference as you review.

Babinski reflex Dorsiflexion of the big toe after stimulation of the lateral sole. It is a normal reflex in infants under the age of 6 months, but indicates a *lesion of the pyramidal (corticospinal) tract* in older individuals.

Barlow test *Developmental dysplasia of the hip* is present if the femoral head moves in and out of the back of the acetabulum while exerting pressure from the front.

Blumberg's sign Transient pain in the abdomen after approximated fingers pressed gently into abdominal wall are suddenly withdrawn—rebound tenderness; associated with *peritoneal inflammation.*

Braxton Hicks contractions Irregular painless uterine contractions.

Brudzinski sign Flexion of the hip and knee induced by flexion of the neck; associated with *meningeal irritation.*

Brushfield spots Speckling of iris associated with *Down syndrome.*

Chadwick's sign Cyanosis of vaginal and cervical mucosa; associated with *pregnancy.*

Cheyne-Stokes respirations Rhythmic cycles of deep and shallow respiration, often with apneic periods; associated with *central nervous system respiratory center dysfunction.*

Chvostek's sign Facial muscle spasm induced by tapping on the facial nerve branches; associated with *hypocalcemia.*

Coopernail's sign Ecchymoses on the perineum, scrotum, or labia; associated with *fracture of the pelvis.*

Cullen's sign Bluish discoloration of the umbilicus; associated with *acute pancreatitis* or *hemoperitoneum,* especially *rupture of fallopian tube* in ectopic pregnancy.

Doll's eye sign Dissociation between the movements of the head and eyes: as the head is raised the eyes are lowered, and as the head is lowered the eyes are raised; associated with *global-diffuse disorders of the cerebrum.* By contrast, in the evaluation of newborns (whose nervous systems are immature), the irises normally remain in midline despite the rotation of the head.

Fluid wave Transmission across the abdomen of a wave induced by snapping the abdomen; associated with *ascites.*

Goldstein's sign Wide distance between the great toe and the adjoining toe; associated with *cretinism* and *trisomy 21.*

Harlequin sign In the newborn infant, reddening of the lower half of the laterally recumbent body and blanching of the upper half, due to a *temporary vasomotor disturbance.*

Hegar's sign Softening of the fundus of the uterus; associated with the *first trimester of pregnancy.*

Homans' sign Pain behind the knee, induced by dorsiflexion of the foot; associated with peripheral vascular disease, especially *venous thrombosis* in the calf (*not* a diagnostic test itself).

Kehr's sign Severe pain in the left upper quadrant, radiating to the top of the shoulder; associated with *splenic rupture.*

Kernig's sign Inability to extend the leg when sitting or lying with the thigh flexed on the abdomen; associated with *meningeal irritation.*

Knie's sign Unequal dilation of the pupils; associated with *Graves' disease.*

Kussmaul's respirations Paroxysmal air hunger; associated with acidosis, especially *diabetic ketoacidosis.*

Lasègue's sign Straight leg raising with hip flexed and knee extended will elicit sciatic pain associated with *herniated lumbar disk.*

Lhermitte's sign Sudden electric shock–like sensation along the spine on flexion of the head caused by *trauma* to the cervical spine, *multiple sclerosis, cervical cord tumor,* or *spondylosis.*

McBurney's sign Tenderness at McBurney's point (located two thirds of the distance from the umbilicus to the anterior-superior iliac spine); associated with *appendicitis.*

Murphy's sign Pain on taking a deep breath when pressure is applied over location of the gallbladder; a sign of *gallbladder disease.*

Ortolani maneuver Manual procedure performed to rule out the possibility of congenital dysplasia of the hip. A "click" sound sometimes is heard if *hip dysplasia* is present; on assessment, the head of the femur can be felt (or heard as a click) as it slips forward in the acetabulum and slips back when pressure is released and the legs are returned to their original position.

Osler's sign Small painful erythematous swellings in the skin of the hands and feet; associated with bacterial endocarditis.

Psoas sign Pain induced by hyperextension of the right thigh while lying on the left side; associated with *appendicitis.*

"Setting sun" sign Downward deviation of the eyes so that each iris appears to "set" beneath the lower lid, with white sclera exposed between it and the upper lid; associated with *increased intracranial pressure* or irritation of the *brainstem;* also seen in *hydrocephalus.* Seen occasionally for brief periods in normal infants.

Simian crease Transverse palmar or plantar crease; associated with *Down syndrome.*

Tinel's sign Tingling sensation felt from light percussion on the radial side of the palmaris longus tendon; associated with *carpal tunnel syndrome.*

Trendelenburg sign When child bears weight on the affected hip, the pelvis tilts downward on the unaffected side instead of upward, as it should; associated with *developmental dysplasia of the hip.*

Trousseau's sign Carpopedal spasm develops when BP cuff is inflated above systolic pressure for 3 minutes; associated with *hypocalcemia.*

Williamson's sign Markedly diminished blood pressure in the leg as compared with that in the arm on the same side; associated with *pneumothorax* and *pleural effusions.*

APPENDIX E

Complementary and Alternative Therapies

Complementary and alternative therapies can be integrated into the treatment plan for many conditions, including the following.

Condition	Complementary/Alternative Therapies
Anxiety (see also **Chapter 8, Table 8.15**)	*Herbals:* St. John's wort Tea: chamomile, peppermint Valerian *Diet/Nutrition:* *Eliminate:* caffeine, alcohol, tobacco, sugar *Lifestyle:* Exercise *Mind-Body Interventions:* Biofeedback Cognitive behavioral therapy Deep breathing Group therapy Meditation Relaxation response *Bioelectromagnetic Therapies:* Energy healing *Alternative Systems of Care:* Acupuncture *Hands-on Healing Techniques:* Massage
Arthritis	*Herbals:* Ginger concentrate Topical: capsaicin *Diet/Nutrition:* Weight loss Vitamins C and E *Lifestyle:* Exercise *Mind-Body Interventions:* Cognitive behavioral therapy; biofeedback Tai chi, qi gong, yoga *Pharmacological and Biological Treatments:* Glucosamine sulfate *S*-adenosylmethionine (SAMe) *Bioelectromagnetic Therapies:* Static magnet therapy

Continued

Condition	Complementary/Alternative Therapies
	Alternative Systems of Care: Acupuncture, acupressure Ayurveda Traditional Chinese medicine *Hands-on Healing Techniques:* Physical therapy
Asthma	*Herbals:* Grapeseed extract Guaifenesin *Diet/Nutrition:* Have: omega-3 fatty acids; onions, garlic; vitamins C, E; zinc *Avoid:* milk, egg, wheat, sulfites, aspirin Reduce: sodium intake *Mind-Body Interventions:* Biofeedback Yoga breathing techniques *Alternative Systems:* Acupuncture Ayurveda Chinese herbals *Hands-on Healing Techniques:* Massage
Coronary artery disease	*Diet/Nutrition:* *Eliminate:* tobacco, caffeine, alcohol Low fat, vegetarian Vitamins C, E, B_6, B_{12}, folic acid *Lifestyle:* Dr. Dean Ornish program *Mind-Body Interventions:* Relaxation and stress management Guided imagery Treat for depression (anger/hostility management)
Depression (see also **Chapter 8, Table 8.15**)	*Herbals:* St. John's wort *Diet/Nutrition:* Folic acid, vitamins B_{12} and C, thiamine, niacin *Lifestyle:* Exercise, relaxation, stress reduction *Mind-Body Interventions:* Biofeedback Cognitive behavioral therapy Meditation Spiritual approaches Tai chi, qi gong *Bioelectromagnetic Therapies:* Light therapy (for seasonal affective disorder [SAD]) *Alternative Systems of Care:* Acupuncture *Hands-on Healing Techniques:* Massage
Diabetes	*Herbals:* Garlic Green tea Fenugreek *Diet and Nutrition/Lifestyle:* Regular exercise Weight loss Diet: high fiber; low simple sugars and fats; potassium; Ornish diet, onion, cold-water fish Alpha-lipoic acid Biotin Chromium Flaxseed oil Vitamins C, B_3, B_6, B_{12}, E

Condition	Complementary/Alternative Therapies
Gastroesophageal reflux disease	*Herbals:* Licorice Raspberry tea Caraway *Diet and Nutrition/Lifestyle:* Weight loss Small meals Don't lie down for 2 hr pc Elevate HOB 6 in. *Avoid:* onions, spicy foods, peppermint, caffeine, alcohol (although white wine may ↑ gastric emptying)
Other gastrointestinal problems	
Constipation	*Herbals:* Aloe, cascara, senna
Diarrhea (antibiotic-induced)	*Diet:* Yogurt
Indigestion	*Herbals:* Peppermint oil
Peptic ulcer	*Herbals:* Licorice (may cause sodium concentration and counteract antihypertensive medications)
Headache (migraine)	*Herbals:* Feverfew (**caution**: ↑ risk of postoperative bleeding and stomach upset if also on NSAIDs) Ginger (dried) *Diet and Nutrition/Lifestyle:* Vitamin B_2 (riboflavin) *Avoid:* chocolate, cheese, beer, red wine, dairy, wheat *Mind-Body Interventions:* Relaxation therapy Biofeedback Guided imagery Meditation Stress management Tai chi, yoga
Hypercholesterolemia	*Herbals:* Garlic cloves Chinese red yeast rice *Diet and Nutrition/Lifestyle:* Exercise, weight loss Fruits/vegetables: 5–7 servings/daily (for bioflavonoids and beta-carotene) Fiber Mediterranean diet Vegetarian diet Soy protein Very low fat (Ornish diet) *Mind-Body Interventions:* Modifying type A behavior: ↓: stress, hostility, time urgency, competitiveness ↑: sleep pattern Relaxation therapy *Alternative Systems of Care:* Ayurveda Traditional Chinese medicine
Hypertension	*Herbals:* Garlic, ginseng dried root, hawthorn *Diet and Nutrition/Lifestyle:* DASH diet; fiber, potassium, low sodium; reduce caffeine Weight loss Aerobic exercise Quit smoking Coenzyme Q10 (CoQ10) Alcohol intake <3 drinks/day

Continued

Condition	Complementary/Alternative Therapies
	Calcium, magnesium Reduce sugar intake Check for heavy metals, such as lead *Mind-Body Interventions:* Anger prevention/management Guided imagery Music therapy Tai chi, yoga *Alternative Systems of Care:* Ayurveda Traditional Chinese medicine
Irritable bowel syndrome	*Herbals:* Peppermint Chamomile tea, fennel tea, raspberry tea Sage Garlic Lemon balm *Diet and Nutrition/Lifestyle:* Charcoal (for excess gas) Fiber Food allergy: identify/eliminate most common (dairy, grain) Lactase (if lactose intolerance) *Lactobacillus acidophilus* Reduce refined sugar in diet *Mind-Body Interventions:* Cognitive behavioral therapy Treat depression; psychotherapy Exercise Progressive muscle relaxation Biofeedback Stress management *Alternative Systems of Care:* Acupuncture Ayurveda Traditional Chinese medicinal herbals
Musculoskeletal problems	*Herbals:* Arnica ointment/gel (topical) Tiger balm (topical) Salicylate ointment Aloe gel Curcumin (anti-inflammatory) Lavender Camphor *Diet and Nutrition/Lifestyle:* Regular exercise Stretching, conditioning; warm-up exercises Bioflavonoids: citrus Calcium (bone, muscle injury) Magnesium (muscle spasm, injury) Vitamin C (connective tissue and muscle damage) Vitamin E (muscle damage); topical for scars Bursitis: Vitamin B_{12} Fibromyalgia: vitamin B_1, magnesium, vitamin E *Mind-Body Interventions:* Guided imagery Tai chi, yoga, qi gong Music therapy *Alternative Systems of Care:* Acupuncture, acupressure Cupping; massage, oil

Condition	Complementary/Alternative Therapies
Upper respiratory infections	*Herbals:* Echinacea (dried root or tea) (**Caution:** may interfere with immunosuppressant medications) Garlic cloves Horseradish Slippery elm tea *Diet and Nutrition/Lifestyle:* *Avoid* exhausting exercise; bedrest Drink large amounts of fluids Gargle: salt water and vinegar Hot water with lemon juice and honey *Mind-Body Interventions:* Social support Stress management *Alternative Systems of Care:* Ayurveda Acupuncture Cupping Traditional Chinese medicine *Hands-on Healing Techniques:* Percussion
Urinary tract infections	*Diet/Nutrition:* Large amounts of low-sugar juices, water (2 L/day) Cranberry juice Blueberry juice *Lifestyle:* Urinate after intercourse (women)

Adapted from Sierpina, VS: *Integrative Health Care: Complementary and Alternative Therapies for the Whole Person.* FA Davis, Philadelphia, 2001.

Index: Content Related to NCLEX-RN® Test Plan

Four General Client Needs and Six Client Subneeds (With Detailed Knowledge, Skills, and Abilities)

The following outline of content (nursing knowledge, skills, and abilities) is organized in terms of **four categories of client need:** *Safe, Effective Care Environment* (SECE), *Health Promotion and Maintenance* (HPM), *Psychosocial Integrity* (PsI), and *Physiological Integrity* (PhI). Included in the outline of topics are **six** numbered **client subneeds** and corresponding task statements. These items are derived from a study of nursing tasks and are *used in the development of the NCLEX-RN® test plan.*

Students who have taken and evaluated their performance on the **Pre-Tests** or **Final Tests** in this book will find this outline a useful guide for a concentrated review of specific problem topics. **Repeat NCLEX-RN® test takers** will also find this outline to be a useful guide for review of their problem areas. Refer to the pages listed in the right column for review of content in a particular topic.

The shaded areas and **bold-faced** topics and *italics* for subtopics are directly linked to the **official NCLEX-RN® Test Plan.**

Continued

Continued

Continued

APPENDIX F

For an index to *questions* relating to each client need/subneed, see **Appendix G.**

APPENDIX G

Index: Questions Related to Client Needs/Subneeds

Use this index to locate *practice questions* throughout the book for each *client need and subneed* that is tested on the NCLEX-RN®.

Questions Related to Client Needs and Subneeds

	Safe, Effective Care Environment				Physiological Integrity			
Chapter	1. Management of Care *Question #*	2. Safety and Infection Control *Question #*	3. Health Promotion and Maintenance *Question #*	4. Psychosocial Integrity *Question #*	5. Basic Care and Comfort *Question #*	6. Pharmacological and Parenteral Therapies *Question #*	7. Reduction of Risk Potential *Question #*	8. Physiological Adaptation *Question #*
Ch 1: Pre-Test 1 (1-75)	60	29, 65, 71	8, 12, 13, 16, 20, 23, 26, 27, 30, 32, 34, 36, 38, 40, 44, 46, 57	2, 35, 39, 45, 69, 72	49, 52, 55, 59	9, 37, 41, 56, 73, 74	1, 3, 7, 10, 14, 17, 25, 47, 50, 51, 54, 62, 66, 68, 70, 75	4, 5, 6, 11, 15, 18, 19, 21, 22, 24, 28, 31, 33, 42, 43, 48, 53, 58, 61, 63, 64, 67
Ch 1: Pre-Test 2 (1-75)	27, 56, 68		1, 23, 35, 52, 59, 62, 67, 72, 73	14, 71	4, 12, 48, 64	28, 39, 44, 46, 61	3, 6, 8, 10, 11, 15, 20, 21, 26, 30, 32, 40, 49, 54, 57, 63, 65, 66, 70	2, 5, 7, 9, 13, 16, 17, 18, 19, 22, 24, 25, 29, 31, 33, 34, 36, 37, 38, 41, 42, 43, 45, 47, 50, 51, 53, 55, 58, 60, 69, 74, 75
Ch 3: Safe, Effective Care Environ-ment (1-75)	1, 2, 3, 4, 5, 8, 10, 11, 12, 14, 15, 16, 17, 18, 19, 20, 21, 24, 25, 27, 28, 29, 35, 39, 42, 46, 47, 50, 51, 55, 57, 62, 63, 67, 68, 69, 70, 71, 72, 73	6, 7, 9, 13, 22, 23, 26, 30, 31, 32, 33, 34, 36, 37, 38, 40, 41, 43, 45, 48, 49, 52, 53, 54, 56, 58, 59, 60, 61, 64, 66, 74, 75					44	65
Ch 4: Child-bearing Family (1-100)			4, 7, 8, 11, 12, 13, 18, 23, 29, 31, 32, 33, 35, 36, 37, 43, 47, 49, 50, 51, 53, 54, 56, 57, 62, 63, 64, 65, 69, 70, 71, 77, 79, 80, 83, 84, 87, 89, 90, 91, 97	9	45, 46, 48, 61, 88	5, 6, 20, 28, 40, 59, 68, 75, 76, 81, 98, 99	3, 14, 16, 17, 19, 25, 30, 34, 38, 39, 41, 42, 44, 55, 60, 67, 73, 74, 78, 82, 85, 86, 94	1, 2, 10, 15, 21, 22, 24, 26, 27, 52, 58, 66, 72, 92, 93, 95, 96, 100

Ch 5: Pediatric (1-100)	26, 44, 55, 56, 92, 98	30, 31, 59, 60, 70, 71, 73	8, 10, 13, 15, 23, 24, 33, 45, 47, 48, 77, 79, 82, 87, 88, 99	21, 22, 66	9, 52, 63, 80, 94	2, 3, 6, 11, 28, 37, 38, 40, 41, 42, 50, 67, 68, 84, 85	1, 5, 12, 14, 16, 17, 18, 19, 20, 27, 29, 32, 34, 39, 49, 51, 53, 57, 61, 62, 65, 69, 72, 74, 76, 81, 83, 86, 90, 91, 95, 96, 97, 100	4, 7, 25, 35, 36, 43, 46, 54, 58, 64, 75, 78, 89, 93
Ch 6: Care of Adult (1-105)	29, 56, 72, 105	1, 21, 28, 42, 63, 84	55, 68, 81, 82	48, 80	7, 8, 31, 49, 52, 102	5, 27, 47, 87	2, 3, 4, 6, 9, 13, 14, 16, 26, 30, 34, 35, 36, 38, 39, 40, 41, 44, 50, 58, 64, 69, 70, 71, 73, 76, 77, 78, 79, 86, 88, 90, 93, 94, 96, 97, 99	10, 11, 12, 15, 17, 18, 19, 20, 22, 23, 24, 25, 32, 33, 37, 43, 45, 46, 51, 53, 54, 57, 59, 60, 61, 62, 65, 66, 67, 74, 75, 83, 85, 89, 91, 92, 95, 98, 100, 101, 103, 104
Ch 7: Geriatric (1-50)	15	29, 41, 43	1, 8, 9, 16, 19, 25, 26, 34, 38, 39	30, 31, 37, 44, 45	2, 3, 6, 24, 36, 40, 42	4, 27, 28, 49, 50	12, 14, 17, 21, 22, 23, 33, 48	5, 7, 10, 11, 13, 18, 20, 32, 35, 46, 47
Ch 8: Pharmacological (1-93)						1, 2, 3, 4, 5, 6, 7, 8, 9, 10, 11, 12, 13, 14, 15, 16, 17, 18, 19, 20, 21, 22, 23, 24, 25, 26, 27, 28, 29, 30, 31, 32, 33, 34, 35, 36, 37, 38, 39, 40, 41, 42, 43, 44, 45, 46, 47, 48, 49, 50, 51, 52, 53, 54, 55, 56, 57, 58, 59, 60, 61, 63, 64, 65, 66, 67, 68, 69, 70, 71, 72, 73, 74, 75, 76, 77, 78, 79, 80, 81, 82, 83, 84, 85, 86, 87, 88, 89, 90, 91, 92, 93	62	

Continued

Questions Related to Client Needs and Subneeds

	Safe, Effective Care Environment				Physiological Integrity			
Chapter	1. Management of Care *Question #*	2. Safety and Infection Control *Question #*	3. Health Promotion and Maintenance *Question #*	4. Psychosocial Integrity *Question #*	5. Basic Care and Comfort *Question #*	6. Pharmacological and Parenteral Therapies *Question #*	7. Reduction of Risk Potential *Question #*	8. Physiological Adaptation *Question #*
Ch 9: Nutrition (1-25)					1, 2, 3, 4, 5, 6, 7, 8, 9, 10, 11, 12, 13, 14, 15, 16, 17, 18, 19, 20, 21, 22, 23, 24, 25			
Ch 10: Psycho-social (1-50)	12, 13, 25, 32, 33, 42, 45	6, 24	1, 28	2, 3, 4, 7, 8, 11, 14, 16, 19, 20, 22, 23, 29, 31, 34, 41, 43, 44, 46, 47, 49, 50	36	5, 9, 10, 18, 26, 30, 38, 39, 40	15, 17, 21, 37, 48	27, 35
Ch 11: Common Procedures (1-73)	1	25, 45, 47	11				2, 3, 4, 5, 6, 7, 8, 9, 10, 12, 13, 14, 15, 16, 17, 18, 19, 20, 21, 22, 23, 24, 26, 27, 28, 29, 30, 31, 32, 33, 34, 35, 36, 37, 38, 39, 40, 41, 42, 43, 44, 46, 48, 49, 50, 51, 52, 53, 54, 55, 56, 57, 58, 59, 60, 61, 62, 63, 64, 65, 66, 67, 68, 69, 70, 71, 72, 73	
Ch 12: Final Test 1 (1-75)			1, 3, 6, 9, 10, 11, 12, 14, 19, 21, 25, 27, 28, 31, 36, 43, 45, 47, 49, 50, 52, 55, 56, 58, 60, 61, 65, 69, 72, 75	16, 22, 63, 71	7, 17	23, 33, 37, 51, 53, 57, 59, 62, 68, 70	5, 30, 34, 42, 44, 48, 54, 66, 73	2, 4, 8, 13, 15, 18, 20, 24, 26, 29, 32, 35, 38, 39, 40, 41, 46, 64, 67, 74
Ch 12: Final Test 2 (1-75)	7, 11	10, 20, 41, 52, 57, 60, 65	30, 37, 48, 63, 72	15	13, 27, 31, 32, 35, 36, 42, 45, 61	21, 26, 39, 40, 47, 50, 53, 54, 55, 62, 67, 68, 73, 74	2, 3, 4, 6, 8, 17, 18, 19, 22, 23, 28, 29, 34, 38, 44, 51, 64, 71, 75	1, 5, 9, 12, 14, 16, 24, 25, 33, 43, 46, 49, 56, 58, 59, 66, 69, 70

APPENDIX H

Reduction of Risk Potential: Index to Diagnostic Tests and Procedures

This is an important area to review because it is a **subcategory** of the **NCLEX-RN®** Test Plan that is often tested. Refer also to **Chapter 11.** The tests below are listed in chronological order by Chapter number.

Diagnostic Tests and Procedures	Page(s)
Chapter 4 Childbearing Family	
Huhner	123
Rubin's	123
Hysterosalpingogram	123
Creatinine clearance	131, 162
STI tests	134, 136
PAP smear	134
TB test	136
Anti-Rh titer	124, 134, 136, 140, 151, 175, 215
Sickle cell	134, 136
Multiple marker screen	136
Indirect Coombs' test	139, 151
Amniocentesis	140, 142, 143, 161, 162
Glucose tolerance test	136, 142
Nonstress test (NST)	142, 143, 161
Sonography	135, 142, 143, 151, 159, 161, 162, 185
X-ray pelvimetry	185
Phosphatidylinositol	143
Nitrazine test	150, 170
HCG levels	134, 151
Amniography	151
Urethral discharge Gram stain	136, 154
VDRL	155, 156
Smears: cervical, labial, vaginal	134, 155
STS (serologic test for syphilis)	155, 156
• TPI	156
• FTA	156
Roll-over test	158
DIC screening	160
Daily fetal movement count (DFMC)	161
Contraction stress test (CST)	143, 161
Biophysical profile (BPP)	143, 162, 180
Oxytocin challenge test	161
Lecithin-sphingomyelin ratios	143, 162, 176, 179

Continued

Index

Note: Page numbers followed by *f* refer to figures; page numbers followed by *t* refer to tables.

C

D

E

F

G

J

K

L

M

O

S

T

U

V

W

X

Y

Z